Prenatal and Postnatal Care

A Woman-Centered Approach

Prenatal and Postnatal Care

A Woman-Centered Approach

Edited by

Robin G. Jordan, Janet L. Engstrom, Julie A. Marfell, and Cindy L. Farley

WILEY Blackwell

This edition first published 2014 © 2014 by John Wiley & Sons, Inc.

Editorial offices: 1606 Golden Aspen Drive, Suites 103 and 104, Ames, Iowa 50010, USA
The Atrium, Southern Gate, Chichester, West Sussex, PO19 8SQ, UK
9600 Garsington Road, Oxford, OX4 2DQ, UK

For details of our global editorial offices, for customer services and for information about how to apply for permission to reuse the copyright material in this book please see our website at www.wiley.com/wiley-blackwell.

Library of Congress Cataloging-in-Publication Data

Prenatal and postnatal care : a woman-centered approach / edited by Robin G. Jordan, Janet L. Engstrom, Julie A. Marfell, Cindy L. Farley.
     p. ; cm.
   Includes bibliographical references and index.
   ISBN 978-0-470-96047-9 (paper : alk. paper)—ISBN 978-1-118-76681-1 (ePub)—ISBN 978-1-118-76687-3 (Mobi)—ISBN 978-1-118-76690-3 (ePdf)
   I. Jordan, Robin G., 1954– editor of compilation.   II. Engstrom, Janet L., editor of compilation.
III. Marfell, Julie A., editor of compilation.   IV. Farley, Cindy L., editor of compilation.
   [DNLM: 1. Neonatal Nursing.   2. Patient-Centered Care.   3. Pregnancy–physiology.   4. Pregnancy Complications–nursing.   5. Women's Health. WY 157.3]
   RJ254
   618.92'01–dc23
                    2013024996

A catalogue record for this book is available from the British Library.

Wiley also publishes its books in a variety of electronic formats. Some content that appears in print may not be available in electronic books.

Cover design by Nicole Teut

Set in 10.5/12.5 pt Minion by Toppan Best-set Premedia Limited
Printed and bound in Singapore by Markono Print Media Pte Ltd

4   2016

To Larry for providing me with space, time, love, and unwavering support during the long birth of this text.
To Francie, Amy, and Debi for your love, humor, and friendship that carry me through many an adventure.
—Robin G. Jordan

For Jack. Thank you for everything.
—Janet L. Engstrom

To my husband Steve for his constant support in all my efforts.
To my son Jesse and my daughter Rose, who inspire me every day to make the world a better place.
To all the nurse practitioners out there providing pregnancy health care. I hope that this book serves as a resource to help you provide woman-centered care during pregnancy and the postpartum period.
—Julie A. Marfell

To my loving companion Larry Gerthoffer, my sister Becky Doherty, my mother Carol Farley, and my children Kyle and Katy McEvoy.
Thank you for the humor, support, and faith that see me through all my endeavors.
—Cindy L. Farley

Contents

About the editors   xix

Contributors   xxi

Reviewers   xxiii

Foreword   xxv

Preface   xxvii

Part I Physiological foundations of prenatal and postnatal care   3

1 Reproductive tract structure and function   5
  Patricia W. Caudle

  Anatomy of the female reproductive system   6
    External genitalia   6
    Internal genitalia   8
  Menstrual cycle physiology   11
    Beginnings   11
    Onset of puberty   13
    The hypothalamic–pituitary–ovarian axis   13
    Menstrual cycle phases   13
  Resources for women   18
  Resources for health-care providers   18
  References   18

2 Conception, implantation, and embryonic and fetal development   19
  Patricia W. Caudle

  Introduction   20
  Conception and implantation   20
  The placenta   21
    Beginnings and structure   21
    Chorionic and amnionic membranes   22
    The umbilical cord   23
    Placental functions   23
  The embryo   27
    Organogenesis   28
  The fetus   29
  Summary   30
  Resources for health-care professionals   32
  Resources for women, their families, and
    health-care professionals   32
  References   32

3 Maternal physiological alterations during pregnancy   34
  Patricia W. Caudle
  Introduction   34

Hematologic system adaptations   34
  Blood changes   35
Cardiovascular changes   37
  Changes to the heart   37
  Vascular adaptations   37
  Changes in blood pressure   37
  Supine hypotensive syndrome   37
Respiratory adaptations   38
  Anatomical changes   38
  Adaptations in pulmonary function   38
Renal adaptations   38
  Anatomical changes   39
  Renal function   39
Gastrointestinal adaptations   39
  Anatomical adaptations   39
  Gastrointestinal function changes   40
  Liver and biliary adaptations   40
Metabolic changes   40
  Basal metabolic rate   41
  Carbohydrate metabolism   41
  Protein metabolism   41
  Fat metabolism   41
  Leptin and ghrelin   41
  Insulin   41
Skin changes   42
  Pigment changes of the skin   42
  Vascular changes of the skin   42
  Connective tissue changes   42
  Sebaceous and sweat gland changes   42
Hair and nail changes   42
Immunologic changes   43
  Fetus as allograft   43
  *Disorders related to immunologic changes
    in pregnancy*   44
Neurological and sensory changes   45
Musculoskeletal adaptations   45
Endocrine changes   46
  Anatomical changes   46
  Pituitary function changes   46
  Thyroid function changes   47
  Adrenal function changes   47
Summary   47
Resources for women and their families   48
Resources for health-care providers   48
References   48

Part II Preconception and prenatal care   49

4 Preconception care   51
  Victoria L. Baker
  Introduction   51

Challenges to providing preconception care   51
Benefits of preconception care   52
Evidence supporting preconception care   52
Content of preconception care   53
  Risk assessment and screening   53
  Preconception counseling   57
  Preconception care for women with
    chronic diseases   61
  Additional considerations   64
  Preconception care for men   65
Summary   66
Resources for women and their families   66
Resources for health-care providers   67
  Tools for screening   68
  Consumer brochures for the office setting   68
References   69

5   Prenatal care: Goals, structure,
    and components   73
    Carrie S. Klima

Introduction   74
A brief history of prenatal care   74
Current goals for prenatal care   75
  Initial and continuing risk assessment   76
  Health promotion   76
  Medical and psychosocial interventions and
    follow-up   76
  Updates to the "content of prenatal care"   77
Structure of prenatal care   77
  The schedule of prenatal visits   78
  How much prenatal care is enough?   78
  What happens in prenatal care?   79
  Integrating quality into prenatal care   79
A new model of prenatal care:
  CenteringPregnancy   80
  Making group prenatal care work   81
Components of prenatal care   81
  Assessment   81
  Physical assessment   85
  Laboratory   85
  Diagnostic testing   87
  Preventative care   88
  Health promotion and education   90
  Health education throughout pregnancy   94
Summary   95
Resources for women and their families   97
Resources for health-care providers   97
References   97

6   Nutrition during pregnancy   99
    Robin G. Jordan and Julie A. Paul

Introduction   100
Understanding food units   100
Size of food servings   100
Prenatal nutrition and health outcomes   100
  Fetal origins of disease hypothesis   102
  Prenatal flavor learning   103

Nutritional needs in pregnancy   103
  Fluid intake   103
Macronutrients: Total energy   103
Macronutrients: Fats   103
  Omega-3 fatty acids   104
Macronutrients: Carbohydrates   105
  Protein   105
Micronutrients   105
  Iron   105
  Folate   106
  Calcium and vitamin D   107
Weight gain in pregnancy   107
  Overweight and obesity in pregnancy   108
  Underweight in pregnancy   108
Food safety during pregnancy   109
  Food-borne infections   110
  Alcohol, caffeine, and artificial sweeteners   110
Factors influencing nutritional intake   111
  Resource availability   111
  Culture and family   111
Making a nutritional assessment   112
  Using resources   112
Counseling for optimal prenatal nutrition   114
Special issues in nutrition   116
  Adolescent pregnancy   116
  Pregnant vegetarians and vegans   117
  Eating disorders   118
  Pica   119
Summary   120
Resources for women and their families   121
Resources for health-care providers   121
References   121

7   Pregnancy diagnosis and gestational age
    assessment   125
    Janet L. Engstrom and Joyce D. Cappiello

Introduction   126
Early pregnancy diagnosis and gestational age
  assessment   126
Pregnancy diagnosis   127
  Presumptive signs of pregnancy   127
  Probable signs of pregnancy   128
  Positive signs of pregnancy   132
Gestational age assessment   133
  Terminology used to describe gestational age   133
  Devices used to calculate the gestational age   136
  Methods of estimating the gestational age   137
Counseling for pregnancy diagnosis   140
  Counseling after a negative pregnancy test   141
  Counseling after a positive pregnancy test   141
  Options counseling for unintended pregnancy   141
  Providing evidence-based information about
    pregnancy options   143
Summary   145
Resources for women and their families   145
Resources for health-care providers   145
References   145

8   Risk assessment and risk management in
    prenatal care   149
    Robin G. Jordan

    Introduction   149
    Process and purpose of risk assessment   149
    Benefits of risk assessment   150
    Limitations   150
        Poor predictive value   150
        Lack of precision   150
        Nonmodifiable risk factors   150
    Disadvantages of risk assessment and
        risk management   150
        Unnecessary interventions   150
        *Normalization of technology and illusion of
            risk control*   151
        Labeling women as high risk   151
    Misapplication of risk assessment and
        risk management   151
        Introduction of actual risk   152
        *Increase in financial, physical, and
            emotional costs*   152
        Birth fear   153
    Perspective of risk and risk screening   153
    Explaining risk to women   153
    Potential problems of risk miscommunication   154
        Informed compliance   154
        Illusion of choice   154
    Informed consent   154
    Resources for health-care providers and
        women and their families   157
    References   157

9   Prenatal genetic counseling, screening,
    and diagnosis   160
    Robin G. Jordan and Janet L. Engstrom

    Introduction   160
    Family history and risk evaluation   161
    Genetic screening procedures offered to all
        pregnant women   161
        Screening options for neural tube defects 161
        Screening options for trisomy 21 and trisomy 18 162
        Cystic fibrosis (CF) screening   165
    Ethnicity-based genetic screening   165
        Additional genetic disease carrier screening 167
    Diagnostic prenatal genetic testing procedures   167
        Amniocentesis   168
        Chorionic villus sampling   168
        Percutaneous umbilical blood sampling   168
    Developments in genetic testing options   168
    Scope of practice considerations   169
    Ethical considerations in genetic screening   169
    Communicating about genetic testing and risk
        during prenatal care   170
        Pretest counseling   170
    Psychosocial effects in genetic testing   170
        *Prenatal genetic testing and the tentative
            pregnancy*   171

    Perspective on genetic counseling during
        prenatal care   171
    Summary   173
    Resources for women and their families   173
    Resources for health-care providers   173
    References   173

10 Assessment of fetal well-being   176
    Jenifer Fahey

    Introduction   176
    Physiological principles and indications for
        antenatal fetal surveillance   177
    Scope of practice considerations   177
    Antenatal fetal testing methods   178
        Fetal movement counts (FMCs)   178
        Nonstress test   180
        Contraction stress test   183
        Amniotic fluid volume assessment   183
        The biophysical profile (BPP) and modified BPP 183
        Doppler velocimetry   187
    Education and counseling   188
    Cultural, personal, and family considerations   188
    Health disparities and vulnerable populations   189
    Legal and liability issues   189
    Summary   190
    References   191

11 Common discomforts of pregnancy   193
    Robin G. Jordan

    Overview   193
    Back pain and pelvic girdle pain   194
        Assessment   195
        Relief and preventative measures   195
    Bleeding gums   196
        Assessment   196
        Relief and preventative measures   196
    Breast tenderness   196
        Assessment   197
        Relief and preventative measures   197
    Carpal tunnel syndrome (CTS)   197
        Assessment   197
        Relief and preventative measures   198
    Cervical pain   198
    Constipation   198
        Assessment   198
        Relief and preventative measures   198
    Dizziness/Syncope   199
        Assessment   199
        Relief and preventative measures   199
    Edema   200
        Assessment   200
        Relief and preventative measures   200
    Emotional changes   200
        Assessment   201
        Relief and preventative measures   201
    Fatigue   201
        Assessment   201
        Relief and preventative measures   201

Flatulence   201
  Assessment   201
  Relief and preventative measures   202
Headache   202
  Assessment   202
  Relief and preventative measures   202
Heartburn   203
  Assessment   203
  Relief and preventative measures   203
Heart palpitations   204
  Assessment   204
  Relief and preventative measures   204
Hemorrhoids   204
  Assessment   204
  Relief and preventative measures   204
Increased warmth and perspiration   204
Leukorrhea   205
  Assessment   205
  Relief and preventative measures   205
Leg cramps   205
  Assessment   205
  Relief and preventative measures   205
Nasal congestion and epistaxis   206
  Nasal congestion   206
  Epistaxis   206
Nausea and/or vomiting during pregnancy   207
  Assessment   207
  Relief and preventative measures   207
Ptyalism   209
  Assessment   210
  Relief and preventative measures   210
Restless leg syndrome (RLS)   210
  Assessment   210
  Relief and preventative measures   210
Round ligament pain   211
  Assessment   211
  Relief and preventative measures   211
Shortness of breath   211
  Assessment   212
  Relief and preventative measures   212
Skin changes   212
  Hyperpigmentation   212
  Vascular changes   213
Hair and nail changes   213
  Assessment   213
  Relief and preventative measures   213
Sleep disturbances   214
  Assessment   214
  Relief and preventative measures   214
Supine hypotension syndrome (SHS)   215
  Assessment   215
  Relief and preventative measures   215
Urinary frequency   215
  Assessment   215
  Relief and preventative measures   215
Urinary incontinence   216
  Assessment   216
  Relief and preventative measures   216

Varicosities (legs/vulva)   216
  Leg varicosities   216
  Vulvar varicosities   217
Visual changes   219
  Subjective data gathering   219
  Assessment   219
  Relief and preventative measures   220
Resources for health-care providers and women
  and their families   220
References   220

12 Medication use during pregnancy   223
    Mary C. Brucker and Tekoa L. King
Introduction   224
Pharmacologic terms   224
Types of pharmaceutical agents   224
Prescriptive authority   224
Governmental oversight of pharmaceutical
  agents   225
The prescription: Essential components   225
Drugs and pregnancy   226
Teratology   227
  Etiology of birth defects   228
  Mechanisms of teratogenic drugs   228
  Identification of a teratogen   229
  FDA categories for drugs in pregnancy   229
  Selected teratogens   231
Pharmacokinetics in pregnancy   231
Rational use of drugs in pregnancy   234
Summary   234
Resources for women and their families   236
References   236

13 Substance use during pregnancy   238
    Daisy J. Goodman, Alane B. O'Connor, and
    Kelley A. Bowden
Risks of perinatal substance abuse   238
Prevalence of prenatal substance abuse   239
Definitions   239
Historical approaches to maternal substance use   240
Harm reduction approach to prenatal
  substance use   240
Position statements on prenatal substance use   240
Comorbid conditions and prenatal substance use   241
  Psychiatric disease   241
  Medical risks   241
Commonly abused substances and pregnancy
  implications   241
  Alcohol   241
  Nicotine   242
  Cocaine   243
  Opioids   243
  Benzodiazepines   243
  Marijuana   244
  Amphetamines/Methamphetamines   244
  Designer drugs   244
Screening for prenatal substance abuse   244
  Screening tools   245

Brief intervention and treatment | 246
Smoking cessation during pregnancy | 246
   The 5 A's and the 5 R's model of smoking
     cessation | 246
   Bupropion (Zyban®, Wellbutrin®) | 246
   Nicotine replacement therapy | 246
   Varenicline (Chantix®) | 246
Care of pregnant women with substance
   use disorders | 247
   Antepartum assessment | 248
Referral to treatment | 249
Opioid replacement therapy in pregnancy | 249
   Methadone | 250
   Buprenorphine | 250
   Treatment with methadone vs. buprenorphine | 250
   Breastfeeding and medication-assisted
     treatment counseling | 251
Communication and coordination of care | 251
Neonatal abstinence syndrome | 252
   Assessment and treatment of neonatal
     abstinence syndrome | 252
   Breastfeeding and neonatal abstinence
     syndrome | 252
   Long-term implications of neonatal
     abstinence syndrome | 252
Postpartum care | 253
   Breastfeeding and substance use | 253
Cultural considerations | 254
Personal and family considerations | 256
Scope of practice considerations | 256
Summary | 256
Resources for health-care providers | 256
Resources for women and their families | 256
References | 256

14   Social issues in pregnancy | 261
Nena R. Harris

Introduction | 261
Poverty | 262
   Interdisciplinary care | 263
Incarceration | 264
Intimate partner violence during pregnancy | 265
Pregnancy and a history of childhood
   sexual abuse | 266
   Assessing for childhood sexual abuse | 266
   Providing care | 268
Summary | 268
Resources for health-care providers | 270
Resources for women and their families | 270
References | 271

15   Exercise, recreational and occupational
issues, and intimate relationships
in pregnancy | 274
Meghan Garland

Exercise in pregnancy | 274
   Physiological changes during pregnancy
     and exercise | 274

Benefits of exercise in pregnancy | 275
Motivating women to exercise in pregnancy | 276
Exercise activities | 277
Exercise guidelines | 277
General advice for exercising in pregnancy | 278
Summary | 279
Environmental exposures in pregnancy | 279
   Making an environmental exposure
     assessment | 280
   Metals and metalloids | 280
   Organic solvents | 282
   Pesticides | 283
   Endocrine-disrupting chemicals | 283
   Reducing exposures | 283
   Summary | 284
Sexuality in pregnancy | 284
   Pregnancy influences on sexuality | 284
   Sexual activities during pregnancy | 285
   Sexual history | 285
   Counseling | 285
   Summary | 286
Working during pregnancy | 286
   Shift work | 286
   Heavy lifting and long work hours | 286
   Noise exposure | 287
   Psychosocial stress | 287
   Pregnancy discrimination in the workplace | 287
   Data gathering and counseling | 287
   Summary | 288
Resources on pregnancy and environmental
   exposure for women | 288
Resources on pregnancy and environmental
   exposure for health-care providers | 288
Resource on work during pregnancy
   for women | 288
References | 288

16   Psychosocial adaptations in pregnancy | 291
Cindy L. Farley

Introduction | 292
Maternal attachment and adaptation | 292
   Bowlby and Ainsworth | 293
   Kennell and Klaus | 293
   Brazelton | 294
   Rubin | 294
   Lederman | 297
Sibling adaptation and attachment | 301
Partner adaptation and attachment | 302
   Male partners | 303
   Lesbian partners | 304
Body image | 305
Childbirth confidence | 306
   Self-efficacy and childbirth | 306
Summary | 308
Resources for women and their families | 308
Resources for health-care providers | 309
References | 309

17   Health education during pregnancy   312
     Lisa Hanson, Leona VandeVusse, and
     Kathryn Shisler Harrod

     Introduction   312
     Sources and quality of consumer childbirth
       education   312
     Prenatal visit approach to individual childbirth
       education   314
     Class education and group prenatal care   314
     Developmental considerations in prenatal health
       education   314
       Adolescents   314
       Adult education principles   315
     Issues integral to prenatal education   315
       *Literacy, health literacy, written materials,
         and reading level*   316
       Prenatal health education guidelines   316
     Prioritizing prenatal education needs   316
       Responding to questions   317
       Discussing health and safety issues   317
       Anticipatory guidance   317
       Providing anticipatory guidance   317
     Trimester-based approaches to prenatal
       education   317
     Cultural considerations   321
     Health disparities and vulnerable populations   321
     Documentation of teaching   321
     Summary   321
     Resources for health-care providers and women   322
     Resources for women and their families   323
     References   323

18   Assessment and care at the onset of labor   325
     Amy Marowitz

     Introduction   325
     Determining the onset of labor   325
     Timing of admission to the birth setting   326
     What is "false labor"?   326
     Determining active labor   327
     Anticipatory guidance during the prenatal period   327
     Data collection   327
       General   328
     Plan of care   328
       Self-care   329
     Sleep and rest   329
     Coping strategies and comfort measures for
       early labor   330
     Ambulation in early labor   330
     Summary   330
     References   332

Part III   Common complications
of pregnancy   333

19   Bleeding during pregnancy   335
     Robin G. Jordan
     Introduction   335

     Bleeding during the first half of pregnancy   335
     Evaluation   336
       Problem-focused history   336
       Physical exam   336
       Laboratory evaluation   337
       Diagnostic testing   337
     Subchorionic hemorrhage or hematoma   337
     Leiomyomas   337
     Spontaneous pregnancy loss   337
       Differential diagnosis   338
       Diagnosis and management   339
       Early pregnancy loss follow-up care   340
       *Early pregnancy loss and family
         considerations*   340
       Recurrent pregnancy loss   341
       *Potential problems of unexplained early
         pregnancy bleeding*   341
     Ectopic pregnancy   341
       Clinical presentation   342
       Diagnosis and management   342
     Gestational trophoblastic disease   343
       Potential problems   344
       Presentation   344
       Diagnosis and management   344
     Early pregnancy bleeding and scope of
       practice considerations   344
     Bleeding during the second half of pregnancy   345
     Placenta previa   345
       Potential problems   345
       Presentation   346
       Differential diagnoses   346
     Placental abruption   346
       Potential problems   347
       Presentation   347
     Diagnosis and management of bleeding in
       the second half of pregnancy   348
     Scope of practice considerations in later
       pregnancy bleeding   348
     Family considerations in later pregnancy
       bleeding   348
     Summary   348
     Resources for women and their families   348
     References   350

20   Amniotic fluid and fetal growth disorders   352
     Victoria H. Burslem and Cindy L. Farley

     Introduction   353
     Amniotic fluid dynamics   353
     Normal placentation and fetal development   354
     Amniotic fluid disorders   354
       Oligohydramnios   354
       Polyhydramnios   357
     Fetal growth disorders   358
       Determination of growth disorders   358
     Intrauterine growth restriction   359
       Assessment and management   360
     Summary   362

Resources for women and their families   363
Resources for health-care providers   363
References   363

21   Preterm labor and birth   365
Robin G. Jordan

Introduction   365
Social and racial disparities   366
Physiology of preterm birth   366
Complications related to prematurity   367
Risk factors for preterm birth   367
Predicting preterm birth   368
    Fetal fibronectin (fFN) testing   368
    Cervical length measurement   368
Diagnosing preterm labor   368
Management of women with preterm labor   368
Preterm birth prevention   369
    Nutrition   369
    Smoking cessation   370
    Interpregnancy interval   370
    Treating infections   370
    Disturbed sleep and fatigue   371
Progesterone therapy   371
Cerclage   371
Summary   371
Resources for women and health-care
    providers   373
References   373

22   Hypertensive disorders in pregnancy   375
Robin G. Jordan

Introduction   375
Classification of hypertensive disorders
    of pregnancy   375
Chronic hypertension   375
Gestational hypertension   376
Preeclampsia–eclampsia   376
Preeclampsia superimposed on chronic
    hypertension   377
Preeclampsia   377
    Pathophysiology of preeclampsia   377
    Potential problems due to preeclampsia   378
    Risk factors for developing preeclampsia   378
    Diagnostic evaluation   379
    Management of women with preeclampsia   380
HELLP syndrome   382
Atypical presentation preeclampsia   382
Prediction of preeclampsia   383
Prevention of preeclampsia   383
Long-term sequelae of preeclampsia   383
Risk management issues in the office setting   384
Interprofessional practice issues   384
Summary   384
Resources for women and their families   384
Resources for health-care providers   384
References   385

23   Gestational diabetes   387
Kimberly K. Trout

Introduction   387
Pathophysiology and potential problems of
    gestational diabetes   387
Prenatal screening and diagnosis of GDM   388
    One-hour oral glucose tolerance testing   389
    Two-hour oral glucose tolerance testing   389
    Screening for women at high risk for GDM   390
Management of gestational diabetes   390
    Dietary intervention   390
    Exercise therapy   391
    Blood glucose monitoring   391
Oral medications for GDM   392
    Glyburide   392
    Metformin   392
Insulin therapy   392
Fetal surveillance and timing of birth   392
    Labor and birth   393
Postpartum follow-up   393
Scope of practice issues   394
Perspective on GDM risk   394
Resources for women and their families   395
Resources for health-care providers   395
References   395

24   Other complications in pregnancy:
    Multiple gestation, post-term
    pregnancy, hyperemesis, and
    abdominal pain   397
Tonya B. Nicholson

Abdominal pain in pregnancy   398
    Appendicitis   399
    Cholylithiasis   399
    Abdominal trauma   399
Hyperemesis gravidarum (HG)   399
    Etiology and risk factors   400
    Complications of hyperemesis gravidarum   400
    Evaluation   400
    Care and management   400
Multifetal pregnancy   401
    Care of women with multifetal gestation   402
    Assessing fetal growth   402
    Fetal surveillance   402
    Nutritional counseling   403
    Anticipatory guidance   403
Post-term pregnancy   403
    Overview   403
    Complications associated with post-term
        pregnancy   404
    Prevention, intervention, and management
        options   404
Resource for health-care providers   406
Resources for women and their families   406
References   407

25   Perinatal loss and grief   409
      Robin G. Jordan

      Introduction   409
      Stillbirth   409
      Breaking the news   410
      Care and management of women with stillbirth   410
      Grieving and emotional care after perinatal loss 411
          Cultural considerations   412
      Physical care after stillbirth   413
      Follow-up   413
      Interconception and subsequent pregnancy care   413
      Summary   414
      Resources for women and their families   415
      Resources for health-care providers   415
      References   415

Part IV   Postnatal care   417

26   Physiological alterations
      during the postnatal period   419
      *Kimberly A. Couch and
      Karen DeCocker-Geist*

      Introduction   419
      Uterus   419
      Lochia   420
      Cervix   420
      Vagina   420
      Labia and perineum   420
      Additional maternal alterations during the
          postpartum period   421
          Endocrine changes   421
          Cardiovascular system   421
          Renal system   421
          Gastrointestinal tract   421
      Summary   421
      Resource for women   422
      Resource for health-care provider   422
      References   422

27   Components of postnatal care   423
      *Tia P. Andrighetti and
      Deborah Brandt Karsnitz*

      Introduction   423
      Assessment of maternal physical and emotional
          adjustment   425
          Review of birth experience   426
          Family adaptation   426
          Infant feeding   428
      Activity/Exercise   428
      Diet and nutrition   429
          Weight loss   429
      Lochia   430
      Afterbirth pain   430
      Perineal discomfort   431
      Diureseis/Diaphoresis   431
      Constipation/Hemorrhoids   431
      Sexuality   431

      Resumption of menses and ovulation   432
      Contraception   432
      Postpartum physical examination   433
          Breast exam   433
          Abdominal exam   433
          Costovertebral angle tenderness (CVAT)   434
          Perineal exam   434
          Vaginal and uterine exam   434
          Rectal exam   434
          Leg exam   435
      Postpartum depression and domestic
          violence screening   435
      Postnatal warning signs   435
      Cultural considerations   435
      Health disparities and vulnerable populations   436
      Scope of practice considerations   437
      Legal issues   438
      Summary   438
      Resources for women   439
      Resources for health-care providers   439
      References   439

28   Common complications during the
      postnatal period   441
      Deborah Brandt Karsnitz

      Introduction   441
      Postpartum morbidity and mortality   442
      Postpartum cultural considerations   442
      Postpartum disorders   443
          Puerperal fever (pyrexia)   443
          Puerperal infection (postpartum infection) 443
          Wound infection   445
          Delayed or late postpartum hemorrhage   445
          Postpartum hematoma   446
          Subinvolution   446
          Postpartum preeclampsia–eclampsia   446
          Postpartum thrombophlebitis   447
          Postpartum thyroiditis   447
          Postpartum mood and anxiety disorders   448
          Postpartum blues   449
          Postpartum depression   449
          Postpartum psychosis   451
          Generalized anxiety disorder   451
          Obsessive-compulsive disorder   451
          Panic disorder   451
          Post-traumatic stress disorder   451
      Summary   457
      Resource for women and their families   458
      Resource for health-care providers   458
      References   458

29   Contraception   462
      Patricia Aikins Murphy and Leah N. Torres

      Introduction   462
      Postpartum care and return to fertility
          after childbirth   463

Considerations in selecting a postpartum
  contraceptive method   463
Contraceptive methods   465
Tier one methods   466
  Permanent methods   466
  *Long-acting reversible contraceptive
    (LARC) methods*   467
Tier two methods   469
  Combined hormonal contraceptives (CHCs)   469
  Progestin-only contraceptives   470
  Lactational amenorrhea method (LAM)   472
Tier three methods   472
  Barrier methods   472
  Other methods   474
Emergency contraception   474
Summary   475
Resources for women and health-care providers   476
References   476

30 Lactation and breastfeeding   478
    Marsha Walker

Introduction   478
Breastfeeding as a public health issue   479
The unique properties of human milk   480
Nutritional properties of human milk   480
  Defense agents in human milk   482
Maternal and infant anatomy and physiology
  of lactation and breastfeeding   482
Promoting and supporting breastfeeding   483
The basics of breastfeeding support and
  assessment   484
  Position   484
  Latch   487
Milk production   489
Breastfeeding patterns   489
Assessing intake   490
Care of the breastfeeding mother   491
  Nutrition for nursing mothers   491
  Contraception   492
  Smoking   492
  Alcohol and illicit drugs   493
  Medications and breastfeeding   493
  Employed nursing mothers   493
Summary   494
Resources for women and health-care providers   495
References   495

31 Common breastfeeding problems   499
    Marsha Walker

Introduction   499
Common infant-related breastfeeding problems   499
  Fussy baby   499
  Sleepy baby   500
  Slow weight gain   501
  Preterm and late preterm infants   502
Common maternal breastfeeding problems   503
  Sore nipples   503
  Management of sore nipples   505

Breast engorgement   506
  Plugged ducts   506
Mastitis   507
Abscess   507
Low milk supply   508
Summary   510
Resources for women and their families   511
Resources for health-care providers   511
References   511

Part V Management of common
health problems during the prenatal
and postnatal periods   515

32 Respiratory disorders   517
    Janyce Cagan Agruss

Introduction   517
Respiratory physiology and pregnancy   517
Asthma   517
  Potential problems   518
  Differential diagnosis   518
  *Common clinical presentation and
    data gathering*   518
  Management of asthma during pregnancy   518
  Scope of practice considerations   520
Influenza   521
Upper respiratory infection   521
Pneumonia   522
Summary   523
Resource for health-care providers   523
References   523

33 Hematological and thromboembolic
    disorders   525
    Julie A. Marfell

Introduction   525
Anemia   525
  Physiological changes in pregnancy   525
Iron-deficiency anemia   526
Hemoglobinopathies   529
  Hemoglobin S   529
  Thalassemia   529
Folate deficiency   530
Vitamin B$_{12}$ deficiency   530
Unexplained maternal anemia   530
Bleeding disorders   531
  Thrombocytopenia   531
  Inherited bleeding disorders   531
Coagulopathies during pregnancy   531
Summary   534
Resource for women and their families   534
Resources for health-care providers   534
References   534

34 Urinary tract disorders   536
    Rhonda Arthur and Nancy Pesta Walsh

Introduction   536

Urinary tract infection   536
  Prevalence and risk factors   536
  Pathophysiology   537
  Common pathogens   537
  Asymptomatic bacteriuria   537
  Acute cystitis   537
  Acute pyelonephritis   538
Evaluation   538
  Health history   538
  Physical examination   538
  Laboratory testing   538
Care of women with urinary tract infections   538
Recurrent UTI   540
Care of women with suspected acute
  pyelonephritis   540
Nephrolithiasis   541
  Evaluation   541
  Care of women with suspected nephrolithiasis 541
Summary   541
Resources for women   542
Resource for health-care providers   542
References   542

35 Gastrointestinal disorders   544
  Audra C. Malone and Karen DeCocker-Geist
Introduction   544
Gastroenteritis   544
  Evaluation and management   544
  Scope of practice issues   545
Intraheptic cholestasis of pregnancy   545
  Scope of practice issues   546
Cholecystitis   546
  Evaluation and management   546
  Scope of practice issues   547
Appendicitis   547
  Evaluation and management   547
  Scope of practice issues   547
Summary   548
Resource for women and their families   548
References   548

36 Obesity   549
  Cecelia M. Jevitt
Introduction   549
Overview   549
Prevalence   550
Health disparities and cultural considerations   550
Personal and family considerations   550
Obesity physiology   551
Potential problems associated with obesity in
  childbearing women   551
Management of pregestational obesity   552
  Nondiscriminatory language   552
  Assessment of the obese pregnant woman   552
Management principles   553
Nutrition   554
Weight loss concerns   554

Physical activity   554
Comfort measures   554
Bariatric surgery   555
Scope of practice considerations   555
Legal and liability issues   555
Intrapartum and postpartum issues   556
Summary   556
Resources for women and their families   556
Resources for health-care providers   556
References   558

37 Endocrine disorders   560
  Elizabeth Gabzdyl
Introduction   560
Thyroid disorders in pregnancy   560
  Thyroid physiology in pregnancy   560
Diagnosing thyroid disorders   561
Overt hypothyroidism   562
  Maternal and fetal risks   562
  Clinical presentation   562
  Laboratory testing, diagnosis, and management 562
Subclinical hypothyroidism   563
Screening for hypothyroidism in pregnancy   563
Preconception care of a woman with
  hypothyroidism   564
Hyperthyroidism   564
  Maternal and fetal risks   564
  Clinical presentation   564
  Laboratory testing, diagnosis, and management 564
  Scope of practice considerations   565
Subclinical hyperthyroidism   565
Thyroid storm   565
Postpartum thyroiditis   565
  Laboratory evaluation, diagnosis, and
    management   565
Pregestational diabetes   566
  Classifications   566
  Perinatal risks of pregestational diabetes 567
  Preconception counseling and care of women
    with pregestational diabetes 567
Summary   567
Resources for women and health-care providers   567
References   568

38 Neurological disorders   570
  Tonya B. Nicholson
Introduction   570
Care of the pregnant woman
  with seizure disorders   570
Care of pregnant women with headache   573
  Tension-type headaches   574
  Migraine headaches   574
  Nonpharmacological headache management   574
  Pharmacological treatment of migraine headaches 575
  Postpartum headaches   576
  Cluster headaches   576
Care of pregnant women with multiple sclerosis   577

Summary   577
Resources for women and their families   578
References   578

39 Dermatological disorders   580
    Gwendolyn Short and Elizabeth
    Powell Holcomb
    Introduction   580
    Atopic dermatitis   580
        Assessment   581
        Differential diagnoses   581
        Treatment and management   581
    Prurigo of pregnancy   581
        Assessment   581
        Differential diagnoses   581
        Treatment and management   582
    Pruritic urticarial papules and plaques
        of pregnancy   582
        Assessment   582
        Differential diagnoses   583
        Treatment and management   583
    Pruritic folliculitis of pregnancy   583
        Assessment   583
        Differential diagnosis   583
        Treatment and management   583
    Pemphigoid gestationis   583
        Assessment   584
        Differential diagnosis   584
        Treatment and management   584
        Collaboration, consultation, and referral   585
    Impetigo herpetiformis   585
        Assessment   585
        Differential diagnosis   585
        Treatment and management   585
        Collaboration, consultation, and referral   585
    Intrahepatic cholestasis of pregnancy   585
        Assessment   586
        Differential diagnoses   586
        Treatment and management   586
        Collaboration, consultation, and referral   586
    Summary   587
    Resources for health-care providers   587
    References   588

40 Infectious diseases   589
    Jacquelyne Brooks and Elizabeth A. Parr
    Introduction   589
    Cytomegalovirus   590
        Potential problems   590
        Clinical presentation and assessment   590
        Management   591
        Prevention   591
    Group B Streptococcus   592
        Potential problems   592
        Assessment   592
        Management   592
    Hepatitis infections   593

        Hepatitis A   593
        Hepatitis B   594
        Hepatitis C   596
    Parvovirus B19   597
        Potential problems   597
        Assessment   597
        Management   597
    Rubella   597
        Presentation and assessment   598
        Management   598
        Prevention of rubella and CRS   599
    Toxoplasmosis   599
        Potential problems   599
        Clinical presentation and assessment   599
        Management   601
        Prevention   602
    Varicella   602
        Potential problems   602
        Clinical presentation and assessment   602
        Management   603
    Summary   603
    Resources for women   604
    Resources for health-care providers   604
    References   604

41 Sexually transmitted infections and
    common vaginitis   608
    Meghan Garland and Barbara P. Brennan
    Introduction   608
    Sexually transmitted bacterial infections   609
        Chlamydia trachomatis   609
        Neisseria gonorrhoeae   609
        Syphilis   610
    Sexually transmitted viral infections   610
        Herpes simplex   610
        Human papillomavirus   612
    Fungal infection   613
        Vaginal candidiasis   613
    Sexually transmitted parasitic infection   613
        Trichomonas vaginalis   613
    Sexually transmitted bacterial infection   614
        Bacterial vaginosis   614
    Partner treatment of an STI   616
    Legal requirements for reporting STI diagnosis   616
    Psychosocial impacts of STI diagnosis   616
        Effects on the individual   616
        STI prevention within relationships   617
    Summary   618
    Resources for health-care providers   619
    Resource for women and partners   619
    References   619

42 Psychological disorders   621
    Heather Shlosser
    Overview   621
    Depression during pregnancy   621
        Potential problems of prenatal depression   623

Screening for prenatal depression   623
Management of prenatal depression   623
Bipolar disorder in pregnancy   625
Signs and symptoms of bipolar disorder   625
Management of pregnant women with
*   bipolar disorder*   626
Generalized anxiety disorder (GAD)   626
Screening for GAD   627
Management of GAD   627

Scope of practice considerations   627
Summary   628
Resources for women and their families   629
Resources for health-care providers   629
References   629

Index   **631**

About the editors

Robin G. Jordan received her certificate in midwifery from the University of Medicine and Dentistry of New Jersey in 1982, after earning her MSN from Case Western Reserve University. In 2006, she was awarded a PhD in Health Sciences from Touro University. Dr. Jordan started the first hospital-based nurse-midwifery service in the greater Northern Michigan area. She has experience in attending childbearing women in the hospital, Birth Center, and home settings. Dr. Jordan was a longstanding faculty member of Frontier Nursing University developing and teaching the Antepartum Care course series for midwifery and nurse practitioner students. She currently teaches maternal-child health nursing at North Central Michigan College. She writes for various publications on antepartum care topics and is coauthor of the Fourth Edition of *Clinical Practice Guidelines for Midwifery and Women's Health*. Dr. Jordan serves as a Senior Project Consultant for the American College of Nurse Midwives updating and developing ACNM documents. Dr. Jordan is also part of a team of educators writing curricula for the new Doctorate of Midwifery degree.

Janet L. Engstrom is a certified nurse-midwife and women's health nurse practitioner. She completed her midwifery and nurse practitioner education at the University of Illinois at Chicago, where she was also a longstanding faculty member and Program Director for the Nurse-Midwifery and Women's Health Care Nurse Practitioner programs. She is currently the Associate Dean for Research at Frontier Nursing University. She is also a professor and researcher at Rush University in Chicago and conducts research examining human milk feeding for premature infants with the Rush Mothers' Milk Club. She has taught women's health care and research methods for over 30 years and has won numerous awards for her teaching and research.

Julie A. Marfell, DNP, APRN, FNP-BC, FAANP, has been a family nurse practitioner and nurse educator for eighteen years. She graduated from the Doctorate of Nursing Program at Rush University in 1994. Dr. Marfell is the Associate Dean for Family Nursing at Frontier Nursing University, having implemented and led the community-based Family Nurse Practitioner Program at Frontier since 1999. Dr. Marfell has presented and published on multiple topics related to health care and nursing education. She currently serves on the Board of Directors for both the National Organization of Nurse Practitioner Faculties and the Kentucky Coalition of Nurse Practitioners and Nurse Midwives. Dr. Marfell continues to provide health care to families as an FNP in a primary care setting.

Cindy L. Farley, CNM, PhD, FACNM, studied midwifery at Emory University. She earned her BSN and PhD from the Ohio State University and her MN from Emory University. She is currently Adjunct Associate Professor at Georgetown University in the Nurse-Midwifery/ Women's health Nurse Practitioner (WHNP) program and Professor in the midwifery programs of the Midwifery Institute of Philadelphia University. She serves as a locum tenens clinician for the midwifery practice at Pomerene Hospital, Millersburg, Ohio, home of the largest Amish and Anabaptist population in the world. Additionally, she takes midwifery students to Haiti to work with the nongovernmental organization (NGO), Midwives for Haiti, working toward building the Haitian midwifery work force and saving lives of Haitian mothers and babies. Dr. Farley serves as a legal expert on selected cases involving midwifery care and is coauthor of the Third and Fourth Editions of *Clinical Practice Guidelines for Midwifery and Women's Health*. Dr. Farley has been active in working toward the development of a Doctorate of Midwifery, as part of an American College of Nurse-Midwives ad hoc committee writing doctoral competencies and as part of a think tank of midwifery educators and stakeholders writing curricula for this innovative new degree.

Contributors

Janyce Cagan Agruss, PhD, APRN, FNP-BC
Rush University, College of Nursing
Chicago, IL

Tia P. Andrighetti, DNP, CNM
Frontier Nursing University
Hyden, KY

Rhonda Arthur, DNP, CNM, WHNP-BC, APRN-BC
Frontier Nursing University
Hyden, KY

Victoria L. Baker, PhD, MSPH, CNM
Frontier Nursing University
Hyden, KY

Kelley A. Bowden, MS, RN
Maine Medical Center
Portland, ME

Barbara P. Brennan, DNP, FNP-BC
Frontier Nursing University
Hyden, KY

Jacquelyne Brooks, MS, CNM, WHNP-BC
Frontier Nursing University
Hyden, KY

Mary C. Brucker, PhD, CNM, FACNM
Georgetown University
Washington, DC
Baylor University
Dallas, TX

Victoria H. Burslem, MSN, CNM
Midwifery Institute of Philadelphia University
Philadelphia, PA

Joyce D. Cappiello, PhD, APRN, FNP-BC, FAANP
ROE Consortium
Boston, MA
University of New Hampshire
Durham, NY

Patricia W. Caudle, DNSc, CNM, FNP-BC
Frontier Nursing University
Hyden, KY

Kimberly A. Couch, DNP, CNM
Frontier Nursing University
Hyden, KY

Karen DeCocker-Geist, DNP, CNM
Frontier Nursing University
Hyden, KY

Janet L. Engstrom, PhD, APN, CNM, WHNP-BC
Frontier Nursing University
Hyden, KY
Rush University, College of Nursing
Chicago, IL

Jenifer Fahey, MSN, MPH, CNM
University of Maryland
Baltimore, MD

Cindy L. Farley, PhD, CNM, FACNM
Georgetown University
Washington, DC

Elizabeth Gabzdyl, DNP, APN, CNM
College of Nursing
University of Illinois at Chicago
Chicago, IL

Meghan Garland, MSN, CNM
Frontier Nursing University
Hyden, KY

Daisy J. Goodman, DNP, CNM, WHNP-BC
Dartmouth Hitchcock Medical Center
Frontier Nursing University
Hyden, KY

Lisa Hanson, PhD, CNM, FACNM
Marquette University, School of Nursing
Milwaukee, WI

Nena R. Harris, PhD, CNM, FNP-BC
Frontier Nursing University
Hyden, KY

Kathryn Shisler Harrod, PhD, APNP, CNM, FACNM
Aurora Health Care Marquette University
Marquette University, School of Nursing
Milwaukee, WI

Elizabeth Powell Holcomb, PhD, FNP-BC
Frontier Nursing University
Hyden, KY

Cecelia M. Jevitt, PhD, CNM, FACNM
Yale University, School of Nursing
New Haven, CT

Robin G. Jordan, PhD, CNM, FACNM
North Central Michigan College
Petoskey, MI
Frontier Nursing University
Hyden, KY, USA

Deborah Brandt Karsnitz, DNP, CNM, FACNM
Frontier Nursing University
Hyden, KY

Tekoa L. King, MPH, CNM, FACNM
Journal of Midwifery and Women's Health
University of California, San Francisco
San Francisco, CA

Carrie S. Klima, PhD, CNM, FACNM
College of Nursing
University of Illinois at Chicago
Chicago, IL

Audra C. Malone, DNP, FNP-BC
Frontier Nursing University
Hyden, KY

Julie A. Marfell, DNP, APRN, FNP-BC, FAANP
Frontier Nursing University
Hyden, KY

Amy Marowitz, DNP, CNM
Frontier Nursing University
Hyden, KY

Patricia Aikins Murphy, DrPH, CNM, FACNM
University of Utah, College of Nursing
Salt Lake City, UT

Tonya B. Nicholson, DNP, CNM, WHNP-BC
Frontier Nursing University
Hyden, KY

Alane B. O'Connor, DNP, FNP
Dartmouth Medical School
Hanover, NH
Vanderbilt University, School of Nursing
Nashville, TN

Elizabeth A. Parr, MSN, CNM
Midwifery Institute of Philadelphia University
Philadelphia, PA

Julie A. Paul, DNP, CNM
Frontier Nursing University
Hyden, KY

Heather Shlosser, DNP, FNP-BC, PMHNP-BC
Frontier Nursing University
Hyden, KY

Gwendolyn Short, DNP, MPH, ARNP, FNP-BC
Frontier Nursing University
Hyden, KY

Leah N. Torres, MD
University of Utah School of Medicine
Salt Lake City, UT

Kimberly K. Trout, PhD, APRN, CNM
University of Pennyslvania
Philadelphia, PA

Leona VandeVusse, PhD, CNM, FACNM
Marquette University, School of Nursing
Milwaukee, WI

Marsha Walker, RN, IBCLC
National Alliance for Breastfeeding Advocacy
Weston, MA

Nancy Pesta Walsh, DNP, RN, CNP, FNP-BC
Frontier Nursing University
Hyden, KY

Reviewers

Anne Z. Cockerham, PhD, CNM, WHNP-BC
Frontier Nursing University, Hyden, KY

Karen DeCocker-Geist, DNP, CNM
Frontier Nursing University, Hyden, KY

Mary Dawn Hennessy, PhD, CNM
University of Illinois at Chicago, Chicago, IL

Deborah Brandt Karsnitz, DNP, CNM, FACNM
Frontier Nursing University, Hyden, KY

Karen Kavanaugh, PhD, RN, FAAN
Wayne State University, Detroit, MI

Barbara McFarlin, PhD, CNM, RDMS, FACNM
University of Illinois at Chicago, Chicago, IL

Claudia Sittler, MS, CNM, WHNP-BC
University of Illinois at Chicago, Chicago, IL

Foreword

A woman-centered approach to health care is provided within the context of the woman as the authoritative knower. Women have unique needs; therefore, the care must be integrated and tailored to fit the specific situation of each woman. This requires care that it is not only comprehensive but also detailed and focused to meet each woman's individualized needs and lived experience. This model of care respects the woman's perspective and includes her input as a significant part of assessment, diagnosis, treatment, and evaluation. Her agency in the process is valued and encouraged.

Prenatal and Postpartum Care: A Woman-Centered Approach provides comprehensive content for clinicians who provide care for women. The attention to details too often overlooked is a critical component of each topic because it ensures that the many, and sometimes disparate, needs and conditions of women who are pregnant or in the postpartum period are recognized and addressed. It is the responsibility of clinicians providing care to women during pregnancy and postpartum to present women with the wide range of information and services available to them so that each woman is able to make informed choices about her health care and that of her growing fetus.

The authors of this text are respected experts in their fields, and each brings their specialized knowledge as nurse-midwives and nurse practitioners to the content. Clinicians will find that this book contains essential and comprehensive content that provides the basis to attend to the many facets important for a healthy pregnancy and postpartum. This knowledge will allow clinicians to provide care that is woman centered in its breadth and depth. This book is an important contribution to all of the clinicians who provide prenatal and postpartum care and to all of the women who receive their care.

Kerri Durnell Schuiling
PhD, CNM, NP,
FACNM, FAAN

Frances E. Likis
DrPH, NP, CNM,
FACNM, FAAN

Preface

Women-centered prenatal and postnatal care

The birth of a baby is a major life-changing event for a woman and her family. A woman transforms into a mother, and a family is created. Optimal care not only focuses on the physical process but also on the emotional experience of pregnancy and the postpartum period. The context of a woman's culture, life experiences, social roles, and physical and mental health status on the childbearing experience influence her choices and outcomes.

This book both describes and challenges current prenatal and postnatal care practices. Prenatal care visits within the current pathology-centered model of care are brief and focused on testing, legalities, and reimbursement. Too often this approach emphasizes the needs of the provider within the office setting rather than the woman's needs during pregnancy. Postnatal care is often limited in scope and connection at a time when the new family needs guidance and support from professionals as well as family members. This is a disservice to women and their families. Opportunities to promote health and well-being for the woman and her family during pregnancy, birth and beyond are being missed in contemporary practice.

The woman herself and her unique needs are the rightful focus of prenatal and postnatal care. "Woman-centered care" is the term used to describe a philosophy of maternity care that is based on the needs and preferences of the woman and her family. This care emphasizes the importance of informed choice, continuity of care, active participation, best care practices, provider responsiveness, and accessibility. Pregnancy, childbirth, and the postpartum period are the start of family life; these periods are not just a series of isolated clinical episodes packaged as "global prenatal care." A full account of the meaning and values that each woman brings to her experience of motherhood should be included in care.

The fundamental principles of woman-centered care encompass the following tenets:

- Women are cocreators of their maternity care with their health-care providers.
- Women have the right to informed choice in the options available to them during pregnancy, labor, birth, and the postnatal period, including the place of birth, who provides care, and where care is provided.

- Women have the ultimate authority over the key decisions that affect the content and progress of their care.
- Women are provided care that supports their optimal health and that of their baby.

Prenatal and postnatal care provided within the context of the woman's own experience, focused on both the life-changing nature of the pregnancy experience as well as physical adaptations and needs, leads to improved maternal and infant outcomes. The views, beliefs, and values of the woman, her partner, and her family in relation to her care and that of her baby are sought and respected at all times. Adequate time is spent in providing optimal prenatal and postnatal care with kindness, respect, and dignity.

The need for this text

A growing body of scientific evidence supports physiological childbearing for healthy pregnant women at low risk for complications. Several decades of escalating pregnancy and birth medicalization have shown that interventions applied on a large scale and without medical indication lead to significant negative iatrogenic consequences. A prime example of this is the increase in elective induction of labor and the associated rise in the birth rate of late preterm babies. However, care supporting physiological labor and birth care does not begin with the first contraction; rather it begins with the first prenatal appointment and continues into the postpartum period. Too much faith is placed in technology and too little faith is placed in human connection and caring. This book brings balance to the fore; it adds a wholistic framework from which to enter into dialogue with the woman who presents for care. Midwives, nurse practitioners and other prenatal and postnatal health-care providers, and students with common practice foundations in providing holistic care, emphasizing patient education and health maintenance in the context of an ongoing relationship, will find this book useful.

The editors of this book are experienced educators of midwives, nurse practitioners, medical students, and other health-care providers. We have found that many available obstetrical and maternity care texts offer limited content on prenatal and postnatal care. Additionally, an appreciation of the effects of the mind–body connection and the background social dynamics of the pregnant woman and her family on her overall health and child-bearing experience has been lacking. This appreciation, in addition to a solid understanding of normal child-bearing processes, will increase health-care providers' competency in supporting the normal and recognizing the abnormal. This text provides a breadth and depth of knowledge on normal pregnancy and postpartum processes and care not found in other texts.

We are extremely fortunate to many highly regarded contributors to this text. All contributing authors have a background in clinical practice and are established content experts in their field. Most of our contributors are also educators, bringing an understanding of the needs of students to the text.

This book was written as a resource for all those interested in providing woman-centered prenatal and postnatal care. While aspects of this care are timeless and do not change, certain elements of prenatal and postnatal

care are refined as new evidence is incorporated into existing bodies of knowledge. Health-care providers are responsible for their ongoing learning in the field and should read critically and widely among the many resources available to them. Evidence-based health care encompasses psychosocial and cultural aspects of care and so is applied in a mutual dialogue and determination with each individual woman.

The authors, editors, and publisher have made every effort to assure accuracy of information as this book goes to press. Nevertheless, they are not responsible for errors, omissions, or outcomes related to the application of this information in the clinical setting. This is at the health-care provider's own discretion.

Robin G. Jordan
Janet L. Engstrom
Julie A. Marfell
Cindy L. Farley

Prenatal and Postnatal Care

A Woman-Centered Approach

Part I

Physiological foundations of prenatal and postnatal care

1

Reproductive tract structure and function

Patricia W. Caudle

Relevant terms

Adrenarche—initiation of increased adrenal androgens
Ampulla—wider end of the fallopian tube
Atresia—degeneration and absorption of immature follicles
Cervix—lower portion of the uterus
Clitoris—erogenous organ with erectile tissue covered by labia minora
Coitus—sexual intercourse
Cornua—both sides of the upper outer area of the uterus where the fallopian tubes join the uterus
Ectropion—visible columnar cells at the cervical os
Endocervical canal—passageway within the cervix to the inner uterus
Endometrium—lining of the uterus
Escutcheon—pubic hair
Fimbriae—fingerlike projections of the ampulla of the fallopian tube
First polar body—other half of the product of division of the primary oocyte
Fornix (fornices)—spaces around the cervix in the vagina
Fourchette—area immediately below the introitus
Gonadarche—period when ovaries begin to secrete sex hormones
Gonadostat—gonadotropin-releasing hormone pulse generator
Granulosa cells—cells lining an ovarian follicle that become luteal cells after ovulation
Ground substance—mucopolysaccharide between smooth muscle and collagen of the cervix
Hart's line—line of change where skin transitions to smoother, moist skin
Hegar's sign—softening and compressibility of the uterine isthmus
Hymen—membranous ring of tissue at the introitus
Introitus—opening to the vagina
Isthmus—uterine "neck" between cervix and body
Labia majora—two rounded folds of adipose tissue covered with pubic hair
Labia minora—folds of tissue between the labia majora

Lactobacilli—normal bacterial flora of the vagina
Leptin—hormone secreted by fat cells that plays a key role in appetite and metabolism
Meatus—opening of the urethra
Menarche—initiation of menses
Metaplasia—normal replacement of one cell type with another
Mittelschmerz—pain upon ovulation
Myometrium—middle, muscular layer of the uterus
Mucin—glycosylated proteins that form mucus that acts as lubricant and protectant
Nulliparous—a woman who has never had a child
Oogenesis—transformation of oogonia into oocytes
Oogonia—primordial female germ cells
Os—opening of the cervix
Parous—woman who has had a child
Peritoneum—thin membrane around abdominal organs that covers the bladder, uterus, and rectum
Rectouterine pouch—fold of peritoneum between the uterus and the rectum
Rectovaginal septum—tissue between the rectum and vagina
Rugae—thin ridges of tissue like an accordion that allow for expansion in the vagina
Squamocolumnar junction (SCJ)—where squamous cells and columnar cells meet on the cervix
Thelarche—breast development
Vagina—musculomembranous tube from the introitus to the cervix
Vasovagal response—bradycardia and syncope caused by stretching the cervical canal
Vesicouterine pouch—fold of peritoneum between the bladder and the uterus
Vesicovaginal septum—tissue between the bladder and the vagina
Vestibule—area inside the labia minora where openings of the urethra and the vagina are found
Vulva—external female genitalia
Zona pellucida—membrane surrounding the plasma membrane of the oocyte

Prenatal and Postnatal Care: A Woman-Centered Approach, First Edition. Edited by Robin G. Jordan, Janet L. Engstrom, Julie A. Marfell, and Cindy L. Farley.
© 2014 John Wiley & Sons, Inc. Published 2014 by John Wiley & Sons, Inc.

Anatomy of the female reproductive system

An understanding of the anatomy of the female reproductive system is essential in caring for women. It is important to be able to recognize normal structures and to appreciate that there is a wide variation of normal among women.

External genitalia

The vulva is a term designated for the external genitalia of the female. The vulva includes the mons pubis, labia majora and minora, clitoris, vestibule, hymen, urinary meatus, and Skene and Bartholin glands. Figure 1.1 and Figure 1.2 illustrate the external genitalia and its development from embryonic structures.

The mons pubis is the cushion-like area over the pubic bone. In the adult woman, the mons is covered with curly, coarse pubic hair called the escutcheon. The pubic hair distribution is usually triangular but may extend up toward the umbilicus in a diamond shape in women who have higher levels of serum androgens.

The labia majora consist of two rounded folds of adipose tissue covered with pubic hair that extend from the mons to the perineum on either side of the vaginal opening. The labia minora, found between the majora, are thinner, pinkish in color, and hairless (Bickley, 2009). The labia majora have the same position and general structure as the male scrotum and arise from the same tissues during embryonic development.

The labia minora have two folds above where it divides to descend on either side of the vestibule, ending at the fourchette just below the introitus, or the opening to the vagina. The upper fold forms the prepuce over the clitoris and the lower fold is the frenulum of the clitoris. The clitoris is an erogenous organ with erectile tissue. The clitoris is exquisitely sensitive in most women and is the primary source of sexual pleasure.

The vulva refers to the external genitals of the female.

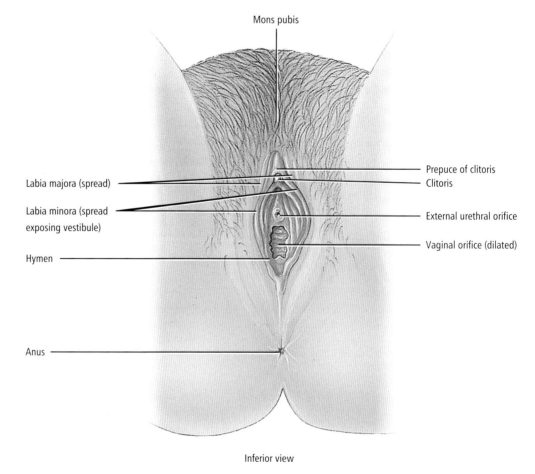

Figure 1.1.　External female genitalia. From Tortora, G. J., & Derrickson, B. (2013). *Principles of anatomy & physiology* (13th ed.). Hoboken, NJ: John Wiley & Sons, Inc.

The external genitals of male and female embryos remain undifferentiated until about the eighth week.

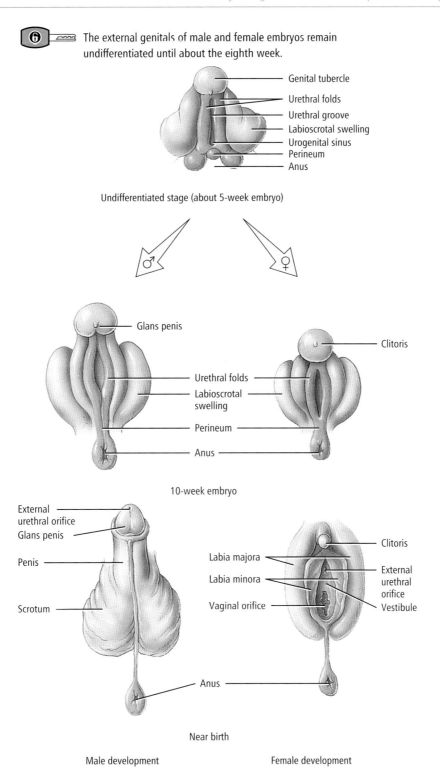

Figure 1.2.   Development of external genitalia from embryonic structures. From Tortora, G. J., & Derrickson, B. (2013). *Principles of anatomy & physiology* (13th ed.). Hoboken, NJ: John Wiley & Sons, Inc.

The vestibule is that area inside the labia minora where the openings to the urethra, vagina, and Skene's and Bartholin's gland ducts are found. The urethra is just above the vaginal opening and below the pubic arch. The vaginal introitus is rimmed with the hymen or its tags. Bartholin glands are located at either side of the lower portion of the introitus. The ducts for these glands open near the hymenal ring at 5 and 7 o'clock. Skene's glands and ducts are found near the urethral meatus. Hart's line is the line of change in the vestibule where vulvar skin transitions to smoother, moister skin around the urethral meatus and the introitus.

Below the vulva is the perineal body and anal opening. These structures can be examined as part of the external genitalia examination. Underlying these structures are the superficial muscles of the perineum and anal sphincter. The superficial muscles most often affected by childbirth include the bulbocavernosus muscle, the superficial transverse perineal muscle, and the external and internal anal sphincters. These structures, with the exception of the internal anal sphincter, converge on the central tendon of the perineum found between the introitus and the anus. The central tendon is part of the perineal body that may tear or be cut during birth (Fig. 1.3).

Internal genitalia

The vagina is a musculomembranous tube that gives access to the cervix for coitus and serves as the birth canal. The lower third of the vagina is supported and fixed by the pubococcygeus muscles of the levator ani group. The upper portion of the vagina and the cervix are supported by the cardinal and uterosacral ligaments. This portion of the vagina is capable of amazing expansion to accommodate birth. Vaginal rugae allow for elasticity and expansion. Vaginal length is about 7–10 cm, depending on genetics, parity, age, and estrogen effect (Summers, 2012). The spaces around the cervix within the vagina are called the anterior, posterior, and lateral fornices.

The rectum supports the middle of the posterior vaginal wall. The anterior vaginal wall offers some support to the bladder (Summers, 2012). The principle innervations for the vagina are the pudendal nerve and the inferior hypogastric plexus, both of which derive from sacral nerve (S) 2–4. Lymph drainage for the vagina is to the para-aortic nodes.

The vagina is lubricated by an epithelial glycoprotein coat and transudate, cervical mucus from the endocervical columnar epithelium, and fluids from the Bartholin and Skene glands (Summers, 2012). The milieu of the

The perineum is a diamond-shaped area that includes the urogenital triangle and the anal triangle.

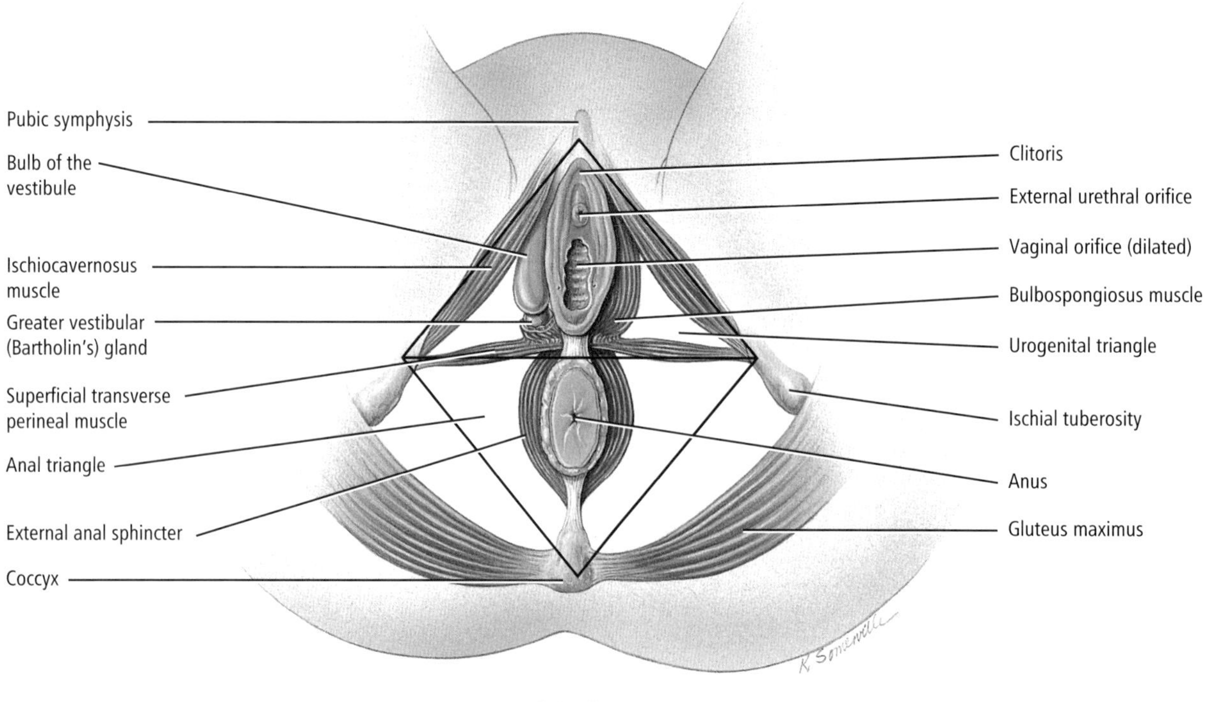

Pubic symphysis
Bulb of the vestibule
Ischiocavernosus muscle
Greater vestibular (Bartholin's) gland
Superficial transverse perineal muscle
Anal triangle
External anal sphincter
Coccyx

Clitoris
External urethral orifice
Vaginal orifice (dilated)
Bulbospongiosus muscle
Urogenital triangle
Ischial tuberosity
Anus
Gluteus maximus

Inferior view

Figure 1.3.   Superficial muscles of the perineum. From Tortora, G. J., & Derrickson, B. (2013). *Principles of anatomy & physiology* (13th ed.). Hoboken, NJ: John Wiley & Sons, Inc.

vagina is acidic and presents a barrier to many bacteria. The pH is normally between 4.0 and 4.5 in women of childbearing age and is maintained by the estrogen effect on the epithelial glycoprotein coat and lactobacilli (normal bacterial flora of the vagina) (Clark et al., 2012). Vaginal secretions increase during pregnancy due to increased vascularity.

The lower portion of the vagina is separated from the urinary bladder by the vesicovaginal septum, and is separated from the rectum by the rectovaginal septum. The rectovaginal septum is at risk for lacerations and tears in the event of an operative birth. The upper vagina, around the cervix, is separated from the rectum via a fold of the peritoneum (thin membrane around abdominal organs that covers the uterus, bladder, and rectum) called the rectouterine pouch or pouch of Douglas. There is a similar, smaller pouch in front of the cervix and behind the bladder called the vesicouterine pouch. This area must be incised and the bladder brought forward during cesarean birth (Cunningham et al., 2010).

The cervix is the lower, narrow part of the pear-shaped uterus that protrudes into the vagina (Fig. 1.4). About half of the cervix is within the vaginal canal. This part of the cervix has an external os followed by a passageway to the uterus called the endocervical canal. The canal ends at the internal os that opens into the uterine cavity. The size and shape of the cervix varies with parity, age, and the amount of estrogen and progesterone available. The cervix of a nulliparous woman is smaller and the external os is smaller and more circular than the cervix of a parous woman, which is wider and the external os is slit-like and more open. The length of the cervix plays a role in cervical integrity during pregnancy.

The blood supply to the cervix arrives via the uterine arteries that derive from the internal iliac arteries. The cervical branches of the uterine arteries are located at 3 and 9 o'clock to the cervical os. Venous blood drains to the hypogastric venous plexus.

The cardinal and uterosacral ligaments support the cervix and upper vagina. The cardinal ligament attaches

After ovulation, a secondary oocyte and its corona radiata move from the pelvic cavity into the infundibulum of the uterine tube. The uterus is the site of menstruation, implantation of a fertilized ovum, development of the fetus, and labor.

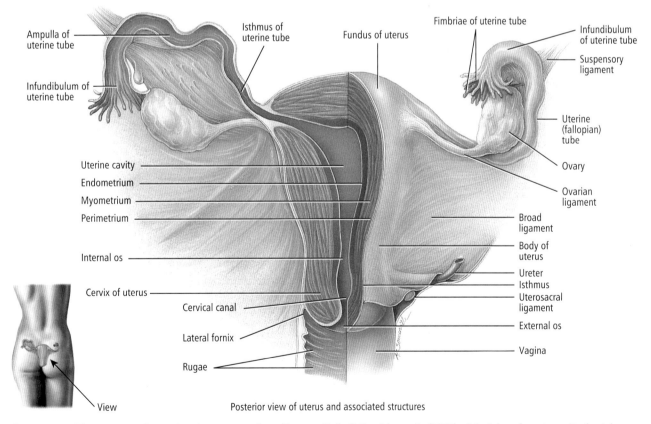

Figure 1.4. The uterus and associated structures. From Tortora, G. J., & Derrickson, B. (2013). *Principles of anatomy & physiology* (13th ed.). Hoboken, NJ: John Wiley & Sons, Inc.

to either side of the cervix and extends laterally to attach to connective tissue called the parametrium. The uterosacral ligament attaches to the posterior cervix and extends posteriorly to attach to the fascia of the sacrum. The main nerve supply to the cervix derives from the hypogastric plexus and follows the uterosacral ligament to the posterior cervix. Since there are sensory, sympathetic, and parasympathetic nerve fibers within the endocervical canal, any instrumentation through the cervical os has the potential for causing a vasovagal response in some women. Conversely, the external cervix has fewer sensory nerve endings, making small external biopsies less painful for women.

The structure of the cervix is complex. It is composed of collagenous connective tissue (smooth muscle and elastic tissue) and ground substance, a mucopolysaccharide. There is a much smaller percentage of smooth muscle in the cervix than in the uterine fundus. The cervix during pregnancy is extraordinarily strong and remains closed as the uterine contents increase in size and volume. Near the end of the pregnancy, the cervix softens and becomes distensible, allowing the fetus to be expelled. This dramatic change requires enzyme activity, an increase in cervical water content, hormonal changes, and an increase in prostaglandins (Blackburn, 2013). After birth, the dilated cervix will shorten and become firmer, so that by 1 week postpartum, the os is dilated to only 1 cm.

Histologically, the cervix has two cell types: the columnar cells that line the endocervical canal and the opening of the cervix, and the squamous epithelium that covers the outside of the cervix. Over 90% of lower genital tract cancers occur where these two cell layers meet at the squamocolumnar junction (SCJ) ("Histology of the Normal Cervix," 2012).

Columnar cells secrete mucin (a glycosylated protein that forms mucus that acts as lubricant and protectant) and have a reddened papillary appearance. The squamous epithelium is smooth and pink. At menarche, higher levels of estrogen cause glycogenation and other changes in the squamous epithelium. These changes and the increasing acidity in the vagina cause the squamous cells to migrate and cover the columnar cells. Metaplasia of the squamous and columnar cells occurs at the SCJ. This makes this area highly susceptible to invasion by human papilloma virus, hyperplasia, and dysplasia. Metaplasia occurs throughout a woman's childbearing years; over time, the SCJ will migrate into the endocervical canal. The SCJ is the most important area for collection of cell samples for the Pap test.

Columnar cells are visible at the cervical os during adolescence, pregnancy, and when women use oral contraceptive pills because of the higher levels of estrogen during these events. This is often referred to as ectropion. Columnar cells produce cervical mucus that changes according to the hormones secreted during the menstrual cycle. During the late follicular phase and ovulation, when estrogen levels are highest, the mucus is clear, stretchy, slick, thin, and abundant. It will facilitate sperm passage from the vagina into the uterus (Hatcher & Namnoum, 2009). Under the influence of progesterone during the luteal phase, the mucus becomes scant, thick, pasty, and opaque. One of the important effects of progestin-only contraceptives is the thickening of the cervical mucus that serves as a barrier to sperm.

Mucus from the columnar cells of the endocervical canal becomes thick and forms a mucous plug during pregnancy. This plug helps to prevent the passage of bacteria into the uterus. Increased vascularity and swelling of the cervix during early pregnancy will cause a bluish coloring called Chadwick's sign.

The uterine cervix is connected to the body of the uterus by the isthmus. This segment of the uterus will soften and become compressible during early pregnancy, a feature specific to pregnancy known as Hegar's sign.

The body or corpus of the uterus (Fig. 1.4) is the most dynamic portion of the uterus. Here, the innermost lining, or endometrium, responds to ovarian hormones every month, building in preparation for implantation, then sloughing as menses if pregnancy does not occur. This is also where implantation and gestation take place and where the powerful forces of labor are generated (Behera, 2012). An adult woman's uterus is about 2–3 in. long before any pregnancies have occurred. After pregnancy and recovery, the range is 3.5–4 in. The weight of the nonpregnant uterus ranges from 1.7 to 2.8 oz, depending on parity (Cunningham et al., 2010). During pregnancy, the muscles of the uterus hypertrophy and the weight will increase to about 38.8 oz by 40 weeks' gestation. This hypertrophy does not extend to the cervix, which contains much less muscle tissue.

Attached to both sides of the upper, outer portion of the uterus, known as the cornua, are the fallopian tubes, round ligaments, and ovarian ligaments. The body of the uterus, unlike the cervix, is mostly muscle tissue. Inside the uterus, the anterior and posterior walls lie very close to each other, forming a slit-like space (Cunningham et al., 2010). Within this space is the very active endometrium, the first of three layers within the uterine corpus (Behera, 2012). The endometrial cyclic response to hormones is explained later in this chapter.

The middle layer of the uterus is the myometrium. This layer is composed of smooth muscle united by connective tissue and makes up most of the uterine bulk. The outermost layer is the perimetrium, a thin layer of epithelial cells (Behera, 2012). The myometrium contains four layers of muscles with blood vessels coursing through each layer. The inner layer of muscle fibers is composed of spirals on the long axis of the uterus. The middle layers of muscle fibers have interlacing fibers that form a figure eight around the many blood vessels. When the placenta is expelled after birth, the empty uterus contracts and the muscles of this layer become "living ligatures" that help halt the blood flow. The outer two layers of muscle fibers are smooth muscle in bundles of 10–50 overlapping cells interspersed with connective tissue and ground substance that transmit contractions during labor (Blackburn, 2013, p. 115). Interestingly, the layers of the myometrium arise from different embryonic locations, so they respond to uterine stimuli in different ways. However, the result is a rhythmic contractile force that propels the fetus toward the cervical opening regardless of the fetal presentation.

The uterine blood supply comes to the uterus from the internal iliac artery via the ovarian and uterine arteries. These arteries feed the arcuate, radial, basal, and spiral arteries. The spiral arteries of the endometrium change during the menstrual cycle. If pregnancy does not occur during the cycle, the spiral arteries constrict, the endometrial matrix breaks down, and menses occurs (Behera, 2012). There is extensive collateral circulation that is enhanced during pregnancy. This arterial system is very efficient in supplying nutrients and oxygen to the growing uteroplacental unit and fetus, but if hemorrhage occurs, this interconnected system of vessels makes control of the bleeding difficult (Cunningham et al., 2010).

There are two sets of lymphatics within the uterine body. One set drains into the internal iliac nodes and the other ends in the para-aortic lymph chain (Cunningham et al., 2010). The nerve supply to the uterus is derived mostly from the sympathetic nervous system and partly from the parasympathetic system. The parasympathetic system fibers derive from sacral nerves 2, 3, and 4. The sympathetic system ultimately comes from the aortic plexus just below the sacral promontory. Sensory fibers from the uterus derive from the 11th and 12th thoracic nerve root and carry the pain signals from contractions of labor to the central nervous system. The sensory nerves from the cervix and upper vagina move through the pelvic nerves to sacral nerves 2, 3, and 4. The primary nerve of the lower vagina is the pudendal nerve.

The fallopian tubes (Fig. 1.4) extend from the upper sides the uterus. These oviducts vary from 8 to 14 cm in length (Cunningham et al., 2010). There are four parts: the interstitial segment that extends from the uterine cavity through the myometrium, the isthmus or narrow portion that begins at the external uterine wall and stretches to the wider ampulla that is over the ovary, and

the fimbriae along the border of the ampulla. The fimbriated ampulla opens into the abdominal cavity with one longer projection that reaches closer to or touches the ovary. The smooth muscle and ciliated cells within the tubes contract rhythmically all the time. At ovulation, these contractions become stronger and more frequent in order to move the ovum toward the uterine lining. Fertilization, if it occurs, will typically happen in the ampulla (Blackburn, 2013).

The ovaries reside on either side of the uterus and are attached to the ovarian ligament that extends to and attaches to the cornua. Other ligaments help support the ovaries and serve as conduits for vessels and nerves. The top layer of the ovary contains oocytes and developing follicles. The core of the ovary is composed of connective tissue, blood vessels, and smooth muscle. Ovaries vary in size but typically are approximately 2.5–5 cm long and 1.5–3 cm wide, giving them an almond shape (Cunningham et al., 2010, p. 29). Ovaries are sometimes palpable during the bimanual examination of the adnexa during pelvic examination (Bickley, 2009).

Menstrual cycle physiology

The menstrual cycle occurs regularly in most women from menarche to menopause with some expected irregularity during the first year after menarche and the years of perimenopause. It is regulated by complex interactions between the hypothalamus, the pituitary gland, the ovaries, and the uterus. This section will highlight the hormonal changes and how these changes affect the ovary and the uterine lining.

Beginnings

The gender of an embryo is determined at the time of fertilization. The male contribution of an X chromosome combined with the female contributed X chromosome produce the basis for a unique female human. Before the seventh week of gestation, the gonads of male and female embryos look the same. It is not until the tenth week after fertilization that primordial germ cells called oogonia can be detected along the genital ridge in females (Molina, 2010; Moore, Persaud, & Torchia, 2013). By 7 months of gestation, all of the oogonia have been transformed into primary oocytes and no new oogonia are formed. At birth, a female newborn will have an average of 200,000–400,000 follicles on the two ovaries (Blackburn, 2013, p. 8). Each follicle contains a primary oocyte that has already begun the first meiotic division (Moore et al., 2013). At puberty, only about 10% or 40,000 of these early follicles will remain due to atresia. Of these, only about 400–500 will develop into a primary follicle (Blackburn, 2013).

Oogenesis is the sequence of events that transforms the oogonia into an oocyte ready to be fertilized. In early fetal life, oogonia divide via mitosis to form primary oocytes. By birth, the primary oocytes have begun the first meiotic division but the process is arrested and remains that way until just before ovulation, when the first meiotic division is completed. At this division, a secondary oocyte receives the bulk of the cytoplasm and the first polar body is formed. At ovulation, the secondary oocyte begins its second meiotic division but the process is arrested and does not resume unless the secondary oocyte is fertilized by a sperm (Blackburn, 2013; Moore et al., 2013 The process of oogenesis is depicted in Figure 1.5.

At term, the gonadotropin-releasing hormone pulse generator, or gonadostat, is at work in the fetus. The gonadostat responds to high levels of maternal estrogen from the placenta by releasing low levels of gonadotropin-releasing hormone. After birth, when maternal estrogens are removed, the gonadotropins follicle-stimulating hormone (FSH) and luteinizing hormone (LH) are released from the newborn's pituitary gland (Deneris &

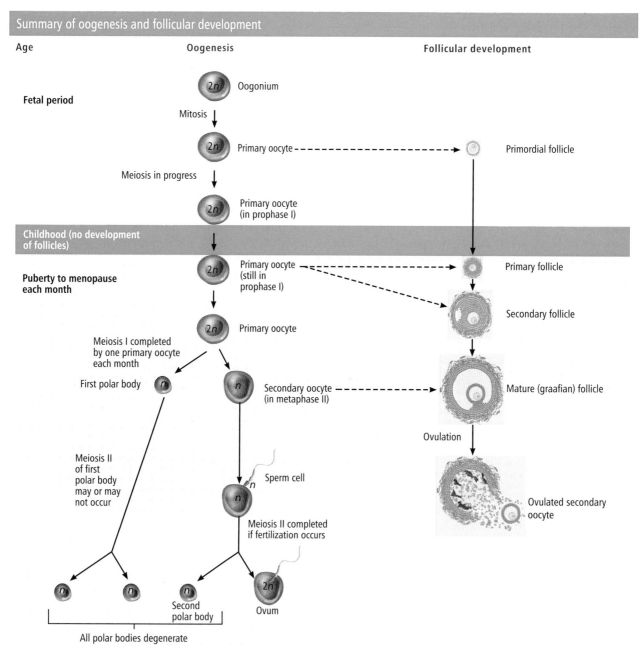

Figure 1.5. Oogenesis. From Tortora, G. J., & Derrickson, B. (2013). *Principles of anatomy & physiology* (13th ed.). Hoboken, NJ: John Wiley & Sons, Inc.

Huether, 2010). During infancy and childhood, estrogen levels are very low and gonadotropin secretion is restrained in a positive feedback fashion.

Onset of puberty

When a girl is 8–12 years old, the gonads begin to produce estrogen and puberty begins with thelarche (breast development). Estrogen production begins in response to complex interrelated changes involving the central nervous system, hypothalamus, pituitary, and ovary. Onset of these changes is influenced by genetics, general health, nutrition, geographic location, exposure to light, and body weight (Deneris & Huether, 2010; Schuiling & Low, 2006). It is thought that increasing body fat and leptin allow maturation. Reproductive maturation involves the central nervous system and the endocrine system in a sequence of changes that will lead to menarche.

The first in the sequence of events that will lead to reproductive maturation is the release of gonadotropin-releasing hormone from the hypothalamus that will cause the release of FSH and LH from the pituitary. These hormones will induce gonadarche and adrenarche, and the hormones from the gonads and adrenal glands stimulate the development of secondary sexual characteristics such as breast growth, pubic and axillary hair growth, and changes in the vagina (Bickley, 2009; Deneris & Huether, 2010). These changes also set the stage for the first ovulation and first ovulatory menstrual period. Figure 1.6 illustrates the sequence for the beginning of hormonal stimulation of the ovary and the beginning negative and positive feedback loops.

The average age for menarche in the United States varies according to population, race, socioeconomic conditions, and nutrition. Among well-nourished white females, the average age at menarche is 12.55 (American College of Obstetricians and Gynecologists [ACOG], American Academy of Pediatrics, 2006, p. 2). Black females begin a little earlier at about 12.06 years, and Hispanic females experience menarche around age 12.25. Table 1.1 describes the characteristics of the normal menstrual cycle.

Once menarche and ovulatory cycles are established, puberty is complete and the female is able to reproduce physiologically; however, social and cultural norms influence reproductive behaviors and choices once physical reproductive maturity is achieved. Throughout the childbearing years, the hypothalamic–pituitary–ovarian (HPO) axis and the uterus go through cycles in production of hormones and changes in the endometrial lining.

The hypothalamic–pituitary–ovarian axis

Once established, the menstrual cycle continues based on feedback mechanisms between the hypothalamus, pituitary, and the ovary. The hypothalamus is a pearl-sized organ at the base of the brain near the optic chiasm. The cells of the hypothalamus synthesize and secrete many releasing hormones that act upon the pituitary and other endocrine glands. It is responsible for regulating thirst, sleep, hunger, libido, and many endocrine functions (Deneris & Huether, 2010). The hypothalamus responds to lower serum levels of estrogen near the end of a cycle by secreting an FSH-releasing factor that will travel to the nearby pituitary gland and stimulate the release of FSH. FSH will stimulate the growth of follicles on the ovary, with one follicle becoming dominant for each cycle. Later, when the follicle releases enough estrogen, the hypothalamus will secrete an LH-releasing hormone that will travel to the pituitary and stimulate the release of LH.

The pituitary gland is located in the sella turcica, below the hypothalamus and optic chiasm. It has a stalk connecting it to the hypothalamus and two lobes, anterior and posterior. The anterior lobe synthesizes and secretes FSH, LH, and many other hormones that affect specific target organs. Figure 1.6, depicts the early HPO axis with feedback loops.

The ovaries are the target organs for the gonadotropins secreted by the anterior pituitary. They are located on either side of the uterus, suspended by the ovarian ligament. They are covered in follicles, each with the potential for growing and releasing an ovum. Figure 1.7 shows the ovarian surface and the stages of the follicle.

The functioning of the HPO axis is dependent on feedback loop control. The most common form of feedback control is negative feedback. This occurs when rising hormone serum levels cause a decrease in another hormone (Brashers & Jones, 2010). The other form of feedback control is positive feedback, where rising levels of one hormone causes a rise in another. These feedback mechanisms help to keep the hormones within normal ranges.

The hormones involved in the menstrual cycle include the gonadotropin-releasing hormones from the hypothalamus, the gonadotropin-stimulating hormones from the pituitary, and the ovarian hormones from the ovary (Table 1.2).

Menstrual cycle phases

There are two parts to the menstrual cycle that occur simultaneously. To help clarify what is happening in each part, this section will separate the ovarian cycle and the endometrial cycle.

Ovarian cycle

There are three phases of the ovarian cycle: the follicular phase, ovulation, and the luteal phase. The follicular

Hormones from the anterior pituitary regulate ovarian function, and hormones from the ovaries regulate the changes in the endometrial lining of the uterus.

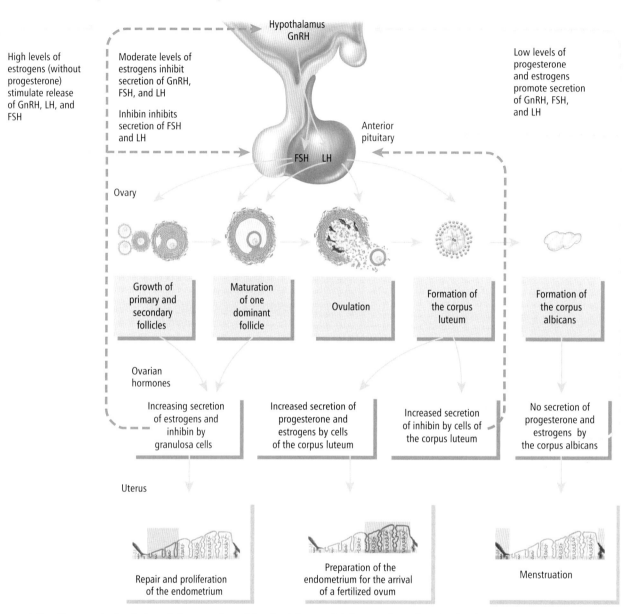

Figure 1.6.   Hormonal stimulation of the gonads and feedback loops. GnRH, gonadotropin-releasing hormone. From Tortora, G. J., & Derrickson, B. (2013). *Principles of anatomy & physiology* (13th ed.). Hoboken, NJ: John Wiley & Sons, Inc.

phase begins on the first day of menses and is more variable than the luteal phase. It typically lasts 10–14 days (Rosen & Cedars, 2011). However, it may last anywhere from 10 to 17 days (Hatcher & Namnoum, 2008). The luteal phase is the most predictable in length because of the life span of the corpus luteum. It lasts 14 days unless pregnancy occurs and the life of the corpus luteum continues.

The follicular phase actually begins during the last days of the previous cycle when decreasing estrogen and inhibin deliver a negative feedback signal to the hypothalamus and pituitary. This signal stimulates the

hypothalamus to release an FSH-releasing factor that stimulates the anterior pituitary to release FSH. The primordial follicles on the ovary each contain an oocyte and a layer of granulosa cells that will respond to the FSH. It is thought that there is at least a 3-month period of stimulation to recruit a dominant follicle for one ovulation (Blackburn, 2013). It is this one "primed" follicle that responds to the FSH first and begins to grow before other follicles on the ovaries that may respond. This follicle takes in more FSH than the others and grows more rapidly. Within this dominant or primary follicle, the oocyte begins to grow and the zona pellucida is formed

Table 1.1 Normal Menstrual Cycle Characteristics

Menarche (average age)	
White	12.55 years
Black	12.06 years
Hispanic	12.25 years
Menstrual cycle length	
First year of menses	32.2 days (range 20–60 days)
Typical menstrual cycle length during the years between menarche and menopause	21–45 days
Flow length	
First year	2–7 days
Typical length	4–6 days (less than 2 or more than 8 considered abnormal)
Flow amount	20–80 mL (second day heaviest)

Adapted from: American College of Obstetricians and Gynecologists (ACOG), American Academy of Pediatrics (2006), Blackburn (2013), Hatcher and Namnoum (2009).

Table 1.2 Hormones of the Menstrual Cycle

Hypothalamus	Follicle-stimulating hormone releasing factor Gonadotropin-releasing factor Luteinizing hormone-releasing factor
Pituitary	Follicle-stimulating hormone Luteinizing hormone
Ovary	Progesterone Estrogen Testosterone Inhibin Activin Follistatin

Adapted from: Molina (2010).

and grows between the oocyte and the granulosa cells (Rosen & Cedars, 2011). Just before ovulation, the corona radiata will form around the zona pellucida. As these changes progress, some of the follicles that had started to respond to FSH but did not fully mature undergo atresia (Molina, 2010).

During the follicular phase, the ovary and the primary follicle are secreting both estrogen and progesterone, with estrogen being produced in higher amounts. FSH stimulates the granulosa cells of the dominant follicle to produce much higher levels of estrogen and to upregulate LH receptors within the follicle cells (Molina, 2010). The higher levels of estrogen cause positive feedback

stimulation of the hypothalamus and pituitary that result in a rise in LH. Near the end of the follicular phase, estrogen will peak causing LH to surge and reach its highest level about 12–24 hours before ovulation (Blackburn, 2013). The higher levels of LH are a very reliable signal of impending ovulation. LH detection kits are available to help couples determine when ovulation occurs (Hatcher & Namnoun, 2009).

LH has other functions. It stimulates ovarian tissue in a way that increases androgen levels and enhances the libido (Hatcher & Namnoun, 2009). It stimulates the remaining granulosa cells of the ruptured follicle to become lutein cells so that the corpus luteum is formed. LH is also responsible for stimulating the oocyte to resume meiosis (Molina, 2010).

Ovulation occurs after a surge and peak level of LH, but there are several factors that facilitate the extrusion of the ovum from the follicle. As the follicle and oocyte have grown, the oocyte has shifted to one side of the follicle. When estrogen begins to decrease, the follicle swells and prostaglandins, proteolytic enzymes, and smooth muscle contractions cause the follicular wall to burst open and the ovum is extruded (Blackburn, 2013). The phenomenon of mittelschmerz or pain upon ovulation is thought to be due to the rupture of the follicle and the release of the ovum and surrounding fluid that can irritate the abdominal lining.

After ovulation, the remaining cells of the follicle are revascularized and transformed into the corpus luteum (Molina, 2010). The corpus luteum continues to secrete estrogen and progesterone, but now progesterone is produced in higher amounts. Progesterone will cause changes in the endometrium and suppress new follicular growth. It will peak between 7 and 8 days after the rapid increase of LH. This highest level of progesterone corresponds with the time of implantation, if fertilization has occurred (Hatcher & Namnoun, 2009). If implantation occurs, the corpus luteum is maintained by the human chorionic gonadotropin secreted by the conceptus so that progesterone levels are maintained.

If fertilization has not occurred, the corpus luteum begins involution and estrogen, progesterone, and inhibin levels will fall (Blackburn, 2013). Cellular changes during involution will result in a small scar on the ovary called the corpus albicans (Molina, 2010). The decrease in the ovarian hormones causes a negative feedback stimulation of the hypothalamus and pituitary and the process begins all over again.

Endometrial cycle

The endometrial cycle has three phases: proliferative, secretory, and menstrual. These phases correspond with events occurring in the ovarian cycle. Proliferative changes in the endometrial lining occur under the

The ovaries are the female gonads; they produce haploid oocytes.

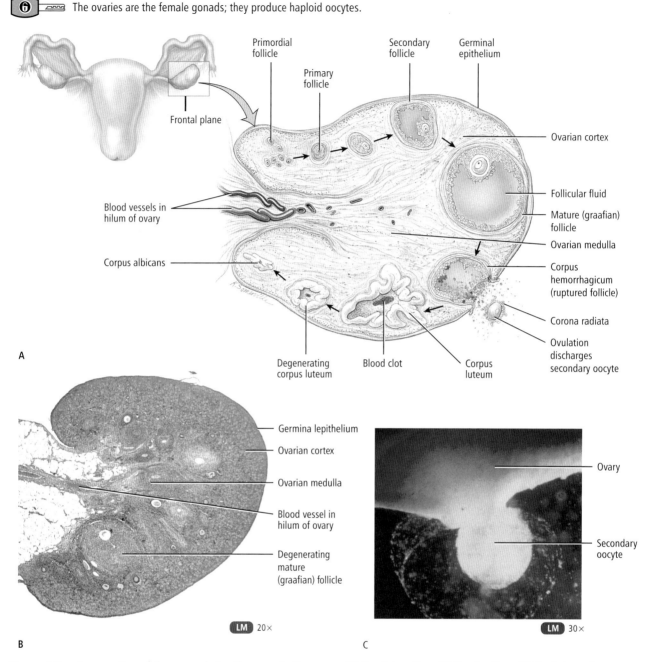

Figure 1.7.   Cross section of the ovary during the reproductive years. (A) Frontal section. (B) Hemisection. (C) Ovulation of a secondary oocyte. From Tortora, G. J., & Derrickson, B. (2013). *Principles of anatomy & physiology* (13th ed.). Hoboken, NJ: John Wiley & Sons, Inc.

influence of estrogen during the corresponding follicular phase. During this phase, there is hyperplasia of the endothelial cells and growth of the stroma within the endometrium (Blackburn, 2013; Molina, 2010). The endometrial height will reach 3–5 mm during this phase (Rosen & Cedars, 2011).

After ovulation, when the corpus luteum begins producing more progesterone, the secretory phase begins. During this time, the epithelial cells accumulate glyco-gen, become more tortuous, and the spiral arteries coil. Capillary permeability of the stroma increases and prostaglandins are produced (Rosen & Cedars, 2011). If fertilization occurs, the secretory endometrium begins transformation to decidual tissue and will be 5–10 mm deep when implantation begins (Blackburn, 2013).

If fertilization does not occur, then the endometrium degenerates and the menstrual phase begins. The corpus luteum atrophies, estrogen and progesterone production

Estrogens are the primary ovarian hormones before ovulation; after ovulation, both progesterone and estrogens are secreted by the corpus luteum.

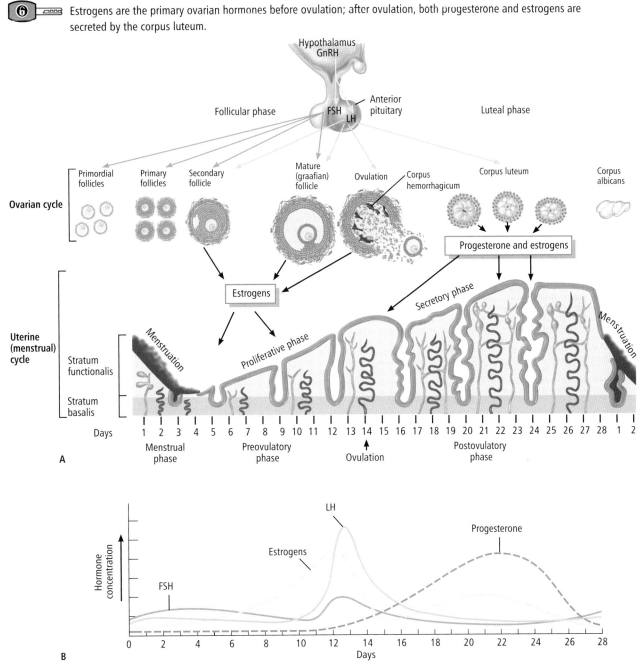

Figure 1.8.   Changing hormone levels during the menstrual cycle. (A) Hormonal regulation of changes in the ovary and uterus. (B) Changes in concentration of anterior pituitary and ovarian hormones. From Tortora, G. J., & Derrickson, B. (2013). *Principles of anatomy & physiology* (13th ed.). Hoboken, NJ: John Wiley & Sons, Inc.

decreases, and prostaglandins are released. Prostaglandins cause vasoconstriction and other changes that lead to ischemia and necrosis of the secretory structures. At the same time, there is the breakdown of proteins within the superficial layer and sloughing. Rupture of capillaries during sloughing leads to bleeding. Bleeding and myometrial contractions help remove the degenerated endometrium (Molina, 2010).

Menses typically lasts 4–6 days, but may be considered normal if all of a woman's cycles are consistently between 2 and 8 days in length. The prostaglandins released will cause contractions, ischemia, and pain in some women. Rising estrogen of the new cycle will induce clot formation to limit blood loss (Hatcher & Namnoun, 2009). Figure 1.8 illustrates the endocrine changes, ovarian cycle, and endometrial cycle in one chart.

The menstrual cycle is a complex and wondrous phenomenon that ensures the continuation of the human race. Most of the time, all of the components work in harmony and there is no need to intervene. The story of embryonic and fetal development that occurs in the uterus is continued in Chapter 2.

Case study

A 23-year-old G1P0 woman presents for her initial prenatal visit.

SUBJECTIVE: She reports her last normal menses as 3 months ago with a typical bleeding pattern of 5–6 days. She reports brief mid-cycle pain each month, which she attributes to release of an ovum; she felt this pain 2.5 months ago on her right side. She says she is quite attuned to her body because she and her partner have been trying to get pregnant for the last 8 months. She had a day of spotting about 2 months ago that concerns her. The spotting has not recurred.

OBJECTIVE: The uterine fundus is palpable at the symphysis pubis abdominally. Fetal heart tones of 158 are obtained with a Doppler. Bimanual exam reveals a grapefruit-sized globular uterus and a slight tenderness but no enlargement in the right ovarian area.

ASSESSMENT: This woman has a 12-week intrauterine pregnancy with historical features that suggest mittelschmerz and implantation bleeding, both of which are normal physiological events.

PLAN: Reassurance is provided that all findings are normal at this point and that the size of the uterus is consistent with her last normal period 3 months ago. Education regarding physiology is given, along with all the routine aspects of the initial prenatal visit.

Resources for women

Menstruation and the Menstrual Cycle Fact Sheet: http://www.womenshealth.gov/publications/our-publications/fact-sheet/menstruation.cfm

Resources for health-care providers

Association of Reproductive Health Professionals: http://www.arhp.org/topics/pregnancy

Reproductive Anatomy & Physiology: http://www.columbia.edu/itc/hs/pubhealth/modules/reproductiveHealth/anatomy.html

References

American College of Obstetricians and Gynecologists (ACOG), American Academy of Pediatrics. (2006). Menstruation in girls and adolescents: Using the menstrual cycle as a vital sign. ACOG Committee Opinion No. 349. *Obstetrics and Gynecology, 108,* 1323–1328.

Behera, M. (2012). Uterine anatomy. In *Medscape Reference.* Last updated 7/14/11. Retrieved from http://emedicine.medscape.com/article/1949215-overview

Bickley, L. (2009). *Bates' guide to physical examination and history taking* (10th ed.). Philadelphia: Wolters Kluwer/Lippincott Williams & Wilkins.

Blackburn, S. (2013). *Maternal, fetal, & neonatal physiology: A clinical perspective* (4th ed.). Maryland Heights, MO: Elsevier.

Brashers, V., & Jones, R. (2010). Mechanisms of hormonal regulation. In K. McCance, S. Huether, V. Brashers, & N. Rote (Eds.), *Pathophysiology: The biologic basis for disease in adults and children* (6th ed., pp. 781–812). Maryland Heights, MO: Mosby/Elsevier.

Clark, M., Rodriguez, A., Gage, J., Herrero, R., Hildesheim, A., Wacholder, S., . . . Schiffman, M. (2012). A large, population-based study of age-related associating between vaginal pH and human papillomavirus infection. *BMC Infectious Diseases, 12,* 33. Retrieved from http://www.biomedcentral.com/1471-2334/12/33

Cunningham, F., Leveno, K., Bloom, S., Hauth, J., Rouse, D., & Spong, C. (2010). *Williams obstetrics* (23rd ed.). New York: McGraw-Hill Medical.

Deneris, A., & Huether, S. (2010). Chapter 22. Structure and function of the reproductive systems. In K. McCance, S. Huether, V. Brashers, & N. Rote (Eds.), *Pathophysiology: The biologic basis for disease in adults and children* (6th ed., pp. 781–812). Maryland Heights, MO: Mosby/Elsevier.

Hatcher, R., & Namnoum, A. (2008). The menstrual cycle. In R. Hatcher, J. Trussell, A. Nelson, W. Cates, F. Stewart, & D. Kowal (Eds.), *Contraceptive technology* (19th ed.). New York: Ardent Media, Inc.

Hatcher, R., & Namnoum, A. (2009). The menstrual cycle. In R. Hatcher, J. Trussell, A. Nelson, W. Cates, F. Stewart, & D. Kowal (Eds.), *Contraceptive technology* (19th ed.). New York: Ardent Media, Inc.

Histology of the normal cervix. (2012). *Practice Management: American Society for Colposcopy and Cervical Pathology (ASCCP).* Retrieved from http://www.asccp.org/PracticeManagement/Cervix/HistologyoftheNormalCervix/tabid/5842/Default.aspx

Molina, P. E. (2010). Chapter 9. Female reproductive system. In P. E. Molina (Ed.), *Endocrine physiology.* Retrieved from http://www.accessmedicine.com/content.aspx?aID=6170103

Moore, K., Persaud, T., & Torchia, M. (2013). *Before we are born: Essentials of embryology and birth defects* (8th ed.). Philadelphia: Elsevier/Saunders.

Rosen, M., & Cedars, M. (2011). Chapter 13. Female reproductive endocrinology and infertility. In D. Gardner & D. Shoback (Eds.), *Greenspan's basic & clinical endocrinology* (9th ed.). Retrieved from http://www.accessmedicine.com/content.aspx?aID=8405598

Schuiling, K., & Low, L. (2006). Women's growth and development across the life span. In K. Schuiling & F. Likis (Eds.), *Women's gynecologic health* (pp. 21–37). Boston: Jones and Bartlett.

Summers, P. (2012). Vaginal anatomy. In *Practice Management: American Society for Colposcopy and Cervical Pathology (ASCCP).* Retrieved from http://www.asccp.org/practicemanagement/vagina/vaginalanatomy/tabid/7488/default.aspx

2

Conception, implantation, and embryonic and fetal development

Patricia W. Caudle

Relevant terms

Acrosome reaction—a process that exposes small openings in the head of the sperm that allows it to penetrate the ovum membrane and release its contents

Active transport—movement across a semipermeable membrane against a concentration gradient

Allantois—small appendage of the umbilical vesicle

Angiogenesis—process by which new vessels form from existing vessels

Apoptosis—programmed cell death

Blastocyst—third stage of the conceptus development; postmorula

Capacitation—removal of the glycoprotein coat from the head of the sperm

Chorion—outer membrane that surrounds the embryo/fetus and becomes the fetal part of the placenta

Chorion frondosum—villi at embryonic pole that extend into the decidua; will develop into the placenta

Chorion leave—smooth chorion that will fuse and disappear

Chorionic villi—projections from the cytotrophoblast to the syncytiotrophoblast that eventually become an arteriocapillary venous network that supplies the embryo

Cleavage—replication process of cells

Cloacal membrane—future site of the anal opening in the embryo

Coelom—cavity that fills with a nutrient lake for molecular exchange between the mother and the embryo

Corona radiata—first layer of the ovum

Cytotrophoblast—inner layer of the trophoblast

Decidual reaction—cellular and vascular changes in the endometrium at implantation

Diploid—contains 46 chromosomes

Ectoderm—outermost layer of the developing embryo

Endoderm—innermost layer of the developing embryo

Extraembryonic somatic mesoderm—layer of mesoderm that will combine with trophoblast to form the chorion

Facilitated transport—movement across a semipermeable membrane that needs a transporter but no energy

Gametes—ovum and sperm

Gastrulation—formation of the germ layers of the embryo

Haploid—contains 23 chromosomes

Hydatidiform mole—abnormal proliferation of the conceptus that can become malignant

Implantation bleeding—loss of a small amount of blood from the uterine lining during implantation

Lacunae—small spaces or "lakes" within the syncytiotrophoblast

Lanugo—fine, soft hair that covers the fetus

Lipolysis—breakdown of fat molecules

Mesenchymal—cells that can differentiate into many different cell types

Mesoderm—middle layer of the developing embryo

Morula—mulberry-like group of cells, second phase of conceptus cellular development, postzygote

Neurulation—formation of the neural tube

Notochordal—rodlike structure that helps organize the nervous system and becomes part of the vertebra and axial skeleton

Oligohydramnios—less than normal amount of amniotic fluid

Oocyte—ovum

Oogonia—primitive ovum

Organogenic—process by which endoderm, mesoderm, and ectoderm develop into internal organs

Peptide—synthesized from protein

Pinocytosis—carrier molecule is required to engulf molecules and move it across the placental barrier

Prenatal and Postnatal Care: A Woman-Centered Approach, First Edition. Edited by Robin G. Jordan, Janet L. Engstrom, Julie A. Marfell, and Cindy L. Farley.
© 2014 John Wiley & Sons, Inc. Published 2014 by John Wiley & Sons, Inc.

Placenta accreta—abnormal attachment of the trophoblast to the endometrium

Polyhydramnios—excessive amniotic fluid

Precursors—building blocks or chemicals used to make another chemical

Primitive streak—line of epiblast cells through the middle of the back of the embryo

Pulmonary hypoplasia—poor fetal lung growth

Quickening—fetal movement first felt by the mother

Sacrococcygeal teratoma—cystic tumor with tissue from all three embryonic germ layers

Simple diffusion—movement across a semipermeable membrane from higher to lower concentration

Somites—segmental mass of mesoderm occurring in pairs along the notochord, which develop into vertebrae and muscles

Steroid—synthesized from cholesterol

Syncytiotrophoblast—outer layer of the conceptus that sends out fingerlike extensions that take in uterine cells as it invades the endometrium

Teratogen—any substance that can disrupt the development of an embryo

Velamentous insertion—umbilical blood vessels insert into the placenta via the amniotic membrane and are not protected by Wharton's jelly

Vernix caseosa—cheesy coating on the fetus that protects the skin

Wharton's jelly—gelatinous connective tissue of the umbilical cord

Zona pellucida—second layer of the ovum

Zygote—first cell created by fusion of ovum and sperm

Introduction

Estrogen produced by the ovarian follicle begins the preparation of the endometrial lining for a potential pregnancy. When the follicle extrudes the ovum, the *corpus luteum* develops and begins to produce more progesterone (literally progestation). This hormone causes the endometrium to become very receptive to implantation should conception occur. This chapter will outline conception, implantation of the *conceptus* into the receptive uterine lining, and the development of the embryo/fetus and placenta. For purposes of consistency, embryonic and fetal age is based on the estimated time of fertilization unless otherwise stated.

Conception and implantation

Conception or fertilization occurs near the open end of the fallopian tube typically within 24 hours of ovulation. In order for conception to occur, about 1000 sperm must be in the fallopian tube when the ovum arrives. It takes that many sperm to produce the enzymes needed for one sperm to fertilize the egg (Stables & Rankin, 2010). During the journey through the cervix and uterus to the fallopian tube, the sperm undergoes capacitation so that when it passes through the corona radiata (the first layer of the ovum), it can begin the acrosome reaction (small openings of the head that releases the contents) and bind to the zona pellucida, which is the second layer of the ovum (Blackburn, 2013). The enzymes that have been released by the other sperm help to remove obstructing cells and allow one sperm to penetrate the zona pellucida and enter the ovum. The entire sperm will be taken into the oocyte or ovum. Once the sperm has entered the ovum cytoplasm, a zonal reaction occurs to prevent another sperm from entering. The sperm will determine the gender of the embryo by contributing either an X (for female) or a Y (for male) sex chromosome.

Within a few hours, the haploid (containing 23 chromosomes) gametes (ovum and sperm) will unite within the ovum to form a complete diploid (containing 46 chromosomes) cell called the zygote, the first cell of a human being. All the information to make a human being is within the zygote. Each cell that develops from this first cell will move and take shape according to the programming of the DNA (deoxyribonucleic acid) from each parent. Cells will change in order to make different tissues and changing cells will influence each other. There will be migrations of cells to form different organs. Apoptosis will occur so that cavities are formed and excessive growth does not occur (Stables & Rankin, 2010). It is a complex and marvelous chain of events.

The zygote begins to move toward the uterus and the cell begins the replication process or cleavage. In about 30 hours, there are two cells (Benirschke, 2009). By about 3 days, a morula made of 12–32 cells enters the uterine cavity (Moore, Persaud, & Torchia, 2013). Fluid accumulates in the morula, forming a blastocyst. The blastocyst is protected from the mother's immune system by the *zona pellucida*, the covering for the blastocyst (Blackburn, 2013). About 5 days after fertilization, a 58-cell blastocyst will shed the zona pellucida and secrete substances that help to make the uterine lining even more receptive to implantation. These substances include human chorionic gonadotropin (hCG).

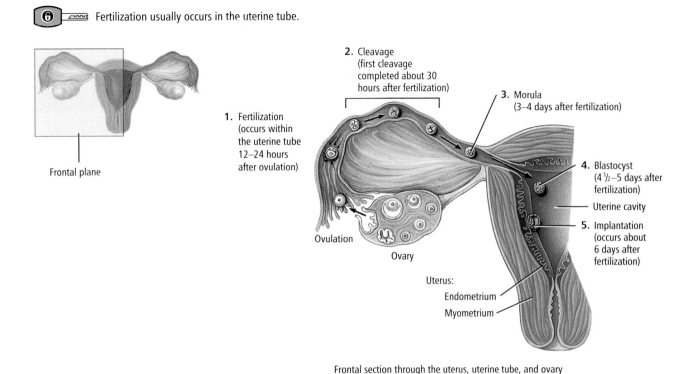

6 ⚿ Fertilization usually occurs in the uterine tube.

2. Cleavage
(first cleavage
completed about 30
hours after fertilization)

3. Morula
(3–4 days after fertilization)

1. Fertilization
(occurs within
the uterine tube
12–24 hours
after ovulation)

4. Blastocyst
(4 ½–5 days after
fertilization)

Uterine cavity

5. Implantation
(occurs about
6 days after
fertilization)

Ovulation

Ovary

Uterus:
Endometrium
Myometrium

Frontal plane

Frontal section through the uterus, uterine tube, and ovary

Figure 2.1.   Cleavage and travel of the conceptus to the uterus.

Spontaneous pregnancy losses that occur during the first 2 weeks are typically caused by chromosomal abnormalities or by failure of the blastocyst and the syncytiotrophoblast to produce enough hCG to maintain the corpus luteum as it produces progesterone. Figure 2.1 depicts the cleavage and travel of the conceptus through the fallopian tube to the uterine implantation site.

About 6–10 days after ovulation, implantation of the blastocyst into the estrogen- and progesterone-primed endometrium begins (Liu, 2009). Most implantations occur on the upper posterior uterine segment closest to the follicle that released the egg. The blastocyst will adjust itself so that the embryonic pole is closest to the endometrial lining (Blackburn, 2013). It will embed entirely into the endometrium where it has adhered itself.

The embryonic disc appears and during the second week, it will develop the ectoderm, endoderm, and mesoderm layers that will later form all the body systems of the embryo. Structures outside the embryonic disc form the amniotic cavity, the amnion, the umbilical cord beginnings, and the chorionic sac.

The placenta

Beginnings and structure

Encircling the blastocyst are trophoblast cells that begin the invasion process by projecting into the uterine lining

to reach maternal blood vessels. These cells will form the placenta. Once adhered to the endometrium, the trophoblast cells differentiate into two layers. The outer layer is the syncytiotrophoblast, which is a multinuclear protoplasm mass that sends out the fingerlike extensions that take in uterine cells as it invades the endometrium. This layer of the trophoblast secretes both peptide and steroid hormones important to the maintenance of the pregnancy. The inner layer of the trophoblast has distinct cells and is called the cytotrophoblast. These cells secrete peptide hormones needed for the pregnancy.

The syncytiotrophoblast grows and begins to develop small spaces called lacunae that will fill with serum from mother's spiral arteries as the invasion progresses. This fluid will nourish the trophoblast. The maternal arteries become fully dilated and a low-resistance, low-pressure continuous flow is established (Cunningham et al., 2010). Communication between the lacunae and uterine vessels begins uteroplacental circulation. The remodeling of the spiral arteries is an important step in establishing optimal circulation and nourishment for the embryo/fetus. Chronic disorders of pregnancy, such as preeclampsia or intrauterine fetal growth restriction, or both, can result from incomplete dilation of the spiral arteries at this stage in development (Blackburn, 2013).

The projections from the cytotrophoblast into the syncytiotrophoblast mass become chorionic villi. These protrusions develop through three stages to become a functioning arteriocapillary venous network that supplies the embryo. Fetal blood begins to circulate by about 21 days after fertilization within the villi. An exchange via diffusion between the maternal and embryonic circulations begins, but the blood from each does not mingle (Stables & Rankin, 2010). More about the cardiovascular development and transfer of nutrients and gases between mother and fetus is presented later in this chapter.

Recall that the endometrium is changing under the influence of the progesterone that has been secreted by the corpus luteum. This secretory endometrial lining must be primed for the conceptus to be able to implant. Correct timing is essential. One mechanism for some types of emergency contraceptive pills is to increase the amount of estrogen available, thereby preventing the development of a secretory endometrium and disrupting the implantation process (Moore et al., 2013).

A decidual reaction (cellular and vascular changes in the endometrium at implantation) occurs around the conceptus after it has embedded into the primed endometrium. This reaction provides an area for the conceptus that is protected from the maternal immune system (Moore et al., 2013). If this reaction is abnormal, then *placenta accreta* (abnormal attachment of the trophoblast to the myometrium) or ectopic pregnancy may occur. The *decidua basalis* is directly under the trophoblast and is compressed. The villi at the embryonic pole extend into the decidua basalis and become the *chorion frondosum* that develops into the placenta. The *decidua capsularis* and *decidua vera (or parietalis)* are over the trophoblast. The decidua capsularis will disappear as the embryo develops. The decidua vera will fuse with the *chorion laeve* (smooth chorion) and disappear as products of conception fill the uterine cavity.

Implantation bleeding, the loss of a small amount of blood from the uterine lining at implantation, occurs when the invasion of the uterine lining causes an abrupt opening in arterioles or veins. This occurs so frequently that it is considered physiological or a normal variant. The appearance of this bleeding occurs at about the same time a menstrual period is anticipated and can be incorrectly interpreted as the last menstrual period. This can affect how the pregnancy is dated, so a careful menstrual history is warranted.

The placenta at term is round and discoid, about 8 in. or 20 cm in diameter (Stables & Rankin, 2010). The maternal surface is formed by about 20 cotyledons (lobes) attached to the decidua via septa connected to the grooves between the cotyledons. Each lobe contains one main stem villi and its many branches. The fetal side is grayish white and covered by the amnion membrane.

Chorionic and amnionic membranes

At about 14 days, the implanted ovum is visible on the endometrium as a polyp-like protrusion. The embryo, amnion, and yolk sac cavities are within the cytotrophoblast layer. The developing embryo at about 14 days is connected inside the trophoblast via a stalk that will become part of the umbilical cord. The stalk is part of the mesoderm, one of three layers of the developing embryo. The ectoderm is part of the amniotic sac epithelium. The endoderm is opposite the ectoderm and beside the yolk sac (Benirschke, 2009). As the embryo grows, it will fold, making the endoderm the innermost portion of the embryo. Eventually, the embryo is surrounded by the amnion and the amniotic fluid (AF).

The yolk sac provides nutrition for the early embryo. As the embryo folds, the yolk sac is enclosed and becomes the primitive gut, nourishing the conceptus (Benirschke, 2009; Blackburn, 2013). The cytotrophoblast cells encircle the extraembryonic coelom, a cavity that fills with a nutrient lake for molecular exchange between the mother and the embryo (Beall & Ross, 2009). The coelom disappears by the end of the first trimester and the amniotic fluid-filled cavity surrounds the fetus.

One layer of the extraembryonic mesoderm is the extraembryonic somatic mesoderm. This layer will combine with the two layers of the trophoblast to form the chorion and the chorionic sac. Within the chorion, the embryo, amniotic sac, and umbilical vesicle are attached to the chorion by the connecting stalk that will become the umbilical cord.

The amniotic sac will enclose the embryo and cells from the amniotic membrane will eventually cover the umbilical cord (Benirschke, 2009). The amniotic sac lies against but does not normally adhere to the entire chorionic membrane by about 12 weeks. There are no blood vessels in the amnion except in rare instances of velamentous insertion (where blood vessels insert or grow into the amniotic membrane). The amniotic membrane is made up of ectodermal epithelial cells, thin connective tissue, and macrophages.

AF fills the amniotic sac around the embryo. It protects the embryo/fetus from trauma and most bacteria, allows for fetal movement and growth, and facilitates lung and limb development (Beall & Ross, 2009). The amount of AF increases steadily between 10 and 30 weeks then slows. Between 36 and 38 weeks, AF begins to decrease normally. At 41 weeks of gestation, AF begins to decrease more rapidly.

Excessive AF, known as polyhydramnios, can occur when the fetus has anencephaly or esophageal atresia, which prevents swallowing of AF, or when the mother has diabetes. Complications of polyhydramnios include placental abruption, uterine dysfunction, and postpartum hemorrhage.

Oligohydramnios, or below normal AF, can occur when there is an obstruction to fetal urine flow, renal agenesis, or other fetal anomalies; chronic leakage of AF; or rupture of the amniotic membrane. Chronic reduction in AF can cause fetal pulmonary hypoplasia or can increase the risk for infection.

Functions of the amniotic fluid

- Protects the embryo/fetus from trauma
- Is a barrier to most bacteria
- Allows for fetal movement and growth
- Facilitates lung and limb development
- Reflects fetal kidney function
- Provides thermoregulation
- Aids in gastrointestinal maturation

The umbilical cord

The connecting stalk is the earliest appearance of the umbilical cord. As the embryo folds during the fourth week, the umbilical cord begins to form and the amnion cells near it develop into the covering for the cord (Moore et al., 2013). Once fetoplacental circulation is established, two umbilical arteries within the cord carry deoxygenated blood away from the fetus to the placenta and mother. The placental barrier between the mother and the fetus is very thin and allows substances, but not blood, to move back and forth between the mother and the fetus. One umbilical vein within the cord brings oxygen and nutrients back to the fetus from the placenta and mother. These three umbilical vessels are surrounded by Wharton's jelly, a gelatinous connective tissue. This protective coating does not cover the entire umbilical cord when there is a velamentous insertion.

The umbilical cord is usually between 12 and 35 in. or 30 and 90 cm long (Moore et al., 2013). If it is too long, there is danger that it will coil around the fetus, tighten, and cut off oxygen and nutrient flow. A true knot in the umbilical cord can be created through fetal movement and is found in about 1 in 100 pregnancies, but only causes problems for 1 in 2000. A longer cord can prolapse with the rupture of amnionic membranes, be occluded by the fetal presenting part, and cause loss of oxygen and nutrients to the fetus. About 1 in 20 umbilical cords are abnormally short (Beall, 2012). The cause of shorter cords is unknown; however, shortened cords may be an indication of decreased fetal movement, placental abruption, or disruption in a part of the cord. A shortened cord can affect fetal descent and expulsion, although there are data that indicate that a vaginal delivery can happen if the cord is as short as 13 cm or 5.125 in.

Placental functions

The placenta and umbilical cord move substances such as nutrients, gases, drugs, and wastes between the mother and the fetus. In addition to the transport of substances, the placenta serves as the organ for gas exchange and waste removal and as an endocrine gland for the fetus. It metabolizes glycogen, cholesterol, and fatty acids for energy, and synthesizes and secretes both steroid and peptide hormones (Moore et al., 2013). The placenta can also detoxify some substances (Adams & Koch, 2010). Shortly after the baby is born, the extraordinary placenta is expelled from the uterus as waste.

Sociocultural uses of the placenta

The American health-care system has often treated the placenta as biohazardous waste material, although placentas have been harvested for medical or commercial use. In some cultures, the placenta is used in rituals designed to honor or protect the mother and the baby, such as burying it under a tree. Two alternative trends are emerging with regard to the placenta: (1) lotus birth in which the umbilical cord is not severed at birth and the cord and placenta are kept with the baby until natural separation occurs; and (2) placental encapsulation in which the placenta is steamed, dehydrated, ground, and placed into capsules for ingestion in the postpartum period by the mother with reputed effects of enhanced milk supply and prevention of depression. Health-care providers should discuss the woman's preferences for the disposal or use of the placenta in the prenatal period.

Placental transport

By the third week after fertilization, the embryo has developed a vascular network and fetal circulation begins by about day 21 (Moore et al., 2013). The embryonic circulation is separated from maternal circulation by a thin membrane often called the placental barrier.

The four main modes of transport for substances across the placental membrane are simple diffusion (movement from higher to lower concentration), facilitated diffusion (movement that needs a transporter but no energy), active transport (movement against a concentration gradient that requires energy), and pinocytosis (carrier molecule is required to engulf the molecule and move it across the placental barrier) (Blackburn, 2013; Moore et al., 2013). Most drugs cross the placenta via simple diffusion (Adams & Koch, 2010). Table 2.1 lists the four modes of transport and gives a few examples of substances that are transported via each mode.

Table 2.1   Four Main Transport Mechanisms

Mode of transport	Examples of materials transported
Simple diffusion	Oxygen, CO_2, carbon monoxide, H_2O, most drugs, steroids, electrolytes, anesthetic gases
Facilitated diffusion	Glucose (facilitated by insulin), cholesterol, triglycerides, phospholipids
Active transport	Amino acids, vitamins, transferrin (carries iron to fetus), iodine, calcium
Pinocytosis	Immunoglobulin G

Adapted from: Adams, M., & Koch, R. (2010). *Pharmacology: Connections to nursing practice.* Upper Saddle River, NJ: Pearson; Cunningham, F., Leveno, K., Bloom, S., Hauth, J., Rouse, D., & Spong, C. (2010). *Williams obstetrics* (23rd ed.). New York: McGraw Hill Medical.

Table 2.2   Transplacental Infections

Viruses	Varicella zoster, Coxsackie, parvovirus (B19), cytomegalovirus, rubella, human immunodeficiency virus, polio virus
Bacteria	*Treponema pallidum* (syphilis), listeriosis, *Borrelia* (Lyme disease)
Protozoa	Toxoplasmosis

Adapted from: Cunningham, F., Leveno, K., Bloom, S., Hauth, J., Rouse, D., & Spong, C. (2010). *Williams obstetrics* (23rd ed.). New York: McGraw Hill Medical; Moore, K., Persaud, T., & Torchia, M. (2013). *Before we are born: Essentials of embryology and birth defects* (8th ed.). Philadelphia: Elsevier/Saunders.

There are several factors that affect substance transfer across the placenta (Adams & Koch, 2010):

1. High maternal plasma level of the specific substance can affect transfer. Higher maternal plasma levels will mean that more of the substance is available for transfer to the fetus.
2. Lipid-soluble substances cross the placental barrier better and more rapidly than do water-soluble substances.
3. The smaller the molecule, the more readily it crosses the placenta. Alcohol, for instance, is a very small molecule and crosses readily. Heparin is a very large molecule and does not cross.
4. Protein binding can make the substance too large to cross.
5. Ionized drugs do not cross as easily as unionized drugs. An example of this is how nicotine crosses and reaches higher concentrations in the fetus. Nicotine is a weak base and maternal serum is slightly more acid than fetal serum. Once in the fetus, nicotine becomes ionized in a higher pH environment and will not cross the placenta back to mother. So, plasma levels of nicotine are higher in the fetus than in the mother.
6. If uteroplacental blood flow is compromised, drugs or other substances can stay in the fetus for a long time. This increases the risk for more serious fetal side effects. In fact, the rate of maternal or fetal blood flow through the villous spaces will affect diffusion.
7. The stage of fetal development makes a difference. Before implantation, drug exposure will either destroy the blastocyst or it will not be affected at all. During organ development between weeks 3 and 8, the developing organs may be damaged by drugs. This is also the time when the risk for abortion is highest. During the fetal phase, weeks 9–40, drugs will be in the fetal system for a longer period of time due to immature metabolism and excretion processes. Exposure at this time, however, does not cause severe malformations. Instead, there may be delayed growth or organ function problems.
8. Some substances are metabolized by the placenta before they can cross the placenta membrane and much smaller amounts reach the fetus.

Some viruses, bacteria, and protozoa cross the placenta to infect the fetus. Table 2.2 lists the infectious agents that may cross the placental barrier and affect the fetus.

Placental endocrine synthesis and secretion

The placenta uses precursors such as cholesterol, estrogen, or protein to synthesize both peptide and steroid hormones. The peptide hormones include, but are not limited to, hCG, human placental lactogen (also called human chorionic somatomammotropin), human chorionic adrenocorticotropin (ACTH), corticotrophin-releasing hormone, relaxin, and inhibin. The steroid hormones include estrogen and progesterone.

hCG is essential to pregnancy. It is produced by both the syncytiotrophoblast and cytotrophoblast for the first 5 weeks of pregnancy, thereafter, by the syncytiotrophoblast and fetal kidneys. It is detectable in maternal serum and urine by 7–9 days after ovulation and is used for pregnancy tests. Maternal plasma levels of hCG double every 31–35 hours until around 63–70 days (Liu, 2009). Plasma levels then decline until about 16 weeks to remain the same until birth.

Maternal serum levels of hCG are used clinically for pregnancy testing and for diagnosis of various pregnancy abnormalities in the early weeks of pregnancy. Levels of hCG that are too high indicate multiple fetuses, fetal hemolytic disease, hydatidiform mole, or Down syndrome. Levels that are too low or that do not double in 2 days can indicate spontaneous abortion or ectopic pregnancy. hCG is also used in combination with other substances such as estriol and alpha-fetoprotein to screen for other fetal abnormalities.

The functions of hCG include maintenance of the corpus luteum; maintenance of the development of spiral arteries in the myometrium and formation of syncytiotrophoblast; acting as a luteinizing hormone to stimulate the male embryonic/fetal testicle to secrete testosterone; stimulation of the maternal thyroid gland; promotion of secretion of relaxin (peptide hormone) from the corpus luteum; and it may promote vasodilation and smooth muscle relaxation of the uterus (Moore et al., 2013). In maintaining the corpus luteum, hCG also prevents menses. It is synthesized without any contribution from the fetus, so maternal serum levels will remain high long after fetal demise (Blackburn, 2013).

Human placental lactogen is synthesized in the syncytiotrophoblast and can be measured in maternal serum at about 3 weeks. Its actions include maternal lipolysis (breakdown of fat for energy), increased maternal insulin resistance that facilitates protein synthesis and availability of amino acids and glucose to the fetus, angiogenesis (embryo blood vessel formation), and increased synthesis and availability of lipids (Blackburn, 2013). This is the placental hormone most involved in keeping a constant flow of glucose and amino acids going to the fetus.

ACTH is important for fetal lung maturation and plays a role in the timing of labor and birth. Corticotropin-releasing hormone (CRH) is produced in the placenta, membranes, and decidua. CRH acts to increase ACTH secretion from the trophoblast, causes smooth muscle relaxation in blood vessels and in the uterus until late in pregnancy, and facilitates maternal immunosuppression. Near term, a rise of CRH from the fetus and the placenta contributes to the genesis of labor.

Relaxin is produced in the corpus luteum, decidua, and the placenta. It acts to quiet the myometrium, facilitate the decidual reaction, remodel collagen, and soften the cervix (Blackburn, 2013). Relaxin also mediates hemodynamic changes of pregnancy and softens ligaments and cartilage in the skeletal system.

Inhibin is another glycoprotein produced by the trophoblast. It acts with sex steroid hormones to decrease the secretion of follicle-stimulating hormone from the pituitary, thereby stopping ovulation during pregnancy.

There are three major estrogens including estrone, estradiol, and estriol. In pregnancy, estriol is the major estrogen. Estriol is synthesized in the placenta from precursors from the maternal and fetal adrenal glands. Dehydroepiandrosterone sulfate (DHEA-S) is synthesized from cholesterol in the fetal adrenal glands, and it is an essential precursor to placental synthesis of estrogen (Blackburn, 2013). During pregnancy, estrogen production increases about 1000 times that seen in nonpregnant women at ovulation (Cunningham et al., 2010). Lower than normal maternal serum levels of estriol are seen when the fetus is anencephalic or has adrenal hypoplasia. Additionally, fetal demise can occur because the fetal pituitary is not releasing ACTH or the fetal adrenal glands are not functioning (Blackburn, 2013). Maternal serum and AF estriol levels, along with other substances, are also used to screen for Down syndrome, trisomy 18, and neural tube defects.

Estrogen in pregnancy has many functions. Estrogens induce the proliferation and secretory phase of the endometrium, stimulate phospholipid synthesis, enhance prostaglandin production, and trigger uterine contractions. Estrogens also promote myometrial vasodilation, increase uterine blood flow, prepare the breasts for breastfeeding, affect the maternal renin–angiotensin system, stimulate the liver to produce globulins, and increase fetal lung surfactant production (Blackburn, 2013; Liu, 2009).

Progesterone is secreted by the corpus luteum early in pregnancy. It is not until about 8–10 weeks that progesterone is synthesized and secreted by the placenta. The precursor for progesterone synthesis is cholesterol. Maternal serum levels of this steroid hormone increase steadily throughout the pregnancy so that by term, 250 mg/day is being produced (Liu, 2009). This is about 10 times the amount produced by the corpus luteum during the luteal phase of the menstrual cycle.

Progesterone is essential for preparation of the endometrium for implantation; maintenance of a quiescent uterus through relaxation of the smooth muscle; inhibition of uterine prostaglandin development, thereby delaying cervical softening; inhibition of the cell-mediated immune system to help prevent rejection of the conceptus; reduction of CO_2 sensitivity in the maternal respiratory center; inhibition of prolactin secretion; relaxation of maternal smooth muscle in the gastrointestinal and urinary systems; and elevation of maternal temperature. Additionally, it is important in creating thicker cervical mucus and a mucous plug that serve as a barrier to infectious agents trying to enter the uterus (Blackburn, 2013; Liu, 2009). Unlike estrogen, the fetus is not necessary for the production of progesterone and maternal serum levels of this hormone will remain high long after fetal demise (Blackburn, 2013). Table 2.3 summarizes the placental hormones and their functions.

Table 2.3 Placental Hormones and Their Functions

Human chorionic gonadotropin (hCG)	Maintains the corpus luteum Promotes vasodilation and relaxation of the uterus Stimulates the male testicle to secrete testosterone Stimulates maternal thyroid Promotes secretion of relaxin
Human placental lactogen (hPL)	Maternal lipolysis Increases maternal insulin resistance Angiogenesis Increases synthesis of lipids
Human chorionic adrenocorticotropin (ACTH)	Promotes fetal lung maturation Plays role in timing of labor
Corticotrophin-releasing hormone	Acts to increase ACTH secretion from the trophoblast Causes smooth muscle relaxation in blood vessels and uterus Facilitates maternal immunosuppression Near term contributes to genesis of labor
Relaxin	Quiets the myometrium Facilitates decidual reaction Remodels collagen Helps soften the cervix Affects cartilage of maternal skeletal system
Inhibin	Acts with other hormones to decrease release of follicle-stimulating hormone, which stops ovulation
Dehydroepiandrosterone sulfate (DHEA-S)	Essential precursor to placental synthesis of estrogen
Estrogen	Acts to prepare the endometrium for pregnancy Stimulates phospholipid synthesis Enhances prostaglandin production Promotes uterine vasodilation Prepares breasts for breastfeeding Increases fetal lung surfactant production
Progesterone	Essential for preparation of the endometrium for implantation Maintains quiescent uterus Inhibits prostaglandin development Inhibits maternal cell-mediated immune system Reduces CO_2 sensitivity in maternal respiratory center Inhibits prolactin secretion Relaxes maternal smooth muscle Causes increase in maternal temperature Increases cervical mucus and formation of mucous plug

Adapted from: Cunningham, F., Leveno, K., Bloom, S., Hauth, J., Rouse, D., & Spong, C. (2010). *Williams obstetrics* (23rd ed.). New York: McGraw Hill Medical; Liu, J. (2009). Endocrinology of pregnancy. In R. Creasy, R. Resnik, & J. Iams (Eds.), *Creasy and Resnik's maternal-fetal medicine: Principles and practice* (6th ed., pp.111–123). St. Louis, MO: Saunders/Elsevier; Blackburn, S. (2013). *Maternal, fetal, and neonatal physiology: A clinical perspective* (4th ed.). Maryland Heights, MO: Saunders/Elsevier.

The embryo

Gastrulation (formation of germ layers of the embryo) changes the embryo from a two-layer disc to a three-layer disc. The three layers include the ectoderm, mesoderm, and endoderm. These layers form the basis for all tissues and organs that will develop as the embryo grows. Gastrulation begins with the appearance of the primitive streak from the tail through the middle of the back of the embryo to the head (Moore et al., 2013). Cells from the primitive streak and its derivatives will migrate away and form the mesoderm until about the fourth week. Near the tail end of the primitive streak, the cloacal membrane develops. This is the future site of the anal opening. Figure 2.2 shows how the primitive streak appears and lengthens.

Gastrulation involves the rearrangement and migration of cells from the epiblast.

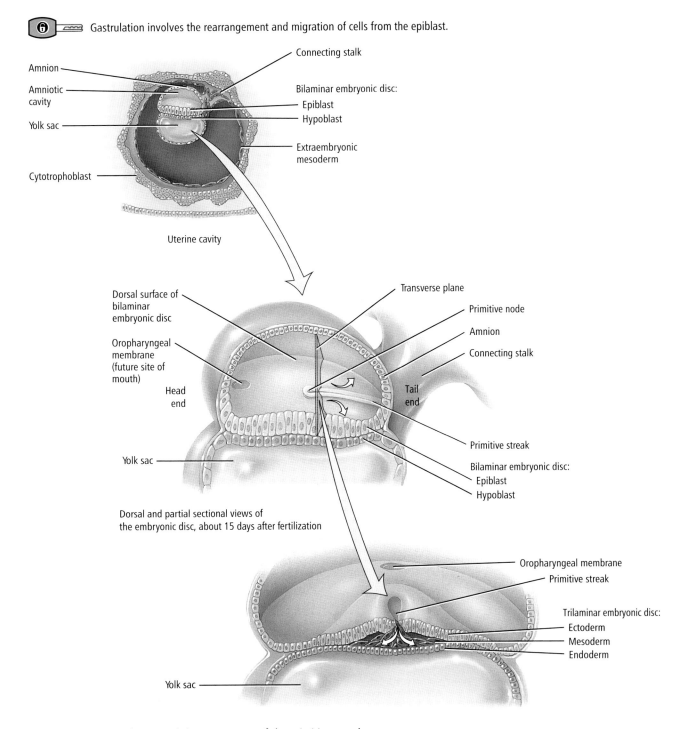

Figure 2.2.   Gastrulation and the appearance of the primitive streak.

Parts of the primitive streak that do not degenerate can give rise to a sacrococcygeal teratoma, a cystic tumor that contains tissues from all three germ layers (Hamilton, 2012). These tumors can be surgically removed from the neonate without any lasting effect.

Mesenchymal cells from the primitive node move toward the head and form the notochordal process and canal. The notochord is a rodlike structure that helps organize the nervous system and later becomes part of the vertebral column and axial skeleton. As the vertebra develops around the notochord, it will degenerate until only remnants are left in the nucleus pulposus between bony vertebrae. The notochord grows between the ectoderm and the endoderm and stops at the prechordal plate. Before it degenerates, the notochord will cause a thickening of the ectoderm and the formation of the neural plate by the end of week 4. This is where the central nervous system and retina begin (Moore et al., 2013). On either side of the notochord, somites (segmental mass of mesoderm occurring in pairs along the notchord) develop, which give rise to the skeleton, muscles, and some of the skin. As the somites develop, they can be used to estimate the age of the embryo (Blackburn, 2013). Near the prechordal plate, layers of ectoderm and endoderm meet and form the oropharyngeal membrane, which will become the mouth.

Mesenchymal cells migrate to the sides of the primitive streak and fuse with the extraembyonic mesoderm that is part of the amnion and umbilical vesicle. These cells also migrate toward the head and form the cardiogenic mesoderm where the heart will begin development at the end of the third week. The allantois is a small appendage of the umbilical vesicle that attaches to the connecting stalk. It is involved with blood formation and the development of the urinary bladder. The blood vessels of the allantois become the arteries and vein of the umbilical cord (Moore et al., 2013).

Neurulation is complete at the end of week 4. About day 18, a neural groove and neural folds appear in the neural plate. These early neural folds are the first signs of brain development. Later, the neural folds fuse to form the neural tube that will separate from the surface ectoderm. The edges of the ectoderm will then fuse over the neural tube, becoming the skin of the back. A neural crest forms between the neural tube and the ectoderm (Moore et al., 2013). Neural crest cells migrate and change into spinal ganglia and autonomic nervous system ganglia. These cells also form the ganglia for cranial nerves V, VII, IX, and X; sheaths for peripheral nerves; the pia mater; and arachnoid mater. This is the time that neural tube defects occur, including anencephaly and meningocele due to failure of primary neurulation, and spina bifida due to failure of secondary neurulation (Jallo, 2011).

The embryo's first nourishment is from maternal blood via diffusion through the chorion, extraembryonic coelom, and umbilical vesicle. At the beginning of the third week, blood vessel formation begins in the extraembyonic mesoderm of the umbilical vesicle and connecting stalk (Moore et al., 2013). At the same time, new blood vessels are being formed in the chorion so that by day 21 postfertilization, the early uteroplacental circulation is functional. At about the same time, the intraembryonic coelom is dividing into the pericardial, pleural, and peritoneal cavities.

Blood formation within the embryo does not begin until week 5. The heart and large vessels develop in the pericardial cavity and the heart begins to beat on day 21 or 22 (Moore et al., 2013). The cardiovascular system is the first system in the embryo to function.

Organogenesis

The fourth to eighth week for the embryo is the period of organogenesis. All the main organ systems begin to develop during these weeks. This is the time when the embryo is most vulnerable to teratogens. As development proceeds, the embryo begins to look more like a unique human being.

These transformative 4 weeks begin with the folding of the embryo so that the flat trilaminar disc becomes a curved cylinder (Moore et al., 2013). The curve is toward the connective stalk and umbilical vesicle. Figure 2.3 depicts the folding of the embryo.

Once folding is complete, the three layers—ectoderm, mesoderm, endoderm—begin to divide, migrate, aggregate, and differentiate in precise patterns to form organs.

Germ layers and organogenesis

Ectoderm—central and peripheral nervous systems, muscle, the skin, hair and nails, mammary glands, pituitary gland, and tooth enamel

Mesoderm—connective tissue, cartilage, bone, striated and smooth muscle, heart, blood, lymphatic system, kidneys, ovaries, testes, spleen, adrenal glands

Endoderm—lining of the gastrointestinal, urinary and respiratory tracts, linings of the ear, parts of the pancreas, and thyroid

---

The fourth week of development will produce somites and the neural tube will be open. The pharyngeal arches are visible and the embryo curves more head to tail (Moore et al., 2013). The heart pumps blood even though it has not yet developed chambers. The forebrain causes an elevation of a portion of the head and there is a

The notochordal process develops from the primitive node and later becomes the notochord.

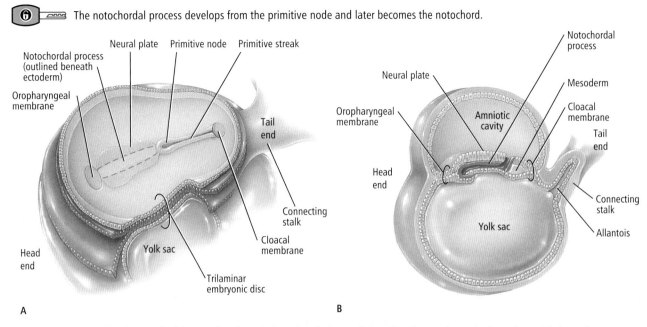

Figure 2.3. Notochord growth. (A) Dorsal and partial sectional views of the trilaminar embryonic disc, about 16 days after fertilization. (B) Sagittal section of the trilaminar embryonic disc, about 16 days after fertilization.

tail-like structure opposite the head. Arm buds are seen on either side of the upper embryo. Otic pits are visible where the ears will be, and a thickening on either side of the head marks where the future eye lenses will be. The leg buds become visible at the end of the fourth week.

During week 5, growth of the head is more rapid than other parts due to the development of the brain and facial features. The embryo is bent in a way that the face will touch the cardiac prominence. Mesonephric ridges appear that will become the kidneys.

The embryo begins slight movements during week 6 and will reflex to touch. Digital rays, the first stages of fingers and hands, appear. The legs develop about 4–5 days after the hands. The auricles for the ears begin to be visible. The retinal pigment for the eyes is present. The head is large and the trunk begins to straighten. The intestines enter the peritoneal cavity near the end of the umbilical cord and an umbilical hernia occurs to give room for the intestine (Moore et al., 2013). At the end of week 6, the embryo is about 22–24 mm in length (Cunningham et al., 2010).

The limbs develop more rapidly during the seventh week. Digital rays become hand plates and the arms and legs become longer. This is also the time when the primordial gut and umbilical vesicle shrink to form the omphaloenteric duct (Moore et al., 2013).

During the last week of organogenesis, fingers are webbed, toes are still digital rays, and the scalp veins become visible and form a band around the head. By the end of the eighth week, digits of the hands and feet have grown longer and the webs are gone. Coordinated movements of all four limbs are seen. The femurs are the first bones to begin to ossify. The tail-like structure has disappeared. The head is still larger than the remainder of the body, but its features are human. The neck is visible, eyelids are closing, and auricles are nearing their final shape. The auricles are low on the head. Sex identification is not yet possible. The fetus will be 10–12 weeks old before it becomes clear that it is either a male or a female. This distinction cannot be made reliably by ultrasound at this stage.

The fetus

The end of week 8 and the beginning of week 9 marks the beginning of the fetal period. The fetal period is a time of rapid growth and differentiation of the systems that have been formed during the preceding 8 weeks. By convention, the main changes in the fetus are considered to occur every 4–5 weeks (Moore et al., 2013).

From weeks 9–12, the fetus doubles its crown to rump length. At 9 weeks, the eyes are wide set, the ears low on the head, and the eyelids are fused. The legs are short and thighs are small. The intestines are seen at the end of the umbilical cord until week 10. The intestines will be completely in the peritoneal cavity by week 11. Urine formation and micturition begin during this period. The fetus begins to swallow AF that contains the urine. Fetal wastes are passed via fetal blood circulation to the mother through the placental membrane. By the end of week 12, the arm length reaches the proportional length they will maintain in relation to the body. The legs are still growing.

During weeks 13–16, the head is smaller in relation to the remainder of the body and the legs are longer. Limb movements as seen via ultrasound are coordinated by week 14. Slow eye movements are seen at 14 weeks and scalp hair has begun to grow. By 16 weeks, ovaries are present in female fetuses and contain ovarian follicles with oogonia (primitive ovum). Sixteen weeks is also the time when fetal bones are visible by ultrasound and the eyes are closer together and look forward. At week 14, the fetal crown–rump length has grown to about 7 cm.

The time period between 17 and 20 weeks marks rapid growth. This is the time that fetal movements can be felt by the mother (quickening). The skin at this stage is covered with vernix caseosa, which protects the skin. The skin is also covered with lanugo, which helps hold the vernix caseosa to the skin. Eyebrows are visible. In females, the uterus is differentiated and formed. In the male, the testes have started migrating toward the scrotum from the posterior abdominal wall. Brown fat for heat generation begins to be deposited in the subcutaneous area (Moore et al., 2013).

Increased weight gain and a more proportional fetus are seen in weeks 21–25. Rapid eye movements and blink-startle responses become evident between weeks 21 and 23 (Moore et al., 2013). Lung development is nearing completion. Surfactant begins to be secreted from the walls for the lungs at 24 weeks. This fluid will help maintain open alveoli, and it is essential for newborn breathing to begin and continue after birth. Fingernails are seen at 24 weeks (Moore et al., 2013).

Between 26 and 29 weeks, the fetus has the potential to survive if it is born prematurely. Its central nervous system has matured enough to direct regular breathing motions and to control body temperature (Moore et al., 2013). The eyelids open and close at 26 weeks and toenails are visible. Brown fat has accumulated and skin wrinkles are smoothed.

Fetal pupils react to light at 30–38 weeks, skin is pink and smooth, and arms and legs become plump. By 35 weeks, the grasp reflex is present and the nervous system is mature enough to function. The abdomen is as wide as the head and the breasts protrude from the chest wall in both boys and girls. Growth begins to slow, although more brown fat is added during the last weeks before birth (Moore et al., 2013). The fetus at 30 weeks weighs about 1800 g or just under 4 lb (Cunningham et al., 2010). Fetal growth may be assessed by ultrasound, magnetic resonance imaging (MRI), or fetal monitoring.

The baby is expected to be born at about 266 days after fertilization or 280–283 days after the mother's last normal menstrual period (Moore et al., 2013). It is estimated that about 12% of babies are born after the expected date of birth (EDB) (Moore et al., 2013). The average baby will weigh about 3400 g at birth. Figure 2.4 is a timetable of human embryonic and fetal development.

Birth defects have the potential for occurring at many times during embryonic growth and development. Table 2.4 lists vulnerable periods and the defects that can occur.

Summary

There is much more to be learned about the development of a human being from the single-celled zygote. The synthesis of the various cells that grow, produce substances that sustain life, migrate to form organs and tissue, or die away to form hollows and spaces is complex and wondrous. It is easy to see that disruption during any stage can cause a cascade of changes that can lead to birth defects or death. It is important that healthcare professionals respect and protect the mother and the embryo/fetus and educate women and their families to enhance the health of mothers and their growing babies.

Case study

Susan is a 21-year-old primigravida at 12 weeks' gestation here for her second prenatal visit.

SUBJECTIVE: She reports that she has recently seen a television program where a mother-to-be sits near a speaker so that her fetus can listen to Mozart music. Susan asks if she should be doing this for her baby.

OBJECTIVE: Physical findings are normal.

ASSESSMENT: Susan is asking good questions stimulated by media information.

PLAN: Explain that fetal hearing begins at around 24–25 weeks. Studies have shown that the fetus can distinguish the mother's voice from other sounds during the third trimester. Studies have also shown that the father's voice and music can be heard by the fetus at about 28 weeks. Encourage Susan and her husband to talk with the fetus as it is growing. This will enhance bonding and it will help both parents to get used to having this new individual in their lives. They can also expose the fetus to music, but using loud speakers or even earphones on the mother's abdomen is not necessary.

Embryonic folding converts the two-dimensional trilaminar embryonic disc into a three-dimensional cylinder.

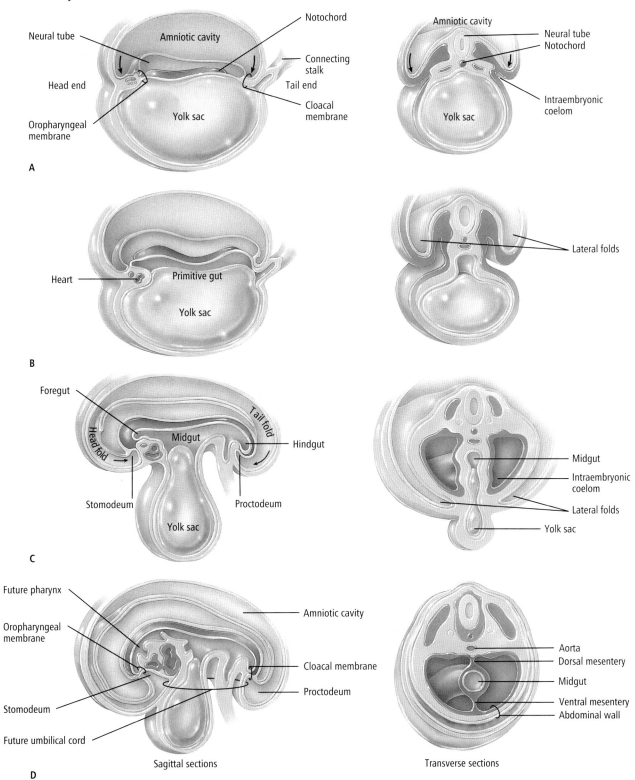

Figure 2.4. Folding of the embryo: (A) 22 days, (B) 24 days, (C) 26 days, and (D) 28 days.

Table 2.4 Vulnerable Periods in Embryonic and Fetal Growth and Development

Timing	Physiological events	Potential vulnerabilities
Weeks 1 and 2	Dividing zygote, implantation, bilaminar embryo	Not susceptible to teratogenesis; spontaneous loss may occur, often due to genetic malfunction early in process
Week 3	Neurological system and cardiac system development begins	Anencephaly; neural tube defects; truncus arteriosis, atrial septal defect or ventricular septal defects may occur near the end of this week of development
Week 4	Brain and nervous system, arms, and later in the week, legs; end of week: ears, eyes	Neural tube defects, heart defects, upper and lower limb defects; low set or deformed ears and deafness; malformed eyes, cataracts, glaucoma
Week 5	Brain and nervous system, heart, arms, legs, ears, eyes, mouth	Same as week 4 and add cleft lip
Week 6	Same as week 5; add tooth enamel and hard palate near the end of week 6	Same as week 5; add enamel hyperplasia and staining; cleft palate near end of week 6
Week 7	Same as week 6; add genitalia	Masculinization of female genitalia may occur at this point
Week 8	Same as week 7; end of this week marks the end of organogenesis	Ears and hearing at risk; eye deformities at week 4; tooth enamel, hard palate, and female genitalia still at risk
Week 9	Brain, hard palate, female genitalia at risk	Brain development deficiencies major threat; hearing still at risk; other major congenital anomalies become less of a threat; functional defects and minor anomalies still possible
Week 16	Brain	Mental retardation; functional defects and minor anomalies continue
Weeks 32–38	Focus on growth and development	Functional and minor anomalies may occur in the central nervous system, ears, eyes, teeth, palate, and external genitalia

Adapted from: Moore, K., Persaud, T., & Torchia, M. (2013). *Before we are born: Essentials of embryology and birth defects* (8th ed.). Philadelphia: Elsevier/Saunders.

Resources for health-care professionals

An interactive visual tool for understanding conception, embryonic, and fetal development, *The Visible Embryo*, is available at http://www.visembryo.com/baby/index .html

The following are web-based animations of various segments of conception and embryonic development:

Implantation from beginning to day 13: http://www .youtube.com/watch?NR=1&feature=endscreen&v =YcxQDkMpj6w

Gastrulation including the mesoderm, primitive streak, and notochord growth: http://www.youtube.com/ watch?v=iHmBIJs77ZQ&feature=endscreen&NR=1

Resources for women, their families, and health-care professionals

Fetal Development Timeline: http://www.babycenter. com/0_fetal-development-timeline_10357636.bc

This Web site from the University of Michigan Medical School (1999) depicts the embryonic period during weeks 3–8: http://www.med.umich.edu/lrc/course pages/m1/embryology/embryo/05embryonicperiod .htm

References

Adams, M., & Koch, R. (2010). *Pharmacology: Connections to nursing practice*. Upper Saddle River, NJ: Pearson.

Beall, M.(2012). Umbilical cord complications. In *Medscape Reference*. Retrieved from http://emedicine.medscape.com/article/262470- overview#aw2aab6b3

Beall, M., & Ross, M. (2009). Amniotic fluid dynamics. In R. Creasy, R. Resnik, & J. Iams (Eds.), *Creasy and Resnik's maternal-fetal medicine: Principles and practice* (6th ed., pp. 47–49). St. Louis, MO: Saunders/Elsevier.

Benirschke, K. (2009). Normal early development. In R. Creasy, R. Resnik, & J. Iams (Eds.), *Creasy and Resnik's maternal-fetal medicine: Principles and practice* (6th ed., pp. 37–44). St. Louis: Saunders/ Elsevier.

Blackburn, S. (2013). *Maternal, fetal, and neonatal physiology: A clinical perspective* (4th ed.). Maryland Heights, MO: Elsevier.

Cunningham, F., Leveno, K., Bloom, S., Hauth, J., Rouse, D., & Spong, C. (2010). *Williams obstetrics* (23rd ed.). New York: McGraw Hill Medical.

Hamilton, C.(2012). Cystic teratoma clinical presentation. In *Mediscape Reference*. Retrieved from http://emedicine.medscape.com/article/281850-clinical

Jallo, G.(2011). Neural tube defects. In *Medscape Reference*. Retrieved from http://emedicine.medscape.com/article/1177162-overview

Liu, J. (2009). Endocrinology of pregnancy. In R. Creasy, R. Resnik, & J. Iams (Eds.), *Creasy and Resnik's maternal-fetal medicine: Principles and practice* (6th ed., pp. 111–123). St. Louis, MO: Saunders/Elsevier.

Moore, K., Persaud, T., & Torchia, M. (2013). *Before we are born: Essentials of embryology and birth defects* (8th ed.). Philadelphia: Elsevier/Saunders.

Stables, D., & Rankin, J. (Eds.). (2010). *Physiology in childbearing* (3rd ed.). Edinburgh, UK: Bailliere Tindall/Elsevier.

3

Maternal physiological alterations during pregnancy

Patricia W. Caudle

Relevant terms

Anabolic—construction of molecules for storage
Anagen—growing phase of the hair growth cycle
Catabolism—breakdown of molecules for energy
Cytokines—molecule messengers that regulate responses to inflammation
Epulis—localized vascular swelling of gums between teeth
Fas/FasL—cell membrane proteins that can activate cellular apoptosis
Fibrinolysis—breakup and removal of excess fibrin
Hyperplasia—increased number of normal cells in normal tissue
Linea alba—line from the umbilicus to the symphysis
Linea nigra—darkened linea alba seen in pregnancy
Lipolytic—breakdown of fat
Lordosis—increased inward curve of the lumbar and cervical spine
Melasma—tan or brown discoloration of areas of the facial skin
Neural tube defects—birth defects of the brain and spinal cord

PCO$_2$—partial pressure of carbon dioxide in the blood
Pedunculated—attached via a stalk
Pica—a craving for nonfood substances
Placentation—development of the placenta
Platelet-derived growth factor—protein that regulates blood vessel formation and growth
Pytalism—excess salivation
Resorption—osteoclasts break down bone and release calcium
Semiallograft—transplanted tissue that is half-maternal genetic material
Telangiectasias—small dilated blood vessels near the skin surface
Telogen—resting phase of the hair growth cycle
Thrombocytes—platelets
Thromboxane—a prostaglandin
Tissue factor—substance that initiates clotting
Trigone—the triangular region of the bladder wall muscle tissue with angles that correspond with ureter and urethra openings

---

Introduction

This chapter outlines physiological changes and adaptations experienced by the pregnant woman as her body accepts, accommodates, and maintains a pregnancy to term. Virtually every body system is affected by remarkable hormonal, anatomical, physiological, and biochemical changes that occur from fertilization through parturition.

Hematologic system adaptations

Maternal physiological changes in the hematologic system include increases in blood and plasma volume,

---

Prenatal and Postnatal Care: A Woman-Centered Approach, First Edition. Edited by Robin G. Jordan, Janet L. Engstrom, Julie A. Marfell, and Cindy L. Farley.
© 2014 John Wiley & Sons, Inc. Published 2014 by John Wiley & Sons, Inc.

Prenatal and Postnatal Care: A Woman-Centered Approach, First Edition. Edited by Robin G. Jordan, Janet L. Engstrom, Julie A. Marfell, and Cindy L. Farley.
© 2014 John Wiley & Sons, Inc. Published 2014 by John Wiley & Sons, Inc.

and increases in the number of red blood cells (RBCs) and white blood cells (WBCs). These changes lead to increased nutritional requirements for iron and folate. In addition, pregnancy is a hypercoagulable state where changes in specific clotting factors, fibrin and fibrino-lytic activities, occur.

Blood changes

Blood is composed of plasma, RBCs and WBCs, plate-lets, and many smaller molecules with numerous func-tions. During pregnancy, blood volume increases by 30% to 50% (Stables & Rankin, 2010). The major compo-nents, plasma and the RBC mass, increase at different rates and through different mechanisms. The more rapid increase in plasma volume causes hemodilution. This hemodilution lowers the hemoglobin, hematocrit, and RBC count per milliliter. These changes do not affect the mean corpuscular volume or mean corpuscular hemo-globin concentration in a normal pregnancy (Kilpatrick, 2009). Table 3.1 delineates the changes in hematologic laboratory parameters during pregnancy.

Red blood cells

The RBC mass will increase by 20–30% by the end of a normal pregnancy (Monga, 2009). This increase occurs because of increased production of RBCs, secondary to increased production of RBCs in the bone marrow. Human placental lactogen (hPL), progesterone, and pro-lactin have been identified as the hormones of pregnancy that stimulate an increase in erythropoiesis (Monga, 2009).

Table 3.1 Changes in Hematologic Laboratory Parameters during Pregnancy

Red blood cells (RBCs)	Increase ~30–35%
Hematocrit	Decreases ~3–5%
Hemoglobin	Decreases 2–10%
White blood cells	Increase 8% (much higher in labor)
Serum ferritin	Decreases
Serum iron	Decreases
Total iron-binding capacity	Increases
Transferrin saturation	Decreases
RBC folate	Decreases
Iron	Decreases
Transferrin	Increases

Adapted from: Blackburn, S. (2013). *Maternal, fetal, and neonatal physiology* (4th ed., pp. 218, 220). Maryland Heights, MO: Elsevier.

White blood cells

Total WBC count increases during pregnancy, ranging from about 5000 to about 15,000 per cubic millimeter (Blackburn, 2013). Most of the increase is in the numbers of neutrophils. Neutrophils function as the first WBC responders in the body's reaction to an infectious or inflammatory process. The WBC count may rise to as high as 30,000 per cubic millimeter during labor and birth without infection. This increase mimics a similar rise in WBCs seen during aerobic exercise.

Plasma

Plasma volume begins to increase as early as 6–8 weeks' gestation (estimated gestational age [EGA]). By about 32 weeks' EGA, plasma volume will have increased 45–50% higher than nonpregnant levels (Monga, 2009). This increase helps to meet increased maternal metabolic needs, to circulate blood within the dilated uterine vascular system, to provide nutrients to the growing conceptus, and to protect the mother against the conse-quences of blood loss during labor and birth. Plasma expands because the production of nitric oxide, a potent vasodilator synthesized from the endothelium of the blood vessel walls, is enhanced and leads to vasodilation, causing the renin–angiotensin–aldosterone system (RAAS) to induce sodium and water retention (Monga, 2009). In addition, human chorionic gonadotropin (hCG) stimulates the thirst centers of the hypothalamus, leading to an increased sensation of thirst and intake of water and other fluids (Blackburn, 2013).

Plasma volume is higher in multiple gestations or when the fetus is larger (Stables & Rankin, 2010). However, increased levels of plasma also occur with hydatidiform mole so the fetus is not the sole reason for plasma increases (Monga, 2009).

Iron requirements

An increase in RBC production and a growing fetus and placenta requires increased iron intake and absorp-tion. It is estimated that the pregnant woman needs 500 mg of extra iron during pregnancy. This includes 300 mg that is used by the fetus and about 200 mg that is needed for normal daily use and loss (Monga, 2009). To meet this need, maternal iron stores are mobilized and increased absorption of dietary iron from the intes-tines occurs (Stables & Rankin, 2010). Progesterone mediates a slowed peristalsis in the small intestine and colon, which enhances iron absorption (Kelly & Savides, 2009).

Many women enter pregnancy with iron stores in the low normal range because of menstrual blood loss. The demands of pregnancy will further deplete these stores, even though there is no menses during the 9 months of the pregnancy (Kilpatrick, 2009). Routine iron supplementation, however, is not routinely recommended until the iron stores are below normal.

The transfer of iron from mother to fetus occurs via active transport through serum transferrin at the placenta. If maternal iron stores are low, then the placenta develops more transferrin receptors (Kilpatrick, 2009). This mechanism helps assure iron transfer to the fetus, even when the mother has limited iron for herself.

Folate requirements

Folate is a water-soluble B vitamin that helps tissues grow and function properly. During pregnancy, folate requirements increase from 50 to 300–500 µg/day because of the growing fetus, the increased maternal RBC mass, and the increased uterine size (Kilpatrick, 2009; Stables & Rankin, 2010). Studies have demonstrated that adequate folate intake, both before and during early pregnancy, will significantly reduce the occurrence of neural tube defects (NTDs).

Changes in clotting factors

Blood also contains substances to help prevent hemorrhage through clotting and, at the same time, substances that assure that blood stays in liquid form. During pregnancy, factors that promote hemostasis and fibrinolysis are enhanced (Cunningham et al., 2010). This adaptation helps control bleeding when there is an increased risk for hemorrhage with implantation and placental development, and again during the third stage of labor when the placenta detaches. Paradoxically, prevention of hemorrhage comes with an increased risk for thrombus formation in the uteroplacental and intervillous circulations, and the deep veins of the legs and pelvis.

The changes that occur to enhance hemostasis are many and complex. Not every component of the hemostatic system increases. For instance, the platelet count during pregnancy decreases slightly, but stays within the same range as the count for nonpregnant women. This decrease has been attributed to hemodilution and increased platelet aggregation in response to increased production of the prostaglandin thromboxane A_2 (Vera, 2011). Platelets are non-nucleated cells synthesized by the bone marrow that play an important role in hemostasis. When there is an injury to a blood vessel, platelets are the first to respond. They work through aggregation, adhesion, and through releasing histamine, serotonin, and platelet-derived growth factor (PDGF). Once released, these substances enhance the enlargement of the platelet plug, activate the coagulation cascade, support the fibrin mesh that develops to further strengthen the plug, and PDGF stimulates smooth

muscle blood vessel walls to help healing (Lockwood & Silver, 2009; Stables & Rankin, 2010).

Progesterone stimulates an increase in tissue factor (TF) (substance that initiates clotting) in the amniotic fluid, decidua, and endometrium (Lockwood & Silver, 2009). During pregnancy, fibrinogen doubles, and clotting factors VII, VIII, IX, and X and the von Willebrand factor all increase. Prothrombin and factor V do not change, and factor XI actually declines slightly. There are decreased anticoagulantion and fibrinolysis; however, the clotting time is about the same. All these adaptations serve to control the bleeding that occurs when the placenta detaches. In fact, a fibrin matrix is established in spiral arteries early in pregnancy that will cause a fibrin mesh to form very quickly over the placenta site. Fibrinolytic activity decreases until about an hour after delivery. These changes and others are summarized in Table 3.2.

Table 3.2   Changes in Coagulation Factors in Pregnancy

Platelets	Decrease slightly but within normal prepregnancy limits
Fibrin deposits	Increased
Tissue factor (TF)	Found in amniotic fluid, decidua, and endometrium
Fibrin–fibrinogen complexes	Increased
Plasminogen-activated inhibitors	Increased
Fibrinogen	Increased
Fibrinolysis	Decreased
Coagulation factor I	Increased
Coagulation factor VII	Increased (10 times normal)
Coagulation factor VIII	Increased (doubles)
Coagulation factor X	Increased
von Willebrand factor	Increased
Activated partial thromboplastin time (aPTT)	Decreased
Prothrombin time (PT)	Decreased
Bleeding time	Unchanged
Protein S (coagulation inhibitor)	Decreased
Fibrin degradation products	Increased
D-dimer (marker for fibrinolysis)	Increased

Adapted from: Blackburn, S. (2013). *Maternal, fetal, and neonatal physiology* (4th ed., pp. 221–223). Maryland Heights, MO: Elsevier; Cunningham, F., Leveno, K., Bloom, S., Hauth, J., Rouse, D., & Spong, C. (2010). *Williams obstetrics* (23rd ed.). New York: McGraw Hill Medical.

Cardiovascular changes

The heart and vascular system undergo profound changes beginning as early as 5 weeks' gestation. Typically, women with healthy hearts seldom report concerns associated with these changes. There are several signs and symptoms that occur, however, that mimic cardiovascular disease, creating a diagnostic dilemma for the health-care provider. Up to 4% of pregnant women will have unrecognized cardiovascular disease; this is emerging as a contributor to maternal morbidity and mortality (Mohamad, 2013). Table 3.3 lists the functional signs and symptoms seen in pregnancy.

Changes to the heart

The ventricular muscle mass increases during the first trimester and the left atrial diameter increases as the blood volume increases (Monga, 2009). Cardiac output, a measure of functional capacity of the heart, increases by 30–50%, with about half of this increase occurring by 8 weeks' gestation (Blackburn, 2013, p. 269). The increase

Table 3.3 Signs and Symptoms of a Normal Pregnancy That Mimic Heart Disease

Dyspnea	Progesterone effect on breathing centers causing increased respiratory rate
Fatigability	Response to increased metabolic demand
Dependent edema	Venous pressure from gravid uterus, lower colloid osmotic pressure
First heart sound louder	Early closure of mitral valve
Split S_2	Expected at about 30 weeks of gestation
S_3	Heard in 90% of pregnant women
Systolic flow murmur	Heard in 95% of pregnant women; begins ~12–20 weeks and disappears about 1 week after birth
Left lateral displacement of the point of maximal impulse	Gravid uterus pressing upward on diaphragm and heart
Mammary souffle	Continuous murmur from mammary vessels, heard best in second intercostal space

Adapted from: Monga, M. (2009). Maternal cardiovascular, respiratory, and renal adaptation to pregnancy. In R. Creasy, R. Resnik, & J. Iams (Eds.), *Creasy and Resnik's maternal-fetal medicine: Principles and practice* (6th ed., pp. 103–104). St. Louis, MO: Saunders/Elsevier.

in cardiac output comes from increases in both stroke volume and heart rate. Stroke volume causes most of the early rise in cardiac output and then declines as the pregnancy nears term. Maternal heart rate begins to increase at 5 weeks' gestation and reaches a maximum increase of about 15–20 beats per minute by 32 weeks' gestation. Increased cardiac output is needed to support the 10-fold increase in uterine blood flow (500–800 mL/min) and the 50% increase in blood flow to the kidneys (Monga, 2009). Blood flow is also increased to the breasts and the skin. These adaptations explain the flow murmurs and other changes in signs and symptoms listed in Table 3.3.

Vascular adaptations

Collagen throughout the vascular system softens, resulting in increased compliance and decreased vascular resistance beginning around 5 weeks' gestation. Vasodilation occurs as the result of the relaxant effects of progesterone and prostaglandin (Monga, 2009). The low-resistance uteroplacental circulation acts like an arteriovenous connection, thereby contributing to lowered vascular resistance. In addition, there is an increased production of endothelial relaxant factors such as nitric oxide that contribute to lowered vascular resistance. All of these changes contribute to decreased venous resistance that will slow the speed of venous flow and contribute to stasis of the blood, thereby increasing the risk for deep vein thrombosis in pregnancy. These changes also contribute to an increased sensitivity to autonomic blockade—such as that produced by epidural anesthesia. When this anesthesia is administered to pregnant women, a sudden drop in blood pressure often occurs (Monga, 2009).

Changes in blood pressure

Normally, arterial blood pressure decreases in pregnancy when the arteries relax and peripheral vascular resistance decreases. This decrease in blood pressure begins at about the seventh week of pregnancy and persists until around 32 weeks, when it begins to rise to prepregnancy levels (Monga, 2009).

Maternal position affects blood pressure measurements. In fact, blood pressure decreases 5–10 mmHg systolic and 10–15 mmHg diastolic when a pregnant woman lies on her left side (Monga, 2009, p. 102). Serial blood pressures taken with the pregnant woman sitting with her feet on the floor are the best for monitoring for any abnormal changes in blood pressure during pregnancy.

Supine hypotensive syndrome

Supine hypotensive syndrome occurs in a small percentage of pregnant women but deserves mention. Lying flat on the back in the supine position after about 30 weeks' gestation can cause the weight of the gravid uterus to compress the vena cava. When the vena cava is compressed, it will limit the amount of blood that can return to the heart. This reduction in stroke volume causes a decrease in cardiac output and a drop in blood pressure (Cunningham et al., 2010). The changes in the mother's cardiovascular system can cause her to feel faint and can lead to a drop in fetal heart rate. Very rarely, loss of consciousness can occur. Women naturally tend to turn to the side when they feel this sensation and no harm is caused by this temporary state. It can be a problem during an office visit when a woman is lying on her back for an examination or during labor if she is immobile and supine. Helping her roll to her side to relieve the pressure of the gravid uterus will restore blood flow and blood pressure.

Respiratory adaptations

Pregnancy causes less stress on the respiratory system than on the cardiovascular system; however, there are significant adaptations. Although some women may complain of shortness of breath, respiratory exchange is more efficient during pregnancy. The primary changes occur in lung volume and ventilation as the oxygen demands of maternal metabolism and the fetoplacental unit increase. These changes begin early in pregnancy.

Anatomical changes

Estrogen and the increasing blood volume of pregnancy will cause capillary engorgement that will lead to swelling and increased mucous production in the nose, sinuses, eustachian tubes, and middle ears. At the same time, progesterone causes a relaxation of veins and increased pooling that further contributes to mucous membrane swelling. The result is increased incidence of pregnancy rhinitis, epistaxis, serous otitis, and congested sinuses (Stables & Rankin, 2010).

The hormone relaxin causes increased pliability of cartilage in the chest, allowing for an increase in chest circumference. As the gravid uterus increases in size, the diaphragm raises about 4 cm, the thoracic circumference increases about 6 cm, and the costal angle widens (Cunningham et al., 2010, p. 121; Whitty & Dombrowski, 2009). There is also an increase in thoracic breathing and more diaphragmatic movement (Whitty & Dombrowski, 2009). Most of the chest wall changes persist after pregnancy.

Adaptations in pulmonary function

Increased maternal progesterone affects respiratory rate, respiratory drive, and total pulmonary resistance. Progesterone reduces pulmonary airflow resistance and

Table 3.4   Respiratory Parameter Changes in Pregnancy

Total lung capacity	Decreased by 4%
Inspiratory capacity	Increased by ~300 mL
Expiratory reserve capacity	Decreased by ~200 mL
Residual volume	Decreased by 20%
Tidal volume	Increased by 40%
Minute ventilation	Increased by 40%
O_2 consumption	Increased by 50%
Total pulmonary resistance	Reduced

Adapted from: Stables, D., & Rankin, J. (Eds.).(2010). *Physiology in childbearing* (3rd ed., p. 256). Edinburgh, UK: Bailliere Tindall/Elsevier; Whitty, J., & Dombrowski, M. (2009). Respiratory diseases in pregnancy. In R. Creasy, R. Resnik, & J. Iams (Eds.). *Creasy and Resnik's maternal-fetal medicine: Principles and practice* (6th ed., pp. 927–931). St. Louis. MO: Saunders/Elsevier.

stimulates the respiratory center of the brainstem to increase the respiratory rate. It also lowers the threshold to carbon dioxide (CO_2) and increases the sensitivity of chemoreceptors to CO_2. An increased metabolic rate increases oxygen requirements and consumption (Monga, 2009). The combined effect is mild hyperventilation and mild respiratory alkalosis that occurs as the mother "blows off" CO_2 and decreases the carbon dioxide partial pressure in blood (PCO_2). Progesterone has also been implicated in the increase in carbonic anhydrase in RBCs that helps in CO_2 transfer and a decrease in PCO_2 (Stables & Rankin, 2010). A reduced maternal PCO_2 facilitates the movement of CO_2 waste from the fetus to the mother and enhances the release of oxygen from the mother to the fetus (Cunningham et al., 2010).

There are several pulmonary function parameters that are changed as adaptation to pregnancy occurs. Table 3.4 lists these parameters. It is important to note that increased oxygen requirements and adaptations in pulmonary function make respiratory diseases such asthma and pneumonia potentially much more serious in pregnancy (Whitty & Dombrowski, 2009).

Renal adaptations

The renal and urinary systems undergo dramatic change in response to pregnancy. The kidneys must adjust to increased blood and extracellular fluid volume, and increased maternal and fetal wastes. There are changes related to hormonal effects, pressure from the gravid uterus, and from cardiovascular adaptations (Blackburn, 2013).

Anatomical changes

The kidneys grow in volume and length during pregnancy due to an increase in renal vascular and interstitial growth (Monga, 2009). The kidneys and ureters dilate when the gravid uterus grows enough to compress the ureters at the pelvic rim and slow urine flow. The right ureter is more greatly affected either because of the right-sided rotation of the uterus or because of the cushioning provided to the left ureter by the sigmoid colon (Cunningham et al., 2010). Ureter dilation may also be a consequence of progesterone, relaxin, and nitric oxide effects that relax smooth muscle; however, most studies support uterine compression as the most likely cause of these changes (Monga, 2009). Dilation of the kidneys and ureters increases the potential for urine stasis and infection. Hydroureter may persist for 3–4 months after birth.

The bladder begins adaptive changes at about 12 weeks of gestation (Cunningham et al., 2010). By then, hyperemia (increased blood flow) and hyperplasia (increased number of normal cells in normal arrangement) of the muscle and connective tissue will cause elevation of the bladder trigone and increase the susceptibility to bladder infection. There is reduced bladder capacity and increased incidence of incontinence during the third trimester related to pressure on the bladder from the gravid uterus. In addition, pressure from the fetal presenting part may slow blood and lymph drainage, causing the base of the bladder to swell and become more prone to infection (Cunningham et al., 2010).

Renal function

Renal plasma flow increases 60–80% by midpregnancy then decreases to about 50% above prepregnancy rates by term (Monga, 2009, p. 105). Lateral lying positions increase venous return and renal plasma flow; the left lateral lying position is best for enhancing renal plasma flow (Blackburn, 2013). These position changes will lead to increased urine flow and nocturia.

Glomerular filtration rate (GFR) increases significantly within 2 weeks after conception and is 50% higher than prepregnancy levels by 12 weeks' gestation (Cunningham et al., 2010, p. 123). This and the weight of the growing uterus on the bladder explain the urinary frequency experienced by women during the first weeks of pregnancy. The increase in GFR causes increased creatinine clearance and decreased serum creatinine, blood urea nitrogen, and serum osmolarity (Cunningham et al., 2010; Monga, 2009).

Renal tubular function also changes in pregnancy. The most impressive tubular function change is the reabsorption of sodium. Sodium retention is promoted by increased levels of estrogen, deoxycorticosterone, and the increased activity of the RAAS (Monga, 2009). Sodium retention is also enhanced by maternal sitting or standing. Interestingly, although sodium is retained during pregnancy, the serum levels of sodium decrease slightly due to hemodilution (Cunningham et al., 2010).

Two other important electrolytes are significantly affected by renal tubular function changes in pregnancy. Potassium is retained, but like sodium, serum levels slightly decrease due to increased plasma volume (Cunningham et al., 2010). Calcium excretion increases while total serum calcium decreases related to a decrease in plasma albumin (Monga, 2009). Further discussion of maternal and fetal calcium physiology is found in the musculoskeletal section of this chapter.

Glucose excretion increases, causing glycosuria in about 15% of normal pregnancies (Cunningham et al., 2010). Increased glycosuria will increase susceptibility to urinary tract infection.

Uric acid excretion is increased and serum uric acid levels decrease between 8 and 24 weeks of gestation. The serum levels begin to rise to near prepregnancy levels by term. Clinically, an increased plasma uric acid level can be a sign of preeclampsia (Monga, 2009).

About two-thirds of the weight gain in pregnancy is retained fluid related to the changes in renal tubular function. About 6 L of body water is retained in extracellular areas and 2 L is gained in intracellular spaces. Plasma increases account for only about one-quarter of the increase in extracellular fluid (Monga, 2009). The allocation of fluid is described as about 3.5 L for amniotic fluid, fetus, and placenta; and about 3 L for maternal blood volume, breasts, and uterus (Cunningham et al., 2010). Clinically, fluid retention of more than 1.5 L is seen as dependent edema (Blackburn, 2013). Fluid seeps into interstitial spaces of the lower extremities because of increased venous hydrostatic pressure below the uterus when the gravid uterus places pressure on the inferior vena cava and pelvic vessels (Cunningham et al., 2010).

Gastrointestinal adaptations

Gastrointestinal (GI) changes related to pregnancy and pregnancy hormones cause discomforts that are experienced in most normal pregnancies. Occasionally, these changes mimic more serious conditions and require careful assessment.

Anatomical adaptations

The GI system is displaced upward and back by the growing uterus. This change will move the appendix as high as the right upper quadrant, causing the pain of appendicitis to be much higher in the abdomen than expected (Cunningham et al., 2010). In most pregnancies, however, the change in location and the compression of the stomach and bowel is well tolerated.

Gastrointestinal function changes

The primary cause of changes in the function of the GI tract in pregnancy is progesterone. This hormone relaxes smooth muscle, thereby causing decreased lower esophageal sphincter tone and slowing of peristalsis and intestinal transit time. A relaxed lower esophageal sphincter will allow for reflux of stomach contents into the lower esophagus, resulting in heartburn, especially when pressure from the growing uterus is exerted against the stomach. The advantages of slowed transit time are the increased absorption of water, vitamin B_{12}, some amino acids, iron, and calcium (Blackburn, 2013; Kelly & Savides, 2009). The disadvantage is a dryer, harder stool and increased incidence of constipation, straining at stool, and hemorrhoids.

In the mouth, the gums respond to increased estrogen by becoming hyperemic, friable, and softer (Cunningham et al., 2010; Stables & Rankin, 2010). Some women will develop one or more epulis, a localized vascular swelling of the gums. These changes increase maternal risks for gingivitis and periodontal disease. There is no evidence that pregnancy increases tooth decay or tooth loss, although this belief is expressed in common folklore.

Progesterone is an appetite stimulant leading to increased food intake to meet metabolic needs. This may be part of the reason for food cravings, including pica, a craving for things such as clay, starch, or other substances with no nutritional value (Stables & Rankin, 2010). However, sociocultural background is a strong influence on eating behaviors.

Ptyalism or excess salivation can occur in pregnancy. Most often this is related to a reluctance to swallow saliva when a woman is troubled by nausea and vomiting of pregnancy (Blackburn, 2013). Nausea and vomiting of pregnancy, a common occurrence, has been linked to hCG, estrogen, elevated T4, altered motility related to progesterone, the emotional and psychological state of the mother, and reflux (Blackburn, 2013; Kelly & Savides, 2009). However, the exact cause is unknown; the phenomenon of nausea and vomiting has multiple determinants. The nausea probably increases some of the food aversions commonly observed in pregnancy.

Liver and biliary adaptations

Anatomically, the liver is displaced up and back as the uterus grows. The liver does not change in size and blood flow to the liver is unchanged. The production of proteins and enzymes by the liver does change. Plasma

Table 3.5 Liver Function Changes in Pregnancy

Albumin	Decreased
Alkaline phosphatase	Increased (also produced in placenta)
Aspartate transaminase (AST)	Slight decrease due to hemodilution
Alanine transaminase (ALT)	Slight decrease due to hemodilution
Bilirubin (conjugated, unconjugated)	Unchanged
Gamma-glutamyl transpeptidase (GGT)	Slight decrease due to hemodilution
Total protein	Decreased

Adapted from: Cunningham, F., Leveno, K., Bloom, S., Hauth, J., Rouse, D., & Spong, C. (2010). *Williams obstetrics* (23rd ed., p. 1261). New York: McGraw Hill Medical.

proteins, including albumin, decrease in pregnancy, in part, because of hemodilution. Newer studies indicate that the rise in alpha-fetoprotein may cause a drop in serum albumin levels (Williamson & Mackillop, 2009). The production of fibrinogen and coagulation factors VII, VIII, IX, and X is increased under the influence of estrogen. Progesterone stimulates an increase in cytochromic P450 isoenzymes, a group of enzymes that assist in the metabolism of organic substances and are important in the body's processing of many drugs. Thyroxine-binding and corticosteroid-binding globulins increase as estrogen levels increase (Nader, 2009a, 2009b). Serum alkaline phosphatase (ALP) increases due to placental production, while other liver enzymes are slightly decreased or stay the same (Williamson & Mackillop, 2009). Table 3.5 lists the changes in liver function tests during pregnancy.

The gallbladder is affected by progesterone-induced slowed peristalsis that will cause an increased bile volume, bile stasis, and increased cholesterol saturation (Williamson & Mackillop, 2009). These changes increase the risk for gallstone formation. The two most common indications for nonobstetric surgery in pregnant women are acute appendicitis and acute biliary disease.

Metabolic changes

The maternal metabolism adjusts to ensure that glucose, protein, and fat are metabolized in a way that will meet the energy needs of the mother, the uteroplacental unit, and the fetus. To better understand this adaptation, several different components involved in the process will be described.

Basal metabolic rate

By the end of a normal pregnancy, the maternal metabolic rate has increased eight times the nonpregnancy rates (Blackburn, 2013). This requires an average of an additional 300 kcal/day, generally starting in the second trimester. Most of this energy is needed for the growth of the fetus, placenta, uterus, and breasts. Some energy is set aside, stored as fat to be used during the last weeks of pregnancy when the fetus is growing more rapidly (Blackburn, 2013).

The first half of pregnancy is dominated by an anabolic state (construction of complex molecules for storage) (Blackburn, 2013). The mother eats more, moves around less, and protein and fat substrates are stored. Weight gain during this half of pregnancy is due to fat storage and the synthesis of protein into growing tissues. During this anabolic state, insulin is also increased and acts like a growth hormone, facilitating the processes of growth.

Catabolism (breakdown of complex molecules for energy) occurs during the second half of pregnancy. Lipolytic (the breakdown of fat) activity is increased and pregnancy hormones cause insulin resistance. hPL, produced by the placenta, has anti-insulin and lipolytic properties that help the mother change from glucose usage for energy to lipid usage for energy (Blackburn, 2013). This change leads to "accelerated starvation" (Cunningham et al., 2010). When a woman is not pregnant and deprived of food, it takes about 24–36 h before she has used all the glucose-based energy and begins to burn fat. When a woman is pregnant, lipolysis will occur in about 12 h.

Carbohydrate metabolism

Serum glucose levels during fasting are lower in pregnancy than in the nonpregnant state. After eating, serum glucose and insulin levels are higher for a longer time in pregnancy. Higher levels of insulin cause a suppression of glucagon and maternal insulin resistance increases as the pregnancy advances. Insulin resistance in the maternal skeletal muscle and adipose tissue is mediated by progesterone, estrogen, hPL, and possibly by free fatty acids released by lipolysis (Cunningham et al., 2010).

Protein metabolism

Protein is essential to tissue building in pregnancy. Amino acids and protein are used by the placenta and fetus. These substances are also diverted to the liver for gluconeogenesis. Consequently, serum amino acid and serum protein levels are lower in pregnancy (Blackburn, 2013). At the same time, urinary excretion of protein by-products does not change. This indicates that maternal muscle breakdown is not used to meet fetal needs (Cunningham et al., 2010).

Table 3.6   Lipid and Lipoprotein Levels in the Third Trimester

Cholesterol	267 ± 30 mg/dL
LDL-C	136 ± 33 mg/dL
HDL-C	81 ± 17 mg/dL
Triglycerides	245 ± 73 mg/dL

Adapted from: Cunningham, F., Leveno, K., Bloom, S., Hauth, J., Rouse, D., & Spong, C. (2010). *Williams obstetrics* (23rd ed., p. 114). New York: McGraw Hill Medical.

Fat metabolism

Lipids, lipoproteins, and apolipoproteins increase in maternal serum during pregnancy. These increases are due to lipolysis and decreased lipoprotein lipase action in fat tissue. Estradiol and progesterone effects on the liver also contribute to these changes (Cunningham et al., 2010). Interestingly, these increases are not associated with vascular endothelial dysfunction in healthy pregnant women. Table 3.6 lists the changes expected in cholesterol, triglycerides, and lipoproteins in pregnancy.

Leptin and ghrelin

Leptin is produced and secreted by maternal fat cells and the placenta (Blackburn, 2013). This peptide hormone helps regulate appetite and enhances energy use. It also contributes significantly to fetal growth and development. Maternal serum leptin is two to four times higher than in nonpregnant women (Cunningham et al., 2010). Leptin is increased even more in women with preeclampsia and gestational diabetes (Blackburn, 2013). Low leptin levels have been detected during spontaneous abortion.

Ghrelin is a hormone secreted by maternal fat cells and the placenta that also has a role in fetal growth. Maternal serum levels of this hormone increase during the first half of pregnancy and decrease during the second half when insulin resistance increases. A similar decrease in ghrelin is seen in metabolic syndrome in nonpregnant individuals (Cunningham et al., 2010).

Insulin

Insulin is a polypeptide hormone produced and secreted by the beta cells of the islet of Langerhans of the endocrine pancreas. It is secreted in response to increased serum glucose, amino acids, free fatty acids, GI hormones, and the parasympathetic nervous system stimulation of the beta cells. It functions to facilitate glucose entry into cells (Brashers & Jones, 2010, p. 713).

Pregnant women with normal glucose tolerance will have an increase in insulin in response to estrogen-induced, increased hepatic glucose production and the increase in serum glucose produced after a meal. Insulin will facilitate the movement of glucose into maternal muscle and fat cells and will suppress further liver production of glucose. Late in pregnancy, insulin resistance increases and more insulin is produced. If a woman is obese or has an abnormal glucose tolerance before pregnancy, her pancreas may not be able to produced the amount of insulin needed to overcome the insulin resistance induced by pregnancy hormones, and gestational diabetes can result (Moore & Catalano, 2009).

Skin changes

The skin is the body's largest organ. Skin functions as a barrier to infection and ultraviolet radiation; it also retains body fluids, regulates body temperature, and produces vitamin D. Skin contains touch and pressure receptors and nociceptors that transmit pain sensation. Skin is part of the integumentary system, which also includes hair, nails, sebaceous glands, and sweat glands. The entire integumentary system is changed during pregnancy. Specifically, there are changes in pigment, vascular supply, and connective tissue of the skin; hair growth; nail structure; and in the sebaceous and sweat gland functions.

Pigment changes of the skin

Estrogen and progesterone produced during pregnancy will stimulate the production of melanocyte-stimulating hormone (MSH). The most frequently seen manifestations of increased MSH are hyperpigmentation of the areolae, genital skin, axillae, inner thighs, and the linea alba (line that extends from the xiphoid to the symphysis pubis), which becomes the linea nigra during pregnancy. Freckles and moles will also darken. These pigment changes are also seen in women taking oral contraceptives. Pigment changes usually fade after pregnancy or when oral contraceptives are discontinued; however, women with darker skin are more likely to have persistent hyperpigmentation (Blackburn, 2013).

Melasma or the "mask of pregnancy" occurs as a result of increased MSH in about 70% of pregnant women (Rapini, 2009). This patch of hyperpigmentation is distributed over the forehead, cheeks, and bridge of the nose in a symmetric pattern. About 30% of women affected will have persistent melasma months to years after delivery. Exposure to sunlight will exacerbate the hyperpigmentation. Sunscreen should be routinely used to decrease the discoloration.

Vascular changes of the skin

The hormones of pregnancy cause vasodilation and the proliferation of capillaries in the skin and can result in the development of telangiectasias (small dilated blood vessels near the skin surface) and palmar erythema. These changes help in thermoregulation by dissipating the heat generated by the fetus, increased maternal metabolic rate, and the thermogenic effects of progesterone (Blackburn, 2013).

Connective tissue changes

Estrogen, relaxin, and adrenocorticoids, along with stretching, contribute to *striae gravidarum*, commonly known as stretch marks. The hormones are thought to relax collagen adhesiveness and facilitate the formation of mucopolysaccharide substance that will develop a separation of collagen fibers. Increased cortisol during pregnancy causes the striae to be purplish in color. The usual locations for striae are over the abdomen, breasts, thighs, and buttocks where skin is stretched by the growing fetus, enlarged breast tissue, and weight gain. Striae become prominent by 6–7 months of gestation and are most prevalent in younger, Caucasian women (Blackburn, 2013). The more severe striae occur in teenagers, women with maternal family history of striae, women who are obese or who gain more than 30 lb, or women with large babies (Rapini, 2009). Interestingly, there is an increased incidence of pelvic relaxation among women who have moderate to severe striae.

Skin tags are another connective tissue phenomenon seen in pregnant women. These tags are soft, pedunculated growths that are the same color of the surrounding skin or are hyperpigmented. They appear on the neck, face, axillae, groin, and between and under the breasts (Blackburn, 2013; Rapini, 2009). Skin tags will usually disappear after birth; however, sometimes they persist, particularly among obese women.

Sebaceous and sweat gland changes

Sebaceous glands secrete more sebum during pregnancy secondary to increased ovarian and placental androgens (Blackburn, 2013). Apocrine sweat glands found in the axillae, scalp, face, abdomen, and genital area have decreased activity during pregnancy related to hormonal changes (Blackburn, 2013; Nicol & Huether, 2010). Eccrine sweat glands that are distributed over the body have an increased activity during pregnancy. This activity increases under the influence of increased thyroid activity, increased maternal metabolic rate, and increased fetal-produced heat. Their main function is to secrete sweat that will evaporate and help dissipate heat.

Hair and nail changes

During pregnancy, estrogen causes an increased number of hairs to remain in the anagen phase (growing phase), and a decreased number enter the telogen phase (resting phase). When pregnancy hormones are removed after the birth of the placenta, the number of hairs that enter the telogen phase increases, resulting in hair loss. This hair loss is called telogen effluvium and can also occur after surgery, illness, crash dieting, or other stressful life events (Rapini, 2009). Hair loss after giving birth is expected and is easily distinguished from alopecia of other causes. This hair loss will generally resolve by 9 months postpartum without treatment.

Changes in the nails are uncommon in pregnancy; however, phenomena such as transverse grooves, increased brittleness, separation of the nail bed at the toe or fingertip, and whitish discoloration have been reported. These changes are benign and will disappear during the postpartum period (Blackburn, 2013; Rapini, 2009).

Immunologic changes

Pregnancy requires changes in the immune system of the mother. In order to accept and maintain a pregnancy to term, some innate, humoral, and cell-mediated immunologic functions must be altered. This section will outline those changes and explain how these alterations may increase risks for infection or provide remission for some autoimmune conditions for the mother.

Fetus as allograft

The fetus is a semiallograft (an allograft is transplanted tissue; "semi" refers to the fact that fetal tissue carries half of mother's genetic material) that is not rejected by the mother's immune system. Even though half of the genetic material in the fetus is from the father, in most cases, the mother's immune system does not reject the foreign antigens on fetal cells. Several possible theories explain this phenomenon (Mor & Abrahams, 2009): The placenta is a barrier; the mother's immune system is suppressed; there is a cytokine shift; there is an absence of major histocompatibility complex (MHC) class I molecules on the conceptus; and there is a local immune suppression mediated by Fas/FasL (Fas ligands are cell membrane proteins that can activate cellular apoptosis). More recently, another theory has been proposed. Pregnancy protein 13 (PP13), produced by the trophoblast, has been identified as an agent that diverts the mother's immune system so that the paternal antigen will be established and grow (Kliman et al., 2011).

The placenta as barrier theory has been discounted; the placenta acts as only a partial barrier to selected substances. In fact, fetal cells can cross into maternal blood and have been found in maternal circulation or organs years after pregnancy (Cunningham et al., 2010). Cell-free fetal DNA also enters the maternal system and

new laboratory tests can isolate fetal DNA from a maternal venous blood sample and perform a limited number of genetic tests on the DNA.

Systemic immune suppression does not fully explain how the conceptus is accepted. How could mothers have lived to give birth through the millennia if they could not defend themselves against bacteria and viruses? Today, the best argument against this theory is that women with human immunodeficiency virus (HIV) infection do not progress into AIDS during pregnancy (Mor & Abrahams, 2009).

Another theory has been that pregnancy is anti-inflammatory in nature, which causes abnormal shifts in cytokines, the molecular messengers that regulate responses to inflammation. This can contribute to spontaneous pregnancy loss or preeclampsia. Newer information demonstrates that pregnancy actually occurs in three different phases with regard to maternal immune response: invasion of the trophoblast and placentation requiring a strong inflammatory response; a quiet anti-inflammatory state where the fetus is growing; and renewed inflammatory response with an increase of immune cells migrating into the uterus to promote contractions, birth, and the rejection of the placenta (Mor & Abrahams, 2009).

Another theory is that there is no MHC class I antigen on the trophoblast, so the mother's immune system does not recognize the foreign antigens. In fact, the placenta does express human leukocyte antigens (HLA-C, HLA-G, and HLA-E). These are subsets of MHC antigens. So, fetal tissues are capable of initiating a maternal T-cell response (Mor & Abrahams, 2009). Interestingly, women who have HLAs similar to those of the father of the baby will not produce the immune substances necessary to prevent rejection of the fetus (Cunningham et al., 2010). This can explain different pregnancy outcomes for the same woman with a new partner.

The theory that there are specific immune suppressor cells that would recognize the paternal antigens that are removed from the mother's system through cell death by the Fas/Fas ligand system is still being investigated (Mor & Abrahams, 2009). In addition, a subset of T lymphocytes called T regulatory cells has been identified as being able to control other T cells that would attack paternal antigens. These are both possible explanations for the survival of the fetal allograft.

It is also important to recognize that several cells of the innate immune system have been identified at the site where the trophoblast implants, including natural killer (NK) cells, macrophages, and dendritic cells. So this part of the mother's immune system does respond to the conceptus. These noncytotoxic NK cells contribute to angiogenesis (growth of new blood vessels) and implantation (Mor & Abrahams, 2009). Macrophages clean out dead cells and debris, while dendritic cells help with early implantation. These activities are crucial to placentation and the immune adjustments necessary for a successful pregnancy.

Disorders related to immunologic changes in pregnancy

During pregnancy, T-helper cells (Th1) and T-cytotoxic cells (Tc) are suppressed. This has been identified as a reason for remission of maternal autoimmune disorders such as rheumatoid arthritis, multiple sclerosis, and autoimmune thyroiditis (Blackburn, 2013; Stables & Rankin, 2010). Suppression of Th1 has also been implicated in the increased susceptibility to viruses, *Candida albicans*, and other organisms. In fact, yeast vulvovaginitis occurs more often in pregnant women due to increased estrogen and the changes in the cell-mediated immune response. This cell-mediated immune response, along with the changes in the lungs and heart, has also been identified as an explanation for the severity of H1N1 influenza during pregnancy (Centers for Disease Control and Prevention, 2011). Systemic lupus erythematosis (SLE) that is not complicated by kidney disease remains stable during pregnancy due to the upregulation or increases in Th2 that is normally seen in pregnancy (Blackburn, 2013). Unfortunately, the disease will often flare within 6–8 weeks after birth.

There are four inflammatory markers that are increased during pregnancy. These include leukocyte ALP, C-reactive protein, erythrocyte sedimentation rate (due to increased plasma globulins and fibrinogen), and complement factors C_3 and C_4 (Cunningham et al., 2010). This should be taken into consideration when interpreting laboratory measures of these markers during pregnancy.

Some spontaneous abortions are a result of immune system changes in pregnancy. Immunologic factors that have been implicated in spontaneous abortion include infection; increased Th1 activity against the trophoblast; an immune-related failure of the corpus luteum to produce progesterone; HLAs similar to those of the father; and, in women with SLE, antiphospholipid antibodies that prevent the development of the placenta (Blackburn, 2013; Cunningham et al., 2010). Recurrent (more than three) spontaneous abortions have been linked with the presence of NK cells like those found in the periphery rather than the noncytotoxic NK cells usually found in the decidua (Blackburn, 2013).

Preterm labor and birth can result from infection that triggers the innate immune system to release inflammatory cytokines, interleukin, and tumor necrosis factors. These cytokines increase the production of prostaglan-

din that will stimulate contractions. At the same time, enzymes that cause a weakening of the fetal membranes are released and the membranes may rupture prematurely (Cunningham et al., 2010). About 25–40% of preterm births occur because of intrauterine infection (Cunningham et al., 2010).

Preeclampsia is specific to pregnancy and is a complex chronic disorder that affects many maternal systems. Evidence suggests that preeclampsia has an immunologic component. In fact, preeclampsia has some of the same cellular changes seen in graft rejection including reduced HLA-G on the trophoblast, an increase in Th1 rather than suppression, more immune complexes, increased fibronectin, increased inflammatory cytokines, changes in complement, and the absence of PP13 (Blackburn, 2013; Kliman et al., 2011).

Unlike the cell-mediated and innate immune systems, the humoral system in pregnancy does not change significantly. However, maternal antibodies can have an effect on the fetus. Humoral immunity occurs when immunoglobulins (Ig) or antibodies are produced by B lymphocytes (plasma cells) in response to a specific antigen. There are five classes of Ig: IgG, IgM, IgE, IgA, and IgD. IgA and IgG are of particular interest during pregnancy. IgA normally protects body surfaces. Its primary benefit in pregnancy is that it is secreted in breast milk and serves to protect the newborn from GI infections through passive immunity (Rote, 2010). IgG is also present in breast milk; however, its primary function occurs due to its smaller size and ability to cross the placenta. IgG provides passive immunity to the fetus from infections for which the mother has antibodies (Rote, 2010).

There are potential problems for the newborn related to IgG crossing the placenta. Women with Graves's disease have thyroid-stimulating IgG that may cross the placenta and cause hyperthyroidism in about 1% of newborns of women with this disorder (Cunningham et al., 2010, p. 1129). Similarly, women with myasthenia gravis have antibodies against acetylcholine receptors that may cross the placenta and cause transient treatable muscular weakness in the newborn that will last about 2–6 weeks (Cunningham et al., 2010, p. 1173).

A more frequently encountered disorder related to the placental transfer of IgG is rhesus (Rh) incompatibility. This example of isoimmunization has the potential for causing severe hemolytic disease in the fetus. In order to develop IgG antibodies against Rh-positive RBCs, the maternal system must be exposed to the antigen. This means that Rh-positive RBCs must have entered the mother's system, either from an earlier pregnancy or from transfusion. Once the IgG to Rh antigen is established, it can cross the placenta to the fetus, recognize fetal Rh-positive RBCs as foreign, mount an attack, and destroy the fetal RBCs. The formation of this antibody occurs only among women with an Rh-negative blood type. The resulting IgG that passes to the fetus is harmful only to the fetus who has inherited Rh-positive RBCs from the father. The Rh antigen that is most associated with Rh incompatibility and fetal hemolytic disease is Du (Blackburn, 2013; Cunningham et al., 2010). For this reason, passive immunization has been developed that prevents humoral production of antibodies in women who receive Rh-positive RBCs from the fetus.

Other RBC antigen incompatibilities exist including, but not limited to, anti-c, anti-Kell, Kidd, and Duffy. For this reason, RBC antibody titers are drawn from pregnant women during the first prenatal visit.

ABO incompatibility can also cause newborn hemolytic disease. However, this form of isoimmunization causes a very mild hemolysis and jaundice due to the increased bilirubin release when the RBC is destroyed. Unlike Rh isoimmunization, this incompatibility does not worsen with each pregnancy. The reason ABO incompatibility is less severe is that most of the anti-A and anti-B antibodies from women with O-type blood are IgM type and are too large to cross the placenta (Blackburn, 2013; Cunningham et al., 2010). If a woman has an O-negative blood type and her fetus is A positive, the Rh and ABO incompatibility can both occur. However, the mother's natural anti-A antibody will recognize and destroy fetal RBCs that may enter her system before these cells can cause an antibody response against the Rh positive factor (Blackburn, 2013).

Neurological and sensory changes

Pregnant women experience changes in their ability to concentrate and to remember. These changes have been attributed to pregnancy hormones (Stables & Rankin, 2010). Sleep patterns are also altered. During the first trimester, women tend to sleep longer at night and nap during the day if their schedules allow. This is a response to fatigue brought on by increased metabolism and progesterone effects. Progesterone has sedative effects and estrogen has stimulant effects (Blackburn, 2013). As the pregnancy advances and these placental hormones increase, sleep patterns are altered. Most pregnant women report difficulty falling asleep, staying asleep, and poor quality of sleep beginning around the twelfth week of gestation (Cunningham et al., 2010). Studies have shown that the hormones of pregnancy change both rapid eye movement (REM) and nonrapid eye movement (NREM) sleep. Specifically, progesterone seems to enhance NREM, while estrogen and cortisol decrease REM sleep (Blackburn, 2013).

Sleep during the second trimester improves. An active fetus, increased minor discomforts of pregnancy, a growing uterus that prohibits position change, and decreased REM sleep combine to make most pregnant women complain of sleep disturbances during the last weeks of pregnancy (Cunningham et al., 2010).

Eye changes during pregnancy include corneal edema, decreased corneal sensitivity, decreased intraocular pressure, and transient loss in accommodation (Blackburn, 2013). Corneal edema and decreased sensitivity has been attributed to fluid retention. Decreased intraocular pressure is due to increased aqueous outflow and the effects of progesterone, relaxin, and hCG (Blackburn, 2013). Pregnancy is not a good time for a woman to be measured for new contact lenses or eyeglasses. The changes in the eyes will resolve after birth.

Estrogen-induced swollen membranes will affect the sense of smell, and in some women, the sense of hearing (Stables & Rankin, 2010). The diminished sense of smell will affect taste and can lead to food aversions.

Musculoskeletal adaptations

The enlarging uterus changes the maternal center of gravity. The spine adjusts by increasing lordosis. At the same time, there is increased mobility of the sacroiliac, sacrococcygeal, and pubic joints related to changes in the cartilage brought about by relaxin and progesterone (Blackburn, 2013). Changes in the low back and pelvis can cause low-back discomfort, aching, numbness, and tingling in the legs as the pregnancy progresses. Changes in the cervical spine, along with slumping of the shoulders and upper back due to heavier breasts, can stretch the ulnar and median nerves, causing tingling discomfort in the arms and hands.

The growing fetus needs calcium for the formation and calcification of the skeleton and teeth. Calcium demands are the greatest in the third trimester of pregnancy. Much of the calcium needed is drawn from the maternal skeleton. At the same time, the absorption of calcium from the maternal intestine doubles and urinary excretion is decreased. Changes in calcium concentration require changes in parathyroid hormone, magnesium, phosphate, vitamin D, and calcitonin physiology. Lowered calcium or magnesium levels have a negative-feedback effect that increases calcitonin and parathyroid hormone release. Parathyroid hormone acts on bone resorption, intestinal absorption, and kidney reabsorption of calcium and phosphate (Cunningham et al., 2010). Parathyroid hormone plasma levels increase steadily as the fetus draws more calcium for bone growth. At the same time, increased maternal glomerulofiltration rate (GFR) and increased plasma volume cause a lower serum calcium level. In addition, estrogen will block the action of parathyroid hormone. All these factors combine to cause "physiological hyperparathyroidism" in pregnancy (Cunningham et al., 2010, p. 128).

Vitamin D is either ingested or obtained via synthesis in sun-exposed skin. During pregnancy, the kidney, decidua, and placenta change vitamin D to 1,25-dihdroxyvitamin D_3. This compound enhances calcium resorption and intestinal absorption of calcium during pregnancy (Cunningham et al., 2010).

Calcium serum levels begin to fall after fertilization regardless of maternal diet (Stables & Rankin, 2010). Calcium levels may be compromised by increased ingestion of phosphate. Too much phosphate will limit calcium absorption in the intestine and increase calcium urinary excretion. Foods high in phosphorus include chips and colas; these foods are commonly consumed as part of American diets.

Endocrine changes

Like other systems, the endocrine glands undergo changes during pregnancy that support fetal growth and pregnancy maintenance. This section is limited to an outline of the changes that occur in the pituitary, thyroid and adrenal glands, and hormones. The changes in the parathyroid and the endocrine pancreas have been described earlier in this chapter. The changes in the gonads are explained in Chapter 2.

Anatomical changes

Physiological pituitary growth occurs in normal pregnancies. In fact, the pituitary will grow to 135% of its original size (Nader, 2009b). Very rarely, the enlargement will be big enough to increase intracranial pressure or put pressure on the optic chiasm. This may cause headaches or vision changes that will resolve after birth.

The thyroid gland will also increase in size during pregnancy as a result of increased vascularity and some hyperplasia of normal gland cells. Significant enlargement, however, may be a sign of iodine deficiency or other thyroid abnormalities (Nader, 2009b). The adrenal glands do not change in size.

Pituitary function changes

The pituitary has two lobes, anterior and posterior, and each lobe secretes hormones in response to the secretion of releasing hormones from the hypothalamus. Table 3.7 lists the hormones secreted by the anterior and posterior lobes of the pituitary.

In pregnancy, the most dramatic change in anterior pituitary function is that it secretes 10 times more prolactin (Nader, 2009b). The lactotrophs (cells that secrete

Table 3.7 Pituitary Hormones

Anterior pituitary	Target organs
Growth hormone	Bone, muscle
Adrenocorticotropic hormone (ACTH)	Adrenal cortex
Thyroid-stimulating hormone (TSH)	Thyroid gland
Gonadotropic hormones (FSH, LH, and ICSH)	Testis, ovary
Melanocyte-stimulating Hormone (MSH)	Skin
Prolactin	Mammary glands
Posterior pituitary	**Target organs**
Antidiuretic hormone (ADH)	Kidney tubules
Oxytocin (OT)	Uterine smooth muscle, mammary glands

Adapted from: Brashers, V., & Jones, R. (2010). Mechanisms of hormonal regulation. In K. McCance & S. Huether (Eds.), *Pathophysiology: The biologic basis for disease in adults and children* (6th ed., pp. 696–725). St. Louis, MO: Mosby/Elsevier.

prolactin) are stimulated by estrogen and account for most of the cellular growth of the pituitary. Prolactin prepares the breasts for breastfeeding and will maintain breast milk production for the duration of the lactation period.

Pituitary growth hormone secretion decreases beginning in the second trimester when placental growth hormone is produced (Nader, 2009b). Thyroid-stimulating hormone (TSH) secretion decreases slightly in the first 12 weeks under the influence of hCG. TSH levels then become static as the pregnancy progresses. Adrenocorticotropic hormone (ACTH) secretion increases, reaching its highest level during labor (Blackburn, 2013).

The posterior pituitary function also changes. The threshold for the release of antidiuretic hormone (ADH) is reset so that the decline in plasma osmolarity can occur. However, the amount of ADH released is not changed (Nader, 2009b). Also, thirst is stimulated by lower levels of osmolarity in pregnant women than in nonpregnant women.

The second posterior pituitary hormone, oxytocin, is increased during pregnancy and spikes during labor to stimulate uterine contractions. Oxytocin does not start labor but is necessary to sustain the contractions needed for birth. Oxytocin continues to be elevated during lactation and is released when a neural impulse is triggered by suckling. This surge of oxytocin causes contractions of the myoepithelial cells surrounding the mammary alveoli and the smooth muscle of the mammary ductal system, resulting in milk ejection (Nader, 2009b).

Oxytocin is also an important facilitator of the bonding process. Oxytocin is an evolutionary substance unique to mammals and has significance other than parturition and breastfeeding. The importance of oxytocin in regard to social recognition, pair bonding, and other social behaviors has been investigated. Oxytocin release appears to promote feelings of security in women, promotes bonding with the newborn, and leads to improved mental health and social outcomes (Uvnäs-Moberg, 1998).

Thyroid function changes

The thyroid gland increases production of thyroid hormones in pregnancy. Increased estrogen causes the liver to produce more thyroxine-binding globulin (TBG) early in pregnancy. As thyroxine (T_4) is bound to TGB, there is a decrease in free T_4 that results in stimulation of the hypothalamus to release thyroxine-releasing hormone and, in response, the anterior pituitary is stimulated to release TSH (Nader, 2009a). This series of events is an example of a negative-feedback con trol loop.

At the same time, the thyroid is being stimulated by hCG, which acts like TSH. By 12 weeks of gestation, hCG has reached serum levels that inhibit pituitary production of TSH (Nader, 2009a). Free serum T_4 peaks at around the same time that hCG peaks (Cunningham et al., 2010). Thyroid clearance of iodine increases threefold. Free and total T_3 increases. All these changes in thyroid function lead to an increase in maternal basal metabolic rate by about 25% during the second half of pregnancy (Stables & Rankin, 2010).

There are significant changes in the thyroid laboratory testing parameters during pregnancy. The laboratory tests that provide the best clinical information for the evaluation of thyroid function in pregnancy are the third-generation TSH and free T_4 levels (Nader, 2009a).

Adrenal function changes

The adrenal cortex, after stimulation by ACTH, releases glucocorticoids (primarily cortisol), mineralocorticoids (primarily aldosterone), and adrenal androgens and estrogens (Brashers & Jones, 2010). Serum ACTH is lower in early pregnancy but begins to increase as pregnancy progresses. Serum cortisol is increased in pregnancy, and much of it is bound by cortisol-binding globulin that is three times higher during pregnancy. This causes the total cortisol levels to rise significantly. Aldosterone levels increase 20-fold during late pregnancy (Nader, 2009b). This increase is necessary because of the antagonistic effects of progesterone including increased sodium excretion (Cunningham et al., 2010). Adrenal testosterone increases in pregnancy because of increased sex hormone-binding globulin produced by the liver (Nader, 2009b).

Corticotropin-releasing hormone (CRH) and ACTH are produced by the placenta and increase significantly during the last weeks of pregnancy. CRH is implicated as a trigger to begin labor (Blackburn, 2013). Both hormones are considered very important to the initiation of labor (Cunningham et al., 2010). In addition, the fetal adrenal gland secretes high levels of cortisol and dehydroepiandrosterone sulfate (DHEA-S). These substances cause an increase in the production of maternal estriol that will enhance uterine muscle gap junctions and facilitate the development of oxytocin receptors within uterine tissue in preparation for rhythmic, uniform contractions.

Summary

Virtually all maternal body systems undergo changes during pregnancy that are necessary for maternal adaptation and fetal growth and development. Understanding the physiology foundational to these changes is imperative for health-care professionals caring for pregnant women and their babies. Differentiating normal changes from potential or real abnormalities and being able to interpret laboratory findings accurately depend on knowledge of these miraculous, complex adaptations.

Case study

Rhonda is a 22-year-old primigravida at 8 weeks of gestation at her initial prenatal visit.

SUBJECTIVE: Rhonda reports that she has been dizzy on standing at three different times in the past week. She says she is eating regularly and has no previous cardiac or neurological concerns.

OBJECTIVE: Vital signs and heart sounds are normal. Rhonda is oriented and has appropriate affect.

ASSESSMENT: Hemodynamic instability of early pregnancy.

PLAN: The health-care provider explains that progesterone, a hormone of pregnancy, has increased in Rhonda's body and it will cause the blood vessels to dilate or widen. This change helps get more blood and nutrients to the baby but lowers blood pressure, and it can slow the return of blood to her brain, leading to dizziness. Rhonda is encouraged to avoid standing for a long time, to get up slowly from sitting or lying down positions, and to avoid hot baths that will dilate the blood vessels further. Reassurance is given that this symptom usually resolves by the end of the first trimester and danger signs are reviewed.

Resources for women and their families

Pregnancy Week by Week: http://www.medicinenet.com/pregnancy/article.htm

Resources for health-care providers

Physiology of Pregnancy: http://www.glowm.com/?p=glowm.cml/section_view&articleid=103

Seasonal Flu Vaccine Safety and Pregnant Women: http://www.cdc.gov/flu/protect/vaccine/qa_vacpregnant.htm

References

Blackburn, S. (2013). *Maternal, fetal, and neonatal physiology: A clinical perspective* (4th ed.). Maryland Heights, MO: Elsevier.

Brashers, V., & Jones, R. (2010). Mechanisms of hormonal regulation. In K. McCance & S. Huether (Eds.), *Pathophysiology: The biologic basis for disease in adults and children* (6th ed., pp. 696–725). St. Louis, MO: Mosby/Elsevier.

Centers for Disease Control and Prevention (2011). Seasonal influenza: Pregnant women and influenza. Last updated October 24, 2011. Retrieved from http://www.cdc.gov/flu/protect/vaccine/pregnant.htm

Cunningham, F., Leveno, K., Bloom, S., Hauth, J., Rouse, D., & Spong, C. (2010). *Williams obstetrics* (23rd ed.). New York: McGraw Hill Medical.

Kelly, T., & Savides, T. (2009). Gastrointestinal disease in pregnancy. In R. Creasy, R. Resnik, & J. Iams (Eds.), *Creasy and Resnik's maternal-fetal medicine: Principles and practice* (6th ed., pp. 1041–1042). St. Louis, MO: Saunders/Elsevier.

Kilpatrick, S. (2009). Anemia and pregnancy. In R. Creasy, R. Resnik, & J. Iams (Eds.), *Creasy and Resnik's maternal-fetal medicine: Principles and practice* (6th ed., pp. 869–872). St. Louis, MO: Saunders/Elsevier.

Kliman, H., Sammar, M., Gimpel, Y., Lynch, S., Milano, K., Pick, E., . . . Gonen, R. (2011). Placental protein 13 and decidual zones of necrosis: An immunologic diversion that may be linked to preeclampsia. *Reproductive Sciences*. Published online before print October 11, 2011. doi:10.1177/1933719111424445.

Lockwood, C., & Silver, R. (2009). Coagulation disorders in pregnancy. In R. Creasy, R. Resnik, & J. Iams (Eds.), *Creasy and Resnik's maternal-fetal medicine: Principles and practice* (6th ed., pp. 828–829). St. Louis, MO: Saunders/Elsevier.

Mohamad, T. N. (2013). Cardiovascular disease and pregnancy. Retrieved from http://emedicine.medscape.com/aricle/162004-overview

Monga, M. (2009). Maternal cardiovascular, respiratory, and renal adaptation to pregnancy. In R. Creasy, R. Resnik, & J. Iams (Eds.), *Creasy and Resnik's maternal-fetal medicine: Principles and practice* (6th ed., pp. 101–107). St. Louis, MO: Saunders/Elsevier.

Moore, T., & Catalano, P. (2009). Diabetes in pregnancy. In R. Creasy, R. Resnik, & J. Iams (Eds.), *Creasy and Resnik's maternal-fetal medicine: Principles and practice* (6th ed., pp. 954–956). St. Louis, MO: Saunders/Elsevier.

Mor, G., & Abrahams, V. (2009). The immunology of pregnancy. In R. Creasy, R. Resnik, & J. Iams (Eds.), *Creasy and Resnik's maternal-fetal medicine: Principles and practice* (6th ed., pp. 87–93). St. Louis, MO: Saunders/Elsevier.

Nader, S. (2009a). Thyroid disease and pregnancy. In R. Creasy, R. Resnik, & J. Iams (Eds.), *Creasy and Resnik's maternal-fetal medicine: Principles and practice* (6th ed., pp. 995–1011). St. Louis, MO: Saunders/Elsevier.

Nader, S. (2009b). Other endocrine disorders of pregnancy. In R. Creasy, R. Resnik, & J. Iams (Eds.), *Creasy and Resnik's maternal-fetal medicine: Principles and practice* (6th ed., pp. 1015–1026). St. Louis, MO: Saunders/Elsevier.

Nicol, N., & Huether, S. (2010). Structure, function and disorders of the skin. In K. McCance & S. Huether (Eds.), *Pathophysiology: The biologic basis for disease in adults and children* (6th ed., pp. 1644–1679). St. Louis, MO: Mosby/Elsevier.

Rapini, R. (2009). The skin and pregnancy. In R. Creasy, R. Resnik, & J. Iams (Eds.), *Creasy and Resnik's maternal-fetal medicine: Principles and practice* (6th ed., pp. 1123–1126). St. Louis, MO: Saunders/Elsevier.

Rote, N. (2010). Adaptive immunity. In K. McCance & S. Huether (Eds.), *Pathophysiology: The biologic basis for disease in adults and children* (6th ed., pp. 217–251). St. Louis, MO: Mosby/Elsevier.

Stables, D., & Rankin, J. (Eds.). (2010). *Physiology in childbearing* (3rd ed.). Edinburgh, UK: Bailliere Tindall/Elsevier.

Uvnäs-Moberg, K. (1998). Oxytocin may mediate the benefits of positive social interaction and emotions. *Psychoneuroendocrinology*, 23(8), 819–835.

Vera, E. (2011). Thrombocytopenia in pregnancy. Medscape reference. Last updated October 5, 2009. Retrieved from http://emedicine.medscape.com/article/272867-overview

Whitty, J., & Dombrowski, M. (2009). Respiratory diseases in pregnancy. In R. Creasy, R. Resnik, & J. Iams (Eds.), *Creasy and Resnik's maternal-fetal medicine: Principles and practice* (6th ed., pp. 927–931). St. Louis, MO: Saunders/Elsevier.

Williamson, C., & Mackillop, L. (2009). Diseases of the liver, biliary system and pancreas. In R. Creasy, R. Resnik, & J. Iams (Eds.). *Creasy and Resnik's maternal-fetal medicine: Principles and practice* (6th ed., pp. 1059–1075). St. Louis: Saunders/Elsevier.

Part II

Preconception and prenatal care

4

Preconception care

Victoria L. Baker

Relevant terms

Chronic disease—diseases of long duration and often characterized by slow progression of the illness

Interconception care—a package of health-care and ancillary services provided to a woman and her family from the time of birth of one child to the conception of the next child

Periodic health evaluation— health-care visit to provide health guidance, screening, and preventive health services

Preconception care—a set of interventions that aim to identify and modify biomedical, behavioral, and social risks to a woman's health or pregnancy outcome through prevention and management, emphasizing those factors that must be acted on before conception or early in pregnancy to have maximal impact

Risk factor—any attribute, characteristic, or exposure of an individual that increases the likelihood of developing a disease or injury (World Health Organization, 2012)

Screening—examination of asymptomatic people to classify them as likely or unlikely to have the disease that is the object of screening

---

Introduction

Preconception care consists of "a set of interventions that aim to identify and modify biomedical, behavioral, and social risks to a woman's health or pregnancy outcome through prevention and management, emphasizing those factors which must be acted on before conception or early in pregnancy to have maximal impact" (Centers for Disease Control and Prevention (CDC),

2006c). The introduction of preconception care occurred much later than prenatal care. The concept of prenatal care was developed at the end of the nineteenth century and expanded during the early decades of the twentieth century (Alexander & Kotelchuck, 2001). The evidence supporting the efficacy of prenatal care was published in the 1970s and its content well defined since 1989 (Hood, Parker, & Atrash, 2007). In contrast, a description of preconception care was first published in 1978 and the idea became more widespread in the 1980s (Freda, Moos, & Curtis, 2006). General recommendations for preconception care were first presented by a national working group convened by the CDC in 2006 (CDC, 2006c). However, clinical guidelines for preconception care have yet to be developed at the national level (CDC, personal communication, 2012). Although preconception care has been widely discussed over the past three decades, the concept has yet to be routinely incorporated into practice because "most providers do not provide preconception care, most consumers do not ask for it, and most insurers to do not pay for it" (Atrash, Jack, & Johnson, 2008).

Challenges to providing preconception care

There are many challenges to the widespread implementation of preconception services. One particular challenge is payment for preconception services. The CDC recommendations for preconception care include coverage of preconception care by third-party payers, particularly for low-income women (CDC, 2006c). There are several policy initiatives that integrate preconception care into the continuum of women's health services for users of Medicaid and Health and Human Services family planning clinic grants (Title X) (Gold & Alrich, 2008), Maternal Child Health Bureau block grants (Title V) (Kent & Streeter, 2008), and private insurance (Rosenbaum, 2008). The Affordable Care Act of 2010 includes recommendations to cover preconception services as part of a routine well-woman visit as a proposed "preventive service" for which third-party payers may not impose copayments (Health Resources and Services Administration (HRSA), n.d.).

Consumer demand also presents a challenge to the widespread implementation of preconception care. Many women of reproductive age do not know about the service or its potential benefits, and many do not engage in behaviors prior to conception that improve pregnancy outcomes (Anderson, Ebrahim, Floyd, & Atrash, 2006). For example, fewer than 40% of women reported receiving preconception counseling from their primary care provider (Frey & Files, 2006). Likewise, studies suggest that many women who are planning a pregnancy do not engage in behaviors known to improve pregnancy outcomes such folic acid supplementation and abstinence from alcohol and tobacco (Chuang et al., 2010; Crozier et al., 2009).

Consumer demand and payment for preconception care continue to be challenges to providing services. Thus, the current recommendation is that preconception care be integrated into routine well-woman primary care visits during the interconception period. For example, preconception care should start during the postpartum period with the goal of helping a woman achieve improved health before she conceives another child.

Benefits of preconception care

The concept of addressing factors that affect pregnancy outcomes before conception has obvious appeal as a preventative strategy since many pathophysiological pathways begin early in pregnancy, sometimes before a woman knows she has conceived. Evidence supports a number of interventions that improve pregnancy outcomes and should be initiated in the preconception period such as folate supplementation, which has been shown to reduce birth defects (Wehby & Murray, 2008). The adoption of behaviors that benefit overall health, such as achieving a healthy weight, may also improve pregnancy outcomes when adopted during the preconception period (Siega-Riz, Siega-Riz, & Laraia, 2006). Preconception control of chronic diseases such as diabetes can also improve pregnancy outcomes. Genetic counseling can provide important information for parents about their risk of having a child with a genetic disorder.

Information on the avoidance of teratogens such as alcohol or medications can prevent such exposures during a pregnancy.

Increased use of preconception care also supports efforts to eliminate health disparities in birth outcomes. For example, low birth weight (LBW) disproportionally affects African American infants. Some factors implicated in the etiology of LBW are amenable to intervention during the preconception period. Supplementation with a multivitamin appears to benefit all women and their babies by reducing LBW rates and thereby reducing health disparities (Burris, Mitchell, & Werler, 2010). Additional evidence supports the use of interventions to reduce LBW by using the intervention during the interconception period (Loomis & Martin, 2000; Lu et al., 2010).

The "Life Course Perspective" (Lu & Halfon, 2003) supports the idea of offering care during the preconception period to improve pregnancy outcome and to reduce racial and ethnic health disparities in pregnancy outcomes. This model conceptualizes health as developing over the course of an individual's life, with early physical and psychosocial experiences, including experiences *in utero*, influencing outcomes later in life. This approach works particularly well in understanding pregnancy outcomes, which are often rooted in exposures and experiences from long before the pregnancy occurs. The life course perspective highlights the need for preconception care, intervening to improve pregnancy outcomes as early as possible in the life course of both mother and child.

Evidence supporting preconception care

Studies focusing on a number of aspects of preconception care have demonstrated effectiveness, such as folic acid supplementation, elimination of alcohol use, vaccination, diabetes management, treatment of sexually transmitted infections, management of hypthroidism, management of maternal phenylketonuria, weight control, tobacco cessation, and, when necessary, selection of medications that can be safely used during pregnancy (CDC, 2006c). Several studies have shown the effects of preconception visits on changing health behaviors, such as increased physical activity, weight loss, folate supplementation (Cena et al., 2008; Scholl, 2008), and improved diet (Cena et al., 2008). Periconception multivitamin use may reduce preterm births and small-for-gestational-age infants (Catov, Bodnar, Ness, Markovic, & Roberts, 2007). Women who have preconception care visits are more likely to initiate prenatal care early (Liu, Liu, Ye, & Li, 2006).

Content of preconception care

The preconception visit is basically a periodic health evaluation with added components for any woman of reproductive age. These components of care can be grouped into three areas: risk assessment and screening, health promotion and counseling, and interventions (Public Health Service Expert Panel on the Content of Prenatal Care, 1989). National guidelines for the clinical content of preconception care have not yet been published, although expert groups have published recommendations (Fig. 4.1).

Risk assessment and screening

The components of risk assessment during preconception care include a health history, physical examination, and laboratory data. Preconception screening checklists are available from various organizations such as the American College of Obstetricians and the March of Dimes to aid health-care providers in performing a complete risk evaluation and appropriate counseling. Links to these resources are found in the Resources for Women and Their Families section of this chapter. Topic areas to be covered include diet and exercise, lifestyle, substance use, medications, family and personal medical and genetic history, home environment, and personal reproductive health history.

History

A complete medical, family, obstetrical, and social history should be obtained. The areas of nutrition, occupation, environment, and lifestyle habits are of particular impor-

tance during the preconception visit. Health-care providers may find it helpful to use a template for the health history that is specific to the preconception period such as the templates provided by the March of Dimes or the Wisconsin Perinatal Association. Links to these organizations are provided in the Resources for Women and Their Families section of this chapter.

Physical examination

Physical examination should follow the health-care provider's protocol for a periodic health evaluation. It should include measurement of height and weight to determine the body mass index (BMI).

Laboratory examination

Laboratory testing is similar to the testing performed during pregnancy (see Chapter 5) with a focus on identifying conditions that can be treated before pregnancy. Testing for immunity to rubella, varicella, and hepatitis B is performed so that women who are not immune to these diseases can be vaccinated before becoming pregnant. Testing for syphilis, gonorrhea, and chlamydia are performed so that the diseases can be treated and eradicated before pregnancy. Pap smear screening is recommended since treatment for abnormal cytology is ideally performed before pregnancy. Additional screening tests are performed as indicated based on risk factors for the condition.

Substance use and abuse

Screening for substance use and abuse in the preconception period is essential. Asking questions about the use and abuse of tobacco, alcohol, and illicit substances provides the opportunity to counsel women and offer interventions to promote cessation before pregnancy. Thus, all women should be asked frankly about the use of tobacco and illicit substances. However, laboratory screening for illicit drug use is not recommended unless indicated (Lanier & Ko, 2008). Women should also be screened for alcohol use by using a validated alcohol screening tool (United States Preventive Services Task Force (USPSTF), 2004). Resources for screening for substance abuse are provided in the Resources for Health-Care Providers section of this chapter and in Chapters 5 and 13.

Mental health issues

The preconception period offers an opportunity for early detection of psychological disorders and in-depth discussion of their management during pregnancy. The USPSTF recommends screening all adults for depression using a validated tool (e.g., two-question screen for depression) where appropriate mental health services are

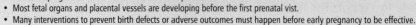

COLORADO
CLINICAL GUIDELINES
COLLABORATIVE

Guideline for Preconception and Interconception Care
Why should women, menarche to menopause, have preconception screening?
• Half of all preganacies in the United States are unplanned.
• Most fetal organs and placental vessels are developing before the first prenatal vist.
• Many interventions to prevent birth defects or adverse outcomes must happen before early pregnancy to be effective.

Colorado Department
of Public Health
and Envionment

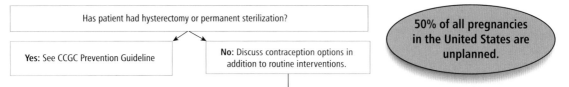

Has patient had hysterectomy or permanent sterilization?

50% of all pregnancies in the United States are unplanned.

Yes: See CCGC Prevention Guideline

No: Discuss contraception options in addition to routine interventions.

Factors	Recommendations
Folic Acid	All women should take a multi-vitamin with **0.4 mg (400 mcg) of folic acid daily**. This can reduce severe anomalies by 46%. Preconception intake of folic acid is crucial because neural tube development is essentially complete by 4 weeks after conception (6 weeks from last menstrual period). Women with a seizure disorder or history of neural tube defects should take 4.0 mg/day.
Body Weight* **(Ideal = 18.5–24.9)**	**Underweight** (BMI = 18.4 and below) assess for eating, malabsorption and/or endocrine disorder. Counsel patients that are at risk for an IUGR infant. **Overweight** (BMI = 25.0–29.9) offer specific strategies to decrease caloric intake and increase physical activity. **Overweight** (BMI = 25.0–29.9) **and one additional risk factor**, test for glucose intolerance with a FBS or a 2 Hour OGTT with a 75 gram glucose load. (**Additional risk factors:** physical inactivity, family history of DM, HTN, CVD, dyslipidemia, history of gestational diabetes or a previous 9 lb. baby, polycystic ovary syndromen, insulin resistance, IGT or high risk ethnicity [African American, Native American, Latina, Asian American or Pacific Islander]). **Obesity** (BMI = 30.0 and above) increases the risk for hypertension, gestational diabetes, C-section and incision complications.
Smoking*	**ASK:** Do you currently smoke or use any form of tobacco? **ADVISE:** for the health of the pregnancy. **REFER:** to Quitline (1–800–784–8669) or access other community-based resources. Infant mortality could be reduced by 10% if smoking were eliminated. Associated with increased risk of miscarriage, premature rupture of membranes, preterm delivery, abruption, intra-uterine fetal demise, low birth weight, and SIDS. Smoking accounts for the highest proportion of preventable problems in pregnant women.
Alcohol & Drugs*	**ASK:** When was the last time you had more than 3 drinks in one day? (positive = in the past 3 months) How many drinks do you have per week? (positive = more than 7) Have you used drugs other than those required for medical reasons (illicit or prescription drug misuse) in the past year? Do a brief intervention to address hazardous or harmful use of alcohol or drugs; refer for more intensive treatment, if indicated. Discuss contraception options. Pregnancy should be delayed until individuals are alcohol and drug free. Alcohol is a teratogen. **COUNSEL:** *No amount of alcohol is considered safe during pregnancy.*
Chlamydia	Screen sexually active women <25 years (CDC recommends at least annually). High risk women[‡] of ANY age should be screened annually.
STIs & Other Infectious Diseases	Women at risk[‡] for gonorrhea, HIV, TB, syphilis and Hepatitis B should be screened and treated.
Immunizations*	Women should be up to date on all immunizations. Check and document immunization status for MMR, varicella, TdaP, HPV and Hepatitis B.
Psychosocial Risks*	**ASK:** Over the past 2 weeks, have you felt down, depressed or hopeless? Over the past 2 weeks have you felt little interst or pleasure in doing things? If yes, use validated screening tool such as Edinburgh Postpartum Depression scale or PHQ-9. Treat or refet to specialist if indicated. Assess for intimate partner violence. **ASK:** Do you feel safe? If no, or ambivalent response, refer to the Colorado Coalition Against Domestic Violence (www.ncadv.org), a safe house and/or law enforcement.
Reproductive History	History of preterm delivery, stillbirth, recurrent pregnancy loss or uterine anomaly should be evaluated for modifiable risk factors. Women with a prior C-section should be counseled wait at least 15 months before next conception. Postpartum women with a history of gestational diabetes should be screened for diabetes using a 2 hour OGTT with a 75 gram glucose load. After the postpartum period, perform a FBS every 1 to 3 years.
Family & Genetic History	Assess for genetic disorders, congenital malformations, mental retardation, and ethnicity of woman and partner. Refer to March of Dimes checklist.
Environmental/ Occupational Exposures	Consider household, environmental and occupational exposures. Refer women with soil and/or water hazard concerns to the local health department for soil and water testing. Refer women with household or workplace exposure concerns to an occupational medicine specialist for modification of exposures.
Medical, Psychiatric History & Medications	See back page for specific conditions, appropriate testing, counseling and treatment.

*See CCGC guidelines for: *Adult Cardiovascular Disease and Stroke Prevention; Adult Diabetes Care; Adult Obesity; Alcohol and Substance Use Screening, Brief Intervention, Referral to Treatment; Depression Disorder in Adults; Gestational Diabetes; Immunizations; Preventive Health Recommendations; and Tobacco Cessation and Secondhand Smoke Exposure.*
[‡]See United States Preventive Services Task Force (USPSTF) definitions for high risk.

Assess for specific health conditions and contraception choices (review side two of this document).

This guideline is adapted from the AJOG Supplement, December 2008 and CDC Proceedings of the Preconception Headlth and Health Care Clinical, Public Health and Consumer Workgroup Meetings, June 2006, and USPSTF Recommendations 2009. The guideline is designed to assist the clinician in preconception and interconception care. It is not intended to replace a clinician's judgement or establish a protocol for all patients. For references and additional copies of the guideline go to www.coloradoguidelines.org or call 720–297–1681. Supported by Grant No. B04MC1 1264 from the Maternal and Child Health Bureau (Title V, Social Security Act). Health Resources & Services Administration, Department of Health and Human Services.
Final 12/18/09

Figure 4.1. Colorado clinical guidelines for preconception and interconception care.

Condition	Counsel	Tests	Contraindicated Medications[§]	Contraception[†]
Asthma*	Women with poor control of their asthma should use contraception until it is well controlled.	See CCGC Asthma Guideline.	No restrictions.	**Safe:** all methods.
Cardiovascular Disease*	Pregnancy is a stressor on the cardiovascular system. Discuss potential life-threatening risks especially with pulmonary hypertension. Contraception should be strongly recommended when pregnancy is contraindicated.	Consult with a Cardiac Specialist.	Find an alternate medication for ACE inhibitors and Coumadin beyond 6 weeks gestation.	**Safe:** Copper IUD, sterilization, LNG IUD, ETG implant, DMPA, and POPs. **Avoid:** estrongen containing methods.
Depression*	Screening prior to pregnancy allows for treatment and control of symptoms that may help prevent negative pregnancy and family outcomes.	Use PHQ-9 or other validated test to monitor.	Paroxetine.	**Safe:** all methods.
Diabetes*	Three-fold increase risk of birth defects, which may be reduced with good glycemic control prior to conception. Women with poor glycemic control should use effective birth control.	Patients should demonstrate goog control of blood sugars with HgbA1c <6.5. Use effective contraception. See CCGC Diabetes Guideline.	ACF Inhibitors, Statins.	**Safe:** all mehods (including those with estrogen) are safe for women who are <35 years, non-smokers and no hypertension or vascular disease. **Avoid:** estrogen methods for all other women.
HIV	HIV may be life-threatening to the infant if transmitted. Antiretroviral can reduce the risk of transmission, but the risk is still about 2%.	Refer to specialist.	Efavirenz (Sustiva®).	**Safe:** all mehods in HIV-infected women who do not have AIDS. Antiretroviral therapy may interfere with hormonal methods. Concomitant use of condoms is strongly recommended.
Hypertension*	Increased maternal and fetal risk during pregnancy, especially pre-eclampsia. Discuss importance of finding alternative to ACE inhibitor prior to pregnancy.	Women with HTN of several years' should be assessed for ventricular hypertrophy, retinopathy and renal disease. Consult with a Cardiac Specialist.	ACE Inhibitors.	**Safe:** all mehods (including those with estrogen) for women who are <35 years, non-smokers and have controlled hypertension (by way of meds or lifestyle changes). **Avoid:** estrogen methods for all other women.
Obesity*	Use effective contraception until ideal body weight (BMI=18.5–24.9) is achieved. Offer specific strategies to decrease caloric intake and increase physical activity. For bariatric surgery, avoid pregnancy until weight stabilization and wait 1–2 years after surgery before conceiving.	Screen for diabetes with either a FBS or a 2 hour OGTT with a 75 grarn glucose load. Refer to page 1 for risk factors.	Weight loss medications should not be used during pregnancy.	**Safe:** all methods.
Renal Disease	Counsel to achieve optimal control of condition prior to conception. Discuss potential life-threatening risks during pregnancy. Contraception should be strongly recommended to those who do not desire pregnancy.	Consult with Renal Specialist.	Find alternative to ACE Inhibitors if at risk of pregnancy.	**Safe:** Copper IUD and LNG IUD, ETG implant, DMPA, sterilization.
Seizure Disorder	Counsel on potential effects of seizures and seizure medications on pregnancy outcomes. Patients should take 4 mg of folic acid per day for at least 1mouth prior to conception.	Whenever possbile, monotherapy in the lowest therapeutic dose should be prescribed.	Valproic Acid (Depakote®).	**Safe:** all methods. Certain anticonvulsants decrease levels of steroid hormones and may decrease contraceptive efficacy.
SLE & Rheumatoid Arthritis	Disease should be in good control prior to pregnancy.	Evaluate for renal function and end-organ disease.	Cyclophosphamide.	**Safe:** Progestin only methods and IUDs.
Thyroid Disease	Proper dosage of thyroid medications prior to conception for normal fetal development. Iodine intake 150 mcg per day.	TSH should be <3.0 prior to pregnancy. Free T4 should be normal.	Redioactive iodine.	**Safe:** all methods.

Other Common Health Conditions	Counsel	Contraception[†]
Uterline Fibroids, Nulligravity, Tension Headaches, History of Ectopic Pregnancy, Fibrocystic Breast or Family History of Breast Cancer, Breastfeeding, and Healthy Women Age >35 years	Reassure patient that these conditions do not generally effect pregnancy. History of ectopic pregnancy: advise to seek care immediately upon conception.	**Safe:** all methods. Progestin only methods and IUDs may be used immediately psst-partum and in breastfeeding women.

*See CCGC guideline
[†]Contraception column based on ACOG Practice Bulletin No 73, *Use of Hormonal Contraception in Women with Coexisting Medical Conditions, June 2006, and The World Healt organization, Medical Eligibility Criteria for Contraceptive Use,* 2008 update.
[§]See Paysicians' Desk Reference® (PDR) for comprehensive medications list.

Other Medical Conditions Where Special Counseling Is Recommended
Bipolar Disorder, Migraine Headaches, Phenylketonuria, Schizophrenia.
Contraception key

Barrier Methods: Latex condoms, diaphragm with spermicide, and sponge have a high failure rate with typical use (20–30 pregnancies per 100 women in one year): encourage more effective methods. Condoms are the only contraceptive method that also prevent STIs. When used correctly and consistently, they reduce the risk of infection by 99%. **COC:** Combined Oral Contraceptives *(contains estrogen and progestin)*. **DMPA:** Depot Medroxyprogesterone Acetate *(progestin only)*. **ETG Implant:** Etonogestrel Implant *(progestin only)*.	**LNG IUD:** Levonorgestrel intrauterine device *(progestin only)*. **Patch:** Combined contraceptive patch *(contains estrogen and progestin)*. **POP:** Progestin only pills *(sometimes referred to as the "mimi-pill")*. **Progestin-Only Emergency Contraception:** May be safely used in any woman of reproductive age; there is no medical condition that predudes its use. **Ring:** Combined vaginal ring *(contains estrogen and progestin)*.

This guideline is adapted from the AJOG Supplement, December 2008 and CDC Proceedings of the Preconception Heath and Health Care Clinical, Public Health and Consumer Workgroup Meeting, June 2006. The guideline is designed to assist the clinician in preconception and interconception care. It is not intended to replace a clinician's judgment or establish a protocol for all patients. For references and adcitional copies of the guideline go to www.coloradoguidelines.org or call 720–297–1681. Supported by Grant NO.B04MC11264 from the Maternal and Child Health Bureau (Title V, Social Securty Act), Health Resources & Services Administration, Department of Health and Human Services.

Final 12/18/09

Figure 4.1. *(Continued)*

available (O'Connor, Whitlock, Beil, & Gaynes, 2009). Additional disorders, such as obsessive–compulsive disorder, post-traumatic stress disorder, anxiety disorders, or bipolar disorder, particularly in the presence of a family history of any of these conditions, may be detected during this visit (Frieder, Dunlop, Culpepper, & Bernstein, 2008). Women should also be screened for intimate partner violence and major psychosocial stressors (Lu, 2007).

Genetics

Preconception is an ideal time to screen for genetic conditions. Couples at risk for having an offspring with a genetic condition have the opportunity to receive genetic counseling and carefully consider whether they wish to plan a pregnancy or consider alternatives such as adoption, surrogacy, or donor sperm or eggs. Preconception counseling also provides couples the opportunity to consider what types of genetic testing, if any, they will perform during the pregnancy (Solomon, Jack, & Feero, 2008).

A genetic screening history in the preconception period should mirror genetic screening in prenatal care. A three-generation medical and ethnic family history should be obtained from both the woman and the person who will be the biological father of the child. These data can identify areas of risk for any potential offspring and indicate the need for referral for genetic testing. Couples with a family history of developmental delay, congenital anomalies, or other known or suspected genetic conditions should be referred for genetic counseling. An obstetrical history of two or more miscarriages prompts testing for potentially contributory genetic conditions such as chromosomal abnormalities or hereditary thrombophilia (Solomon et al., 2008). Women can be offered serum screening for cystic fibrosis or ethnicity-related genetic conditions (see Chapter 9), enabling them to make reproductive decisions prior to pregnancy.

Medications

Regularly used prescription and over-the-counter (OTC) medications and supplements should be reviewed. Teratogenic medications should be discontinued in the preconception period when possible. The risks and benefits to the woman and the potential pregnancy and fetus should be balanced when making these decisions. Any medication not clearly needed should be discontinued (Cragan et al., 2006).

Environmental and occupational exposures

Environmental exposures are not always obvious; however, they can affect conception and the subsequent pregnancy (see Chapter 15). History questions should address potential exposures in a person's residence, workplace, and community, including type of work, diet, and use of household agents (McDiarmid, Gardiner, & Jack, 2008; McDiarmid & Gehle, 2006). Some toxins of concern in pregnancy can be investigated when history suggests possible environmental exposures (see Fig. 4.2). Women who use well water should have the water tested for safety. If there is concern about exposure to a potential toxic waste site, the Environmental Protection Agency lists the location of known toxic waste sites on their Web site (U.S. Environmental Protection Agency, n.d.). A history of previous lead exposure should prompt more specific questions related to lead exposure and possibly to testing blood lead levels (McDiarmid et al., 2008). Substantial consumption of high-mercury fish or other exposure to mercury might prompt a mercury blood level examination (Agency for Toxic Substances and Disease Registry (ATSDR), n.d. a). Exposures to chemicals should be investigated individually. The ATSDR provides an updated, online database (ATSDR, n.d. b). The database can be searched by agent, providing the clinician with current information including data on reproductive effects. Occupational health specialists might be consulted for toxins related to specific jobs or activities.

Infections

Some infections can impact pregnancy outcomes by directly affecting the fetus or because they are more dangerous to women during pregnancy. A number of infections are subclinical and screening allows detection and treatment before pregnancy. For example, treatment of syphilis and malaria preconceptionally can reduce stillbirths (Bhutta et al., 2011). Health-care providers should discuss with women and their partners what risks they have for these infections and the recommendations for screening (see Table 4.1). In cases where screening is recommended during pregnancy but not during routine well-women care, an argument can be made to test in the preconception period, such as in the case of screening for human immunodeficiency virus (HIV). Knowledge of HIV status may change a couple's reproductive plans or contraceptive choices. Or, if the couple decides to attempt a pregnancy, the risk of transmission to the fetus can be reduced by detection and treatment in the preconception period.

Certain infections may be prevented with vaccination; therefore, immunity screening and vaccination are appropriate for varicella, rubella, hepatitis B, and human papillomavirus. Depending on costs and client history, vaccination might be ordered without first screening for immunity.

Other infections are of particular concern during pregnancy but do not lend themselves to preconception

Preconception Occupational/Environmental History Check List

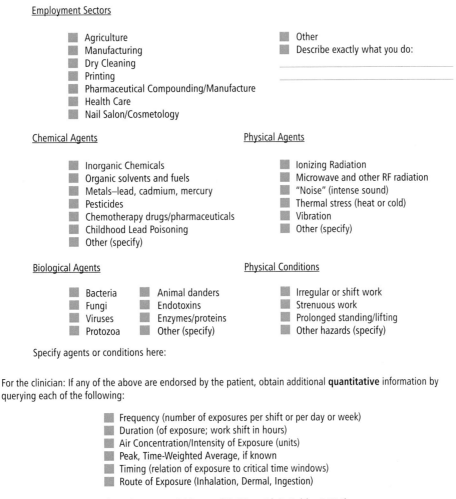

For the patient: Indicate by checking any of the boxes below, the sector in which you work and if you come in contact with any of the listed agents.

Employment Sectors

- Agriculture
- Manufacturing
- Dry Cleaning
- Printing
- Pharmaceutical Compounding/Manufacture
- Health Care
- Nail Salon/Cosmetology

- Other
- Describe exactly what you do:

_____

_____

Chemical Agents

- Inorganic Chemicals
- Organic solvents and fuels
- Metals–lead, cadmium, mercury
- Pesticides
- Chemotherapy drugs/pharmaceuticals
- Childhood Lead Poisoning
- Other (specify)

Physical Agents

- Ionizing Radiation
- Microwave and other RF radiation
- "Noise" (intense sound)
- Thermal stress (heat or cold)
- Vibration
- Other (specify)

Biological Agents

- Bacteria
- Fungi
- Viruses
- Protozoa

- Animal danders
- Endotoxins
- Enzymes/proteins
- Other (specify)

Physical Conditions

- Irregular or shift work
- Strenuous work
- Prolonged standing/lifting
- Other hazards (specify)

Specify agents or conditions here:

For the clinician: If any of the above are endorsed by the patient, obtain additional **quantitative** information by querying each of the following:

- Frequency (number of exposures per shift or per day or week)
- Duration (of exposure; work shift in hours)
- Air Concentration/Intensity of Exposure (units)
- Peak, Time-Weighted Average, if known
- Timing (relation of exposure to critical time windows)
- Route of Exposure (Inhalation, Dermal, Ingestion)

Figure 4.2.   Preconception occupational/environmental history (McDiarmid & Gehle, 2006).

detection and treatment. Evidence does not support preconception treatment of the following infections, perhaps because of reinfection: group B strep, asymptomatic bacteriuria, and parvovirus.

Periodontal disease has been linked to preterm birth. While evidence is lacking on the effect of preconception treatment of periodontal infections on subsequent pregnancies, such treatment is advocated as it influences the overall health of the woman (Boggess & Edelstein, 2006). Some infections present danger to a pregnancy such as cytomegalovirus and toxoplasmosis, but there is no vaccine or treatment. Those women not immune to these infections should be instructed on avoidance measures.

Preconception counseling

The purpose of preconception care counseling is to improve health behaviors and health status to optimize

perinatal outcomes. Adequate counseling covers a wide range of topics and takes time to perform. Written material summarizing the essential components of the information should be provided so that the material can be reviewed later. The woman's or couple's current healthcare practices should be explored and recommendations should be within the context of their cultural health beliefs and practices. Listening is as important as speaking when counseling on healthy behaviors (Rollnick, Miller, & Butler, 2008).

Diet

A healthy diet provides multiple health benefits when preparing for pregnancy. Eating is an activity wrapped in cultural beliefs and practices, and dietary counseling must take into account the particular beliefs and practices of the individual, as well as the influence of their

Table 4.1 United States Preventive Services Task Force (USPSTF) Recommendations for Screening for Selected Infections of Particular Concern in Pregnancy

Infection	Recommendations with grades* for screening	Risk factors
Chlamydia	Pregnancy (A) Adult women and 24 or younger (A) Women, 25 or older, with risk factors (A)	History of chlamydial or other sexually transmitted infection New or multiple sexual partners Inconsistent condom use Exchanging sex for money or drugs
Gonnorhea	Pregnancy (B) Adult women with risk factor(s) (B) Adult women without risk factors (D)	History of chlamydial or other sexually transmitted infection New or multiple sexual partners Inconsistent condom use Exchanging sex for money or drugs
Hepatitis B	Pregnancy (A) Adults (D)	NA
Hepatitis C	Adults (D) Adults with risk factors (I)	Current or past intravenous drug use Transfusion before 1990 Dialysis Being a child of an HIV-infected mother
Herpes simplex virus (HSV)	Pregnant women (D) Adults (D) Adolescents (D)	NA
Human immunodeficiency virus (HIV)	Pregnant women (A) Adolescents or adults with risk factors (A) Adolescents or adults without risk factors (C)	Men who have had sex with men after 1975 Men and women having unprotected sex with multiple partners Past or present injection drug users Men and women who exchange sex for money or drugs or have sex partners who do Individuals whose past or present sex partners were HIV infected, bisexual, or injection drug users Persons being treated for sexually transmitted diseases (STDs) History of blood transfusion between 1978 and 1985 Persons who request an HIV test
Syphilis	Women with risk factors (A) Women without risk factors (D)	Men who have sex with men and engage in high-risk sexual behavior Commercial sex workers Persons who exchange sex for drugs
Tuberculosis	Adults with risk factors recommended by CDC (2011b) (no current USPSTF recommendation)	Contacts of persons with active TB disease or HIV Immigrant from endemic country (most countries in Latin America and the Caribbean, Africa, Asia, Eastern Europe, and Russia) Live where active TB disease is more common such as a homeless shelter, migrant farm camp, prison or jail, or some nursing homes Inject illegal drugs

*Grades for recommendations used by the USPSTF:
A, high certainty of benefit without harm from this test.
B, high certainty of benefit of this test; moderate certainty test is not harmful.
C, no recommendation.
D, recommendation against this test.
I, insufficient evidence to recommend for or against this test.
USPSTF recommendations available at http://www.uspreventiveservicestaskforce.org.

family and community. The preconception period provides an opportunity for women to consider the value of healthy behaviors.

Some evidence suggests that anovulatory infertility may respond to dietary changes (Chavarro, Rich-Edwards, Rosner, & Willett, 2007). The recommended dietary changes are very similar to healthy adult eating, including higher intake of low glycemic carbohydrates such as whole grain products, five to seven daily portions of fruits and vegetables, and the consumption of lean proteins. Some women may ask how to improve their chances of conceiving either a girl or a boy. Evidence suggests that diet does not influence gender outcome (Cramer & Lumey, 2010).

Caffeine intake of >200 mg daily in early pregnancy is linked with an increase in the miscarriage rate, with a fivefold increase when the caffeine comes from sources other than coffee. More than 250 mg of caffeine daily also reduces female fertility (Practice Committee of the American Society for Reproductive Medicine in collaboration with the Society for Reproductive Endocrinology and Infertility, 2008). Thus, couples should be advised to minimize or eliminate their caffeine intake.

Supplementation

Folic acid supplementation may be the best known of interventions specific to the preconception visit. The benefits of supplementation in reducing neural tube defects (NTDs) have been well documented for many years (Scholl, 2008). This effective intervention is fairly inexpensive and simple to implement. However, only about 40% of reproductive age women in the United States take folic acid supplements (Carter, Lindsey, Petrini, & Prue, 2004). Many women are not aware of the importance of folic acid supplements in preventing birth defects (Kannan, Menotti, Scherer, Dickinson, & Larson, 2007). Women with no health risks for NTD should be advised to take 0.4–1.0 mg folic acid daily for at least 2–3 months prior to conception and throughout pregnancy and postpartum (CDC, 2012). This is an amount found in a typical prenatal vitamin. Women with health risks, including epilepsy, insulin-dependent diabetes, obesity with BMI >35, family history of NTD, or belonging to a high-risk ethnic group require increased dietary intake of folate-rich foods and daily supplementation with 4 mg of folic acid. This supplementation should begin 2–3 months prior to conception and continue until 12 weeks postconception, when the dose is lowered to 0.4 mg (Wilson et al., 2007).

Women in their reproductive years should be informed that the excessive use of vitamin A shortly before and during pregnancy could cause birth defects. The upper limit for supplementation of vitamin A (as retinol/ retinyl esters) is 8000 IU/day prior to or during pregnancy.

Weight

Maintaining a normal BMI supports conception. Women who are underweight or overweight should receive dietary counseling to improve their diet and to achieve a normal BMI (Chavarro et al., 2007; Practice Committee of the American Society for Reproductive Medicine in collaboration with the Society for Reproductive Endocrinology & Infertility, 2008). Evidence supports intense counseling for obese adults to assist in weight loss (USPSTF, 2003).

Exercise

Regular exercise has many benefits for a woman's health and is not harmful while attempting to conceive. Women who exercise during pregnancy have faster labors and fewer LBW babies. The preconception period is an opportunity to counsel women on the importance of initiating regular physical activity.

Substance use and abuse

As a substance of both use and abuse, alcohol use is an important subject to address in the preconception period. Fetal alcohol spectrum disorder refers to the range of effects from fetal exposure to maternal alcohol. No safe levels of alcohol have been established in pregnancy, which is a particular problem for women who conceive unplanned pregnancies and drink before they become aware of conception (Floyd, Ebrahim, Tsai, O'Connor, & Sokol, 2006). Preconception counseling should clearly describe the risk of any alcohol consumption during pregnancy. Women should be advised that more than two alcoholic drinks daily can reduce female fertility (Practice Committee of the American Society for Reproductive Medicine in collaboration with the Society for Reproductive Endocrinology and Infertility, 2008). For women planning to conceive, preconception counseling may reduce their consumption of alcohol (e.g., Tough, Tofflemire, Clarke, & Newburn-Cook, 2006).

Helping women quit tobacco use may be the single most useful clinical intervention to improve health over a lifetime. In addition, both active and passive smoking interfere with female and male fertility (Practice Committee of the American Society for Reproductive Medicine, 2008; Practice Committee of the American Society for Reproductive Medicine in collaboration with the Society for Reproductive Endocrinology and Infertility, 2008), so the cessation message may be more acceptable in a preconception visit. Tobacco addiction is powerful and the list of detrimental effects to health and to pregnancy outcome is quite lengthy. In the preconception period, clinicians should describe the overall health risks of tobacco use and its effects on pregnancy (Floyd et al., 2008). Brief interventions in an office setting can make a difference for all adults and for pregnant women in attempts to quit tobacco use. The "5 As" model of smoking cessation is commonly used (see Chapters 5 and 13). Women who express a desire to quit tobacco should be offered help with developing a plan to quit smoking, referrals to support groups and quit lines, and appropriate medical treatments (Fiore et al., 2008).

About 4% of pregnant women and 10% of women between 15 and 44 years old report the use of illicit substances such as marijuana, cocaine, inhalants, hallucinogens, and heroin (Floyd et al., 2008). Outcomes such as LBW, placental abruption, and perinatal mortality are linked to cocaine use, and lower intelligence test scores are linked to marijuana exposure *in utero* (Floyd et al., 2008). Marijuana use is also linked to decreased fertility (Practice Committee of the American Society for Reproductive Medicine in collaboration with the Society for Reproductive Endocrinology and Infertility, 2008). During a preconception care visit, information on the effects of substances on pregnancy and on the fetus should be provided, and referrals for treatment should also be provided (Floyd et al., 2008).

Conception

Many couples need basic information about the process of conception. Women should be informed that conception is most likely during the 6 days before ovulation, with ovulation occurring in the middle (around day 14) of a typical menstrual cycle. However, the timing of ovulation varies widely within and between women and cannot be determined by simply keeping a calendar, even in women with regular cycles. Monitoring cervical mucus produces better results, with coitus timed for peak cervical mucus production. The frequency of intercourse that optimizes conception is about every 1–2 days during the fertile period, although couples should not try to follow a coital schedule that creates tension in the relationship. Couples should also be aware that regular intercourse outside of the fertile period is also important and that ejaculation about twice a week will help optimize the number and quality of sperm. If a couple has not conceived after 12 months of attempting pregnancy, they should be offered an evaluation for infertility.

Preparation for pregnancy and childbirth

Some decisions about childbirth are best considered before pregnancy. Several different kinds of health-care providers offer care during pregnancy and childbirth in the United States including Certified Nurse-Midwives,

Certified Professional Midwives, Family Practice Physicians, and Obstetricians. Prenatal care and birth services can be provided in the home, birth centers, and hospitals. Investigating services congruent with a woman's preferences, her risk evaluation, and that are covered by her health-care insurance can be done well before pregnancy. Preconception visits with such health-care providers offer women an opportunity to find someone suited to her needs before conception.

Breastfeeding choices are often not discussed with women until pregnancy, but there are advantages to encouraging women to consider this decision earlier. The preconception period offers an opportunity to provide information on the improved health outcomes associated with breastfeeding for both infants and mothers. Support from lay and professional educators and social networks increase breastfeeding rates (Meedya, Fahy, & Kable, 2010), and the preconception period provides the opportunity to identify such support. Longer time with the intention to breastfeed and self-efficacy in breastfeeding also increase breastfeeding rates (Meedya et al., 2010).

Infections

Many infections can affect pregnancy. In addition to screening and vaccination recommendations, healthcare providers should counsel about avoiding infections when women might be pregnant. Toxoplasmosis, cytomegalovirus, and listeriosis are infections typically asymptomatic in women and devastating to the fetus. They can cause cerebral palsy, mental retardation, stillbirth, blindness, hearing loss, epilepsy, and other sequelae. Screening for immunity is not recommended for these infections. Information on how to avoid these infections should be provided and includes frequent and thorough hand washing, no sharing of utensils, careful cleaning of food and utensils, thorough cooking of meat, and not cleaning cat litter boxes (or using gloves and a mask). These precautions are particularly important for women with frequent exposure to young children, such as preschool teachers (Coonrod et al., 2008; Ross, Jones, & Lynch, 2006).

Environmental exposure to toxins

Preconception counseling should include recommendations to avoid common environmental exposures of particular concern in pregnancy such as exposure to mercury and bisphenol A (BPA).

Mercury is a neurotoxin of particular concern for the developing fetus. Women should be counseled to avoid consumption of fish known to have higher mercury levels, such as shark, swordfish, king mackerel, and tile fish. Fishes of moderate mercury levels such as tuna should be consumed in moderation, limiting consumption to not more that 3 oz twice a week.

BPA has emerged recently as a potential exposure of concern for the developing fetus as well as infants and children. This agent is found in canned food packed in epoxy (white plastic container liners) and in plastic bottles stamped "7." Thus, women should be advised to avoid these foods until more is known about their effects (McDiarmid et al., 2008). The use of household insecticides and pesticides should be discouraged as they have been linked with adverse effects such as an increase in NTDs, reduced childhood cognitive development, and an increase in childhood cancers (Red et al., 2011).

Vaccinations

Several considerations particular to the preconception period determine which vaccinations should be offered. Many vaccines are contraindicated in pregnancy or their safety is undetermined, but immunity to these diseases can prevent the infections most likely to harm the developing fetus. In addition, the changes in immune response during pregnancy make many infections more dangerous to the woman during pregnancy, even when not transmitted to the fetus. In some cases, treatment for infections is a problem in pregnancy. Thus, the preconception period is the best time to offer these vaccinations, before a fetus can be affected and before the changes in immunity that accompany pregnancy occur in the woman.

All considerations and recommendations for routine vaccination apply during the preconception period. The CDC's Advisory Committee on Immunization Practices provides general guidance on the principles and logistics of vaccine administration (CDC, 2011a), with specific recommendations for pregnancy (CDC, 2007a). Table 4.2 provides information on the CDC recommendations for vaccinations during the preconception period and during pregnancy.

Preconception care for women with chronic diseases

In addition to routine preconception care, women with chronic diseases merit additional consideration since they may be at increased risk of unfavorable pregnancy outcomes and they may not be aware of those risks (Chuang, Velott, & Weisman, 2010; Murphy et al., 2010). In some cases, limited data are available about a particular disease and its associated risks during pregnancy. Preconception counseling should include counseling on any risks to pregnancy and fetal outcomes specific to a diagnosis, as well as risks to the woman associated with the physiological alterations that accompany pregnancy. Generally, an effort should be made to achieve optimum

health and chronic disease control before conception. Nurse practitioners and midwives should refer women with chronic diseases to a maternal-fetal medicine specialist to explore these issues (Menard & Goodnight, 2009). Table 4.3 summarizes preconception care recommendations for women with chronic diseases.

Cancer survivors

Survivors of cancer have specific concerns about pregnancy. Both men and women typically want to know about whether their cancer treatment will affect their fertility. For females, premature ovarian failure occurs in one-third of cancer survivors of reproductive age but varies depending on the type of cancer and its treatment. Some measures can be taken at the time of cancer treatment to preserve fertility, such as cryopreserving a woman's oocytes (Grady, 2006; Ruhl & Moran, 2008). Women also worry that the physiological changes associated with pregnancy such as the elevated hormone levels may increase their risk of a cancer recurrence. Carriers of the breast cancer genes (BRCA1 and BRCA2) who are breast cancer survivors do experience higher recurrence rates by age 40 if they have been pregnant (Grady, 2006). However, the risk is not increased in many other cancers.

Any chronic health issue resulting from cancer and its treatment may have an effect on pregnancy, such as heart disease resulting from radiation damage (Ruhl & Moran, 2008). Radiation treatment may increase rates of miscarriage, stillbirth, preterm birth, and LBW infants. However, there does not appear to be an increased risk of childhood cancer among the offspring of cancer survivors (Grady, 2006). Women who wish to become pregnant should discuss their desire with their oncology specialist to determine their risk of a recurrence and the optimal timing of the pregnancy.

Chronic hypertension

Women with chronic hypertension can experience a worsening of hypertension during pregnancy and have higher rates of preeclampsia, eclampsia, cardiac decomposition, and renal compromise. These risks should be addressed in preconception counseling.

The preconception period offers an opportunity to improve control of hypertension. If medications are necessary, a single medication regimen is the optimal approach if the blood pressure can be controlled (Menard & Goodnight, 2009). However, angiotensin-converting enzyme inhibitors and angiotensin-receptor blockers are contraindicated during pregnancy, and diuretics and some beta-blockers should be avoided if possible. Baseline renal function, presence of ventricular hypertrophy, and retinopathy should be assessed during the

Table 4.2 Characteristics of Routine and Other Vaccinations Relevant to Preconception Care

Vaccines routinely recommended for adults	Vaccine contraindicated or safety undetermined in pregnancy	Serious sequelae of the disease	
		Can be worse in pregnancy	Fetal
Hepatitis A (CDC, 2006b; Panda, Panda, & Riley, 2010)	√		
Hepatitis B (CDC, 2006a; Lu, 2007; Panda et al., 2010)			√
Human papilloma virus (HPV) (Ault, 2003; CDC, 2010a)		√	√
Influenza (inactivated) (CDC, 2010c; Lu, 2007; Zimmerman & Middleton, 2007)		√	
Influenza (live attenuated influenza vaccine [LAIV], live attenuated virus) (CDC, 2010c; Lu, 2007)	√	√	
Measles, mumps, rubella (MMR, live attenuated viruses) (CDC, 1998; Lu, 2007)	√		√
Meningococcal (MCV4, conjugate) (CDC, 2005)	√		
Pneumococcal (CDC, 1997, 2010d; Zimmerman, Middleton, Burns, Clover, & Kimmel, 2007)	√		
Polio (CDC, 2000)	√	√	
Tetanus-diphtheria (Td) (CDC, 2008c, Lu, 2007)	Approved after first trimester	√ (diphtheria)	
Tetanus-diphtheria-pertussis (Tdap) (CDC, 2008c)	√	√ (diphtheria)	
Varicella (live attenuated virus) (CDC, 2007b, Lu, 2007).	√	√	√

Other Vaccines	Vaccine Contraindicated or Safety Undetermined in Pregnancy	Serious sequelae of the disease	
		Can be worse in pregnancy	Fetal
Anthrax (CDC, 2010e)	√	√	
BCG (live attenuated virus) (CDC, 1996; Mnyani, 2011)	√		√
Japanese encephalitis (CDC, 2010b)	√		√
Meningococcal (CDC, 2005)			
Rabies (CDC, 2008a)			
Typhoid (parenteral and oral, live attenuated virus) (CDC, 1994)	√		
Vaccinia (smallpox, live attenuated virus) (CDC, 2001)	√	√	√
Yellow fever (live attenuated virus) (CDC, 2010f)	√		√
Zoster (shingles, live attenuated virus) (CDC, 2008b; Zimmerman et al., 2007)	√	√	√

Based on Advisory Committee on Immunization Practices guidelines (CDC, 2007a, 2011a, 2011b), the Coonrod's group recommendations on immunizations in preconception care (2008), and as otherwise noted.

Table 4.3 Preconception Care for Women with Selected Chronic Medical Conditions

Medical condition	Preconception care content
All women	Provide general preconception care. Stabilize condition, optimal maternal health. Recommend contraception appropriate for pregnancy intention and medical condition. Discontinue teratogenic medications. Discuss potential effect of condition on pregnancy and offspring. Discuss potential effect of pregnancy on long-term health of woman.
Cancer survivors	Achieve stable remission. Address potential effects on fertility and pregnancy. Address potential recurrence with pregnancy.
Cardiac disease	New York Heart Association Class 2 or more, left heart obstruction, prior cardiac event, ejection fraction <40% → high risk for cardiac event in pregnancy Correct structural lesion prior to conception Baseline echocardiogram Conversion from warfarin for chronic anticoagulation
Chronic hypertension	Address increased rates in pregnancy of preeclampsia/eclampsia, central nervous hemorrhage, cardiac decompensation, renal deterioration, preterm delivery, intrauterine growth restriction, placental abruption, fetal demise. Attempt single-agent control of hypertension (<150/100). Angiotensin-converting enzyme inhibitors and angiotensin-receptor blockers are contraindicated during pregnancy and should be discontinued while attempting conception. Assess baseline renal function, presence of ventricular hypertrophy, and retinopathy.
Dermatology	Avoid conception on isotretinoin. Avoid conception 1–2 years following etretinate.
Diabetes	Multidisciplinary team Good glycemic control prior to pregnancy Treatment of diabetic complications
Epilepsy	Address possibility of increased seizures in pregnancy. Address possibility of increased congenital anomalies with seizures, even when no medications. Address other adverse pregnancy outcomes associated with seizure disorders. Withdraw or reduce anticonvulsant medication where possible.
HIV	Transmission counseling Low viral load, highly active antiretroviral therapy (HAART) after the first trimester
Mental health disorders	Depression, anxiety screens Intimate partner violence screen Identify social support Major psychosocial stressors
Obesity	Diabetes screen Cardiovascular screening/sleep apnea assessment Weight reduction Delay pregnancy 1–2 years following obesity surgery
Phenylketonuria	Dietary control of phenylalanine levels (<6 mg/dL × 3 months)
Rheumatoid arthritis	May prolong time to conception Risk of postpartum flare Review teratogenicity of methotrexate or other medications. Discontinue before conception. Men should be advised that leflunomide, sulfasalazine, and cyclophosphamide can reduce their fertility.
Sickle cell disease	Genetic counseling for transmission Baseline renal, pulmonary, cardiac function
Thrombobophilia	Assess need for prophylaxis in pregnancy or postpartum period Conversion from warfarin for chronic anticoagulation Early identification of pregnancy
Thyroid condition	Control of thyroid levels Anticipate increase in thyroid medications during pregnancy if hypothyroid condition is present

Source: Frieder et al., 2008; Grady, 2006; Lu, 2007; Mahmud & Mazza, 2010.

preconception period. This often requires referral to medical specialists.

Diabetes

Preconception care for women with diabetes has been shown to reduce rates of perinatal mortality and congenital malformation (Dunlop et al., 2008). Several sets of international guidelines are available for preconception care of diabetic women. Diabetes management for women of reproductive age by a multidisciplinary team, treatment of diabetes complications, and good glycemic control is essential to improving pregnancy outcomes. Medications must be carefully evaluated for teratogenic potential and changed accordingly, and statins should be discontinued. Glycemic control is extremely important and the hemoglobin A1C should be kept as close to normal levels as possible (American Diabetes Association (ADA), 2012). Some guidelines also recommend that thyroid function be monitored for women with type I diabetes (Mahmud & Mazza, 2010). Preconception counseling should address the increased fetal risks in women with poor glycemic control.

Epilepsy

Seizure disorders can worsen in pregnancy, and both seizures and the medications used to control them can adversely affect pregnancy outcomes. Although no evidence exists to show that preconception care influences pregnancy outcomes in women with epilepsy (Winterbottom, Smyth, Jacoby, & Baker, 2008), some interventions make sense. Women should be aware of the possibility of increased seizures in pregnancy and of increased congenital anomalies with seizures, even when no medications are used. Information should be provided about other adverse pregnancy outcomes associated with seizure disorders, such as spontaneous abortion, LBW, and developmental disabilities. To minimize these risks, anticonvulsant medication choices should be reviewed for teratogenicity and changed, withdrawn, or reduced when possible.

HIV infection

Preconception care specific to women living with HIV infection should focus on achieving optimal health before conception, using medications that present few risks to the fetus, conceiving without infecting the sexual partner, and preventing transmission to the fetus (Coonrod et al., 2008; Lampe, 2006). Artificial insemination using her partner's sperm offers the safest method of conception in serodiscordant couples (Panel on Treatment of HIV-Infected Pregnant Women and Prevention of Perinatal Transmission, 2011). Women who are HIV positive should be referred to an HIV specialist for care

before and during pregnancy. Ideally, care should be provided by an interprofessional team led by an infectious disease specialist (see Chapter 40).

Thyroid disorders

Uncontrolled hyperthyroidism and hypothyroidism are each associated with increased maternal and neonatal morbidity. Both conditions are treatable, and treatment improves pregnancy outcomes dramatically (American College of Obstetricians and Gynecologists (ACOG), 2002; Dunlop et al., 2008). Women with hypothyroidism should be informed of the need for increased thyroid replacement (Dunlop et al., 2008). Those with hyperthyroidism may experience remission in pregnancy (Casey & Leveno, 2006). Preconception goals should include counseling on risks and control of thyroid levels with medication (see Chapter 37).

Mental illness

Psychiatric disorders can complicate pregnancies and adversely affect both mental health and pregnancy outcomes. Relapses and diagnoses of mood and anxiety disorders, including depression, are more common during pregnancy. Depression and anxiety during pregnancy have been linked to self-injury, suicide, substance abuse, impaired family relationships, preterm birth, LBW, and long-term developmental, cognitive, and behavioral impairment in children. Bipolar disorder presents even more challenges with teratogenic medications, frequent exacerbations for women who discontinue their medications in pregnancy, and high rates of postpartum exacerbations. Schizophrenia offers many challenges as well, with the highest rates of exacerbation in pregnancy and high risks for fetal malformation and demise. Psychosis in pregnancy can lead to abuse of the fetus or neonate as well as inability to recognize the onset of labor.

Several interventions can help women with mental illness in the preconception period. They should receive counseling on the potential for teratogenic effects of medications, symptom exacerbations, and effects on pregnancy outcomes. Medications should be assessed for safety in pregnancy, and alternative treatments considered, such as other medications or psychotherapy. Many women will also want to learn about whether their condition has a genetic component and can be transmitted to their offspring. Help in identifying social support and inclusion of friends or family in preconception care is particularly important for these women.

Additional considerations

There are a number of conditions that require special consideration for preconception care. These conditions include a history of pregnancy complications, prior pregnancy loss, and women with disabilities.

Prior pregnancy history

For women who have had a pregnancy complication, the interconception period offers a unique time frame to address risks before the next pregnancy is conceived. Risk assessment should include a careful history of the previous pregnancy, including outcomes such as preterm birth, LBW, or fetal demise. Information about events, diagnoses, or health behaviors that may have contributed to the outcomes should be obtained. For example, if a woman had a previous preterm birth, the possibility of asymptomatic infections such as periodontal disease or sexually transmitted infections should be considered.

A comprehensive health history should be obtained and assessed for factors that may have contributed to an unfavorable pregnancy outcome. These factors and their potential contribution to subsequent pregnancy complications should be discussed with women during the interconception period (Lu et al., 2006; Stubblefield et al., 2008). For example, the probable contribution of smoking to LBW or of substance abuse to placental abruption should be clarified, always in a respectful and caring way. While it may be easier to avoid such delicate topics, women do not always know of the links between behavior and outcomes and deserve to know this information as they make decisions for the future. The long-term implications of pregnancy complications, such as gestational diabetes, should be presented to women in the interconception period, with recommendations for possible changes, such as improved diet or weight reduction (Lu et al., 2006). Some pregnancy outcomes, such as preterm birth and LBW, have an increased risk of recurring in subsequent pregnancies, and women should be aware of these increased risks (Lu et al., 2006; Stubblefield et al., 2008). Chronic illnesses and mental illnesses often have exacerbations or a higher prevalence in pregnancy or the postpartum period (Lu et al., 2006). The implications of a cesarean birth for subsequent pregnancies should be addressed (Stubblefield et al., 2008), particularly in light of the controversy around vaginal birth after cesarean birth (Cunningham et al., 2010).

The interconception period is also an excellent time to discuss choices made during the previous pregnancy. For example, topics such as the woman's breastfeeding experience should be discussed, assessing problems or successes from previous attempts. Satisfaction with the choice of health-care provider and site of birth can also be assessed, helping the woman to evaluate the various influences on her birth experience.

Prior pregnancy loss

A woman with a previous pregnancy loss should be carefully evaluated. Women who take longer than 6 months to move through acute feelings of grief and return to activities of daily life should be evaluated for complicated grief or depression. Both men and women may experience disenfranchised grief, which occurs when cultural norms do not recognize the loss of a pregnancy as a significant source of grief for the couple. Thus, grief should be carefully evaluated and openly discussed with every couple who has experienced a pregnancy loss.

The preconception period offers an opportunity to discuss what factors may have contributed to the pregnancy loss and to modify the factors that can be changed. The optimum timing of a subsequent pregnancy depends on the health of the woman and the emotional state of the couple. This period is also a good time to evaluate the social support available to the couple (Moore, Parrish, & Black, 2011).

Disabilities

Preconception counseling for women with disabilities should include an assessment of whether her condition will affect her ability to care for her child (Smeltzer, 2007). This assessment must be performed objectively, without preconceived notions, since women with disabilities often encounter negative attitudes when they wish to start a family (Ruhl & Moran, 2008; Thierry, 2006). As with other families, no assumptions should be made about the couple's desire for genetic counseling. Indeed, some couples view a referral for genetic counseling as an intervention taken to eliminate individuals with disabilities (Ruhl & Moran, 2008; Smeltzer, 2007; Thierry, 2006). The potential impact of the woman's disability on pregnancy should be explored carefully as with any chronic disease, including the risks of exacerbation of the disabling condition or the risk of an unfavorable pregnancy outcome (Ruhl & Moran, 2008; Thierry, 2006). Possible barriers to access to care should also be considered when planning care for a woman with a disability.

Preconception care for men

Men's health also matters in the preconception period. Sperm plays a critical role in successful conception. In addition to their biological contribution to the pregnancy, men influence the health of their female partners during pregnancy. These influences can be negative (e.g., sexually transmitted infections, tobacco use in the home) or positive (e.g., emotional and financial support). However, scant attention has been paid to the appropriate content of care for men considering conceiving with their partners. Despite the lack of guidelines, preconception care for men should mirror care for women with a focus on risk assessment, counseling, and vaccination.

Risk assessment and screening

Men should have a comprehensive history, physical exam, and laboratory testing. Screening for sexually transmitted infections in those at risk is essential. BMI is also of particular importance in the preconception period since obesity is associated with reduced fertility. Medical conditions that might impair sperm quality, such as diabetes mellitus, obesity, varicocele, and sexually transmitted infections, should be addressed. Medication use should be carefully evaluated since some medications can affect sperm quality or increase risk to the fetus. Social history should consider occupational and environmental exposures, including materials used in hobbies. A three-generation family history should be obtained, with particular attention to sex-linked and autosomal recessive disorders.

Counseling

Men should be encouraged in health-promoting behaviors at routine health visits. In a visit with preconception as an added component, the following data on male reproduction should be discussed as applicable.

Male preconception counseling points

- Tobacco, heavy drinking, marijuana, cocaine, and metabolic steroids have all been linked to impaired sperm quality or infertility.
- Zinc and folic acid have been shown to protect sperm from DNA damage.
- Obesity is associated with reduced male fertility.
- Chronic inflammation, such as with periodontal infections, can damage sperm.
- While data on the relationship between stress and infertility are inconclusive, reducing stress in a man's life will likely improve his family relationships as he prepares for a new family member.
- Avoid exposure to occupational and environmental toxins that may affect fertility. Exposures can be evaluated using material data safety sheets, which are available online (CDC, n.d.).
- Men should be vaccinated against all infectious diseases that might be transmitted to their pregnant partner or their new infant, such as hepatitis B or varicella. Follow the CDC guidelines for adults (CDC, 2011a, 2011b) (See Table 4.2).

Source: Frey, Navarro, Kotelchuck, & Lu (2008).

Summary

Preconception care has great potential to improve pregnancy outcome and the long-term health of families. Preconception care is likely to have the greatest impact when it is integrated into routine primary care and well-woman health visits. The period between pregnancies is especially important to provide health-promoting and disease-preventing services as it allows changes in health and lifestyle to begin long before the conception of the next pregnancy.

Resources for women and their families

About midwives. American College of Nurse-Midwives: http://www.midwife.org/index.asp?sid=7

Baby Friendly Hospital Initiative USA (2011). Baby friendly hospitals and birth centers: http://www.baby friendlyusa.org/find-facilities

Centers for Disease Control and Prevention (2011). Breastfeeding: http://www.cdc.gov/breastfeeding/re sources/index.htm

Choosing a caregiver. Childbirth Connection: http://www.childbirthconnection.org/article.asp?Clicked Link=247&ck=10158&area=27

Choosing a place of birth. Childbirth connection: http://www.childbirthconnection.org/article.asp?Clicked Link=252&ck=10145&area=27

Folic acid: Helping to ensure a healthy pregnancy. Podcasts by the Centers for Disease Control and Prevention (2008): http://www2c.cdc.gov/podcasts/player .asp?f=7552 (English), http://www2c.cdc.gov/pod casts/player.asp?f=7553 (Spanish).

Interconception Care Project of California: http://everywomancalifornia.org/content_display.cfm ?contentID=221&categoriesID=18

Immunization recommendations and guidelines. Advisory Committee on Immunization Practices (ACIP) of the Centers for Disease Control and Prevention (CDC) (2012): http://www.cdc.gov/vaccines/recs/ acip/default.htm#recs

La Leche League. Excellent source of information on and support for breastfeeding: http://www.lalecheleague .org/

March of Dimes. Excellent source of information on pregnancy and preconception for both consumers and providers: http://www.marchofdimes.com

Patient Page. More than 100 topics in English and Spanish. American Congress of Obstetricians and Gynecologists:http://www.acog.org/For_Patients.aspx

Preconception health. Centers for Disease Control and Prevention: http://www.womenshealth.gov/pregnancy/ before-you-get-pregnant/preconception-health.cfm

Case study

Twyla is a 23-year-old African American woman who is seeing her nurse practitioner for her a routine well-woman visit. When obtaining her health history, the nurse practitioner learns that Twyla recently married and is thinking of becoming pregnant in the next year. The nurse practitioner quickly recognizes the opportunity to expand this routine well-woman visit to include preconception care to help Twyla be in the best health possible before becoming pregnant.

Before proceeding with her routine well-woman exam, the nurse practitioner reviews Twyla's health and family history and learns that she has never been pregnant and has used combined oral contraceptive pills for the past 4 years. She has no chronic medical conditions, has never had surgery or been hospitalized, reports no reproductive health problems, and has received all of the recommended immunizations. Her family history reveals hypertension in both of her parents and adult onset diabetes in her mother. There are no known genetic disorders in either her or her husband's families, but Twyla is unsure of whether she has been tested to determine whether she is a carrier for the sickle cell gene. Twyla reports drinking two to three alcoholic beverages on weekends and smokes 10 cigarettes a day. She denies using any illicit substances or taking any medications except for the occasional use of ibuprofen 400 mg for headaches. She has had all of the routine childhood and adolescent immunizations. Twyla works as an elementary school teacher. Her husband is healthy without chronic diseases and works as a software engineer.

During Twyla's gynecological examination, the nurse practitioner obtains a cervical specimen to be sent for testing for chlamydia. After the exam is complete, the nurse practitioner suggests that Twyla have the following laboratory tests today: complete blood count, blood type and Rh factor, testing for hemoglobin S (sickle cell), hepatitis B surface antigen, and HIV status. The nurse practitioner recommends that Twyla begin taking a daily multivitamin/multimineral supplement that contains at least 400 mcg folic acid daily and continue the supplement throughout the preconception period and pregnancy. Twyla is encouraged to quit smoking as soon as possible, and the nurse practitioner provides a referral to a smoking cessation program and offers to prescribe a medication to help Twyla quit before becoming pregnant. The nurse practitioner also recommends that Twyla discontinue alcohol use in the month that she plans to begin attempting pregnancy and abstain throughout her pregnancy. Twyla is also encouraged to use acetaminophen instead of ibuprofen for her headaches and to avoid OTC medications and unnecessary dietary supplements or botanical preparations. Brief dietary counseling is provided. When Twyla asks about obtaining more information about how to conceive and what to expect during pregnancy, the nurse practitioner recommends sources with high-quality information such as the Web sites of the CDC, Office of Women's Health, March of Dimes, and the American College of Nurse-Midwives "Share with Women" Web site.

Toxic substances portal. Agency for Toxic Substances and Disease Registry (n.d.): http://www.atsdr.cdc.gov/toxprofiles/index.asp

Resources for health-care providers

Baby-friendly hospitals and birth centers. Baby Friendly Hospital Initiative USA: http://www.babyfriendlyusa.org/find-facilities

Baby Friendly Hospital Initiative. World Health Organization: http://www.who.int/nutrition/publications/infantfeeding/9789241594950/en/index.html

Breastfeeding. Centers for Disease Control and Prevention: http://www.cdc.gov/breastfeeding/resources/index.htm

Clinical practice recommendations. ADA (2012): http://professional.diabetes.org/ResourcesForProfessionals.aspx?cid=84160

Drinking and reproductive health: A Fetal Alcohol Spectrum Disorders prevention tool kit. American Congress of Obstetricians and Gynecologists: http://www.acog.org/About_ACOG/ACOG_Departments/Tobacco__Alcohol__and_Substance_Abuse/Drinking_and_Reproductive_Health_Tool_Kit_for_Clinicians

Folic acid recommendations. Centers for Disease Control and Prevention: http://www.cdc.gov/ncbddd/folicacid/recommendations.html

Guidelines for vaccinating pregnant women. Centers for Disease Control and Prevention: http://www.cdc.gov/vaccines/pubs/preg-guide.htm

Helping patients who drink too much: A clinician's guide. United States Department of Health and Human Services (HHS) (2005). Rockville, MD: National Institutes of Health. National Institute on Alcohol Abuse and Alcoholism. NIH Publication No. 07-3769. Available online at: http://pubs.niaaa.nih.gov/

publications/Practitioner/CliniciansGuide2005/clinicians_guide.htm

Info for breastfeeding advocates/health-care professionals. Baby Friendly Hospital Initiative USA: http://www.babyfriendlyusa.org

Interconception Care Project of California: http://everywomancalifornia.org/content_display.cfm?contentID=221&categoriesID=18

Preconception screening and counseling checklist, March of Dimes: http://health.utah.gov/mihp/pdf/preconceptool.pdf

Preconception care. American College of Obstetrician Gynecologists: http://mail.ny.acog.org/website/PreconBooklet.pdf

Routine prenatal care (includes recommendations for preconception care content). Institute for Clinical Systems Improvement (ICSI) (2010). In the Agency for Healthcare Research and Quality National Guideline Clearinghouse: http://www.guideline.gov/content.aspx?id=24138

Smoking cessation during pregnancy: A clinician's guide to helping pregnant women quit smoking (includes health education pamphlets). ACOG (2011): http://www.acog.org/About_ACOG/ACOG_Departments/Tobacco__Alcohol__and_Substance_Abuse/NEW_Prenatal_Smoking_Clinician_s_Guide

Toxic substances portal. Agency for Toxic Substances and Disease Registry: http://www.atsdr.cdc.gov/toxprofiles/index.asp

What is preconception care? Centers for Disease Control and Prevention: http://www.cdc.gov/ncbddd/preconception

Pregnancy. National Center on Birth Defects and Developmental Disabilities of the Center for Disease Control and Prevention: http://www.cdc.gov/ncbddd/index.html

Preconception care questions and answers. Professionals Center for Disease Control and Prevention: http://www.cdc.gov/ncbddd/preconception/QandA_providers.htm

Materials and publications. This includes a preconception history form with rationales for each question for sale. Wisconsin Association for Perinatal Care: http://www.perinatalweb.org/index.php?option=com_content&task=view&id=23&Itemid=41

Tools for screening

Alcohol screening history tools. Boulware, L. E., Barnes, G. J., Wilson, R. F., Phillips, K., Maynor, K., Hwang, C., . . . & Daumit, G. L. Value of the periodic health evaluation. Evidence report/technology assessment No. 136. AHRQ Publication No. 06-E011. Rockville, MD: Agency for Healthcare Research and Quality: http://archive.ahrq.gov/downloads/pub/evidence/pdf/phe/phe.pdf

Depression screening history (two-question). US Preventive Services Task Force (USPSTF) (2009). Screening for depression in adults: Recommendation statement: http://www.uspreventiveservicestaskforce.org/uspstf09/adultdepression/addeprrs.htm

Genetic screening history for preconception. Solomon, B., Jack, B., & Feero, W. (2008). The clinical content of preconception care: Genetics and genomics. *American Journal of Obstetrics and Gynecology, 199*(6 Suppl. 2), S340–S344. Table 2.

Occupational/environmental exposure screening history. McDiarmid, M., & Gehle, K. (2006). Preconception brief: Occupational/environmental exposures. *Maternal and Child Health Journal, 10*(5 Suppl.), S123–S128.

Periodic examination history. American College of Obstetricians and Gynecologists Committee on Gynecologic Practice (2011). ACOG Committee Opinion No. 483: Primary and preventive care: Periodic assessments. Source: Practice. *Obstetrics & Gynecology, 117*(4), 1008–1015.

Preconception screening history. March of Dimes (n.d.). Preconception screening and counseling checklist: http://health.utah.gov/mihp/pdf/preconceptool.pdf

Preconception screening history. Wisconsin Association for Perinatal Care (n.d.). Healthcare provider reference to "Becoming a Parent Preconception Checklist": http://www.perinatalweb.org/images/stories/PDFs/Materials%20and%20Publication/peconception%20checklist_2013_locked.pdf

Consumer brochures for the office setting

Preconception care: A guide to optimizing pregnancy outcomes. American College of Obstetricians and Gynecologists: http://www.health.ny.gov/publications/2026.pdf

Birth defects prevention materials, including information on diabetes and folate supplementation in English and Spanish. Centers for Disease Control and Prevention: http://www2a.cdc.gov/ncbddd/faorder/orderform.htm

Women, Infants, and Children Publications – resources of WIC clinics. Order form for Breastfeeding: A magical bond of love health education brochure. Food and Nutrition Services of the US Department of Agriculture: http://www.fns.usda.gov/wic/publications.htm

Zwanger Worden (2006). Becoming pregnant? Begin with ZwangerWijzer: http://www.zwangerwijzer.nl/pdfbestanden/ZwangerWijzer%20NL-Engels.pdf. An internet-based preconception questionnaire which can be purchased for use with patients. Validated in Landkroon, de Weerd, van Vliet-Lachotzki, and Steegers (2010).

References

Agency for Toxic Substances and Disease Registry (ATSDR). (n.d. a). Public health statement: Mercury. Toxic substances portal. Retrieved from http://www.atsdr.cdc.gov/ToxProfiles/tp46-c1-b.pdf

Agency for Toxic Substances and Disease Registry (ATSDR). (n.d. b). Toxic substances portal. Retrieved from http://www.atsdr.cdc.gov/toxprofiles/index.asp

Alexander, G. R., & Kotelchuck, M. (2001). Assessing the role and effectiveness of prenatal care: History, challenges, and directions for future research. *Public Health Reports, 116*, 306–316.

Algorithms from Interconception Care Project of California. (2009). Preconception Health Council of California. Retrieved from http://everywomancalifornia.org/content_display.cfm?contentID=221&categoriesID=18

American College of Obstetricians and Gynecologists (ACOG). (2002). ACOG Practice Bulletin. Thyroid disease in pregnancy. *Obstetrics & Gynecology, 79*(2), 171–180.

American College of Obstetricians and Gynecologists. (2011). Smoking cessation during pregnancy: A clinician's guide to helping pregnant women quit smoking. Retrieved from http://www.acog.org/About_ACOG/ACOG_Departments/Tobacco__Alcohol__and_Substance_Abuse/NEW_Prenatal_Smoking_Clinician_s_Guide

American College of Obstetricians and Gynecologists Committee on Gynecologic Practice. (2011). ACOG Committee Opinion No. 483: Primary and preventive care: Periodic assessments. Source: Practice. *Obstetrics & Gynecology, 117*(4), 1008–1015.

American Congress of Obstetricians and Gynecologists. (n.d.). Drinking and reproductive health: A fetal alcohol spectrum disorders prevention tool kit. Retrieved from http://www.acog.org/About_ACOG/ACOG_Departments/Tobacco__Alcohol__and_Substance_Abuse/Drinking_and_Reproductive_Health_Tool_Kit_for_Clinicians

American Diabetes Association (ADA). (2012). Clinical practice recommendations. Retrieved from http://professional.diabetes.org/ResourcesForProfessionals.aspx?cid=84160

Anderson, J., Ebrahim, S., Floyd, L., & Atrash, H. (2006). Prevalence of risk factors for adverse pregnancy outcomes during pregnancy and the preconception period—United States, 2002–2004. *Maternal and Child Health Journal, 10*(5 Suppl.), S101–S106.

Atrash, H., Jack, B., & Johnson, K. (2008). Preconception care: A 2008 update. *Current Opinion in Obstetrics & Gynecology, 20*(6), 581–589.

Ault, K. A. (2003). Human papillomavirus infections: Diagnosis, treatment, and hope for a vaccine. *Obstetrics and Gynecology Clinics of North America, 30*(4), 809–817.

Bhutta, Z., Yakoob, M., Lawn, J., Rizvi, A., Friberg, I., Weissman, E., . . . Goldenberg, R. (2011). Stillbirths: What difference can we make and at what cost? *Lancet, 377*(9776), 1523–1538.

Boggess, K. A., & Edelstein, B. L. (2006). Oral health in women during preconception and pregnancy: Implications for birth outcomes and infant oral health. *Maternal Child Health Journal, 10*, S169–S174.

Boulet, S. L., Johnson, K., Parker, C., Posner, S. F., & Atrash, H. (2006). A perspective of preconception health activities in the United States. *Maternal Child Health Journal, 10*, S13–S20.

Boulware, L. E., Barnes, G. J., Wilson, R. F., Phillips, K., Maynor, K., Hwang, C., & Daumit, G. L., . . . Daumit, G. L. (2006). Value of the periodic health evaluation. Evidence report/technology assessment No. 136. AHRQ Publication No. 06-E011. Rockville, MD: Agency for Healthcare Research and Quality. Retrieved from http://archive.ahrq.gov/downloads/pub/evidence/pdf/phe/phe.pdf

Burris, H., Mitchell, A., & Werler, M. (2010). Periconceptional multivitamin use and infant birth weight disparities. *Annals of Epidemiology, 20*(3), 233–240.

Carter, H., Lindsey, L. L. M., Petrini, J. R., & Prue, C. (2004). Use of vitamins containing folic acid among women of childbearing age—United States, 2004. *MMWR. Morbidity and Mortality Weekly Report, 54*(36), 847–848.

Casey, B. M., & Leveno, K. J. (2006). Thyroid disease in pregnancy. *Obstetrics and Gynecology, 108*(5), 1283–1292.

Catov, J., Bodnar, L., Ness, R., Markovic, N., & Roberts, J. (2007). Association of periconceptional multivitamin use and risk of preterm or small-for-gestational-age births. *American Journal of Epidemiology, 166*(3), 296–303.

Cena, E., Joy, A., Heneman, K., Espinosa-Hall, G., Garcia, L., Schneider, C., . . . Zidenberg-Cherr, S. (2008). Learner-centered nutrition education improves folate intake and food-related behaviors in nonpregnant, low-income women of childbearing age. *Journal of the American Dietetic Association, 108*(10), 1627–1635.

Centers for Disease Control and Prevention (CDC). (n.d.). NIOSH pocket guide to chemical hazards. Retrieved from http://www.cdc.gov/niosh/npg

Centers for Disease Control and Prevention (CDC). (1994). Typhoid immunization: Recommendations of the Advisory Committee on Immunization Practices (ACIP). *MMWR. Morbidity and Mortality Weekly Report, 43*(RR14), 1–7. Retrieved from http://www.cdc.gov/mmwr/PDF/rr/rr4314.pdf

Centers for Disease Control and Prevention (CDC). (1996). The role of the BCG vaccine in prevention and control of tuberculosis in the United States: A joint statement by the Advisory Council for the Elimination of Tuberculosis and the Advisory Committee on Immunization Practices. *MMWR. Morbidity and Mortality Weekly Report, 45*(RR4), 1–18. Retrieved from http://www.cdc.gov/mmwr/PDF/rr/rr4504.pdf

Centers for Disease Control and Prevention (CDC). (1997). Prevention of pneumococcal disease: Recommendations of the Advisory Committee on Immunization Practices (AIC). *MMWR. Morbidity and Mortality Weekly Report, 46*(RR8), 1–24. Retrieved from http://www.cdc.gov/mmwr/PDF/rr/rr4608.pdf

Centers for Disease Control and Prevention (CDC). (1998). Measles, mumps, and rubella—Vaccine use and strategies for elimination of measles, rubella, and congenital rubella syndrome, and control of mumps: Recommendations of the Advisory Committee on Immunization Practices (AIC). *MMWR. Morbidity and Mortality Weekly Report, 47*(RR8), 1–21. Retrieved from http://www.cdc.gov/mmwr/PDF/rr/rr4708.pdf

Centers for Disease Control and Prevention (CDC). (2000). Poliomyelitis prevention in the United States: Recommendations of the Advisory Committee on Immunization Practices (AIC). *MMWR. Morbidity and Mortality Weekly Report, 49*(RR5), 1–14. Retrieved from http://www.cdc.gov/mmwr/PDF/rr/rr4905.pdf

Centers for Disease Control and Prevention (CDC). (2001). Vaccinia (smallpox) vaccine: Recommendations of the Advisory Committee on Immunization Practices (AIC), 2001. *MMWR. Morbidity and Mortality Weekly Report, 50*(RR10), 1–26. Retrieved from http://www.cdc.gov/mmwr/PDF/rr/rr5010.pdf

Centers for Disease Control and Prevention (CDC). (2005). Prevention and control of meningococcal disease: Recommendations of the Advisory Committee on Immunization Practices. *MMWR. Morbidity and Mortality Weekly Report, 54*(RR7), 1–21. Retrieved from http://www.cdc.gov/mmwr/PDF/rr/rr5407.pdf

Centers for Disease Control and Prevention (CDC). (2006a). A comprehensive immunization strategy to eliminate transmission of hepatitis B virus infection in the United States: Recommendations of the Advisory Committee on Immunization Practices (ACIP). Part II Immunization of adults. *MMWR. Morbidity and Mortality Weekly Report*, *55*(RR16), 1–23. Retrieved from http://www.cdc.gov/mmwr/PDF/rr/rr5516.pdf

Centers for Disease Control and Prevention (CDC). (2006b). Prevention and control of hepatitis A through active or passive immunization: Recommendations of the Advisory Committee on Immunization Practices. *MMWR. Morbidity and Mortality Weekly Report*, *55*(RR7), 1–23. Retrieved from http://www.cdc.gov/mmwr/PDF/rr/rr5507.pdf

Centers for Disease Control and Prevention (CDC). (2006c). Recommendations to improve preconception health and health care—United States: A report of the CDC/ATSDR Preconception Care Work Group and the Select Panel on Preconception Care. *MMWR. Morbidity and Mortality Weekly Report*, *55*(RR6), 1–23. Retrieved from http://www.cdc.gov/mmwr/PDF/rr/rr5506.pdf

Centers for Disease Control and Prevention (CDC). (2007a). Guidelines for vaccinating pregnant women: From recommendations of the Advisory Committee on Immunization Practices. Bethesda, MD: Centers for Disease Control and Prevention. Retrieved from http://www.cdc.gov/vaccines/pubs/downloads/b_preg_guide.pdf

Centers for Disease Control and Prevention (CDC). (2007b). Prevention of varicella: Recommendations of the Advisory Committee on Immunization Practices (ACIP). *MMWR. Morbidity and Mortality Weekly Report*, *56*(RR4), 1–40. Retrieved from http://www.cdc.gov/mmwr/PDF/rr/rr5604.pdf

Centers for Disease Control and Prevention (CDC). (2008a). Human rabies prevention: United States, 2008: Recommendations of the Advisory Committee on Immunization Practices (ACIP). *MMWR. Morbidity and Mortality Weekly Report*, *57*(RR3), 1–28. Retrieved from http://www.cdc.gov/mmwr/preview/mmwrhtml/rr5703a1.htm

Centers for Disease Control and Prevention (CDC). (2008b). Prevention of herpes zoster: Recommendations of the Advisory Committee on Immunization Practices (ACIP). *MMWR. Morbidity and Mortality Weekly Report*, *57*(RR5), 1–30. Retrieved from http://www.cdc.gov/mmwr/PDF/rr/rr5705.pdf

Centers for Disease Control and Prevention (CDC). (2008c). Prevention of pertussis, tetanus, and diphtheria among pregnant and postpartum women and their infant: Recommendations of the Advisory Committee on Immunization Practices (ACIP). *MMWR. Morbidity and Mortality Weekly Report*, *57*(RR4), 1–41. Retrieved from http://www.cdc.gov/mmwr/PDF/rr/rr5704.pdf

Centers for Disease Control and Prevention (CDC). (2010a). FDA licensure of bivalent human papillomavirus vaccine (HPV2, Cervarix) for use in females and updated HPV vaccination recommendations from the Advisory Committee on Immunization Practices (ACIP). *MMWR. Morbidity and Mortality Weekly Report*, *59*(20), 624–629. Retrieved from http://www.cdc.gov/mmwr/PDF/wk/mm5920.pdf

Centers for Disease Control and Prevention (CDC). (2010b). Japanese encephalitis vaccine: Recommendations of the Advisory Committee on Immunization Practices (ACIP). *MMWR. Morbidity and Mortality Weekly Report*, *59*(RR1), 1–27. Retrieved from http://www.cdc.gov/mmwr/pdf/rr/rr5901.pdf

Centers for Disease Control and Prevention (CDC). (2010c). Prevention and control of influenza with vaccines: Recommendations of the Advisory Committee on Immunization Practices (ACIP), 2010. *MMWR. Morbidity and Mortality Weekly Report*, *59*(RR8), 1–61. Retrieved from http://www.cdc.gov/mmwr/PDF/rr/rr5908.pdf

Centers for Disease Control and Prevention (CDC). (2010d). Updated recommendations for prevention of invasive pneumococcal disease among adults using the 23-valent pneumococcal polysaccharide vaccine (PPSVS23). *MMWR. Morbidity and Mortality Weekly Report*, *59*(34), 1102–1106. Retrieved from http://www.cdc.gov/mmwr/pdf/rr/rr5906.pdf

Centers for Disease Control and Prevention (CDC). (2010e). Use of anthrax vaccine in the United States: Recommendations of the Advisory Committee on Immunization Practices (ACIP), 2009. *MMWR. Morbidity and Mortality Weekly Report*, *59*(RR6), 1–36. Retrieved from http://www.cdc.gov/mmwr/pdf/rr/rr5906.pdf

Centers for Disease Control and Prevention (CDC). (2010f). Yellow fever vaccine: Recommendations of the Advisory Committee on Immunization Practices (ACIP). *MMWR. Morbidity and Mortality Weekly Report*, *59*(RR7), 1–12. Retrieved from http://www.cdc.gov/mmwr/PDF/rr/rr5907.pdf

Centers for Disease Control and Prevention (CDC). (2011a). General recommendations of immunization: Recommendations of the Advisory Committee on Immunization Practice. *MMWR. Morbidity and Mortality Weekly Report*, *60*(2), 1–61. Retrieved from http://www.cdc.gov/vaccines/pubs/ACIP-list.htm

Centers for Disease Control and Prevention (CDC). (2011b). Recommended adult immunization schedule: United States 2011. *MMWR. Morbidity and Mortality Weekly Report*, *60*(4), 1–61. Retrieved from http://www.cdc.gov/vaccines/pubs/ACIP-list.htm

Centers for Disease Control and Prevention (CDC). (2012). Folic acid helps prevent neural tube defects. http://www.cdc.gov/Features/FolicAcid/

Chavarro J. E., Rich-Edwards J. W., Rosner B., & Willett W.C. (2007). Diet and lifestyle in the prevention of ovulatory disorder infertility. *Obstetrics & Gynecology*, *110*(5), 1050–58.

Chuang, C., Velott, D., & Weisman, C. (2010). Exploring knowledge and attitudes related to pregnancy and preconception health in women with chronic medical conditions. *Maternal and Child Health Journal*, *14*(5), 713–719.

Chuang, C., Weisman, C., Hillemeier, M., Schwarz, E., Camacho, F., & Dyer, A. (2010). Pregnancy intention and health behaviors: Results from the Central Pennsylvania Women's Health Study cohort. *Maternal and Child Health Journal*, *14*(4), 501–510.

Coonrod, D., Jack, B., Boggess, K., Long, R., Conry, J., Cox, S., . . . Dunlop, A. (2008). The clinical content of preconception care: Immunizations as part of preconception care. *American Journal of Obstetrics and Gynecology*, *199*(6 Suppl. 2), S290–S295.

Cragan, J., Friedman, J., Holmes, L., Uhl, K., Green, N., & Riley, L. (2006). Ensuring the safe and effective use of medications during pregnancy: Planning and prevention through preconception care. *Maternal and Child Health Journal*, *10*(5 Suppl.), S129–S135.

Cramer, J., & Lumey, L. (2010). Maternal preconception diet and the sex ratio. *Human Biology*, *82*(1), 103–107.

Crozier, S. R., Robinson, S. M., Borland, S. E., Godfrey, K. M., Cooper, C., Inskip, H. M., & SWS Study Group. (2009). Do women change their health behaviours in pregnancy? Findings from the Southampton Women's Survey. *Paediatric and Perinatal Epidemiology*, *23*, 446–453.

Cunningham, F. G., Bangdiwala, S., Brown, S. S., Dean, T. M., Frederiksen, M., Rowland Hogue, C. J., . . . Zimmet, S. C. (2010). National Institutes of Health consensus development conference statement: Vaginal birth after cesarean: New insights. *Obstetrics & Gynecology*, *115*(6), 1279–1295.

Dunlop, A., Jack, B., Bottalico, J., Lu, M., James, A., Shellhaas, C., . . . Prasad, M. (2008). The clinical content of preconception care: Women with chronic medical conditions. *American Journal of Obstetrics and Gynecology*, *199*(6 Suppl. 2), S310–S327.

Fiore, M. C., Jaen, C. R., Baker, T. B., Bailey, W. C., Benowitz, N. L., & Wewers, M. E., . . . Wewers, M. E. (2008). Treating tobacco use and dependence: 2008 update. *Clinical Practice Guideline*. Rockville,

MD: U.S. Department of Health and Human Services, Public Health Service. Retrieved from http://www.ncbi.nlm.nih.gov/books/NBK63952.

Floyd, R., Ebrahim, S., Tsai, J., O'Connor, M., & Sokol, R. (2006). Strategies to reduce alcohol-exposed pregnancies. *Maternal and Child Health Journal, 10*(5 Suppl.), S149–S151.

Floyd, R., Jack, B., Cefalo, R., Atrash, H., Mahoney, J., Herron, A., . . . Sokol, R. (2008). The clinical content of preconception care: Alcohol, tobacco, and illicit drug exposures. *American Journal of Obstetrics and Gynecology, 199*(6 Suppl. 2), S333–S339.

Freda, M. C., Moos, M. K., & Curtis, M. (2006). The history of preconception care: Evolving guidelines and standards. *Maternal Child Health Journal, 10*(Suppl. 1), 43–52.

Frey, K., Navarro, S., Kotelchuck, M., & Lu, M. (2008). The clinical content of preconception care: Preconception care for men. *American Journal of Obstetrics and Gynecology, 199*(6 Suppl. 2), S389–S395.

Frey, K. A., & Files, J. A. (2006). Preconception healthcare: What women know and believe. *Maternal Child Health Journal, 10,* S73–S77.

Frieder, A., Dunlop, A., Culpepper, L., & Bernstein, P. (2008). The clinical content of preconception care: Women with psychiatric conditions. *American Journal of Obstetrics and Gynecology, 199*(6 Suppl. 2), S328–S332.

Gold, R. B., & Alrich, C. (2008). Role of Medicaid Family Planning Waivers and Title X in enhancing access to preconception care. *Women's Health Issues: Official Publication of the Jacobs Institute of Women's Health, 18S,* S47–S51.

Grady, M. (2006). Preconception and the young cancer survivor. *Maternal and Child Health Journal, 10*(5 Suppl.), S165–S168.

Health Resources and Services Administration (HRSA). (n.d.). Women's preventive services: Required health plan coverage guidelines. Retrieved from http://www.hrsa.gov/womensguidelines

Hood, J. R., Parker, C., & Atrash, H. (2007). Recommendations to improve preconception health and health care: Strategies for implementation. *Journal of Women's Health, 16*(4), 454–457.

Institute for Clinical Systems Improvement (ICSI) (2010). Routine prenatal care. Retrieved from the Agency for Healthcare Research and Quality National Guideline Clearinghouse http://www.guideline.gov/content.aspx?id=24138

Kannan, S., Menotti, E., Scherer, H., Dickinson, J., & Larson, K. (2007). Folic acid and the prevention of neural tube defects: A survey of awareness among Latina women of childbearing age residing in southeast Michigan. *Health Promotion Practice, 8*(1), 60–68.

Kent, H., & Streeter, N. (2008). Title V strategies to ensure a continuum of women's health services. *Women's Health Issues: Official Publication Of The Jacobs Institute Of Women's Health, 18S*(2008), S67–S73.

Lampe, M. A. (2006). Human immunodeficiency virus-1 and preconception care. *Maternal Child Health Journal, 10,* S193–S195.

Landkroon, A., de Weerd, S., van Vliet-Lachotzki, E., & Steegers, E. (2010). Validation of an internet questionnaire for risk assessment in preconception care. *Public Health Genomics, 13*(2), 89–94.

Lanier, D., & Ko, S. (2008). Screening in primary care settings for illicit drug sse: Assessment of screening instruments—A supplemental evidence update for the U.S. Preventive Services Task Force. Evidence Synthesis No. 58, Part 2. AHRQ Publication No. 08-05108-EF-2. Rockville, MD: Agency for Healthcare Research and Quality. January 2008. Retrieved from http://www.uspreventiveservicestaskforce.org/uspstf08/druguse/drugevup.pdf

Liu, Y., Liu, J., Ye, R., & Li, Z. (2006). Association of preconceptional health care utilization and early initiation of prenatal care. *Journal Of Perinatology: Official Journal Of The California Perinatal Association, 26*(7), 409–413.

Loomis, L. W., & Martin, M. W. (2000). The Interconception Health Promotion Initiative: A demonstration project to reduce the incidence of repeat LBW deliveries in an urban safety net hospital. *Family & Community Health, 23*(3), 1–16.

Lu, M. (2007). Recommendations for preconception care. *American Family Physician, 76*(3), 397–400.

Lu, M., Kotelchuck, M., Culhane, J., Hobel, C., Klerman, L., & Thorp, J. (2006). Preconception care between pregnancies: The content of internatal care. *Maternal and Child Health Journal, 10*(5 Suppl.), S107–S122.

Lu, M. C., & Halfon, N. (2003). Disparities in birth outcomes: A life course perspective. *Maternal and Child Health Journal, 7*(1), 13–30.

Lu, M. C., Kotelchuck, M., Hogan, V., Jones, L., Wright, K., & Halfon, N. (2010). Closing the Black-White gap in birth outcomes: A life course approach. *Ethnicity & Disease, 20*(1 Suppl. 2), 62–76.

Mahmud, M., & Mazza, D. (2010). Preconception care of women with diabetes: A review of current guideline recommendations. *BMC Women's Health, 105.*

March of Dimes. (n.d.). Preconception screening and counseling checklist. Retrieved from http://health.utah.gov/mihp/pdf/preconceptool.pdf

Marmot, M. G., Shipley, M. J., Hemingway, H., Head, J., & Brunner, E. J. (2008). Biological and behavioural explanations of social inequalities in coronary heart disease: The Whitehall II study. *Diabetologia, 51*(11), 1980–1988.

McDiarmid, M., & Gehle, K. (2006). Preconception brief: Occupational/environmental exposures. *Maternal and Child Health Journal, 10*(5 Suppl.), S123–S128.

McDiarmid, M., Gardiner, P., & Jack, B. (2008). The clinical content of preconception care: Environmental exposures. *American Journal of Obstetrics and Gynecology, 199*(6 Suppl. 2), S357–S361.

Meedya, S., Fahy, K., & Kable, A. (2010). Factors that positively influence breastfeeding duration to 6 months: A literature review. *Women and Birth: Journal of the Australian College of Midwives, 23*(4), 135–145.

Menard, M., & Goodnight, W. (2009). The role of specialists in providing preconception health care and guidance to women with chronic medical conditions. *North Carolina Medical Journal, 70*(5), 445–448.

Mnyani, C. N. (2011). Tuberculosis in pregnancy. *British Journal of Obstetrics and Gynaecology: An International Journal of Obstetrics and Gynaecology, 118*(2), 226–231.

Moore, T., Parrish, H., & Black, B. (2011). Interconception care for couples after perinatal loss: A comprehensive review of the literature. *The Journal Of Perinatal & Neonatal Nursing, 25*(1), 44–51.

Murphy, H., Temple, R., Ball, V., Roland, J., Steel, S., Zill-E-Huma, R., . . . Skinner, T. (2010). Personal experiences of women with diabetes who do not attend pre-pregnancy care. *Diabetic Medicine: A Journal of the British Diabetic Association, 27*(1), 92–100.

O'Connor, E. A., Whitlock, E. P., Beil, T. L., & Gaynes, B. N. (2009). Screening for depression in adult patients in primary care settings: A systematic evidence review. *Annals of Internal Medicine, 151,* 793–803. Retrieved from http://www.uspreventiveservicestaskforce.org/uspstf09/adultdepression/addeprart.pdf

Panda, B., Panda, A., & Riley, L. E. (2010). Selected viral infections in pregnancy. *Obstetrics and Gynecology Clinics of North America, 37*(2), 321–331.

Panel on Treatment of HIV-Infected Pregnant Women and Prevention of Perinatal Transmission. (2011). Recommendations for use of antiretroviral drugs in pregnant HIV-1-infected women for maternal health and interventions to reduce perinatal HIV transmission in the United States. Retrieved from http://aidsinfo.nih.gov/contentfiles/PerinatalGL.pdf

Practice Committee of the American Society for Reproductive Medicine (2008). Smoking and infertility. *Fertility and Sterility*, *90*, S254–S259.

Practice Committee of the American Society for Reproductive Medicine in collaboration with the Society for Reproductive Endocrinology and Infertility. (2008). Optimizing natural fertility. *Fertility and Sterility*, *90*(5 Suppl.), S1–S6.

Public Health Service Expert Panel on the Content of Prenatal Care. (1989). *Caring for our future: The content of prenatal care*. Bethesda, MD: National Institutes of Health. Retrieved from http://www.eric.ed.gov/PDFS/ED334018.pdf

Red, R. T., Richards, S. M., Torres, C., & Adair, C. D. (2011). Environmental toxicant exposure during pregnancy. *Obstetrical & Gynecological Survey*, *66*(3), 159–169.

Rollnick, S., Miller, W. R., & Butler, C. C. (2008). *Motivational interviewing in health care: Helping patients change behavior*. New York: Guilford.

Rosenbaum, S. (2008). Women and health insurance: Implications for financing preconception health. *Women's Health Issues*, *18*(6 Suppl.), S26–S35.

Ross, D., Jones, J., & Lynch, M. (2006). Toxoplasmosis, cytomegalovirus, listeriosis, and preconception care. *Maternal and Child Health Journal*, *10*(5 Suppl.), S187–S191.

Ruhl, C., & Moran, B. (2008). The clinical content of preconception care: Preconception care for special populations. *American Journal of Obstetrics and Gynecology*, *199*(6 Suppl. 2), S384–S388.

Scholl, T. (2008). Maternal nutrition before and during pregnancy. Nestlé Nutrition Workshop Series. Paediatric Programme, 6179–6189.

Siega-Riz, A. M., Siega-Riz, A. M., & Laraia, B. (2006). The implications of maternal overweight and obesity on the course of pregnancy and birth outcomes. *Maternal Child Health Journal*, *10*, S153–S156.

Smeltzer, S. (2007). Pregnancy in women with physical disabilities. *Journal of Obstetric, Gynecologic, and Neonatal Nursing: JOGNN/NAACOG*, *36*(1), 88–96.

Solomon, B., Jack, B., & Feero, W. (2008). The clinical content of preconception care: Genetics and genomics. *American Journal of Obstetrics and Gynecology*, *199*(6 Suppl. 2), S340–S344.

Stubblefield, P. G., Coonrod, D. V., Reddy, U. M. Sayegh, R., Nicholson, W., Rychlik, D. F., & Jack, B. W. (2008). The clinical content of preconception care: Reproductive history. *American Journal of Obstetrics and Gynecology*, *199* (6 Suppl. 2), s373–S383.

Thierry, J. M. (2006). The importance of preconception care for women with disabilities. *Maternal Child Health Journal*, *10*, S175–S176.

Tough, S., Tofflemire, S., Clarke, M., & Newburn-Cook, C. (2006). Do women change their drinking behaviors while trying to conceive? An opportunity for preconceptionl counseling. *Clinical Medicine & Research*, *4*(2), 97–105.

United States Department of Health and Human Services (HHS). (2005). Helping patients who drink too much: A clinician's guide. Rockville, MD: National Institutes of Health. National Institute on Alcohol Abuse and Alcoholism. NIH Publication No. 07-3769. Retrieved from http://pubs.niaaa.nih.gov/publications/Practitioner/CliniciansGuide2005/clinicians_guide.htm

United States Preventive Services Task Force (USPSTF). (n.d.). Recommendations. Retrieved from http://www.uspreventiveservicestaskforce.org/uspstf/uspsobes.htm

United States Preventive Services Task Force (USPSTF). (2003). Screening for obesity. Retrieved from http://www.uspreventiveservicestaskforce.org/3rduspstf/alcohol/alcomisrs.htm

United States Preventive Services Task Force (USPSTF). (2004). Screening and behavioral counseling interventions in primary care to reduce alcohol misuse. Retrieved from http://www.uspreventiveservicestaskforce.org/3rduspstf/alcohol/alcomisrs.htm

United States Preventive Services Task Force (USPSTF). (2009). Counseling and interventions to prevent tobacco use and tobacco-caused diseases among adults and pregnant women: U.S. Preventive Services Task Force reaffirmation recommendation statement. *Annals of Internal Medicine*, *150*, 551–555. Retrieved from http://www.uspreventiveservicestaskforce.org/uspstf09/tobacco/tobaccors2.pdf

U.S. Environmental Protection Agency. (n.d.). National priorities list sites in the United States. Retrieved from http://www.epa.gov/superfund/sites/npl/index.htm

Wehby, G. L., & Murray, J. C. (2008). The effects of prenatal use of folic acid and other dietary supplements on early child development. *Maternal Child Health Journal*, *12*, 180–187.

Wilson, R. D., Johnson, J. A., Wyatt, P., Allen, V., Gagnon, A., Langlois, S., . . . Kapur, B. (2007). Preconceptional vitamin/folic acid supplementation 2007: The use of folic acid in combination with a multivitamin for the prevention of neural tube defects and other congenital anomalies. *Journal Obstetrics & Gynaecology of Canada*, *29*(12), 1003–1026.

Winterbottom, J., Smyth, R., Jacoby, A., & Baker, G. (2008). Preconception counselling for women with epilepsy to reduce adverse pregnancy outcome. *Cochrane Database Of Systematic Reviews (Online)*, *3*, CD006645.

Wisconsin Association for Perinatal Care (n.d.). Healthcare provider reference to "Becoming a Parent Preconception Checklist". Retrieved from http://www.perinatalweb.org/images/stories/PDFs/Materials%20and%20Publication/peconception%20checklist_2013_locked.pdf

World Health Organization (WHO). (2012). Risk factors. Retrieved from http://www.who.int/topics/risk_factors/en

Zimmerman, R. K., & Middleton, D. B. (2007). Vaccines for persons as high risk, 2007. *The Journal of Family Practice*, *56*(2), S38–S36.

Zimmerman, R. K., Middleton, D. B., Burns, I. T., Clover, R. D., & Kimmel, S. R. (2007). Routine vaccines across the life span, 2007. *The Journal of Family Practice*, *56*(2), S18–S37.

5

Prenatal care: Goals, structure, and components

Carrie S. Klima

Relevant terms

Ballantyne, John—(1862–1923) a Scottish obstetrician credited with founding modern prenatal care; his book, *A Manual of Antenatal Pathology and Hygiene* published in 1902, established recognition of the fetal period being influenced by the prenatal health of the mother.

Breckinridge, Mary—(1881–1965) an American nurse-midwife and founder of the Frontier Nursing Service, an organization that provided care to rural and underserved Appalachian women and their families for decades and continues to educate nurse-midwives and nurse practitioners to work in rural and underserved areas. Mrs. Breckinridge imported the British style nurse-midwife and demonstrated the value of the nurse who was also educated as a midwife.

Children's Bureau—the first federal agency devoted to the welfare of children, signed into law in 1912 by William Howard Taft in response to grassroots efforts led by nurse Lillian Wald. Early agency issues were maternal and infant mortality; its work continues today with child abuse and neglect as leading modern-day concerns.

Dick-Read, Grantly—(1890–1959) a British obstetrician and leading advocate of natural childbirth who published his opinions in a widely read book, *Childbirth without Fear*. He was ostracized by his colleagues for his support of unmedicated birth.

Feminist movements—social reform efforts advocating for women's rights. First-wave feminism (1880s–1940s) secured the right to vote and property rights for women; second-wave feminism (1960s–1980s) focused on reproductive

rights and social equality; third-wave feminism ideology (1990s–present) embraces diversity and change.

Gaskin, Ina May—(1940–present) a self-taught American midwife who popularized midwifery through her book *Spiritual Midwifery*, recounting her experiences of birth at a commune called The Farm in Tennessee. She continues to work tirelessly to promote maternal and infant health through midwifery care.

Lamaze, Fernand—(1891–1957) a French obstetrician noted for developing psychoprophylaxis, a method of childbirth preparation and pain management popularized through the book *Thank You, Dr. Lamaze* written by consumer Marjorie Karmel in 1959.

Naegele, Franz Karl—(1778–1851) a German obstetrician who developed a general rule for dating pregnancies; taught maternity care at Heidelberg University. His textbook for midwives ran for 14 editions. A pelvic dimension, the Naegele obliquity, also carries his name.

Rising, Sharon Schindler—(1940–present) founder of the CenteringPregnancy movement in 1993; changed the care paradigm by taking pregnant women out of the exam room and placing them into a group setting for assessment, education, and community building. Over 300 practices use this emerging group model of prenatal care; it has been applied to other populations as well.

Sheppard–Towner Maternity and Infancy Protection Act—an act of Congress in 1921 that provided federal funds to states for maternity and child health care; passed in response to the Children's Bureau finding that 80% of all mothers did not receive any prenatal care at that time.

Prenatal and Postnatal Care: A Woman-Centered Approach, First Edition. Edited by Robin G. Jordan, Janet L. Engstrom, Julie A. Marfell, and Cindy L. Farley.
© 2014 John Wiley & Sons, Inc. Published 2014 by John Wiley & Sons, Inc.

Introduction

Prenatal care, also referred to as antenatal care, begins "when conception is first considered and continues until labor begins" (Public Health Service. Expert Panel on the Content of Prenatal Care, 1989, p. 10). During the prenatal period, health promotion, risk assessment, and targeted interventions are processes used by prenatal health-care providers with the cooperation of women and their families to optimize the health and well-being of mothers and babies (Public Health Service. Expert Panel on the Content of Prenatal Care, 1989). While prenatal care has been commonly practiced for more than a century, it has changed little since its initial focus on the detection of preeclampsia/eclampsia in pregnant women. This medical model of pregnancy care was the standard for almost a century before the first scientific review of prenatal care was published in 1989.

A brief history of prenatal care

In 1843, the association between albuminuria and eclampsia was discovered, followed by the conclusion that the presence of proteinuria, edema, and convulsions were related to a common pathology of pregnancy. It was not until the invention of the sphygmomanometer in the late 1800s that blood pressure was included in the triad of symptoms commonly held to signify preeclampsia. Concurrently, in Scotland, Dr. John Ballantyne was advocating that obstetrics and midwifery broaden their focus of care from the processes of labor and birth to the antenatal period. He recommended routine antenatal visits and suggested that infections could be transmitted from mother to baby, and that environmental substances such as heavy metals and nicotine might adversely affect the fetus. He advocated for the first antenatal beds within hospitals and is commonly referred to as the "father" of prenatal care (Ballantyne, 1923; Dunn, 1993). In the early 1900s, the United States saw similar trends developing in antenatal surveillance for maternal complications, including the routine measurement of blood pressure in pregnancy; however, this practice did not become widespread until 20 years later (Merkatz & Thompson, 1990). In the United States, prenatal care was initially introduced to decrease infant morbidity and mortality and was promoted by social reformers and public health nurses in the early 1900s. An early program in Boston provided self-care information and emotional support by visiting nurses to women enrolled at the Boston Lying-in Hospital. Similar programs began in Baltimore, where the diagnosis of syphilis was emphasized in addition to content on personal hygiene, rest, and diet. In 1917, the Maternity Center Association (MCA) was opened in New York City, providing prenatal care that included a physical exam by a physician, visits with public health nurses at home and at the Center, and an educational emphasis on preparation for labor, birth, and infant care. The MCA reported that the outcomes for almost 9000 women over a 3-year period included a 30% reduction in neonatal death and a 21.5% reduction in maternal mortality. These early attempts at prenatal care were seen by many as a way to address the high rates of maternal and neonatal morbidity and mortality of that time (Merkatz & Thompson, 1990).

During the ensuing decades of the early 1900s, The Children's Bureau was formed to oversee efforts to decrease infant mortality. In 1921, the Sheppard–Towner Maternity and Infancy Protection Act was passed, providing funding for pregnancy education, well-baby clinics, and visiting nurse services for pregnant and postpartum women and their infants. In 1925, the Children's Bureau published prenatal care standards, which included maternal history, physical exam, and educational content for pregnancy and birth. Current-day practices differ only slightly from these early standards and point to the fact that little has changed in the structure and content of prenatal care over the last century.

Innovations to the care of childbearing women were few over the following decades. The discovery of the Rh antigen in 1940 provided insight into a common cause of fetal/infant morbidity and mortality. The immune globulin RhoGAM® was developed in 1963 preventing Rh isoimmunization disease and dramatically reducing morbidity and mortality for infants of Rh negative mothers (Merkatz & Thompson, 1990). An estimated 10,000 babies' lives are saved each year with Rh prophylaxis; Rh isoimmunization has been virtually eradicated in the developed world today. The development and widespread use of antibiotics during World War II, along with improved hygienic techniques during birth, led to a drastic reduction in puerperal or childbed fever—a form of septicemia that claimed many women's lives shortly after childbirth. Blood replacement products emerged during the same era and saved many women from death due to postpartum hemorrhage. After World War II, an emphasis on technology ensued, leading to the invention of ultrasound for visualization of the fetus and the introduction of electronic fetal monitoring. Both technologies were developed for use in high-risk pregnancies; however, both became commonplace by the 1970s.

Medications became more commonly prescribed for pregnant women with the introduction of diethylstilbestrol (DES) in the 1940s to prevent miscarriage. It was not until 1971 that the Food and Drug Administration (FDA) determined that DES was contraindicated for the prevention of miscarriage and in fact had long-term consequences such as genital cancers and reproductive tract anomalies in female offspring and epididymal cysts in male offspring. Another drug with tragic consequence was thalidomide, primarily used in European countries. Thalidomide was touted as a sedative and antiemetic, making pregnant women a potential market for this drug given the common pregnancy discomforts of insomnia, nausea, and vomiting. However, it was quickly recognized to be a teratogen, resulting in significant morbidity, mortality and major limb deformities in affected fetuses. These medications were introduced into practice without long-term studies of their effectiveness and safety for mothers and babies; the tragic outcomes pointed to the need for a more careful approach to the introduction of technologies and therapies during pregnancy (Chalmers, 1986). This is a cautionary tale, however, since most drugs are not tested on pregnant women and the long-term effects are not known until the drugs have been in widespread use for a period of time.

There were profound changes occurring in maternity care in the United States in the 1900s. The early twentieth century saw the advent of social changes that essentially moved the care of women from home to the hospital for birth. Hospitals were being built in large cities to provide care for the sick and dying; these institutions also allowed opportunities for medical education. The automobile provided mobility and transport to hospitals. Physicians began a campaign designed to discredit and replace traditional midwives who had been the maternity care providers for thousands of immigrant women, and this care now took place in hospitals. Scientific advances such as anesthesia and twilight sleep made hospital birth more attractive to many women. Many hospitals, especially in urban areas, developed clinics to care for the large numbers of indigent, immigrant women who had arrived in the United States in the previous decades. This shift from home to hospitals and from midwives to physicians contributed to the medicalization of pregnancy and childbirth that occurred during the twentieth century (Rooks, 1997).

The Childbirth Education movement, perhaps as a response to the growing medicalization of pregnancy and childbirth, began with Grantly Dick-Read and the publication of *Childbirth without Fear* in the 1940s and continued with other methods of prepared childbirth such as Lamaze and the Bradley method. All of these prepared childbirth education models focused upon the psychosocial needs of the mother, infant, and family, and sought to offer families methods to become active participants in the pregnancy and birth experience. During the second-wave feminist movement of the 1960s–1980s, childbirth preparation became more popular and was an adjunct to the traditional prenatal care that was provided

mainly by physicians. It was also during this time that both direct-entry midwifery and nurse-midwifery were beginning to grow, and nurse-midwives and direct-entry midwives were providing alternatives to the prevailing medical model of prenatal care (Rooks, 1997). Mary Breckinridge brought nurse-midwifery care to the Appalachian mountains of rural Kentucky in the 1920s with British trained midwives who traveled to homes by horseback, giving rise to the local legend that babies were brought in saddlebags. Ina May Gaskin was instrumental in the growth and professionalization of the direct-entry midwife in the United States; these midwives are the primary providers offering prenatal, labor, and birth care to women choosing out-of-hospital birth settings.

Current goals for prenatal care

In 1989, "Caring for Our Future: The Content of Prenatal Care" (CPC) was published. This landmark document was the result of a multidisciplinary panel convened by the Department of Health and Human Services to scientifically evaluate the current state of prenatal care. The goals of this Expert Panel group were to "understand, explain and define the content of prenatal care" (Public Health Service. Expert Panel on the Content of Prenatal Care, 1989, p. ii). All aspects of care were reviewed, including the prenatal visit schedule and frequency of visits, the evidence for common prenatal care practices, and the health education and psychosocial content of care during pregnancy. The resulting work created objectives for prenatal care for women, infants, and families; recommendations for maintaining certain care practices; identified practices for which there was little evidence to support their efficacy; and created a broader, more comprehensive view of prenatal care (Public Health Service. Expert Panel on the Content of Prenatal Care, 1989).

The Expert Panel also identified the goals of prenatal care for the mother, fetus/infant, and family (Table 5.1). For the first time, the goals of prenatal care were expanded to include goals for the infant and family for the first year of life. This expansion of prenatal care challenges prenatal care providers to move beyond simply identifying women at risk for medical and pregnancy-related conditions to providing effective and timely education to pregnant women and their families as they prepare for the birth of their infant and the nurturing of that infant to maturity.

Second, while the panel identified that prenatal care was a "cornerstone of healthcare delivery in our society" (Public Health Service. Expert Panel on the Content of Prenatal Care, 1989), it was often accessed too late to mitigate medical, obstetrical, and psychosocial risk

Table 5.1 Goals of Prenatal Care

Mother	Fetus/infant	Family
Increase well-being before, during, and after pregnancy; improve self-image and self-care	Increase well-being	Promote family development
Reduce mortality and morbidity, fetal loss, unnecessary interventions	Reduce preterm birth, intrauterine growth restriction, congenital anomalies, and failure to thrive	Reduce unintended pregnancy
Reduce health risks to subsequent pregnancies and overall health	Promote healthy growth and development	Reduce child neglect and family violence
Promote the development of parenting skills	Reduce child abuse and neglect, preventable acute and chronic illness, extended hospital stays after birth	

Adapted from: Public Health Service. Expert Panel on the Content of Prenatal Care. (1989). Caring for our future, the content of prenatal care: A report of the Public Health Service Expert Panel on the Content of Prenatal Care. Washington, DC: Department of Health and Human Services.

factors that are present in the first trimester of pregnancy. Therefore, preconception care, provided to women as part of comprehensive reproductive and primary care, was promoted to achieve optimal health status of the woman at the time of conception. However, preconception care is not often sought by women since half of all pregnancies in the United States, are unintended and many women have difficulty accessing services due to lack of insurance or limited availability of preconception care providers or services in their communities (Centers for Disease Control and Prevention (CDC), 2006).

Three basic components of prenatal care were identified: (1) initial and continuing risk assessment, (2) health promotion, and (3) medical and psychosocial interventions and follow-up. The Expert Panel acknowledged that while the focus on medical complications during pregnancy was important, expanding prenatal interventions to address psychosocial concerns such as stress, healthy behaviors, and financial concerns can have a positive effect on pregnancy outcomes and the family after birth. Growing evidence points to the relationship between psychosocial stressors and medical complications such as hypertension and preterm delivery (Lu,

Tache, Alexander, Kotelchuck, & Halfon, 2003; MacKey, Williams, & Tiller, 2000). These complex problems require interprofessional collaborative approaches to address the medical and psychosocial issues that complicate the pregnancies of women in the United States and across the globe.

Initial and continuing risk assessment

Risk assessment is a dynamic process that begins preconceptionally or at the first prenatal visit and continues throughout pregnancy (Public Health Service. Expert Panel on the Content of Prenatal Care, 1989). Risk assessment "enables the prenatal care provider to determine whether the woman, her fetus or infant, or the family are at increased risk of failing to achieve the objectives of prenatal care and should provide a basis for intervention" (Public Health Service. Expert Panel on the Content of Prenatal Care, 1989, p. 13).

Health promotion

Health promotion includes the education and counseling activities that are intended to assist the woman to attain, maintain, and enhance health; to support healthful behaviors; to increase knowledge about pregnancy, birth, and parenting; and to empower women to take an active role in their care during pregnancy. Individual and group sessions, as well as interpersonal interactions among women and their health-care providers, can enhance health promotion during pregnancy (Public Health Service. Expert Panel on the Content of Prenatal Care, 1989).

Medical and psychosocial interventions and follow-up

Medical and psychosocial interventions refer to care strategies planned to cure or ameliorate identified risk factors or conditions diagnosed by the prenatal health-care team. These interventions can be medically based, such as the treatment of an infection, or can address a psychosocial issue such as intimate partner violence (IPV) identified during pregnancy. Any treatment for an identified prenatal problem should always be evaluated for efficacy, improvement in symptoms, and amelioration of any adverse effects upon maternal and child health (Public Health Service. Expert Panel on the Content of Prenatal Care, 1989). This follow-up is a critical aspect of providing prenatal care.

The Expert Panel recognized that the traditional "one-size-fits-all" prenatal care package does not adequately address the needs of all women. For example, the health education needs of nulliparous women are usually different from those of parous women; and women with medical or psychosocial risk factors can have an increased need for surveillance when compared to healthy, low-risk women. Creating individualized, targeted, and appropriate prenatal care and education has the potential to deliver optimal care to the individual woman and her family in a cost-effective manner. A standard prenatal record was recommended to allow for the smooth transfer of health information across health systems during pregnancy as well as for the collection and analysis of data across populations (Public Health Service. Expert Panel on the Content of Prenatal Care, 1989). Electronic health records hold the promise of easier portability of health information from the office to the hospital, as well computer applications that provide decision support for the health-care provider.

Lastly, the panel identified that there was insufficient evidence to support many of the prenatal care practices that were common throughout pregnancy, while other care practices lacked rigorous evaluation. Recognizing that new prenatal care practices will be developed, it was recommended to systematically evaluate prenatal care practices and policies for efficacy, cost, outcomes, and patient satisfaction (Public Health Service. Expert Panel on the Content of Prenatal Care, 1989).

Updates to the "content of prenatal care"

In 2005, an update to the CPC was completed, with a review of relevant literature since the original publication (Gregory, Johnson, Johnson, & Entman, 2006). The decades after the publication of CPC have seen the introduction of many new prenatal care practices especially in genetic and laboratory screening and technological advances in antenatal fetal assessment. However, despite these advances, there has not been a significant improvement in the pregnancy-related morbidity and mortality for women and their infants (Hamilton, Martin, & Ventura, 2009; Lu et al., 2003).

One example of significant change in prenatal care practices since the CPC was originally published is in the diagnosis, treatment, and prevention of maternal–child transmission (MCT) of HIV. Routine screening for all pregnant women for HIV is now recommended, and new treatment modalities and perinatal care practices have been effective in decreasing MCT. Rapid testing is now available, and current recommendations suggest an opt-out approach to testing, with the goal of universal HIV testing for all pregnant women.

Similarly, the ensuing decades have witnessed an increase in knowledge related to genetic diseases and options for testing to identify women and their offspring at risk for these disorders. Identification of risks for genetically transmitted disorders ideally occurs prior to the pregnancy, which then allows for careful pregnancy planning, including use of reproductive technologies for

selected genetic conditions. With the advent of first-trimester screening and sequential screening in the first and second trimesters, adequate counseling for women and their families regarding their individualized risk for genetic disorders is important. Counseling for genetic screening for women and families is complex and requires providers to be knowledgeable about risks, screening, testing, and referrals, and to be sensitive to the beliefs and preferences of the individual (March of Dimes Foundation, 2003–2012).

Preterm labor and birth is another area in which advances have been made with regard to risk assessment and preventive treatments during pregnancy. The measurement of cervical length in the second trimester via transvaginal ultrasound or the CerviLenz® device, progesterone therapy for selected women with risk factors for preterm labor and birth, and laboratory testing for fetal fibronectin are new technologies that require appropriate counseling about options, including benefits, harms, and efficacy (Norwitz, Phaneuf, & Caughey, 2011).

Structure of prenatal care

In 1925, the first published prenatal care guidelines proposed a visit schedule recommending that pregnant women be seen by a physician every month for the first 6 months, then biweekly until the last month of pregnancy when visits should occur weekly (U.S. Department of Labor: Children's Bureau, 1925). There was no information provided as to how this schedule was determined other than it "was only by intelligent compromise that such a group of physicians agree on what was essential for inclusion in the standards of prenatal care" (U.S. Department of Labor: Children's Bureau, 1925, p. iii). Present-day prenatal care visit practices have changed little in regard to recommendations for when and how frequently women should engage in prenatal care (Lockwood & Lemons, 2007). Despite the urging of the Expert Panel that the number and timing of visits should be reevaluated, prenatal care most often continues to reflect the 1925 guidelines.

There are many professional, governmental, and public health organizations that contribute to the current-day recommendations for the care of women and their families during the prenatal period. Professional organizations include the American Congress of Obstetrics and Gynecology (ACOG), the American Academy of Pediatrics (AAP), the American College of Family Physicians (ACFP), and the American College of Nurse-Midwives (ACNM). Government agencies include the Agency for Healthcare Research and Quality (AHRQ), the U.S. Preventive Services Task Force (USPSTF), and the CDC (see "Resources for Health-Care Providers"). In 1983, ACOG and the AAP published the first guidelines for perinatal care, which summarized goals for prenatal care and provided clinicians with recommendations for care throughout the prenatal, intrapartum, postpartum, and neonatal periods for women, children, and their families. Regular updates have continued with the most recent guidelines published in 2012 (American Academy of Pediatrics and American College of Obstetricians and Gynecologists). The visit schedule promotes the initiation of prenatal care within the first trimester, with monthly visits occurring every month until 28 weeks when biweekly visits are suggested. Weekly visits are recommended beginning at 36 weeks until birth (Lockwood & Lemons, 2007). While the visit schedule has remained virtually unchanged, the recommendations for prenatal care content now reflect the scientific and technological advances that have evolved to become common and accepted prenatal care practices.

The schedule of prenatal visits

Evidence suggests that the preconception visit can mitigate selected maternal health, nutritional, and behavioral concerns prior to pregnancy (Johnson et al., 2006). However, over half of all pregnancies are unplanned, resulting from contraceptive failures or the failure to use contraception. Thus, the concept of preconception care needs to be introduced to all women of childbearing age during primary care or well-woman health-care encounters. Prenatal care initiated in the first trimester can result in improved health outcomes for the mother and the infant. There are differences in recommendations with the Expert Panel advocating for prenatal care to begin within the first 2 months of pregnancy (Public Health Service. Expert Panel on the Content of Prenatal Care, 1989), and ACOG/AAP recommending that care begin in the first 3 months of pregnancy (Lockwood & Lemons, 2007); however, the rationale for this difference is unclear. Latest statistics indicate that 71% of women begin prenatal care in the first trimester of pregnancy, although this varies by age, race, and ethnicity (U.S. Department of Health and Human Services, Health Resources and Services Administration, Maternal and Child Health Bureau, 2011).

The Expert Panel recommended that care should be tailored to meet the medical, psychosocial, and educational needs of women. Women experiencing their first pregnancy are expected to have greater educational needs than multiparous women; however, all women require ongoing risk assessment (Public Health Service. Expert Panel on the Content of Prenatal Care, 1989). The Expert Panel suggested that fewer visits, with more emphasis on education and health promotion, were appropriate for

Table 5.2 Prenatal Visit Schedule

	Expert Panel on Content of Prenatal Care (1989)*	American Academy of Pediatrics and American College of Obstetricians and Gynecologists (2012)
	Preconception visit	Preconception visit
First visit	6–8 weeks	Prior to 12 weeks
Second visit	Within 4 weeks	16 weeks
Third visit	14–16 weeks	20 weeks
Fourth visit	24–28 weeks	24 weeks
Fifth visit	32 weeks	28 weeks
	32–38 weeks (childbirth classes)	
Sixth visit	36 weeks	30 weeks
Seventh visit	38 weeks	32 weeks
Eighth visit	40 weeks	34 weeks
Ninth visit	41 weeks	36 weeks
Tenth visit		37 weeks
Eleventh visit		38 weeks
Twelfth visit		39 weeks
Thirteenth visit		40 weeks

Adapted from: Bloch, Dawley, and Suplee (2009), Lockwood and Lemons (2007), Public Health Service. Expert Panel on the Content of Prenatal Care (1989).
*Low-risk, primiparous women.

low-risk women. It was postulated that women who received education about pregnancy, healthy behaviors, and symptoms of pregnancy complications would require fewer visits, utilize community resources when appropriate, and be well prepared for birth and parenting (Public Health Service. Expert Panel on the Content of Prenatal Care, 1989; Walker & Koniak-Griffin, 1997) (see Table 5.2). The World Health Organization recommends a minimum of four prenatal visits (World Health Organization, 2013); however, less than half of women worldwide achieve this goal due to harsh disparities between developed and developing nations.

How much prenatal care is enough?

What constitutes enough prenatal care? In the late 1960s, data collection regarding the timing of the initiation of prenatal care and the number of prenatal visits began with the addition of this information to the Certificate of Live Birth. Subsequently, there have been several attempts to determine how best to measure the adequacy of prenatal care. Such information can be used to assist researchers and policy makers in the assessment of the sufficiency of prenatal care resources, the effectiveness of prenatal care in addressing morbidities and mortalities, and the identification of areas for research and changes in health policies. ACOG recommends that care begins in the first trimester (prior to 12 weeks) completing 12–14 visits throughout the pregnancy with a minimum of 9 visits to be considered adequate (Alexander & Kotelchuck, 1998; Lockwood & Lemons, 2007; Stringer, 1998). The Kessner Index, developed in the 1970s with support from the Institute of Medicine (IOM), considers in what trimester care was initiated, how many prenatal visits were attended, and when the infant was born (Alexander & Kotelchuck, 1998; Bloch et al., 2009; Stringer, 1998). Care was deemed to be adequate if the number of prenatal visits at delivery met or exceeded ACOG recommendations, while inadequate care was defined as less than 50% of the adequate visit criteria (Stringer, 1998). Later, the Adequacy of Prenatal Care Utilization (APNCU) Index was developed by Kotelchuck, proposing separate assessments based upon when prenatal care was initiated and how many visits occurred between initiation and delivery. The number of visits is compared to the number of expected visits based upon ACOG recommendations to evaluate adequacy (Kotelchuck, 1994; Stringer, 1998). All of these indices are commonly used in research and evaluation of prenatal care, but they address the quantity, not the quality of care.

What happens in prenatal care?

The focus upon how many prenatal care encounters a woman receives only provides a snapshot of the quantity of care. While some evidence suggests that more prenatal care visits may result in improved outcomes for mothers and infants, the quality of the prenatal care also has an influence on the health and psychosocial outcomes for women and families. The Expert Panel examined the content of care and developed a framework for organizing prenatal care based upon available evidence. Their recommendations for risk assessment included assessment of maternal blood pressure and laboratory studies. Interventions that resulted in improved maternal and/ or infant outcomes included avoidance of substance abuse, nutritional information, appropriate weight gain in pregnancy, vitamin/mineral supplementation, and breastfeeding support and advice (Public Health Service. Expert Panel on the Content of Prenatal Care, 1989). Ideally, the provision of appropriate health promotion content during pregnancy supports changes in maternal behavior. For example, if a pregnant woman who smokes is provided with information regarding the dangers of smoking and is given resources to curtail or quit smoking, the expectation is that she will either stop or attempt to stop smoking. However, health behaviors are complex and change is based on more than knowledge.

Providing all the recommended health information and verifying the woman's understanding during prenatal care visits is challenging in the current model of prenatal care due to time constraints in the clinical setting. An early study, which looked at a large population of almost 1000 women, found that only 32% of women reported receiving all the recommended prenatal advice (Kogan, Alexander, Kotelchuck, Nagey, & Jack, 1994). Another study with the same population found that women who did not receive all the recommended health advice during pregnancy were at higher risk for delivering a low-birth-weight (LBW) baby (Kogan, Alexander, Kotelchuck, & Nagey, 1994). In today's health-care environments, some of the essential prenatal education is provided by support staff or through written or electronic media sources.

Integrating quality into prenatal care

In 2001, the IOM released a landmark report focusing on the changes needed in our health-care system to improve safety and quality across all health-care settings. Their recommendations were intended to serve as a framework to be used by the government, health insurers, health-care providers, and consumers as they prepared for a twenty-first century health-care system. Their recommendations included the following:

- *Safe*—avoiding injuries to patients from the care that is intended to help them
- *Effective*—providing services based on scientific knowledge to all who could benefit and refraining from providing services to those not likely to benefit (avoiding underuse and overuse, respectively)
- *Patient centered*—providing care that is respectful of and responsive to individual patient preferences, needs, and values and ensuring that patient values guide all clinical decisions
- *Timely*—reducing waits and sometimes harmful delays for both those who receive and those who give care
- *Efficient*—avoiding waste, including waste of equipment, supplies, ideas, and energy
- *Equitable*—providing care that does not vary in quality because of personal characteristics such as gender, ethnicity, geographic location, and socioeconomic status (Institute of Medicine, 2001).

While the recommendations of the IOM for improving the quality of care are not complex, the ability of the health-care system to adapt to the needed changes has been poor. Despite evidence about the quantity and the quality of prenatal care, perinatal morbidity and mortality statistics have not significantly improved, and in many sectors, undesirable outcomes have actually increased (CDC, 2013a). For example, more than half a million premature infants (<37 weeks' gestational age) are born each year in the United States, and the overall preterm birth rate of 12.7% represents a 36% increase over the last 20 years (Hamilton et al., 2009). There are substantial health disparities associated with prematurity, LBW, and maternal health outcomes such as pregnancy weight gain; for example, in African Americans, the preterm birth rate is 18.3%, while the Hispanic rate is 12.2%, and the white rate is 11.7%. African American women are about two to three times more likely to have inadequate weight gain and LBW infants during pregnancy when compared with white women (Hamilton et al., 2009) Disparities in the quality of prenatal care have also been found based upon race/ethnicity, income, and prenatal provider type (Gavin, Adams, Hartmann, Benedict, & Chireau, 2004). Latina women and African American women report discussing recommended prenatal care content less often than white women (Kogan, Alexander, Kotelchuck, & Nagey, 1994; Vonderheid, Montgomery, & Norr, 2003; Vonderheid, Norr, & Handler, 2007). These variations in the quality of prenatal care have been linked to an increase in the risk of LBW, prematurity, and infant mortality (Kogan, Alexander, Kotelchuck, & Nagey, 1994).

More recently in 2011, an evaluation by the United States Preventative Services Task Force (USPSTF) examined critical, evidence-based health recommendations specifically for women, within the context of upcoming health-care reform and expansion of health-care benefits to all Americans. The recommendations that directly relate to prenatal care include

- screening for gestational diabetes in pregnant women between 24 and 28 weeks of gestation and at the first prenatal visit for pregnant women identified to be at high risk for diabetes
- counseling on sexually transmitted infections for sexually active women annually
- providing the full range of FDA-approved contraceptive methods, sterilization procedures, and patient education and counseling for women with reproductive capacity
- offering comprehensive lactation support, counseling, and costs of renting breastfeeding equipment; a trained provider should provide counseling services to all pregnant women and to those in the postpartum period to ensure the successful initiation and duration of breastfeeding

- screening and counseling for interpersonal and domestic violence; screening and counseling involve elicitation of information from women and adolescents about current and past violence and abuse in a culturally sensitive and supportive manner to address current health concerns about safety and other current or future health problems
- advising at least one well-woman preventive care visit annually for adult women to obtain the recommended preventive services, including preconception and prenatal care; the committee also recognizes that several visits may be needed to obtain all necessary recommended preventive services, depending on a woman's health status, health needs, and other risk factors (Institute of Medicine, 2011).

A new model of prenatal care: CenteringPregnancy

CenteringPregnancy is a group model of prenatal care that was developed and implemented in 1993 by Sharon Schindler Rising, a nurse-midwife. The ensuing decades have seen a rapid uptake of this group model among obstetrical providers, including midwives, obstetricians, nurse practitioners, and family medicine physicians. CenteringPregnancy builds upon the Expert Panel recommendations and combines the essentials of risk assessment, education, and support and bundles prenatal services into a cohesive model of care (Rising, 1998; Rising, Kennedy, & Klima, 2004). In CenteringPregnancy, 8–12 women with similar due dates are invited to join a group after their initial prenatal visit. Women learn self-care skills such as measuring their own weight, blood pressure, and gestational age, and then recording this information in their medical record. This self-assessment is followed by a short individual assessment with their prenatal care provider in the group space and includes assessment of fundal height, fetal position and presentation, fetal heart sounds, and maternal well-being. Concerns and questions are brought to the group for discussion. Healthy snacks and opportunities for socializing among group participants build community and provide peer support for all members.

Group care changes the paradigm of traditional health care and builds upon the recommendation of the IOM for redesigning health care. Groups are patient centered as the group directs conversations to issues that are important and relevant to their lives and experiences. Groups are efficient for women, their providers, and health systems. They are planned well in advance so that women know when all their prenatal appointments will be and health centers can utilize individual exam room space for seeing other patients. Groups are efficient since health-care providers need to convey important information only once and other prenatal care services such as social work and lactation support can be bundled into the group setting. Groups always start and end on time so the time is productive for the women and the prenatal care provider. One participant remarked "We came at the same time, we left at the same time and something happened the whole time we were there."

CenteringPregnancy has been shown to make a difference in prenatal outcomes; however, a recent Cochrane Review highlights the early and evolving nature of the evidence base in this area (Homer et al., 2012). In the largest randomized controlled trial (RCT) to date, over 1000 women enrolled in group care had a 33% reduction in premature birth when compared to women in individual care (Ickovics et al., 2007). When African American women were evaluated in this study, their premature birth rate was 41% lower than those enrolled in individual care. Women in groups were more satisfied with their care, initiated breastfeeding more frequently and felt better prepared for labor, birth, and parenting (Ickovics et al., 2007). A retrospective analysis found that adolescents enrolled in group care had increased attendance at health-care visits, lower rates of preterm birth and LBW babies, and were more satisfied with their care (Grady & Bloom, 2004). When the model was implemented in a large urban public health setting, women in groups were found to have higher rates of attendance at prenatal care visits, improved pregnancy weight gain, and higher satisfaction with care. This study also evaluated the prenatal care provider's experience with the group model and found that providers believed the model to be an effective model for patient education and provided the opportunity for learning and social support (Klima, Vonderheid, Norr, & Handler, 2009).

Making group prenatal care work

As group care changes how health care is delivered, system change is necessary and health-care providers and support staff require training to become facilitative leaders. Experience suggests that involving all key stakeholders within an organization helps to create a climate of change that supports CenteringPregnancy. The Centering Healthcare Institute (CHI) is the nonprofit organization that supports health-care systems and providers to adapt to a new model of group care. Health-care providers and staff who plan to facilitate group care must attend training sessions to learn group skills and facilitative leadership, and to gain practical experience in conducting CenteringPregnancy groups. Health systems must adapt to changes in scheduling systems and work duties, and may even adapt physical space to accommodate groups. The 13 Essential Elements, created to define

Table 5.3   13 Essential Elements of CenteringPregnancy (Centering Healthcare Institute, 2013)

- Health assessment occurs within the group space.
- Participants are involved in self-care activities.
- Groups are conducted in circle.
- Opportunities for socialization are provided.
- Groups honor the contributions of each member.
- A facilitative leadership style is used.
- Group size is optimal to promote the process.
- Groups are stable but not rigid.
- There is stability of group leadership.
- Each session has an overall plan.
- Attention is given to core content; emphasis may vary.
- Involvement of support people is optional.
- There is ongoing evaluation of outcomes.

Reproduced with Permission from the Centering Healthcare Institute.

the group health-care experience, reflect the recommendations of the Expert Panel on Prenatal Care as well as the recommendations for health-care redesign from the IOM (see Table 5.3).

Components of prenatal care

Assessment

Assessment during the prenatal period refers to the collection of medical, nutritional, obstetrical, psychosocial, and family histories, as well as physical assessment of the mother and fetus. Laboratory studies collected at the initial and subsequent prenatal visits assess selected aspects of maternal and fetal health at the onset of prenatal care, as well as affirmation of ongoing wellness and early detection of pathology. Physical assessment of the mother is comprehensive and includes a physical exam along with a detailed exam of the reproductive system at entry into prenatal care. Episodic physical assessment occurs at subsequent prenatal visits and focuses on pregnancy-related changes, overall physical well-being with special attention to potential signs of pregnancy complications. Targeted physical assessments are performed whenever there are signs and symptoms of emerging problems or coexisting disorders. Additionally, assessment of the fetus is ongoing throughout the pregnancy. Ultrasound screening is commonly performed during early pregnancy to verify viable intrauterine pregnancy, confirm or assign gestational age, assess fetal anatomy, and measure fetal growth and development. Lastly, assessment of past and current psychosocial issues, including mental health status, substance abuse, and environmental issues such as housing, socioeconomic concerns, and safety, is addressed at entry into care and at each subsequent visit. Risk assessment is integral to each prenatal encounter to evaluate the presence or absence of factors or conditions associated with adverse perinatal outcomes for the mother and or fetus/infant (Merkatz & Thompson, 1990). Risk assessment may also improve the quality of care for women and families, and align prenatal care resources to women so that they receive the appropriate levels of care based upon their individualized risk status (Merkatz & Thompson, 1990).

While risk assessment is an important component of prenatal care, there is no standardized system that accurately predicts individual risk. The evaluation of risk is confounded due to complexity of numerous variables, their interactions with each other, and the fact that some conditions may be more highly associated with adverse outcomes than others. Concentrating prenatal resources solely on women with risk factors may adversely affect women who have been deemed low risk. Other women can experience an adverse outcome without any identifiable risk factors. Some conditions, such as tobacco abuse, are well studied with known sequelae; however, not every woman who smokes experiences these adverse outcomes. Other conditions, such as maternal obesity, may be less well studied or do not have easily implemented interventions to address the identified risks (Enkin et al., 2000; Merkatz & Thompson, 1990). Risks that involve long-standing habits or lifestyle preferences require a readiness to make behavior change on the part of the woman and persistent effort in creating and maintaining this behavior change. Refer to Chapter 8, "Risk Assessment during Pregnancy," for further detail.

Health history: Initial visit

Ideally, the maternal history is obtained at a preconception visit so that health conditions and health behaviors that can adversely affect pregnancy are identified, discussed, and ameliorated. The Expert Panel on Prenatal Care reviewed all components of the health history and reviewed the scientific evidence for the components of the health history that may impact maternal and fetal pregnancy outcome. With few exceptions, reviewing the health history on all women at the onset of prenatal care is an important activity and is an integral component of evaluating risk status and planning for comprehensive care. The health history not only provides a snapshot of past and current health status but also identifies health behaviors that can negatively impact the pregnancy and can be impacted during the pregnancy. Knowledge of the health history allows health-care providers to tailor the care in pregnancy to specific health risks and educational opportunities (see Table 5.4).

Pregnancy dating is an important activity during the first prenatal visit and the menstrual history is a critical

component of this assessment. Ascertaining the normal last menstrual period (LMP) is the first step in determining the gestational age. The reliability of this measure can be affected by maternal recall, history of irregular menses, recent contraceptive use, lactation, or medication use. In the early 1880s, German obstetrician Dr. Franz Karl Naegele determined that the mean gestational age of human pregnancy was 280 days or 40 weeks and suggested that the estimated delivery date (EDD) could be established by subtracting 3 months, adding 1 week, and 1 year to the date of the first day of the LMP. Ninety percent of all women with a known LMP will deliver by the forty-first week using Naegele's rule. Mean human gestation length has been estimated at ranges between 281 and 287 days with the average being 283 days, somewhat greater than the estimate based upon Naegele's rule (Merkatz & Thompson, 1990). Accurate dating of the pregnancy is critical to the identification of a reliable estimated date of birth (EDB), accurately interpreting selected prenatal genetic laboratory screening, effectively caring for women who experience premature labor or post-term pregnancy, and eliminating risks associated with procedures and interventions (Merkatz & Thompson, 1990). For example, a misdated pregnancy may erroneously indicate that a pregnancy is post-term and requires induction of labor. Gestational age wheels are commonly used by health-care providers to calculate the estimated gestational age of the pregnancy; however, slight variations among wheels are common and the wheels are based on a standard 28-day menstrual cycle. More recently, numerous electronic methods of calculating the gestational age of the pregnancy have become available. With the advent of electronic medical records, gestational age can be determined by the computer based upon clinical data. Similarly, many Internet-based applications exist that compute gestational age based upon maternal clinical data. Ultrasound is recommended when the LMP is unknown or unreliable. Ultrasound fetal age estimations are a more accurate measure of gestational age when performed early in the pregnancy.

The *pregnancy history* will identify any previous pregnancy-related conditions that can impact the current pregnancy. When eliciting the pregnancy history, it is important to explore the circumstances of all pregnancy losses, gestational age at which they occurred, what precipitated the loss, and what, if any, evaluation occurred after the loss such as genetic testing or autopsy. This information will highlight the potential risk for chromosomal abnormalities, premature labor, or other pregnancy conditions likely to recur. Any operative procedures such as cesarean section should be evaluated along with the indications for the surgery, the conduct of the

Table 5.4 Medical and Psychosocial Prenatal History Content

Content	Evidence of efficacy from content of prenatal care (1989 & update 2005)	Health information collected
Sociodemographic	Good	Name, age, racial/ethnic group, relationship status, insurance status, emergency contact information
Menstrual history	Good	Menarche, date of last menstrual period (LMP), regularity, frequency and length of menses, length and character of LMP, bleeding or spotting since LMP
Past pregnancy history	Good	Gravidity, parity, history of live births, miscarriage (<20 weeks), fetal loss (circumstances), stillbirths (circumstances) and living children; history of ectopic pregnancy; pregnancy outcomes; type of birth (vaginal birth, operative vaginal birth, cesarean section, vaginal birth after cesarean section [VBAC]); history of infertility and any infertility treatments
Contraceptive history	Not studied	Previous method use, date of last use
Sexual history	Not studied	Onset of sexual activity, number of partners, current partner, past/current partner behavior risks, sexual practices, use of safer sex practices; history of sexually transmitted infections of self and partner, including treatment
Medical/surgical history	Good	Preexisting chronic or episodic maternal medical conditions, especially those that may adversely affect the current pregnancy. These include but are not limited to hypertension, diabetes, thyroid disease, cardiac disease, blood disorders, respiratory illness, and gastrointestinal disorders. Past and current treatments should be obtained. Surgical history includes all relevant surgeries that may impact pregnancy, especially any uterine surgery.
Infection history	Good	Common childhood illness; communicable diseases; sexually transmitted infections
Family/genetic history	Good	Three-generation family pedigree; medical history in first-degree relatives, especially for conditions with familial tendencies such as diabetes; mental, behavioral cognitive problems, atypical physical features or problems, chromosomal abnormalities, single-gene conditions, consanguinity
Nutrition	Good	Overall dietary history, access to food, vitamin/mineral supplementation, special dietary concerns, vegetarianism, fish intake, exposure to teratogens or infectious agents
Smoking	Good	Onset, amount, exposure to second-hand smoke
Alcohol	Good	Onset, amount, duration of use, type of alcohol, family history, dependence. Screening tools are available.
Illicit drugs	Good	Type of drug and how it is used; onset, duration, and amount; related behaviors such as sex for drugs or needle-sharing
Social support	Fair	Multiple measures, depression, family, relationship
Stress	Fair	Multiple measures, acute versus chronic, coping and support resources, external resources, amenable to interventions, community stressors, financial resources
Intimate partner violence	Good	History, current abuse, type and severity, resources, children, readiness for intervention, safety plan
Mental health	Not studied	History or current mental illness, past and current treatment, medications, safety, potential for self-harm or harm to others
Teratogen exposure	Good	Environmental, occupational, medication, herbs, home, pets
Occupational	Fair	Type of work, heavy lifting, repetitive work tasks, hours per day per week, exposure to chemical or environmental hazards
Activity/exercise	Good	Exercise, type and frequency, resources for increasing activity level, limitations

labor, and any complications arising from the operative intervention. A history of infertility treatments and assisted reproductive technologies can alert the provider to an increased risk for multifetal pregnancy.

Sexual history provides an opportunity to evaluate risk for sexually transmitted infections and sexual practices that can continue to increase risk for the mother and fetus. The sexual history should be elicited with a nonjudgmental approach and should include the following four P's:

1. *Partners*—number and gender, health behavior of partners such as substance abuse, condom use, length of current sexual relationship
2. *Practices*—sexual practices and safer sex practices will determine the woman's current risk status and can indicate need for additional screening for sexually transmitted infections
3. *Protection*—Are condoms regularly used? Her perception of her own risk status should be explored. Does she have concerns about exposure to STI or partner's risk factors?
4. *Previous history*—Explore the history of past STI and treatments. Does she currently have symptoms? Was her partner treated (CDC, n.d.)?

The *infection history* will identify preexisting immunity and risks for infection during the pregnancy and will also identify the need for immunization during and after pregnancy. Depending on the history of childhood disease and immunization, a pregnant woman may have immunity to infections, may be at risk for infections, or may require targeted education to avoid infectious diseases during the pregnancy. Planning for postpartum immunizations will help women decrease their risk of selected infectious diseases throughout the lifespan and particularly during future pregnancies.

Family history encompasses the evaluation for medical conditions that can place the pregnant woman at a higher risk during pregnancy and may require additional screening and/or evaluation during pregnancy. For example, a woman with a strong family history of diabetes may be at higher risk for diabetes or gestational diabetes and may require additional screening (Lockwood & Lemons, 2007). An important component of the family history is the genetic history. Histories that are significant for familial or hereditary diseases will alert the provider to the need for additional counseling, testing, or referral to a genetic counselor. Women should be provided with accurate information regarding personalized risk, screening, pregnancy options, benefits and harms of testing options, and any potential outcomes related to the particular genetic problem (Merkatz & Thompson, 1990). While genetic issues can be complex,

all prenatal care providers should be able to discuss basic genetic counseling and testing and to perform a basic three-generation pedigree with genetic history. Numerous resources exist for health-care providers to become more proficient regarding the genetic components of prenatal care, such as the March of Dimes and the International Society of Nurses in Genetics (ISONG).

Nutritional history not only provides an assessment of the current diet and nutritional status of a pregnant woman but can also identify areas of dietary deficiencies that may be amenable to interventions. For example, sufficient intake of folic acid during the periconceptional period reduces the incidence of neural tube defects (Gregory et al., 2006; Lockwood & Lemons, 2007). The nutritional history also identifies dietary practices that can impact the pregnancy. For example, women who eat a vegan diet may require information about additional sources of protein, vitamins, and minerals to meet the recommended allowances for pregnancy. Women who report consuming foods that can negatively impact pregnancy, such as eating certain fish species, raw meat, or certain cheeses, may be at increased risk for exposure to toxins or infectious diseases and need targeted information to make the necessary dietary changes (Gregory et al., 2006). A review of maternal diet can also indicate the need to supplement the diet with vitamins and minerals. Guidelines from the USPHTF as well as the IOM outline dietary recommendations for pregnant women based upon age (Lockwood & Lemons, 2007).

The *psychosocial history* explores the life and work concerns of a pregnant woman and can highlight areas for support, education, and additional resources. Stress and lack of social support can impact pregnancy outcomes, so it is important to elicit the woman's perceptions of stress and her coping mechanisms, as well as her support systems. This is accomplished through dialogue and open-ended questioning throughout the pregnancy; tools can be used to quantitatively measure stress and coping. Perceived stress can result from many aspects of life such as family, work, or relationships. Financial concerns can also lead to additional stressors such as housing and basic resources like food. The psychosocial history will provide direction for targeted resources that may be needed. It is not uncommon that multiple resources will be needed to address multiple concerns. It is important for prenatal care providers to become familiar with community resources and agencies that can provide necessary services to women during pregnancy. The Expert Panel recommended that the psychosocial history take place at the initial visit and then regularly updated at each subsequent prenatal visit (Public Health Service. Expert Panel on the Content of Prenatal Care, 1989).

Health history: Subsequent visit

At each subsequent visit, the prenatal care provider should assess the woman for signs and symptoms associated with common pregnancy problems. Changes in lifestyle, circumstances, exposures, and recent illness should also be assessed. Prior to term, symptoms of premature labor, vaginal bleeding, or leakage of amniotic fluid should be assessed at each visit. Common pregnancy changes and discomforts should be explored. A review of the psychosocial history should be completed with special attention to violence, depression, and substance use if applicable.

Physical assessment

Initial visit

A general physical examination should be conducted on all women at the first prenatal visit. Since pregnancy affects all body systems, each system should be evaluated and the findings recorded (Gabbe et al., 2012; Public Health Service. Expert Panel on the Content of Prenatal Care, 1989). Measuring height and weight on all women is beneficial, along with calculation of the body mass index (BMI). Prepregnancy weight is important as it will guide the recommendations for weight gain during the pregnancy. Blood pressure, pulse, and respirations should be measured on all women at the initial visit. A pelvic exam to assess for uterine size is especially important in early pregnancy, before 12–14 weeks, and can help in confirming gestational age (Gabbe et al., 2012). Clinical pelvimetry, although commonly done at the initial visit, was studied by the Expert Panel and was found to have poor evidence supporting its efficacy (Public Health Service. Expert Panel on the Content of Prenatal Care, 1989). However, it may be useful to assess pelvic adequacy in late pregnancy or during labor. Auscultation of the fetal heart sounds with a handheld Doppler ultrasound device can begin at 11–12 weeks of gestation, although the heart sounds may be heard earlier depending upon maternal habitus and the position of the uterus. Assessment of the location of the fundal height can begin when the uterus becomes an abdominal organ sometime after the twelfth week of pregnancy. The measurement of the fundal height provides information regarding the growing uterus; however, its accuracy is limited by the skill of the practitioner, maternal characteristics such as the status of the maternal bladder or abdominal adiposity, and the angle of the examination table. The most common way to measure fundal height is to place a tape measure on the superior border of the symphysis pubis and to bring the tape measure across the contour of the maternal abdomen, in the midline, to the top of the fundus. Using this method, the centimeters should approximately equal the weeks of gestation after 20 weeks' gestation (Varney, Kriebs, & Gegor, 2004).

Subsequent visits

At each subsequent visit, maternal blood pressure and weight should be obtained. Weight gain since the last visit and since the onset of pregnancy can inform the woman and her provider about the adequacy and pattern of weight gain. Fundal height in centimeters is measured at each visit along with locating and counting the fetal heart rate. Assessment of maternal perception of fetal movement usually begins in the second trimester and is determined at each visit. Auscultation of the fetal heart rate using a handheld Doppler ultrasound device can begin as early as 11 weeks and at 16 to 20 weeks if using a fetoscope (Gabbe et al., 2012; Public Health Service. Expert Panel on the Content of Prenatal Care, 1989). Beginning in the third trimester, Leopold's maneuvers are performed. These maneuvers are a series of abdominal examinations that can help the prenatal care provider determine the fetal lie, presentation, position, and engagement of the fetal presenting part into the pelvis (Varney et al., 2004). The abdominal exam can also assist the health-care provider in estimating the fetal weight. Routine cervical examination is not recommended until the forty-first week of pregnancy by the Expert Panel but may be appropriate earlier in women at risk for premature labor (Gabbe et al., 2012; Public Health Service. Expert Panel on the Content of Prenatal Care, 1989). The Expert Panel found insufficient evidence to recommend routine urine screening for protein and glucose at each prenatal visit in the absence of symptoms of preeclampsia or infection (Public Health Service. Expert Panel on the Content of Prenatal Care, 1989).

Laboratory

Routine laboratory studies were evaluated by the Expert Panel, and most of these tests were found to be an important component to prenatal care and risk assessment. Routine laboratory screening at the first prenatal visit was important in the diagnosis of anemia, certain infections, and determination of the Rh factor. Subsequent to the Expert Panel, recommendations for additional laboratory studies have been suggested due to new evidence of their association with improved pregnancy outcomes. Numerous organizations and professional organizations contribute to the recommendations for laboratory testing during pregnancy. Not all types of testing are available to all women due to geographic location, financial resources, or site of care. Current recommendations for routine laboratory studies and the appropriate timing are found in Table 5.5.

Table 5.5 Recommended Laboratory Studies in Pregnancy

Laboratory study	When	Population to be screened	Recommended by whom	Evidence
Hemoglobin or hematocrit	Initial, 24–28 weeks, and 36 weeks in selected populations	All	EPPC	Good
Blood type and Rh factor*	Initial	All	EPPC	Good
Rubella titer	Initial	All	EPPC	Good
Urine dipstick for protein and glucose	Initial	All	EPPC	Good
Tuberculosis	Initial	Some	EPPC	Fair
Gonorrhea	Initial and 36 weeks	Under age 25 and those at risk	EPPC USPHTF	Good B
Chlamydia[†]	Initial and 36 weeks	Under age 25 and those at risk	EPPC, USPHTF	Good B, C
Syphilis[‡]	Initial and 24–28 weeks	All	EPPC USPHTF	Good A
Urine culture for asymptomatic bacteriuria	12–16 weeks or first visit	All	USPHTF	A
Hepatitis B	Initial	All	EPPC USPHTF	Good A
HIV (opt out)	Initial	All	EPPC USPHTF	Good A
Pap smear	Initial	Age 21 and over, every 1–3 years dependent upon age and past screening	ACOG	Good
Herpes[§]	Initial	Selected populations	EPPC	Fair
Varicella	Initial based upon history	Selected populations	EPPC	Fair
Hemoglobinopathies	Initial	Selected populations	EPPC	Good
Toxoplasmosis	Initial	Selected populations	EPPC	Good
Illicit Drug Screen (offered)	Initial	All	EPPC	Good

Recommended by either the Expert Panel on Prenatal Care (EPPC), United States Preventative Health Task Force (USPHTF), or ACOG. EPPC labeled evidence as good, fair, and poor, USPHTF rates evidence as A, B, C with A being the highest level of evidence.
*The Expert Panel did not include blood type, but it is routinely assessed on all pregnant women in the United States.
[†]Chlamydia is now routinely tested concurrently with gonorrhea. In selected populations, rescreening at 36 weeks may be indicated.
[‡]Syphilis may be repeated in selected populations at 24–28 weeks.
[§]The USPHTF recommends against screening asymptomatic women at any time during pregnancy.

Genetic screening

Prenatal genetic screening has expanded significantly since the Expert Panel reviewed the scientific literature. Some genetic screening is routinely offered to all women, while other tests are offered to selected groups based upon racial or ethnic heritage, age, or other risk factors. All discussions regarding genetic testing should be based upon the principles of shared decision making with the woman and/or her family. Informed consent is necessary to assure that the pregnant woman understands the voluntary nature of genetic testing, the purpose of the test, the limitations of the test, what she will do with the information, and what the implications are for herself, her baby and future pregnancies (March of Dimes Foundation, 2003–2012) (see Table 5.6). Prenatal genetic testing is reviewed in more detail in Chapter 9.

Table 5.6 Recommended Genetic Screening Testing to Be Offered during Pregnancy

Disease or condition	Genetic screening test	Offer	Timing	Comments
Trisomy 21, 18	Pregnancy-associated plasma protein A (PAPP-A) and free human chorionic gonadotropin (hCG)	All	First trimester between 11 and 13 weeks	May be done in conjunction with nuchal translucency
Neural tube defects	Maternal serum alpha-fetoprotein (MSAFP) (if PAPP-A and hCG were done in first trimester) QUAD screen (MSAFP, unconjugated estriol, hCG, and inhibin-A	All	15–21 weeks	May be done alone or in conjunction with first-trimester screening
Hemoglobinopathies: sickle cell disease	Hemoglobin electrophoresis	African American and African descent	Initial prenatal visit	
Hemoglobinopathies: thalassemia	Complete blood count (CBC)	Southeast Asian, Mediterranean, and Hispanic	Initial prenatal visit	Hemoglobin electrophoresis dependent upon the results of CBC
Cystic fibrosis	Carrier screening	All	First trimester	More sensitive with certain ethnic groups. More complex testing required if + family history. Partner will need testing if positive.
Tay–Sachs disease	Carrier screening	Ashkenazi Jewish, Cajun, French Canadian	First trimester	
Canavan's disease	Carrier Screening	Ashkenazi Jewish	First trimester	
Familial dysautonomia	Carrier screening	Ashkenazi Jewish	First trimester	

Sources: ACOG Practice Bulletin Screening for Fetal Chromosomal Abnormalities Number 17, January 2007. *Obstetrics and Gynecology, 109*(1), 217–227;
ACOG Committee Opinion Number 442, October 2009. Preconception and Prenatal Carrier Screening for Genetic Diseases in Individuals of Eastern European Jewish Descent. Retrieved April 12, 2013 http://www.acog.org/~/media/Committee%20Opinions/Committee%20on%20Genetics/co442.pdf?dmc=1&ts=20120503T1524205976;
ACOG Committee Opinion Number 486, April 2011. Update on Carrier Screening for Cystic Fibrosis. Retrieved April 12, 2013 http://www.acog.org/Resources%20And%20Publications/Committee%20Opinions/Committee%20on%20Genetics/Update%20on%20Carrier%20Screening%20for%20Cystic%20Fibrosis.aspx.
ACOG Recommendations for Carrier Screening (Gregory et al., 2006).

Diagnostic testing

Diagnostic testing in prenatal care was not evaluated by the Expert Panel; however, the use of diagnostic testing has increased significantly over the last decade. Ultrasound is the most commonly used diagnostic test in pregnancy and can provide information about many normal events as well as abnormal processes, First-trimester ultrasound is an accurate way to confirm the viability of an intrauterine pregnancy with the identification of a fetus with cardiac activity and confirm that the pregnancy is implanted in the uterus instead of an extrauterine site. A frequent use of ultrasound is the confirmation of gestational age; it can also be also be used to accurately estimate gestational age and establish an EDD in the absence of a reliable LMP (Gabbe et al., 2012). Ultrasound also plays a role in genetic screening with the evaluation of nuchal translucency. Specially trained personnel can measure the neck of the fetus and identify abnormalities; when coupled with genetic serum screening, ultrasound can identify a fetus at risk for several trisomies, allowing for an earlier diagnosis than other available methods.

After the first trimester, ultrasound can be used as a screening exam for structural abnormalities at 18–20 weeks of gestation. Ultrasound can also play a role in evaluating the fetal anatomy, placental position and implantation, amniotic fluid volume, and fetal growth as needed by clinical indications. Abnormalities identified on a standard ultrasound may require additional information, such as a fetal echocardiogram to more closely examine the structure and function of the fetal heart. Doppler studies can evaluate the placental blood flow and abnormalities, which may indicate a compromised blood flow to the placenta and fetus (Gabbe et al., 2012; Lockwood & Lemons, 2007). Fetal well-being may also be evaluated with ultrasound by using the biophysical profile. The purpose of antenatal surveillance of the fetus is to identify pregnancies at risk for stillbirth, decrease the risk of intrauterine fetal demise, and prevent unnecessary intervention in pregnancies in which there is no benefit to the cessation of the pregnancy through intervention (Lockwood & Lemons, 2007). Increased risk to the fetus is identified through the maternal history, such as a previous fetal demise, a maternal condition such as hypertension, reports of decreased maternal perception of fetal movement, or a prolonged pregnancy. The assessment of fetal well-being is reviewed in detail in Chapter 10.

Preventative care

Prenatal care is a form of preventative care in many respects. Goals include prevention of adverse pregnancy outcomes through the identification of risk factors, treatment of ongoing health issues, and utilization of health education and preventive health practices to adjust to pregnancy changes and to prepare for a new baby. Most preventative care focuses upon maternal care needs but can provide for improved health outcomes for infants as well. One such example is immunization.

Immunization

Immunizations not only provide immunity for women for vaccine-preventable illnesses but can provide passive immunity for the newborn. While the most opportune time to evaluate for the immunization needs of women is during the preconception period, many vaccines are safe to administer during pregnancy and are recommended to promote optimal maternal health. Live virus vaccines are contraindicated during pregnancy, but can be given in the immediate postpartum period, even if breastfeeding. The CDC maintains the most current listing of recommended immunizations for women during and after pregnancy (see Fig. 5.1).

Oral health

Recent evidence suggests that poor oral health may increase the risk of preterm delivery. Periodontal disease has been identified as an independent risk factor for preterm birth (Gregory et al., 2006) Encouraging good oral health including regular brushing and flossing, as well as cleaning and treatment of dental caries, is an important preventative health practice during pregnancy. Women should be encouraged to visit the dentist early in pregnancy. During pregnancy, it is safe to receive shielded dental X-rays, have local anesthesia if needed,

and to use antibiotics that are safe in pregnancy, as needed for dental procedures. Tetracycline and related antibiotics should never be used during pregnancy as they can cause permanent tooth staining in infants exposed during pregnancy. Pregnant women may notice that their gums can bleed more easily during regular tooth brushing, and this observation can prompt questions regarding oral health during regular prenatal visits (Lockwood & Lemons, 2007).

Mental health

Mental health issues are an important component of the prenatal care. Maternal stress has been linked to prematurity as well as poor infant health outcomes (Loomans et al., 2012). A woman's ability to cope with the changes related to pregnancy, transition to parenthood, and new motherhood will directly impact her health as well as her new baby. In the last decade, it has been recognized that depression throughout the perinatal period is more common than originally thought and contributes to morbidity and mortality for childbearing families. Major depression during pregnancy and up to 6 months postpartum affects up to 10–15% of all childbearing women (Melzer-Brody, 2011). Screening of all women during pregnancy as well as the postpartum period is now recommended. There are a number of tools developed to measure depression, some specifically during the perinatal period. These include the Edinburgh Postnatal Depression Scale (EPDS) and the Postpartum Depression Screening Scale (PDSS); other scales used during the perinatal period but designed for use with the general population include the Beck Depression Inventory (BDI), the Centers for Epidemiological Studies-Depression (CES-D), and the Patient Health Questionnaire (PHQ-9). Regardless of the screening tool used, all women should have screening done at least once during the pregnancy and once in the postpartum period. Scores indicating depression should be shared with women and referrals for mental health services should be offered when indicated. While there is controversy about treatment modalities due to safety concerns in pregnancy for some medications, some women with significant depression may require pharmacological treatment as well as individual or group counseling.

Intimate partner violence

IPV includes "physical, sexual or psychological harm by a current or former partner or spouse" and affects women of all races and ethnicities and all socioeconomic groups (CDC, 2013b). Violence against women can escalate during pregnancy, making women more vulnerable to both physical and psychological abuse. It is recommended that all women be screened for IPV during the

Immunization & Pregnancy

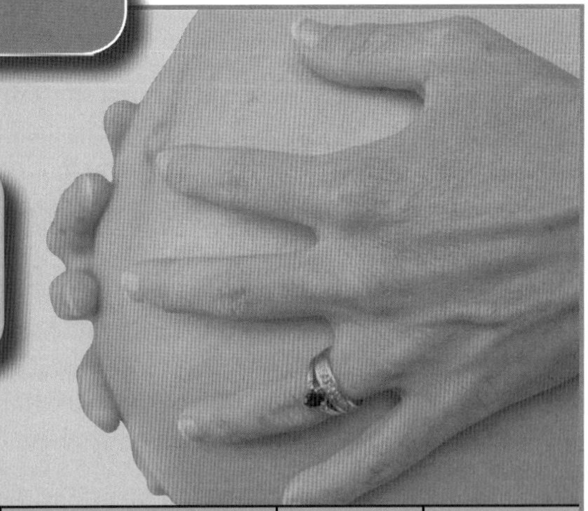

Vaccines help keep a pregnant woman and her growing family healthy.

Vaccine	Before pregnancy	During pregnancy	After pregnancy	Type of Vaccine	Route
Hepatitis A	Yes, if at risk	Yes, if at risk	Yes, if at risk	Inactivated	IM
Hepatitis B	Yes, if at risk	Yes, if at risk	Yes, if at risk	Inactivated	IM
Human Papillomavirus (HPV)	Yes, if 9 through 26 years of age	No, under study	Yes, if 9 through 26 years of age	Inactivated	IM
Influenza TIV	Yes	Yes	Yes	Inactivated	IM, ID (18-64 years)
Influenza LAIV	Yes, if less than 50 years of age and healthy; avoid conception for 4 weeks	No	Yes, if less than 50 years of age and healthy; avoid conception for 4 weeks	Live	Nasal spray
MMR	Yes, avoid conception for 4 weeks	No	Yes, give immediately postpartum if susceptible to rubella	Live	SC
Meningococcal: • polysaccharide • conjugate	If indicated	If indicated	If indicated	Inactivated Inactivated	SC IM
Pneumococcal Polysaccharide	If indicated	If indicated	If indicated	Inactivated	IM or SC
Tetanus/Diphtheria Td	Yes, Tdap preferred	Yes, Tdap preferred if 20 weeks gestational age or more	Yes, Tdap preferred	Toxoid	IM
Tdap, one dose only	Yes, preferred	Yes, preferred	Yes, preferred	Toxoid/ inactivated	IM
Varicella	Yes, avoid conception for 4 weeks	No	Yes, give immediately postpartum if susceptible	Live	SC

For information on all vaccines, including travel vaccines, use this table with www.cdc.gov/vaccines

Get an answer to your specific question by e-mailing cdcinfo@cdc.gov or calling 800-CDC-INFO (232-4636) • English or Spanish

National Center for Immunization and Respiratory Diseases
Immunization Services Division

CDC

CS226523B 10/2011

Figure 5.1. Immunizations and pregnancy. Available at http://www.cdc.gov/vaccines/pubs/downloads/f_preg_chart.pdf

first prenatal visit and once each trimester or whenever IPV is suspected based on history or physical examination (CDC, 2013b). A brief set of questions has been used successfully to assist prenatal providers in identifying women who may be experiencing IPV:

- In the last year have you been hit, slapped, kicked, or physically hurt by someone?
- Since you have been pregnant, have you been hit, slapped, kicked, or physically hurt by someone?
- Has anyone ever forced you to have sex with them?
- Are you afraid of your partner or anyone else?

These questions should be asked in private without a partner present, and if positive responses are elicited, further evaluation is required. The prenatal care provider can provide a safe environment to explore the issue, reassure that this abuse is not her fault, and assess for her current and future safety. IPV is a complex situation and leaving an abusive partner may not be immediately feasible or preferred by the woman. Referrals to local resources are critical including counseling and shelters.

Health promotion and education

Perhaps at no other time in a woman's life will she have the unique motivation for making health behavior changes as during pregnancy. It is also a time when health behavior changes can have the most impact by improving maternal health, creating a healthier environment for the developing fetus, and setting the stage for maintenance of healthy behaviors after pregnancy. When the Expert Panel reviewed the evidence regarding the health promotion topics with a positive effect on maternal and neonatal outcomes, nutrition and smoking cessation were found to be the two most likely behaviors to improve with counseling (Public Health Service. Expert Panel on the Content of Prenatal Care, 1989).

Nutrition

Nutritional information during pregnancy includes not only dietary information regarding calorie needs, vitamin and mineral requirements, and food safety but also information on appropriate weight gain during pregnancy. During pregnancy, the energy needs of women increase, especially in the second and third trimesters. Protein intake needs increase by about 20% and most vitamin and mineral needs increase, some significantly. For example, iron, folic acid, and vitamin D needs double during pregnancy (Gabbe et al., 2012). While a well-balanced diet can meet most of the increased dietary requirements, it is fairly common for women to take a prenatal vitamin and mineral supplement. Optimally, this supplement will begin in the preconception period

to provide adequate folic acid intake at the time of conception. Women who present with preexisting nutritional deficiencies such as iron deficiency anemia may need additional supplementation. A nutritional assessment begins with a discussion regarding a woman's typical diet, cultural food preferences, special dietary practices, and food resources. The health-care provider should provide nutritional information so that the woman understands the increased dietary needs of pregnancy. For example, the calcium needs during pregnancy significantly increase, so identifying dietary sources of calcium will allow women to alter their diets. Similarly, as iron deficiency is common among women of childbearing age, providing information regarding foods that have high iron content will be helpful. Food safety is important during pregnancy as it can prevent transmission of food-borne illnesses that can cause poor maternal and fetal outcomes.

A common way to evaluate maternal nutritional status is by calculation of the BMI. In 2010, the IOM revised guidelines that tailored recommendations for weight gain during pregnancy to the maternal BMI and nutritional status at the onset of pregnancy (Table 5.7) (Rasmussen et al., 2009). In resource-poor countries, maternal nutrition is commonly focused upon increasing maternal calories and supplementation due to poor food resources and food quality. However, in the United States, it is more common for a woman to begin her pregnancy overweight or obese, thereby increasing her risk of complications. Similarly, women may gain more than the recommended weight during pregnancy, which increases their risk for pregnancy complications and chronic illnesses.

General nutritional guidelines for all women during pregnancy include the following:

- Eat a wide variety of foods—a well-balanced diet will help to meet all the daily requirements.
- Increase foods that are high in fiber, such as fruits, vegetables, and foods made with whole grains.
- Eat three meals per day, with healthy snacks in between meals.
- Drink eight glasses of water per day (64 oz/day).
- Gain the recommended amount of weight.
- Use supplements if needed.
- Avoid foods that may increase risk for mother/baby.
- Prepare foods safely.

The United States Department of Agriculture (USDA) sponsors for the Women, Infants, and Children (WIC) nutrition program. This program provides supplemental nutrition for pregnant and lactating women, allowing for the addition of healthy foods to meet the needs for increased protein, calcium, fiber, and calories in

Table 5.7 IOM Recommended Pregnancy Weight Gain (Rasmussen, Yaktine, & Committee to Reexamine IOM Pregnancy Weight Guidelines, Institute of Medicine, Research Council, 2009)

Prepregnancy BMI category	Total weight gain (lb)	Weight gain, first trimester (lb)	Weight gain, second and third trimesters (lb/week)
Underweight: BMI < 18.5	28–40	5	1–1.3
Normal weight: BMI 18.5–24.9	25–35	2–5	0.8–1
Overweight: BMI 35–29.9	15–25	0–2	0.5–0.7
Obese (all classes): BMI ≥ 30	11–20	0–1	0.4–0.6

low-income women. Women who qualify for this program should be directed to enroll in services. Maternal nutrition during pregnancy is covered in further detail in Chapter 6.

Substance abuse

Culture, relationships, and genetics all play a significant role when exploring substance abuse among women. While women report a lower incidence of substance abuse than men, once initiated, women are just as likely to develop substance abuse disorders (Center for Substance Abuse Treatment, 2009). Women are more relationship oriented and are more likely to abuse substances if their partner is a substance abuser or if they have a past history of trauma or abuse. During pregnancy, it is possible that women may reduce or abstain from addictive substances; however, if they are unwilling or unable, serious consequences may ensue due to the fetal and maternal of effects of tobacco, alcohol, or illicit substances (Center for Substance Abuse Treatment, 2009). Additionally, substance abuse is often underreported by women, particularly for fears related to child custody. Overall, how substance abuse affects the woman and her pregnancy will depend on the type of substance or substances used, how long and how frequently she uses the substance, and what, if any, comorbidities are present. For example, women who drink alcohol are also more likely to smoke cigarettes. Mental health issues can coexist with substance use and should be assessed by the health-care provider.

Tobacco use

Experts all agree that there is benefit to counseling pregnant women about the risks of smoking and that smoking cessation programs during pregnancy can decrease the incidence of premature labor and LBW infants (Gregory et al., 2006; Merkatz & Thompson, 1990; Public Health

Service. Expert Panel on the Content of Prenatal Care, 1989). The adverse effects of smoking in pregnancy are well documented and include an increased risk of ectopic pregnancy, spontaneous abortion, LBW, abruptio placentae, placenta previa, and prematurity. The toxic chemicals in cigarettes as well as carbon monoxide are thought to be responsible for a lack of oxygen to the fetus as well as the neurobehavioral and cognitive effects frequently observed in the children of women who smoked during pregnancy (Surgeon General, 2010). Smoking cessation programs can be effective in pregnancy as women are usually highly motivated to change behaviors that are linked to poorer health outcomes in their infants. However, tobacco addiction is difficult to overcome and the relapse rate is high after pregnancy (Gregory et al., 2006).

Many resources exist to assist prenatal providers to help their patients to quit smoking during pregnancy. Each state has a telephone quit line that links women to resources for quitting, including access to printed materials, support from telephone counselors, and information on the prevention of relapse. Health-care providers should give the National Quitline Number 1-800-QUIT NOW to all women who smoke during pregnancy. While not all states offer all services, those with access to telephone-based counseling have been shown to be more effective (American College of Obstetricians and Gynecologists, 2010, 2011a; Surgeon General, 2010). Additionally, there are many quit smoking Web sites and applications for mobile devices that can be used as cessation aids. Targeted and effective smoking cessation counseling can and should occur during prenatal care. ACOG and the CDC have developed self-instructional educational programs and toolkits that provide information and support regarding effective counseling techniques. The 5 A's is one such program that is effective in counseling women regarding smoking cessation during pregnancy (Table 5.8).

Table 5.8 The 5 A's for Smoking Cessation

Ask	Always ask women about their current smoking status at each visit.
Advise	Advise the woman to quit smoking and provide information about the health and economic benefits of quitting for her, her baby, and her family.
Assess	Assess whether the woman is willing to make a quit attempt within the next 30 days.
Assist	Assist the woman with her quit attempt by providing information and resources for smoking cessation, and referrals to smoking cessation counseling and quit lines.
Arrange	Arrange to follow up with the woman within a week of her planned quit attempt. Follow up on her progress at each visit and offer continued support, information, and other resources as needed.

Sources: American College of Obstetricians and Gynecologists (2011a); Five Major Steps to Intervention (The "5 A's"). Agency for Healthcare Research and Quality, Rockville, MD. Retrieved from http://www.ahrq.gov/professionals/clinicians-providers/guidelines-recommendations/tobacco/5steps.html; Treating tobacco use and dependence: 2008 update. Tobacco use and dependence guideline panel. Rockville, MD: U.S. Department of Health and Human Services.

Currently, there is insufficient evidence to suggest that pharmacotherapies are effective and safe for use in pregnancy. It is not recommended that nicotine replacement products or antidepressants be used as therapies for smoking cessation during pregnancy (American College of Obstetricians and Gynecologists, 2010, 2011a). Alternative therapies such as meditation, hypnosis, and acupuncture have been used with some success in smoking cessation. While there is insufficient evidence regarding the effectiveness of these alternative therapies, there are thought to be few risks with their use (American College of Obstetricians and Gynecologists, 2010).

Alcohol use

Alcohol has been associated with a number of adverse pregnancy outcomes. The CDC estimates that one out of eight women consume some alcohol while pregnant and that each year, 40,000 babies are born affected by fetal alcohol spectrum disorders (FASDs) (CDC, 2013c). Women who consume alcohol regularly during pregnancy are at increased risk for spontaneous abortion, abruptio placentae, and infection. Similarly, the fetus is at an increased risk of LBW, intrauterine growth restriction, congenital anomalies, preterm birth, and neonatal

depression (Merkatz & Thompson, 1990). Alcohol-related neurodevelopmental disorders (ARNDs) and alcohol-related birth defects (ARBDs) are syndromes incorporating a wide range of findings consistent with maternal alcohol use; no safe amount of alcohol use has been determined. Therefore, women should be advised to abstain from alcohol use during pregnancy. Alcohol dependence can develop with regular use, making it difficult for women to stop drinking without assistance from prenatal care providers and mental health specialists. Helping women identify that they may have an alcohol problem is the first step in addressing alcohol dependence in pregnancy. The T-ACE Questionnaire is a tool especially for women that can help them identify alcohol-related problems.

T-ACE questionnaire

T—Tolerance: How many drinks does it take to make you feel high? (>2 drinks = 2 points)
A—Annoyed: Have people annoyed you by criticizing your drinking? (yes = 1 point)
C—Cut down: Have you ever felt you ought to cut down on your drinking? (yes = 1 point)
E—Eye-opener: Have you ever had a drink first thing in the morning to steady your nerves or get rid of a hangover? (yes = 1 point)

A score of 2 or greater indicates the need for further assessment and referral (American College of Obstetricians and Gynecologists, 2011b). Alternatively, the National Center on Alcohol Use and Alcoholism suggests that women are at risk for alcohol-related problems if they consume more than seven drinks per week or more than three drinks per occasion, or any drinking by women who are pregnant or may become pregnant. During pregnancy, women who report they are unable to stop drinking should be offered a referral to a substance abuse treatment provider or facility (American College of Obstetricians and Gynecologists, 2011b).

Illicit drugs

Addressing substance abuse during pregnancy can have a positive effect on maternal and fetal outcomes. Drugs of abuse present special challenges for women in pregnancy. Not only do most illicit drugs have significant effects on the developing fetus and increase the risk of LBW and prematurity, the illegal nature of the substances also places the woman at risk of difficulties with law enforcement. In some states, pregnant women who abuse illegal drugs can be detained or can face custody issues after the birth if an infant tests positive for illicit drugs. In some states, drug testing is mandatory during pregnancy and providers can be required to report documented substance abuse (Dailard & Nash, 2000). It is incumbent upon the health-care provider to know the laws of the state regarding testing and reporting of women who may be suffering from a substance abuse disorder.

Screening for drugs of abuse during pregnancy is a complicated issue as women may not want to admit they are abusing drugs due to illegality or understand negative consequences related to admitting to substance use. Similarly, they may be under the influence of an addictive substance and fear the effects of withdrawal, or may not be at the point where they are ready to seek help, even though they may understand the risks to themselves or their baby. All women should be screened for substance abuse in pregnancy, although there is no consensus as to which modality of screening is most effective. There is some evidence that self-report questionnaires may elicit more accurate information than face-to-face interviews (Center for Substance Abuse Treatment, 2009). Screening identifies women who may require a more thorough assessment for an addictive disorder. A common screening tool for substance abuse is the "5 P's." There is a correlation between smoking and substance abuse, and women are more likely to abuse drugs and alcohol during pregnancy if they smoked in the month prior to pregnancy. A "yes" response to any item on the 5 P's suggests a need for a more thorough assessment.

The 5 P's screening tool for substance abuse
(Center for Substance Abuse Treatment, 2009)

Peers—Do any of your friends have a problem with drug or alcohol use?

Partner—Does your partner have a problem with alcohol or drugs?

Parents—Did either of your parents ever have a problem with alcohol or drugs?

Past use—Before you knew you were pregnant, how often did you drink beer, wine, wine coolers, or liquor? *Not at all, rarely, sometimes, or frequently?*

Present use—In the past month, how often did you drink beer, wine, wine coolers, or liquor? *Not at all, rarely, sometimes, or frequently?*

Smoke—How many cigarettes did you smoke in the month prior to pregnancy?

Currently, routine toxicology screening is not recommended for pregnant women. However, certain mater-

nal behaviors and pregnancy complications are often associated with substance use and can alert the healthcare provider that further evaluation is warranted. Women with late entry into care, lack of compliance with scheduled visits, or no prenatal care can indicate substance abuse. Preterm labor, placental abruption, precipitous labor, unexplained stillbirth, and intrauterine growth restriction have all been linked to substance abuse. If testing is warranted, the woman should be informed, but in most states, consent is not required. However, the clinician should understand that, ethically, the woman has a right to this information as well as a right to refuse such testing. Coercive or punitive strategies for unacceptable maternal behaviors deny a woman's right to privacy and bodily integrity and are not in the best interest of helping the woman or her baby. Testing can be accomplished through urine screening, hair analysis, or by testing the infant. However, accuracy of the results depends upon the drug used and the timing of the last administration (Center for Substance Abuse Treatment, 2009; Lockwood & Lemons, 2007).

Women who are unable to discontinue substance use during pregnancy will need intensive treatment, most likely as an inpatient, although there are few residential treatment centers that accept pregnant women. Certain drugs of abuse like heroin are highly addictive and require careful detoxification to prevent maternal and fetal complications. Depending on what substances are used during pregnancy, some infants will require detoxification after birth and require extended hospitalization. Prenatal care provides a unique opportunity to provide services and support to women with addictive disorders. Women during pregnancy are often highly motivated to change unhealthy behaviors and want to do what is best for themselves and their infants. Further information about substance abuse during pregnancy is provided in Chapter 13.

Exercise

Exercise in pregnancy is encouraged and can assist women to achieve healthy weight gain goals, and benefits overall health and well-being. While all women can benefit from moderate exercise for 30 minutes each day, some activities may increase risk to the mother and/or the fetus and should be avoided. Exercise that has a risk for falling, abdominal trauma, or high contact sports should be avoided. Exercise patterns may change as the pregnancy progresses, and the enlarging abdomen will necessitate alterations in routine exercise regimens.

Women should be encouraged to "listen" to their bodies and discontinue or decrease exercise intensity if they begin to experience any of the following:

- vaginal bleeding
- dyspnea prior to exertion
- dizziness
- headache
- chest pain
- muscle weakness
- calf pain or swelling
- preterm labor
- decreased fetal movement
- amniotic fluid leakage (Lockwood & Lemons, 2007; Merkatz & Thompson, 1990).

While these recommendations apply to most pregnant women, some women may be counseled to avoid exercise during pregnancy. More detailed information on exercise during pregnancy is provided in Chapter 15.

Working and pregnancy

Women throughout the world routinely work during pregnancy. For the majority of women, there are few risks for adverse health outcomes from continuing work during the pregnancy and there can be benefits of working; however, certain workplaces or occupations may pose risks or may require certain accommodations during pregnancy. There is a wide range of potential exposures to workplace substances and their effects on pregnancy and reproductive outcomes. Women who may be exposed to hazardous chemicals, cytotoxic drugs, ionizing radiation, gases, and minerals like lead need to consult their workplace for evaluation of potential exposures to determine whether it is safe to continue to work in these areas. Material safety data sheets (MSDSs) are documents containing information and instructions on hazardous materials present in the workplace; MSDSs contain details about hazards and risks relevant to the substance, requirements for its safe handling, and actions to be taken in the event of fire, spill, or overexposure. It should be noted, however, that few of these substances will have data on effects during pregnancy, so a cautious approach is indicated. The Occupational Safety and Health Administration (OSHA) requires that this information is available at the workplace. OSHA is an excellent resource for workers and providers and can assist in determining workplace risk during pregnancy (see "Resources for Women and Families").

The type of work performed, hours worked, and the workplace environment can all contribute to a woman's tolerance of work throughout the pregnancy. Women who work in jobs in which there is repetitive lifting, climbing, stooping, or bending should have their work duties evaluated for continued safety throughout the pregnancy. In 1984, the American Medical Association developed recommendations for limiting certain types of work activities during pregnancy, which included limiting repetitive bending, climbing, or heavy lifting (more than 23 kg) and limiting standing to no more than 30 min/h at 32 weeks (Merkatz & Thompson, 1990). However, occupations vary a great deal in terms of required activities and will need to be considered on an individual basis for recommendations regarding continuation, alteration, or discontinuation of that specific job.

Some women will want to stop working prior to the onset of labor due to fatigue and difficulty with the physical demands of advancing gestation. It is common that women can be considered eligible for a pregnancy leave at 38 weeks' gestation. In the United States, women do not enjoy generous paid maternity benefits and often have short periods of paid leave or no leave at all. The Family Medical Leave Act (FMLA) was enacted in 1993 and provides for unpaid leave of up to 12 weeks for women due to pregnancy. The Pregnancy Discrimination Act (PDA) (1978) prohibits discrimination based on pregnancy when it comes to any aspect of employment, including hiring, firing, pay, job assignments, promotions, layoff, training, fringe benefits such as leave and health insurance, and any other term or condition of employment. Pregnant women who experience a medical complication related to pregnancy must be treated as any other employee with a short-term disability and must be offered light duty, alternate assignments, or disability leave (Equal Employment Opportunity Commission, 1978).

Health education throughout pregnancy

Health education during pregnancy is important for maternal health and psychosocial well-being and helps to prepare for transition to parenthood. The challenge in prenatal care is how to incorporate the necessary health education, with ongoing physical and risk assessment, within the prevailing prenatal care system. Health education may not be a priority or is limited due to the time constraints of prenatal care providers. While women who attend CenteringPregnancy groups have extensive health education as a major component of prenatal care, women in traditional individual care will need additional resources to meet their ongoing educational needs. In order to obtain in-depth and comprehensive health education, it may be necessary for women to attend classes outside of their regularly scheduled visits or to seek outside resources, such as books and online resources. Prenatal care providers should be familiar with common consumer resources for their clients (see "Resources for Women and Families"). The Expert Panel recommended health promotion content be provided based upon the needs of women

Table 5.9 Health Education Topics throughout Pregnancy

First trimester	Second trimester	Third trimester
Counseling to promote healthy behaviors and avoidance of teratogens	Counseling to promote healthy behaviors and avoidance of teratogens	Counseling to promote healthy behaviors and avoidance of teratogens
Nutritional information, recommended weight gain, referrals for WIC if appropriate	Nutritional information, healthy weight goals	Nutritional information, healthy weight goals
Safety such as seatbelts, work safety, food safety	Physiological and emotional changes in pregnancy	Physiological and emotional changes in pregnancy
Safer sex practices	Common pregnancy discomforts and recommendations	Common pregnancy discomforts and recommendations
Physiological and emotional changes in early pregnancy	Fetal growth and development, anticipated fetal movement	Fetal growth and development, anticipated fetal movement
Common pregnancy discomforts and recommendations	Preparation for common screening and diagnostic tests, such as genetic screening, ultrasound	Preparation for common screening and diagnostic tests, such as group B strep screening
Exercise	Danger signs to report and how to contact provider	Danger signs to report and how to contact provider
Expected prenatal care including content and frequency of visit	Signs and symptoms of preterm labor	Signs and symptoms of preterm labor
Preparation for common screening and diagnostic tests, such as genetic screening	Breastfeeding promotion	Breastfeeding promotion, preparation, breastfeeding class
Danger signs to report and how to contact provider	Birth preparation, available educational opportunities	Labor and birth preparation, childbirth education class, visit to birth place, birth plan
Explanations of philosophy of care of the prenatal providers, scope of practice, and place of birth		Preparation for baby, car seat, infant feeding, newborn care
Explanation of community resources for pregnant and parenting families		Preparation for parenting, roles, support, pediatric care and provider, parenting class, sibling adjustment
		Signs and symptoms of labor, when to notify provider, when and how to arrive at place of birth
		Postpartum changes, postpartum depression, activity, plan of care during postpartum period
		Contraceptive plans
		Post term pregnancy expectations

Sources: Lockwood and Lemons (2007), Merkatz and Thompson (1990), Public Health Service. Expert Panel on the Content of Prenatal Care (1989).

throughout the pregnancy. Early pregnancy concerns will be different from those at the end of pregnancy. Anticipatory guidance is critical so that women will know what to expect at each stage of pregnancy. This will help them to identify common changes and discomforts and alert them to danger signs that may indicate the need for evaluation. Preparing for labor and birth and early parenting is important to help promote a successful transition to parenthood and ensure that women have appropriate resources and information (Table 5.9). Health education during pregnancy is reviewed in further detail in Chapter 17.

Summary

Prenatal care has the potential to affect the health of a woman, her infant, and her family in a positive way. Current trends in health care emphasize the importance of evidence-based care to achieve improved health outcomes. Pregnancy and childbirth care represents one of the largest expenditures of health-care dollars for both public and private insurers, yet despite this significant expenditure, the United States ranks well below other developed and some developing countries in maternal and child health outcomes. Recent efforts like the Transforming Maternity Care Movement have identified that the current system of maternity care is procedure intensive and costly, and that overuse is contributing to excessive harm and costs. Conversely, preventative care is underused and misunderstood by many prenatal care providers. Significant disparities exist in maternal and infant outcomes, and little to no progress in improving outcomes has been made despite significant expenditure. Lastly, childbearing women lack choice in their health-care provider, place of birth, and childbirth experience due to institutional policies, reimbursement issues, and provider availability and preferences. Prenatal care providers have a unique opportunity to change how women and families experience pregnancy and birth. Transforming Maternity Care is a group of over 100 experts in maternity health care and health policy brought together to create a blueprint for achieving a safer, cost-effective and woman-centered prenatal care system. They recommend the following:

1. Each woman is engaged as a partner in her own care and education during pregnancy; she receives affirmation and practical support for her role as the natural leader of her care team to the extent that she so desires and is encouraged to provide input to shape her own care.
2. Each woman's preferences are known, respected, and matched with individually tailored care that meets her needs and reflects her choices during pregnancy, delivered by a care team whose composition is also customized based on her needs and preferences.
3. Each woman has access to complete, accurate, up-to-date, high-quality information, decision support, and education to help ensure that she feels emotionally and psychologically prepared to make decisions during her pregnancy, and confident about her birth care options and choices well in advance of the onset of labor.
4. Education and care during pregnancy are designed and delivered to be empowering to women, emphasizing a climate of confidence.
5. Education and care during pregnancy include support for breastfeeding; most women make decisions about infant feeding well before they give birth.
6. Each pregnant woman receives personalized coaching and has access to high-quality resources for comprehensive health promotion, disease prevention, and improved nutrition and exercise for optimal wellness during her pregnancy.
7. Care during pregnancy is available when needed and can be accessed in a time and place that is convenient and accessible for each woman, and balanced with concerns for value and efficiency.
8. Care during pregnancy acknowledges the social context in which pregnancy occurs for each woman and includes opportunities for social networking and access to adequate professional and peer support during pregnancy (Cook Carter et al., 2010).

These changes may not be easy but are necessary to improve the health of families and communities. Prenatal care is over 100 years old with many traditional aspects that remain important today, but it is time to integrate the current evidence into best care practices for women and families throughout pregnancy and birth.

Case study

Roxie is a 17-year-old G2 P0010 Caucasian who presents at 16 weeks for her second prenatal visit and her first CenteringPregnancy group visit. She is a bit embarrassed to be here after her miscarriage 6 months ago and says "I guess I didn't decide on the pill soon enough!" This Centering group consists of Roxie and seven other teens. An overview of genetic screening test options with the teens is planned as they are all between 14 and 16 weeks pregnant.

After the belly checks, weigh-ins, and blood pressures are done, the facilitator opens by saying this is their group, they can determine what needs they have and would like to address in the group setting, would anyone care to start? A long awkward pause ensues. Roxie then blurts out, "My grandma says that beer is okay while you are pregnant, it relaxes you. Is that right?" Lexie, a 15 year old at 14 weeks pregnant, mumbles just loud enough for the group to hear "Duh."

SUBJECTIVE: It is important to understand that a group is more than the sum of its parts and that individual needs must be addressed, but the group needs must also be assessed. Individual contributions within the group are considered for what these messages communicate about the pregnant woman but also for their influence on the emotional climate of the group.

OBJECTIVE: Roxie has indicated insecurity through her words and gestures, while Lexie has exhibited oppositional behavior. This can be a reflection of normal group formation as individuals deal with uncertainty regarding their role within a newly forming group.

ASSESSMENT: Initial group formation is in process; health education regarding alcohol consumption during pregnancy is requested and needed.

PLAN: Set a positive and welcoming tone for the group, including a discussion of group norms for respectful behavior. Invite suggestions from the group as well as make suggestions as the facilitator. Emphasize that the goals of the group include education, support for and from each other, and a healthy pregnancy, labor, and birth for each woman culminating with a healthy, beautiful baby. Address Roxie's question with education and discussion. Watch Lexie and the others for negative reactions, but these typically settle out as the group goes through its initial phase of formation. Continue with the planned education regarding prenatal genetic testing.

Resources for women and their families

American Pregnancy Association: http://www.american
pregnancy.org/

Childbirth Connection for Women: http://www.child
birthconnection.org/home.asp?Visitor=Woman

March of Dimes: http://www.marchofdimes.com/

Occupational Safety and Health Administration
(OSHA): http://www.osha.gov/

Resources for health-care providers

Agency for Healthcare Research and Quality (AHRQ):
http://www.ahrq.gov/

American Academy of Pediatrics (AAP): http://
www.aap.org/en-us/Pages/Default.aspx

American College of Family Physicians (ACFP): http://
www.aafp.org/online/en/home.html

American College of Nurse-Midwives: http://www
.midwife.org/

American Congress of Obstetricians and Gynecologists:
http://www.acog.org/

Centering Healthcare Institute: https://www.centering
healthcare.org/index.php

Centers for Disease Control and Prevention: http://www
.cdc.gov/

Childbirth Connection for Health Professionals: http://
www.childbirthconnection.org/home.asp?Visitor
=Professional

Transforming Maternity Care: http://transform.child
birthconnection.org/

United States Department of Agriculture (USDA) sponsors for the Women, Infants, and Children (WIC)
Nutrition Program: http://www.fns.usda.gov/wic/

U.S. Preventive Services Task Force (USPSTF): http://
www.ahrq.gov/clinic/uspstfix.htm

References

Alexander, G. R., & Kotelchuck, M. (1998). Quantifying the adequacy
of prenatal care: A comparison of indices. *Public Health Reports*,
111, 408.

American Academy of Pediatrics and American College of Obstetricians and Gynecologists. (2012). *Guidelines for perinatal care* (7th
ed.). Elk Grove Village, IL: Author.

American College of Obstetricians and Gynecologists. (2010).
Smoking cessation during pregnancy. *Obstetrics and Gynecology*,
116, 1241–1244. Report No.: Committe Opinion #471.

American College of Obstetricians and Gynecologists. (2011a).
Smoking Cessation during Pregnancy Self-instructional Guide and
Tool Kit. ACOG, Washington DC.

American College of Obstetricians and Gynecologists. (2011b). Women
and at risk alcohol use: Screening and intervention. *Obstetrics and
Gynecology*, *118*, 383–388. Report No.: Committee Opinion # 496.

Ballantyne, J. W. (1923). An address on the new midwifery: Preventive
and reparative obstetrics. *British Medical Journal*, *1*, 617.

Bloch, J., Dawley, K., & Suplee, P. (2009). Application of the Kessner
and Kotelchuck prenatal care adequacy indices in a pre-term birth
population. *Public Health Nursing*, *26*(5), 449.

Center for Substance Abuse Treatment. (2009). *Substance abuse treat-
ment: Addressing the specific needs of women*. Rockville, MD:
Substance Abuse and Mental Health Services Administration
(US). Report No.: Treatment Improvement Protocol (TIP) Series,
No. 51.

Centering Healthcare Institute. (2013). (https://www.centeringhealth
care.org/pages/centering-model/elements.php). Essential Elements
of Centering [Internet].

Centers for Disease Control and Prevention (CDC). (n.d.) A guide to
taking a sexual history. Publication # 99-8445. Atlanta, GA: Department of Health and Human Services. Retrieved from http://
www.cdc.gov/std/treatment/SexualHistory.pdf

Centers for Disease Control and Prevention (CDC). (2013a). National
Vital Statistics System. Retrieved from http://www.cdc.gov/nchs/
nvss.htm

Centers for Disease Control and Prevention (CDC). (2013b). Injury
Center: Violence Prevention. Retrieved from http://www.cdc.gov/
violenceprevention/intimatepartnerviolence/index.html

Centers for Disease Control and Prevention (CDC). (2013c). Facts
about FASD. Retrieved from http://www.cdc.gov/NCBDDD/fasd/
facts.html

Centers for Disease Control and Prevention (CDC). (2006). Proceedings of the Preconception Health and Health Care Clinical, Public
Health, and Consumer Workgroup Meetings. Atlanta, GA: Department of Health and Human Services.

Chalmers, I. (1986). Minimizing harm and maximizing benefit during
innovation in healthcare: Controlled or uncontrolled experimentation? *Birth (Berkeley, Calif.)*, *13*, 155–164.

Cook Carter, M., Corry, M., Delbanco, S., Clark-Samazan Foster, T.,
Friedland, R., Gabel, R., . . . Jolivet, R. (2010). 2020 vision for a
high-value, quality maternity care system. *Women's Health Issues*,
20(1 Suppl.), S7. Jacobs Institute of Women's Health.

Dailard, C., & Nash, E. (2000). State's responses to substance abuse
among pregnant women. New York: Alan Guttmacher Institute.
Report No.: Volume 3: Number 6.

Dunn, P. (1993). Dr. John Ballantyne (1861–1923) Perinatologist
extraordinary of Edinburgh. *Archive of Diseases in Childhood*, *68*, 66.

Enkin, M., Keirse, M., Neilson, J., Crowther, C., Duley, L., Hodnett, E.,
& Hofmeyr, J. (2000). *A guide to effective care in pregnancy and
childbirth* (3rd ed.). Oxford: Oxford University Press.

Equal Employment Opportunity Commission. (1978). Pregnancy
Discrimination Act [Internet].

Gabbe, S., Niebyl, J., Simpson, J., Landon, M., Galan, H., Jauniaux, E.
& Driscoll, D. (2012). *Obstetrics: Normal and problem pregnancies*
(6th ed.). Philadelphia: Elsevier Saunders.

Gavin, N. I., Adams, E. K., Hartmann, K. E., Benedict, M. B., &
Chireau, M. (2004). Racial and ethnic disparities in the use of
pregnancy-related health care among Medicaid pregnant women.
Maternal and Child Health Journal, *8*, 113.

Grady, M. A., & Bloom, K. C. (2004). Pregnancy outcomes of adolescents enrolled in a CenteringPregnancy program. *Journal of Midwifery and Women's Health*, *49*(5), 412–420.

Gregory, K. D., Johnson, C. T., Johnson, T. R., & Entman, S. S. (2006).
The content of prenatal care. Update 2005. *Women's Health Issues*,
16(4), 198–215.

Hamilton, B. E., Martin, J. A., & Ventura, S. J. (2009). Births: Preliminary
data for 2007. National vital statistics reports. Web release: National
Center for Health Statistics. Released March 18, 2009. 57(12).

Homer, C. S. E., Ryan, C., Leap, N., Foureur, M., Teate, A., & Catling-
Paull, C. J. (2012). Group versus conventional antenatal care for

women. *Cochrane Database of Systematic Reviews*, (11), CD007622. doi:10.1002/14651858.CD007622.pub2

Ickovics, J. R., Kershaw, T. S., Westdahl, C., Magriples, U., Massey, Z., Reynolds, H., & Rising, S. S. (2007). Group prenatal care and perinatal outcomes: A randomized controlled trial. *Obstetrics and Gynecology*, 110(2 Pt. 1), 330–339.

Institute of Medicine. (2001). *Crossing the quality chasm*. Washington, DC: National Academy Press.

Institute of Medicine. (2011). *Clinical preventive services for women: Closing the gaps*. Washington, DC: National Academy of Sciences.

Johnson, K., Posner, S. F., Biermann, J., . . . Curtis, M. G. (2006). Recommendations to improve preconception health and health care: United States: a report of the CDC/ATSDR Preconception Care work group and the Select Panel on Preconception Care. *MMWR. Morbidity and Mortality Weekly Report*, 55, 1–23.

Klima, C., Vonderheid, S. C., Norr, K. F., & Handler, A. (2009). CenteringPregnancy in a public health clinic. *Journal of Midwifery and Women's Health*, 54(1), 27–34.

Kogan, M. D., Alexander, G. R., Kotelchuck, M., & Nagey, D. A. (1994). Relation of the content of prenatal care to the risk of low birth weight. maternal reports of health behavior advice and initial prenatal care procedures. *JAMA: The Journal of the American Medical Association*, 271(17), 1340–1345.

Kogan, M. D., Alexander, G. R., Kotelchuck, M., Nagey, D. A., & Jack, B. W. (1994). Comparing mothers' reports on the content of prenatal care received with recommended national guidelines for care. *Public Health Reports*, 109(5), 637–646.

Kotelchuck, M. (1994). Adequacy of prenatal care utilization index: Its US distribution and its association with low birth weight. *American Journal of Public Health*, 84(1), 1486.

Lockwood, C., & Lemons, J. (Eds.). (2007). *Guidelines for perinatal care*. Washington, DC: American Academy of Pediatrics & American College of Obstetricians and Gynecologists.

Loomans, E. M., van Dijk, A. E., Vrijkotte, T. G., van Eijsden, M., Stronks, K., Gemke, R. J., & Van den Bergh, B. R. (2012). Psychosocial stress during pregnancy is related to adverse birth outcomes: Results from a large multi-ethnic community-based birth cohort. *The European Journal of Public Health*, 23(3), 485–491.

Lu, M. C., Tache, V., Alexander, G. R., Kotelchuck, M., & Halfon, N. (2003). Preventing low birth weight: Is prenatal care the answer? *The Journal of Maternal-fetal and Neonatal Medicine*, 13(6), 362–380.

MacKey, M. C., Williams, C. A., & Tiller, C. M. (2000). Stress, pre-term labour and birth outcomes. *Journal of Advanced Nursing*, 32(3), 666–674.

March of Dimes Foundation. (2003–2012). Genetics and Your Practice.

Melzer-Brody, S. (2011). New insights into perinatal depression: Pathogenesis and treatment in pregnancy and postpartum. *Dialogues in Clinical Neuroscience*, 13(1), 90.

Merkatz, I., & Thompson, J. E. (Eds.). (1990). *New perspectives on prenatal care*. New York: Elsevier.

Norwitz, E., Phaneuf, L., & Caughey, A. (2011). Progesterone supplementation and the prevention of preterm birth. *Obstetrics and Gynecology*, 40(2), 60.

Public Health Service. Expert Panel on the Content of Prenatal Care. (1989). Caring for our future, the content of prenatal care: A report of the Public Health Service Expert Panel on the Content of Prenatal Care. Washington, DC: Department of Health and Human Services.

Rasmussen, K., Yaktine, A., & Committee to Reexamine IOM Pregnancy Weight Guidelines, Institute of Medicine, Research Council. (2009). *Weight gain during pregnancy: Reexamining the guidelines*. Washington, DC: National Academies Press.

Rising, S. S. (1998). Centering pregnancy. An interdisciplinary model of empowerment. *Journal of Nurse-Midwifery*, 43(1), 46–54.

Rising, S. S., Kennedy, H. P., & Klima, C. S. (2004). Redesigning prenatal care through CenteringPregnancy. *Journal of Midwifery and Women's Health*, 49(5), 398–404.

Rooks, J. (1997). *Midwifery and childbirth in America*. Philadelphia: Temple University Press.

Stringer, M. (1998). Issues in determining and measuring adequacy of prenatal care. *Journal of Perinatology: Official Journal of the California Perinatal Association*, 18(1), 68.

Surgeon General. (2010). 2010 Surgeon General's Report on Smoking-How tobacco smoke causes disease: The biology and behavioral basis for smoking-attributable disease. Washington, DC: Centers for Disease Control.

U.S. Department of Health and Human Services, Health Resources and Services Administration, Maternal and Child Health Bureau. (2011). Child Health USA 2011. Rockville, MD: U.S. Department of Health and Human Services.

U.S. Department of Labor: Children's Bureau. (1925). Standards of Prenatal Care. Washington, DC: U.S. Government; Report No.: 153.

Varney, H., Kriebs, J., & Gegor, C. (2004). *Varney's midwifery* (4th ed.). Sudbury, MA: Jones & Bartlett.

Vonderheid, S. C., Montgomery, K. S., & Norr, K. F. (2003). Ethnicity and prenatal health promotion content. *Western Journal of Nursing Research*, 25(4), 388–404.

Vonderheid, S. C., Norr, K. F., & Handler, A. S. (2007). Prenatal health promotion content and health behaviors. *Western Journal of Nursing Research*, 29, 258.

Walker, D. S., & Koniak-Griffin, D. (1997). Evaluation of a reduced-frequency prenatal visit schedule for low-risk women at a free-standing birth center. *Journal of Nurse-Midwifery*, 42, 295–303. doi:10.1016/S0091-2182(97)00027-X

World Health Organization. (2013). Antenatal care (At least 4 visits). Retrieved from http://www.who.int/gho/urban_health/services/antenatal_care_text/en/index.html

6

Nutrition during pregnancy

Robin G. Jordan and Julie A. Paul

Relevant terms

Adequate intake (AI)—reference value set for nutrient levels when sufficient scientific evidence is not available

Body mass index (BMI)—a measure of weight in kilograms divided by height in meters squared. BMI is considered a reliable indicator of total body fat. BMI status categories include underweight, healthy weight, overweight, and obese. During pregnancy, only the prepregnant BMI is relevant to weight gain guidelines.

Calorie density—a measurement of energy provided by foods relative to the amount of food (kilocalorie per gram)

Dietary reference intake (DRI)—standardized nutrient level for populations used to set nutritional goals

Fats—one of the three macronutrients

Fiber—nondigestible carbohydrates and lignin that are found in plants that are beneficial to gastrointestinal function

Food-borne illness—illness resulting from the consumption of food contaminated with pathogenic bacteria (e.g., *Escherichia coli*), viruses (e.g., norovirus), or parasites (e.g., *Toxoplasma gondii*)

Food insecurity—the limited or uncertain availability of nutritionally adequate and safe foods

Fortification—the addition of one or more essential nutrients to a food item, whether or not it is normally contained in the food

Macronutrients—dietary components that provide energy. Macronutrients are proteins, fats, and carbohydrates.

Micronutrients—dietary nutrients required in small quantities that orchestrate a range of physiological functions

Monounsaturated fatty acids (MUFAs)—have one double bond. Plant sources of an unsaturated fatty acid (UFA) include nuts and vegetable oils such as canola, olive, safflower and sunflower oils.

Omega-3 PUFAs—essential fatty acids obtained only in the diet, such as eicosapentaenoic acid (EPA) and

docosahexaenoic acid (DHA) found primarily in fish and shellfish; also called n-3 fatty acids

Omega-6 PUFAs—essential fatty acids found only in the diet, such as linoleic acid; primary sources are liquid vegetable oils such as soybean, corn, and safflower oil; also called n-6 fatty acids

Ovo-lacto vegetarians—those persons following a diet that does not include meat, poultry, or fish/seafood but does contain eggs and dairy foods

Polyunsaturated fatty acids (PUFAs)—have two or more double bonds and are generally liquid at room temperature

Portion size—the amount of food chosen to be eaten at one sitting

Recommended daily allowance (RDA)—levels of nutrient intake advised by experts based on sufficient scientific evidence

Requirement—the lowest intake of a nutrient to qualify for a specific criterion of adequacy

Saturated fatty acids—have no double bond and are generally solid at room temperature. Typically found in animal products such as meat and milk, and coconut and palm oils

Serving size—a standardized specific amount for the five food groups set by the United States Department of Agriculture (USDA)

Tolerable upper intake levels (TULs)—a set of values reflecting the highest average daily nutrient intake that is likely to pose no risk of toxicity to almost all individuals in that particular life stage and gender group

Trans-fatty acids—unsaturated fatty acids that have one or more isolated double bonds; typically found in hydrogenated vegetable oils such as baked goods, snack foods, fried foods, and margarine

Vegans—those persons following a diet that does not include meat, poultry or fish/seafood, dairy, eggs, or honey

Vegetarians—those following a diet that does not include meat, poultry, or fish/seafood

---

Prenatal and Postnatal Care: A Woman-Centered Approach, First Edition. Edited by Robin G. Jordan, Janet L. Engstrom, Julie A. Marfell, and Cindy L. Farley.

Introduction

Nutrition plays a major and long-lasting role in maternal and child health. Nutrient needs typically increase more during pregnancy than during any other stage of an adult woman's life. An increase in select nutrients is required during the prenatal period for fetal development and growth of maternal tissue that support human gestation. Healthy eating behaviors during pregnancy enable optimal gestational nutrition and weight gain, both of which are linked to positive birth outcomes and the reduction of perinatal complications. The association between maternal nutrition and birth outcome is complex and is influenced by many biological, socioeconomic, and demographic factors, which vary widely in different populations.

Pregnancy nutrition is often viewed in isolation rather than in a broader context of a woman's overall health and nutritional status. There is a growing movement promoted by the World Health Organization to view nutrition using the life-course approach, which considers prenatal nutritional influences on adult health status. Understanding the relation between maternal nutrition and birth outcomes may provide a basis for developing nutritional interventions that will improve birth outcomes and long-term quality of life and reduce mortality, morbidity, and health-care costs. Providers of prenatal care must understand the complex relationship between maternal nutritional status and health outcomes to provide comprehensive and effective dietary guidance to pregnant women. This chapter provides foundational information on nutritional needs during pregnancy; impact of nutrition on maternal, child, and adult health; assessment of nutritional status; and nutritional counseling and modification strategies.

Understanding food units

Nutrition experts have produced a set of standards that define the amounts of energy, nutrients, and other dietary components that best support health based on scientific evidence. These recommendations are called dietary reference intake (DRI), the general term for a set of reference values used for planning and assessing nutrient intake for healthy people. DRIs reflect the collaborative efforts of scientists in the United States and Canada and take into account the amount of nutrients needed to promote health and to prevent chronic diseases whenever possible.

There are two sets of values used as DRIs that help set nutritional goals for individuals. The recommended daily allowance (RDA) is the foundation of the DRI. The RDA recommends the average daily intake that is sufficient to meet the nutrient requirements of nearly all healthy individuals in each age and gender group. RDAs are based on scientific evidence with an emphasis on human experiments. The adequate intake (AI) values were established whenever scientific evidence was insufficient to generate an RDA, using scientific findings as much as possible. Some nutrients have an RDA and others have AI. Both the RDA and AI are nutrient reference values set by experts to promote optimal health during various life stages.

The United States Department of Agriculture (USDA) has established food guides based on DRIs to help individuals build healthy diets. The USDA Food Guide is a plan that builds a diet recommending specific daily amounts of food from each of the major five food groups (Table 6.1). An understanding of this foundational content enables health-care providers to make accurate dietary assessments and recommendations during pregnancy.

Size of food servings

The trend in the United States has been toward consuming larger food portions, contributing to an increasing obese population in all age groups. Many people are not aware of what constitutes a serving of a particular food item. The serving size of a given food is the amount recommended by the USDA. The USDA has moved toward using food measures based on weight in ounces or amounts in cups of food rather than "servings" of food. Fruits, vegetables, and milk are measured in 1-cup servings, and whole grains, meats, and beans are measured in 1-oz. servings. People often confuse the "serving" recommendation to mean "portions" with no regard to size. For example, 6–11 servings of whole grains are recommended daily during pregnancy. The USDA indicates that one serving equals 1 oz, which translates into one slice of bread or ½ cup of rice or pasta.

The USDA food guides provide guidance on food selections and serving and portion sizes that will provide adequate amounts of nutrients for a healthy pregnancy diet (Table 6.2).

Prenatal nutrition and health outcomes

Maternal nutrition plays a crucial role in influencing fetal development and birth outcomes. Poor pregnancy nutrition is linked with adverse conditions, such as fetal growth restriction (FGR), preterm birth, low birth weight, preeclampsia, gestational diabetes (GDM), and certain congenital anomalies (Abu-Saad & Fraser, 2010; Ramakrishnan, Grant, Goldenberg, Zongrone, & Martorell, 2012). Some of these adverse outcomes have

Table 6.1 Food Groups and Subgroups

Food group	Subgroup and examples
Vegetables	Dark-green vegetables: all fresh, frozen, and canned dark-green leafy vegetables and broccoli, cooked or raw: for example, broccoli; spinach; romaine; collard, turnip, and mustard greens Red and orange vegetables: all fresh, frozen, and canned red and orange vegetables, cooked or raw: for example, tomatoes, red peppers, carrots, sweet potatoes, winter squash, and pumpkin Beans and peas: all cooked and canned beans and peas: for example, kidney beans, lentils, chickpeas, and pinto beans; does not include green beans or green peas (see additional comment under protein foods group) Starchy vegetables: all fresh, frozen, and canned starchy vegetables: for example, white potatoes, corn, and green peas Other vegetables: all fresh, frozen, and canned other vegetables, cooked or raw: for example, iceberg lettuce, green beans, and onions
Fruits	All fresh, frozen, canned, and dried fruits and fruit juices: for example, oranges and orange juice, apples and apple juice, bananas, grapes, melons, berries, and raisins
Grains	Whole grains: All whole grain products and whole grains used as ingredients: for example, whole-wheat bread, whole grain cereals and crackers, oatmeal, and brown rice Enriched grains: All enriched refined-grain products and enriched refined grains used as ingredients: for example, white breads, enriched grain cereals and crackers, enriched pasta, and white rice
Dairy products	All milks, including lactose-free and lactose-reduced products and fortified soy beverages, yogurts, frozen yogurts, dairy desserts, and cheeses. Most choices should be fat-free or low-fat. Cream, sour cream, and cream cheese are not included due to their low calcium content.
Proteins	All meat, poultry, seafood, eggs, nuts, seeds, and processed soy products. Meat and poultry should be lean or low-fat. Beans and peas are considered part of this group, as well as the vegetable group, but should be counted in one group only.

Adapted from: http://www.cnpp.usda.gov/Publications/DietaryGuidelines/2010/PolicyDoc/Chapter5.pdf.

Table 6.2 Serving Size Guidelines and Needs in Pregnancy

Food	Amount per day	Food group serving size	Comments
Grains	6 oz	✓ 1 oz is a serving ✓ 1 slice of bread ✓ 1 cup of dry cereal ✓ ½ cup of cooked rice, pasta, or cereal	✓ Eat whole wheat bread and pasta for more fiber and nutrients. ✓ Choose low-sugar cereals.
Vegetables	2–3 cups	✓ Most vegetables = ½ cup ✓ 1 cup greens like lettuce or spinach	✓ Select various color vegetables.
Fruits	2 cups	✓ 1 cup fresh fruit or 100% fruit juice ✓ ½ cup dried fruit ✓ A single piece of fruit	✓ Choose whole fruit instead of juice more often.
Dairy	3–4 cups	✓ 1.5 oz natural cheese ✓ 2.0 oz processed cheese ✓ 1 cup milk ✓ 1 cup yogurt ✓ 1 cup fortified soymilk	✓ Choose low-fat or skim milk and yogurt.
Protein foods	5–6 oz	✓ ¼ cup beans ✓ 1 oz meat, poultry, seafood, shellfish ✓ 1 egg ✓ 1 tbs peanut or other nut butters	✓ Eat seafood twice per week. ✓ Select lean meats and poultry.
Oils	6 tsp	✓ 1 tsp vegetable oil ✓ 1½ tsp mayonnaise ✓ 2 tsp French dressing	✓ Use vegetable oils rather than solid fats like butter or lard.

lifelong consequences for growth and development and quality of life in offspring.

Nutrition prior to and during the first trimester of pregnancy is especially important as it may affect placental function and significantly influence pregnancy outcome (Ramakrishnan et al., 2012). The placenta is the interface between the maternal–fetal circulations and optimal placental functioning is critical for adequate fetal nutrition and oxygenation and, consequently, fetal growth. In turn, placental ability to supply nutrients to the fetus depends on the size, morphology, blood supply, and transport ability (Belkacemi, Nelson, Desai, & Ross, 2010). During normal pregnancy, the placenta undergoes physiological changes that are regulated by angiogenic factors, hormones, and nutrient-regulated genes, to maximize efficiency for the progressively increasing fetal demand for nutrients (Stables & Rankin, 2009). Changes in these factors caused by undernutrition, especially in early pregnancy, can significantly alter nutrient availability to the fetus for the entire pregnancy. Animal studies indicate that low nutrient intake during placental development suppresses cell proliferation and vascular development (Redmer, Wallace, & Reynolds, 2004), explaining the higher incidence of low birth weight in those women with insufficient weight gain during pregnancy.

Fetal origins of disease hypothesis

Prenatal nutrition affects not only fetal growth and development—evidence indicates it also has a significant influence on adult health. Several decades ago, physician and professor David Barker showed for the first time that people born at low birth weight are at greater risk of developing coronary heart disease. In 1995, the British Medical Journal named this the "Barker hypothesis," which is now widely accepted. Evidence from both epidemiological studies in humans and experimental ones in animals indicates that prenatal maternal nutrition has long-lasting consequences and sensitizes the offspring to the development of several chronic diseases.

Prenatal flavor learning

The perception of flavor is moderated by three senses that act synergistically: chemosensory irritation, taste, and smell. Chemosensory irritation refers to oral perceptions of food or beverages such as burning (e.g., with hot peppers), fizziness (carbonated beverages), or coolness (menthol). For taste, there are five primary categories: sweet, salty, bitter, sour and umami, or savory (Bachmanov & Beauchamp, 2007). Taste buds are present in the fetus by 7–8 weeks, with evidence of receptor cell maturity by 16 weeks. There is evidence that by the third trimester, fetuses have demonstrated innate preference for sweets by increasing fetal swallowing of amniotic fluid after injection of sweet substances into the amniotic fluid. Conversely, bitter substances have been shown to decrease fetal swallowing (Blackburn, 2012). From an evolutionary perspective, there is an advantage to preferring sweets (often rich in calories to support growth) and to avoiding bitter substances (many bitter plants are poisonous).

The largest factor in flavor perception is usually the sense of smell. Specific chemical compounds called odorants are detected by olfactory receptor cells in the epithelium of the nasal cavity, with transmission of impulses to the olfactory bulb, a structure located at the anterior end of the brain. Projections from the olfactory bulb extend to the prepyriform cerebral cortex, the amygdala (part of the limbic system, known as the emotional center of the brain), and the hypothalamus. These connections directly impact the hypothalamic–pituitary–adrenocortical axis. These projections explain why the memory of certain odors can produce intense emotions and even engender a stress response of the sympathetic nervous system (Herz, 1998). In the fetus, ciliated olfactory receptor cells are present by 11 weeks' gestation, with evidence of odor molecules stimulating fetal odor receptors by the third trimester of pregnancy (Blackburn, 2012). Strong odors such as garlic have been easily detected in amniotic fluid (Mennella, Johnson, & Beauchamp, 1995).

In an early study on prenatal flavor learning, pregnant women were randomly assigned to consume either 300 mL of carrot juice or water for 4 days/week for three consecutive weeks in their last trimester of pregnancy. After the infants' birth, when mothers began to supplement their infant's diet with solid foods months later, infants were videotaped while eating cereal mixed with water on one test day and cereal mixed with carrot juice on another test day. The videotapes of the feedings were reviewed by independent raters who were blinded to the experimental conditions of the study. Those infants who had prenatal exposure to the carrot flavor were more likely to accept carrots when compared with infants who had no prenatal exposure to the carrot flavor (Mennella, Jagnow, & Beauchamp, 2001). Cell biologists have been able to identify the specific neuroanatomic changes that occur in olfactory bulb glomeruli in mice pups with *in utero* exposure to odorants from metabolites of the mother's diet, with subsequent preferences for the odorants by mice pups after parturition (Todrank, Heth, & Restrepo, 2011).

There is evidence in humans that flavor learning continues postnatally with breastfeeding (Beauchamp & Mennella, 2009). This has been postulated as another factor contributing to the improved health status of the breastfed infant, as a variety of flavors are encountered from mother's milk, compared to the monotonous flavors found in commercial formula.

Contributed by Kimberly Trout, CNM, PhD.

In particular, links are well established between reduced birth weight and increased risk of coronary heart disease, diabetes, hypertension, and stroke in adulthood (Fall, 2005; Vieau, 2011). In addition, infants born with FGR are at high risk for physical and mental impairments in later life (Institute of Medicine [IOM], 2007).

Prenatal flavor learning

Recent research has suggested that flavor preferences start *in utero* based on what the mother consumes. Exposure to a variety of healthy food flavors starting *in utero* and early infancy can modulate children's flavor preferences with the potential to improve lifelong health (Esposito, Fisher, Mennella, Hoelsher, & Huang, 2009). Adding the concept of pre- and postnatal flavor learning to nutrition education, health-care providers can empower pregnant and breastfeeding women to influence their child's future nutritional health by eating a large variety of healthy food.

Nutritional needs in pregnancy

The need for most nutrients increases during pregnancy to meet pregnancy demands. The pregnant woman's basal metabolic rate (BMR) is elevated to produce maternal pregnancy components; fetal growth needs increase during pregnancy and the body stores fat to prepare for lactation. Increased nutrient intake is needed to account for these amazing physiological activities.

Fluid intake

Fluid requirements increase during pregnancy to approximately 3 L/day, primarily due to the increase in blood volume, production of amniotic fluid, and increase in BMR. This translates into approximately 8–12 8-oz glasses per day. Adequate fluid intake also prevents urinary tract infection and constipation. The fluid needs are even higher in warm weather or during periods of exercise. Pregnant women should be encouraged to drink fluids regularly throughout the day rather than wait to feel thirst.

High consumption of sugary drinks during pregnancy has been associated with an increased risk of GDM, (Chen, Hu, Yeung, Willett, & Zhang, 2009), preterm birth (Englund-Ögge et al., 2012), and obesity in offspring (Phelan et al., 2011). Consumption of high-sugar drinks such as sodas, and some sports drinks and fruit drinks, should be discouraged during pregnancy, and women should be informed of the rationale behind these recommendations. The ready availability of prepackaged and high-sugar fluids contributes to reduced water consumption. Adequate water consumption should be promoted.

Strategies to increase water consumption

Inform women of the pregnancy benefits of adequate water consumption:

- decreases constipation, swelling, headache, risk of urinary tract infection, heartburn, cramping
- prevents dehydration
- promotes adequate blood volume to carry fetal nutrients
- aids digestion
- regulates body temperature.

Flavor water with lemon or lime.
Set a timer to drink water.
Bring a water bottle to work and keep it filled and nearby.
Fill a large pitcher with daily water amount to drink during the day.

Macronutrients: Total energy

Caloric recommendation in pregnancy should be based upon trimester and the woman's prepregnancy body mass index (BMI). During the first trimester, there is no increased energy cost associated with a singleton pregnancy in a woman who is of normal weight or higher (Rasmussen, Yaktine, & Committee to Reexamine IOM Pregnancy Weight Guidelines, Institute of Medicine, National Research Council, 2009). Weight gain during the first trimester is relatively minimal, ranging from 0 to 4 lb. Some women may gain no weight because extreme nausea, vomiting, or fatigue prevents them from eating their normal diet, while others may add a few pounds to their frame because of increased hunger, fluid retention, or reduced physical activity. Generally speaking, women need to increase caloric intake by 340 kcal/day during the second trimester and 450 kcal/day during the third trimester for a singleton pregnancy. Women with a BMI in the underweight range should increase their caloric intake in the first trimester by approximately 150 cal/day.

Macronutrients: Fats

Fats are a type of lipid and are sources of vitamins and concentrated calories and contribute to the healthy development of cells. Fats are essential components of a healthy prenatal diet. An RDA or AI has not been established for fats as a group; however, the recommendation is for fats to make up 20–35% of the total daily caloric intake (IOM, 2010). An evaluation of the type of fats frequently consumed by the pregnant women should be done during the nutritional intake history. Monounsaturated fats (olive, canola, peanut oils) and polyunsaturated fats (flaxseed, corn oils) should predominate in the diet, while saturated (coconut oil, lard) and trans fats (packaged baked goods, chip snacks) should be limited.

Omega-3 fatty acids

The three main omega-3 fatty acids are alpha-linolenic acid (ALA), eicosapentaenoic acid (EPA), and docosahexaenoic acid (DHA). ALA comes from plants and is found in vegetable, flaxseed, walnut, canola, and soybean oils. ALA is the most common omega-3 fatty acid in the Western diet. ALA is a dietary essential fatty acid; we must eat it because our bodies cannot make it and use it to form the functionally essential omega-3 fatty acids, EPA and DHA. Although the American diet contains the recommended amount of ALA, it is not well converted to EPA and DHA. Therefore, preformed EPA and DHA are required for optimal health in most people, especially during periods of rapid growth and development such as pregnancy and in the first year of life. EPA and DHA are known as the "long-chain" or marine omega-3 fatty acids since they are mainly found preformed in fish and fish oils. EPA and DHA have significant health benefits; however, both are especially low in the American diet.

Perinatal outcomes

The major benefits for infants are in brain and eye development and improved developmental outcomes. The significance of DHA for fetal brain and eye development is widely recognized. DHA is important for the structure, growth, and development of the fetal central nervous system and the retina. Comprising roughly 30% of fetal brain weight, DHA is a major part of fetal neural tissue, and it maintains good neurotransmitter function. Adequate levels of maternal DHA during pregnancy and breastfeeding have been linked with improved infant and childhood cognitive development (Hibbeln, Davis, & Steer, 2007; McCann & Ames, 2005).

The fetus and nursing newborn acquires DHA from its mother. DHA accrues rapidly in the brain during the third trimester and the first 6 weeks of life. DHA naturally occurs in human milk, and omega-3 supplementation during pregnancy and lactation increases levels of DHA in breast milk as well as in infants. Since Food and Drug Administration (FDA) approval in 2002, infant formula is supplemented with DHA to support optimal brain and eye development.

Emerging research suggests that prenatal DHA supplementation reduces the risk for early preterm birth. A review of observational studies, randomized trials, and meta-analyses of the association between fish oil and preterm birth reported a correlation in between fish intake during pregnancy and a modest increased length of gestation (Makrides, Duley, & Olsen, 2006). Omega-3 supplementation is associated with a significantly lower rate of early preterm birth (<34 weeks' gestation) compared with controls (Horvath, Koletzko, & Szajewska, 2007).

Recommendations for omega-3 intake in pregnancy

The European Perinatal Lipid Intake (Perlip) Group along with other experts in omega-3 research recommended a minimal intake of 200 mg of DHA per day during pregnancy and lactation. The National Institute of Health (NIH) recommended a daily intake of 300 mg DHA per day. There are no specific recommendations for EPA. Higher intakes (up to 1 g/day of DHA and 2.7 g/ day total long-chain polyunsaturated fatty acid [LC-PUFA]) have been shown in randomized trials to have no significant adverse effects in pregnancy (Makrides et al., 2006). It is reasonable to advise women to take in 200–300 mg/day.

Helping women to sort through and understand complex nutritional information is a key component of prenatal nutritional counseling. A conflicting set of messages confronts pregnant women regarding fish consumption: "eat more fish because it is promotes healthy fetal brain development," and "eat less fish because it contains mercury." Mercury is a neurotoxin that is detrimental for brain development *in utero* and throughout early childhood. The main sources of mercury are coal-burning power plants and chemical facilities, which emit mercury to the atmosphere; from the air, it is deposited on water bodies. It enters the food chain via bacteria that convert it into methyl mercury, and then it bioaccumulates along the food chain so that large, predatory fish have the highest levels. Fish are the primary sources of essential omega-3 fatty acids documented to improve maternal, neonatal, and childhood health. Pregnant women eat less than the recommended servings of fish (Lando, Fein, & Choinière, 2012). To reduce food-borne exposure, pregnant women should follow U.S. Environmental Protection Agency (EPA) and state-specific fish consumption guidelines (Table 6.3).

Fish oil supplements are typically purified and free of harmful levels of mercury, polychlorinated biphenyls (PCBs), and dioxins. Cod liver oil is not the best supplement for pregnant mothers due to high levels of vitamin A. Although it is possible for pregnant women to achieve recommended DHA intake via supplements or fortified foods, most experts recommend regular fish consumption when possible (Cetin & Koletzko, 2008).

A risk–benefit analysis confirmed that the childhood cognitive benefits from maternal fish and shellfish consumption far outweigh potential risks due to environmental contaminants (Environmental Protection Agency (EPA), 2007). The U.S. Departments of Agriculture and

Table 6.3 EPA and FDA Advice to Pregnant Women about Eating Fish

- Fish contains omega-3 fatty acids that promote fetal brain and retinal development.
- Consume two servings (12 oz) of fish per week.
- Supplement with fish oil if fish is not eaten.
- Avoid eating shark, swordfish, king mackerel, and tilefish (also known as golden bass or golden snapper), which contain high levels of mercury.
- Canned chunk light tuna has less mercury and can be eaten twice per week. Limit albacore ("white") tuna to 6 oz per week.
- Remove skin and surface fat from fish before cooking.
- Check local and state advisories on safety of recreationally caught fish. Information on advisories can be found at http://www.epa.gov/fishadvisories/.

of Health and Human Services agree and suggest that pregnant and breastfeeding women should eat no less than 8 oz of seafood a week to ensure the best possible brain and eye development for their babies. The World Health Organization recommends that health-care providers inform pregnant women that eating a variety of fish helps to improve fetal and neonatal brain development and not eating fish may deprive the baby of this health benefit (WHO, 2011). Pregnant women need to be informed that they can safely eat cooked seafood regularly, provided they eat fish within the EPA guidelines and follow local recommendations for recreationally caught fish.

Macronutrients: Carbohydrates

The primary source of fuel for fetal growth and development is glucose, a substrate primarily related to the amount and type of carbohydrate in the maternal diet. Carbohydrates occur in two different forms: simple and complex. Simple carbohydrates are broken down quickly by the body into glucose to be used as energy. Simple carbohydrates are found naturally in foods such as fruits, milk, and milk products. They are also found in processed and refined foods such as candy, table sugar, syrups, and soft drinks.

Complex carbohydrates, also known as starches, are found in some cereals, whole grain foods, starchy vegetables like broccoli and corn, and legumes. Overall, complex carbohydrates take longer to digest, are important sources of dietary fiber, and promote satiety for longer periods. All carbohydrates break down into glucose. Complex carbohydrates tend to maintain blood glucose levels more evenly over time, and simple sugars tend to increase blood glucose levels then drop more quickly.

The recommended RDA carbohydrate intake for pregnant women is 175 g/day. Most American women eat enough carbohydrates to meet normal pregnancy requirements. Pregnant women should be advised that low carbohydrate diets are not healthy during pregnancy, though women with GDM (Chapter 23) benefit from a mild restriction on carbohydrates. As with other nutrients, the quality of the carbohydrate food source should be evaluated. The majority of carbohydrate intake should come from complex carbohydrates and naturally occurring sugars rather than processed or refined sugars.

Protein

Protein intake is essential to pregnancy because it forms the structural basis for the new cells and tissues in the mother and fetus. Nitrogen is the primary element in protein that differentiates it from fats and carbohydrates. Protein sources include meat, fish, poultry eggs, dairy products, tofu and other soy products, legumes, nuts, and seeds. The RDA for protein intake during pregnancy and lactation is 71 g/day. The average protein intake for American women ages 20–39 is 74 g/day; thus, protein needs are easily met by most women. Women who choose no-meat diets and those living with food insecurity are at higher risk for protein deficiency.

When evaluating a diet for protein intake, the overall quality of the diet should be taken into account. A woman may have an adequate protein intake, but if her overall caloric intake is low, some of the amino acids from protein are used for energy rather than for building blocks. The quality of the protein should also be evaluated. Low-fat protein sources and food preparation methods should predominate in the prenatal diet.

High-protein prenatal diets in daily excess RDA should be avoided. Observational and experimental animal studies suggest that a consistent high-protein maternal diet raises fetal ammonia levels and can cause harmful effects, such as an increase in spontaneous early pregnancy loss (Kind, Moore, & Davis, 2006) and high blood pressure (Shiell et al., 2001) and altered stress response in offspring (Koski & Hill, 1986).

Micronutrients

Iron

Maternal iron needs nearly double during pregnancy, though the demand for additional iron is not spread evenly throughout pregnancy. In the first trimester, requirements are actually reduced because menstruation has ceased, the demands of the fetus are still small, and the expansion of the maternal red cell mass is not yet significant. The need for additional iron begins early in the second trimester and reaches a peak toward the

Table 6.4   Select Daily Macronutrient and Micronutrient Dietary Reference Intakes in Pregnancy

	Calcium (mg)	Vitamin D (µg)	Iron (mg)	Folate (mcg)	DHA and EPA (mg)	Carbohydrate (g)	Fiber (g)	Protein (g)
14–18 years old pregnant	1300	600	27	400	200–300	175	28	71
19–50 years old pregnant	1000	600	27	400	200–300	175	28	71

Adapted from: Food and Nutrition Board, Institute of Medicine, National Academies.

end of the third trimester. Maternal iron deficiency anemia increases risk for adverse birth outcomes, including low birth weight, perinatal mortality, and may increase risk of preterm birth. Iron needs increase in pregnancy to support the increased maternal red blood cell mass and to build fetal iron stores needed for the first several months of life. The RDA for pregnant women is 27 mg/day, which is the amount of iron commonly found in most prenatal vitamin formulations (Table 6.4).

Iron absorption

Iron absorption refers to the amount of dietary iron that the body obtains and uses from food. Healthy adults absorb about 10–15% of dietary iron, but individual absorption is influenced by several factors. Iron absorption increases when body stores are low. When iron stores are high, absorption decreases to help protect against the toxic effects of iron overload. A woman's body absorbs iron more efficiently during pregnancy, offering a protective effect against anemia.

Iron absorption is also influenced by the type of dietary iron consumed. Dietary iron has two forms: heme iron and nonheme iron. Heme is found in meat, poultry, and fish. Nonheme iron is found in eggs and plant-based foods, such as legumes, vegetables, fruit, grains, nuts, and iron-fortified grain products. Iron utilization from heme iron provides for a higher bioavailability of iron than nonheme sources or from ferrous sulfate iron supplementation (Young et al., 2010). This suggests that pregnant women should be encouraged to eat fish and animal proteins to meet iron needs in pregnancy. Absorption of heme iron from meat proteins is efficient and is not significantly affected by diet. In contrast, lesser amounts of nonheme iron in plant foods is absorbed and is significantly influenced by various food components ingested at the same meal. Meat proteins and vitamin C will improve the absorption of nonheme iron. Tannins, as found in tea and wine, calcium, and some substances found in legumes and whole grains can decrease absorption of nonheme iron (National Institutes of Health (NIH), 2007). Pregnant women should be advised to include foods that enhance nonheme iron absorption, especially when only vegetarian nonheme sources of iron are consumed.

Iron supplementation

Additional iron supplementation could be of particular benefit to low-income or ethnically diverse women who have some of the lowest iron intakes (Bokhari, Derbyshire, Li, & Brennan, 2012). Anemic women with hematocrit levels less than 33% in the first and third trimesters or less than 32% in the second trimester should be supplemented with oral iron preparations and encouraged to consume iron-rich foods. The gastrointestinal side effects of iron supplementation, such as constipation, painful passage of hard stool, and nausea, often prompt women to stop supplementation. Intermittent supplementation of one tablet one to three times per week weekly can reduce side effects and increase acceptance and adherence to supplementation, while still improving anemia (Peña-Rosas, De-Regil, Dowswell, & Viteri, 2012). In addition, intermittent supplementation decreases the number of women with high hemoglobin concentrations during mid and late pregnancy compared with daily regimens. High hemoglobin concentrations may be harmful as they may be associated with an increased risk of preterm birth and low birth weight (Peña-Rosas et al., 2012).

Folate

Folate, or folic acid, is a water-soluble form of vitamin B_9 found in foods such as leafy green vegetables, bananas, lentils, and fortified cereal products. It is well established that adequate folate intake before conception and during the first month after conception reduces the risk of neural tube defects (NTDs). Supplementation of grain products with folic acid was initiated in 1998 by a mandate from the FDA in response to scientific knowledge about NTD prevention. The fortification program has been effective in reducing the incidence of NTD by 70% (Blencowe, Cousens, Modell, & Lawn, 2010). Folic acid taken in the early weeks of pregnancy can reduce risk of oral cleft and cardiovascular anomalies (Goh, Bollano, Einarson, & Koren, 2006). Low levels of folate in early pregnancy are associated with lower placental weight and birth weight, and increased incidence of preeclampsia (Bergen et al., 2012). Expert groups advocate that childbearing age women take folic acid supplements; however, the majority of childbearing age women do not consume folic acid supplements regularly (Tinker, Cogswell, Devine, & Berry, 2010). Women should consume 400 mcg of folate prior to and during pregnancy (IOM, 2010). Most prenatal vitamin formulations have at least 400 mcg of folic acid.

Calcium and vitamin D

The growing fetus requires adequate calcium for skeletal growth and development. Fetal calcium levels exceed maternal levels, indicating active transport of calcium across the placenta (Stables & Rankin, 2009). The high fetal demand for calcium during pregnancy is facilitated by a maternal increase in calcium absorption ability during pregnancy. The RDA for elemental calcium is 1000 mg/day in pregnant and lactating women 19–50 years of age and 1300 mg for pregnant girls 14–18 years old (IOM, 2010).

Many childbearing age women in the United States do not consume the DRI for calcium. Women at risk for lower calcium intake include adolescents, those who are lactose intolerant, women following a vegetarian diet, and women with low income. Vegetarians might absorb less calcium than omnivores because they consume more plant products containing oxalic and phytic acids (IOM, 2010). Women who chronically consume very low amounts of calcium (<500 mg/day) may be at risk for increased bone loss during pregnancy (Hacker, Fung, & King, 2012). Women who begin pregnancy with adequate daily intake may not need additional calcium, but women with suboptimal intakes (<500 mg) require additional amounts to meet both maternal and fetal bone needs.

Rich natural sources of well-absorbed calcium include milk, yogurt, and cheese. Calcium content varies slightly by fat content; the more fat, the less calcium the food contains. Some vegetables such as kale, broccoli, and Chinese cabbage contain calcium. Calcium-fortified foods like orange juice and cereals are also excellent sources.

Vitamin D, a fat-soluble molecule acquired through exposure to sunlight or diet, has been identified as a steroid hormone precursor that modulates long-term programming of human health. Vitamin D helps the body use calcium and maximizes fetal bone growth (Young et al., 2012). There is a wide divergence of recommendations for prenatal vitamin D intake. The commonly followed guidelines issues by the NIH (2011) and IOM (2011) recommend 600 IU daily during pregnancy. The Endocrine Society supports a daily intake of 4000-IU vitamin D_3 to achieve a circulating 25-hydroxyvitamin D of 40–60 ng/mL (100–150 nmol) during pregnancy (Hollis & Wagner, 2013).This more current recommendation takes into account both observational and randomized controlled trial data. Research is ongoing in this area to reach consensus on recommendations. It is espe-

cially important to ensure adequate vitamin D intake during the winter months and for women with dark pigmented skin since sunlight helps the body synthesize vitamin D. Prenatal vitamin formulations typically contain between 400 and 600 mg vitamin D.

Weight gain in pregnancy

Once pregnancy is confirmed, monitoring gestational weight gain is incorporated as part of the prenatal care regimen. At the first prenatal visit, prepregnancy BMI is calculated using previously measured weights and heights or self-reported prepregnancy weight to establish the appropriate weight gain range. The weight gain range serves as the woman's weight gain goal. The total amount of weight gained in normal-term pregnancies varies considerably among women. As pregnancy progresses, protein, fat, water, and minerals are deposited in the fetus, placenta, amniotic fluid, uterus, mammary gland, blood, and adipose tissue. The products of conception placenta, fetus, and amniotic fluid comprise approximately 35% of the total pregnancy weight gain (Pitkin, 1976). Normal fetal growth is relatively uniform until the mid-second trimester. At term, there is much greater variation in fetal weight.

Average pregnancy weight gain distribution

- 6–8 lb   Baby
- 1.5 lb   Placenta
- 2 lb   Amniotic fluid
- 2 lb   Uterus growth
- 2 lb   Breast growth
- 8 lb   Added and body fluids
- 7 lb   Added muscle and fat stores

Source: Rasmussen et al. (2009).

As American women of childbearing age have become heavier, recommendations have been reexamined to achieve a balance between the risks due to overweight or obese status and fetal growth needs. The IOM issues pregnancy weight gain recommendations based on prepregnancy weight (Table 6.5). Recommended weight gains for short women and for individual racial and ethnic groups are the same as those for the whole population. Women who gain weight within the IOM guidelines are more likely to have better maternal and infant outcomes (Siega-Riz et al., 2009). The pattern of gestational weight gain, like total gestational weight gain, is

Table 6.5   IOM Recommendations for Total and Rate of Weight Gain during Pregnancy by Prepregnancy BMI

Prepregnancy BMI category	Optimal weight gain (lb)	Weight gain, first trimester (lb)	Weight gain, second and third trimesters (lb/week)
Underweight: BMI <18.5	28–40	5	1–2
Normal weight: BMI 18.5–24.9	25–35	2–5	1–2
Overweight: BMI 35–29.9	15–25	0–2	1/2–2/3
Obese: BMI ≥30	11–20	0–1	1/2

highly variable, even among women with good pregnancy outcomes.

Weight gain higher than the recommendations is linked with the same prenatal, intrapartum, and postpartum complications as prepregnancy obesity such as preeclampsia and macrosomia (see Chapter 36, "Obesity"). Excess weight gain during pregnancy and failure to lose weight after pregnancy are important and identifiable predictors of long-term obesity and weight-related complications in women later in life. More than half of American women gain excessive weight in pregnancy (Herring, Rose, Skouteris, & Oken, 2012; Ludwig & Currie, 2010). Women should be counseled preconceptually and at the first prenatal visit on their optimal range of weight gain during pregnancy.

Overweight and obesity in pregnancy

Approximately 30% of reproductive age women in the United States are overweight, while another 30% are obese (Ogden, Caroll, Bit, & Flegal, 2012). Maternal overweight or obesity status prior to pregnancy is linked with increased risks for pregnancy complications such as GDM and preeclampsia (Chu et al., 2007), NTDs, oomphalocele, and cardiac anomalies (Rasmussen, Chu, Kim, Schmid, & Lau, 2008). Maternal obesity doubles the risk of stillbirth and neonatal death (Kristensen, Vestergaard, Wisborg, Kesmodel, & Secher, 2005). Women who are overweight or obese before pregnancy are more likely to exceed the IOM's recommended maximum weight gain for their body size. The issues related to pregnancy obesity are covered in detail in Chapter 36.

Underweight in pregnancy

The percentage of women who started their pregnancy underweight is approximately 6–7% in white women, 4–5% in black women, and 3–4% in Hispanic women

(Reinold, Dalenius, Brindley, Smith, & Grummer-Strawn, 2011). Women who begin their pregnancy underweight as defined by a BMI of less than 18.5 have a greater risk of neonatal morbidity, preterm delivery (Zhong, Macones, Zhu, & Odibo, 2010), placental abruption, and infant low birth weight and FGR (Deutsch, Lynch, Alio, Salihu, & Spellacy, 2010; Kosa et al., 2011; Rasmussen & Yaktine, 2009). Regardless of BMI, pregnant women who gain inadequate amounts of weight face increased risks of preterm birth and low birth weight (Abu-Saad & Fraser, 2010).

Screening for additional risk factors such as smoking, tobacco and alcohol abuse, and the presence of an eating disorder should be done since these are often coexisting comorbidities in women who are underweight and malnourished (Harris, 2010). Additional factors that may promote inadequate weight gain include nausea and vomiting, food aversions, lactose intolerance, cultural food practices, minimal resources (such as poverty), poor prepregnancy diet, and excessive physical activity.

Strategies to improve weight gain begin with the development of a nutrition plan. Underweight pregnant women should take a multivitamin and mineral supplementation and should receive regular nutritional counseling during prenatal care. The optimal weight gain for women who start pregnancy underweight is between 28 and 40 lb. A goal of 1–2 lb/week can be encouraged.

Advice for achieving a healthy weight gain in pregnancy

Women will be more likely to achieve and maintain a healthy weight before, during, and after pregnancy if they

- eat breakfast
- eat fiber-rich foods such as oats, beans, peas, lentils, grains, seeds, fruits and vegetables, as well as whole grain bread and pastas, and brown rice
- eat low-fat proteins such as fish, lean meat, and skim milk
- eat at least five portions of various fruits and vegetables daily
- eat a low-fat diet and avoid increasing fat intake
- eat as little as possible of fried food; drinks and desserts high in added sugars (such as cakes, pastries, and fizzy drinks); and other foods high in fat and empty calories (such as fast foods)
- monitor portion size of meals and snacks
- make activities such as walking, cycling, swimming, aerobics, and gardening part of daily life
- minimize sedentary activities, such as sitting for long periods watching television, at a computer, or playing video games.

Sources: NICE, IOM.

Food safety during pregnancy

What is safe to eat and what should not be consumed during pregnancy can be an area of confusion for both women and health-care providers. Pregnant women are at an increased risk for getting some food-borne infections because of the hormonal changes that occur during pregnancy. While such changes are necessary for the survival of the fetus, they also suppress the mother's immune system, thereby increasing the chance of infection from certain food-borne pathogens. All pregnant women should be provided with information on food safety and foods to avoid. Table 6.6 contains a list of foods and beverages that should be avoided during pregnancy.

Safe food handling

- Wash hands frequently.
- Wash fruits and vegetables before eating or preparation.
- Wash kitchen surfaces, cutting boards, and utensils before and after food preparation, especially after contact with raw meat or poultry.
- Separate raw meat, poultry, and seafood from other foods.
- Cook food to proper temperatures.
- Refrigerate foods quickly to prevent harmful bacteria from proliferating.
- Refrigerate all perishable foods at or below 40°F.
- Reheat leftover foods to 165°F before eating.

Table 6.6 Foods and Beverages to Avoid during Pregnancy

Food to avoid	Rationale	Do not consume
Alcohol	Drinking during pregnancy, especially in the first few months of pregnancy, may result in negative behavioral or neurological consequences in the offspring.	Beer, wine, mixed drinks
Raw fish	Raw or undercooked fin and shellfish are more likely to contain parasites and bacteria than foods made from cooked fish.	Sushi; sashimi; raw or undercooked oysters, clams, and mussels; scallops; ceviché.
Raw eggs	Raw eggs can contain salmonella and other food-borne illness-causing bacteria. The CDC estimates that one egg in 20,000 may be contaminated.	Cookie dough, fresh eggnog, Hollandaise sauce, Béarnaise sauce, homemade mayonnaise and ice cream, mousse, meringue, tiramisu made with uncooked eggs
Raw milk	Some cheeses are made with unpasteurized milk. These cheeses are typically produced and sold locally. Potential pathogens are *Listeria* and *E. coli*.	Raw milk such as goat's milk cheeses like chèvre; queso fresco, Brie, Camembert; soft blue-veined cheeses, such as Danish blue, gorgonzola, and Roquefort
Raw sprouts	Bacteria can get into the sprout seeds through cracks in the shell before the sprouts are grown. Once this occurs, these bacteria are nearly impossible to wash out.	Alfalfa, clover, radish sprouts in salads or on sandwiches
Unpasteurized juice	Unpasteurized juices may contain harmful bacteria such as *E. coli*. Unpasteurized juices must have a warning on the label.	Unpasteurized apple cider, health-food store juices, juice bar juices.
Smoked meats and seafood including pâté	Possible source of *Listeria*	Refrigerated smoked seafood like whitefish, salmon, and mackerel; meat fish and vegetable pâté
Unheated lunch meats, hot dogs	Possible source of *Listeria*; to eat safely, these meats should be reheated until steaming hot.	
Excessive caffeine	Possible increased risk of miscarriage	>200 mg caffeine: about two 8 oz cups of coffee

Food-borne infections

Certain organisms can cross the placenta and cause fetal infection. Infection can result in miscarriage, stillbirth, preterm birth, fetal infection, and neonatal illness. Examples of pathogens of special concern to pregnant women are *Listeria monocytogenes*, *Toxoplasma gondii*, *Brucella* species, *Salmonella* species, and *Campylobacter jejuni.*

Listeriosis is a form of infection that may result when foods containing the bacteria *L. monocytogenes* are consumed. *L. monocytogenes* is widely found in soil, groundwater, plants and animals. *L. monocytogenes* is often carried by humans and animals, and has the ability to survive unfavorable conditions, including refrigeration temperatures, food preservatives, and conditions with little or no oxygen. It is easily destroyed by cooking. Once in the bloodstream, *Listeria* bacteria can travel to any site, but seem to prefer the central nervous system and the placenta. The fetus is unusually prone to listeriosis and infection can cause early pregnancy loss, stillbirth, or infection of the neonate and significant health problems. There is an estimated 14-fold increase in the incidence of listeriosis among pregnant women compared to nonpregnant adults, with pregnant women accounting for approximately one-third all cases (Pouillot, Hoelzer, Jackson, Henao, & Silk, 2012).

Listeriosis is more common in the third trimester, and signs and symptoms are easily missed. A nonspecific flu-like illness with symptoms such as fever, chills, headache, muscle aches, and backaches is the most common presentation. Foods typically associated with listeriosis have a long shelf life and are eaten without further cooking (Lorber, 2010). Outbreaks have involved foods such as coleslaw, Mexican-style soft cheeses, milk, pâté, pork tongue, hot dogs, processed meats, and deli salads. To avoid infection from *L. monocytogenes*, pregnant women are advised to practice safe food handling procedures, avoid eating soft cheeses and other foods made from raw milk, unpasteurized milk, raw or undercooked seafood, refrigerated, smoked or precooked seafood, deli seafood salads, and hot dogs, luncheon meats, deli meats, and pâté unless reheated to steaming hot before serving (USDA, 2009).

Toxoplasmosis, the infection caused by the parasite *T. gondii*, can be passed to humans by water, dust, soil, or through eating contaminated foods. It is estimated that 1.5 million people in the United States become infected with *T. gondii* each year (USDA, 2009). Most individuals do not experience symptoms and will develop a protective resistance to the parasite. However, if a woman not previously exposed to *T. gondii* first acquires the parasite a few months before or during pregnancy, she may pass the organism to the fetus. This could result in stillbirth, fetal death, or neonatal health problems such as eye or brain damage. Symptoms in the baby may not be visible at birth but can appear months or even years later.

Toxoplasmosis most often results from eating raw or undercooked meat, especially pork, and wild game meat, eating unwashed fruits and vegetables, cleaning a cat litter box, or handling contaminated soil (Lindsay & Dubey, 2011). To avoid infection from *T. gondii*, it is important that pregnant women practice safe food handling procedures. Meat should be cooked to an internal temperature of 145°F with a 3-minute rest time as this kills *T. gondii* (Centers for Disease Control and Prevention [CDC], 2011). Pregnant women should also wash hands often, especially after handling animals or working in the garden, and have a family member clean the litter box or wear gloves during the task if they own a cat.

Campylobacteriosis is an infection caused by consuming food or water that contains the bacteria *C. jejuni or Campylobacter coli*. It is a very common cause of diarrhea accompanied by fever in the United States. These organisms are found in the intestinal tracts of animals, especially chickens, and in untreated water. People are infected most often by consuming raw unpasteurized milk and raw milk products, raw or undercooked poultry or meat, and raw shellfish (CDC, 2011). Maternal campylobacteriosis infection can be transmitted to the fetus through the placenta. Consequences of fetal infection include abortion, stillbirth, or preterm birth. Maternal symptoms usually appear within 2–5 days after eating the contaminated food and include fever, stomach cramps, muscle pain, diarrhea, nausea, and vomiting. The diagnosis is established by stool culture and is treated with erythromycin. To avoid campylobacteriosis, pregnant women are advised to practice safe food handling procedures, to consume only pasteurized milk and milk products, and to thoroughly cook meat, poultry, and shellfish (CDC, 2011).

Alcohol, caffeine, and artificial sweeteners

No safe level of alcohol consumption during pregnancy has been established. All pregnant women should be counseled to abstain from drinking alcoholic beverages. Many women are concerned about alcohol intake in early gestation before they knew they were pregnant. During conception and for about 2 weeks thereafter, most cells of the conceptus are not yet committed to a specific developmental program. One damaged cell can be replaced by another, and normal development will usually ensue, although the embryo will not survive if too many cells are damaged or killed. This is known as the "all or none" period where the fetus is generally not susceptible to teratogens (Cragan et al., 2006). Women who ingested

Caffeine content of select coffee brands		
Coffee	**Serving size (fl oz)**	**Caffeine (mg)**
Dunkin' Donuts Coffee with Turbo Shot	Large, 20	436
Starbucks Coffee	Venti, 20	415
Starbucks Coffee	Grande, 16	330
Panera Frozen Mocha	16.5	267
Starbucks Coffee	Tall, 12	260
Starbucks Caffè Americano	Grande, 16	225
Panera Coffee	Regular, 16.8	189
Starbucks Espresso Frappuccino	Venti, 24	185
Dunkin' Donuts Coffee	Medium, 14	178
Starbucks Caffè Mocha	Grande, 16	175
Starbucks Iced Coffee	Grande, 16	165
Dunkin' Donuts Cappuccino	Large, 20	151
Starbucks—Caffè Latte, Cappuccino, or Caramel Macchiato	Grande, 16	150
Starbucks Espresso	Doppio, 2	150
Keurig Coffee K-Cup, all varieties	1 cup, makes 8	75–150
Starbucks Doubleshot Energy Coffee, can	15	146
Starbucks Mocha Frappuccino	Venti, 24	140
Starbucks VIA House Blend Instant Coffee	1 packet, makes 8	135
McDonald's Coffee	Large, 16	133
Seattle's Best Coffee—Iced Latte or Iced Mocha, can	9.5	90
Starbucks Frappuccino Coffee, bottle	9.5	90
International Delight Iced Coffee	8	76

December 2012. Most of the information was obtained from company Web sites. Serving sizes are based on commonly consumed portions or the amount of the leading-selling container size. For example, beverages sold in 16- or 20-oz bottles were counted as one serving.

alcohol in the first few weeks of pregnancy should be offered reassurance regarding this early exposure.

High caffeine intake during pregnancy is associated with an increased risk of spontaneous miscarriage and low birth weight (Weng, Odouli, & Li, 2008). Caffeine intakes greater than 200 mg/day are discouraged (March of Dimes [MOD], 2012). Average caffeine content of brewed coffee is 188 mg for 16 oz, with a range of 143–300 mg (McCusker, Goldberger, & Cone, 2003), although caffeine content can vary widely among different type of beans used within one brand. Women should be counseled of the different caffeine contents of various coffee brands and encouraged to reduce serving size.

Carbonated sodas contain between 18 and 48 mg/12-oz can, whereas energy drinks have higher caffeine content of 33–75 mg/8.4 oz (McCusker, Goldberger, & Cone, 2006).

Very few studies have investigated whether regular intakes of foods containing artificial sweeteners are safe during pregnancy. Moderate intake of alternative sweeteners that are classified by the FDA as "generally recognized as safe" within acceptable daily intakes is considered safe in pregnancy. Alternative sweeteners that are generally recognized as safe include aspartame, sucralose, neotame, and stevia. Saccharin should be avoided during pregnancy because of possible slow fetal clearance (Shwide-Slavin, Swift, & Ross, 2012). Daily intake of artificially sweetened soft drinks may increase the risk of preterm birth; however, more study is needed before conclusive recommendations can be made (Englund-Ögge et al., 2012).

Factors influencing nutritional intake

Resource availability

There are significant differences in food choices in different socioeconomic classes that lead to both under- and overnutrition. Class differences in diet are of particular concern with respect to health inequalities. Women with nutritional deficits are often found in low socioeconomic populations and commonly involve multiple nutrients (Fall et al., 2003). Food insecurity is associated with risk of greater than recommended weight gain during pregnancy and pregnancy complications such as diabetes mellitus (Laraia, Siega-Riz, & Gundersen, 2010).

Culture and family

Traditions, beliefs, and values are among the main factors that influence food preference, mode of food preparation, and nutritional status. The shaping of food choices takes place in the home, which typically reflects cultural preferences and norms. Diverse cultural components of behavior have significant impacts on patterns of eating irrespective of socioeconomic status. Many cultures have food beliefs, customs, or proscriptions specific to pregnancy that are considered important to maternal–fetal, physical, emotional, and spiritual health. Some food beliefs may have a negative impact on nutrition. For example, based on beliefs that foods have certain "hot and cold" properties with specific maternal and fetal effects, many women from India and Pakistan avoid nutritious food such as beef, eggs, or citrus fruits during pregnancy (Shahid, Ahmed, Rashid, Kahn, & Rehman, 2011). Foods from all cultures can enable a healthy pregnancy diet, and nutritional advice should be provided within the context of the woman's cultural preferences.

Making a nutritional assessment

A dietary assessment is essential to inform the midwife or NP about the pregnant woman's diet that forms a foundation for prenatal nutritional intervention. At the initial prenatal visit, the woman's attitudes toward weight gain, physical activity, and nutrition during pregnancy should be assessed and individualized advice provided based on this assessment. Simple dietary assessments, such as 24-hour diet recalls and food records and checklists, can be used by the health-care provider to evaluate diet and nutrient intakes throughout pregnancy. A complete nutritional assessment includes relevant history, relevant physical examination, and laboratory testing. An assessment of nutritional status begins with taking an accurate history of factors that can influence eating behaviors and nutrition. Much of this information is obtained during routine questioning at the first prenatal visit (Table 6.7). Historical risk factors for inadequate nutrition during pregnancy include adolescence, smoking or other substance use, brief interconceptual period, multiple gestation, high or low BMI, restrictive diet patterns, bariatric surgery, and social issues such as homelessness, poverty, or domestic violence. A focused nutritional history is then obtained.

After the general history is taken, a more specific history regarding diet is obtained in order to make a complete evaluation and relevant plan for pregnancy nutrition (Table 6.8). Starting the Conversation (STC) is a validated, efficient eight-item screening tool designed for assessment and counseling in busy clinical settings to identify dietary patterns and readiness to make changes (Paxton, Strycker, Toobert, Ammerman, & Glasgow, 2011) (Fig. 6.1). Depending on the woman's responses

Table 6.7	Historical Assessment of Nutritional Influences
Relevant medical history	✓ Preexisting conditions such as diabetes or cardiovascular disease ✓ Bariatric surgery ✓ Anemia or other nutritional deficiencies ✓ Past or current eating disorder ✓ Food allergies or intolerances
Psychosocial and personal history	✓ Tobacco, alcohol, or substance use ✓ Current exercise and activity patterns ✓ Economic status and resources ✓ Living situation and family structure ✓ Family or intimate partner violence ✓ Support systems ✓ Prior history of depression and current emotional health ✓ Feelings about pregnancy ✓ Educational level ✓ Cognitive level ✓ Ethnic/cultural group and food preferences ✓ English language proficiency
Past and current pregnancies	✓ Parity and outcome, especially prior history of preterm birth or low-birth-weight infant ✓ Gestational diabetes ✓ Interconceptional interval ✓ Breastfeeding history ✓ Weight gain pattern in prior pregnancy ✓ Presence of nausea and vomiting, heartburn, constipation

to the questions and readiness to change, appropriate advice for dietary improvement and guidance with goal setting can be provided. To facilitate the counseling session, responses are organized into three columns. The left column indicates the healthiest dietary habits; the center column indicates less healthy habits; and the right column indicates the least healthy practices. Responses in the left column are scored 0, and responses in the center column and right column are scored 1 and 2, respectively. Total scores range from 0 to 14, with higher scores reflecting poor diet habits and lower scores healthy diet habits.

The physical exam to assess nutritional status includes parameters evaluated at the first prenatal visit. The determination of weight and BMI status is done first. The remainder of the exam includes skin, hair, nails, mucosa, heart, thyroid, and screens for signs of nutritional deficiencies (Table 6.9).

Using resources

Specific dietary information delivered through a multimedia method can improve dietary behaviors (Neville,

Table 6.8 Components of a Detailed Nutritional History

Topic	Questions
Food resources	Does the family run out of food before there is money to buy more?
Food assistance programs	Does the family receive food stamps? Utilize community food pantries? Is she enrolled in the WIC program?
Food preparation and cooking resources	Who purchases and prepares the family food? Does the family have a working refrigerator, stove, oven, and freezer?
Eating away from home	How often does she eat away from home? What types of foods? Fast food?
Usual eating pattern	What are the typical patterns of eating meals and snacks? Describe a typical day. Does she skip meals?
Cultural/ethnic/religious food practices	What types of foods does she eat and how are they prepared? Does she have specific cultural food beliefs related to pregnancy?
Dietary supplements	Does she take vitamin supplements and herbal preparation? How often and in what doses?
Dieting practices	Has she dieted frequency in the past, gained and lost weight? What diet methods were used?
Detailed diet history	This can be done with screening tools (like STC; see Fig. 6.1) and/or a 1- to 3-day food diary to be brought at the next visit.

Starting The Conversation: Diet

(Scale developed by: the Center for Health Promotion and Disease Prevention, University of North Carolina at Chapel Hill, and North Carolina Prevention Partners)

Over the past few months:

		Less than 1 time	1–3 times	4 or more times
1.	How many times a week did you eat fast food meals or snacks?	☐ 0	☐ 1	☐ 2

		5 or more	3–4	2 or less
2.	How many servings of fruit did you eat each day?	☐ 0	☐ 1	☐ 2
3.	How many servings of vegetables did you eat each day?	☐ 0	☐ 1	☐ 2

		Less than 1	1–2	3 or less
4.	How many regular sodas or glasses of sweet tea did you drink each day?	☐ 0	☐ 1	☐ 2

		3 or more times	1–2 times	Less than 1 time
5.	How many times a week did you eat beans (like pinto or black beans), chicken, or fish?	☐ 0	☐ 1	☐ 2

		1 time or less	2–3 times	4 or more times
6.	How many times a week did you eat regular snack chips or crackers (not low-fat)?	☐ 0	☐ 1	☐ 2
7.	How many times a week did you eat desserts and other sweets (not the low-fat kind)?	☐ 0	☐ 1	☐ 2

		Very little	Some	A lot
8.	How much margarine, butter, or meat fat do you use to season vegetables or put on potatoes, bread, or corn?	☐ 0	☐ 1	☐ 2

SUMMARY SCORE (sum of all items): _____

Figure 6.1. Starting the Conversation: diet instrument. Source: Widen, E., & Siega-Riz, A. M. (2010). Prenatal nutrition: A practical guide for assessment and counseling. *Journal of Midwifery & Women's Health, 55,* 540–549. doi:10.1016/j.jmwh.2010.06.017.

O'Hare, & Milat, 2009). The instant feedback and tailored approach provided with Internet-based technologies can improve nutritional self-efficacy and nutritional knowledge. MyPlate is an illustrative and interactive tool provided by the USDA that helps women analyze dietary habits and provides daily recommendations for healthy eating during pregnancy based on individual BMI, physical activity level, and gestational age (Table 6.10) (see "Resources for Women and Families"). The tool provides an individualized estimate of nutrients needed by food groups and the daily amount recommended in cups or ounces for each food group. This type of information may be more practically usable than the general advice given by many clinicians of simply encouraging an additional 300 cal/day. Women can see how their food choices compare to what they need during pregnancy and can develop printable daily menu plans specific to pregnancy needs. Additionally, MyPlate uses a visual plate icon to "measure" the relative portion sizes of the food groups women should eat at a meal they have planned, thus enhancing knowledge of appropriate servings and portion size.

The Food Tracker on the ChooseMyPlate.gov Web site analyzes and provides nutrient output for consumers. Women can enter food data themselves and evaluate areas of adequacy and those areas that need improvement. This self-assessment can help empower women to evaluate nutritional choices and make changes during pregnancy as needed and monitor their progress (see "Resources for Women and Families). Some women do not have access to computer technologies to obtain information and thus rely on the clinician to provide resources. The Food Tracker can be used in an office setting to enter a woman's information and provide resources to print and take home. Additionally, midwives and NPs can create packets of printed materials on pregnancy nutritional needs and strategies for healthy eating and weight control.

The Women, Infants, and Children's (WIC) program, frequently referred to as WIC, is a supplemental food and nutrition program for pregnant and postpartum women and children under the age of 5 years old. Through the WIC program, financial assistance in purchasing food, counseling and information on healthy eating, breastfeeding support and information, and referrals to health care and other community resources are available. All prenatal health-care providers should be familiar with program services provided and to facilitate enrollment for eligible women. Women who need more comprehensive dietary guidance such as those with diabetes, obesity, and who follow restrictive diets benefit from referral to a dietitian who can help them meet pregnancy nutritional needs.

Counseling for optimal prenatal nutrition

Detailed and personalized advice on weight gain and food selection can help women attain pregnancy weight goals. A lack of advice and support from health-care professionals leads women to seek information for themselves from potentially unregulated sources (Brown & Avery, 2012). Pregnant women often receive a wealth of sometimes conflicting advice on what constitutes an optimal diet. Health professionals are often cited as the trusted source of nutrition and weight management advice for these women, and therefore, it is very important that the advice offered is consistent and evidence based and able to counter any conflicting advice that they may receive from family, friends, and the media. Advice women receive from health care providers during the course of prenatal care regarding weight gain, diet, and exercise is brief and is generally not related to weight management during pregnancy (Brown & Avery, 2012). Specific information on dietary improvements and lifestyle interventions during prenatal care reduce maternal gestational weight gain and improve outcomes for both mother and baby. Interventions focused on personal diet are the most effective and are associated with reductions in maternal

Table 6.9   Clinical Signs of Nutritional Status

Body area	Signs of adequate nutrition	Signs of inadequate nutrition
Weight	Normal for height, body build	Overweight or underweight
Hair	Shiny, firm, not easily plucked	Stringy, brittle, sparse
Skin	Smooth, good color	Rough, dry, scaly, petechiae, pale, bruised
Oral membranes	Reddish/pink	Mucosa swollen, boggy tissue
Gums	Pink, no swelling or bleeding	Spongy, bleeds easily, inflamed, gums receding
Teeth	No cavities, no pain	White unfilled black caries, absent teeth, worn surfaces, malpositioned teeth
Eyes	Bright, clear, no sores, moist	Pale conjunctiva, dryness, redness
Nails	Firm, pink	Brittle, ridged, spoon-shaped

Table 6.10 USDA MyPlate Pregnancy Food Plan for a 26-Year-Old Woman Who Is 5 ft 4 in., 145 lb at 12 Weeks' Gestation Who Has Approximately 30 Minutes of Moderate Physical Activity Daily

Calories	Allowance = 2600 per day		
Food groups	Food group amount	"What counts as . . ."	Tips
Grains	9 oz/day	1 oz of grains	
		1 slice of bread (1 oz) ½ cup cooked pasta, rice, or cereal 1 oz uncooked pasta or rice 1 tortilla (6-in. diameter) 1 pancake (5-in. diameter) 1 oz ready-to-eat cereal (about 1 cup cereal flakes)	Eat at least half of all grains as whole grains. Substitute whole grain choices for refined grains in breakfast cereals, breads, crackers, rice, and pasta. Check product labels—is a grain with "whole" before its name listed first on the ingredients list?
Vegetables	3½ cups/day	1 cup of vegetables	
		1 cup raw or cooked vegetables 1 cup 100% vegetable juice 2 cups leafy salad greens	Include vegetables in meals and in snacks. Fresh, frozen, and canned vegetables all count. Add dark-green, red, and orange vegetables to main and side dishes. Use dark leafy greens to make salads. Beans and peas are a great source of fiber. Add beans or peas to salads, soups, side dishes, or serve as a main dish.
Fruits	2 cups/day	1 cup of fruit	
		1 cup raw or cooked fruit 1 cup 100% fruit juice ½ cup dried fruit	Select fresh, frozen, canned, and dried fruit more often than juice; select 100% fruit juice when choosing juice. Enjoy a wide variety of fruits and maximize taste and freshness by adapting your choices to what is in season. Use fruit as snacks, salads, or desserts.
Dairy	3 cups/day	1 cup of dairy	
		1 cup milk 1 cup fortified soymilk (soy beverage) 1 cup yogurt 1½ oz natural cheese (e.g., cheddar) 2 oz processed cheese (e.g., American)	Drink fat-free (skim) or low-fat (1%) milk. Choose fat-free or low-fat milk or yogurt more often than cheese. When selecting cheese, choose low-fat or reduced-fat versions.
Protein foods	6½ oz/day	1 oz of protein foods	
		1 oz lean meat, poultry, seafood 1 egg 1 tbs peanut butter ½ oz nuts or seeds ¼ cup cooked beans or peas	Eat a variety of foods from the protein food group each week. Eat seafood in place of meat or poultry twice a week. Select lean meat and poultry. Trim or drain fat from meat and remove poultry skin.
Oils	8 tsp/day	1 tsp of oil	
		1 tsp vegetable oil (e.g., canola, corn, olive, soybean) 1½ tsp mayonnaise 2 tsp tub margarine 2 tsp French dressing 8 large olives	Choose soft margarines with zero trans fats made from liquid vegetable oil rather than stick margarine or butter. Use vegetable oils (olive, canola, corn, soybean, peanut, safflower, sunflower) rather than solid fats (butter, shortening). Replace solid fats with oils rather than adding oil to the diet. Oils are a concentrated source of calories, so use oils in small amounts.

Source: USDA Super tracker; https://www.supertracker.usda.gov/myplan.aspx.

gestational weight gain and improved perinatal outcomes (Thangaratinam et al., 2012). It is essential for women to be provided with specific dietary information, guidance, and support throughout the course of prenatal care to achieve pregnancy weight gain goals.

Strategies to promote optimal pregnancy nutrition

- Provide positive feedback on healthful dietary practices.
- Share findings on dietary areas of adequacy/excess/ deficiency.
- Share specific nutrient information on how much is taken in now and what is needed daily.
- Provide information on how that nutrient is useful to the fetus.
- Provide specific suggestions for change with examples.
- Assess diet and weight gain at each visit.

Special issues in nutrition

Adolescent pregnancy

Adolescence represents the second major growth phase in an individual's life. The additional energy and nutrient demands of pregnancy place adolescents at nutritional risk. Adolescent mothers tend to follow a social path of poor performance in school. Pregnant teens are more likely to have a background of poverty, be a member of an ethnic minority, and engage in smoking, alcohol, and substance abuse, placing them at further risk for poor pregnancy outcomes. Adolescents may not have adequate knowledge of nutrition and their present-focused orientation may inhibit them from easily linking current behaviors such as eating poorly to later outcomes. Poor dietary habits are common among adolescent girls, and many enter pregnancy with suboptimal iron status, unhealthy weight, and low intake of several key nutrients. Teens are more likely than adults to consume energy-dense, micronutrient-poor diets and to experience adverse pregnancy outcomes such as low birth weight (Baker et al., 2009).

Assessment

In addition to the routine history and physical examination noted earlier, the evaluation of a pregnant teen's nutritional status includes menstrual age, or the number of years since onset of menarche. Teen who conceive within 2 years of menarche are at highest risk for poor pregnancy outcomes due to their own biological immaturity. The greater the amount of uncompleted growth at conception, the greater the energy and nutrient needs above those normally required during pregnancy.

Pregnancy nutritional needs

Many pregnant adolescents have diets that provide less than recommended intakes of key nutrients such as calcium and iron. Low calcium intakes are well documented in adolescent girls. Optimal calcium intake and adequate maternal vitamin D status are both needed to maximize fetal bone growth. Improving maternal calcium intake and vitamin D status during pregnancy has a positive effect on fetal skeletal development in pregnant adolescents (Young et al., 2012). Teen pregnancy is associated with osteoporosis later in life (Cho et al., 2012). Adolescence is a critical time of life to accumulate bone for peak bone mass; thus, ensuring adequate calcium intake during pregnancy is important to later health. The DRI is 1300 mg calcium/day for those women 18 years of age or younger who are pregnant or lactating.

Pregnant teens have a high prevalence of anemia. Physiological iron needs are high at this stage of life because of increased requirements for the expansion of the blood volume associated with the adolescent growth spurt and the onset of menstruation. Pregnancy places an addition burden on iron stores, predisposing the pregnant teen to anemia.

Counseling

Pregnancy can motivate many pregnant adolescents to improve their diets to have a healthy baby. Pregnancy provides a window of opportunity for NPs and midwives to educate young women about the importance of healthy eating during pregnancy and to encourage immediate and long-term healthy eating practices. Adolescents who have given birth have higher percentages of total body fat than those who have not given birth (Gunderson et al., 2009), indicating increased weight retention after pregnancy. Prenatal nutrition and activity counseling to promote optimal weight gain can reduce postpartum weight retention. Developing strategies for working with pregnant adolescents can increase compliance and improve outcomes.

Strategies for dietary change in pregnant adolescents

- Establish a relationship with the teen.
- Assess the teen's perspective of her diet.
- Determine the teen's willingness to improve diet.
- Use specific foods rather than nutrients in teaching.
- Use images of food on handouts to display optimal food choices.
- Follow up on diet and physical activity at each visit.
- Provide verbal positive feedback for improvements.

To facilitate dietary change, health-care providers should work within the context of the pregnant adolescent's current eating habits. For example, adolescents often eat fast food and other convenience foods. While these may not be the best options, pregnant adolescents can be assisted to choose healthier foods such as salads and milk instead of French fries and soft drinks when eating at fast food restaurants. Frequent meals and snacking are another common characteristic of adolescent eating behaviors. Working within this habit, pregnant adolescents can be encouraged to carry healthy snacks such as fruits, crackers, or granola bars.

Concrete and practical strategies can help adolescents track nutritional goals. For example, a notebook or a wipe-away board that lists the daily servings of all food groups can be used to mark off the servings she has consumed throughout the day. Adolescents tend to think concretely and can relate to specific foods better than vague nutrients of which they have little knowledge. Providing literature that has food pictures can help young women readily understand healthy food choices.

Most pregnant adolescents live with their immediate or extended family. These relationships can greatly influence not only what the pregnant adolescent eats but also when and under what circumstances. An evaluation of the family food dynamics and meals is important to enable the health care provider to work within the family norms for improving adolescent nutrition. Pregnant adolescents with limited resources should be encouraged to utilize the WIC program to supplement current food sources.

Pregnant vegetarians and vegans

Approximately 5% of the U.S. adult population follows a vegetarian diet and 2% report themselves as vegan (Gallup, 2012). A vegetarian diet typically does not include consumption of animal flesh such as meat, poultry, or fish/seafood. Individuals that further restrict animal protein sources and refrain from eating dairy, eggs, or honey are considered vegan. Vegetarians who avoid flesh yet do eat animal products such as cheese, milk, and eggs, are considered ovo-lacto vegetarians. Vegetarian diets are associated with health advantages including lower blood cholesterol levels, lower risk of heart disease, lower risk of hypertension and type 2 diabetes, and lower levels of obesity and various cancers (Marsh, Zeuschner, & Saunders, 2012). Vegetarian diets tend to be lower in saturated fat and cholesterol and have higher levels of dietary fiber, magnesium, potassium, vitamins C and E, flavenoids, and other phytochemicals (Craig, 2010). However, vegans and some vegetarians may have lower intakes of vitamin B_{12}, calcium, vitamin D, and long-chain fatty acids (Marsh et al., 2012).

The American Dietetic Association considers a vegetarian diet compatible with all life stages including pregnancy and lactation (American Dietetic Association (ADA), 2009). However, few studies have addressed vegetarian diets and pregnancy outcomes. There has been a reported association between vegetarian diet during pregnancy and increased risk of hypospadias (North, Golding, & the ALSPAC Study Team, 2000). As vegetarians have a greater exposure to phytoestrogens than do omnivores, it is possible that phytoestrogens have a deleterious effect on the developing male reproductive system.

In planning vegetarian diets to ensure adequate nutritional intake, iron, protein, B vitamins, vitamin D and calcium, and omega-3 fatty acids are considered nutrients of concern in vegetarian diets (Table 6.11).

Table 6.11   Vegetarian and Vegan Diet Nutrient Sources

Whole grains, breads, cereals
Nine or more servings
Serving = 1 slice of bread, 1/2 bun or bagel
½ cup cooked cereal, rice, or pasta
3/4–1 cup ready-to-eat cereal

Vegetables
Four or more servings
Serving = ½ cup cooked or 1 cup raw vegetables
Choose several dark green vegetables daily.

Fruits
Four or more servings
Serving = ½ cup cooked, 1 cup raw fruits
1 piece of fruit, ¾ cup fruit juice, ¼ cup dried fruit

Legumes, soy products, nondairy milks
Five to six servings
Serving = ½ cup cooked beans, tofu, tahini, or tempeh
8 oz fortified soymilk or other nondairy milk
3 oz meat analogue

Nuts, seeds, wheat germ
One to two servings
Serving = 2 tbs nuts or seeds
2 tbs nut butter, 2 tbs wheat germ

Adapted from Food and Nutrition Board, Institute of Medicine, National Academies.
A reliable source of vitamin B_{12}, such as many prenatal vitamins or fortified nondairy milk or cereal should be included.

Protein

Pregnant vegetarians consume lower levels of protein and higher levels of carbohydrates than pregnant non-vegetarians (Kniskern & Johnston, 2011). Protein needs in pregnancy can be met from plant sources with planning. Dried beans and other legumes, soy products like tofu, nut butters, and eggs are good protein sources toward meeting the 71-g daily protein requirement.

B vitamin

B vitamin deficiency is of particular concern for vegetarians. Women on vegetarian diets have lower serum B_{12} levels than women eating diets that include animal protein (Koebnick et al., 2004). Many foods are fortified with vitamin B_{12} including meat substitute products, soy milks, tofu, cereals, and nutritional yeasts. Four servings daily of B_{12} fortified foods are recommended during pregnancy.

Iron

Iron needs may be greater for those on a vegetarian diet because of less efficient absorption of iron from plant sources. It is difficult for any pregnant woman to meet increased iron needs through diet alone. Therefore, iron supplements or prenatal vitamins containing iron are often required regardless of diet. Vegetarian women should include iron-rich plant foods daily, in addition to taking their prescribed vitamins or supplements. Iron supplements should not be taken at the same time as tea, coffee, or calcium supplements. Dairy products decrease iron absorption and should be avoided. Iron sources include whole and enriched grains, legumes, nuts, seeds, dark green vegetables, dried fruit, beans, lentils, and blackstrap molasses. Including vitamin C-rich foods at meals can increase absorption of iron from these sources.

Calcium

Calcium needs must be met from sources other than dairy. Adequate calcium intake for vegetarians and vegans is 1200–1500 mg/day, higher than for omnivores due to lower calcium absorption in many plant-based calcium sources. Many vegetables contain calcium but may have low bioavailability (e.g., spinach). Other greens with high calcium bioavailability such as kale, broccoli, cabbage, and bok choy should be encouraged. Other excellent sources of calcium include tofu and soy beans, dark green leafy vegetables, beans, figs, sunflower seeds, tahini, almond butter, calcium-fortified nondairy milk, and calcium-fortified cereals and juices. If these foods are included in the diet every day, pregnancy calcium needs are easily met.

Vitamin D

Requirements for vitamin D do not increase during pregnancy. However, vitamin D is of concern for pregnant women who live in northern climates where they may not produce enough. Sunlight is a viable source of vitamin D in warmer climates and during the summer in northern latitudes. Inadequate vitamin D is also a concern for women following vegetarian diets. With the exception of foods such as eggs and salmon with bones, few foods naturally contain vitamin D. Fortified foods include soy milk and some breakfast cereals. Vitamin D is also included in most prenatal vitamin supplements.

Omega-3 fatty acids

DHA and EPA, essential for fetal brain and nervous system development, pose challenges for pregnant vegetarians since they are found primarily in fatty fish. It is important to include adequate amounts of short-chain fatty acids such as ALA found predominantly in chia seeds, flaxseeds, and walnuts. ALA is endogenously converted to long-chain omega-3 fatty acids. Minimal amounts of dietary omega-6 fatty acids, found in vegetable oils and margarines, are essential to optimize conversion to DHA and EPA. Eggs from chickens fed a DHA-rich diet and foods fortified with microalgae-derived DHA are additional food sources.

Women choose a vegetarian diet for many reasons, including religious beliefs, concerns about animal rights, health, and environmental issues. Perhaps because of this awareness, those following a vegetarian diet tend to be well informed about a balanced diet. A thorough diet history and accurate diet counseling in addition to consultation with a dietician will help to optimize pregnancy outcomes.

Eating disorders

Approximately 5–6% of American women suffer from some type of eating disorder (Harris, 2010). Eating disorders are thought to arise from the interplay of genetics, biology, and psychosociocultural factors. Eating disorders are classified as anorexia nervosa, bulimia, or eating disorders not otherwise specified (EDNOS), such as binge eating (Harris, 2010). Anorexia nervosa is diagnosed based on a group of symptoms including unwillingness to maintain body weight at a minimally normal weight for age and height, intense fear of gaining weight or becoming fat, body image disturbances, and amenorrhea for at least three consecutive months (Reiter & Graves, 2010). Bulimia nervosa is often diagnosed based on symptoms such as inaccurate perception of body image, a sense of lack of control during recurrent episodes of binge eating occurring at least two times per week for at least 3 months, use of compensatory behaviors to prevent weight gain (such as self-induced vomiting, misuse of laxatives, enemas or diuretics, and excessive exercise occurring at least two times per week for at least 3 months) (Reiter & Graves, 2010). EDNOS is a diagnosis of exclusion; it involves those who exhibit some symptoms but do not fit the criteria of anorexia or bulimia. Some examples may include binge eating and those individuals with a normal weight but who purge after eating, chew and spit out food rather than swallowing to prevent weight gain, psychiatric impairment related to diet pills and diuretics, or obsessive preoccupation with cosmetic surgery to deal with shape and weight issues (Reiter & Graves, 2010).

There is a correlation between severity of the eating disorder and the incidence of pregnancy-associated morbidities. Women with eating disorders have a greater likelihood of miscarriage and cesarean sections (Harris, 2010). Infants born to women with eating disorders have an increased risk of stillbirth, low birth weight, low Apgar scores, infant microcephaly, breech presentation, and cleft lip and palate (Bulik et al., 2009; Harris, 2010).

It is not uncommon for eating disorders to go unnoticed in pregnancy. Pregnancy may be a strong motivator to change eating habits as up to 70% of women have improved symptoms during pregnancy (Harris, 2010). Early detection of eating disorders in pregnancy can minimize complications. Women with eating disorders may present with the following risk factors: severe anxiety, body dissatisfaction, food obsession, negative affectivity, exercise obsession, and depressive symptoms (Harris, 2010; Reiter & Graves, 2010; Stice, Marti, & Durant, 2011). The presence of hyperemesis gravidarum, lack of weight gain over two consecutive visits, unexplained electrolyte disorders, and dental erosion can be cues to prompt further history and evaluation for eating disorders (Harris, 2010).

Screening for eating disorders during the initial history is routinely done for all pregnant women (Harris, 2010). Specific areas of inquiry include reproductive history, history of amenorrhea lasting longer than 3 months, eating habits, exercise history, history of frequent weight loss and gain, and prior history of eating disorders. Screening tools designed to detect eating disorders can be used in those women who need further assessment. SCOFF is one such screening tool used by clinicians in general practice.

SCOFF tool to screen for eating disorders

S—Do you make yourself *sick* because you are uncomfortably full?
C—Do you worry about loss of *control* over your eating?
O—Have you recently lost *one* stone (14 lb) in 3 months?
F—Do you believe you are *fat* although others say you are thin?
F—Would you say *food* predominates your life?

One point is given for each "yes" answered and a score of 2 or more indicates the presence of an eating disorder is likely (Harris, 2010).

Successful strategies to assist women with eating disorders include care from the same midwife or NP throughout her entire pregnancy whenever possible. This will provide some consistency and allow for a trusting relationship to develop. An increased prenatal visit schedule will allow for small goal setting and increase the likelihood of success (Harris, 2010). Discussing appropriate food portions and necessary nutrients and vitamins of her choice may increase the likelihood of appropriate weight gain. Potential obstacles may arise as a consequence to reintroduction of food and the physiological changes of pregnancy affecting the gastrointestinal system. Pregnant women identified with an eating disorder may also benefit from referral to a nutritionist and a mental health-care provider.

Pica

Pica is derived from the Latin word for magpie, a bird known for its unusual and indiscriminate eating habits. It is defined as the compulsive and purposeful intake of nonnutritive substances that the consumer does not define as food for greater than a 1-month duration (Lopez, Langini, & Pita de Portela, 2007; Young, 2010). Women with pica ingest products such as ice (pagophagia—70% of pica practices), dirt/clay (geophagia—18% of pica), corn starch (amylophagia), soap (4% of pica practices), charcoal, ash, paper, chalk, cloth, baby powder, coffee grounds, eggshells, and nail polish (Lopez et al., 2007; Mills, 2007; Young, 2010). The etiology of pica is poorly understood. Certain nutrient deficiencies such as zinc, iron, and calcium may play a role in the development of pica (Mills, 2007; Young, 2010). Pica may be initiated by individuals who enjoy the taste, texture, and smell of the substance ingested (Mills, 2007). Cultural beliefs may determine why some women consume nonnutritive substances. Pica may also be a psychological and behavioral response to stress, a habit or disorder, or a manifestation of an oral fixation (Mills, 2007).

Pica appears to be more common in African American women, women living in rural areas, and those with a family history of pica (Mills, 2007). Complications vary based on the type of pica practices. Pica is associated with iron deficiency anemia, though it is unclear whether iron deficiency anemia is a result of pica or may be a predisposing factor to pica. Pica can lead to heavy metal poisonings (especially lead), alimentary canal damage, and excessive pregnancy weight gain (especially starch ingestion) (Young, 2010). Other potential complications include nutrient deficiencies, constipation, electrolyte imbalances, gastrointestinal disturbances, parasitic infections, dental complications, gestational hyperglycemia, and metabolic disturbances.

Pica is a condition that often goes unreported and undiagnosed primarily because of embarrassment and guilt. A nonjudgmental, understanding, and culturally supportive environment can facilitate reporting of pica.

The substance and amount consumed should be identified and counseling, education, and nutritional management for all women practicing pica provided.

Summary

Pregnancy is a critical time in human development and outcomes can be strongly influenced by prenatal nutrition. Facilitating early prenatal care appointments allow for the best opportunity to assess nutritional habits and status and to institute dietary modifications, thus improving perinatal outcomes. It is imperative for midwives and NPs to have the knowledge and resources to be able to provide women with relevant information on prenatal diet choices and influences on pregnancy and fetal health. It is also critical to prioritize adequate time during prenatal care visits to evaluate and address nutrition throughout pregnancy. Promoting healthy diet and lifestyle choices can influence the long-term health of both the mother and her offspring.

Case study

Katie is a 25-year-old G1P0 at 10 weeks' gestation presenting for her first prenatal visit. Her past medical and current health history are within normal. Katie lives with her best friend from high school and works full time as an administrative secretary in a large office complex. This is an unplanned pregnancy with her boyfriend of 9 months, and she indicates that she plans to keep the baby and that they are working through how they will handle this together. Katie indicates it is a supportive relationship, though she feels a high level of stress about being pregnant and facing an uncertain future. She is 5 ft 8 in. tall with a prepregnant weight of 121 lb. She goes to the gym three times a week, works out with weights, and does an aerobic circuit. She denies illegal substance use, is a nonsmoker, and drinks alcohol socially about three to four times per week but has had none since she found out she was pregnant. She reports extreme fatigue and mild nausea intermittently during the day for the last 3 weeks, though she has not vomited. Katie states that she does feel better after she eats but has not changed her eating habits since she became pregnant. Both she and her roommate cook when they are home; however, she eats breakfast and lunch out most days of the week and eats dinner out about three to four nights per week. Katie is very trim, athletic, and enjoys fashionable clothing and going out with her friends. She voices concern about pregnancy body changes and feels she can limit those changes by limiting her dietary intake. Katie

indicates none of her friends have had babies and she "doesn't know much about being pregnant."

At this visit, her weight is 122 lb. Urine dip is +1 for ketones. She brings a 3-day diet history with her and indicates this is a typical diet for her.

Day 1	Day 2	Day 3
Morning:	Morning:	Morning:
Large coffee with 2 tbs soy milk	Large coffee with 2 tbs soy milk	Large coffee with 2 tbs soy milk
Low-fat bran muffin	½ bagel	Low-fat lemon muffin
Afternoon:	Afternoon:	Afternoon:
½ tuna sandwich, handful potato chips, diet soda	Small Caesar salad with bulgar wheat, apple, diet soda	½ turkey sandwich, handful potato chips, diet soda
Low-fat energy bar	Low-fat energy bar	Low-fat energy bar
Evening: green salad with two chopped eggs, tomatoes, carrots and pine nuts, vitamin water	Evening: spaghetti with tomato sauce, small green salad, vitamin water	Evening: bowl of raisin bran cereal with skim milk, handful of oyster crackers
Snack: three saltine crackers	Snack: 2 hardboiled eggs	Snack: 1 hardboiled egg

A physical examination was done which was within normal limits.

ASSESSMENT: Katie's BMI is 18.4 and is in the underweight category. She has gained 1 lb thus far; however, scale differences between home and the office make this gain amount uncertain. Her diet reveals deficiency in calories, protein, calcium, iron, and other major nutrients and long periods without caloric intake. Katie values a thin appearance, which may make change challenging for her. She needs dietary information on optimal pregnancy diet and weight gain.

PLAN: Time was spent talking with Katie about her feelings about the pregnancy, about gaining weight, and pregnancy-related changes to her body. She indicated a strong desire to have a healthy baby and a willingness to change her dietary habits. A chart on the distribution of baby weight during pregnancy was provided and discussed. Katie was advised that her BMI indicated she is underweight and that she should gain between 28 and 40 lb. The findings of her diet history were reviewed and Katie was informed that her diet needs to increase in calories, calcium, protein, complex carbohydrates and fiber, iron, and omega-3 fatty acids. Food sources and the role of each nutrient during pregnancy were discussed. Katie was informed that gaining adequate weight and eating regularly during pregnancy would help reduce her risk of a preterm birth. Katie's lifestyle and food preferences were reviewed. Katie readily agreed that she would be able to increase her calorie and protein intakes with foods she enjoyed eating. Increasing calcium intake would be more challenging for her since she did not like milk. She liked Greek yogurt and indicated she would have some daily between meals and would drink soy milk daily with meals. She was advised that she is entering a period of gestation where calcium is needed for rapid fetal bone growth. This information helped to provide Katie with a connection between her diet and fetal needs. A multivitamin with 300 mg DHA and EPA and 30 mg iron was prescribed. Lists of food high in iron, calcium, and complex carbohydrates were used to jointly create a sample meal plan for the week and were given to Katie to use as resources. She was also provided with the MyPlate Web address to create her own plan and to track her progress. A revisit appointment was made for 2 weeks to review her lab work and to evaluate her diet and weight gain. A joint goal to gain between 2 and 4 lb by the next visit was established. Katie was encouraged to bring her boyfriend or her roommate to visits with her as she may need continued encouragement to achieve adequate weight gain. Ongoing care will include regular discussions about her diet habits, education related to nutrients and fetal health, and weight gain assessments. A referral to nutritional services may be considered as needed.

Resources for women and their families

From the USDA, a widely used interactive Web site for pregnant women on healthy eating during pregnancy called MyPlate: http://www.choosemyplate.gov/pregnancy-breastfeeding.html

A printable brochure on pregnancy nutrition from the International Food Information Council, Healthy Eating during Pregnancy Brochure: http://www.foodinsight.orgResourcesDetail.aspxtopic Healthy_Eating_During_Pregnancy http://www.foodinsight.org/Resources/Detail.aspx?topic=Healthy_Eating_During_Pregnancy

This USDA Web site allows women to enter food eaten and to receive an evaluation of nutrient intake. USDA Interactive Dietary Food Tracker: https://www.supertracker.usda.gov/foodtracker.aspx

Resources for health-care providers

USDA National Nutrient Database: http://www.nal.usda.govfnicfoodcompsearch http://ndb.nal.usda.gov/

U.S. Environmental Protection Agency: Local and state information on safety of recreationally caught fish can be found: http://www.epa.gov/fishadvisories/ http://water.epa.gov/scitech/swguidance/fishshellfish/fishadvisories/index.cfm

USDA Interactive Dietary Reference Intake and Estimated Energy Requirement Calculator: http://fnic.nal.usda.govinteractiveDRI http://fnic.nal.usda.gov/fnic/interactiveDRI/

Information on the supplemental food and nutrition program, WIC: http://www.fns.usda.gov/wic

A CDC Web site with consumer information on food safety during pregnancy: http://www.cdc.gov/pregnancy/infections.html

References

Abu-Saad, K., & Fraser, D. (2010). Maternal nutrition and birth outcomes. *Epidemiologic Reviews, 32*, 5–15.

American Dietetic Association (ADA). (2009). Position of the American Dietetic Association: Vegetarian diets. *Journal of the American Dietetic Association, 109*, 1266–1282.

Bachmanov, A. A., & Beauchamp, G. K. (2007). Taste receptor genes. *Annual Review of Nutrition, 27*, 389–414.

Baker, P., Wheeler, S., Sanders, T., Thomas, J., Hutchinson, C., Clarke, K., . . . Poston, L. (2009). A prospective study of micronutrient status in adolescent pregnancy. *The American Journal of Clinical Nutrition, 89*(4), 1114–1124. doi:10.3945/ajcn.2008.27097

Beauchamp, G. K., & Mennella, J. A. (2009). Early flavor learning and its impact on later feeding behavior. *Journal of Pediatric Gastroenterology and Nutrition, 48*, S25–S30.

Belkacemi, L., Nelson, D. M., Desai, M., & Ross, M. G. (2010). Maternal undernutrition influences placental-fetal development. *Biology of Reproduction, 83*(3), 325–331. doi:10.1095/biolreprod.110.084517

Bergen, N., Jaddoe, V., Timmermans, S., Hofman, A., Lindemans, J., Russcher, H., . . . Steegers, E. (2012). Homocysteine and folate concentrations in early pregnancy and the risk of adverse pregnancy outcomes: The Generation R Study. *BJOG: An International Journal of Obstetrics and Gynaecology, 119*, 739–751. doi:10.1111/j.1471-0528.2012.03321.x

Blackburn, S. T. (2012). Chapter 15: Neurologic, muscular and sensory systems. In *Maternal, fetal & neonatal physiology* (4th ed.). Maryland Heights, MO: Elsevier, Inc.

Blencowe, H., Cousens, S., Modell, B., & Lawn, J. (2010). Folic acid to reduce neonatal mortality for neural tube defects. *International Journal of Epidemiology, 39*(Suppl. 1), i110–i121. doi:10.1093/ije/dyq028

Bokhari, F., Derbyshire, E., Li, W., & Brennan, C. (2012). Can an iron-rich staple food help women to achieve dietary targets in pregnancy? *International Journal of Food Sciences and Nutrition* [serial on the Internet], *63*(2), 199–207.

Brown, A., & Avery, A. (2012). Healthy weight management during pregnancy: What advice and information is being provided. *Journal of Human Nutrition and Dietetics* [serial on the Internet], *25*(4), 378–387.

Bulik, C. M., Holle, A. V., Siega-Riz, A. M., Torgersen, L., Lie, K. K., Hamer, R. M., . . . Reichborn-Kjennerud, T. (2009). Birth outcomes in women with eating disorders in the Norwegian mother and child cohort study. *International Journal of Eating Disorders, 42*(1), 9–18.

Centers for Disease Control and Prevention (CDC). (2011). Vital signs: Incidence and trends of infection with pathogens transmitted commonly through food—Foodborne diseases active surveillance network, 10 U.S. sites, 1996–2010. *MMWR. Morbidity and Mortality Weekly Report, 60*(22), 749–755.

Cetin, I., & Koletzko, B. (2008). Long chain omega-3 fatty acid supply in pregnancy and lactation. *Current Opinion in Clinical Nutrition and Metabolic Care, 11*, 207–302.

Chen, L., Hu, F. B., Yeung, E., Willett, W., & Zhang, C. (2009). Prospective study of pre-gravid sugar-sweetened beverage consumption and the risk of gestational diabetes mellitus. *Diabetes Care, 32*(12), 2236. doi:10.2337/dc09-0866

Cho, G., Shin, J., Yi, K., Park, H., Kim, T., Hur, J., & Kim, S. (2012). Adolescent pregnancy is associated with osteoporosis in postmenopausal women. *Menopause (New York, N.Y.), 19*(4), 456–460.

Chu, S. Y., Callahan, W. M., Kim, S. Y., Schmid, C. H., Lau, J., England, L. J. & Dietz, P. M. (2007). Maternal obesity and risk of gestational diabetes mellitus. *Diabetes Care, 30*(8), 2070–2076.

Cragan, J. D., Friedman, J. M., Holmes, L. B., Uhl, K., Green, N. S., & Riley, L. (2006). Ensuring the safe and effective use of medications during pregnancy: Planning and prevention through preconception care. *Maternal and Child Health Journal, 10*(Suppl. 1), 129–135.

Craig, W. J. (2010). Nutrition concerns and health effects of vegetarian diets. *Nutrition in Clinical Practice, 25*(6), 613–620.

Deutsch, A., Lynch, O., Alio, A., Salihu, H., & Spellacy, W. (2010). Increased risk of placental abruption in underweight women. *American Journal of Perinatology, 27*(3), 235–240.

Englund-Ögge, L., Brantsæter, A. L., Haugen, M., Sengpiel, V., Khatibi, A., Myhre, R., . . . Jacobsson, B. (2012). Association between intake of artificially sweetened and sugar-sweetened beverages and preterm delivery: A large prospective cohort study. *The American Journal of Clinical Nutrition, 96*, 552–559.

Environmental Protection Agency (EPA). (2007). *Proceedings of the 2007 National Forum on Contaminants in Fish.* Retrieved from http://www.epa.gov/waterscience/fish/forum/2007/

Esposito, L., Fisher, J. O., Mennella, J. A., Hoelsher, D. M., & Huang, T. T. (2009). Developmental perspectives on nutrition and obesity from gestation to adolescence. *Preventing Chronic Disease, 6*(3), 1–11.

Fall, C. (2005). Fetal and maternal nutrition. In S. Stanner (Ed.), *Cardiovascular disease: Diet, nutrition and emerging risk factors. The report of a British Nutrition Foundation Task Force* (pp. 177–195). Oxford: Blackwell Science.

Fall, C. H., Yajnik, C. S., Rao, S., Davies, A. A., Brown, N., & Farrant, H. J. (2003). Micronutrients and fetal growth. *The Journal of Nutrition, 133*(5 Suppl. 2), 1747S–1756S.

FAO/WHO. (2011). *Report of the joint FAO/WHO expert consultation on the risks and benefits of fish consumption.* Rome and Geneva: Food and Agriculture Organization of the United Nations; World Health Organization. Retrieved from http://www.fao.org/docrep/014/ba0136e/ba0136e00.pdf

Gallup. (2012). Retrieved from http://www.gallup.com/poll/156215/consider-themselves-vegetarians.aspx

Goh, Y. I., Bollano, E., Einarson, T. R., & Koren, G. (2006). Prenatal multivitamin supplementation and rates of congenital anomalies: A meta-analysis. *Journal of Obstetrics and Gynaecology Canada, 28*(8), 680–689.

Gunderson, E., Striegel-Moore, R., Schreiber, G., Hudes, M., Biro, F., Daniels, S., & Crawford, P. B. (2009). Longitudinal study of growth and adiposity in parous compared to nulligravid adolescents. *Archives of Pediatrics and Adolescent Medicine, 163*(4), 349–356.

Hacker, A. N., Fung, E. B., & King, J. C. (2012). Role of calcium during pregnancy: Maternal and fetal needs. *Nutrition Reviews, 70*(7), 397–409.

Harris, A. A. (2010). Practical advice for caring for women with eating disorders during the prenatal period. *Journal of Midwifery and Women's Health, 55*(6), 579–586.

Herring, S. J., Rose, M. Z., Skouteris, H., & Oken, E. (2012). Optimizing weight gain in pregnancy to prevent obesity in women and children. *Diabetes, Obesity and Metabolism, 14*(3), 195–203.

Herz, R. S. (1998). Are odors the best cues to memory? A cross-modal comparison of associative memory stimuli. *Annals of the New York Academy of Sciences, 855*, 670–674.

Hibbeln, J. R., Davis, J. M., & Steer, C. (2007). Maternal seafood consumption in pregnancy and neurodevelopmental outcomes in childhood (ALSPAC Study). *Lancet, 369*, 578–585.

Hollis, B. W., & Wagner, C. L. (2013). Vitamin D and pregnancy: Skeletal effects, nonskeletal effects, and birth outcomes. *Calcified Tissue International, 92*(2), 128–139.

Horvath, A., Koletzko, B., & Szajewska, H. (2007). Effect of supplementation of women in high risk pregnancies with long chain polyunsaturated fatty acids on pregnancy outcomes and growth measures at birth: Meta-analysis of randomized controlled trials. *The British Journal of Nutrition, 98*(2), 253–259.

Institute of Medicine (IOM). (2010). Food and Nutrition Board, National Academies. *Dietary reference Intakes Tables and*

Application. Retrieved from http://www.iom.edu/Activities/Nutrition/SummaryDRIs/DRI-Tables.aspx

Institute of Medicine (US) (IOM). (2007). Committee on Understanding Premature Birth and Assuring Healthy Outcomes. 11 Neurodevelopmental, health, and family outcomes for infants born preterm. In R. E. Behrman & A. S. Butler (Eds.), *Preterm birth: Causes, consequences, and prevention.* Washington, DC: National Academies Press (US). Retrieved from http://www.ncbi.nlm.nih.gov/books/NBK11356/

Kind, K. L., Moore, V. M., & Davies, M. J. (2006). Diet around conception and during pregnancy–Effects on fetal and neonatal outcomes. *Reproductive Biomedicine Online, 12*(5), 532–541.

Kniskern, M. A., & Johnston, C. S. (2011). Protein dietary reference intakes may be inadequate for vegetarians if low amounts of animal protein are consumed. *Nutrition, 27*(6), 727–730.

Koebnick, C., Hoffmann, I., Dagnelie, P. C., Heins, U. A., Wickramasinghe, S. N., Ratnayaka, I. D., . . . Leitzmann, C. (2004). Long-term ovo-lacto vegetarian diet impairs vitamin B-12 status in pregnant women. *The Journal of Nutrition, 134*(12), 3319–3326.

Kosa, J. L., Guendelman, S., Pearl, M., Graham, S., Abrams, B., & Kharrazi, M. (2011). The association between pre-pregnancy BMI and preterm delivery in a diverse Southern California population of working women. *Maternal and Child Health Journal, 15*, 772–781.

Koski, K. G., & Hill, F. W. (1986). Effect of low carbohydrate diets during pregnancy on parturition and postnatal survival of the newborn rat pup. *The Journal of Nutrition, 116*, 1938–1948.

Kristensen, J., Vestergaard, M., Wisborg, K., Kesmodel, U., & Secher, N. J. (2005). Pre-pregnancy weight and the risk of stillbirth and neonatal death. *BJOG: An International Journal of Obstetrics and Gynaecology, 112*, 403–408. doi:10.1111/j.1471-0528.2005.00437.x

Lando, A. M., Fein, S. B., & Choinière, C. J. (2012). Awareness of methylmercury in fish and fish consumption among pregnant and postpartum women and women of childbearing age in the United States. *Environmental Research, 116*, 85–92.

Laraia, B. A., Siega-Riz, A. M., & Gundersen, C. (2010). Household food insecurity is associated with self-reported pregravid weight status, gestational weight gain, and pregnancy complications. *Journal of the American Dietetic Association, 110*(5), 692–701.

Lindsay, D. S., & Dubey, J. P. (2011). *Toxoplasma gondii*: The changing paradigm of congenital toxoplasmosis. *Parasitology, 9*, 1–3.

Lopez, L. B., Langini, S. H., & Pita de Portela, M. L. (2007). Maternal iron status and neonatal outcomes in women with pica during pregnancy. *International Journal of Gynaecology and Obstetrics, 98*, 151–163.

Lorber, B. (2010). *Listeria monocytogenes.* In G. L. Mandell, J. E. Bennett, & R. Dolin (Eds.), *Principles and practice of infectious diseases* (7th ed.). Philadelphia: Churchill Livingstone.

Ludwig, D. S., & Currie, J. (2010). The association between pregnancy weight gain and birthweight: A within-family comparison. *The Lancet, 376*(9745), 984–990.

Makrides, M., Duley, L., & Olsen, S. F. (2006). Marine oil, and other prostaglandin precursor, supplementation for pregnancy uncomplicated by pre-eclampsia or intrauterine growth restriction. *Cochrane Database of Systematic Reviews,* (3), CD003402. doi:10.1002/14651858.CD003402.pub2

March of Dimes. (2012). *Eating and nutrition.* Retrieved from http://www.marchofdimes.com/pregnancy/nutrition_caffeine.html

Marsh, K., Zeuschner, C., & Saunders, A. (2012). Health implications of a vegetarian diet: A review. *American Journal of Lifestyle Medicine, 6*(3), 250–267.

McCann, J. C., & Ames, B. N. (2005). Is docosahexaenoic acid, an n-3 long chain polyunsaturated fatty acid, required for development of normal brain function? An overview of evidence from cognitive and behavioral tests in human and animals. *The American Journal of Clinical Nutrition, 82*, 281–295.v.

McCusker, R. R., Goldberger, B. A., & Cone, E. J. (2003). Caffeine content of specialty coffees. *Journal of Analytical Toxicology, 27*, 520–522.

McCusker, R. R., Goldberger, B. A., & Cone, E. J. (2006). Caffeine content of energy drinks, carbonated sodas, and other beverages. *Journal of Analytical Toxicology, 30*, 112–114.

Mennella, J. A., Jagnow, C. P., & Beauchamp, G. K. (2001). Prenatal and postnatal flavor learning by human infants. *Pediatrics, 107*(6), E88–E93.

Mennella, J. A., Johnson, A., & Beauchamp, G. K. (1995). Garlic ingestion by pregnant women alters the odor of amniotic fluid. *Chemical Senses, 20*(2), 207–209.

Mills, M. E. (2007). More than food: The implications of pica in pregnancy. *Nursing for Women's Health, 11*(3), 266–273.

National Institutes of Health (NIH). (2007). *Dietary Supplement Fact Sheet—Iron.* Retrieved from http://ods.od.nih.gov/factsheets/Iron-HealthProfessional/

National Institutes of Health (NIH). (2011). *Dietary Supplement Fact Sheet—Vitamin D.* Retrieved from http://ods.od.nih.gov/factsheets/VitaminD-HealthProfessional/

Neville, L. M., O'Hare, B., & Milat, A. J. (2009). Computer-tailored dietary behavior change interventions: A systematic review. *Health Education Research, 24*(4), 699–720.

North, K., Golding, J., & the ALSPAC Study Team. (2000). A maternal vegetarian diet in pregnancy is associated with hypospadias. *BJU International, 85*, 107–113.

Ogden, C. L., Caroll, M. D., Bit, B. K., & Flegal, K. M. (2012). *Prevalence of obesity in the United States 2009–2010.* NCHS data brief no. 82. Hyattsville, MD: National Center for Health Statistics.

Paxton, A. E., Strycker, L. A., Toobert, D. J., Ammerman, A. S., & Glasgow, R. E. (2011). Starting the Conversation: Performance of a brief dietary assessment and intervention tool for health professionals. *American Journal of Preventive Medicine, 40*(1), 67–71.

Peña-Rosas, J. P., De-Regil, L. M., Dowswell, T., & Viteri, F. E. (2012). Intermittent regimes of iron supplementation during pregnancy. Cochrane Summaries.

Phelan, S., Hart, C., Phipps, M., Abrams, B., Schaffner, A., Adams, A., & Wing, R. (2011). Maternal behaviors during pregnancy impact offspring obesity risk. *Experimental Diabetes Research, 2011*, 985139. doi:10.1155/2011/985139

Pitkin, R. M. (1976). Nutritional Support in Obstetrics and Gynecology*. *Clinical Obstetrics and Gynecology, 19*(3), 489–513.

Pouillot, R., Hoelzer, K., Jackson, K. A., Henao, O. L., & Silk, B. J. (2012). Relative risk of listeriosis in Foodborne Diseases Active Surveillance Network (FoodNet) sites according to age, pregnancy, and ethnicity. *Clinical Infectious Diseases, 54*(Suppl. 5), S405–S410.

Ramakrishnan, U., Grant, F., Goldenberg, T., Zongrone, A., & Martorell, R. (2012). Effect of women's nutrition before and during early pregnancy on maternal and infant outcomes: A systematic review. *Paediatric and Perinatal Epidemiology, 26*, 285–301. doi:10.1111/j.1365-3016.2012.01281.x

Rasmussen, K. M., & Yaktine, A. L. (2009). *Committee reexamine IOM pregnancy weight guidelines; Institute of Medicine; National Research Council.* Retrieved from http://www.nap.edu/catalog.php?record_id=12584

Rasmussen, K. M., Yaktine, A. L., & Committee to Reexamine IOM Pregnancy Weight Guidelines, Institute of Medicine, National Research Council. (2009). *Weight gain during pregnancy: Reexamining the guidelines.* The National Academies Press.

Rasmussen, S. A., Chu, S. Y., Kim, S. Y., Schmid, C. H., & Lau, J. (2008). Maternal obesity and risk of neural tube defects: A meta-analysis. *American Journal of Obstetrics and Gynecology, 198*(6), 611–619.

Redmer, D. A., Wallace, J. M., & Reynolds, L. P. (2004). Effect of nutrient intake during pregnancy on fetal and placental growth and vascular development. *Domestic Animal Endocrinology, 27*(3), 199–217.

Reinold, C., Dalenius, K., Brindley, P., Smith, B., & Grummer-Strawn, L. (2011). *Pregnancy Nutrition Surveillance 2009 Report*. Atlanta: U.S. Department of Health and Human Services, Centers for Disease Control and Prevention. Retrieved from http://cdc.gov/pednss/pnss_tables/pdf/national_table21.pdf

Reiter, C. S., & Graves, L. (2010). Nutrition therapy for eating disorders. *Nutrition in Clinical Practice, 25*(2), 122–136.

Shahid, A., Ahmed, M., Rashid, F., Kahn, M. W., & Rehman, M. (2011). Pregnancy and food; women beliefs and practices regarding food during pregnancy—A hospital based study. *Professional Medical Journal, 18*(2), 189–194. Retrieved from http://www.theprofesional.com/article/2011/vol-18-no-2/004-Prof-1709.pdf

Shiell, A. W., Campbell-Brown, M., Haselden, S., Robinson, S., Godfrey, K. M., & Barker, D. J. P. (2001). High-meat, low-carbohydrate diet in pregnancy: Relation to adult blood pressure in the offspring. *Hypertension, 38*, 1282–1288. doi:10.1161/hy1101.095332

Shwide-Slavin, C., Swift, C., & Ross, T. (2012). Nonnutritive sweeteners: Where are we today? *Diabetes Spectrum, 25*(2), 104–110.

Siega-Riz, A. M., Viswanathan, M., Moos, M. K., Deierlein, A., Mumford, S., Knaack, J., . . . Lohr, K. N. (2009). A systematic review of outcomes of maternal weight gain according to the Institute of Medicine recommendations: Birthweight, fetal growth, and postpartum weight retention. *American Journal of Obstetrics and Gynecology, 201*, 339 e1–339 e14.

Stables, D., & Rankin, J. (2009). *Physiology in childbearing with anatomy and related biosciences* (3rd ed.). Edinburgh: Elsevier.

Stice, E., Marti, C. N., & Durant, S. (2011). Risk factors for onset of eating disorders: Evidence of multiple risk pathways from an 8-year prospective study. *Behaviour Research and Therapy, 49*, 622–627.

Thangaratinam, S., Rogozińska, E., Jolly, K., Glinkowski, S., Roseboom, T., Tomlinson, J. W., . . . Khan, K. S. (2012). Effects of interventions in pregnancy on maternal weight and obstetric outcomes: Meta-analysis of randomised evidence. *BMJ: British Medical Journal, 344*.

Tinker, S. C., Cogswell, M. E., Devine, O., & Berry, R. J. (2010). Folic acid intake among U.S. women aged 15–44 years, National Health and Nutrition Examination Survey, 2003–2006. *American Journal of Preventive Medicine, 38*(5), 534–542.

Todrank, J., Heth, G., & Restrepo, D. (2011). Effects of *in utero* odorant exposure on neuroanatomical development of the olfactory bulb and odour preferences. *Proceedings of the Royal Society B: Biological Sciences, 278*(1714), 1949–1955.

USDA. (2009). Food Safety. Retrieved from http://www.fda.gov/Food/FoodSafety/FoodContaminantsAdulteration/Pesticides/ucm114992.htm

Vieau, D. (2011). Perinatal nutritional programming of health and metabolic adult disease. *World Journal of Diabetes, 2*(9), 133–136.

Weng, X., Odouli, R., & Li, D.-K. (2008). Maternal caffeine consumption during pregnancy and the risk of miscarriage: A prospective cohort study. *American Journal of Obstetrics and Gynecology, 198*, 279.e1–279.e8.

Young, B. E., McNanley, T. J., Cooper, E. M., McIntyre, A. W., Witter, F., Harris, Z. L., & O'Brien, K. O. (2012). Maternal vitamin D status and calcium intake interact to affect fetal skeletal growth in utero in pregnant adolescents. *The American Journal of Clinical Nutrition, 95*(5), 1103–1112. doi:10.3945/ajcn.111.023861

Young, M. F., Griffin, I., Pressman, E., McIntyre, A. W., Cooper, E., McNanley, T., . . . O'Brien, K. O. (2010). Utilization of iron from an animal-based iron source is greater than that of ferrous sulfate in pregnant and nonpregnant women. *The Journal of Nutrition, 140*(12), 2162–2166.

Young, S. L. (2010). Pica in pregnancy: New ideas about an old condition. *Annual Review of Nutrition, 30*, 403–422.

Zhong, Y., Macones, G., Zhu, F., & Odibo, A. (2010). The association between prepregnancy maternal body mass index and preterm delivery. *American Journal of Perinatology, 27*(4), 293–298.

7

Pregnancy diagnosis and gestational age assessment

Janet L. Engstrom and Joyce D. Cappiello

Relevant terms

Amenorrhea—the absence of menstruation; suggestive of pregnancy in a woman of reproductive age who has a history of regular menstrual cycles

Basal body temperature—temperature upon awakening, before rising or engaging in any activity or consuming any food or beverage

Chadwick's sign—bluish discoloration of the vagina that occurs during pregnancy

Dickinson's sign—softening of the uterus in the area of implantation; creates a sensation of inconsistency in the uterus during a bimanual exam, described as a feeling of "furrows and grooves"

Endocrine pregnancy test—biochemical measurement of the pregnancy-related hormone human chorionic gonadotropin (hCG), sometimes called a "beta-hCG" because the test targets the beta subunit of the hormone

Estimated date of delivery or estimated due date (EDD), also known as the estimated date of birth (EDB) and estimated date of confinement (EDC)—approximate date that a woman is expected to give birth, calculated as 280 days from the first day of the last menstrual period or 266 days from the date of conception

Fetal heart activity or fetal heart sounds—fetal heart activity can be observed using real-time ultrasound; fetal heart sounds can be heard by using a handheld Doppler ultrasound unit or auscultated using a fetoscope

Fetoscope—modified stethoscope used to auscultate fetal heart sounds; the stethoscope has a headpiece that is placed against the examiner's frontal bones to facilitate the transfer of the faint sounds of the fetal heartbeat

Fundal height measurements—distance between the uppermost border of the symphysis pubis and the uppermost border of the uterine fundus measured in centimeters; used to assess fetal growth and to determine whether the size of the uterus is appropriate for the gestational age of the pregnancy

Gestational age—estimated duration of the pregnancy in weeks from the first day of the last menstrual period

Gestational weeks—number of completed weeks since the first day of the last menstrual period, also known as menstrual weeks

Goodell's sign—softening of the uterine cervix during pregnancy

Hegar's sign—softening and compressibility of the lower uterine segment during pregnancy

Jacquemin's sign—bluish or violet discoloration of the vaginal mucosa near the urethra

Ladin's sign—a small spot of softening in the anterior center of the lower uterine segment

Leopold's maneuvers—a series of maneuvers used to palpate the fetus through the mother's abdomen to assess fetal size, position, and presentation

McDonald's sign—ability to move the uterus and cervix toward each other during a bimanual exam due to softening of the lower uterine segment during pregnancy

Positive sign of pregnancy—findings directly attributable to the fetus that can be detected by the health-care provider; considered "absolute" proof of pregnancy

Presumptive sign of pregnancy—maternal physiological and anatomical changes that can be observed or palpated by a health-care provider, suggestive of pregnancy but not diagnostic

Probable sign of pregnancy—physiological changes that a woman experiences or notices, suggestive of pregnancy but not diagnostic

Postconceptional weeks—terminology used by embryologists (but not in clinical practice) to describe the age of the embryo or fetus; the calculation is based on the actual date of conception: postconceptional weeks are 2 weeks less than the number of gestational weeks

Quickening—perception of the first fetal movement by the mother, also known as "feeling life"

Prenatal and Postnatal Care: A Woman-Centered Approach, First Edition. Edited by Robin G. Jordan, Janet L. Engstrom, Julie A. Marfell, and Cindy L. Farley.
© 2014 John Wiley & Sons, Inc. Published 2014 by John Wiley & Sons, Inc.

Introduction

The diagnosis of pregnancy remains an important life event for women and their families. Pregnancy diagnosis and the decisions that accompany the confirmation of a pregnancy have ramifications for a woman and her family's physical, psychosocial, and economic well-being. Although the woman's health and that of her developing fetus are the primary concern when a pregnancy is identified, the diagnosis also raises important moral, ethical, legal, social, and personal questions that must be carefully considered and addressed by the woman in a relatively short period of time.

The diagnosis of pregnancy also begins a process of establishing the duration of the pregnancy and estimating the date of birth, known as the gestational aging or "dating" the pregnancy. Many of the clinical signs used to diagnose pregnancy are also used to estimate gestational age and the probable date of birth, known as the estimated date of delivery or estimated due date (EDD), also known as the estimated date of birth (EDB), or previously as the estimated date of confinement (EDC). The estimated date of birth (EDB) is the preferred term. Knowledge of the gestational age is essential to almost all aspects of prenatal care so accurate estimation of the gestational age is an important component of prenatal care.

This chapter presents the clinical, biochemical, and biophysical methods of diagnosing pregnancy and establishing gestational age. Also described are the health, psychosocial, and economic considerations that must be addressed at the time of pregnancy diagnosis. The appropriate counseling that should accompany pregnancy testing and confirmation of a pregnancy are also discussed.

Early pregnancy diagnosis and gestational age assessment

Pregnancy raises a number of health issues and decisions so early diagnosis of a pregnancy is ideal. Early pregnancy diagnosis is important for women who decide to terminate the pregnancy because early termination is associated with lower maternal morbidity and mortality and allows women more options in termination procedures. For women who decide to continue the pregnancy, early diagnosis facilitates early entry to prenatal care. Diagnosis of a pregnancy provides the opportunity to advise women to avoid potential teratogens and to minimize unnecessary exposures such as alcohol, tobacco, and illicit drugs. For women with preexisting medical conditions such as diabetes, seizure disorders,

and hypertension, early pregnancy diagnosis facilitates management of these conditions and the selection of medications most compatible with pregnancy.

Early pregnancy diagnosis also facilitates the accurate assessment of gestational age. Indeed, calculation of the gestational age and EDB begin at the time of pregnancy diagnosis because gestational age is essential to many aspects of routine prenatal care. For example, the timing and interpretation of many screening and diagnostic procedures depend on knowledge of the gestational age. Most notable is the need for accurate dating of the pregnancy to determine when to perform blood and ultrasound testing for genetic screening as well as for more invasive testing such as chorionic villi sampling and genetic amniocentesis. Knowledge of the gestational age is also required to know when to perform procedures such as screening for diabetes or administering Rh immune globulin.

The appropriate diagnosis and treatment of pregnancy complications such as preterm labor and postterm pregnancy also depend on an accurate assessment of the gestational age. In the case of preterm labor, decisions about whether to use medications such as tocolytics and antenatal steroids or to transport a mother to a regional perinatal center are dependent upon knowledge of the gestational age. Knowledge of the gestational age is also essential to the identification of pregnancy problems that cause the uterus to be abnormally large or small such as fetal growth restriction, fetal macrosomia, amniotic fluid volume disorders, multiple gestations, and hydatidiform mole. Knowledge of the gestational age is also essential to the correct timing of procedures such as the induction of labor and scheduled cesarean birth. If health-care providers do not have an accurate assessment of gestational age in these situations, they may overlook important pregnancy complications and fail to intervene when indicated, or they may intervene inappropriately.

Finally, knowledge of gestational age is essential to providing relevant and timely health education throughout pregnancy. A woman's need for information varies through the various stages of pregnancy. Early in pregnancy, teaching focuses on the avoidance of teratogens, nutrition, a healthy lifestyle, and the warning signs and symptoms of early pregnancy complications such as miscarriage and ectopic pregnancy, whereas the teaching later in pregnancy focuses on the preparation for labor, birth, breastfeeding, and parenting as well as the recognition of the complications associated with more advanced pregnancy such as preterm birth. Thus, early pregnancy diagnosis with concurrent and ongoing assessment of gestational age is a cornerstone of prenatal care.

Pregnancy diagnosis

Over the past three decades, the diagnosis of pregnancy has changed dramatically with the introduction of readily available sensitive and specific pregnancy tests and easy access to real-time ultrasonography. Although modern biochemical pregnancy tests and biophysical methods of identifying a pregnancy have greatly advanced pregnancy care, assessment of the clinical signs and symptoms of pregnancy remain an important component of prenatal care. In fact, the diagnosis of pregnancy usually begins with a woman's recognition of subjective symptoms associated with pregnancy such as the absence of menstrual bleeding at the anticipated time or a cluster of symptoms such as nausea, vomiting, and fatigue.

Although no single subjective symptom or cluster of symptoms is absolutely diagnostic of pregnancy, documentation of clinical signs and symptoms augments the information gleaned from biochemical pregnancy tests and biophysical assessments such as ultrasound. Women's reports of pregnancy-related symptoms provide opportunities to teach women about the normal physiological changes that occur during pregnancy. Many of these symptoms are associated with some discomfort, so women's reports of these symptoms provide the opportunity to teach women about measures to mitigate the symptoms. This also provides the opportunity to determine whether the symptoms are within the range of normal or indicative of a pregnancy complication or other health problem.

Knowledge of the signs and symptoms of pregnancy also enables health-care providers to consider the possibility of pregnancy when women seek care for symptoms that they attribute to other health problems. For example, women occasionally seek care for a symptom such as amenorrhea or nausea, thinking that the symptom is related to a normal physiological event such as menopause or a serious health problem such as cancer. Health-care providers must be vigilant in their differential diagnosis to exclude pregnancy as a cause of the symptoms in women of childbearing age, even in women at the extreme ends of the reproductive years. Indeed, for many of the symptoms described in this chapter, pregnancy should be at the top of the list of differential diagnoses in women of childbearing age.

Historically, the signs and symptoms of pregnancy have been organized into three categories: presumptive, probable, and positive. Presumptive signs are those noted by the woman and are considered "subjective" symptoms of pregnancy. Probable signs are those that can be observed or palpated by the health-care provider and are considered "objective" signs of pregnancy.

Table 7.1   Signs and Symptoms of Pregnancy

Category	Defining characteristic of the category	Sign or symptom
Presumptive signs	Physiological changes that the woman experiences or notices Subjective sensations or assessments noted by the woman Suggestive but not diagnostic of pregnancy	Amenorrhea Breast changes Vaginal changes Skin changes Nausea and vomiting Urinary frequency Fatigue Fetal movement
Probable signs	Maternal physiological and anatomical changes that can be observed or palpated by a health-care provider on exam Objective findings on clinical exam Suggestive but not diagnostic of pregnancy	Enlargement of the abdomen Vaginal changes Cervical changes Uterine changes Palpation and ballottement of the fetus Basal body temperature elevation Endocrine pregnancy tests
Positive signs	Findings directly attributable to the fetus that can be detected by the health-care provider Considered "absolute" proof of pregnancy Diagnostic of pregnancy	Detection of the embryo or fetus by ultrasound or X-ray Identification of fetal heart activity Detection of fetal movement by the examiner

Positive signs of pregnancy are those that can be directly attributed to the fetus such as seeing the embryo on ultrasound or hearing the fetal heart beat. The positive signs of pregnancy are the only signs that are considered "absolute" proof of pregnancy. These presumptive, probable, and positive signs of pregnancy are summarized in Table 7.1.

Presumptive signs of pregnancy

The presumptive signs of pregnancy are symptoms and findings that are perceived by the woman. These subjective symptoms are the least accurate method of diagnosing pregnancy because they can have a variety of causes other than pregnancy. The subjective symptoms include amenorrhea, breast changes, vaginal symptoms, skin changes, and other subjective sensations.

Amenorrhea

Amenorrhea, or the absence of menstruation, is strongly suggestive of a pregnancy in women with a history of regular menstrual cycles. However, amenorrhea is less predictive of pregnancy in women with preexisting amenorrhea, irregular menstrual cycles, lactating women, or perimenopausal women. Additionally, a number of pregnant women have some bleeding early in pregnancy that can be mistaken for menses and can delay the diagnosis of pregnancy.

Breast changes

There are a number of breast changes that occur during pregnancy. Enlargement of the breasts is one of the earliest symptoms of pregnancy, occurring as early as the fourth week after the last menstrual period (LMP). Tenderness, throbbing, stretching, tingling, and fullness of the breasts are also common in the early weeks of pregnancy. Other changes include enlargement and increased pigmentation of the nipples and areola with increased protuberance of the Montgomery glands. Secretion of colostrum or milk occurs in some women but is more likely to occur in multiparous women and tends to occur later in pregnancy, usually during mid- to late gestation.

Vaginal changes

During pregnancy, women often notice an increase in the normal vaginal discharge, a symptom known as leukorrhea. The increased discharge is odorless and not irritating, and is not indicative of any inflammatory or infectious process.

Skin changes

Skin changes that may be noted during pregnancy include increased pigmentation in areas such as the nipple, areola, axilla, genitals, and the line down the center of the abdomen and around the umbilicus—an area known as the linea nigra. Many women also experience changes in pigmentation on the face, known as cholasma. Other skin changes include the appearance of striae, most often on the abdomen and breasts, but they may also appear on the buttocks and thighs. Changes in the vasculature of the skin include vascular spiders and palmar erythema. However, these changes are often not noted until later in pregnancy.

Subjective sensations

Women may notice many other subjective sensations commonly associated with pregnancy such as nausea and vomiting, urinary frequency, and fatigue. The prevalence of these symptoms varies widely among women, limiting their usefulness in pregnancy diagnosis. When they occur, they tend to be the most pronounced in the early weeks of pregnancy.

Another notable maternal subjective sensation is fetal movement. Although long considered a hallmark of pregnancy, maternal perception of fetal movement is classified as a subjective sensation and is therefore only a presumptive sign of pregnancy. The first perception of fetal movement or "quickening" is a pivotal event in the pregnancy and an important milestone in maternal role development and attachment to the fetus. Historically, quickening was thought to reflect the moment at which the fetus became alive or showed signs of life (Engstrom, 1985b). The maternal perception of fetal movement is still often termed "feeling life." In the era before biochemical and biophysical methods of diagnosing pregnancy were widely available, quickening was often a woman's only method verifying of the existence of a pregnancy. Although quickening remains an important and notable pregnancy event for women, its role in the diagnosis of pregnancy has lessened with the advent of modern chemical and biophysical tests since fetal movement perception varies widely among women. Quickening usually occurs between 15 and 22 weeks of gestation, but has been reported much earlier and later in gestation by both nulliparous and multiparous women (Andersen, Johnson, Barclay, & Flora, 1981; Engstrom, 1985b; Gillieson, Dunlap, Nair, & Pilon, 1984; Herbert, Bruninghaus, Barefoot, & Bright, 1987; Hertz et al., 1978; Jimenez, Tyson, & Reisch, 1983; Kraus & Hendricks, 1964; O'Dowd & O'Dowd, 1985; Rawlings & Moore, 1970; Thiery, 1986).

Probable signs of pregnancy

The probable signs of pregnancy are maternal physiological and anatomical changes that can be detected by the health-care provider. Although the probable signs of pregnancy are more objective, observable, and verifiable than the subjective sensations reported by women, the probable signs of pregnancy are still not absolute signs of pregnancy. Thus, even in the presence of several clinically detectable signs, the pregnancy must still be verified by another method. There are several probable signs of pregnancy: enlargement of the abdomen, vaginal changes, cervical changes, uterine changes, ballottement of the fetus, palpation of the fetus, maternal basal body temperature (BBT) elevation, and endocrine pregnancy tests.

Enlargement of the abdomen

Enlargement of the maternal abdomen is one of the classic signs of pregnancy. However, the uterus is usually not palpable through the maternal abdomen until about 12 weeks of gestation. Although the pattern of enlargement of the pregnancy is generally predictable, there is variation among women. Additionally the ability to accurately assess the size of the uterus through the maternal abdomen may be hindered by the amount of adipose tissue and the strength of the musculature of the women's abdomen as well as by the skill of the examiner. Another limitation of using abdominal enlargement as a sign of pregnancy is that any abdominal mass can be mistaken for the uterus and, periodically, a woman will experience enlargement of the abdomen due to a cancerous or noncancerous tumor and mistakenly assume that the enlargement is due to pregnancy. For example, uterine fibroids can cause substantial abdominal enlargement and can be mistaken for a pregnancy.

Vaginal changes

Vaginal changes noted during early pregnancy include a change in the color of the vaginal mucosa. The change usually begins in the anterior lower portion of the vagina, close to the vaginal opening. The change begins in the area of a venous plexus and is described as a bluish or purplish spot known as Jacquemin's sign (McDonald, 1908). The location of this color change is depicted in Figure 7.1. Over time, the dusky blue or violet color change spreads from the lower anterior vaginal wall to the entire vaginal mucosa. This color change is known as Chadwick's sign (Munsick, 1986). The color changes in the vagina occur early in pregnancy, as early as 6 weeks of gestation (McDonald, 1908).

Cervical changes

Cervical changes noted in pregnancy are the changes in cervical color and consistency. Similar to the vagina, the cervix becomes bluish purple or violet color in appearance. The softening of the cervix is remarkable and is known as Goodell's sign (Munsick, 1986). A classic description of cervical consistency is that the nonpregnant cervix is as firm as the tip of the nose, whereas the pregnant cervix is as soft as the cheek or lips. The softening of the cervix begins on the lateral sides first at 3 o'clock and 9 o'clock. These areas of softening are described as grooves along the sides of the cervix. These grooves appear early but eventually disappear as the remainder of the cervix softens.

Uterine changes

The uterus undergoes a number of changes during pregnancy. One of the first changes noted is the softening of the lower uterine segment. The softening is known as Ladin's sign and begins as a single soft spot in the center of the anterior aspect of the lower uterine segment (Munsick, 1986). The softening spreads throughout the lower uterine segment and is called Hegar's sign (Spreet,

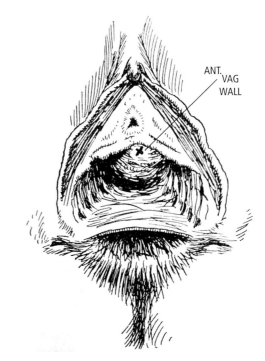

Figure 7.1.   Jacquemin's sign of pregnancy. From McDonald, E. (1908). The diagnosis of early pregnancy. *American Journal of Obstetrics and Diseases of Women and Children, 57,* 323–346.

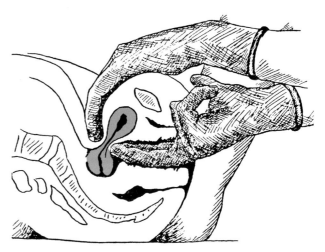

Figure 7.2.   Hegar's sign of pregnancy. From McDonald, E. (1908). The diagnosis of early pregnancy. *American Journal of Obstetrics and Diseases of Women and Children, 57,* 323–346.

1955). The softening of the lower uterine segment is readily detectable upon bimanual pelvic examination and is so pronounced that the lower segment can easily be compressed, giving the impression that there is no lower uterine segment whatsoever—just a cervix and the corpus of the uterus (McDonald, 1908). The softening and compressibility of the lower uterine segment is illustrated in Figure 7.2.

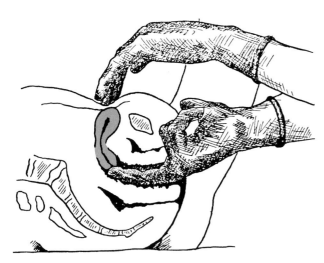

Figure 7.3.   McDonald's sign of pregnancy. From McDonald, E. (1908). The diagnosis of early pregnancy. *American Journal of Obstetrics and Diseases of Women and Children, 57,* 323–346.

Uterine size and shape on bimanual examination	
4–5 weeks	Pear
6 weeks	Juice orange
8 weeks	Navel orange
12 weeks	Grapefruit

The softening of the lower segment also makes this area of the uterus more flexible and acts like a hinge, enabling the examiner to bend the uterus so that the fundus and the cervix move toward each other, a finding known as McDonald's sign (Munsick, 1986). McDonald's sign is illustrated in Figure 7.3.

Other areas of the uterus also demonstrate softening. The body of the uterus also softens during pregnancy. The first area of softening in the body of uterus is the area in which implantation occurred. This area of softening is surrounded by areas of the firmness and creates a sensation of "furrows and grooves" to the examiner, a sign known as Dickinson's sign (McDonald, 1908; Munsick, 1985). Although present in most women, these changes are subtle and may not be easily palpated by the novice examiner.

The uterus also demonstrates changes in size and shape. The nonpregnant uterus is described as being shaped like a flattened pear, with the narrowest diameter in the sagittal plane (anterior–posterior). The first change in the shape and size of the uterus occurs at the site of implantation; the uterus enlarges asymmetrically in that area. Shortly thereafter, the uterus increases in the anterior–posterior diameter becoming pear shaped by 4–5 weeks of gestation. The uterus continues to enlarge and become rounder through the first trimester of pregnancy, acquiring the shape and size of a juice orange by 6 weeks of gestation, a navel orange by 8 weeks, and a grapefruit by 12 weeks (Fox, 1985; Margulies & Miller, 2001).

The uterus can be palpated by the examiner through the maternal abdomen at approximately 12 weeks of gestation. Initially, the uterine fundus is located immediately above the symphysis pubis. Subsequently, the uterine fundus is located approximately halfway between the symphysis pubis and umbilicus at 16 weeks of gestation, at the umbilicus at about 20 weeks, about halfway between the umbilicus and the xiphisternum at 28 weeks, and at the xiphisternum at 36 weeks (Andersen et al., 1981; Engstrom, 1988). However, there is a wide variation among women in when the uterine fundus reaches these landmarks due to anatomic differences among women, the adiposity and muscularity of the maternal abdomen, and the size of the uterus (Andersen et al., 1981; Beazley & Underhill, 1970; Engstrom, 1988; Jimenez et al., 1983).

Location of the uterine fundus during pregnancy	
12 weeks	At the symphysis pubis
16 weeks	About halfway between the symphysis pubis and umbilicus
20 weeks	At the umbilicus
28 weeks	About halfway between the umbilicus and the xiphisternum
36 weeks	At the xiphisternum

Contractions of the uterus, known as Braxton Hicks contractions, can often be detected early in pregnancy. These contractions are painless and are usually not perceptible by the woman until later in pregnancy. The contractions can be palpated early in pregnancy by the health-care provider and are often stimulated by a bimanual or abdominal examination (McDonald, 1908). However, these contractions are subtle and may not be easily palpated by the novice examiner.

Palpation and ballottement of the fetus

Palpation of the fetus by a health-care provider is another probable sign of pregnancy. Even before fetal parts can be palpated, the examiner can "bounce" the fetus between the examiner's hands, a finding known as ballottement. Later, individual fetal parts such as the head, buttocks, back, and extremities are palpable. Although the palpation of the fetus is useful in identifying fetal position and presentation and in estimating fetal weight later in pregnancy, these signs have limited value in pregnancy diagnosis since they occur later in pregnancy and are only detectable once the fetus is large enough to be palpated.

Basal body temperatures

BBTs can be useful in identifying a pregnancy. The basal temperature is the temperature upon first awaking in the morning before any activity. Thus, the temperature must be obtained before the woman arises from bed, ideally after a full night of undisturbed rest. A woman's BBT is influenced by the presence of progesterone, which has a thermogenic effect on body temperature, causing it to increase. Normally, BBTs are lower (below 98°F) during the follicular phase (first half or approximately the first 14 days) of the menstrual cycle when serum progesterone levels are consistently low. Around the time of ovulation, temperatures begin to increase as progesterone is beginning to be produced by the luteinized follicle. Progesterone is produced in large amounts by the corpus luteum after ovulation and body temperature remains elevated throughout the luteal phase (second half or last 14 days of the cycle). In the presence of a pregnancy, the temperature remains elevated throughout the remainder of the pregnancy. The amount of temperature increase associated with ovulation and pregnancy varies but is usually 0.4–0.8°F and postovulatory temperatures are usually above 98°F.

Endocrine pregnancy tests

Modern endocrine pregnancy tests measure the hormone human chorionic gonadotropin (hCG). The tests are often called "beta-hCG" because the tests target the beta subunit of the molecule. The tests can be performed on urine or serum and are classified as qualitative, semiquantitative, and quantitative. Qualitative tests simply detect the presence of hCG and the results are reported as "positive" or "negative," with positive indicating the presence of enough of the hormone to be associated with a pregnancy. There are also semiquantitative urine pregnancy tests that measure hCG in categories of units (IU/L), but these tests are not currently available in the United States (Cole, 2012; Grossman, Berdichevsky, Larrea, & Beltran, 2007). Quantitative tests measure the precise level of hCG in the serum and report the findings in units (IU/L). Thus, serum pregnancy tests are used to diagnose pregnancy and to monitor pregnancy progress

in selected pregnancy complications such as suspected ectopic pregnancy or threatened abortion.

Types of endocrine pregnancy tests		
Type of test	**Type of specimen**	**Characteristics of the test**
Qualitative	Urine	Reported as positive or negative Available over-the-counter and in health-care settings
Semiquantitative	Urine	Reported in categories of units based on the amount of hormone present Available outside of the United States
Quantitative	Serum	Reported in units (IU/L) Available in health-care settings

There are two additional categories of urine pregnancy tests: point-of-care tests used in health-care settings and over-the-counter pregnancy tests used by women in home testing. The promotional materials for both point-of-care and over-the-counter tests claim high sensitivity and specificity and indicate that pregnancy can be detected several days before the missed menstrual period. However, the accuracy of both types of products varies widely (Cervinski et al., 2009; Cole, 2012). When the tests are positive, there is a high probability that a woman is pregnant. False positive tests are uncommon but can occur in a woman who has recently been pregnant and in women with certain cancers and selected medical conditions. In contrast, false negative rates can be high in early pregnancy (Cole, 2012). The tests are most likely to be inaccurate when the level of hCG is the lowest during the first 2–3 weeks after conception (Cervinski et al., 2009; Cole, 2012; Greene et al., 2013). Surprisingly, many commonly used point-of-care pregnancy tests fail to detect pregnancy at the time of the missed menstrual period; the false negative rate at the time of missed menses is 33–60%, depending on the product used (Cervinski et al., 2009; Cole, 2012). Thus, when a woman has a negative test around the time of the missed menstrual period, it is reasonable to perform another pregnancy test 4–7 days later. Four days is selected as the minimum interval between tests because the level of hCG increases exponentially in early pregnancy, nearly doubling every other day. Thus, by 4–7 days, the levels should be substantially increased.

Positive signs of pregnancy

The positive signs of pregnancy are signs that are directly attributed to the fetus and can be detected by the examiner. The positive signs of pregnancy are considered "absolute signs" of pregnancy. There are three positive signs of pregnancy: identification of fetal heart activity, detection of the embryo or fetus by ultrasound or X-ray, and detection of fetal movement by the examiner.

Identification of fetal heart activity

Fetal heart activity can be visualized using real-time ultrasound or by hearing fetal heart sounds using Doppler ultrasound or auscultation. In most settings in the United States, fetal heart sounds are assessed during the prenatal period using a handheld Doppler ultrasound unit. Early in pregnancy, the best place to listen for heart sounds is in the suprapubic area, slightly above the pubic bone in the center of the maternal abdomen. The fetal heart rate is faster than the mother's heart rate and is typically heard at a rate of 110–160 beats per minute. When using a handheld Doppler ultrasound device, fetal heart sounds should be heard by 12 weeks of gestation and are often heard as early as 10 weeks. Real-time ultrasound can also be used to identify fetal heart activity as early as 6 weeks of gestation (Richards, 2012).

Historically, fetal heart sounds, also called fetal heart "tones," were auscultated using a modified stethoscope known as a fetoscope. The fetoscope has a specially modified headpiece added to a stethoscope that provides additional stimulation of the head bones to facilitate the conduction of the sounds through the frontal bones, thereby enabling the health-care provider to hear the faint sounds of early fetal heart activity. The use of the fetoscope is depicted in Figure 7.4. Although the fetoscope is primarily of historic interest in the Unites States, it is still used to assess fetal heart activity in some health-care settings, especially in low-resource settings or when avoidance of technology is desired. Fetal heart sounds are not usually heard with a fetoscope until 15–22 weeks of gestation (Andersen et al., 1981; Engstrom, 1985b; Herbert et al., 1987; Hertz et al., 1978; Jimenez et al., 1983). Later in pregnancy, fetal heart sounds can be auscultated with a regular stethoscope.

Detection of the embryo or fetus by ultrasound or X-ray

Observation of the embryo or fetus by ultrasound or X-ray is a definitive sign of pregnancy. X-ray is rarely

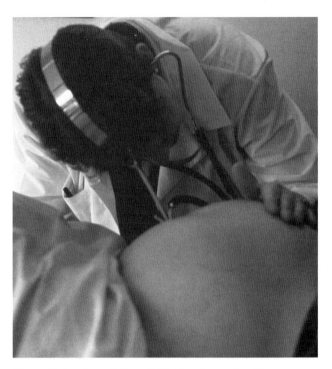

Figure 7.4.   Auscultation of fetal heart sounds with a fetoscope. Photo courtesy of Ginger Michels, MSN, CNM.

used during pregnancy, but ultrasonography is widely used and can detect the gestational sac as early as 4 weeks of gestation (Richards, 2012). The embryo can be observed by 6 weeks of gestation on ultrasound, and embryonic heart activity can also be observed at that time (Richards, 2012).

Detection of fetal movement by the examiner

The third positive sign of pregnancy is detection of fetal movement by the examiner. The fetus is usually not palpable by a health-care provider until the second half of pregnancy. The detection of fetal movement usually occurs during the routine prenatal examination of the pregnant abdomen. The abdomen is systematically palpated using a series of procedures known as Leopold's maneuvers (McFarlin, Engstrom, Sampson, & Cattledge, 1985; Sharma, 2009). All palpation is performed gently using a circular motion with the flat portion of the fingers rather than the tips. To relax the woman's abdominal musculature during the exam, the head of the exam table is raised slightly and the woman's legs are flexed and bent at the knees. The procedures for performing Leopold's maneuvers are depicted in Figure 7.5 and described in the following textbox.

Leopold's maneuvers

First maneuver	Facing the head of the examination table, systematically palpate the uterine fundus to determine which fetal parts are present. The buttocks feel irregular and soft, whereas the head is round and hard. The absence of any part in the area may indicate a transverse lie.
Second maneuver	Facing the head of the examination table, systematically palpate each side of the uterus. Place one hand on each side of the uterus, near the fundus. The examiner's left hand should be placed on the right side of the uterus and the right hand on the left side of the uterus. Hold the left hand stable while palpating with the right hand. Move the hands systematically from the fundus to the symphysis to cover all of the areas. Then, repeat the procedure holding the right hand still while palpating with the left hand along the right side of the uterus. The fetal back is usually along one side of the uterus and the "small parts" (arms and legs) are along the other side. The back feels smooth and firm. The small parts are very irregular and small.
Third maneuver	Facing the head of the examination table, the examiner separates the thumb and fingers of the right hand to form a large "C." Palpate the lateral borders of the uterus immediately above the symphysis pubis to determine whether the head or the buttocks are in the area. The absence of any part in the area may indicate a transverse lie.
Fourth maneuver	Face the foot of the examination table and place both hands along the lateral uterine borders immediately above the symphysis pubis. Gently glide the hands along the fetal presenting part into the pelvis to identify the presenting part and its relationship to the pelvis.

Sources: McFarlin et al. (1985), Sharma (2009).

Gestational age assessment

Once the presence of a pregnancy is confirmed, the gestational age of the pregnancy should be determined. Knowledge of the gestational age is such an important component of prenatal care that gestational age assessment begins at the time of pregnancy diagnosis. At each prenatal visit, the clinician verifies the gestational age and compares the size of the uterus to the calculated gestational age to determine whether uterine size and fetal growth are consistent with the gestational age. The dates of other events such as quickening, hearing the fetal heart sounds for the first time, and when the uterine fundus reaches the level of the umbilicus are also compared to the estimated gestational age to determine whether the timing of these events is consistent with the estimated gestational age.

Terminology used to describe gestational age

In clinical practice, gestational age is usually calculated by using the first day of the woman's LMP. The first day of the LMP is used regardless of the time of day that menstruation started or the amount of menstrual flow. When calculated from the LMP, the duration of human pregnancy is 280 days or 40 completed weeks. The first day of the LMP is used to calculate the number of gestational weeks. Thus, the terms *gestational weeks* or *gestational age* refer to the number of *completed* weeks since the first day of the LMP. Gestational weeks are also known as *menstrual weeks* or *menstrual age* since the counting of weeks begins with the first day of the LMP. Gestational weeks are described in completed weeks and many health-care providers add the number of days in the week to more completely describe the gestational age. For example, a note in the record may indicate 35 weeks, 6 days, or 35[6.] Importantly, the number of gestational weeks is never rounded up to the next week.

Although the phrase "gestational weeks" is the accepted terminology in clinical practice, embryonic development is described in postconceptional weeks, beginning with the date of conception. When postconceptional weeks are used, the duration of pregnancy is 266 days or 38 weeks. Although useful in understanding embryonic development, the terminology of postconceptional weeks is not used in the clinical setting because of the potential confusion with the standard use of gestational weeks. The terminology gestational weeks or gestational age is used when communicating in the clinical setting.

Pregnancy is also sometimes described in months and trimesters. The relationship between gestational weeks, lunar months, and trimesters is depicted in Table 7.2. The terminology surrounding the use of months is fraught with confusion and can easily lead to miscommunication. When months are used to describe pregnancy, the months are lunar months, each consisting of 28 days. Thus, a normal pregnancy is 10 lunar months. Lunar months are shorter than calendar months, so 10 lunar months translates to about 9-1/3 calendar months. For these reasons, health-care providers should avoid using the terminology of months whenever possible.

Pregnancy is also described in trimesters. Surprisingly, the method of dividing the pregnancy into trimester has varied over time. Logically, trimesters should be of equal length, but various schemes have been used in the past.

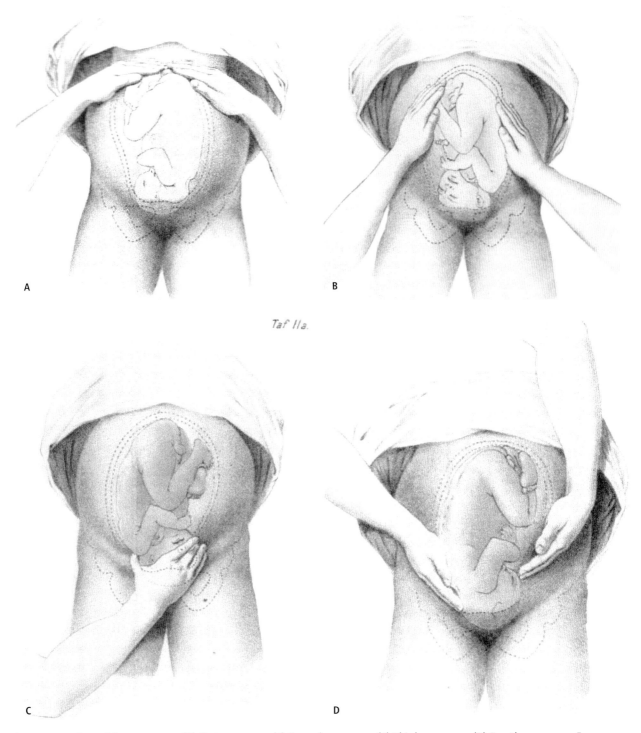

A

B

Taf IIa.

C

D

Figure 7.5. Leopold's maneuvers. (A) First maneuver. (B) Second maneuver. (C) Third maneuver. (D) Fourth maneuver. From: Sharma, J. B. (2009). Evaluation of Sharma's modified Leopold's maneuvers: A new method for fetal palpation in late pregnancy. *Archives of Gynecology and Obstetrics, 279,* 481–487. Used with permission.

Table 7.2 Timing of Events in Gestation

Trimester	Lunar month	Week of gestation	Event
First	1	1	First day of the last menstrual period (LMP) Follicular phase of the menstrual cycle begins.
		2	Follicular phase of the menstrual cycle continues. Ovulation Fertilization of the oocyte (conception) on approximately day 14 of a perfect menstrual cycle
		3	Maternal basal body temperature increase Transport of the conceptus through the fallopian tube and into the uterus Preliminary attachment of the conceptus to the endometrium
		4	Implantation of the conceptus in the endometrium Urine and serum endocrine pregnancy tests (hCG) may be positive. Breast tenderness and fullness may occur.
	2	5	Gestational sac may be observed on ultrasound.
		6	Embryo observed on ultrasound Fetal heart activity observed on real-time ultrasound The uterus becomes more rounded and is approximately the size of a juice orange. Jacquemin's sign may appear between 6 and 12 weeks. Chadwick's sign may appear between 6 and 12 weeks. Goodell's sign may appear between 6 and 12 weeks. Ladin's sign may appear between 6 and 12 weeks. Hegar's sign may appear between 6 and 12 weeks. McDonald's sign may appear between 6 and 12 weeks. Dickinson's sign may appear between 6 and 12 weeks.
		7	
		8	The uterus is the size of a navel orange.
	3	9	
		10	Fetal heart sounds are usually heard with Doppler ultrasound at 10–12 weeks.
		11	
		12	The uterus is the size of a grapefruit. The uterus is palpable at the symphysis pubis.
	4	13	
		14	
Second		15	Quickening usually occurs between 15 and 22 weeks. Fetal heart sounds are first auscultated with a fetoscope between 15 and 22 weeks.
		16	The uterus is about halfway between the symphysis pubis and the umbilicus.
	5	17	
		18	
		19	
		20	The uterus is at about the level of the umbilicus. Fundal height measurements (in centimeters) are approximately equal to the number of gestational weeks from 20 to 36 weeks (±3 cm).
	6	21	
		22	
		23	
		24	

(Continued)

Table 7.2   *(Continued)*

Trimester	Lunar month	Week of gestation	Event
	7	25	
		26	
		27	
		28	The uterus is about halfway between the umbilicus and the xiphisternum.
Third	8	29	
		30	
		31	
		32	
	9	33	
		34	
		35	
		36	The uterus is at the xiphisternum.
	10	37	
		38	
		39	
		40	

Current trimester terminology

First trimester	Week 1 through the end of week 14
Second trimester	Week 15 through the end of week 28
Third trimester	Week 29 through birth

Currently, the recommendation is to divide the pregnancy into three trimesters, each lasting 14 weeks (Cunningham et al., 2010).

Because the terminology surrounding trimesters is varied and each trimester spans a long time period that includes important events and milestones, the terminology trimesters should only be used in the broadest sense such as when discussing how to focus health education or the period of pregnancy when selected pregnancy discomforts and complications are most likely to occur. For example, ectopic pregnancy usually occurs in the first trimester of pregnancy, whereas preeclampsia is most likely to become symptomatic in the third trimester.

Devices used to calculate the gestational age

Gestational age should be calculated at the time of pregnancy diagnosis and verified at each health-care encounter thereafter. Verifying the gestational age at each health-care visit during pregnancy assures that the health-care provider has an accurate assessment of the gestational age at that particular encounter and prevents the problem of carrying forward a calculation error from a previous visit. Although this precaution may seem trivial, an error of even a few days in estimating the gestational age can result in serious health consequences for the mother and the fetus. Thus, verifying the gestational age is an essential part of each health-care encounter during the prenatal period.

There are a number of electronic calculators that can be used to assist health-care providers with the calculation of gestational weeks and the EDB. These devices are available online and as applications for mobile devices such as cellular phones and electronic tablet devices. The electronic calculators are uniformly accurate and are the preferred method of choice for calculating gestational weeks and the EDB (Smout, Seed, & Shennan, 2012).

Gestational weeks can also be calculated using a manual calculator, commonly known as a "wheel" because of its circular design and rotating wheels. There are a number of small, handheld, manual cardboard or plastic devices available, and they are often given to health-care providers as a promotional item advertising maternity care products. Although handy in low-resource settings, the accuracy of these devices varies widely. There are significant differences between the gestational age and EDB calculations made with various devices, as well as differences between health-care providers when using the same device (McParland & Johnson, 1993; Ross, 2003; Smout et al., 2012). The devices also yield different results than electronic calculators, with differences as large as 5 days reported (Ross, 2003). Thus, the use of manual calculators should be avoided except in low-resource settings where there is no access to an electronic calculator. In those settings, all health-care providers should use the same brand of device and verify that they all obtain the same result when using the device. Before selecting a manual calculator, the device should be validated with an electronic calculator to assure its accuracy.

Methods of estimating the gestational age

There are several methods of estimating gestational age including the date of the LMP, the date of conception, the date of a single act of coitus or insemination, the date of a sustained increase in BBT, fundal height measurements, and ultrasound. The timing of these events as well as the timing of the appearance of many of the clinical signs of pregnancy described previously in this chapter are summarized in Table 7.2.

Last menstrual period

The date of the first day of the LMP is the most commonly used method of estimating gestational age and the EDB. When this date is known and the woman has regular menstrual cycles, the estimation of gestational weeks and the EDB is usually accurate. Unfortunately, a substantial number of women are unable to provide an accurate recollection of the date of the LMP. And, even when a woman presents with an accurate LMP, the estimation of the gestational weeks may be inaccurate if the woman has irregular cycles, long cycles, a recent pregnancy, is lactating, or has recently used hormonal contraception.

The standard calculation of the EDB is based on an average pregnancy interval of 280 days and assumes that ovulation and fertilization take place on day 14 of the cycle. The EDB can be calculated using the following procedure, named Naegele's rule (Baskett & Nagele, 2000; Hunter, 2009):

Naegele's rule for calculating the EDB	Example
1. Use the first day of the LMP.	8-10-2014
2. Subtract 3 from the number of months.	5-10-2014
3. Add 7 to the number of days.	5-17-2014
4. Adjust the year if the pregnancy will occur in the next year.	5-17-2015

Naegele's rule is easy to apply and does not require the use of any devices or calculators. However, the calculation provides only one date, the EDB. The calculation does not assist health-care providers during pregnancy with calculating the gestational weeks, information that is needed at each prenatal visit. Thus, gestational weeks must be calculated using a gestational calculator. Additionally, Naegele's calculation does not account for differences in the number of days in the various months throughout the year. Depending on the particular months included in the pregnancy, the difference between the calculation made by Naegele's rule and the calculation of the EDB using 280 days from the LMP can be different by as many as 3 days (McParland & Johnson, 1993; Ross, 2003). For these reasons, Naegele's rule is only used in low-resource settings or when no other method of calculating the EDB is available. Calculations made using Naegele's rule should be verified with a validated electronic or manual gestational calculator.

Because the LMP is essential in calculating gestational weeks, a thorough menstrual history is an essential component of pregnancy diagnosis and the initial prenatal visit. Although many women initially respond that they do not remember the date of the LMP, many can be encouraged to recall the date by simply looking at a calendar or thinking about events at the time of the LMP. The regularity of cycles as well as the normality of the LMP should also be addressed. It is also important to determine whether the woman recently used hormonal contraception, had a recent gestation or lactation, or any other factor that may influence the regularity of menstrual cycles or delay ovulation.

The primary limitation of using the LMP is that many women do not know the precise dates of their LMP (Lynch & Zhang, 2007) and, even when women are reasonably certain of the date, recall has a significant amount of error and the amount of error increases over time (Wegienka & Baird, 2005). Women also tend to preferentially report certain days of the month (days 1, 5, 10, 15, 20,, 25, and 28) and days of the week (Monday and Wednesday) when reporting the date of the LMP (Savitz et al., 2002; Waller, Spears, Gu, & Cunningham, 2000). Even when women are certain of the date of the LMP, the use of the LMP is limited because the actual date of ovulation and conception is unknown (Nakling, Buhaug, & Backe, 2005). The time between the first day of the LMP and ovulation varies widely among women, even in women who have cycles of the same length, and even in the same woman from month to month (Lynch & Zhang, 2007). The calculated gestational age based on the LMP is a relatively good estimate in a woman with regular cycles who is certain of the date of the LMP but will always be limited by the variability in the timing of ovulation. Research has suggested that when the LMP is used to calculate the EDB, the prediction is 1–3 days earlier than the actual EDB (Bergsjo, Denman, Hoffman, & Meirik, 1990; Hoffman et al., 2008; Nakling et al., 2005; Nguyen, Larsen, Engholm, & Moller, 1999; Savitz et al., 2002; Taipale & Hiilesmaa, 2001). This underestimation results in more pregnancies being classified as post-term when the LMP is used rather than when sonographic estimates of gestational age are used (Bergsjo et al., 1990; Hoffman et al., 2008; Savitz et al., 2002; Taipale & Hiilesmaa, 2001). For these reasons, some experts have recommended using ultrasound estimates of gestational age rather than the LMP when the ultrasound estimate is obtained between 6 and 20 weeks of gestation and is performed by a skilled sonographer (Gardosi, 1997; Nakling et al., 2005; Nguyen et al., 1999; Richards, 2012; Taipale & Hiilesmaa, 2001)

Known date of conception

The gestational age of a pregnancy can be most accurately calculated when assisted reproductive technology procedures such *in vitro* fertilization are used to achieve pregnancy. In these cases, the date of conception is certain and can be used to accurately calculate gestational age. The calculation is performed by adding 38 weeks (266 days) to the date of conception.

Occasionally a woman will report a single act of unprotected coitus that led to the pregnancy. However, even when the woman knows the precise date of coitus or insemination, the actual date of conception is unknown because sperm can reside in the female reproductive tract for up to 6 days before fertilizing the egg (Wilcox, Dunson, & Baird, 2000). Thus, estimates made using a single act of coitus or insemination are likely to be accurate within 1 week.

Change in basal body temperature

Occasionally, a woman can provide BBTs from the cycle in which she conceived. Although neither the day of ovulation nor the day of conception can be pinpointed from a BBT graph, the change in temperature associated with ovulation can provide an excellent estimate of the date of conception and is likely to be accurate within 1 week.

Fundal height measurements

Fundal height measurements are a routine part of the prenatal assessment and can be useful in determining whether uterine size is appropriate for the number of gestational weeks. Abnormally large or small fundal height measurements can indicate that gestational age estimation is incorrect or that a fetal growth disturbance, amniotic fluid abnormality, or multifetal gestation is

present (Morse, Williams, & Gardosi, 2009; Roex, Nikpoor, Eerd, Hodyl, & Dekker, 2012). The measurements are approximately equal to the number of gestational weeks between 20 and 36 weeks of gestation. However, there is wide variation in the measurements, so differences of up to 3 cm between the measurements and the number of gestational weeks are considered acceptable. The measurements can be used as a part of the prenatal assessment to corroborate pregnancy dating but are not accurate enough to be used to estimate gestational age except in the very lowest-resource settings (White et al., 2012).

The measurements are also known as symphysis-fundus measurements because the distance between the uppermost borders of the symphysis pubis and the uterine fundus is measured. The measurements should be obtained as follows.

Fundal height measurement

Ask the woman when she last urinated. If it has been more than 30 minutes, ask the woman to empty her bladder.

Place the woman in a supine position with her legs extended and the head of the exam table flat.

Lower the woman's clothing so that the pubic area is exposed. Use a drape or sheet to discreetly cover the area.

Place the tape measure in the midline of the maternal abdomen with the numeric centimeter markings on the tape measure facing the maternal abdomen.

Identify the uppermost border of the symphysis pubis and place the zero mark of the tape measure on that point.

Identify the uppermost border of the uterine fundus and bring the tape measure to that point.

The tape measure should be in contact with the skin of the maternal abdomen throughout the length of the measurement.

Mark the point on the tape measure by tearing, folding, or holding the tape measure at that point.

The measurement procedure is depicted in Figure 7.6 and Figure 7.7. It is important that the measurements be made using the same measurement technique because different measurement techniques have been described in the literature and yield significantly different results (Engstrom, 1985a; Engstrom & Sittler, 1993). Provider bias in obtaining fundal height measurements is also an important problem. When health-care providers can see the numeric centimeter markings on the tape measure, they are likely to record the number as being closer to the number of gestational weeks (Engstrom, Sittler, &

Swift, 1994; Jelks, Cifuentes, & Ross, 2007). Thus, the measurements should be obtained with the numeric centimeter markings facing away from the examiner, toward the maternal abdomen.

Despite the simplicity of the measurement procedures, research indicates that health-care providers have difficulty identifying the uterine fundus accurately (Engstrom, McFarlin, & Sampson, 1993). There can be significant differences in measurements obtained by different health-care providers (Crosby & Engstrom, 1989; Engstrom, McFarlin, & Sittler, 1993). All health-care providers within a single setting should use the same technique to measure fundal height to limit variation.

Maternal bladder fullness is known to increase the fundal height measurement, so women should be asked when they last urinated and if the amount of time is more than 30 minutes, the woman should be asked to

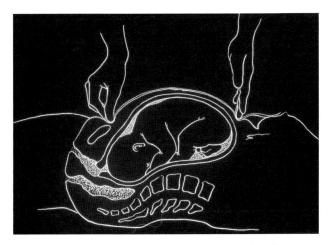

Figure 7.6. Landmarks used to measure fundal height. From Engstrom, J. L., & Sittler, C. P. (1993). Fundal height measurement. Part 1—Techniques for measuring fundal height. *Journal of Nurse-Midwifery, 38,* 5–16.

empty her bladder before the measurement is obtained (Engstrom, Ostrenga, Plass, & Work, 1989; Worthen & Bustillo, 1980). Maternal position during fundal height measurement significantly influences the measurements, so it is important to consistently use the same position for all measurements (Engstrom, Pisceroni, Low, McShane, & McFarlin, 1993). The measurements are closest to the actual number of gestational weeks when the woman is in the supine position with her legs extended (Engstrom et al., 1993). However, the supine position should be avoided for any length of time during pregnancy, so women should only be placed in this position for the time that the measurement requires, and then the head of the exam table should be elevated and the woman's legs bent at the knees.

Fundal height measurements can be plotted on a fundal height growth curve to graphically depict uterine growth during pregnancy. However, there is no standardized growth curve for the United States. Additionally, the limits of normal vary widely on the published curves, so the fundal height growth curves should be used with caution and tested in the clinical setting before adopting their routine use (Engstrom & Work, 1992; Wise & Engstrom, 1985).

Ultrasound

Ultrasound is widely used to estimate gestational age and the technology can provide a very accurate assessment of the gestational age between 6 and 20 weeks of gestation (American College of Obstetricians and Gynecologists (ACOG), 2009; Callen, 2008). The earliest structure visible is the gestational sac. The sac can be identified as early as 4 weeks of gestation (Richards, 2012). Although measurements of the gestational sac can be used to estimate gestational age, the estimates are not as accurate as when other fetal parameters are measured, so gestational

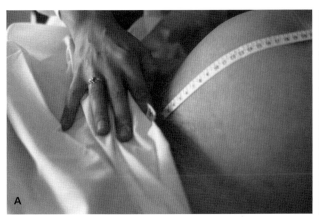
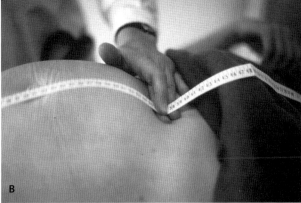

Figure 7.7. Measurement of fundal height. (A) Placement of the zero mark of the tape measure on the uppermost border of the symphysis pubis. (B) Placement of the tape measure at the uppermost border of the uterine fundus in the midline of the maternal abdomen. Photo courtesy of Ginger Michels, MSN, CNM.

sac measurements should not be used as the only method of estimating gestational age (Richards, 2012). Measurements of the embryo and fetus such as crown–rump length, biparietal diameter, head circumference, femur length, and abdominal circumference are the most accurate predictors of gestational age when the measurements are obtained during the first half of pregnancy (ACOG, 2009).

During the first trimester of pregnancy, the crown–rump length of the embryo provides a very accurate estimate of the gestational age. The crown–rump length can be used to accurately estimate gestational age within 5–7 days from 6–12 weeks of gestation. By 13 weeks of gestation, the crown–rump length becomes less accurate, so other fetal parameters such as the fetal biparietal diameter and femur length are used (Richards, 2012). Gestational age assessments made using these parameters can accurately estimate gestational age within 7–10 days from 14 to 20 weeks of gestation (ACOG, 2009; Callen, 2008).

In the second half of pregnancy, the amount of error in the sonographic estimation of gestational age increases rapidly because fetal growth becomes more variable. The error in gestational age assessment increases to about 2–3 weeks from 21 to 30 weeks of gestation. After 30 weeks, the error in gestational age estimates is large, with errors as large as 3–4 weeks. Thus, the timing of ultrasound examinations for gestational aging is extremely important, and when verification of gestational age is needed, it should be requested in the first half of pregnancy.

Accuracy of ultrasound assessment of gestational age

Weeks of gestation	Structures measured for gestational age assessment	Accuracy of gestational age assessments
6–12 weeks	Crown–rump length	±5–7 days
14–20 weeks	Biparietal diameter Head circumference Femur length Abdominal circumference	±7–10 days
21–30 weeks	Biparietal diameter Head circumference Femur length Abdominal circumference	±2–3 weeks
>30 weeks	Biparietal diameter Head circumference Femur length Abdominal circumference	±3–4 weeks

Sources: ACOG (2009), Callen (2008), Richards (2012).

Counseling for pregnancy diagnosis

All counseling about the results of a pregnancy test should be conducted in a neutral manner, with no indication that a positive or negative test is the desired result. For example, statements such as "Congratulations, your test is positive" or "Good news, your test is negative" should never be used when reporting pregnancy results. Rather, the results should simply be delivered in an accurate, clear, and simple manner, and statements should be devoid of any value regarding a "good" or "bad" result. Similarly, all discussions about the women's reproductive options are conducted in a nondirective and noncoercive fashion. Equally important is the confidential nature of any discussion related to pregnancy testing. However, there are some exceptions to confidentiality, such as reporting suspected neglect and abuse if the woman is under the age of consent, and parental notification laws for abortion services in some states, so health-care providers must know state reporting regulations and advise women of any exceptions to confidentiality.

Urine pregnancy test results are reported as positive or negative, with positive indicating the presence of a pregnancy and negative indicating that the woman is not pregnant or the pregnancy is too early to be detected. Although the language of positive and negative test results is very clear to health-care professionals, the meaning of positive and negative tests is not clear to many patients. Additionally, a woman may be so anxious about the test results that she may not completely understand the terminology. When reporting the pregnancy test results to the woman, the ideal language should clarify the meaning of a positive and a negative test. For example, a health-care provider might say, "Your pregnancy test is positive; that means that you are pregnant," or "Your test is negative; that means that you are not pregnant or that the pregnancy is so early that the test may not yet detect the pregnancy."

Many women who visit a health-care facility for pregnancy testing have already performed a home pregnancy test and have an idea of whether they are pregnant or not. These women often seek health care because they are looking for confirmation of the result or are hoping the home test result is incorrect. Research indicates that most women make a decision about their pregnancy within 1 day of receiving pregnancy test results, suggesting that most women already suspect they are pregnant and have some sense of how they feel about the pregnancy prior to taking a test (Finer, Frohwirth, Dauphinee, Singh, & Moore, 2006).

Pregnancy test results should be delivered promptly to the woman; the woman should not be required to sit through counseling or education sessions before receiving the results. After stating the test results, it is beneficial to allow the woman a moment to process the information and to collect her thoughts. Although health-care providers are often tempted to "manage" the situation by providing information and referrals, it is usually helpful to engage in active listening by giving the woman time to reflect on how she feels about the result of the pregnancy test. Nonverbal clues may provide a sense of how the woman feels about the result. If the woman's feelings are not evident, health-care providers can elicit the woman's feelings by asking, "How are you feeling about this?" or "Is this what you were expecting?" or "You seem upset/sad/shocked/happy." Additional areas to explore include the woman's support system and how she expects them to respond to the news of the pregnancy. Neutral comments such as "Tell me more about what is concerning you" or "Many women have mixed feelings about a pregnancy" can often open the conversation and elicit her concerns.

Counseling after a negative pregnancy test

If a pregnancy test is negative and the woman is disappointed, further assessment is warranted. If she desires a pregnancy, this is an ideal time to discuss preconception care. If there is a concern of infertility, the woman's feelings of disappointment should be recognized and a detailed gynecological, reproductive, and health history should be obtained. Counseling to optimize the probability of conceiving should be provided and referrals to fertility specialists should be provided as needed.

If a woman is relieved by a negative test result, this is a "teachable moment" for contraceptive counseling. Following a negative test, women are often highly motivated to use a highly effective method of birth control and to learn about emergency contraception. Both prescription and nonprescription emergency contraceptive products are available. Women should be advised that these products are kept "behind the counter" even though they are available without a prescription.

A negative pregnancy test also provides an opportunity for women to develop a reproductive life plan, as recommended by the Centers for Disease Control and Prevention (CDC), and to educate women as to how their reproductive life plan impacts contraceptive and health-care decision making. Preconception health and reproductive life planning tools for health-care providers can be found on the CDC website (Centers for Disease Control and Prevention (CDC), 2012). Research indicates that women use contraception because it allows them to better care for themselves and their families, to complete their education, or to achieve financial security (Frost & Duberstein, 2012).

Unintended pregnancies are associated with poorer health outcomes both for the mother and the infant, as well as negative social, educational, and economic consequences. The burden of unintended pregnancy is higher in poor women, women with lower educational levels, and women of color (Finer & Henshaw, 2006). Helping women to prevent unintended pregnancies can help women to achieve both their reproductive and life goals (Taylor & James, 2011).

Counseling after a positive pregnancy test

If the woman is pleased with the positive pregnancy results, she should be congratulated and given a referral for early pregnancy care. Essential information that should be provided at the time of pregnancy diagnosis includes the importance of avoiding alcohol, illicit drugs, unnecessary medications, and potential teratogens. Also important is information about the signs and symptoms of early pregnancy complications such as ectopic pregnancy and miscarriage. All women should be advised to immediately start taking a folic acid supplement of 0.4 mg/day (400 µg/day) if she is not already taking a supplement. Referrals for prenatal care should be provided. If the woman's financial resources are limited, the woman should be given information about state Medicaid programs for prenatal care as well as the Women, Infants, and Children (WIC) nutrition program.

Options counseling for unintended pregnancy

Given that 49% of all pregnancies in the United States are unintended (defined as either mistimed or unwanted) and that no significant progress has been made in meeting the Healthy People national public health goal of reducing unintended pregnancy, many women will experience an unintended pregnancy (U.S. Department of Health and Human Services (USDHHS), 2010). Thus, health-care providers should expect to encounter women with unintended pregnancies in a wide variety of clinical settings and be prepared to provide sensitive and nonjudgmental-option counseling.

A woman with a newly diagnosed pregnancy may need support in deciding whether to continue or terminate the pregnancy. If she decides to terminate an early pregnancy, she has the option of medication or surgical aspiration abortion. If continuing the pregnancy, she will have to decide whether she will parent the child or make a plan for an adoption.

The issue of providing comprehensive reproductive health care for a woman with an unintended pregnancy raises personal and professional ethical conflicts for many health-care providers. To effectively facilitate the decision making process for women facing unintended pregnancy, it is helpful for health-care providers to examine their personal beliefs and biases that may interfere with providing woman-centered care. Values clarification enables health-care providers to resolve these conflicts in a way that ensures patient safety and preserves the professional integrity of the provider (Simmonds & Likis, 2005). Resources for values clarification are provided at the end of this chapter.

Additionally, professional midwifery and nursing organizations have articulated ethical guidelines that provide the framework for the professional role of the advanced practice nurse and midwife (as shown in the box below). Finally, health-care providers should remember that they are not personally responsible for ethical consequences of the decisions made by their patients who are exercising their own right to autonomy in decision making (Beal & Cappiello, 2008; Cappiello, Beal, & Hudson-Gallogly, 2011).

Health-care providers can assist women experiencing ambivalence about pregnancy by helping women to identify life circumstances that affect the decision to parent a child at this point in their lives. The decision to continue or terminate a pregnancy is motivated by several interrelated social factors. Women who feel that they cannot continue a pregnancy often report resource limitations such as financial constraints, lack of partner support, and responsibility to others (Finer, Frohwirth, Dauphiness, Singh, & Moore, 2005). A substantial number of women report that having a child would interfere with their ability to care for their existing children, continue their educational plans, or meet their work commitments. Other common reasons that women decide that they cannot continue a pregnancy include not wanting to be single mother, that they are not ready emotionally to have a child, or that they had already completed their childbearing (Finer et al., 2005). Thus, these factors should be explored in the discussion of pregnancy options. Ask the woman to identify her support systems. Many women want to involve a partner, a friend, or a family member in their decision. If a partner or support person is in the waiting room, ask the woman if she wants the person involved in this discussion.

It is important to discuss a timetable for decision making about the pregnancy. Thus, assessment of the gestational age of the pregnancy is essential to determine whether the woman is close to the legal time limit for pregnancy termination. Fortunately, the majority of pregnancies are diagnosed in the first trimester when women can take the time needed to make a decision that is suited to their personal situation.

Professional ethics and standards for reproductive options counseling

The American College of Nurse-Midwives' (ACNM) Code of Ethics emphasizes conflict resolution, respect for human and reproductive rights, and midwives' respect for their own dignity. Midwives follow guidelines in Standard VIII of the Standards for the Practice of Midwifery to incorporate new procedures into their practice, including abortion (ACNM, 2008, 2009).

The American Nurses' Association Code of Ethics for Nurses states that nurses are justified in not participating in some treatments if patient safety is not compromised. The patient may not be abandoned by the nurse until an alternative source of nursing care is available to the patient. Nurses have the obligation to communicate the limitations of their participation in advance so that other arrangements can be made for patient care (American Nurses Association, 2001, 2010).

The Nurse Practitioners in Women's Health (NPWH) mandate that the nurse practitioner promote patient autonomy, dignity, self-determination, and respect patients' reproductive choices, establish a partnership with the patient that facilitates decision making and self-care, and support the patient's right to make her own decisions regarding her health and reproductive choices within the context of her belief system (National Association of Nurse Practitioners in Women's Health (NPWH) and Association of Women's Health, Obstetric and Neonatal Nurses, 2008).

The Association of Women's Health, Obstetric and Neonatal Nurses (AWHONN) promulgates care that is provided in a nonjudgmental and nondiscriminatory manner and that is sensitive to patient diversity and patient preferences whenever possible (Association of Women's Health, Obstetric and Neonatal Nurses (AWHONN), 2009).

The National Organization of Nurse Practitioner Faculties (NONPF) articulates the obligation for educators of nurse practitioners to prevent personal biases from interfering with the delivery of quality care to persons of differing beliefs and lifestyles (National Organization of Nurse Practitioner Faculties (NONPF), 2012, 2013).

The health-care provider must assess if the woman has accurate and adequate information to make an informed decision, and whether she is capable of understanding the information and of making a decision. The possibility that the woman's decision is being coerced or manipulated by someone else must also be explored.

Health-care providers should provide any additional information and service required and, if needed, arrange for counseling appointments. Health-care providers must know what local referral resources are available so that they can provide referrals for care in a seamless manner. It is important to have printed information for counseling services, adoption agencies, abortion services, and prenatal-care providers. Many women need support beyond simply providing the name and contact information of local agencies. Care coordination may take the form of assessing the need for transportation, financial aid, childcare, and other needs (Simmonds & Likis, 2011).

When referring women for counseling and services, it is important to be aware that some clinics have a history of unethical practices in pregnancy counseling. For example, clinics known as "crisis pregnancy centers" are nonprofit organizations established to provide supportive services to pregnant or parenting women. The centers offer free pregnancy testing and ultrasound screening but do not provide a full range of reproductive options. Typically, these centers do not support a woman's autonomy to explore other options beyond parenting or adoption and have been known to provide false and misleading health information to women (United States House of Representatives Committee on Government Reform, 2006).

Generally, health-care issues are considered confidential, but some states require parental notification or parental consent for a teenager to make a decision about a pregnancy. In the case of abortion, many states with parental notification or parental consent laws have judicial bypass arrangements for teenagers that are unable to involve their parents. Health-care providers must be aware of the state policies regarding these matters, and resources to find those regulations are provided at the end of the chapter.

When counseling a woman with an unintended pregnancy, the health-care provider must also determine whether the woman is at risk for intimate partner violence. Approximately one in five women are abused during pregnancy and 40% of pregnant women who have been exposed to abuse report that their pregnancy was unintended, compared to only 8% of nonabused women (Hathaway et al., 2000). Women experiencing abuse in the year prior to and/or during a recent pregnancy are 40–60% more likely than nonabused women to experience complications such as high blood pressure, vaginal bleeding, severe nausea, urinary tract infections, and hospitalization during pregnancy, and are 37% more likely to deliver preterm (Silverman, Decker, Reed, & Raj, 2006).

Suggested steps in pregnancy option counseling

1. Explore how the woman is feeling about the positive test result.
2. Assess for any immediate health concerns.
3. Provide nonjudgmental, nondirective counseling using specific counseling techniques.
4. Address issues of ambivalence.
5. Explore current life circumstances.
6. Help her to identify support systems.
7. Assure that the informed-consent process includes accurate, evidenced-based information about the options of parenting, adoption, and abortion.
8. Assess that she is capable of understanding the information and that her decision making is not coerced.
9. If she is not ready to make a decision, discuss a timetable for decision making after estimating gestational age by LMP/clinical exam and/or ultrasound.
10. Support the woman in her decision making.
11. Provide resources, referrals, and care coordination to quality providers.

Providing evidence-based information about pregnancy options

To provide accurate information and support to women newly diagnosed as pregnant, the health-care provider must be knowledgeable about all reproductive options. The options legally available to all women in the United States include continuation of the pregnancy, termination of the pregnancy, and adoption. Pregnancy care is described throughout the remainder of this textbook. However, many health-care providers have limited knowledge of pregnancy termination procedures and adoption services.

Adoption counseling

Adoption information should be presented in as much detail as possible, including the options of open, closed, familial, and state adoption as well as foster care. Appropriate language to use in discussions about adoption is summarized in the following textbox. Most adoption agencies provide some degree of openness in the adoption process. Openness in adoption can range from simply sharing information between the birth mother and the adoptive family prior to placement to arrangements in which birth mothers choose the adoptive family and maintain ongoing contact once the child is born. It is important that birth mothers work with agencies that support them in creating adoption plans and agreements that are noncoercive, and fully explain her rights and the range of options available to her. Some women are interested in familial adoptions, in which a member of their family assumes the legal rights of the child. It is important to refer women to agencies that can help them navigate the legal and emotional nuances of this process.

Positive language for discussing adoption

Preferred language	Negative language that should *not* be used
Planning an adoption for your child	Giving your child away
Choosing an adoptive family for your child	Putting your child up for adoption
Birth mother, birth father, birth parent	Real or natural parents
Deciding to parent the child	Keeping the child

Adapted from http://www.openadopt.org.

Pregnancy termination counseling

Options for early pregnancy termination include medication and aspiration abortion. Medication abortion has been available since 2000 in the United States. The most commonly used regimen for medication abortion in the United States is mifepristone, followed by misoprostol. Misoprostol is a synthetic prostaglandin that causes uterine contractions and is currently Food and Drug Administration (FDA) approved for use up to 9 weeks of gestation. Oral mifepristone is administered in the office, followed by self-administration of buccal or vaginal misoprostol in the next 24–48 hours at home. The vaginal or buccal routes of administration are typically used as the efficacy rate of misoprostol is slightly reduced with the oral route. The miscarriage-like bleeding event lasts 4–6 hours, followed by 1–3 weeks of spotting. Efficacy rates vary from 93% to 98%. If unsuccessful, a vacuum aspiration is performed. Many women value the privacy that medication abortion provides and perceive it as a less invasive, more "miscarriage-like" event.

Medication abortions have an excellent safety profile, with serious complications occurring in less than 0.5% of cases (Grimes, 2005). Several cases of *Clostridium sordellii* infection, the cause of fatal toxic shock, has been reported in medication abortion as well as miscarriage, childbirth, aspiration, and other non-pregnancy-related events (CDC, 2005). The CDC continues an ongoing monitoring program of all *C. sordellii* infections, and the Food and Drug Administration (2011) has issued an advisory to health-care providers regarding the warning signs of severe toxic shock.

Vacuum aspiration procedures have a high success rate at 99% and are usually completed within minutes. The procedures can be performed up to 14–15 weeks of gestation and allow for sedation if desired. Infection is extremely rare, occurring in less than 1% of procedures (Caitlin, Brothers, Neena, & Beverly, 2004). Another risk is uterine perforation, but this is extremely rare. Vacuum aspiration procedures usually require only one visit, and for women who must travel long distances to find an abortion provider, access issues may be a determining factor in their decision making.

Abortions performed later in pregnancy may use a dilation and evacuation (D & E) procedure. Complication rates are somewhat higher for procedures provided between 13 and 24 weeks than for the first-trimester procedures. General anesthesia, which is sometimes used in abortion procedures at any gestation, carries its own risks. Less than 2% of all abortions are provided after 20 weeks of gestation. The most common indications for later procedures are severe fetal abnormalities or severe medical complications of the mother. Induction or instillation techniques are rarely used (<1% of all abortions).

It is important for health-care providers to be familiar with the current evidence related to abortion care. Many women have misunderstandings about the safety of abortion and its impact on their long-term health. For example, information in the popular media has inaccurately linked abortion to breast cancer and mental health problems. However, research has failed to substantiate a relationship between abortion and breast cancer (Brind, 2007; Tanne, 2007) or depression and mental illness (Adler et al., 1990, 1992; Charles, Polis, Sridhara, & Blum, 2008; Stotland, 1992, 2002, 2007). Similarly, the popular media has carried inaccurate statements about the fetus's ability to experience pain during abortions under 20 weeks' gestation (Lee, Ralston, Drey, Partridge, & Rosen, 2005).

Some health-care providers will perform medication abortion and aspiration abortion procedures as a component of their practice. Abortion care is regulated outside of the usual regulatory process for advanced practice nursing and midwifery. Nurse practitioners and midwives who are interested in expanding their practice to include medication or aspiration procedures must know their state-based scope of practice regulations specific to the provision of abortion services (Taylor, Safriet, Dempsey, Kruse, & Jackson, 2009). Additionally, midwives and nurse practitioners must follow the guidelines of their professional organization on how to add an advanced skill such as medication and aspiration abortion services to their practice.

Summary

Pregnancy diagnosis and gestational aging are essential components of prenatal care. Early and accurate pregnancy diagnosis facilitates subsequent health-care services as well as a woman's personal health behaviors. Pregnancy diagnosis should be accompanied by unbiased, nondirective, and noncoercive counseling about pregnancy options. Early pregnancy diagnosis also provides the opportunity to accurately assess the gestational age, information that is essential to all aspects of prenatal care. Although endocrine pregnancy tests and ultrasonography play increasingly important roles in pregnancy diagnosis and gestational aging, clinical methods of assessing the signs of pregnancy and gestational age remain an important part of prenatal care and can augment the assessments made by biochemical and biophysical methods.

Case study

Anne is a 20-year-old college student who is seen in the office today to discuss contraception.

SUBJECTIVE: Anne reports that she has been using condoms for birth control, but she wants to discuss another method in addition to condoms, adding that she hopes that she is not already pregnant.

OBJECTIVE: The urine pregnancy test is positive. Anne is visibly upset by this news.

ASSESSMENT: Anne is pregnant with an unintended pregnancy.

PLAN: Discuss the pregnancy test results in a neutral manner, "The urine pregnancy test result is positive and that means that you are pregnant." Engage in active listening as Anne responds in disbelief and experiences difficulty in thinking through the ramifications of a pregnancy. Ask her if there is anyone with whom she wishes to discuss this matter. Anne shares that she feels unable to parent a child at this time and wants to talk with her partner. Offer information, counseling, and referrals regarding the options of adoption, terminating the pregnancy, or continuing the pregnancy. The gestational age of the pregnancy is assessed to be 6 weeks; reassure Anne that she has some time to make a decision. Schedule a return visit in 1 week to discuss Anne's decision and make further arrangements for care.

Resources for women and their families

Adoption information: http://www.openadopt.org

Pregnancy Options Workbook: http://www.pregnancy options.info/pregnant.htm

Reproductive Life Plan by the Centers for Disease Control and Prevention: http://www.cdc.gov/preconception/ reproductiveplan.html

Values clarification workshop outline by the Reproductive Health Access Project: http://www.reproductive access.org/integrating_reprohealth/values_clar.htm

Resources for health-care providers

Abortion care toolkit for nurse-midwives, nurse practitioners, and physician assistants: http://www.apc toolkit.org

Adoption information: http://www.openadopt.org

Guttmacher Institute: State policies regarding access and funding for contraceptive and abortion services: http://www.guttmacher.org/statecenter/adolescents .html; http://www.guttmacher.org/statecenter/spibs/ spib_SFAM.pdf; http://www.guttmacher.org/state center/spibs/spib_RICA.pdf; http://www.guttmacher .org/statecenter/spibs/spib_MWPA.pdf

Values clarification: Exploring attitudes toward abortion by the Association of Reproductive Health Professionals: http://core.arhp.org/search/searchDetail.aspx ?itemId=1286

Values clarification guide for health-care professionals: The abortion option by the National Abortion Federation: http://www.prochoice.org/pubs_research/publi cations/downloads/professional_education/abortion _option.pdf

References

Adler, N., David, H., Major, B., Roth, S., Russo, N., & Wyatt, G. (1990). Psychological responses after abortion. *Science*, *248*(6), 41–44.

Adler, N., David, H., Major, B., Roth, S., Russo, N., & Wyatt, G. (1992). Psychological factors in abortion: A review. *The American Psychologist*, *47*(10), 1194–1203.

American College of Nurse-Midwives (ACNM). (2008). *Code of ethics.* Retrieved from http://www.midwife.org/ACNM/files/ccLibrary Files/Filename/000000002732/ACNM%20Code%20of%20 Ethics%2010%202008.pdf

American College of Nurse-Midwives. (2009). *Standards for the practice of midwifery.* Retrieved from http://www.midwife.org/ACNM/ files/ccLibraryFiles/Filename/000000000270/Standards_for_ Practice_of_Midwifery_12_09_001.pdf

American College of Obstetricians and Gynecologists (2009). Ultrasonography in pregnancy. *Obstetrics and Gynecology*, *113*, 451–461.

American Nurses Association. (2001). *Code of ethics for nurses with interpretive statements.* Silver Spring, MD: NursingWorld. Retrieved from http://www.nursingworld.org/MainMenuCategories/Ethics Standards/CodeofEthicsforNurses/Code-of-Ethics.aspx

American Nurses Association. (2010). *Nursing's social policy statement: The essence of the profession* (3rd ed.). Silver Spring, MD: Nursebooks.

Andersen, H. F., Johnson, T. R., Barclay, M. L., & Flora, J. D. (1981). Gestational age assessment. I. Analysis of individual clinical observations. *American Journal of Obstetrics and Gynecology, 139*, 173–177.

Association of Women's Health, Obstetric and Neonatal Nurses (AWHONN). (2009). *Standards for professional nursing practice in the care of women and newborns* (7th ed.). Washington, DC: AWHONN.

Baskett, T. F., & Nagele, F. (2000). Naegele's rule: A reappraisal. *British Journal of Obstetrics and Gynaecology, 107*, 1433–1435.

Beal, M. W., & Cappiello, J. D. (2008). Professional right of conscience. *Journal of Midwifery & Women's Health, 53*, 406–412.

Beazley, J. M., & Underhill, R. A. (1970). Fallacy of the fundal height. *British Medical Journal, 4*, 404–406.

Bergsjo, P., Denman, D. W., Hoffman, H. J., & Meirik, O. (1990). Duration of human singleton pregnancy: A population-based study. *Acta Obstetrica et Gynecologica Scandinavica, 69*, 197–207.

Brind, J. (2007, Summer). Induced abortion and breast cancer risk: A critical analysis of the report of the Harvard nurses study II. *Journal American Physicians and Surgeons, 12*, 38–39.

Caitlin, S., Brothers, L. P., Neena, M. P., & Beverly, W. (2004). Infection after medical abortion: A review of the literature. *Contraception, 70*(3), 183–190.

Callen, P. W. (2008). Measurements frequently used to estimate gestational age and fetal biometry. In *Ultrasonography in obstetrics and gynecology* (5th ed., pp. 1159–1160). Philadelphia: Saunders.

Cappiello, J., Beal, M., & Hudson-Gallogly, K. (2011). Applying ethical practice competencies in the prevention and management of unintended pregnancy. *Journal of Obstetric, Gynecologic, and Neonatal Nursing, 40*(6), 808–816.

Centers for Disease Control and Prevention (2005). *Clostridium sordellii* toxic shock syndrome after medical abortion with mifepristone and intravaginal misoprostol—United States and Canada, 2001–2005. *MMWR. Morbidity and Mortality Weekly Report, 54*, 724.

Centers for Disease Control and Prevention (CDC) (2012). Reproductive life plan tools for health professionals. Retrieved from http://www.cdc.gov/preconception/RLPtool.html

Cervinski, M. A., Lockwood, C. M., Ferguson, A. M., Odem, R. R., Stenman, U. H., Alfthan, H., . . . Gronowski, A. M. (2009). Qualitative point-of-care and over-the-counter urine hCG devices differentially detect the hCG variants of early pregnancy. *Clinica Chimica Acta, 406*, 81–85.

Charles, V., Polis, C., Sridhara, S., & Blum, R. (2008). Abortion and long-term mental health outcomes: A systematic review of the evidence. *Contraception, 78*(6), 436–450.

Cole, L. A. (2012). The hCG assay or pregnancy test. *Clinical Chemistry and Laboratory Medicine, 50*, 617–630.

Crosby, M. E., & Engstrom, J. L. (1989). Inter-examiner reliability in fundal height measurement. *Midwives Chronicle & Nursing Notes, 102*(1219), 254–256.

Cunningham, F. G., Leveno, K. J., Bloom, S. L., Hauth, J. C., Rouse, D. J., & Spong, C. Y. (2010). Prenatal care. In *William's obstetrics* (23rd ed.). New York: McGraw Hill.

Engstrom, J. L. (1985a). *Fundal height and abdominal girth measurements during pregnancy* (Doctoral dissertation). University of Illinois at Chicago, Chicago, IL.

Engstrom, J. L. (1985b). Quickening and auscultation of fetal heart tones as estimators of the gestational interval: A review. *Journal of Nurse-Midwifery, 30*, 25–32.

Engstrom, J. L. (1988). Measurement of fundal height. *Journal of Obstetric, Gynecologic, and Neonatal Nursing, 17*, 172–178.

Engstrom, J. L., McFarlin, B. L., & Sampson, M. B. (1993). Fundal height measurement. Part 4—Accuracy of clinicians' identification of the uterine fundus during pregnancy. *Journal of Nurse-Midwifery, 38*, 318–323.

Engstrom, J. L., McFarlin, B. L., & Sittler, C. P. (1993). Fundal height measurement. Part 2—Intra- and interexaminer reliability of three measurement techniques. *Journal of Nurse-Midwifery, 38*, 17–22.

Engstrom, J. L., Ostrenga, K. G., Plass, R. V., & Work, B. A. (1989). The effect of maternal bladder volume on fundal height measurements. *British Journal of Obstetrics and Gynaecology, 96*, 987–991.

Engstrom, J. L., Piscioneri, L. A., Low, L. K., McShane, H., & McFarlin, B. (1993). Fundal height measurement. Part 3—The effect of maternal position on fundal height measurements. *Journal of Nurse-Midwifery, 38*, 23–27.

Engstrom, J. L., & Sittler, C. P. (1993). Fundal height measurement. Part 1—Techniques for measuring fundal height. *Journal of Nurse-Midwifery, 38*, 5–16.

Engstrom, J. L., Sittler, C. P., & Swift, K. E. (1994). Fundal height measurement. Part 5—The effect of clinician bias on fundal height measurements. *Journal of Nurse-Midwifery, 39*, 130–141.

Engstrom, J. L., & Work, B. A. (1992). Prenatal prediction of small- and large-for-gestational age neonates using fundal height growth curves. *JOGN Nursing, 21*, 486–495.

Finer, L. B., & Henshaw, S. (2006). Disparities in unintended pregnancy in the United States, 1994 and 2001. *Perspectives on Sexual and Reproductive Health, 38*(2), 90–96.

Finer, L. B., Frohwirth, L. F., Dauphiness, L. A., Singh, S., & Moore, A. M. (2005). Reasons U.S. women have abortions: Quantitative and qualitative perspectives. *Perspectives on Sexual and Reproductive Health, 37*(3), 110–118.

Finer, L. B., Frohwirth, L. F., Dauphinee, L. A., Singh, S., & Moore, A. M. (2006). Timing of steps and reasons for delays in obtaining abortions in the United States. *Contraception, 74*, 334–344.

Food and Drug Administration (FDA). (2011). Postmarket drug safety information for patients and providers. Mifeprex (mifepristone) information. Retrieved from http://www.fda.gov/Drugs/DrugSafety/PostmarketDrugSafetyInformationforPatientsandProviders/ucm111323.htm

Fox, G. N. (1985). Teaching first trimester uterine sizing. *Journal of Family Practice, 21*, 400–401.

Frost, J. J., & Duberstein, L. D. (2012). Reasons for using contraception: Perspectives of US women seeking care at specialized family planning clinics. *Contraception, 87*, 465–472. doi:10.1016/j.contraception.2012.08.012

Gardosi, J. (1997). Dating of pregnancy: Time to forget the last menstrual period. *Ultrasound in Obstetrics and Gynecology, 9*, 367–368.

Gillieson, M., Dunlap, H., Nair, R., & Pilon, M. (1984). Placental site, parity, and date of quickening. *Obstetrics and Gynecology, 64*, 44–45.

Greene, D. N., Schmidt, R. L., Kamer, S. M., Grenache, D. G., Hoke, C., & Lorey, T. S. (2013). Limitations in qualitative point of care hCG tests for detecting early pregnancy. *Clinica Chimica Acta, 415*, 317–321.

Grimes, D. A. (2005). Risk of mifepristone abortion in context. *Contraception, 71*, 161.

Grossman, D., Berdichevsky, K., Larrea, F., & Beltran, J. (2007). Accuracy of a semi-quantitative urine pregnancy test compared to serum beta-hCG measurement: A possible screening tool for ongoing pregnancy after medication abortion. *Contraception, 76*, 101–104.

Hathaway, J. E., Mucci, L. A., Silverman, J. G., Brooks, D. R., Mathews, R., & Pavlos, C. A. (2000). Health status and health care use of Massachusetts women reporting partner abuse. *American Journal of Preventive Medicine, 19*(4), 318–321.

Herbert, W. N. P., Bruninghaus, H. M., Barefoot, A. B., & Bright, T. G. (1987). Clinical aspects of fetal heart auscultation. *Obstetrics and Gynecology, 69,* 574–577.

Hertz, R. H., Sokol, R. J., Knoke, J. D., Rosen, M. G., Chik, L., & Hirsch, V. J. (1978). Clinical estimation of gestational age: Rules for avoiding preterm delivery. *American Journal of Obstetrics and Gynecology, 131,* 395–402.

Hoffman, C. S., Messer, L. C., Mendola, P., Savitz, D. A., Herring, A. H., & Hartmann, K. E. (2008). Comparison of gestational age at birth based on last menstrual period and ultrasound during the first trimester. *Paediatric and Perinatal Epidemiology, 22,* 587–596.

Hunter, L. A. (2009). Issues in pregnancy dating: Revisiting the evidence. *Journal of Midwifery & Women's Health, 54,* 1184–1190.

Jelks, A., Cifuentes, R., & Ross, M. G. (2007). Clinician bias in fundal height measurement. *Obstetrics and Gynecology, 110,* 892–889.

Jimenez, J. M., Tyson, J. E., & Reisch, J. S. (1983). Clinical measures of gestational age in normal pregnancies. *Obstetrics and Gynecology, 61,* 438–443.

Kraus, G. W., & Hendricks, C. H. (1964). Significance of the quickening date in determining duration of pregnancy. *Obstetrics and Gynecology, 24,* 178–182.

Lee, S., Ralston, H., Drey, E., Partridge, J., & Rosen, M. (2005). Fetal pain: A systematic multidisciplinary review of the evidence. *Journal of the American Medical Association, 294,* 947–954.

Lynch, C. D., & Zhang, J. (2007). The research implications of the selection of a gestational age estimation method. *Paediatric and Perinatal Epidemiology, 21*(Suppl. 2), 86–96.

Margulies, R., & Miller, L. (2001). Fruit size as a model for teaching first trimester uterine sizing in bimanual examination. *Obstetrics and Gynecology, 98,* 341–344.

McDonald, E. (1908). The diagnosis of early pregnancy. *American Journal of Obstetrics and Diseases of Women and Children, 57,* 323–346.

McFarlin, B. L., Engstrom, J. L., Sampson, M. B., & Cattledge, F. (1985). The concurrent validity of Leopold's maneuvers in determining fetal presentation and position. *Journal of Nurse-Midwifery, 30,* 280–284.

McParland, P., & Johnson, H. (1993). Time to reinvent the wheel. *British Journal of Obstetrics and Gynaecology, 100,* 1061–1062.

Morse, K., Williams, A., & Gardosi, J. (2009). Fetal growth screening by fundal height measurement. *Best Practice & Research Clinical Obstetrics and Gynaecology, 23,* 809–818.

Munsick, R. A. (1985). Dickinson's sign: Focal uterine softening in early pregnancy and its correlation with the placental site. *American Journal of Obstetrics and Gynecology, 152,* 799–802.

Munsick, R. A. (1986). Correct use of Hegar's sign [letter]. *American Journal of Obstetrics and Gynecology, 154,* 691–692.

Nakling, J., Buhaug, H., & Backe, B. (2005). The biologic error in gestational length related to the use of the first day of the last menstrual period as a proxy for the start of pregnancy. *Early Human Development, 81,* 833–839.

National Association of Nurse Practitioners in Women's Health (NPWH) and Association of Women's Health, Obstetric and Neonatal Nurses. (2008). *The women's health nurse practitioner: Guidelines for practice and education* (6th ed.) Washington, DC: AWHONN.

National Organization of Nurse Practitioner Faculties (NONPF). (2012). *Nurse practitioner core competencies.* Retrieved from http:// www.nonpf.com/associations/10789/files/NPCoreCompetencies Final2012.pdf

National Organization of Nurse Practitioner Faculties (NONPF). (2013). *Population-focused nurse practitioner competencies.* Retrieved from http://www.nonpf.org/associations/10789/files/Population FocusNPComps2013.pdf

Nguyen, T. H., Larsen, T., Engholm, G., & Moller, H. (1999). Evaluation of ultrasound-estimated date of delivery in 17,450 spontaneous singleton births: Do we need to modify Naegele's rule? *Ultrasound in Obstetrics and Gynecology, 14,* 23–28.

O'Dowd, M. J., & O'Dowd, T. M. (1985). Quickening—A re-evaluation. *British Journal of Obstetrics and Gynaecology, 92,* 1037–1039.

Rawlings, E. E., & Moore, B. A. (1970). The accuracy of methods of calculating the expected date of delivery for use in the diagnosis of postmaturity. *American Journal of Obstetrics and Gynecology, 106,* 676–679.

Richards, D. S. (2012). Obstetrical ultrasound: Imaging, dating, and growth. In S. G. Gabbe, J. R. Niebyl, H. L. Galan, E. R. M. Jauniaux, M. B. Landon, J. L. Simpson, & D. A. Driscoll (Eds.), *Obstetrics: Normal and problem pregnancies* (6th ed., pp. 166–192). Philadelphia: Elsevier.

Roex, A., Nikpoor, P., Eerd, E. V., Hodyl, N., & Dekker, G. (2012). Serial plotting on customized fundal height charts results in doubling of antenatal detection of small for gestational age fetuses in nulliparous women. *The Australian and New Zealand Journal of Obstetrics and Gynaecology, 52,* 78–82.

Ross, M. G. (2003). Circle of time: Errors in the use of the pregnancy wheel. *Journal of Maternal-Fetal & Neonatal Medicine, 14,* 370–372.

Savitz, D. A., Terry, J. W., Dole, N., Thorp, J. M., Siega-Riz, A. M., & Herring, A. H. (2002). Comparison of pregnancy dating by last menstrual period, ultrasound scanning, and their combination. *American Journal of Obstetrics and Gynecology, 187,* 1660–1666.

Sharma, J. B. (2009). Evaluation of Sharma's modified Leopold's maneuvers: A new method for fetal palpation in late pregnancy. *Archives of Gynecology and Obstetrics, 279,* 481–487.

Silverman, J. G., Decker, M. R., Reed, E., & Raj, A. (2006). Intimate partner violence victimization prior to and during pregnancy among women residing in 26 U.S. states: Associations with maternal and neonatal health. *American Journal of Obstetrics and Gynecology, 195*(1), 140–148.

Simmonds, K., & Likis, F. (2005). Providing options counseling for women with unintended pregnancies. *Journal of Obstetric, Gynecologic, and Neonatal Nursing, 34,* 373–379.

Simmonds, K., & Likis, F. (2011). Caring for women with unintended pregnancies. *Journal of Obstetric, Gynecologic, and Neonatal Nursing, 40,* 794–807.

Smout, E. M., Seed, P. T., & Shennan, A. H. (2012). The use and accuracy of manual and electronic gestational age calculators. *The Australian and New Zealand Journal of Obstetrics and Gynaecology, 52,* 440–444.

Spreet, H. (1955). Alfred Hegar: Hegar's sign and dilators. *Obstetrics and Gynecology, 6,* 679–683.

Stotland, N. (1992). The myth of the abortion trauma syndrome. *Journal of the American Medical Association, 268*(15), 2078–2079.

Stotland, N. (2002). Psychiatric issues related to infertility, reproductive technologies, and abortion. *Primary Care: Clinics in Office Practice, 29*(1), 13–26.

Stotland, N. (2007). Postabortion depression: Clarification. *Psychiatric Times, 24*(12), 31.

Taipale, P., & Hiilesmaa, V. (2001). Predicting delivery date by ultrasound and last menstrual period in early gestation. *Obstetrics and Gynecology, 97,* 189–194.

Tanne, J. H. (2007). Abortion does not raise risk of breast cancer. *British Medical Journal, 334*(76), 923–924.

Taylor, D., & James, A. (2011). An evidence-based blueprint for unintended pregnancy prevention guidelines. *Journal of Obstetric Gynecologic and Neonatal Nurses, 40*, 782–793.

Taylor, D., Safriet, B., Dempsey, G., Kruse, B., & Jackson, C. (2009). Providing abortion care: A professional toolkit for nurse-midwives, nurse practitioners, and physician assistants. Retrieved from http://www.apctoolkit.org/PDFs/APCToolkit_COMPLETE BOOK.pdf

Thiery, M. (1986). Quickening—A re-evaluation [letter]. *British Journal of Obstetrics and Gynaecology, 93*, 892.

United States House of Representatives Committee on Government Reform (2006). False and misleading health information provided by federally funded pregnancy resource centers. Committee on government reform—Minority staff report. Retrieved from http://www.chsourcebook.com/articles/waxman2.pdf

U.S. Department of Health and Human Services (2010). Family planning—Objectives. Retrieved from http://healthypeople.gov/2020/topicsobjectives2020/objectiveslist.aspx?topicid=13

Waller, D. K., Spears, W. D., Gu, Y., & Cunningham, G. C. (2000). Assessing number-specific error in the recall of onset of last menstrual period. *Paediatric and Perinatal Epidemiology, 14*, 263–267.

Wegienka, G., & Baird, D. D. (2005). A comparison of recalled date of last menstrual period with prospectively recorded dates. *Journal of Women's Health, 14*, 248–252.

White, L. J., Lee, S. J., Stepniewska, K., Simpson, J. A., Dwell, S. L. D., Arunjerdja, R., . . . McGready, R. (2012). Estimation of gestational age from fundal height: A solution for resource-poor settings. *Journal of the Royal Society, Interface, 9*, 503–510.

Wilcox, A. J., Dunson, D., & Baird, D. D. (2000). The timing of the "fertile window" in the menstrual cycle: Day specific estimates from a prospective study. *British Medical Journal, 321*, 1259–1262.

Wise, D., & Engstrom, J. L. (1985). The predictive validity of fundal height curves in the identification of small- and large-for-gestational-age infants. *Journal of Obstetric, Gynecologic, & Neonatal Nursing, 14*(2), 87–92.

Worthen, N., & Bustillo, M. (1980). Effect of urinary bladder fullness on fundal height measurements. *American Journal of Obstetrics and Gynecology, 138*, 759–762.

8

Risk assessment and risk management in prenatal care

Robin G. Jordan

Relevant terms

Absolute risk—the probability that an event will occur

Attributable risk—commonly additional adverse events can be attributed to the risk factor itself

Negative predictive value—the true negatives among all those with negative screens; reflects the probability that a negative test reflects not having the underlying condition being tested; a high negative predictive value means that the test only rarely indicates that a person has the condition being tested when they actually do not

Positive predictive value—the true positive among all those with positive screens; reflects the probability that a positive test reflects actually having the underlying condition being tested

Relative risk—estimate of the probability of an adverse event in one group compared to another group

Risk factors—any attribute, characteristic, or exposure of an individual that increases the likelihood of developing a disease or injury

Sensitivity—proportion of positive screens among those known to have the condition being screened for

Specificity—proportion of negative screens among those known not to have the condition being screened for

Soft markers—slight deviations from normal findings on ultrasound that may or may not indicate increased risk for defect or anomaly

---

Introduction

Risk is the likelihood that a particular event will occur. Risk assessment is the clinical process of screening for conditions that could result in adverse perinatal outcomes, for which an intervention would improve the

health outcome for mother or child (Bryers & van Teijlingen, 2010). All prenatal care providers assess a woman's risk status at each visit. Risk assessment guides pregnant women behaviors and health-care provider management, and the appropriateness for continued care in various birth settings. In situations of known risk during pregnancy or birth, successful planning or intervention can improve the likelihood of positive outcomes. Misapplication of the risk assessment can introduce problems that diminish optimal perinatal outcomes, which is contrary to the goal of risk assessment. The appropriate application of the risk assessment process and interpretation and management of risk during prenatal care requires an understanding of normal childbearing physiology; the benefits and limitations of the risk assessment process; and an appropriate appraisal of theoretical, perceived, and actual risk. Health-care providers must also skillfully communicate appropriate evaluations of risk. This chapter will focus on the risk assessment process, limitations and potential problems of risk assessment, and appropriate risk management and communication of childbearing risk to women and their families.

Process and purpose of risk assessment

While risk assessment is ideally started prior to conception, many pregnancies are unplanned and the process is begun at the first prenatal visit. Risk assessment is primarily accomplished via history, the physical exam, and laboratory studies. Subjective and objective data assessment of the woman's medical, psychosocial, nutritional, genetic, occupational, and environmental factors

---

Prenatal and Postnatal Care: A Woman-Centered Approach, First Edition. Edited by Robin G. Jordan, Janet L. Engstrom, Julie A. Marfell, and Cindy L. Farley.
© 2014 John Wiley & Sons, Inc. Published 2014 by John Wiley & Sons, Inc.

is evaluated on an ongoing process throughout prenatal care. Data are gathered at each prenatal visit to evaluate changes in risk status. A woman's risk status can change to a higher risk or a lower risk during prenatal care.

Benefits of risk assessment

Ideally, risk assessment directs each pregnant woman to the best place for her birth, to the most appropriate health-care provider, and allocates appropriate resources to foster optimal maternal and infant outcomes (Jordan & Murphy, 2009). Pregnant women identified at high risk for adverse outcome can be directed to facilities with availability of appropriate specialty care. Women deemed low risk can explore options regarding place of birth and birth attendants.

Identification of risk factors can start the process of working with the woman to improve health-promoting behaviors. Lifestyle issues such as diet, exercise, smoking, and other substance use can be addressed and remediated with education, support, and motivational strategies to change behavior, thus reducing perinatal risk. Knowledge of the presence of risk factors can alert health-care providers to recommend specific measures to evaluate and monitor risk such as laboratory testing and fetal surveillance techniques. Risk information also allows the provider and the woman to be aware and watchful for the development of associated conditions or symptoms in an effort to prevent adverse outcomes.

Limitations

Poor predictive value

The validity of various risk scoring tools is undetermined and the benefit of prenatal risk scoring systems remains undocumented (Davey, Watson, Rayner, & Rowlands, 2011). Many tools are poor predictors of actual outcome. Risk scoring tools to predict preterm birth historically have performed poorly, resulting in higher intervention costs with no significant improvement in perinatal outcome (Berglund & Lindmark, 1999). It is common for women with risk factors to have a normal pregnancy and birth course. Conversely, women with no risk factors can develop complications.

Lack of precision

Definitions of risk factors vary considerably and many are not quantifiable. Research has found many factors associated with increased risk for a particular event; however, the role of these factors in causing the event may be tenuous or nonexistent. For example, a meta-analysis found that unmarried women have higher rates of low-birth-weight infants than married women. This

is an association, not a causation, and a factor that is not amenable to change by provider intervention. The high numbers of "risk factors" included in standard risk assessment forms result in large numbers of women being labeled "at risk." However, many of these so-called risk factors are statistically associated with adverse outcomes, with no evidence of actual causation (Stahl & Hundley, 2003). Women placed in risk categories based on tools with poor predictive value for actual occurrence of adverse event can mislead decisions by health-care providers and pregnant women (Jordan & Murphy, 2009).

Nonmodifiable risk factors

Women may have risk factors that are not amenable to modification such as socioeconomic status, age, and race. It is still important, however, to identify these non-modifiable risk factors so that appropriate screening tools may be offered when available. For example, we may determine that a 40-year-old pregnant woman is at higher risk for fetal anomalies. While we cannot reduce her age or prevent fetal anomalies, we can offer her screening or diagnostic testing to determine if the outcome associated with increased age (anomaly) has occurred.

Disadvantages of risk assessment and risk management

It is clear that identification of risk factors during the course of prenatal care is extremely important to maternal fetal health and to help guide care decisions. The disadvantages and potential problems of inappropriate risk assessment and risk management in childbearing care are not as readily recognized. There has been a broad shift in maternity care over the last several decades toward a focus on potential risk and risk management. We now label many more pregnant women "at risk" than in the past. This has fundamentally altered not only the way in which pregnancy is perceived by women and providers but also how pregnancy and birth are experienced by women.

Unnecessary interventions

The effect of evaluation of risk and use of subsequent interventions can have a profound influence on a woman's course of pregnancy and labor and birth. The proliferation of prenatal testing in pregnancy surveillance has led to prenatal care to serve as a platform for testing as a technologic imperative: "we have the technology; therefore we must use it" (Lock & Koenig, 1998). The use of prenatal ultrasound offers an example. Consider the common situation of a pregnant woman in the last month of pregnancy who has been told by her clinician that she has a "large baby." Ultrasound for evaluation of estimated fetal weight at 38 weeks indicates the baby is over 8 lb. The woman is encouraged to consider labor induction for "impending macrosomia" within the next week to avoid potential intrapartum problems attributed to a large baby at term. Induction of labor prior to the physiological preparation necessary for labor to ensue is associated with an increase in cesarean births (Ehrenthal, Jiang, & Strobino, 2010; Grivell, Reilly, Oakey, Chan, & Dodd, 2012). During labor induction, women are typically tethered to bed with electronic fetal monitoring and intravenous lines, limiting mobility that can contribute to labor dysfunction (Lawrence, Lewis, Hofmeyr, Dowswell, & Styles, 2009; Simkin & O'Hara, 2002). Even though ultrasound is one of the least accurate methods to assess fetal weight (Chauhan, Lutton, Bailey, Guerrieri, & Morrison, 1992; Dudley, 2005), the clinician's advice to proceed with induction prompts the woman to agree to labor induction with known and qualified risks to reduce the possibility of a poorly qualified risk.

Normalization of technology and illusion of risk control

The routine use of childbearing technology has become an expectation of the public and clinicians. Using technology to preempt adverse events may give both women and clinicians a sense of certainty and control over the unknown that may be unfounded. Prenatal ultrasound serves to illustrate these concepts. Despite the fact that no expert obstetrical organization promotes routine ultrasound during prenatal care, many women and clinicians have come to perceive ultrasound examinations as an essential component of routine pregnancy care. Women may feel that their care is substandard if they do not receive at least one ultrasound examination. The vast majority of pregnant women in the United States undergo at least one ultrasound examination with more than half of receiving multiple ultrasounds in the course of prenatal care (Declerq, Sakala, Corry, & Applebaum, 2006). If the fetus can be "seen," women and their providers feel relieved and reassured despite the low positive predictive value of an ultrasound to detect many abnormalities (Baillie, Smith, Hewison, & Mason, 2000). Additionally, it is not uncommon for ultrasound to visualize "soft markers" or findings of undetermined significance, which generates further ultrasound and diagnostic evaluations. While most of these findings are ultimately determined to be of no significance, this causes an increased maternal anxiety and affects developing maternal fetal attachment (Viaux-Savelon et al., 2012).

Labeling women as high risk

Prenatal care providers should be aware that classifying a woman as high risk can produce negative psychological effects. When women are labeled "high risk" during pregnancy, they experience increased anxiety, negative self-perception (Stahl & Hundley, 2003), and increased stress and loss of control (Saxell, 2006). Women with nonmodifiable risk factors, such as age, who are told they are high risk experience increased feelings of guilt, even though no high-risk condition has been detected and nothing can be done about the factor that placed them in the "high risk" category (Handwerker, 1994).

Misapplication of risk assessment and risk management

In many ways, our culture is risk averse, and we believe we can prevent, manage, and control risk. If an adverse event occurs, legal redress is directed at the party perceived as incorrectly managing risk. Risk aversion and obstetrical interests have led to exaggerated perceptions of pregnancy risk and the ability of technology and intervention to reduce risk (Jordan & Murphy, 2009). A reconceptualization of childbearing as potentially pathologic requires routine intervention and invasive surveillance to maintain "safety" has occurred over the last several decades with the rise of technology use in health care. Universal applications of medical intervention once reserved for use for individual indication is now standard obstetrical care as a preemptive strategy to prevent adverse outcomes regardless of a woman's actual risk status. Despite this increased use of medical interventions during childbearing care, maternal and infant outcomes have not appreciably improved in the last decade and outcomes such as preterm birth and low birth weight infants have increased (Martin et al., 2012).

Nocebo ("I shall harm") effects are the inadequately recognized opposite of placebo ("I shall please") effects. It is the absolute belief in a negative outcome. It is argued that nocebo effects are common in contemporary childbearing care practices (Benedetti, Lanotte, Lopiano, & Colloca, 2007; Sakala, 2007). Prenatal visits become an opportunity for women to be reminded of pregnancy risks. Consider such communication such as, "let's get another ultrasound just in case," or "I think your baby is getting large," or "we don't want you going past her due date." This unrecognized negative effect creates a "climate of doubt" rather than instilling confidence in pregnant women regarding their abilities to labor and birth. The cumulative effect of constant focus on potential perinatal problems regardless of actual risk can undermine women's confidence in their ability to maintain health throughout pregnancy and to give birth (Sakala, 2007).

There are a variety of reasons contributing to providers treating pregnancy as in need of nonindicated medical intervention regardless of real risk. Obstetrical care is an area of high liability and health-care provider litigation fears are a real concern. Survey research indicated the vast majority of obstetrician gynecologists have engaged in defensive care practices such as prescribing medication or ordering ultrasound without indication (Studdert et al., 2008). This "risk to the health-care provider" is a distinct factor in obstetrical decision making (Bassett, Iyer, & Kazanjian, 2000). Obstetricians themselves indicate that fear of childbirth has contributed to increased use of technology and, in particular, the escalating cesarean section rate (Klein, 2005). This may be reflected in the reported medical bias toward operative birth as a safe alternative to vaginal delivery (Edwards & Davies, 2001).

Lifestyle issues may create incentives for misapplication of risk evaluations and management decisions. Health-care providers attending to women during childbirth have a lifestyle characterized by unpredictability, less control over personal time, heavy workload, and long hours. The process of labor is generally unknown: when it will start, how long it will be, when it will end, and how the process will unfold. These factors create challenges in other aspects of life. Provider incentives to control patient scheduling and workload, maximize daytime deliveries, allow for more personal time (Barber, Eisenberg, & Grubman, 2011; Peled et al., 2011; Spetz, Smith, & Ennis, 2001), as well as surgical financial incentives (Spetz et al., 2001) have been attributed to increasing use of practices such as nonindicated labor induction and cesarean section.

Some of the following examples used to illustrate the potential problems of misapplication of risk evaluation and management sections are related to labor and birth; however, many decisions related to labor and birth are made during prenatal care. Therefore, an understanding of the association between prenatal application of risk assessment and risk management and childbearing experience and outcomes is vital.

Introduction of actual risk

Surgical cesarean section, once reserved for situations of fetal and or maternal risk, has increased in the United States by more than 40% since 1996 (Martin et al., 2012). This dramatic rise in cesarean birth has not resulted in improved health outcomes. In fact, the overuse of cesarean has recently been linked with unanticipated secondary health problems such as placenta accrete, placenta previa, emergency cesarean hysterectomy, maternal mortality, and a higher rate of uterine rupture in subsequent pregnancies (Howard, 2011; Main et al., 2011; Solheim

et al., 2011). In an effort to eliminate perceived risk of vaginal birth, the use of a major surgical procedure without true indication has caused an increase in real and measurable risk to the mother and the fetus.

Increase in financial, physical, and emotional costs

Routine use of non-evidence-based interventions incurs financial costs to society and is an acute burden to the current health-care system already under financial strain. For example, operative birth requires expensive operating room facilities and personnel and longer hospital stays. There can be a physical cost to women. This can be illustrated by the routine use of continuous electronic fetal monitoring in all laboring women. It is well established that this practice results in immobility, adding to physical discomfort, prolonging labor and operative birth (Alfirevic, Devane, & Gyte, 2006), and fetal heart rate findings that are incorrectly interpreted, causing additional interventions (Santos & Bernardes, 2008).

Emotional costs of attempts to preemptively manage perceived pregnancy and birth risks can be difficult to quantify and easier to set aside as less important. However, childbirth is not only a physical event, but it is also a major emotional and transformative event in a woman's life. Prenatal and birth technology has led to a transfer of authoritative birth knowledge from women themselves to medical professionals (Davis-Floyd, 2001). Reliance on technology can diminish a woman's sense of personal and experiential knowledge of her pregnancy health, instead creating a reliance on external measures to inform her of pregnancy normalcy. Women may wait to obtain results of tests to "prove" all is well before incorporating the pregnancy into her sense of self, creating a delay in the prenatal attachment process (Lawson & Turriff-Janasson, 2006). Survey research indicated that 67% of women reported an abnormal test result during pregnancy, the majority relating to an ultrasound scan and eventually found to be normal. More than half of these women reported being acutely worried and one-quarter were still concerned 5 weeks later (Peterson, Paulitsch, Guethlin, Gensichen, & Albrecth, 2009).

Some experts make compelling arguments that risk assessment has become a way of controlling women's childbirth choices (Tracy, 2006). Women have great trust in expert knowledge and in medical technical measures to provide security and protection from risk during childbearing (Kringeland & Moller, 2006), creating a climate in which women are reluctant to question authoritative decisions. Most women feel little power to challenge medical authority (Crossley, 2007), and pregnancy is an especially vulnerable time for women due to concerns for health and safety of self and fetus and anxiety of the unknown.

Birth fear

Fear of childbirth, or tocophobia, is a relatively new phenomena in contemporary society. Research indicates that women are fearful about normal pregnancy issues such as going past their due date, pain, the labor process, and loss of control (Rouhe, Salmela-Aro, Halmesmäki, & Saisto, 2009). Women learn about childbirth from the media, the medical community, and family and friends, and these sources are also the sources of significant childbirth fear (Munro, Kornelsen, & Hutton, 2009; Sercekus & Okumus, 2007). While alarming information may be disseminated by friends, family, and media, maternity care clinicians also have strong influence on birth fear (Melander & Lauri, 2002). Medical claims about the inherent danger of childbirth are evident in the decline in even expectation for a normal birth of today's women (Reiger & Dempsey, 2006). Escalating interventions and cesarean birth rates are seen as proof that birth is dangerous and frightening. Some anxiety about birth is normal and serves a useful purpose as a prompt for women to seek safety and security. Escalated fear of birth can lead to a woman's reliance on unnecessary interventions (Fenwick, Gamble, Nathan, Bayes, & Hauck, 2009; Nieminen, Stephansson, & Ryding, 2009) to physical labor dysfunction (Laursen, Johansen, & Hedegaard, 2009) and a personal sense of failure (Nilsson & Lundgren, 2007).

Perspective of risk and risk screening

There is a growing awareness among clinicians that maternity care practices should be based on evidence to reduce unintended sequel and to improve maternal satisfaction and perinatal outcomes. Antepartum care is an opportunity for health-care providers to perform realistic and evidence-based appraisals of pregnancy risk and to help women develop an appropriate sense of confidence regarding their health and their childbearing abilities. The underlying belief that childbirth is a normal physiological human function forms the foundation for applying evidence-based care practices to pregnant women. Childbearing is not without risk; however, the translation of theoretical and actual risks into a meaningful probability is essential in order to explain risk assessment to pregnant women and their families in a realistic way.

Risk assessment in pregnancy includes both primary and secondary preventions. For example, primary prevention of gestational diabetes might involve screening women prior to pregnancy and helping them achieve a normal body weight before becoming pregnant.

Secondary prevention would involve screening healthy asymptomatic pregnant women for evidence of abnormal glucose tolerance to detect those who have gestational diabetes. Screening tests and evaluations should be accurate, and accuracy is evaluated by sensitivity, specificity, and predictive value of the screening test. Predicted values are very dependent on the prevalence of the condition of the population being screened. When screening large numbers of asymptomatic women in a population that has a low prevalence of the condition, the number of false positive screens will increase as more and more healthy women are screened. For example, a 5% false positive rate in 100 healthy women will create five false positive diagnoses. The same rate in 10,000 women will create 500 false positive diagnoses. Therefore, it is important to consider the consequences of false positive screen results on healthy women, such as the introduction of additional risk from added stress and invasive procedures.

Explaining risk to women

Clinicians discuss risk or risk factors with pregnant women frequently in the course of prenatal care, and the different ways risk can be expressed and communicated should be understood. In general, risk can be expressed in several ways using the same underlying data. Absolute risk is the probability that an event will occur. Relative risk is an estimate of the probability of an adverse event in one group (for example, with prior cesarean section) relative to another (no prior cesarean section). Attributable risk refers to how many additional adverse outcomes can be attributed to the risk factor.

Choices on how to communicate risk of an event have a strong influence on how women perceive their own risk. The following example illustrates how a realistic understanding of the risk of an adverse event depends on the provider presentation. Consider the following statements when counseling a pregnant woman interested in having a vaginal birth after having a cesarean section (VBAC) in her first pregnancy:

- "Your risk of uterine rupture in this pregnancy is 0.2%." (absolute risk)
- "Your risk of uterine rupture in this pregnancy is 37 times higher than a woman who had no previous cesarean section." (relative risk)
- "VBAC at first birth creates 1.9 additional uterine ruptures for every 1000 cesarean births." (attributable risk)

Each of these statements is based on exactly the same underlying data, but each conveys a different perspective. A woman who is counseled about an adverse event that is 37 times more likely to happen if a particular course of action is taken will most likely interpret her risk as much higher than the woman who is counseled that she has a 2 in 1000 risk of the same adverse event. Additionally, a woman who is advised only of the risks of VBAC and not the risks of cesarean section may view her risks differently and, thus, may view her choices differently.

Women who received the labels of "positive" or "abnormal" test results perceived themselves to be at much higher risk than women who received "negative" or "normal" interpretive results, even when the actual risk numbers are the same. In a study examining risk communication, women who were told their risk of 5/1000 meant "abnormal test result" showed greater interest in further diagnostic testing compared with women who were told the risk of 5/1000 meant "normal test result" (Zikmund-Fisher, Fagerlin, Keeton, & Ubel, 2007). A significant concern is the variation in interpretation of the meaning of judgment terms such as "low risk" or "high risk." To one person, a low risk is equated with a risk of 1%, whereas to a second person, a low risk might be 10%. It is best not to use interpretive labels such as "abnormal" or "high risk" to results that can increase a woman's perception of her risk, and further affects her behavioral intentions to act on that risk. Using numerical risk when available will help women make better informed decisions rather than decisions based on their perceptions as to whether their risk had increased or decreased.

Research indicates that people misinterpret risk when it is stated as a probability with the numerator of 1 (Lipkus, Samsa, & Rima, 2001). For example, some may perceive the risk of 1/250 as greater than 1/25 simply because they see only the larger number. Converting risk probabilities to use standard denominations can facilitate communication and understanding of risk. The Paling Palette is an effective tool that efficiently and effectively communicates risk in an understandable manner using a denominator of 1000, and includes the probability of both adverse event occurring and adverse events not occurring. (Fig. 8.1). For example, when talking with a woman regarding her chances for successful VBAC and her risk of uterine rupture, all risks should be presented numerically with a denominator of 1000. The discussion should include the probability that no adverse effect will occur. This balance presentation of risk perspective can lead to a more realistic appraisal and understanding of potential problems (Table 8.1).

Potential problems of risk miscommunication

Informed compliance

The principles of informed choice may not be applied when tests are considered by clinicians as routine or necessary. Informed compliance is a term that means rather than making a choice, the woman is taking an action to which she has been directed by the provider. Power imbalances in the woman–provider relationship foster a climate where the person doing the informing influences women's actions. This can be illustrated with the common clinical scenario of a pregnant woman at her first prenatal care visit. She is provided literature about the serum quad screen, informed that this is done at 16 weeks of gestation, and instructed to let the clinician know if she has questions. Based on this presentation, she is likely to believe that that all pregnant women should and do have this test, that she would be deviant if she declined, and follow along without a full understanding of the genetic screening test and its implications. In this example, the clinician most likely believes the acts of talking about and given written information regarding the serum quad screen implies an informed client who could then give informed consent to have the test. When women lack full information on the benefits, risks, limitations and implications of tests and procedures, and the freedom to decline without sanction, it is not possible for them to have the opportunity to make an informed choice.

Illusion of choice

Information about risk can also be framed by the clinician toward offering a superior choice over another to avoid clinician-perceived risks. The practice can lead to an "illusion of choice." This concept is illustrated by the situation of a pregnant woman at 38 weeks of gestation assessed by the health-care provider as having a big baby. The woman is offered the choice of labor induction at 38 weeks to avoid potential problems related to suspicion of macrosomia. The discussion focuses on possible fetal risks without quantification of those risks. Importantly, she is not equally informed of the labor induction risks, the relative plasticity of the pelvis in late pregnancy, and the capacity of the fetal head to mold during labor, and therefore, this woman does not have a complete picture of the various risks to judge and weigh for herself. The woman feels she is being offered a decision that empowers her to avoid a potential threat. In reality, the potential for harm by waiting for natural labor may be quite remote, while a decision to induce labor puts her at new and undisclosed yet quantified risks with potential for maternal and fetal harm.

Informed consent

Pregnancy is a unique time in a woman's life when she seeks expert health-care information and opinion, even though she is not experiencing illness. Pregnant women

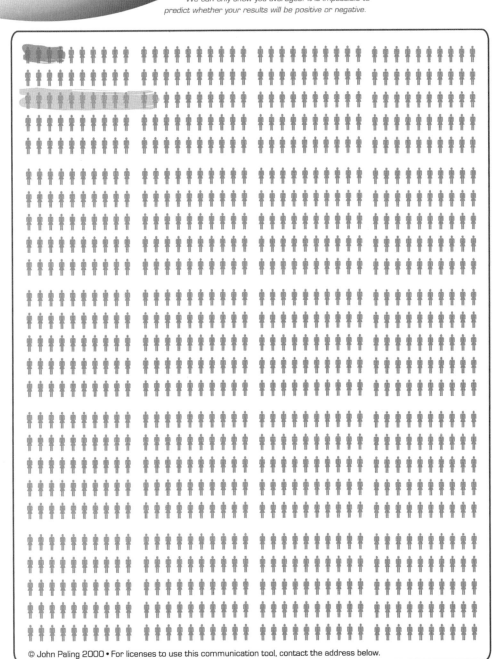

Odds for a _39_ year old woman of producing a child with Down Syndrome or other chromosome abnormality: _12 out of 1,000_

Odds of a woman having a miscarriage as a result of amniocentesis: _4 out of 1,000_

The Risk Communication Institute | 5822 NW 91st Boulevard • Gainesville, FL 32653 • (352) 377-2142
www.trci.info or www.riskcomm.com

Figure 8.1. Paling Palettes ©. Reprinted with permission from J. Paling: The Risk Communication Institute, 2008. Further information available at: http://www.riskcomm.com.

Table 8.1   Principles of Communicating Risk

1. *Provide numeric likelihoods of risks and benefits.* Describing risk with word only can inflate or minimize risk and does not provide enough detail to make an informed decision.
2. *Provide absolute risks, not just relative risks.* Risk perception can be significantly influenced with relative risk.
3. *Keep denominators constant for comparisons.* A single denominator should be chosen for comparisons, preferably, 1 in 1000.
4. *Explain the risk numbers by using visual aids.* These give context as well as achieving understanding for the largest number of patients.
5. *Make the differences between baseline and treatment risks and benefits clear.* Use pictographs to show baseline risks in one color and the risks due to treatment in a different color.
6. *Reduce the amount of information to what is essential when possible.* Clinicians are often motivated to provide women with as much information as possible. However, with excess information, women may not know where to focus their attention and what information should be most important in their decisions.
7. *Provide both positive and negative frames.* People are unduly influenced by whether a treatment is described in positive or negative terms. When possible, describe the risks and benefits using both frames.
8. *Limit using interpretive labels to convey risk information.* Avoid using phrases like "You have a high risk for a certain condition."
9. *Test communications prior to use.* It is critical to test educational materials prior to use to determine understandability and to ensure bias is eliminated in the materials.

Adapted from: Fagerlin and Peters (2011).

trust the health-care system and few women question information provided with the justification of the prenatal tests advised (Dahl, Kesmodel, Hvidman, & Olesen, 2006). It is the responsibility of prenatal health-care providers to provide pregnant women with complete information in an understandable format. Women need to understand all aspects of care offerings so that they can make the best decision for themselves.

Discussions on childbearing risk should culminate in a mutually agreeable decision about how to proceed with the risk information presented. Informed consent is not a signature on a document; it is a process of exchange between a woman and her midwife or nurse practitioner to foster her ability to make the best decision about what to allow to be done to her. Applying informed consent principles to commonly used technology such as non-indicated ultrasound, genetic screening, and elective

induction allows depth of information for an informed decision and permits informed refusal without sanction.

Patient knowledge for informed consent

- The known or possible diagnosis requiring treatment
- The nature and purpose of proposed treatments
- The benefits and risks associated with proposed treatment
- Potential complications and side effects
- Likelihood of treatment success for this patient
- Reasonable alternatives available
- Benefits and risk associated with alternatives

Informed consent not only ensures the protection of a woman against unwanted or unnecessary medical treatment but also promotes her active involvement in her care and planning for the major life event of childbearing (American College of Obstetricians and Gynecologists (ACOG), 2009). The informed consent process requires skillful communication and an understanding of the woman's perspective. Written material is a useful adjunct to promote understanding of conditions, testing, and risk during prenatal care. Most women prefer information to be provided on a face-to-face basis and written material should supplement, not replace, these important discussions (National Institute for Health and Clinical Excellence (NICE), 2010).

Nurse practitioners and midwives must recognize that the inherent inequalities in power and status between the patient and the health-care provider have a great influence on what happens to women during prenatal care. Equalizing the power balance between a pregnant woman and her health-care provider within the context of a caring relationship promotes open dialogue. When women are able to form a trusting relationship with their health-care providers, they are more likely to have increased confidence to ask questions and to make choices about their care, rather than simply being "compliant" (Pairman, 2000). Fostering the transition of authoritative childbirth knowledge from the health-care provider to the pregnant woman should be a prenatal care goal. All women should leave each prenatal encounter feeling that she knows more about what is going on in her body and how to best care for herself than she did before the visit. Validating and affirming a woman's experiential knowledge of pregnancy can empower her to rely less on outsiders' opinions on her pregnancy needs and allow her to make more autonomous care decisions.

Childbearing is not without risk. The risk assessment process is essential to competent and safe prenatal care and guides nurse practitioners and midwives by

Case study

Blanca is a 37-year-old G1P0 woman who is here for her first prenatal visit at 8 weeks of gestation. She is married, works full time as a buyer for a department store, and she and her husband are excited to be pregnant. They have been married for 2 years and have not used birth control. A complete history was taken. She has a body mass index (BMI) of 25.3, eats a varied diet including all food groups, exercises three to four times per week at a local gym, and has no significant health problems. She reports drinking one to two glasses of wine several times per week after work, but has had none since she received a positive pregnancy test. She currently takes a multivitamin with folic acid, and Tylenol as needed for headaches. She reports breast tenderness and daily mild nausea with no vomiting over the last 2 weeks. She expresses concern that she is "high risk" because she is over age 35.

A complete physical exam was done and findings were within normal: BP 122/70; anteverted uterus enlarged to correspond with approximately 8 weeks of gestation.

A discussion ensued about her concerns. It was explained that her physical findings indicate good health and that additional pregnancy risk is often based on age-related disorders such as hypertension and diabetes, which are not a present issue for her. The increased risk of genetic anomalies was discussed. Using the Paling Palette to her risk for Down syndrome

(DS) at 1 in 230 women was explained in both positive and negative frames (1 in 230 chance of a baby with DS, 229/230 that she will not have a baby with DS). At this time, all genetic testing options, including invasive diagnostic testing, were discussed with Blanca. Written information was also provided, and she planned to discuss the choices with her husband before making a firm decision.

She was informed about routine prenatal laboratory testing. The 24-week screening test for gestational diabetes (GDM) was discussed, in particular, as she is a slightly increased risk for GDM due to her age. Routine prenatal care issues such as common discomforts, nutrition, and anticipatory guidance were addressed. She was counseled to abstain from alcohol during pregnancy and the rational was covered.

Her concern about being high risk was further addressed by informing her that neonatal outcomes in healthy women over age 35 are similar to younger women. She was reassured that her physical examination and history reveal no risk factors that place her in a high risk category at this time. She was advised that her pregnancy progress and health will be monitored at each prenatal visit the same as any pregnant women. Blanca was provided with additional routine pregnancy information. At the conclusion of the visit, a return appointment was for 2 weeks to review genetic testing options and decisions as well as her lab work.

delineating consultation and referral patterns. Evaluations of pregnancy risk are ongoing throughout prenatal care and can improve perinatal outcomes in some situations. However, the translation of theoretical and potential risks into reasonable and evidence-based care practices requires a broad understanding of what risk assessment can and cannot do. Transforming risk assessment into universal applications of prenatal surveillance and risk management strategies regardless of actual risk lacks evidence of improved outcomes and introduces new potential for harmful consequences. An awareness of the pitfalls of risk-based pregnancy evaluation and management can assist the clinician in avoiding inappropriate distortion of pregnancy risk and harmful consequences.

Resources for health-care providers and women and their families

The Early Prenatal Risk Assessment Program: A website for women and prenatal care providers initiated by

Canadian prenatal laboratories, health-care professionals, and imaging services: http://www.earlyrisk assessment.com/

The Risk Communication Institute: For health-care professional and consumers, offering visual aids to help communicate risk: http://www.riskcomm.com/

References

Alfirevic, Z., Devane, D., & Gyte, G. M. L. (2006). Continuous cardiotocography (CTG) as a form of electronic fetal monitoring (EFM) for fetal assessment during labour. *CochraneDatabase of SystematicReviews*, (3), CD006066. doi:10.1002/14651858.CD006066

American College of Obstetricians and Gynecologists (ACOG) (2009). Informed consent. *Obstetrics and Gynecology*, *114*, 401–408. ACOG Committee Opinion No. 439.

Baillie, C., Smith, J., Hewison, J., & Mason, G. (2000). Ultrasound screening for chromosomal abnormality: Women's reactions to false positive results. *British Journal of Health Psychology*, *5*, 377–394. doi:10.1348/135910700168991

Barber, E., Eisenberg, D., & Grubman, W. (2011). Type of attending obstetrician call schedule and changes in labor management and outcome. *Obstetrics and Gynecology, 118*(6), 1371–1376.

Bassett, K. L., Iyer, N., & Kazanjian, A. (2000). Defensive medicine during hospital obstetrical care: A byproduct of the technological age. *Social Science and Medicine, 51*, 523–537.

Benedetti, F., Lanotte, M., Lopiano, L., & Colloca, L. (2007). When words are painful: Unraveling the mechanisms of the nocebo effect. *Neuroscience, 147*, 260–271.

Berglund, A., & Lindmark, G. (1999). The usefulness of initial risk assessment as a predictor of pregnancy complications and premature delivery. *Acta Obstetricia et Gynecologica Scandinavica, 78*, 871–876.

Bryers, H. M., & van Teijlingen, E. (2010). Risk, theory, social and medical models: A critical analysis of the concept of risk in maternity care. *Midwifery, 26*, 488–496.

Chauhan, S. P., Lutton, P. M., Bailey, K. J., Guerrieri, J. P., & Morrison, J. C. (1992). Intrapartum clinical, sonographic, and parous patients' estimates of newborn birth weight. *Obstetrics and Gynecology, 79*, 956–958.

Crossley, M. (2007). Childbirth, complications, and the illusion of choice: A case study. *Feminism and Psychology, 17*, 543–563.24.

Dahl, K., Kesmodel, U., Hvidman, L., & Olesen, F. (2006). Informed consent: Attitudes, knowledge and information concerning prenatal examinations. *Acta obstetrica at Gynecologica, 85*, 1414–1419.

Davey, M. A., Watson, L., Rayner, J. A., & Rowlands, S. (2011). Risk scoring systems for predicting preterm birth with the aim of reducing associated adverse outcomes. *Cochrane Database of Systematic Reviews*, (11), CD004902. doi:10.1002/14651858.CD004902.pub4

Davis-Floyd, R. (2001). The technocratic, humanistic, and holistic paradigms of childbirth. *International Journal of Gynecology & Obstetrics, 75*(Suppl. 1), S5–S23.

Declerq, E. R., Sakala, C., Corry, M. P., & Applebaum, S. (2006). Listening to mothers II survey and report. Retrieved from http://www.childbirthconnection.org/article.asp?ck=10396

Dudley, N. J. (2005). A systematic review of the ultrasound estimation of fetal weight. *Ultrasound in Obstetrics and Gynecology, 25*, 80–89. doi:10.1002/uog.1751

Edwards, G., & Davies, N. (2001). Elective cesarean section—The patient's choice? *Journal of Obstetrics and Gynaecology, 21*, 128–129.

Ehrenthal, D. B., Jiang, X., & Strobino, D. M. (2010). Labor induction and the risk of a cesarean delivery among nulliparous women at term. *Obstetrics and Gynecology, 116*(1), 35–42. doi:10.1097/AOG.0b013e3181e10c5c

Fagerlin, A., & Peters, E. (2011). Chapter 7. Quantitative information, In B. Fischoff, N. T. Brewer, & J. S. Downs (Eds.), *Communicating risks and benefits: An evidence-based user's guide*. Washington, DC: FDA Department of Health and Human Services. Retrieved from http://www.fda.gov/downloads/AboutFDA/ReportsManualsForms/Reports/UCM268069.pdf

Fenwick, J., Gamble, J., Nathan, E., Bayes, S., & Hauck, Y. (2009). Pre- and postpartum levels of childbirth fear and the relationship to birth outcomes in a cohort of Australian women. *Journal of Clinical Nursing, 18*(5), 667–677.

Grivell, R. M., Reilly, A. J., Oakey, H., Chan, A., & Dodd, J. M. (2012). Maternal and neonatal outcomes following induction of labor: A cohort study. *Acta Obstetricia et Gynecologica Scandinavica, 91*(2), 198. doi:10.1111/j.1600-0412.2011.01298.x

Handwerker, L. (1994). Medical risk: Implicating poor pregnant women. *Social Science and Medicine, 38*, 665–675.

Howard, B. (2011). The right thing cesarean delivery rate in America: What are the consequences? *Obstetrics and Gynecology, 118*(3), 687–690.

Jordan, R., & Murphy, P. (2009). Risk assessment and risk distortion: Finding the balance. *Journal of Midwifery and Women's Health, 54*(3), 191–200.

Klein, M. (2005). Obstetrician's fear of childbirth: How did it happen? *Birth (Berkeley, Calif.), 32*(3), 207–209.

Kringeland, T., & Moller, A. (2006). Risk and security in birth. *Journal of Psychosomatic Obstetrics and Gynecology, 27*, 185–191.

Laursen, M., Johansen, C., & Hedegaard, M. (2009). Fear of childbirth and risk for birth complications in nulliparous women in the Danish National Birth Cohort. *BJOG: An International Journal of Obstetrics and Gynaecology, 116910*, 1350–1355.

Lawrence, A., Lewis, L., Hofmeyr, G. J., Dowswell, T., & Styles, C. (2009). Maternal positions and mobility during first stage labour. *Cochrane Database of Systematic Reviews*, (2), CD003934. doi:10.1002/14651858.CD003934.pub2

Lawson, K. L., & Turriff-Janasson, I. S. (2006). Maternal serum screening and psychosocial attachments to pregnancy. *Journal of Psychosomatic Research, 60*, 371–378.

Lipkus, I. M., Samsa, G., & Rima, B. K. (2001). General performance on a numeracy scale among highly educated sample [serial online]. *Medical Decision Making: An International Journal of the Society for Medical Decision Making, 21*, 37–44. Retrieved from http://mdm.sagepub.com/cgi/content/abstract/21/1/37?ck=nck

Lock, M., & Koenig, B. (1998). The technological imperative in medical practice: The social creation of "routine" treatment. In M. Lock & D. Gordon (Eds.), *Biomedicine examined* (pp. 465–496). Dordrecht, The Netherlands: Kluwer.

Main, E. K., Morton, C. H., Hopkins, D., Giuliani, G., Melsop, K., & Gould, J. B. (2011). *Cesarean deliveries, outcomes, and opportunities for change in California: Toward a public agenda for maternity care safety and quality*. Palo Alto, CA: CMQCC. Retrieved from http://www.cmqcc.org

Martin, J. A., Hamilton, B. E., Ventura, S. J., Osterman, M. J., Wilson, E. C., & Mathews, T. J. (2012). Births: Final data for 2010. National vital statistics reports, Vol. 60, No. 1. Hyattsville, MD: National Center for Health Statistics.

Melander, H. L., & Lauri, S. (2002). Experiences of security associated with pregnancy and childbirth: A study of pregnant women. *International Journal of Nursing Practice, 8*, 289–296.

Munro, S., Kornelsen, J., & Hutton, E. (2009). Decision making in patient-initiated elective cesarean delivery: The influence of birth stories. *Journal of Midwifery & Women's Health, 54*, 373–379. doi:10.1016/j.jmwh.2008.12.014

National Institute for Health and Clinical Excellence (NICE). (2010). Antenatal Care. Retrieved from http://www.nice.org.uk/nicemedia/live/11947/40115/40115.pdf

Nieminen, K., Stephansson, O., & Ryding, E. L. (2009). Women's fear of childbirth and preference for cesarean section—A cross sectional study at various stages of pregnancy in Sweden. *Acta Obstetricia et Gynecologica Scandinavica, 88*(7), 807–813.

Nilsson, C., & Lundgren, I. (2007). Women's lived experience of fear of birth. *Midwifery, 25*(2), 1–9.

Pairman, S. (2000). Women-centred midwifery: Partners or professional friendships? In M. Kirkham (Ed.), *The midwife-mother relationship* (pp. 207–226). London: Macmillan.

Peled, Y., Melamed, N., Chen, R., Pardo, J., Ben-Shitrit, G., & Yogev, Y. (2011). The effect of time of day on outcome of unscheduled cesarean deliveries. *The Journal of Maternal-Fetal and Neonatal Medicine, 24*, 1051–1054.

Peterson, J., Paulitsch, M., Guethlin, C., Gensichen, J., & Albrecth, J. (2009). A survey on worries of pregnant women—Testing the German version of the Cambridge worry scale. *BMC Public Health, 9,* 490. Retrieved from http://www.biomedcentral.com/1471-2458/9/490

Reiger, K., & Dempsey, R. (2006). Performing birth in a culture of fear: An embodied crisis of late modernity. *Health Sociology Review, 15,* 364–373.

Rouhe, H., Salmela-Aro, K., Halmesmäki, E., & Saisto, T. (2009). Fear of childbirth according to parity, gestational age, and obstetric history. *BJOG: An International Journal of Obstetrics & Gynaecology, 116,* 67–73. doi:10.1111/j.1471-0528.2008.02002.x

Sakala, C. (2007). Letter from North America: Understanding and minimizing nocebo effects in childbearing women. *Birth (Berkeley, Calif.), 34*(4), 348–350.

Santos, C. C., & Bernardes, J. (2008). Differences and consequences in interobserver variation in intrapartum fetal heart rate assessment. *American Journal of Obstetrics and Gynecology, 200*(6), e8.

Saxell, L. (2006). Risk: Theoretical or actual. In L. A. Page & R. McCandlish (Eds.), *The new midwifery: Science and sensitivity in practice* (2nd ed.). Edinburgh: Churchill Livingston.

Sercekus, P., & Okumus, H. (2007). Fears associated with childbirth among nulliparous women in Turkey. *Midwifery, 2592,* 155–162.

Simkin, P., & O'Hara, M. (2002). Nonpharmacologic relief of pain during labor: Systematic reviews of five methods. *American Journal of Obstetrics and Gynecology, 186,* S131–S159.

Solheim, K. N., Esakoff, T. L., Little, S. E., Cheng, Y. W., Sparks, T. N., & Caughey, A. B. (2011). The effect of cesarean delivery rates in the future incidence of placenta previa, placental concrete, and maternal mortality. *The Journal of Maternal-Fetal and Neonatal Medicine, 24*(11), 1341–1346.

Spetz, J., Smith, M. W., & Ennis, S. F. (2001). Physician incentives and the timing of cesarean sections: Evidence from California. *Medical Care, 39,* 536–550.

Stahl, K., & Hundley, V. (2003). Risk and risk assessment in pregnancy—Do we scare because we care? *Midwifery, 10,* 298–309.

Studdert, D., Mello, M., Sage, W., DesRoches, C., Peugh, J., Zapert, K., & Brennan, T. (2008). Defensive medicine among higher risk specialist physicians in a volatile medical environment. *Obstetrical and Gynecological Survey, 60*(11), 718–720.

Tracy, S. (2006). Chapter 11. Risk: Theoretical or actual? In L. Page & R. McCandlish (Eds.), *The new midwifery: Science and sensitivity in practice* (2nd ed.). Philadephia: Elsevier.

Viaux-Savelon, S., Dommergues, M., Rosenblum, O., Bodeau, N., Aidane, E., Philippon, O., Mazet, P. . . . Cohen, D. (2012). Prenatal ultrasound screening: False positive soft markers may alter maternal representations and mother-infant interaction. *PLoS ONE, 7*(1), e30935. doi:10.1371/journal.pone.0030935

Zikmund-Fisher, B. J., Fagerlin, A., Keeton, K., & Ubel, P. A. (2007). Does labeling prenatal screening test results as negative or positive affect a woman's responses? *American Journal of Obstetrics and Gynecology, 197,* 528e1–528e6.

9

Prenatal genetic counseling, screening, and diagnosis

Robin G. Jordan and Janet L. Engstrom

Relevant terms

Alpha-fetoprotein (AFP)—plasma protein produced by the fetus and measured in maternal serum as a marker for risk of neural tube defects

Aneupolidy—abnormal number of chromosomes

Closed neural tube defects—the spinal defect is covered by skin

Confined placental mosaicism—a mosaic abnormality in the placental tissue but not in the fetus or embryo

Detection rate—percentage of those actually affected and called "screen positive" by the test/screen.

False negative rate—number of individuals incorrectly identified as negative, or not having a condition or disease, by a screening test

False positive rate—number of individuals incorrectly identified as positive, or having a condition or disease, by a screening test

Mendelian condition—mutation in a single gene that follows a dominant, recessive or X-linked pattern of inheritance

Nuchal translucency—ultrasound measurement of the fetal neck; used in the screening for Down syndrome

Open neural tube defects—the brain and/or spinal cord are exposed through an opening in the skull or vertebrae

Positive predictive value—percentage of individuals with positive screening test that have the disease or condition

Prenatal diagnosis—making a certain diagnosis of a genetic condition or birth defect prior to birth

Prenatal screening—procedures that identify fetuses at risk for genetic conditions or birth defects prior to birth

Sensitivity—ability of a screening test to correctly identify individuals who have the disease or condition

Specificity—ability of a screening test to correctly identify individuals who do not have the disease or condition

Trisomy 18—an extra copy of chromosome 18 is present; also known as Edwards syndrome

Trisomy 21—an extra copy of chromosome 21 is present; also known as Down syndrome

---

Introduction

Over the last three decades, there have been major advances in the science of genetics and the application of this knowledge to prenatal screening and testing during in pregnancy. The option of screening for and diagnosing genetic disorders and birth defects during pregnancy has become an integral part of prenatal care for women. Genetic screening begins at the first prenatal visit with a comprehensive family history, and all women are offered screening for selected conditions such as neural tube defects (NTDs) and trisomies 18 and 21. The baseline risk of some type of birth defect is 3–4% of all births. The incidence of birth defects is higher for women with selected risk factors, such as family history or increased maternal age. Genetic screening and testing allows women and families to know their risk of a genetic disorder or birth defect and to make decisions regarding pregnancy that is best for them.

The purposes of genetic testing

- Prepare parents for infants with special needs
- Prepare parents for an adverse pregnancy outcome
- Allow parents the opportunity to terminate the pregnancy

The chapter reviews genetic risk screening using the personal health and multigenerational family history as well as the genetic screening procedures offered to all pregnant women. Indications for targeted genetic screening and diagnostic tests for women with specific risk factors are reviewed as well as the indications for referral for genetic counseling. Finally, the essential components of genetic counseling are described including the ethical and social issues as well as strategies for counseling families about their options for genetic testing.

Family history and risk evaluation

A multigenerational family history should be obtained at the first prenatal visit (American College of Obstetricians and Gynecologists (ACOG), 2011). This can be done using a checklist filled out by the woman or by a verbal questioning about whether there is a family history of disorders, conditions, or health problems. Another method of evaluating the family history is the pedigree, which is commonly used by genetic counselors. A pedigree is a visual diagram to evaluate genetic relationships and assess the risk of individuals to develop certain diseases or conditions. This visual form of documenting family health history offers a more comprehensive method of capturing significant health patterns than can be achieved with a narrative description (Wolpert & Speer, 2005). A pedigree includes at least three generations and includes ethnicity, age, age of death if deceased, relevant health history, illness, and age of onset of the condition for each family member. The type of pedigree tool used should be tailored for use in the maternity care setting. The most useful family history includes medical, developmental, and pregnancy outcome information on first-, second-, and third-degree relatives (Table 9.1). Family health pedigrees are documented and analyzed using standard nomenclature and symbols. Many resources are available to create a pedigree for use in the clinical setting.

Table 9.1 Degree of Relationship and Shared Genes

First-degree relatives	Second-degree relatives	Third-degree relatives
50% shared genes	25% shared genes	12.5% shared genes
Children Siblings Parents	Aunts and uncles Nieces and nephews Half siblings Grandparents	Cousins Great-grandparents

Genetic screening procedures offered to all pregnant women

All pregnant women are offered a number of genetic testing and screening procedures. The information about these tests should be presented at the first prenatal visit if the visit occurs during the first 20 weeks of gestation (ACOG, 2007a). Most of the screening tests are noninvasive and provide an estimated risk or risk score for certain birth defects or genetic disorders. Women with a risk above the cutoff are considered screen positive and are at an increased risk of carrying an affected fetus. Women with a risk score below the cutoff are considered screen negative and are not at an increased risk of carrying an affected fetus. These tests are blood tests that involve measurement maternal serum markers that have been associated with selected birth defects and genetic disorders and are known as maternal serum screening. The screening tests measure four or five maternal serum markers and are commonly called "quad" or "penta testing." Based on the results of the tests, the woman's risk of having an affected infant is calculated using an algorithm that factors in information about the woman, including her age, weight, race, and gestational age at the time of the screening, in addition to the amounts of the maternal serum markers. The raw value of the maternal serum markers is converted to a multiple of the median (MoM) that is similar to a standard deviation. Utilizing the MoM allows for comparison of results between patients as well as laboratories. The result is often referred to as "screen positive/screen negative" or "abnormal/normal," with the woman's specific numeric risk provided.

It is imperative that the correct information is used for the calculation to provide the most accurate risk assessment. For example, using a gestational age that is incorrectly calculated by as little as 1 week can change the risk assessment. Thus, whenever there is an abnormal test result for the estimated gestational age, an ultrasound should be performed to confirm gestational age. If there is a discrepancy in gestational age estimated by ultrasound and the last menstrual period of more than 10 days, then the test result must be reinterpreted using the gestational age from the ultrasound (Driscoll & Gross, 2009). Of all women who have a positive serum screening test, only a very small number are carrying a fetus with a NTD or chromosomal abnormality.

Screening options for neural tube defects

NTDs are a complex group of disorders ranging in severity from spina bifida occulta to anencephaly and are one of the most common congenital malformations worldwide. NTDs are caused by a combination of multiple genes and multiple environmental factors and develop in the first 4 weeks of pregnancy, often before a woman may even know that she is pregnant. The incidence of NTDs is approximately 1 per 1000 live births in the United States (National Institute of Child Health and Human Development (NICHHD), 2012). Overall, most women have a low risk of having an infant with an NTD. Regardless of her age, a woman's chance of delivering an infant with an NTD is 1/1000 or 0.1% (NICHHD, 2012). It is well established that adequate folic acid is preventative for NTD, and all childbearing aged and pregnant women are advised to consume 400 mcg folic acid daily (Blencowe, Cousens, Modell, & Lawn, 2010). The introduction of folic acid fortified cereal grains sold in the United States has reduced the incidence of NTDs by approximately 50% (Mills & Signore, 2004).

In the United States, NTD prevalence is highest among Hispanics, followed in descending order by Caucasians, Native Americans, African Americans, and Asians (Centers for Disease Control and Prevention (CDC), 2009; Hendricks, Simpson, & Larsen, 1999). The incidence of NTDs is higher in people of Celtic descent, such as the Welsh, Irish, and Scotch. Areas with a high number of people from these ethnicities such as Boston and the Appalachian region have a higher NTD prevalence.

Risk factors for NTD

Family history of NTD
Maternal obesity
Insulin-dependent diabetes
Maternal hyperthermia in early gestation
Medications (antiseizure medications, warfarin)
Ethnicity/geographic region (Caucasian, United Kingdom, Ireland, Indian Sikhs)
Sources: ACOG (2007a), Lumley, Watson, Watson, and Bower (2001).

Although the history of an NTD in an immediate family member increases a woman's chance of having an infant with an NTD, about 95% of couples who have a fetus affected with an open NTD have a negative family history (ACOG, 2007a). Having a previous infant with an NTD increases the risk of having a second baby with an NTD by 2–3% (ACOG, 2003).

Screening for NTD is offered to all pregnant women presenting for prenatal care prior to 20 weeks of gestation by measuring serum alpha-fetoprotein (AFP), one component of the more comprehensive quad or penta serum screen done in the second trimester (ACOG, 2003) (Table 9.2). The optimal time for NTD screening is at 16–18 weeks of gestation, but screening can be done between 15 and 20 weeks of gestation. Screening is based

on the presence of AFP, a protein made in the fetal liver that can be measured in maternal serum and amniotic fluid. Fetuses with an opening in the skull or spine leak extra AFP into the amniotic fluid. In addition to NTD, fetuses with other openings such as the ventral wall defect gastroschisis can also be identified with serum AFP screening.

Screening options for trisomy 21 and trisomy 18

Antepartum detection of fetal aneuploidy is one of the major goals of prenatal screening. Two of the most commonly encountered aneuploidies are trisomy 18 and trisomy 21.

Trisomy 21, commonly known as Down syndrome, is the most common chromosome anomaly found in newborns and is the most common genetic cause of intellectual disability. Down syndrome occurs in approximately 1 in 691 live births (Parker et al., 2010).

The features of Down syndrome can include variable intellectual disability, hypotonia, distinctive facial features, heart defects, gastrointestinal anomalies, vision and hearing problems, thyroid problems, seizure disorders, increased incidence of leukemia and Alzheimer features, and spine instability. Children with Down syndrome typically accomplish their developmental milestones later than children who do not have Down syndrome. Early intervention programs are effective in assisting children with Down syndrome reach their full potential. Health Supervision Guidelines from the American Academy of Pediatrics can assist health-care providers in planning the specialized care needed for individuals with Down syndrome.

A major risk factor for Down syndrome is increased maternal age. Although older women are at higher risk, the majority of children with Down syndrome are born to women younger than age 35 since the majority of pregnancies occur in younger women. Therefore, all pregnant women presenting for prenatal care prior to 20 weeks of gestation are offered Down syndrome screening.

Trisomy 18, also known as Edwards syndrome, is a chromosomal disorder characterized by severe mental retardation, congenital heart disease, renal malformations, low set ears, and clenched fists. An unknown number of cases spontaneously abort during the first trimester, and at least half of the pregnancies carried to term result in an intrauterine fetal demise. Thirty percent of those born with trisomy 18 die within the first month of life and 90% within the first year. The estimated incidence is 1 per 6000 live births, and the incidence increases with advanced maternal age (Trisomy 18 Foundation, 2013).

Table 9.2 Common Prenatal Genetic Screening Options

Test	Conditions screened	Components	Ideal or required timing	Sensitivity for Down syndrome detection	Benefits and limitations
First-trimester screen	Trisomy 21	• PAPP-A • hCG • NT	Blood test at 9 weeks' gestation NT at 11–13 completed weeks' gestation	Detection 81–85%% False positive 5%	Benefits: Allows for earlier diagnosis Safer and earlier termination choices Limitations: Does not screen for NTD Requires availability of certified technician
Quad screen	NTD Trisomy 18 Trisomy 21	• AFP • hCG • uE3 • DIA	15–20 weeks gestation	Detection 80% False positive 5%	Benefits: Widely available Screens for DS and NTD
Penta screen	NTD Trisomy 18 Trisomy 21	• AFP • hCG • uE3 • DIA • h-hCG	15–20 weeks' gestation	Detection 83% False positive 5%	Limitations: Later diagnosis Later gestation termination risks
Integrated screen	NTD Trisomy 18 Trisomy 21		Blood test #1 at 10–13 weeks' gestation NT at 11–14 weeks' gestation Blood test #2 at 15–20 weeks' gestation	Detection 90–96% False positive 1–2%	Benefits: Highest sensitivity Lowest false positive Screens for NTD Limitations: Later diagnosis Later gestation termination risks Increased maternal anxiety with waiting time between tests

Sources: ACOG (2007a, 2007b), Canick et al. (2006), Palomaki, Lambert-Messerlian, and Canick (2007), Quest Diagnostics (2013). NT, nuchal translucency by ultrasound; AFP, alpha-fetoprotein; hCG, human chorionic gonadotropin; uE3, unconjugated estriol; DIA, dimeric inhibin A; h-hCG, hyperglycosylated human chorionic gonadotropin.

Whereas NTD risk assessment is based on maternal serum AFP measurement alone, trisomy 21 and trisomy 18 risk assessments are based on multiple marker combinations that may include maternal age, AFP, human chorionic gonadotropin (hCG), unconjugated estriol (uE3), pregnancy-associated plasma protein-A (PAPP-A), dimeric inhibin A (DIA), and hyperglycosylated human chorionic gonadotropin (h-hCG). There are several methods of trisomy 21 and trisomy 18 risk screening available in the first and second trimesters (Table 9.2).

First-trimester screening

First-trimester screening is performed between 11 and 13 weeks' gestation and includes a nuchal translucency (NT) measurement by ultrasound and maternal serum measurement of free or total β-hCG and PAPP-A. Women who screen positive are given the option of having a diagnostic test such as an amniocentesis or chorionic villus sampling (CVS) to determine whether the fetus is affected.

First-trimester screening offers several potential advantages over second-trimester screening. When test results are negative, it may help reduce maternal anxiety earlier in pregnancy. If results are positive, this early screening allows women to take advantage of first-trimester prenatal diagnosis by CVS, which can be performed between 10 and 12 weeks' gestation. First-trimester screening also affords women greater privacy and less health risk if they decide to terminate the pregnancy (ACOG, 2007a). First-trimester screening has a slightly better detection rate (82–87%) for Down syndrome compared to the second-trimester maternal serum quad screening (Table 9.2), especially if it is done at 11 weeks' gestation (Malone et al., 2005). Another advantage of first-trimester screening is that the rate of invasive testing decreases (Chasen, McCullough, & Chervenak, 2004). For women who undertake first-trimester screening, second-trimester AFP screening, and/or ultrasound examination should be offered to screen for open NTDs.

Second-trimester screening

In the second trimester, a maternal multiple serum marker screening test is offered to screen for Down syndrome, trisomy 18, and NTDs. This test is commonly known as "quad screening" because four markers are analyzed (Table 9.2). The quad screen detects approximately 79–81% of fetuses with Down syndrome (ACOG, 2007a). The quad screen measures AFP and therefore screens for NTD, with a detection rate of 80–90%, depending on the nature of the defect (Driscoll & Gross, 2009). A more recent screen called the "penta screen" includes measurement of a fifth analyte, h-hCG. This increases the Down syndrome detection rate by 3–4% over the quad screen (Quest Diagnostics, 2013).

Quad and penta screen results can be affected by factors such as race, placental size, maternal weight, and inaccurate pregnancy dating. If pregnancy dating is well established and a quad or penta screen indicates a high level of AFP, this is considered a marker for an increased risk of NTD. If the AFP is low and hCG and inhibin A levels are high, this indicates a higher risk of Down syndrome. This last particular combination of results is not related to accuracy of the gestational age assessment. Genetic counseling and additional testing such as a targeted ultrasound and amniocentesis for diagnosis are typically offered with a positive screen.

Integrated screening

Integrated screening combines both first-trimester NT measurement and first-trimester serum markers *along with* second-trimester quad screen markers (Table 9.2). NT is measured by ultrasound between 11 and 13.6 weeks' gestation and assesses the thickness of soft tissues of the nape of neck of the fetus. Higher thickness measurements are associated with Down syndrome and certain cardiac defects. A risk score is then assigned based on the combined serum and NT scan results in the second trimester. This test provides the highest sensitivity with the lowest false positive rate, limiting the number of invasive amniocenteses done for positive results. The availability of technicians trained in NT measurement may limit access to this test for women in rural and underserved areas. Since the integrated screen measures AFP, it also screens for NTD.

Variations of integrated screening protocols are also available. Serum integrated screen is the same as the integrated screen except the NT measurement is not done. Although the serum integrated screen has a lower detection rate than the integrated screen, it is the test of choice when NT measurement is not available. Sequential integrated screening is a method in which the woman is informed of the part 1 serum screening results instead of waiting for the later components of the screening to issue a risk score (Platt et al., 2004). If the part 1 serum screen is positive, CVS is offered for diagnosis. When the results from part 1 are negative, the second part of the test is completed and markers from parts 1 and 2 are combined to provide risk estimates. Thus, the sequential integrated screen enables earlier diagnosis for women with a first-trimester elevated risk while maintaining a high detection rate. While these options have increased the availability and number of screening options for women, the options can be overwhelming to women if not presented clearly.

Ultrasound for genetic screening

Ultrasonography can be diagnostic for fetal structural defects, such as heart defects or open NTDs. If a serum screening indicates a higher risk for NTD or Down syndrome, a more comprehensive ultrasound is performed to more thoroughly examine fetal anatomy.

Although ultrasound is not diagnostic for fetal chromosome anomalies, recent advances in ultrasound technology have improved the use of ultrasound in detecting so-called soft markers indicating an increased risk for fetal aneuploidy. Ultrasound soft markers such as short long bones, choroid plexus cysts, or increased NT, and structural anomalies such as ventricular septal defects suggest an increased risk of aneuploidy. However, ultrasound also detects findings that have undetermined significance, which generate uncertainty over fetal health and increases maternal anxiety and stress (Ball, Van Riper, Engstrom, & Matheson, 2005; Larsson, Svalenius, Marsal, & Dykes, 2009; Viaux-Savelon et al., 2012). In many cases of soft marker findings or "abnormalities," no actual problem is found (Van den Hof & Wilson, 2005). Experts agree that ultrasound alone has limited utility in genetic screening (ACOG, 2008b; Neilson, 1998; Smith-Bindman, 2001; U.S. Preventive Services Task Force (USPSTF), n.d.). The American College of Radiology (ACR), the American College of Obstetricians and Gynecologists (ACOG), and the American Institute of Ultrasound in Medicine (2007) (AIUM) joint practice guideline on fetal ultrasonography states that "fetal ultrasound should be performed only when there is a valid medical reason" (American College of Radiology (ACR), American College of Obstetricians and Gynecologists (ACOG), and the American Institute of Ultrasound in Medicine (AIUM), 2007, p. 1).

Despite lack of endorsement from the leading professional organizations, it has become commonplace to integrate a fetal anomaly scan ultrasound into prenatal care, usually between 16 and 20 weeks of gestation. This detailed scan systematically examines fetal anatomy for major structural anomalies. The brain, face, spine, heart, lungs, diaphragm, stomach, kidneys, bowel, and the upper and lower limbs are examined. The detection rate of fetal abnormalities can vary widely depending on many factors (from 16% to 85%) (Crane et al., 1994). The detection of major structural anomalies and lethal anomalies by ultrasound is approximately 60% of such cases (Chitayat, Langlois, Wilson, & SOGC Genetics Committee; CCMG Prenatal Diagnosis Committee, 2011).

Health-care providers should be aware that this routine ultrasound is a type of genetic screening. Indeed, in professional and consumer literature, it is termed "the fetal anomaly scan." When offering the fetal anomaly scan, the same approach should be used as with other genetic screening methods. Simply saying, "We're going to get an ultrasound to check on the baby, see if everything is OK," is not informed consent, nor is it full disclosure. Women in the United States have come to expect ultrasound as part of prenatal care and generally see this as a pleasant opportunity to see the baby and discover the fetal sex, and often do not realize that this is a form of genetic screening (Åhman, Runestam, & Sarkadi, 2010; Van der Zalm & Byrne, 2006). When unexpected abnormalities are found, women feel frightened, unprepared, and uninformed (Åhman et al., 2010; Van der Zalm & Byrne, 2006). They experience heighted anxiety and distress (Ball et al., 2005; Kaasen et al., 2010), and normal attachment behaviors can be negatively impacted (Viaux-Savelon et al., 2012). Offering a routine anomaly scan ultrasound procedure should be appropriately framed within the context of genetic screening and information provided to women on the conditions being screened for, detection rate, false positive rate, and any risks and benefits. As with all screening tests, women have the right to accept or decline testing without sanction.

Cystic fibrosis (CF) screening

CF is an inherited disease that affects the respiratory and digestive systems and is one of the more common, life-threatening genetic diseases in the United States. More than 10 million Americans, including 1/29 Caucasian Americans, are asymptomatic carriers of the CF gene (Cystic Fibrosis Foundation, 2012) (Table 9.3). A serum screening test can help detect carriers, who could pass the CF gene to their children. CF is an autosomal recessive condition; therefore, a child must inherit one copy of the abnormal CF gene from each parent to develop symptomatic CF.

While Caucasian Americans are at greatest risk for CF, all pregnant women are offered CF serum screening at the first prenatal visit since it affects all races. Testing is done by serum or saliva samples, and can be done anytime in pregnancy. It is important to include the ethnicity of the individual on the laboratory requisition since detection rates and calculation of carrier risk is dependent on this information.

All pregnant women are offered:

- Down syndrome screen
- Neural tube screen
- CF screen
- Amniocentesis or CVS if she will be age 35 or older at the estimated date of birth or if specific indications for testing exist
- Ultrasound fetal anomaly scan
- Full disclosure and informed consent for any of the above
- Option of no testing

Ethnicity-based genetic screening

There are a number of conditions that have a higher prevalence in individuals of certain ethnic groups. Specific genetic screening procedures are offered based on ethnicity and risk. For example, Tay–Sachs disease is more common in Ashkenazi Jews, French Canadians, and Cajuns; sickle cell disease is more common in individuals of African descent; and beta-thalassemia is more common in Mediterranean populations (Table 9.3). CF is currently one of the only ethnicity-based diseases that is part of routine genetic screening offerings, but there is a strong trend to include testing for more conditions in routine screening panels due to population migration and interethnic marriage (Ross, 2012).

The genetic conditions of concern due to ethnicity are all Mendelian conditions and follow an autosomal recessive pattern of inheritance. Mendelian conditions are single gene or monogenic disorders, meaning that a mutation in one specific gene is associated with a specific disease. Mendelian disorders can follow a dominant or recessive pattern of inheritance. Dominant conditions occur when only one copy of the gene mutation is present. Recessive conditions only occur when an individual has two copies of the gene mutation. A carrier of a recessive condition is an individual who has one normal copy of the gene paired with a copy of the abnormal gene. Carriers of recessive conditions usually do not have features of the condition.

Table 9.3 Ethnicity-Related Diseases: Carrier Frequency and Disease Characteristics

Disease	Ethnicity and carrier frequency	Disease characteristics
Thalassemia	Southeast Asian (Cambodian, Hmong, Thai, Laotian, Vietnamese) 1/4 to 1/60 carrier African American 1/15 to 1/50 carrier Mediterranean (Greek, Italian) 1/20 to 1/50 carrier	• Alpha-thalassemia disease can range from mild to a severe anemia that causes stillbirth. • Mothers of an affected baby may develop serious health problems during the pregnancy. • Beta-thalassemia disease causes severe anemia and poor growth beginning in infancy/early childhood. • Life span is often shortened. • Hemoglobin E/beta-thalassemia disease is a variable condition that causes moderate to severe anemia. • Thalassemia usually cannot be cured.
Sickle cell disease	African American 1/12 carrier	• Blood disorders beginning in infancy/early childhood that cause anemia, bone pain, and frequent serious infections • Life span may be shortened. • Treatment may include frequent hospital stays, medications, and blood transfusions. • Severity varies. Some live without serious illness. • Generally cannot be cured
Cystic fibrosis	Caucasian 1/29 carrier	• Body produces thick mucus in the lungs and in the gastrointestinal (GI) system. • Can lead to severe infections, difficulty absorbing food, poor growth • Life span may be shortened to 30–40 years. • Treatment includes pancreatic enzymes, respiratory treatments.
Tay–Sachs disease	Ashkenazi Jewish 1/30 carrier French Canadian 1/15 to 1/30 carrier Louisiana Cajun 1/27 carrier	• Brain and nervous system disease • Progressive muscle weakness, mental deterioration, and blindness • Death occurs by about 3–5 years of age. • No treatment or cure
Canavan disease	Ashkenazi Jewish 1/40 carrier	• Brain and nervous system disease • Progressive loss of myelin causing muscle weakness, mental deterioration, and seizures • Death usually occurs by 10 years of age. • No treatment or cure
Familial dysautonomia	Ashkenazi Jewish 1/30 carrier	• Disease of the nervous system beginning in infancy • Can lead to pain insensitivity, unstable blood pressure and/or temperature, problems with speech and movement, difficulty swallowing • The average life span is 30 years. • Currently no cure
Spinal muscular atrophy	Caucasian 1/47 carrier Asian 1/59 carrier Ashkenazi Jewish 1/67 carrier	• Severe neuromuscular disease • Rapid progressive muscle weakness and paralysis • The average life span is 2 years. • Death caused by respiratory failure

Sources: Cystic Fibrosis Foundation (2012), Johns Hopkins Medicine (2008), Kaiser Permanente (2010), National Tay–Sachs & Allied Diseases Association (ND), Sugarman et al. (2012).

Mendelian disorders are autosomal or X-linked. Most are autosomal, meaning that they occur on the autosomes. The genes for X-linked conditions are located on the X chromosome and also display a dominant or recessive pattern of inheritance. Males are typically affected with X-linked conditions regardless of whether the condition has a dominant or recessive pattern of inheritance since males have only one X chromosome. Females have two copies of the X chromosome, so X-linked conditions typically follow the classic Mendelian pattern of dominance and recessive inheritance. The exception to this rule is that in the female, one of the X chromosomes in each cell is randomly inactivated. Thus, the chromosome with the gene mutation will be inactivated in approximately half of the female's body cells, meaning that the individual will be less affected by the disease and that the expression of the disease is more variable in women.

Carrier screening for autosomal recessive conditions is important since carrier status can be inherited through generations without knowledge of the condition within the family. Carrier screening for a genetic condition is straightforward if there is a family history of the condition; however, in many instances, carriers identified through screening programs report that there is no family history of the condition. If two individuals are carriers for the same genetic condition, with each pregnancy, there is a 25% chance of having a child with the condition, a 50% chance a child will be a carrier like the parents, and a 25% chance the child will be neither affected nor a carrier of the condition. If both parents are carriers of mutations for the same disease, prenatal diagnostic testing (primarily amniocentesis) is offered to determine if the baby has that recessive disease.

There are numerous conditions with a higher incidence in individuals of Ashkenazi Jewish ancestry. In the past, Tay–Sachs disease was the only condition for which carrier testing was available. The American College of Medical Genetics recommends that carrier screening for the following conditions be offered to individuals who have Ashkenazi Jewish ancestry: CF, Canavan disease, familial dysautonomia, Tay–Sachs disease, Fanconi's anemia (group C), Niemann–Pick disease (type A), Bloom syndrome, mucolipidosis IV, and Gaucher's disease (Gross, Pletcher, & Monaghan, 2008).

Screening for the hemoglobinopathies, such as sickle cell disease, beta-thalassemia, and alpha-thalassemia, is best performed by utilizing a complete blood count (CBC) and a hemoglobin electrophoresis (ACOG, 2007b). Although the SickleDex test is available, hemoglobin electrophoresis is recommended to evaluate for sickle cell disease as the SickleDex test is known to have false negatives. Beta- and alpha-thalassemias are found with relative increased frequency in individuals with

African American ancestry and would be missed if the SickleDex alone is performed. In addition, couples in which one member has a sickle cell trait and the other has a beta-thalassemia trait are at risk of having a child with a sickling disorder (sickle cell/beta-thalassemia) that can be as severe as sickle cell disease.

Additional genetic disease carrier screening

In recent years, the inclusion of fragile X syndrome and spinal muscular atrophy (SMA) carrier screening as population-based screening options has been debated. Neither has been found with an increased frequency in a specific population; however, the carrier rates are similar to other conditions for which screening is readily available and encouraged. Fragile X is a rare familial disorder characterized by mental disability ranging from mild to severe and specific facial features, and may include behavioral problems and seizures. Fragile X affects approximately 1 in 4000 males and 1 in 6000–8000 females (CDC, 2011). The diagnosis of fragile X syndrome often occurs in early childhood, in some instances after additional children who are at risk are born. Women with a family history of fragile X-related disorders, unexplained mental retardation or developmental delay, autism, or premature ovarian insufficiency are candidates for genetic counseling and fragile X carrier screening (ACOG, 2010). SMA is an autosomal neuromuscular disease characterized by rapidly progressive muscle weakness and paralysis. There are different types based on the degree of severity. Babies born with SMA have an average life span of 2 years and death is often caused by respiratory failure. Individuals diagnosed at a later age have less severe symptoms and may have normal life spans. Women with a family history of SMA or SMA-like disease should be offered carrier screening (ACOG, 2009).

The fragile X syndrome and SMA family advocacy communities have advocated for including carrier screening for their respective genetic conditions on a population-based screening basis. However, the current recommendations are for selective, risk-based screening.

Diagnostic prenatal genetic testing procedures

Amniocentesis and CVS are the two most commonly performed diagnostic procedures. Percutaneous umbilical blood sampling (PUBS) and ultrasonography may be indicated in certain circumstances. The advantage of diagnostic testing is that fetal chromosomal complement can be accurately determined. Diagnostic genetic testing is routinely offered to all pregnant women who will be age 35 or older at the time of birth because the risk of having an infant with a chromosomal abnormality and the risk of losing the pregnancy due to a procedure-related complication are the same. Although some organizations advocate that all pregnant women should be offered invasive diagnostic testing regardless of age (ACOG, 2007a), this practice can introduce a higher risk of pregnancy loss and complications in women at low risk for chromosomal abnormalities and may be considered unethical (Chitayat et al., 2011).

Amniocentesis

Amniocentesis was the first prenatal diagnostic procedure to examine fetal chromosomes and involves withdrawing a small amount of amniotic fluid from the amniotic sac. Within the fluid, there are skin and other cells from the fetus. These cells contain the fetal chromosomes that can then be analyzed for structural and numerical chromosomal abnormalities. The procedure involves cleaning the woman's abdomen with an iodine-containing wash, and under ultrasound guidance, a needle is inserted and a small amount of amniotic fluid, about 20 mL, is removed. The amniotic fluid is centrifuged and the cells are grown in culture for the cytogenetic analysis. A small portion of the fluid is used to measure the amount of AFP to screen for open NTDs. If the amniotic fluid alpha-fetoprotein (AFAFP) level is elevated, typically above 2.0 multiples of the median (MoM), the sample is analyzed for the presence of acetylcholinesterase (AChE). The presence of AChE indicates the presence of an open NTD in the fetus.

Amniocentesis is typically performed between 15 and 20 weeks' gestation when the amnion and chorion are fused. Complications are rare and include chorioamnionitis and transient amniotic fluid leakage or spotting. Procedure-related pregnancy loss rates are approximately 1 in 300 to 1 in 500 pregnancies (ACOG, 2007a).

Chorionic villus sampling

CVS is offered to all pregnant women who will be age 35 or older at the time of birth, and who elect to have prenatal diagnosis in first trimester. CVS can diagnose Down syndrome and other chromosomal abnormalities but does not detect NTD. It is performed in the first trimester of pregnancy between 10 and 12–6/7 weeks' gestation and involves removing a small portion of the placenta. There are several approaches to obtain the sample and the location of the placenta determines which method is used. The transcervical approach involves inserting a small catheter through the cervix using ultrasound guidance. A catheter is directed to the placenta and a small amount of suction is applied to remove a small amount of chorionic villi (about 20–25 mg). The transabdominal approach is similar in technique to amniocentesis in that a needle is inserted through the abdomen, under ultrasound guidance, but the needle is directed to the placenta rather than the amniotic fluid. Suction is applied and a small amount of placental tissue is removed. Lidocaine is often used with the transabdominal approach.

A primary benefit of CVS is that it allows for earlier and safer pregnancy termination options. Privacy is also enhanced for women since it can be done before the pregnancy is far advanced. CVS pregnancy loss rates are approximately 1 in 100 to 1 in 300 pregnancies and approach the lower loss rate associated with amniocentesis for experienced clinicians (ACOG, 2007a; Ogilvie & Akolekar, 2013; Tabor, Vestergaard, & Lidegaard, 2009).

Percutaneous umbilical blood sampling

PUBS, or cordocentisis, is a less commonly performed diagnostic test since the risk of complications is significant. Procedure-related risks include fetal bleeding, umbilical cord hematoma, maternal–fetal hemorrhage, and fetal bradycardia. However, in certain circumstances, such as evaluation of hydrops or the need to obtain a specimen of fetal blood, it has a place in the armament of available diagnostic procedures. Under ultrasound guidance, a needle is inserted in the umbilical cord and a small amount of blood is withdrawn.

Developments in genetic testing options

Noninvasive prenatal diagnosis (NIPD)—also termed noninvasive prenatal testing (NIPT)—technologies are rapidly evolving. Plasma cell-free DNA analysis allows for analysis of circulating fetal cells in the maternal bloodstream using a technique called massively parallel shotgun sequencing (MPSS). This technique refers to literally thousands of individual reactions conducted simultaneously by a single machine. NIPT offers detection of fetal trisomies 21, 13 and 18 from maternal plasma, and can be performed as early as 10 weeks of gestation. NIPT offers a higher rate of detection and a lower false positive rate than conventional screening (Sparks et al., 2012). Despite excellent detection and low false positive rates, NIPT should still be regarded as a high performance screening method rather than diagnostic testing, as data demonstrate less than 100% sensitivity and specificity. Currently, the National Society of Genetic Counselors (NSGC) and The American College of Obstetricians Gynecologists Committee on Genetics (2012) recommends that NIPT only be utilized for higher-risk pregnancies and accompanied by counseling from a certified genetic counselor. Neither expert group endorses NIPT as a routine, first-tier test. Follow-up with a conventional diagnostic procedure is recommended, depending on test results (Devers et al., 2013). Women age 35 and over, women with a prior history of a child with a trisomy, ultrasound findings congruent with aneuploidy, or women with a positive first or second trimester serum screen result can be offered NIPT (ACOG, 2012). Clinical data supporting use in a general screening population has been accumulating since these recommendations were issued (Fairbrother, Johnson, Musci, & Song, 2013), and it is likely NIPT will be more offered to all pregnant women in the future. The use of NIPT in a general screening population allows for equal access to a technology that can detect more trisomy cases, avoid false positive results resulting in unnecessary costly and invasive diagnostic testing as compared with conventional prenatal screening tests. The cost of this technology is still relatively expensive when compared with conventional prenatal screening procedures, but is comparable with the costs of amniocentesis. Biotech companies developing these methods hope to eventually provide accurate diagnostic information on whether or not a fetus actually has a trisomy disorder. NIPT may obviate the need for amniocentesis or CVS, both of which are invasive and pose a small risk to the expectant mother and/or fetus.

Chromosomal microarray analysis (CMA) is a genetic test on fetal cells obtained by CVS or amniocentesis that finds small amounts of genetic material that traditional testing such as karyotyping cannot detect. Researchers suggest that this test has the potential to identify potential intellectual disabilities and congenital abnormalities as well as to determine why a pregnancy failed (Reddy, Page, & Saade, 2012). CMA testing is sensitive for many disorders and is currently offered in some large healthcare centers.

Scope of practice considerations

Genetic counselors are health professionals with specialized graduate degrees and experience in the areas of medical genetics and counseling. Referral to a genetic counselor is appropriate for women with more complex personal health and family histories.

Consider referral to a genetic counselor:

- Abnormal serum marker screening results
- Fetal abnormalities on prenatal ultrasound
- Personal or family history of a known or suspected genetic disorder, birth defect, or chromosome abnormality
- Family history of mental retardation of unknown etiology
- Women with a medical condition known or suspected to affect fetal development

---

Women who choose to have diagnostic procedures need to be referred to physicians who are experts in these procedures.

Ethical considerations in genetic screening

It is the responsibility of the prenatal care provider to provide adequate, neutral counseling with full informed consent and to provide follow-up for positive genetic tests (ACOG, 2008a). "Consent" and "informed consent" are not the same. Consent to a procedure or test applies to decisions that are of low risk and cases in which there is one clear best choice (Whitney, McGuire, & McCullough, 2003). Genetic screening and testing are high risk and high stakes for women and families with many choices and possible life altering scenarios. Despite the ethical responsibility to provide informed consent, research indicates that many pregnant women accept the tests offered without being informed of the side effects, complications, and implications of positive test results (Dahl et al., 2011; Press, 2000). Informed compliance, where women receive an explanation of testing procedure with limited or no additional information, is not an ethical practice, yet it is a common prenatal care practice (Ackmann, 2005; van den Berg, Timmermans, Ten Kate, van Vugt, & van der Wal, 2005).

In a commonly accepted definition, informed consent consists of these five components: (1) competence to understand and decide, (2) disclosure of risks and benefits, (3) understanding of information and plans, (4) voluntariness in choosing testing or no testing, and (5) consent or authorizing the choice (Beauchamp & Childress, 2001, p. 79). One study examined 78 studies of prenatal screening and found an overwhelming inadequacy in achievement of informed consent, with healthcare providers consistently failing to meet criteria 2–5 listed earlier (Seavilleklein, 2009). It is a primary responsibility of the prenatal health-care provider to obtain informed consent, not simply consent or informed compliance. It is each woman's individual choice to accept or decline any testing options. Women deserve to have a full understanding of what will happen to them and their fetus before proceeding with any type of testing or treatment.

The power of health-care technology to identify the genetic traits of embryos and fetuses is rapidly increasing. New genetic testing options will continue to bring additional ethical challenges to health-care providers and to women and families. The ability to appropriately manage resolution of ethical dilemmas and conflicts that may result in the consideration of genetic screening and diagnosis testing is an essential skill for prenatal care providers (Lea, Williams, & Donahue, 2005).

Communicating about genetic testing and risk during prenatal care

Pretest counseling

Pretest counseling is perhaps the most important component of offering prenatal genetic testing and screening. The purpose of pretest counseling is to provide full and balanced information on genetic screening options to allow women to make their best personal choice. The principles of nondirective, noncoercive counseling should be employed when talking to women about their screening and testing options. It is important to provide counseling in a manner that empowers women to make decisions that are best for them and their families through information about their risks and options, in a culturally sensitive, confidential manner. When discussing genetic risk and testing choices, women need to know the following to make an informed choice (Hodgson & Gaff, 2013; Lea et al., 2005):

- the condition(s) for which the test is directed
- the women's numerical risk for the condition
- the test to detect the condition
- when and how the test is performed
- risks and benefits of that test
- that a assessment of probability is not a diagnosis
- the meaning of the test results
- the probability for false positive and false negative results
- implications of a positive test result including psychological effects
- clear choice that choosing no testing is an equal option
- that the woman and her partner will be faced with difficult decisions if the results are positive
- how common the abnormalities are and possible consequences for the child
- alternatives after diagnosis
- resources for additional information

The points of discussion cover the principles of informed consent. It is especially important to explain false positives when discussing maternal serum genetic screening options. For example, the quad screen has a false positive rate of 5%. This means that 1 out of 20 women who have the test will have a positive screen yet have a normal baby. Many of these women with positive screens will undergo invasive diagnostic testing yet have a normal baby. All women also need to be aware that a negative screening test does not guarantee the birth of an unaffected baby.

Another consideration to discuss is the question, "What would you do in the event of positive results"? Some women would agree to invasive testing, and others would not want to introduce added risk in a most likely normal pregnancy. Informed consent requires taking the time needed to adequately provide detailed teaching about the implications of genetic screening. Consider this scenario. A woman wants to have the first-trimester screening or quad screen but tells you she would never agree to invasive testing. This is a potential dilemma for her. Would she worry during her entire pregnancy that something was wrong with her baby? Would she feel guilty for not having the test when her care providers thought she should? Since most women who screen positive ultimately are found to have a normal fetus, she will likely worry for nothing. These points are essential to bring up in discussions of genetic testing options to encourage women to fully consider the possible results in making their testing decisions. Discussions on prenatal genetic testing are complex, and providing written material to supplement the discussions will allow women time to integrate the information with their own needs and values.

Psychosocial effects in genetic testing

For contemporary American women living in a high-tech information age, the current pressures and expectations about appropriate maternal behavior, including genetic testing choices, are hard to escape. Information about new procreative technologies and appropriate maternal behavior is available in popular magazines, reality television shows, and popular books for pregnant women and potential mothers. In this context, the domain of maternal responsibilities seems infinitely expandable. The slogan "information is power" has become something of a truism in contemporary American culture. However, information is not neutral; it is often used to empower some people or to justify some interests at the expense of others. Robin Gregg (1993), a sociological researcher in genetic testing issues, states (p. 70):

> Information and knowledge can be used as a tool to maintain their power or to disempower others. Those who wish to control pregnant women's behavior can be empowered by research findings, but the information may not empower pregnant women themselves. In fact, the information may make them feel powerless. In this light, one of the paradoxical things about prenatal tests and procreative technologies is that their existence has created a situation where difficult choices must be made.

Conclusions based on research done by Gregg (p. 69) indicate that

> When the participants made choices about prenatal testing and other procreative technologies, they experienced subtle and overt outside pressures on their choices

and behaviors. They faced advice and comments from strangers, acquaintances, co-workers, family members and health providers. Women felt they had choices, but they were burdened with their own and other people's expectations that they make the "right" choices. *Women in the study experienced feelings of guilt and ambivalence both before and after they made prenatal screening and testing choices.* The women in the study discovered that their prenatal choices were double-edged swords. Though they welcomed the freedom to make prenatal choices, they discovered that these choices were accompanied by social and internal pressures and feelings of ambivalence and guilt.

There are aspects of prenatal testing decision making that are much more complex than for other health issues. First, a woman considering testing must simultaneously weigh and compare several risk figures: (1) her risk of giving birth to an affected child, (2) her risk of having an abnormal test result, and (3) the risk that the test may cause a pregnancy loss. This personal risk assessment is made even more complex because of the value-laden nature of the potential outcomes being weighed. Numerous hypothetical trade-offs and consideration of possible scenarios depending on choices made are required in the process of making a decision. How risks are perceived individually may differ from the way that they are perceived in relationship to each other. Women need to create scenarios on how they might think, feel, act, and respond to the news of a baby with a problem and weigh them against each other. Additionally, the process of making a decision about prenatal testing typically includes at least some discussion with the woman's partner or family members. The negotiation about testing options is likely to involve not only two potentially different perceptions of risk but also two somewhat different sets of attitudes and prior experiences (Gates, 2004).

Prenatal genetic testing and the tentative pregnancy

Genetic testing is a serious undertaking for both women and their health-care providers. In several studies, women who had serum screening and who fully understand the information gained from testing suspended emotional attachment to their fetus pending the results of the testing (Lawson & Turriff-Jonasson, 2006; Rowe, Fisher & Quinlivan, 2009). This disruption in attachment can be significant to the normal process of maternal identity development. Barbara Katz-Rothman (1993) coined the term "tentative pregnancy" to describe this phenomenon in the 1980s with regard to women who underwent amniocentesis and exhibited delayed attachment behaviors. This delay in prenatal attachment may go unrecog-

nized and may be more prevalent with the advent of routine genetic testing offered to all pregnant women.

Women who receive screening information indicating a higher risk for the fetus having Down syndrome describe the waiting time for having an amniocentesis for diagnosis as a time when they repressed the pregnancy (Baillie et al., 2000; Georgsson et al., 2006; Susanne, Sissel, Ulla, Charlotta, & Sonja, 2006). They avoided thinking about the baby and denied their pregnancy in different ways, such as expressing no feelings of happiness about the pregnancy, not disclosing the news of the pregnancy to family or friends, not preparing baby supplies or not thinking about names for the baby. This "time-out" lasted until a normal result from the invasive test was received. Even after a reassuring diagnostic test, some women may exhibit higher levels of anxiety and worry about the health of their fetus, indicating that false positive results can have a lasting effect on pregnant women (Green, Hewison, Bekker, Bryant, & Cuckle, 2004; Sapp et al., 2010). All prenatal health-care providers need to be aware of the ways in which prenatal testing changes women's experiences of pregnancy.

Genetic testing may not offer enough information to make a fully informed decision, thereby making already difficult decisions for women and families even harder. For example, prenatal CF carrier testing can identify couples who are both carriers. When the CF mutations are identified in the parents, prenatal diagnosis can be performed to determine whether a fetus has inherited a CF gene mutation from each parent. Knowing that a fetus has inherited two CF mutations, however, does not predict the severity of CF in the baby. For couples in this situation, the ethical dilemma involves the decision to continue or to end a pregnancy without having knowledge of the severity of the disorder.

Perspective on genetic counseling during prenatal care

Prenatal diagnosis and counseling can be an emotional issue for both the health-care provider and the client. Providers are likely to have an opinion about whether testing is valuable or not, in which situation it is more valuable, what women should do with the results of their tests, and when certain tests should be ordered. The challenge for health-care providers is to stay objective, to inform women all of their potential options, and to provide accurate, objective information regarding what tests are available, as well as the risks and benefits of these tests. To do this, health-care providers must remain current in their knowledge of genetic testing and closely examine personal biases. Pregnancy termination is one of the many choices involved in genetic counseling and testing. This is a topic that will always be debated with strong feelings on both sides of the issue. It is each woman's own choice to have or not have prenatal genetic screening and/or testing and what to do with that information. It is the responsibility of the health-care provider to give appropriate, nonjudgmental, and complete information that fully enables women to make these decisions, and that provides respect and support to women in their right to make decisions that will affect their lives.

Case study

Donna is a 38-year-old G2P0010 woman presenting for her first prenatal visit at 7 weeks' gestation. Her first pregnancy 6 years ago ended at 8 weeks' gestation with a spontaneous abortion. She and her husband have been trying for a pregnancy for the last year and are excited to be pregnant. She is aware there is an increased risk of birth defects in older women and states she "knows she is high risk."

A complete history and physical examination were completed. She has a history of mild asthma controlled with occasional use of an inhaled bronchodilator, and she had an appendectomy at age 22. Her family history is unremarkable. A three-generation genetic pedigree was completed with no factors indicating increased genetic risk. She works part time as a realtor and exercises three to five times weekly. Her physical exam finds a body mass index (BMI) of 22.2, BP 120/66, anteverted uterus compatible with 7 weeks' gestation and normal physical findings.

ASSESSMENT: Donna is a healthy 38-year-old at 7 weeks' gestation.

PLAN: The findings of her history and physical exam were reviewed and Donna was reassured that her primary increase in genetic risk was due to her higher maternal age. The only birth defects that increase in incidence with maternal age are chromosome abnormalities. Since she is healthy and does not have medical conditions such as hypertension or diabetes, her pregnancy is likely to progress normally. At 38 years old, Donna had a 1/149 chance (less than 1%) to have a child with a chromosomal abnormality and approximately 1/180 chance of a child with Down syndrome. A Paling palette tool depicting her chance of a baby with Down syndrome out of 1000 women was used to help facilitate understanding of her age-related genetic risks. Donna stated she was somewhat familiar with Down syndrome and this condition was reviewed for clarification.

Genetic screening options were then offered and explained at this visit. She was informed of NT, serum integrated screen, and serum quad screen with regard to the procedures, test timing, information gained by the tests, false positives, and follow-up for abnormal results. It was stressed that these tests do not diagnose a problem but indicate an increased possibility of a problem. Donna was informed that most women with abnormal results have a normal baby. Ultrasound as a noninvasive means of providing limited screening was also offered.

Because of her age, genetic diagnostic testing choices were also offered and discussed. Amniocentesis and CVS were offered with explanations on the procedure, timing, and information gained and procedure risks. Both procedures involve a small risk of pregnancy loss, estimated at 1/300 to 1/500 for amniocentesis and approximately 1/100 to 1/300 for CVS. Donna was informed that CVS offers the advantage of earlier diagnosis and termination of the pregnancy if that was an option for her. Donna was also advised that the choice of no testing was an equal option and she needs to consider what she would do with the information gained as she considers her choices. After the discussion, Donna indicated that she and her husband were unlikely to terminate the pregnancy regardless of fetal condition. She also stated that she is concerned about the risk of the invasive tests.

She was provided with written information about the screening and diagnostic tests to review at home. Donna was advised to call the office if she decided on the integrated screen or the CVS to ensure that scheduling was done within the appropriate time frame. Her regular prenatal appointment was schedule for 4 weeks from now.

Donna called the office 1 week after her appointment and stated she and her husband decided to do the integrated screen as it offered a high detection rate for Down syndrome with a low false positive rate. She stated they did not want to take the risks of invasive testing and that they wanted to be prepared if the baby had a problem. At her 10-week prenatal appointment, her choices were reviewed and confirmed.

A NT and blood draw for PAPP-A were done when Donna was at 11 weeks' gestation. The second blood draw for AFP, hCG, uE3, and inhibin-A (inhA) was done at 16 weeks' gestation. Results were ready at 17 weeks' gestation. The results came back screen negative with risk for Down syndrome on integrated screening (1 in 270). The AFP result was reported as screen negative at <2.5 MoM. Donna expressed great relief at this news and was excited to start preparing for the baby.

Summary

Offering women genetic testing choices is standard care and allows women and families expanded control over reproduction. The goal of screening is to identify early disease or risk in order to implement preventive therapy and to provide women with information relevant to reproductive decisions. Prenatal genetic tests offer increasingly comprehensive identification of genetic conditions and susceptibilities. It is essential that these testing options be offered with a nondirective approach and full informed consent so women have a full understanding of testing ramifications. For women choosing to undergo prenatal testing, most will get results confirming a normal pregnancy. Some will learn their baby has a defect or developmental condition, and in a small number of cases, testing will yield results that health-care providers are unable to interpret. Prenatal genetic testing offers more information about the unborn fetus yet raises additional questions about what to do with the information. Prenatal health-care providers must be aware of the physical and emotional impact of prenatal genetic testing, and possess the skill to provide true informed consent as well as navigate the ethical dilemmas that may arise. Genetic testing technologies are expanding rapidly and will continue to give women more reproductive choices while creating ethical challenges for new parents.

Resources for women and their families

American College of Nurse Midwives (ACNM) Web site with printable resources on prenatal testing, several also available in Spanish: http://www.midwife.org/Share-With-Women

March of Dimes Web site with information on specific genetic conditions and birth defects as well as testing options: http://www.marchofdimes.com/profession als/medicalresources_pocketfacts.html

U.S. Department of Health and Human Services Web site with information on prenatal genetic tests: http://www.womenshealth.gov/pregnancy/you-are-preg nant/prenatal-care-tests.cfm

Resources for health-care providers

Claire Altman Heine Foundation uses its funding to identify carriers of SMA, support population-based SMA carrier screening, raise awareness of SMA, and educate the public and medical communities about SMA: http://www.clairealtmanheinefoundation. org/

Genetics Home Reference by the NIH offers information on all genetic conditions with guidelines and resources for professionals: http://ghr.nlm.nih.gov/

National Institutes of Health (NIH) Web site devoted to genetic research and educating professionals about genetics: http://www.genome.gov/Education/

National Society for Genetic Counselors Web site, with a resource section for professionals: http://www.nsgc. org/

Victor Center for Jewish Genetic Diseases is dedicated to ensure access to comprehensive genetic education, counseling services, and screenings. There is section for health-care providers: http://www.victorcenters. org/

References

Ackmann, E. A. (2005). Prenatal testing gone awry: The birth of a conflict of ethics and liability. *Indiana Health Law Review*, 2, 199–224.

Åhman, A., Runestam, K., & Sarkadi, A. (2010). Did I really want to know this? Pregnant women's reaction to detection of a soft marker during ultrasound screening. *Patient Education and Counseling*, 81(1), 87–93.

American College of Obstetricians and Gynecologists (ACOG). (2010). Carrier screening for fragile X syndrome. Committee Opinion No. 469. American. *Obstetrics and Gynecology*, 116, 1008–1010.

American College of Obstetricians and Gynecologists (ACOG). (2011). Family history as risk assessment tool. Committee Opinion No. 478. *Obstetrics and Gynecology*, 117, 747–750.

American College of Obstetricians and Gynecologists (ACOG). (2012). Noninvasive prenatal testing for fetal aneuploidy. Committee Opinion No. 545. *Obstetrics and Gynecology*, 120, 1532–1534.

American College of Obstetricians and Gynecologists (ACOG). (2007a). Screening for fetal chromosomal abnormalities. ACOG Practice Bulleting No. 77. *Obstetrics and Gynecology*, 109(1), 217–227.

American College of Obstetricians and Gynecologists. (2007b). Hemoglobinopathies in pregnancy. ACOG Practice Bulletin No. 78. *Obstetrics and Gynecology*, 109, 229–237.

American College of Obstetricians and Gynecologists (ACOG). (July 2003). Neural tube defects. ACOG Practice Bulletin, number 44 (reaffirmed 2011).

American College of Obstetricians and Gynecologists (ACOG). (2008a). Ethical issues in genetic testing. ACOG Committee Opinion No. 410. *Obstetrics and Gynecology*, 111, 1495–1502.

American College of Obstetricians and Gynecologists (ACOG). (2008b). ACOG Practice Bulletin number 98, October 2008 Ultrasonography in pregnancy. Abuhamad AZ, ACOG Committee on Practice Bulletins-Obstetrics. *Obstetrics and Gynecology*, 112(4), 951.

American College of Obstetricians and Gynecologists (ACOG). (2009). Spinal muscular atrophy. ACOG Committee Opinion No. 432. *Obstetrics and Gynecology*, 113, 1194–1196.

American College of Radiology (ACR), American College of Obstetricians and Gynecologists (ACOG), and the American Institute of Ultrasound in Medicine (AIUM). (2007). ACR–ACOG–AIUM practice guideline for the performance of obstetrical ultrasound: Practice guideline, obstetrical ultrasound, p. 1. Retrieved from http://www.acr.org/~/media/F7BC35BD59264E7CBE648F6D1BB8 B8E2.pdf

Baillie, C., Smith, J., Hewison, J., & Mason, G. (2000). Ultrasound screening for chromosomal abnormality: Women's reactions to false positive results. *British Journal of Health Psychology, 5*(4), 377–394.

Ball, J. R., Van Riper, M., Engstrom, J. L., & Matheson, J. K. (2005). Incidental finding of ultrasound markers for Down syndrome in the second trimester of pregnancy. *Journal of Midwifery & Women's Health, 50,* 243–245.

Beauchamp, T. L., & Childress, J. F. (2001). *Principles of biomedical ethics* (5th ed.). New York: Oxford University Press U.S.

Blencowe, H., Cousens, S., Modell, B., & Lawn, J. (2010). Folic acid to reduce neonatal mortality from neural tube disorders. *International Journal of Epidemiology, 39*(Suppl. 1), i110–i121.

Canick, J. A., Lambert-Messerlian, G. M., Palomaki, G. E., Neveux, L. M., Ball, R. H., Nyberg, D. A., . . . D'Alton, M. E. for the First and Second Trimester Evaluation of Risk (FASTER) Trial Research Consortium (2006). Comparison of serum markers in first-trimester Down syndrome screening. *Obstetrics and Gynecology, 108*(5), 1192–1199.

Centers for Disease Control and Prevention (CDC). (2009). Racial/Ethnic differences in the birth prevalence of Spina Bifida—United States 1995–2005. *MMWR. Morbidity and Mortality Weekly Report, 57*(53), 1409–1413.

Centers for Disease Control and Prevention (CDC). (2011). Fragile X syndrome and associated disorders. Retrieved from http://www.cdc.gov/features/fragilex/

Chasen, S. T., McCullough, L. B., & Chervenak, F. A. (2004). Is nuchal translucency screening associated with different rates of invasive testing in an older obstetric population? *American Journal of Obstetrics and Gynecology, 190,* 769–774.

Chitayat, D., Langlois, S., Wilson, R. D., & SOGC Genetics Committee; CCMG Prenatal Diagnosis Committee. (2011). Prenatal screening for fetal aneuploidy in singleton pregnancies. SOGC clinical Practice Guideline No. 261, July 2011. *Journal of Obstetrics and Gynaecology Canada, 33,* 736–750.

Crane, J. P., LeFevre, M. L., Winborn, R. C., Evans, J. K., Ewigman, B. G., Bain, R. P., . . . & McNellis, D. (1994). A randomized trial of prenatal ultrasonographic screening: Impact on the detection, management, and outcome of anomalous fetuses. *American Journal of Obstetrics and Gynecology, 171*(2), 392–399.

Cystic Fibrosis Foundation. (2012). About cystic fibrosis. Retrieved from http://www.cff.org/index.cfm

Dahl, K., Hvidman, L., Jørgensen, F. S., Henriques, C., Olesen, F., Kjaergaard, H., & Kesmodel, U. S. (2011). First-trimester Down syndrome screening: Pregnant women's knowledge. *Ultrasound in Obstetrics and Gynecology, 38,* 145–151. doi:10.1002/uog.8839

Devers, P., Cronister, A., Ormond, K., Facio, F., Brasington, C., & Flodman, P. (2013). Noninvasive prenatal testing/noninvasive prenatal diagnosis: The position of the National Society of Genetic Counselors. *Journal of Genetic Counseling.* doi:10.1007/s10897-012-9564-0

Driscoll, D., & Gross, S. (2009). Screening for fetal aneuploidy and neural tube defects. *Genetics in Medicine, 11*(11), 818–821.

Fairbrother, G., Johnson, S., Musci, T. J., & Song, K. (2013). Clinical experience of noninvasive prenatal testing with cell-free DNA for fetal trisomies 21, 18, and 13, in a general screening population. *Prenatal Diagnosis, 33,* 580–583.

Gates, E. A. (2004). Communicating risk in prenatal genetic testing. *Journal of Midwifery & Women's Health, 49,* 220–227. doi:10.1016/S1526-9523(04)00106-0

Georgsson, S., Öhman, S., Saltvedt, U., Waldenström, C., Grunewald, S., & Olin-Lauritzen, S. (2006). Pregnant women's responses to information about an increased risk of carrying a baby with Down syndrome. *Birth (Berkeley, Calif.), 33*(1), 664–673.

Green, J. M., Hewison, J., Bekker, H. L., Bryant, L. D., & Cuckle, H. S. (2004). Psychological aspects of genetic screening of pregnant women and newborns: A systematic review. *Health Technology Assessment, 8*(33), 1–109.

Gregg, R. (1993). "Choice" as a double-edged sword: Information, guilt and mother-blaming in a high-tech age. *Women & Health, 20*(3), 53–73.

Gross, S. J., Pletcher, B. A., & Monaghan, K. G. (2008). American College of Medical Geneticists (AMCG). Practice Guideline: Carrier screening in individuals of Ashkenazi Jewish decent. *Genetics in Medicine, 10*(1), 54–56.

Hendricks, K. A., Simpson, J. S., & Larsen, R. D. (1999). Neural tube defects along the Texas-Mexico border, 1993–1995. *American Journal of Epidemiology, 149,* 1119–1127.

Hodgson, J., & Gaff, C. (2013). Enhancing family communication about genetics: Ethical and professional dilemmas. *Journal of Genetic Counseling, 22*(1), 16–21.

Johns Hopkins Medicine. (2008). Genetic carrier screening. Retrieved from http://www.hopkinsmedicine.org/fertility/resources/genetic_screening.html

Kaasen, A., Helbig, A., Malt, U. F., Naes, T., Skari, H., & Haugen, G. (2010). Acute maternal social dysfunction, health perception and psychological distress after ultrasonographic detection of a fetal structural anomaly. *BJOG: An International Journal of Obstetrics and Gynaecology, 117*(9), 1127–1138.

Kaiser Permanente. (2010). Ethnicity based genetic screening. Retrieved from http://mydoctor.kaiserpermanente.org/ncal/specialty/genetics/screening_programs/ebsgeneticscreening.jsp

Larsson, A., Svalenius, E., Marsal, K., & Dykes, A. (2009). Parental level of anxiety, sense of coherence and state of mind when choroid plexus cysts have been identified at a routine ultrasound examination in the second trimester of pregnancy: A case control study. *Journal of Psychosomatic Obstetrics and Gynaecology, 30,* 95–100.

Lawson, K. L., & Turriff-Jonasson, S. I. (2006). Maternal serum screening and psychosocial attachment to pregnancy. *Journal of Psychosomatic Research, 60*(4), 371–378.

Lea, D. H., Williams, J., & Donahue, M. P. (2005). Ethical issues in genetic testing. *Journal of Midwifery & Women's Health, 50*(3), 234–240.

Lumley, J., Watson, L., Watson, M., & Bower, C. (2001). Periconceptional supplementation with folate and/or multivitamins for preventing neural tube defects. *Cochrane Database of Systematic Reviews,* (3), CD001056.

Malone, F. D., Canick, J. A., Ball, R. H., Nuberg, D. A., Comstock, C. H., Bukowski, R., D'Alton, M. E., & For the First-and Second-Trimester Evaluation of Risk (FASTER) Research Consortium. (2005). First-trimester or second-trimester screening, or both, for Down's syndrome. *The New England Journal of Medicine, 352,* 2001–2011.

Mills, J. L., & Signore, C. (2004). Neural tube defect rates before and after food fortification with folic acid. *Birth Defects Research Part A: Clinical and Molecular Teratology, 70*(11), 844–845.

National Institute of Child Health and Human Development (NICHHD). (2012). How many people are affected by or are at risk for neural tube defects? *Neural Tube Defects (NTDs).* U.S. National Institutes of Health.

National Tay–Sachs & Allied Diseases Association (ND). (2013). Tay-Sachs Disease. Retrieved from http://www.tay-sachs.org/taysachs_disease.php

Neilson, J. P. (1998). Ultrasound for fetal assessment in early pregnancy. *Cochrane Database of Systematic Reviews,* (4), CD000182. doi:10.1002/14651858.CD000182

Ogilvie, C. M., & Akolekar, R. (2013). Procedure-related pregnancy loss following invasive prenatal sampling: Time for a new approach to risk assessment and counseling. *Expert Review of Obstetrics & Gynecology, 8*(2), 135–142.

Palomaki, G. E., Lambert-Messerlian, G. M., & Canick, J. A. (2007). A summary analysis of Down syndrome markers in the late first trimester. *Advances in Clinical Chemistry, 43*, 177–210.

Parker, S. E., Mai, C. T., Canfield, M. A., Rickard, R., Wang, Y., Meyer, R. E., . . . Correa A., & for the National Birth Defects Prevention Network. (2010). Updated national birth prevalence estimates for selected birth defects in the United States, 2004–2006. *Birth Defects Research. Part A, Clinical and Molecular Teratology, 88(12),* 1008–1016.

Platt, L. D., Greene, N., Johnson, A., Zachary, J., Thom, E., Krantz, D., & First Trimester Maternal Serum Biochemistry and Fetal Nuchal Translucency Screening (BUN) Study Group. (2004). Sequential pathways of testing after first-trimester screening for trisomy 21. *Obstetrics and Gynecology, 104*, 661–666.

Press, N. (2000). Assessing the expressive character of prenatal testing: The choices made or the choices made available. In E. Parens & A. Asch (Eds.), *Prenatal testing and disability rights* (pp. 214–233). Washington, DC: Georgetown University Press.

Quest Diagnostics. (2013). Prenatal screening and diagnosis of neural tube defects, Down syndrome, and Trisomy 18. Retrieved from http://www.questdiagnostics.com/home/physicians/testing -services/condition/genetics.html

Reddy, U. M., Page, G. P., & Saade, G. R. (2012). Two noninvasive approaches to prenatal diagnosis offer promise—But practicality and cost are uncertain. *Birth, 367*(23), 2185–2193.

Ross, L. F. (2012). A re-examination of the use of ethnicity in prenatal carrier testing. *American Journal of Medical Genetics. Part A, 158A*(1), 19–23.

Rothman, B. K. (1993). *The tentative pregnancy: How amniocentesis changes the experience of motherhood.* New York: W.W. Norton.

Rowe, H., Fisher, J., & Quinlivan, J. (2009). Women who are well informed about prenatal genetic screening delay emotional attachment to their fetus. *Journal of Psychosomatic Obstetrics & Gynecology, 30*(1), 34–41.

Sapp, J. C., Hull, S. C., Duffe, S., Zornetzer, S., Sutton, E., Marteau, T. M., & Biesccker, B. B. (2010). Ambivalence toward undergoing invasive prenatal testing: An exploration of its origins. *Prenatal Diagnosis, 30*, 77–82. doi:10.1002/pd.234

Seavilleklein, V. (2009). Challenging the rhetoric of choice in prenatal screening. *Bioethics, 23*, 68–77.

Smith-Bindman, R., Hosmer, W., Feldstein, V. A., Deeks, J. J., & Goldberg, J. D. (2001). Second-trimester ultrasound to detect fetuses with Down syndrome: A meta-analysis. *JAMA: The Journal of the American Medical Association, 285*(8), 1044–1055. doi:10.1001/jama.285.8.1044

Sparks, A. B., Wang, E. T., Struble, C. A., Barrett, W., Stokowski, R., McBride, C., . . . Oliphant, A. (2012). Selective analysis of cell-free DNA in maternal blood for evaluation of fetal trisomy. *Prenatal Diagnosis, 32*, 3–9. doi:10.1002/pd.2922

Sugarman, E., Nagan, N., Zhu, H., Akmaev, V. R., Zhou, Z., Rohlfs, E. M., . . . Allitto, B. A. (2012). Pan-ethnic carrier screening and prenatal diagnosis for spinal muscular atrophy: Clinical laboratory analysis of >72 400 specimens. *European Journal of Human Genetics, 20*(1), 27–32.

Susanne, G. O., Sissel, S., Ulla, W., Charlotta, G., & Sonja, O. L. (2006). Pregnant women's responses to information about an increased risk of carrying a baby with Down syndrome. *Birth (Berkeley, Calif.), 33*(1), 64–73.

Tabor, A., Vestergaard, C. H. F., & Lidegaard, Ø. (2009). Fetal loss rate after chorionic villus sampling and amniocentesis: An 11-year national registry study. *Ultrasound in Obstetrics and Gynecology, 34*, 19–24. doi:10.1002/uog.6377

Trisomy 18 Foundation. (2013). What is Trisomy 18? Retrieved from http://www.trisomy18.org/site/PageServer?pagename=whatisT18 _whatis

U.S. Preventive Services Task Force (USPSTF). (n.d.). *Screening for ultrasonography in pregnancy.* Retrieved from http://www.uspreven tiveservicestaskforce.org/uspstf/uspsuspg.htm

van den Berg, M., Timmermans, D. R., Ten Kate, L. P., van Vugt, J. M., & van der Wal, G. (2005). Are pregnant women making informed choices about prenatal screening? *Genetics in Medicine, 7*(5), 332–338.

Van den Hof, M. C., & Wilson, R. D. (2005). Fetal soft markers in obstetric ultrasound. *Journal of obstetrics and gynaecology Canada: JOGC = Journal d'obstétrique et gynécologie du Canada: JOGC, 27*(6), 592.

Van der Zalm, J. E., & Byrne, P. J. (2006). Seeing baby: Women's experience prenatal ultrasound examination and unexpected fetal diagnosis. *Journal of Perinatology, 26*(7), 403–408.

Viaux-Savelon, S., Dommergues, M., Rosenblum, O., Bodeau, N., Aidane, E., Philippon, O., . . . Cohen, D. (2012). Prenatal ultrasound screening: False positive soft markers may alter maternal representations and mother-infant interaction. *PLoS ONE, 7*(1), e30935. doi:10.1371/journal.pone.0030935

Whitney, S. N., McGuire, A. L., & McCullough, L. B. (2003). A typology of shared decision making, informed consent, and simple consent. *Annals of Internal Medicine, 140*(1), 54–59.

Wolpert, C. M., & Speer, M. C. (2005). Harnessing the power of the pedigree. *Journal of Midwifery and Women's Health, 50*(3), 189–196.

10

Assessment of fetal well-being

Jenifer Fahey

Relevant terms

Acidemia—increased concentration of hydrogen ions in blood (increased acidity of blood); normal, term newborn umbilical cord arterial blood pH is 7.27 ± 0.07

Acidosis—increased concentration of hydrogen ions in tissue (increased acidity of tissue)

Asphyxia—combination of hypoxia and metabolic acidosis. This is due to profound and/or prolonged lack of oxygen. Asphyxia is associated with a risk of brain damage.

Fetal heart rate (FHR) baseline—the baseline FHR is the predominant heart rate during a 10-minute segment rounded to the nearest 5 beats per minute (bpm); normal range of FHR is 110–160 bpm

Fetal heart rate (FHR) variability—baseline variability is defined as fluctuations in the FHR of more than two cycles per minute; the presence of variability is an indicator of fetal oxygenation

Hypoxemia—decreased oxygen content of blood; normal, term fetal scalp blood PO_2 is 21.8 ± 2.6 (mmHg)

Hypoxia—decreased oxygen content in tissue

Negative predictive value—likelihood that if a test is negative, the condition is truly absent in that individual; the nonstress test (NST) has good negative predictive value for fetal acidemia

Oligohydramnios—abnormally low amniotic fluid volume of ≤200–500 mL—diagnosed on ultrasound when the largest pocket of fluid is <2 cm or the amniotic fluid index (AFI) is <5 cm

Parasympathetic nervous system—the part of the autonomic nervous system that usually inhibits or opposes the physiological effects of the sympathetic nervous system; it slows the fetal heart rate

Polyhydramnios—abnormally high amniotic fluid volume—diagnosed on ultrasound when the largest cord-free pocket of fluid is >8 cm or the AFI is ≥25 cm

Positive predictive value—likelihood that if a test is positive, the condition is truly present in that individual. The NST has poor positive predictive value for fetal acidemia

Sensitivity—ability of a test to identify that a condition or disease is present, for example, the ability of the NST to identify the presence of fetal academia; the NST has poor sensitivity for fetal acidemia

Specificity—ability of a test to identify that a condition or disease is absent, for example, the ability of the NST to determine that acidemia is not present; the NST has excellent specificity for acidemia

---

Introduction

One of the primary responsibilities of providers of prenatal care is to monitor fetal well-being, as evidenced by growth and oxygenation. There are multiple techniques and technologies available to assist in this task—from time-honored measures such as measurement of fundal growth and fetal movement counts (FMCs) to the newer, technologically based tests such as ultrasound assessment of fetal breathing movements and Doppler velocimetry. Prenatal care providers will conduct some of these tests, while others are performed by specialists or subspecialists such as perinatologists. In these cases, the primary prenatal care provider is responsible for ensuring that, when necessary, women in their care are appropriately referred for testing and assessment. Often, it is

Prenatal and Postnatal Care: A Woman-Centered Approach, First Edition. Edited by Robin G. Jordan, Janet L. Engstrom, Julie A. Marfell, and Cindy L. Farley.

also the responsibility of the primary prenatal care provider to interpret the results of those tests and to make an appropriate management plan based on the findings. In all cases, the prenatal care provider must be able to educate the woman regarding the indications for testing, testing procedures, test results, and the management plan based on those results. This chapter focuses on those assessment techniques that evaluate fetal circulation and oxygenation starting at approximately 24 weeks' estimated gestational age (EGA) but prior to the onset of labor.

These tests of fetal well-being include:

- FMCs
- nonstress test (NST)
- contraction stress test (CST)
- biophysical profile (BPP)
- amniotic fluid volume or index (AFV or AFI)
- Doppler flow studies.

These tests, which are described in detail in this chapter, are often referred to collectively as "antenatal fetal surveillance" or "antenatal fetal testing." The tests are used to evaluate uteroplacental perfusion and fetal oxygenation to determine whether fetal well-being is compromised. The main goal of antenatal fetal testing is to help providers prolong pregnancy as long as possible to minimize the risks to the neonate from prematurity, but to intervene early enough to prevent fetal death or complications from fetal asphyxia. Included in this chapter is a discussion of each of these testing methods including a description of each test, indications for testing, testing procedures, interpretation of test results, and general management principles. Screening for genetic anomalies and fetal growth assessment are addressed in Chapters 9 and 20. The topic of intrapartum fetal heart rate (FHR) monitoring is outside the scope of this chapter.

Physiological principles and indications for antenatal fetal surveillance

The antenatal fetal tests described in this chapter are used to determine whether there are signs and symptoms of compromised fetal oxygenation, which include:

- redirection of blood flow to preferentially perfuse the fetal heart, adrenal glands, and brain
- decreased fetal movement
- decreased perfusion of the fetal kidneys, which results in decreased fetal urine production
- loss of fetal heart rate accelerations
- development of fetal heart rate decelerations.

Some of these fetal responses are protective and adaptive and allow the fetus to withstand periods of decreased oxygenation without central nervous system damage, while some are signs of deteriorating fetal status.

Determining who should receive antenatal fetal testing beyond those assessments that are part of routine prenatal care is a critical task of the primary provider of prenatal care.

> Current evidence does *not* support the routine use of antepartum fetal testing in uncomplicated pregnancies prior to 41 weeks' EGA (Grivell, Alfirevic, Gyte, & Devane, 2010).

Antenatal fetal testing in a low-risk population has been demonstrated to have low sensitivity and specificity as well as poor positive predictive value for fetal compromise. There is evidence from observational studies, however, that in populations at increased risk of fetal asphyxia, antenatal surveillance may help improve outcomes (Kontopoulos & Vintzileos, 2004). One of the tasks for prenatal care providers, therefore, is to identify those women who may benefit from antenatal fetal testing, and to either conduct this assessment or to refer the woman to receive this assessment.

Table 10.1 includes a list of conditions that are associated with an increased risk of asphyxia and fetal death. Increased fetal surveillance is recommended for women with one or more of these conditions. It must be emphasized, however, that approximately one-third to one-half of fetal deaths after 28 weeks' gestation occur in women without any of these risk factors (Froen et al., 2001; Huang et al., 2000; Yudkin, Wood, & Redman, 1987).

Intrauterine growth restriction significantly increases the risk of intrauterine fetal demise (Flenady et al., 2011). Thus, timely recognition of fetal growth disorders is critical so that an appropriate surveillance and management plan can be put in place. Assessment of fetal growth is covered in Chapter 7 of this book.

There is insufficient evidence at this time to make specific recommendations regarding what type of antenatal fetal testing is best, when this surveillance should start, or how often it should be repeated. A fetal surveillance plan, therefore, must be determined based on individual risk factors and the clinical picture and may require consultation with a specialist.

Scope of practice considerations

Many of the conditions listed in Table 10.1 are conditions that may put the woman's care outside of the scope of independent midwifery or nurse practitioner management. The main role for these providers is to ensure that women are appropriately screened for these

Table 10.1 Conditions Related to an Increased Risk of Fetal Death

Maternal conditions
Pregestational diabetes mellitus
Hypertensive disorders
Thyroid disorders (poorly controlled)
Renal disease
Cardiac disease (cyanotic)
Systemic lupus erythematosus (SLE)
Hemoglobinopathies
Antiphospholipid syndrome
Pregnancy-related conditions
Post-term pregnancy
Decreased fetal movement
Hypertensive disorders of pregnancy
Intrauterine growth restriction
Oligohydramnios
Multiple gestation with growth discrepancy
Isoimmunization
Previous stillbirth
Cholestasis of pregnancy

Data from Signore, Freeman, and Spong (2009).

conditions with a thorough history, appropriate lab work and diagnostic tests, and monitoring of fetal and maternal health status throughout pregnancy. When a pregnancy risk factor is identified, the midwife or NP must make a decision as to whether independent management of the woman is still appropriate or whether consultation, collaborative management, or transfer of care is most appropriate. This decision will be influenced by the practice site, the personnel and facility resources, and by the clinical situation.

It is not unusual for prenatal care providers to conduct testing or to refer women for testing due to a post-term pregnancy (see Chapter 24) and to then make recommendations regarding timing of birth based on the results of those tests.

Antenatal fetal testing methods

Fetal movement counts (FMCs)

Decreased fetal activity is a known response of the fetus to hypoxia and has been demonstrated to be associated with an increased risk of fetal death (O'Sullivan, Stephen,

Martindale, & Heazell, 2009; Sinha, Sharma, Nallaswarmy, Jayagopal, & Bhatti, 2007). The fetus experiencing hypoxia will preferentially perfuse vital organs such as the adrenal glands, heart, and brain. This is accomplished, in part, by decreasing the overall demand for oxygen by decreasing or ceasing movement of the limbs and trunk. In theory, therefore, if a woman at risk for fetal hypoxia conducts daily counts of fetal movements, she can detect a decrease in activity that may indicate compromised fetal oxygenation. Maternal reporting of a decrease in fetal activity can, in turn, allow the provider to conduct additional assessments and intervene in time to avoid fetal injury or death in cases where there is additional evidence of compromised fetal oxygenation. This is the theoretical basis for FMC.

FMC is different from maternal awareness of fetal movement. In this chapter, as in most of the published literature, FMC is defined as a formal process by which a pregnant woman conducts a daily FMC using the same method each time and with specific criteria to determine whether there is decreased fetal movement that should be reported to her provider. FMC is an attractive fetal assessment modality because it is easily taught to women and can be conducted at home without the need for health-care personnel or expensive equipment.

Studies investigating the effectiveness of FMC in reducing the incidence of stillbirth have produced mixed results. Some observational studies have shown a significant decrease in stillbirth rate in women who conducted regular FMCs and reported decreased fetal movement to their health-care providers (Moore & Piacquadio, 1989; Neldam, 1980; Tveit et al., 2009). However, other studies, including the largest study examining the effectiveness of FMC in reducing fetal deaths ($n = 68,654$), showed no effect of FMC on the stillbirth rate (Grant, Valentin, Elbourne, & Alexander, 1989). These studies suggest that part of the failure of FMC to consistently improve outcomes may be related to delays in intervention and to false negative results during additional testing. Authors of a Cochrane systematic review concluded that there are insufficient data to recommend in favor of or against routine FMC for any pregnant women, even those considered at high risk of fetal demise (Mangesi, Hofmeyr, & Smith, 2007).

Part of the difficulty in maximizing the potential effectiveness of FMC is the wide range of normal fetal activity patterns as well as the fact that maternal perception of fetal movement can be highly variable among women and even in the same woman. Studies correlating perceived fetal movement with sonographic evidence of fetal movements demonstrate that women feel only a fraction of the total number of fetal movements and that there is a wide variation from woman to woman in the percentage of fetal movements perceived (Hijazi & East, 2009). There are a variety of factors that affect maternal perception of fetal movement and these are summarized in the following textbox. A woman concentrating on fetal movement is more likely to perceive a higher percentage of her fetus's movements than a woman who is distracted or concentrating on something else.

Factors influencing maternal perception of fetal movement

- Fetal position
- Amniotic fluid volume
- Placental location
- Maternal position
- Maternal attention to fetal movement
- Smoking

A woman asked to conduct formal FMCs must receive clear instructions on the procedures that should be used for counting. There are a number of techniques for conducting FMCs. Some of the most commonly used methods are the following:

1. *Cardiff "count to ten"*—The woman starts counting at the same time each day and records how long it takes for her to count 10 movements. If she does not feel 10 movements in 12 hours or if it takes progressively longer to get to 10 movements (e.g., usually it takes 5 hours and suddenly it is taking >5 hours), she should report decreased fetal movement to the health- care provider (Pearson & Weaver, 1976).
2. *Liston*—similar to Cardiff, but 10 movements should be felt in 6 hours (Liston, Cohen, Mennuti, & Gabbe, 1982).
3. *Moore*—similar to Cardiff and Liston, but 10 movements should be felt in 2 hours (Moore & Piacquadio, 1989).
4. *Sadovsky*—A woman counts how many movements she has in a specific period of time (at the same time every day) and reports to her health-care provider if the number of movements is decreased (Sadovsky & Yaffe, 1973).

There is insufficient evidence to support one method over another, but there is agreement that a woman should only use one method and that she should conduct the counts around the same time of day. Conducting FMC in the early evening in a semireclined position may help improve maternal perception of fetal movement. In women at an increased risk for fetal demise, FMCs should be conducted in addition to and *not* in place of additional fetal surveillance. In other words, FMC should

not be the sole method of antenatal fetal surveillance in pregnancies at increased risk of fetal demise.

Written instructions on the particular FMC technique that is recommended should be provided. These instructions should include a clear threshold for reporting decreased fetal movement, directions on how to proceed if they do not feel the targeted number of fetal movements, and contact numbers. Women should be told that additional evaluation will be needed when she perceives a decrease in fetal movement, but they should also be told that, in most cases, further evaluation will reveal a normal, well-oxygenated fetus. It should be emphasized when providing instructions to women that a complete cessation of movement is never normal and needs to be reported immediately.

A distinction must be made between recommending that women conduct formal FMC and counseling women to be aware of fetal movement. All pregnant women should be counseled to be aware of fetal movement in the third trimester and encouraged to report changes and/or decreases in fetal movement. To avoid unnecessary maternal anxiety, it is important that prenatal care providers educate all pregnant women on normal fetal behaviors and movement patterns. This education should include information on the following:

1. Maternal awareness of fetal movement ("quickening") is not expected to begin until sometime between 16 and 20 weeks' gestation and that primigravidas experience fetal movement a little later than multigravidas.
2. By 26–28 weeks of gestation, women should feel distinct fetal movement several times a day.
3. The fetus has a circadian rhythm that becomes evident in the second trimester and, therefore, will be more active during some portions of the day than others.
4. There are normal variations in the quality of fetal movement with progressive gestational age. In other words, the movement of the 28-week fetus will feel different from the movement at 38 weeks, but the amount of movement should be similar.

A woman who reports decreased fetal movement should receive additional assessment such as a NST and/ or BPP. The ideal timing for this follow-up testing is unknown, but most studies that reported a decreased incidence of fetal death conducted additional testing within 1–12 hours of the decrease in fetal movement. Cessation of fetal movement should be assessed immediately. Despite the commonly held belief that eating or drinking will stimulate fetal movement, low glucose levels have not been associated with a decrease in fetal movement (Velazquez & Rayburn, 2002). Fetal anomalies should be ruled out prior to intervening for decreased fetal movement. The algorithm in Figure 10.1 outlines the steps in the management of decreased fetal movement.

Key points on fetal movement

- Decreased fetal movement is associated with an increased risk of fetal death.
- There are two broad categories of fetal movement monitoring: (1) general maternal awareness of fetal movement patterns in which a woman is informed that by 26–28 weeks of gestation she should feel fetal movement multiple times a day, and that a cessation of fetal movement is never normal; and (2) formal FMC in which a woman is instructed on a particular method of counting in which a specific number of fetal movements are expected during a specific time period. FMCs are conducted using the same technique at least once a day usually at the same time of the day.
- There is insufficient evidence to support a strategy of *routine* FMCs in pregnancy even for women at high risk of fetal demise.
- The benefits of FMC in women with an increased risk for fetal hypoxemia may outweigh the inconvenience, limited evidence, and risks associated with FMC.
- Women who are going to conduct FMC should be taught one clear, consistent method for FMC and given explicit instructions for when and how to notify a health-care provider and seek additional evaluation if she does not experience the targeted number of movements.
- All pregnant women should be educated on the normal parameters of fetal movement and asked to be aware of their baby's movements/patterns of movement.
- All women should be advised to immediately report a complete cessation of fetal movement, a marked decrease in the usual pattern of fetal movement, or a progressive decrease in fetal movement that has occurred over the course of a couple of days.
- In each of the scenarios described above, a woman reporting a decreased FMC or decreased fetal movement should receive immediate evaluation of fetal well-being.

Nonstress test

Selected terms related to fetal heart rate (FHR) monitoring used in this section are defined in at the beginning of the chapter. For a more detailed discussion of this terminology and fetal heart rate pattern interpretations, health-care providers should refer to the report from the 2008 National Institute of Child Health and Human Development Research Planning Workshop (Macones, Hankins, Spong, Hauth, & Moore, 2008).

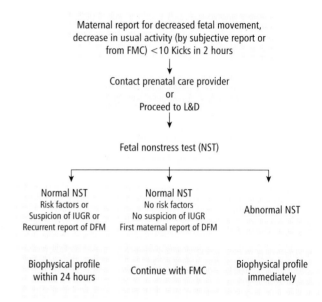

Figure 10.1. Algorithm for the management of decreased fetal movement. IUGR, intrauterine growth restriction; DFM, decreased fetal movement. Adapted from: Liston, R., Sawchuck, D., Young, D., & Fetal Health Surveillance Consensus Committee. (2007). Fetal health surveillance: Antepartum and intrapartum consensus guideline. *Journal of Obstetrics and Gynaecology Canada*, *29*(9), s1–s56.

As gestational age advances and the fetal nervous system develops and matures, the parasympathetic system gains increased influence over fetal heart rate modulation. This neurological maturation results in certain fetal heart rate tracing characteristics, which include a decrease in the average baseline FHR and an appearance of fetal heart rate variability and fetal heart rate accelerations (see textbox "Fetal Heart Rate Accelerations"). Accelerations are abrupt increases in fetal heart rate that usually occur in conjunction with fetal movement.

Fetal heart rate accelerations

The National Institute of Child Health and Human Development (NICHD) has defined the normal amplitude and duration of accelerations as 15 beats per minute (bpm) above baseline lasting at least 15 seconds in a fetus of 32 or more weeks' gestational age and 10 bpm above baseline lasting 10 seconds or more in a fetus at less than 32 weeks' gestational age (Macones et al., 2008). Accelerations lasting 2 minutes or more, but less than 10 minutes, are considered prolonged accelerations. An increase in fetal heart rate above baseline that lasts 10 minutes or more is considered a change in baseline.

Studies have shown that a loss of fetal heart rate accelerations and variability often precede fetal demise due to progressive hypoxia (Cetrulo & Schifrin, 1976; Kodama, Sameshima, Ikeda, & Ikenou, 2009; Low, Pickersgill, Killen, & Derrick, 2001; Pillai & James, 1990). These findings provided hope that antenatal fetal heart rate monitoring would allow the identification of fetuses at risk for demise due to progressive hypoxia with enough time to intervene to prevent fetal death. Based on this, the NST was developed and became widely established as a method of antenatal fetal surveillance. As an increasing body of evidence on the predictive value of the NST has emerged, however, significant limitations to the NST as an independent test of fetal well-being have been identified. These limitations are discussed in more detail later in this chapter.

The NST is conducted using an electronic fetal monitor (EFM) that produces a visual record of the fetal heart rate and uterine contractions. The fetal heart rate is monitored for 20 minutes and then the recorded visual output ("strip") is evaluated for the presence of gestational-age-appropriate FHR accelerations and categorized as reactive or nonreactive.

Reactivity is defined using the following parameters:

Two accelerations of ≥15 bpm above baseline lasting ≥15 seconds in a fetus at ≥32 weeks' EGA

or

Two accelerations of ≥10 bpm above baseline lasting ≥10 seconds in a fetus at <32 weeks' EGA

An example of a reactive NST is provided in Figure 10.2). A reactive NST indicates a well-oxygenated fetus at the moment of testing. The risk of fetal death in the 7 days following a reactive NST is very small (2.3–7 per 1000) (Manning, 2009). It must be kept in mind, however, that this is due in great part to the fact that fetal demise at >28 weeks' EGA is already a relatively rare event occurring at a rate of fewer than 5 per 1000 live births (MacDorman & Kirmeyer, 2009).

If the strip does not meet the criteria for reactivity in the initial 20 minutes of monitoring, the testing can be extended for an additional 20 minutes. If in that

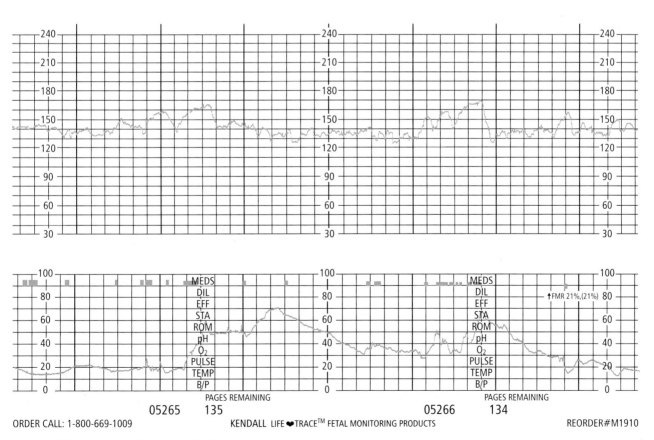

Figure 10.2.   Example of a reactive fetal heart rate monitoring strip.

additional time the strip still does not meet gestational-age-appropriate criteria for reactivity, then the NST is considered nonreactive. A nonreactive strip should be considered an abnormal finding in any fetus >30 weeks' gestational age, and further evaluation is warranted. Similarly, loss of FHR reactivity in a fetus that previously had exhibited FHR accelerations is a finding that warrants further evaluation regardless of gestational age.

The absence of accelerations coupled with the presence of prolonged, late, or repetitive variable FHR decelerations may indicate a fetus that is at increased risk for acute deterioration. In these cases, it may be appropriate to truncate the NST and immediately proceed to ultrasound or other assessment method in a clinical facility able to perform an emergency C-section if indicated. This is particularly important if the decelerations are accompanied by a loss of variability.

Although a reactive NST is a sensitive predictor of a fetus that is adequately oxygenated at the time of testing, a nonreactive NST has very poor positive predictive value for hypoxemia and acidosis. Studies indicate that the NST has low sensitivity (50–62%) for predicting fetal hypoxemia—especially in low-risk populations (Khooshideh, Izadi, Shahriari, & Mirteymouri, 2009; Ocak et al., 1992). Intervention for a nonreactive NST, therefore, must be undertaken with caution especially if the fetus is premature because intervention based solely on a nonreactive NST can lead to an increase in the rate of labor induction, cesarean section, and iatrogenic prematurity without a decrease in perinatal morbidity and mortality.

In an effort to avoid unnecessary interventions, additional testing is often warranted to attempt to determine whether a nonreactive strip is due to compromised fetal oxygenation or due to another, nonhypoxic cause of nonreactivity such as a fetal sleep cycle, maternal sedation, or maternal smoking. These additional testing modalities include the BPP and Doppler velocimetry, both of which are discussed in more detail later in this chapter. Sometimes, there may be identifiable and modifiable maternal conditions, such as acute maternal hypovolemia or maternal seizures that compromise of fetal oxygenation and when these conditions are alleviated, fetal oxygenation may improve. In the presence of these conditions, attention should be focused primarily on efforts to address the underlying cause of fetal compromise and not on additional testing.

In addition to its low predictive value for fetal hypoxia, another limitation of the NST is that it can take a significant amount of time to conduct. Loud external sounds and vibrations—referred to as acoustic or vibroacoustic stimulation (VAS)—have been used to elicit fetal heart rate accelerations. VAS is used to shorten the length of time needed for an NST or to stimulate accelerations in a fetus that has a nonreactive FHR monitoring strip in the initial 20–40 minutes of testing. This type of stimulation has been shown to significantly shorten the average time needed to achieve a reactive NST (Pinette, Blackstone, Wax, & Cartin, 2005). Some experts, however, discourage the use of acoustic stimulation or VAS during antenatal fetal testing, particularly if the fetus at high risk for compromised oxygenation because of concerns regarding safety and falsely reassuring results (Harman, 2009). The reliability of accelerations evoked through acoustic stimulation or VAS to predict adequate fetal oxygenation status has not been demonstrated, especially in the presence of other signs of compromised fetal oxygenation (East et al., 2005). In other words, it cannot be assumed that accelerations stimulated by the use of VAS are equivalent to spontaneous accelerations in predicting a well-oxygenated fetus.

Maternal administration of glucose has also been used in an attempt to decrease both the amount of time needed to achieve a reactive NST and to decrease the rate of nonreactive NSTs. However, research demonstrates that this practice does not achieve either of these goals (Tan & Sabapathy, 2001).

Accelerations of the fetal heart rate can be detected through auscultation (O'Leary, Mendenhall, & Andrinopoulos, 1980). Fetal testing using manual plotting of auscultated accelerations has been proposed as an alternative to the NST (Paine, Johnson, Turner, & Payton, 1986; Paine, Payton, & Johnson, 1986). During an auscultated acceleration test (AAT), the FHR is auscultated and the number of beats in 5 seconds is counted and plotted in a grid that converts the beats in this 5-second period to beats per minute. This is done in alternating 5-second intervals for 3 minutes. If an acceleration of 2 bpm in a 5-second period associated with fetal movement is detected, the AAT is considered reactive. If no acceleration is detected in the first 3-minute period, an attempt is made to elicit fetal movement and the FHR is auscultated for another minute. If no acceleration with movement is detected in this additional minute, the process to elicit fetal movement is repeated and the FHR is auscultated for another 2 minutes. If no acceleration is detected in these additional 3 minutes of auscultation, then the AAT is considered nonreactive. Nonrandomized studies have shown that the AAT produces comparable results to the NST and may be a reasonable alternative to the NST, particularly in settings and/or situations where electronic fetal monitoring is unavailable or impractical.

Key points on nonstress testing

- An acceleration of the fetal heart rate (FHR) is an increase in the fetal heart rate of at least 15 bpm higher than baseline at its peak, and lasting 15 seconds or more from start to finish (10 bpm for 10 seconds or more if EGA is less than 32 weeks).
- Accelerations occur in association with fetal movement.
- The NST is based upon the knowledge that fetal heart rate accelerations are a sign that the fetus that is well oxygenated and neurologically intact.
- A NST is conducted by monitoring fetal heart rate for at least 20 minutes using a continuous EFM to look for FHR accelerations.
- After 20 minutes, the FHR monitoring strip is evaluated to look for accelerations and the test gets classified as reactive or nonreactive:
  - A reactive NST is one where there are two or more EGA-appropriate accelerations of the FHR in a 20-minute period.
    - A reactive NST correlates very highly with a fetus that is not acidotic (high negative predictive value).
  - A nonreactive NST is one in which there is either only one acceleration in a 20-minute period or where there are no accelerations in a 20-minute period.
    - A nonreactive NST correlates poorly (poor positive predictive value) with a fetus who is acidotic.
- If an NST is nonreactive, additional testing is warranted before determining if intervention is warranted.
- The AAT is a reasonable alternative to the NST in settings or situations where electronic fetal monitoring is not available or impractical.

Contraction stress test

A CST or oxytocin challenge test (OCT) is used to evaluate for uteroplacental pathology that may lead to fetal asphyxia or death. It is used primarily to determine the need for delivery in women at high risk for uteroplacental insufficiency. The test should only be performed in a clinical site capable of performing an emergency cesarean section. A CST consists of inducing three uterine contractions in a 10-minute period and seeing whether the fetus develops late or repetitive variable decelerations in response to the contractions. The contractions are induced using either oxytocin or nipple stimulation. Results are interpreted as follows:

1. *Negative (normal)*—absence of late or significant (recurring and deep) variable FHR decelerations.
2. *Positive (abnormal)*—presence of recurrent (present in 50% or more of contractions) late decelerations or significant variable decelerations.

If there are intermittent late or variable decelerations, the CST is considered equivocal. Given the increased

likelihood of compromised uteroplacental function in this situation, especially in a high-risk pregnancy, additional and/or prolonged assessment should be considered.

It is known that uterine tachysystole can cause FHR decelerations even in the absence of underlying fetal or uteroplacental pathology (Stewart et al., 2012). Therefore, if recurrent fetal heart rate decelerations develop during a CST in a woman whose contraction pattern is consistent with tachysystole, the test is also considered equivocal.

Because CSTs are invasive, require prolonged periods of time to conduct, and have the risk of creating complications such as preterm labor (if conducted prior to term) or tachysystole leading to fetal hypoxemia, the CST is not as commonly used as other tests of fetal oxygenation. This is especially true in settings that have other more sensitive testing options such as Doppler velocimetry (Figueras et al., 2003). There are, however, situations in which this test may be particularly useful, such as when a woman at an increased risk for intrapartum fetal hypoxemia has reached term and the healthcare provider is trying to assess whether to proceed with an induction of labor or schedule a cesarean section. Again, it must be underscored that this test should only be undertaken in a place and situation in which a woman can be safely and immediately delivered via cesarean section if necessary.

Amniotic fluid volume assessment

When a fetus is faced with prolonged periods of hypoxemia, one of its adaptive mechanisms is to redistribute cardiac output to selectively perfuse organs essential to survival—the placenta, heart, brain, and adrenal glands. This means that other organs, including the kidneys, have reduced circulation. Decreased renal perfusion results in decreased urine output. Fetal urine makes up the majority of amniotic fluid volume during the end of second trimester and in the third trimester (Brace, 1997). Thus, a decrease in urine output, leads to a decrease in amniotic fluid volume. This chain of events explains why amniotic fluid volume (AFV) can be used to assess fetal oxygenation status.

Amniotic fluid volume is measured using ultrasound and there are multiple methods that are used to quantify AFV. Table 10.2 describes these methods and their interpretation.

Amniotic fluid volume is one of the components of the BPP and the modified BPP described next in this chapter.

The biophysical profile (BPP) and modified BPP

The BPP uses sonography to look for multiple indicators of fetal well-being with the purpose of gaining a more

Table 10.2   Ultrasound Methods to Estimate Amniotic Fluid Volume

Single deepest pocket

With the transducer at a right angle to the uterine contour, measure the vertical dimension of the largest pocket of amniotic fluid (without umbilical cord or fetal extremities/small parts). The horizontal dimension must be at least 1 cm.

Normal	Oligohydramnios	Polyhydramnios
Vertical depth: 2.1–8 cm	Vertical depth: 0–2 cm	Vertical depth: >8 cm

Two-diameter pocket technique

With the transducer at a right angle to the uterine contour, find the largest pocket of fluid (without umbilical cord or fetal extremities/small parts) and calculate the product of the vertical depth multiplied by the horizontal diameter.

Normal 15.1–50 cm^2	Oligohydramios 0–15 cm^2	Polyhydramnios >50 cm^2

Amniotic fluid index (AFI)

Divide the uterus into four imaginary quadrants using the linea nigra for the right and left divisions and the umbilicus for the upper and lower quadrants. Calculate the AFI by measuring the maximum vertical amniotic fluid pocket diameter (without umbilical cord or fetal extremities/small parts) in each quadrant and adding the four measurements together.

Normal 5–25 cm	Oligohydramios 0–5 cm	Polyhydramnios >25 cm

The 2 × 1 cm pocket

The criterion for the biophysical profile (BPP) is to have at least one pocket of fluid with a measurement of 2 × 1 cm.

Data from Chamberlain, P. F., Manning, F. A., Morrison, I., Harman, C. R., & Lange, I. R. (1984). Ultrasound evaluation of amniotic fluid volume. I. The relationship of marginal and decreased amniotic fluid volumes to perinatal outcome. *American Journal of Obstetrics & Gynecology, 150*(3), 245–249; Magann, E. F., Nolan, T. E., Hess, L. W., Martin, R. W., Whitworth, N. S., & Morrison, J. C. (1992). And Measurement of amniotic fluid volume: Accuracy of ultrasonography techniques. *American Journal of Obstetrics & Gynecology, 167*(6), 1533–1537; Rutherford, S. E., Phelan, J. P., Smith, C. V., & Jacobs, N. (1987). The four-quadrant assessment of amniotic fluid volume: An adjunct to antepartum fetal heart rate testing. *Obstetrics & Gynecology, 70*(3 Pt. 1), 353–356; and Manning, F. A., Platt, L. D., & Sipos, L. (1979). Antepartum fetal evaluation: development of a fetal biophysical profile. *American Journal of Obstetrics & Gynecology, 136*(6), 787–795.

accurate evaluation of fetal status than is possible with a single indicator such as FHR reactivity. The BPP is based on the knowledge that, in the absence of an anomaly, a fetus that is well oxygenated and neurologically intact will exhibit certain behavioral characteristics such as gross body movements and breathing movements, have a reactive NST if at an appropriate gestational age, and produce enough urine to have an adequate amount of amniotic fluid. Therefore, the indicators of well-being that comprise the BPP are (1) a reactive NST, (2) fetal breathing, (3) fetal movement, (4) fetal tone, and (5) amniotic fluid volume. Items 1–4 are considered acute measures of fetal oxygenation because they are suppressed as an immediate response to fetal hypoxia, whereas decreased AFV is considered a chronic measure of fetal oxygenation because it takes a prolonged period of hypoxemia to produce oligohydramnios. The BPP as initially described by Manning, Platt, and Sipos (1980) is scored with each of the five components receiving a score of 2 if present and a score of 0 if absent. The maximum score for the BPP is 10/10. The scoring for the Manning et al. method is described in Table 10.3). Vintzileos, Campbell, Igardia, and Nochimson (1983) subsequently proposed a modification to this scoring system that gives a score of 1 when the fetus had some activity in a component but the activity did not meet the criteria to receive a score of 2 as originally described by Manning et al. Vintzielos et al. also added a sixth component to their version of BPP (placental grading), which means that the maximum score for this version of the BPP is 12. The scoring for the Vintzielos et al. method is described in Table 10.4.

There are no large randomized studies of the BPP. However, existing studies (including large observational studies) indicate that the BPP is effective at predicting the absence of fetal acidemia. In other words, the fetus with a BPP of 10/10 (or 8/10 if AFV is normal) has a low (approximately 2%) chance of having acidemia (Manning, Morrison, Lange, Harman, & Chamberlain, 1987). Furthermore, the risk of fetal demise in the week following a normal BPP is less than 1 in 1000 (Manning, Morrison, & Lange, 1985).

The BPP is a less accurate predictor of fetal acidemia. However, studies have established that the risk of perinatal mortality increases significantly as BPP score decreases. One large study found a perinatal mortality rate of 1/1000, 31.3/1000, and 200/1000 for fetuses with BPP scores of 8–10, 6, and 0–4, respectively (Baskett, Allen, Gray, Young, & Young, 1978).

When making management decisions based on BPP results, the health care provider must take the full clinical picture into account. An acute change in maternal status, for example, could mean an acute change in fetal status that would require assessment or intervention regardless

Table 10.3   Biophysical Profile Manning Scoring Criteria

Parameter	Scoring criteria
Movement	
Score 2	≥3 gross body movements in 30 minutes
Score 0	<3 gross body movement in 30 minutes
Tone	
Score 2	≥1 movement of limb from flexion to extension and back to flexion
Score 0	Limb extension with no return to flexion
Breathing	
Score 2	≥30 seconds of sustained fetal breathing movements in 30 minutes
Score 0	<30 seconds of sustained fetal breathing movements in 30 minutes
Amniotic fluid (AF)	
Score 2	≥1 AF pocket measuring ≥2 × 2 cm in two perpendicular planes
Score 0	No AF pockets measuring ≥2 × 2 cm in two perpendicular planes
Fetal heart rate (FHR)	
Score 2	≥2 FHR accelerations of >15 bpm lasting ≥15 seconds in a 40-minute period
Score 0	<2 FHR accelerations of >15 bpm lasting ≥15 seconds in a 40-minute period

Data from Manning, F. A., Platt, L. D., & Sipos, L. (1980). Antepartum fetal evaluation: Development of a fetal biophysical profile. *American Journal of Obstetrics & Gynecology*, 136, 787–795.

of the presence of a normal BPP within the past week. Additionally, when making decisions regarding the optimal timing for birth, maternal indicators for birth may supersede a reassuring BPP. The BPP is less accurate as a positive predictor of fetal acidemia making the clinical context important to decision making. A BPP score of 6, for example, may be managed quite differently in a fetus near term or early term when the risks of a slightly early birth may be outweighed by the risk of progressive fetal hypoxia, whereas a fetus far from term may face greater risks from a preterm birth.

The decision of when to initiate testing and how often to repeat testing depends on the clinical picture. Testing should not begin if a fetus is at a gestational age that

Table 10.4   Biophysical Profile Vintzileos Scoring Criteria

Criteria for scoring biophysical variables according to Vintzileos and coworkers

Nonstress test (NST)

Score 2 (NST 2): five or more FHR accelerations of at least 15 bpm in amplitude and at least a 15-second duration associated with fetal movements (FMs) in a 20-minute period
Score 1 (NST 1): two to four accelerations of at least 15 bpm in amplitude and at least 15-second duration associated with FMs in a 20-minute period
Score 0 (NST 0): one or less acceleration in a 20-minute period

Fetal movements

Score 2 (FM 2): at least three gross (trunk and limbs) episodes of FMs within 30 minutes; simultaneous limb and trunk movements are counted as a single movement.
Score 1 (FM 1): one or two FMs within 30 minutes
Score 0 (FM 0): absence of FMs within 30 minutes

Fetal breathing movements (FBMs)

Score 2 (FBM 2): at least one episode of fetal breathing of at least 60-second duration within a 30-minute observation period
Score 1 (FBM 1): at least one episode of fetal breathing lasting 30–60 seconds within 30 within a 30-minute observation period
Score 0 (FBM 0): absence of fetal breathing of breathing lasting less than 30 seconds within a 30-minute observation period

Fetal tone

Score 2 (FT 2): at least one episode of extension of extremities with return to position of flexion and also one episode of extension of spine with return to position of flexion
Score 1 (FT 1): at least one episode of extension of extremities with return to position of flexion or one episode of extension of spine with return to flexion
Score 0 (FT 0): extremities in extension; FMs not followed by return to flexion; open hand

Amniotic fluid volume

Score 2 (AF 2): fluid evident throughout the uterine cavity; a pocket that measures greater than 2 cm in vertical diameter
Score 1 (AF 1): a pocket that measures less than 2 cm but more than vertical diameter
Score 0 (AF 0): crowding of fetal small parts; largest pocket less than 1 cm in vertical diameter

Placental grading

Score 2 (PL 2): placental grading 0, 1, or 2
Score 1 (PL 1): placenta posterior difficult to evaluate
Score 0 (PL 0): placental grading 3

Maximal score, 12; minimal score, 0

Reprinted from Oyelese, Y. & Vintizileos A. M. (2011). The uses and limitations of the fetal biophysical profile. *Clinics in Perinatology*, *38*, 49, with permission from Elsiever.

would preclude intervention, that is, if the fetus is so far from term that birth would not be an option. In pregnancies where there is an increased risk of stillbirth (see Table 10.1), testing is usually initiated sometime between 32 and 34 weeks of gestation with the exception of testing for postdate pregnancy, which usually begins at 41 weeks of gestation. A BPP profile will often be used to evaluate a report of decreased fetal movement, regardless of gestational age. There is no conclusive research to guide the frequency of BPP testing in pregnancies at risk for fetal compromise. Most clinical sites will conduct testing once or twice weekly. BPPs may be performed on a more frequent basis, especially in the management of the preterm fetus with significant growth restriction who may have a rapid deterioration in status. When to start and how often to repeat a BPP in situations other than postdate pregnancy is a decision that should be made in collaboration with an obstetrician or maternal-fetal medicine specialist. Similarly, women with pregnancies requiring regular BPP testing prior to term should either be referred for medical management or should be managed in collaboration with an obstetrician or perinatologist.

The BPP is performed in a setting that has both electronic fetal monitoring and ultrasound capabilities. In some settings or situations, the NST is conducted first and the results of the NST are used to determine whether a full or modified BPP should be performed (see textbox on BPP). In other settings or situations, the NST may be postponed until after the ultrasound portion of the BPP because, in the presence of all four ultrasound indicators of fetal well-being, the NST may not be necessary. The procedure for the NST is the same during a BPP as when it is done as an independent test. Ultrasound is used to look for the other four components of the BPP—movement, breathing, tone, and amniotic fluid. As soon as a parameter is observed, it can be given a score of 2. Continuous observation for 30 minutes is required before it can be determined that an indicator of well-being is absent and given a score of 0. This is to account for fetal sleep–wake cycles. At the end of the testing, the total score is calculated and interpreted (Table 10.5).

Research has demonstrated that the presence of normal amniotic fluid volume and a reactive NST is as accurate at ruling out fetal acidemia as is a score of 10 on a full BPP (Miller, Rabello, & Paul, 1996). To reduce the amount of time needed to conduct a BPP, it may be acceptable to conduct what is referred to as a "modified" BPP in which only the NST and AFV are obtained. If both of these assessments receive a score of 2, then fetal acidemia can be ruled out, but if one or both of these components receive a score of 0, then the full BPP is warranted (Fig. 10.3).

Table 10.5 Interpretation and Management of Biophysical Score

Test result	Interpretation	Management
10/10 8/10 with normal fluid 8/8 without NST	The risk of fetal asphyxia is very low (1/1000 risk of perinatal death within 1 week if no intervention)	Manage based on obstetric and/or maternal condition and factors
8/10 with abnormal fluid	Potential chronic fetal hypoxia	If membranes are intact and there is no known renal malfunction/ abnormality, delivery is indicated if fetus is term. If <34 weeks' gestation, increased surveillance may be preferred due to risks of prematurity.
6/10 with normal fluid	Equivocal	Repeat test within 24 hours.
6/10 with abnormal fluid	Possible fetal asphyxia	Deliver if fetus term. If <34 weeks' gestation, consider clinical picture and whether increased fetal surveillance to prolong pregnancy is preferable to delivery.
4/10	High likelihood of fetal asphyxia (91/1000 risk of perinatal death if no intervention within 1 week)	Deliver.
2/10	Fetal asphyxia probable	Deliver.
0/10	Fetal asphyxia nearly certain (600/1000 risk of perinatal death within 1 week if no intervention)	Deliver.

Adapted from: Manning, F. A. (1995). Dynamic ultrasound-based fetal assessment: the fetal biophysical profile score. *Clinical Obstetrics & Gynecology, 38*(1), 26–44.

It has also been demonstrated that if the four ultrasound parameters (AFV, movement, breathing, and tone) are present—that is, the BPP score is 8/8—this is also as reliable at ruling out fetal acidemia as the full BPP or the modified BPP (Manning et al., 1987). If all ultrasound parameters receive a score of 2, the NST is not needed. If any parameter receives a 0, the NST should be performed. Similarly, achieving a score of 8/10 by any combination of parameters of the BPP is as effective at establishing fetal well-being as a score of 10/10 as long as the AFV is normal (Alfirevic & Neilson, 2000).

Key points on BPP

- The BPP combines the NST and four ultrasound parameters (movement, tone, breathing movements, and amniotic fluid volume) to evaluate fetal oxygenation status.
- Each of the five parameters receives a score of either 0 or 2 (present or not present).
- A score of 10/10 indicates a fetus that is well oxygenated and has a low likelihood of dying in the 7 days following testing.
- There is no evidence to support routine use of BPP in either low-risk or high-risk pregnancies.
- The decision of whom to test and when to test must be made on a case-by-case basis determined by the clinical situation.
- A modified BPP uses only the NST and the AFV, and a score of 4/4 on the modified BPP is as accurate as a score of 10/10 or 8/10 (if AFV is normal) on the full BPP in determining if a fetus is well oxygenated. If either the NST or the AFV are abnormal, the full BPP is indicated.
- If the fetus is greater than 37 weeks' gestational age, and the score is anything less than 10/10 or 8/10 with normal AFV, then delivery may be indicated.
- A patient at less than 37 weeks of gestation with a BPP of 8/10 with low fluid or with a BPP lower than 8/10 regardless of AFV, should be transferred for medical management or managed in collaboration with a physician.

Doppler velocimetry

Blood flow velocities through maternal and fetal vessels can provide information regarding uteroplacental and fetal status. Ultrasound Doppler velocimetry uses reflected sound waves to measure blood flow through vessels. In antenatal Doppler velocimetry, the flow through specific maternal (uterine artery) and fetal vessels (umbilical artery, middle cerebral artery, ductus venosus) is assessed and the waveforms are analyzed to

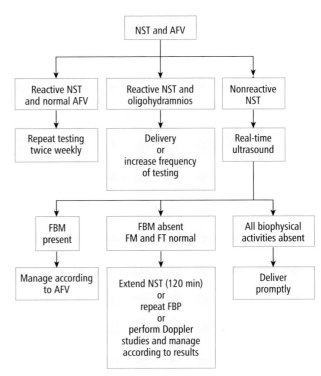

Figure 10.3. Algorithm for the use of modified BPP. AFV, amniotic fluid volume; FBM, fetal breathing movements; NST, nonstress test. Data from Hanley M. L., & Vintizileos A. M. (1988). *Antepartum and intrapartum fetal surveillance of fetal well being. Medicine of the fetus and mother* (2nd ed.). Philadelphia: JB Lippincott, p. 793, and Vintzileos A. M., Fleming A. D., Scorza W. E., Wolf E. J., Balducci J., Campbell W. A., & Rodis J. F. (1991). Relationship between fetal biophysical activities and umbilical cord blood gas values. *American Journal of Obstetrics & Gynecology, 165*(3), 707–713. Reprinted from Oyelese Y., & Vintzileos A. M. (2011). The uses and limitations of the fetal biophysical profile. *Clinics in Perinatology 38*, 61, with permission from Elsevier.

look for disruption in normal flow that is indicative of compromised placental circulation and/or fetal deteriorating status. Proper measurement of Doppler waveforms and interpretation by individuals knowledgeable in the significance of changes in these waveforms is essential to preventing unwarranted interventions and for ensuring that those fetuses with clear evidence of compromised blood flow receive proper follow-up/intervention. The performance of these studies, therefore, is at this time confined mostly to centers that have specialists in maternal–fetal medicine.

Multiple studies have confirmed abnormal Doppler velocimetry of the umbilical artery as an accurate predictor of fetal hypoxia and acidemia (Giles & Bisits, 1993). Therefore, its use for evaluation of pregnancies at high risk for fetal demise has become more widespread. This type of testing is most often used to optimize the timing of birth of fetuses that are preterm and have suspected or confirmed growth restriction and are at high risk for intrauterine demise. The American College of Obstetricians and Gynecologists (ACOG) (1999) does not currently recommend the routine use of Doppler velocimetry in pregnancies other than those affected by fetal growth restriction. It is quite likely that as evidence accumulates regarding effectiveness, Doppler studies will be more frequently used in the surveillance of other high-risk conditions.

Doppler velocimetry of fetal vessels has been used for the monitoring of fetal status in specific high-risk situations such as to evaluate fetal cardiac arrhythmias and to monitor pregnancies with isoimmunization and fetal anemia. Assessment of the uterine artery flow has also been used to detect pregnancies at risk for placental abruption, preeclampsia, and fetal growth restriction (Papageorghiou et al., 2001). Further studies are still needed before this type of test can be used as a routine screening tool for these complications, but the results of existing studies look promising.

Education and counseling

To optimize the effectiveness of any fetal surveillance plan, the pregnant woman must be considered as part of the team and counseled appropriately. All women should be provided with clear instructions on when and how she can contact her prenatal care providers (including after hours and on weekends) should an issue arise that requires immediate attention. All women should also be taught about normal fetal movement/behavior (see the section "Fetal Movement Counts [FMC]") and they should be counseled to be aware of fetal movement starting in the late second trimester (at about 24 weeks) and to immediately report a sudden decrease or cessation of fetal movement.

If a woman is going to undergo antenatal fetal testing, the provider should make sure to explain to her the following:

- indication for testing
- goals of testing
- testing method(s)
- testing frequency/schedule
- alternatives to testing
- potential outcomes of testing (including the possibility of emergent delivery)
- financial costs of testing.

The plan for antenatal testing and the patient education process should be documented in the woman's prenatal care record.

Women and their families may develop unrealistic expectations of what antenatal fetal surveillance can achieve. This can lead to confusion and anger when there is a poor outcome despite reassuring testing, or when emergent surgical birth is conducted but there is no evidence of fetus compromise at birth. Thus, it is especially important that women be counseled on the limitations of antenatal fetal testing. Women need to know that many fetuses that have abnormal testing will have no evidence of compromise upon further testing or upon delivery. Women also need to know that fetal testing provides information on fetal status at the particular moment in time that the testing is conducted. Women must be reminded, therefore, that even if a test is reassuring, an acute event can lead to an acute change in fetal status. Women undergoing antenatal fetal surveillance for a severely growth-restricted fetus are at particular risk for sudden deterioration in fetal status and should be counseled accordingly.

Cultural, personal, and family considerations

Providers should remember that the fetus is a member of the family with whom parents, siblings, grandparents, and others will have bonded even before birth. The determination that a pregnancy is "high risk" and requires increased fetal surveillance is likely to be a source of anxiety and concern for these family members as well as the pregnant woman.

There are some cultural, ethnic, and religious groups that may have restrictions on the use of technology either in general or on particular days of the week. For some of these individuals, the use of EFMs and ultrasound for fetal surveillance may be precluded. The initiation of fetal testing may be an issue that the woman will want to discuss with other family members and possibly with a religious leader before making a decision on whether to consent to testing. Rather than making assumptions on what may or may not be acceptable for a particular person based on their religion or ethnic background, the clinician should ask every woman if she has any concerns or limitations on the use of technology in pregnancy and use her response as a starting point for the conversation.

For women who are uninsured, the need to undergo frequent fetal evaluation can mean a significant expense and one that she and her family may not be able to afford. Providers can help families find a testing site that provides free, reduced-cost or sliding-scale fees. Local health departments may be able to help in identifying such services.

It is important for prenatal care providers to refrain from making unfavorable judgments of families that choose to forgo fetal testing for economic, religious, or other personal issues. Once a woman has received appropriate counseling on the testing, it is her right to determine whether or not she will undergo the tests.

Health disparities and vulnerable populations

There are disparities in risk of perinatal death internationally, with more than 95% of fetal deaths occurring in low-income countries (Cousens et al., 2011). The risk of poor perinatal outcomes is unevenly distributed among racial and ethnic groups in the United States as well. A black woman in the United States, for example, has more than twice the risk of experiencing a fetal death than a white woman (1/87 vs. 1/202) (Willinger, Ko, & Reddy, 2009).

Most of the variation in perinatal death rates between low-income and high-income countries can be attributed to differences in the access to health services and health facilities, particularly at the time of labor, birth, and the immediate postpartum. In the United States, however, the discrepancy in perinatal outcomes is due less to inequalities in access to prenatal and intrapartum health services and more to differences in the prevalence of underlying risk factors including obesity, diabetes, and hypertensive disorders—all of which increase a woman's likelihood of experiencing complications of pregnancy (Willinger et al., 2009). While providers can take steps to ameliorate the effects of these risk factors on the fetus once a woman is already pregnant, the biggest impact on these rates of complications will be achieved by improving the health of women prior to conception.

Legal and liability issues

In their 2010 "Annual Benchmarking Report: Malpractice in Obstetrics," Harvard's Controlled Risk Insurance Company (CRICO) reports the results of an analysis of 800 obstetric claims. Analysis of these claims revealed that birth asphyxia (27%), shoulder dystocia (18%), and intrauterine fetal death (6%) are the three most common types of cases in obstetrics. Among the most common allegations in these cases are that there was a delay in treatment of fetal "distress" and that there was an improper management of pregnancy. The report does not include enough detail on the claims to determine if there were allegations specifically related to antenatal fetal surveillance. An analysis of the cases related to management of pregnancy, however, reveals several common

contributors to claims that are particularly relevant to antepartum fetal surveillance: miscommunication among health-care providers and lack of coordination of care. It is likely, therefore, that in cases involving mismanagement of pregnancy, especially those in which an intrauterine fetal death occurred, issues regarding communication about, and coordination of, antepartum testing may have emerged.

An analysis of diagnosis-related claims drawn not just from the 800 obstetric cases but from the larger pool of over 200,000 cases is especially relevant when considering potential liability issues related to antenatal fetal surveillance. This analysis details the most common issues identified in claims involving injury arising from the outpatient diagnostic process:

- ordering of diagnostic/lab tests
- interpretation of tests
- history/physical and evaluation of symptoms
- referral management.

Follow-up and patient compliance with tests were also raised as recurring concerns in the outpatient diagnosis process.

Many of these issues are similar to those identified by Webster et al. (2008) in the Agency for Healthcare Research and Quality (AHRQ) report on quality and safety problems in the ambulatory care setting:

- Missed or delayed diagnosis
- Delay in proper treatment or preventive services
- Errors or disruptions in communication and information flow processes:
  - ineffective communication between patient/family and health-care provider and among office/clinic staff members
  - problems in the communication chain from patient to primary care provider to specialty or subspecialty referral
  - breakdowns in communication from ambulatory care setting to hospital and from hospital to ambulatory care setting
  - errors in hand-off communications along the continuum of care
  - missing reports from laboratories, imaging and other tests, consultants, procedures, and correspondence.

The following are steps that may help reduce the medicolegal risks related to antenatal fetal surveillance:

- Ensure that women are screened for conditions that may warrant increased antenatal fetal surveillance.
- Establish an appropriate fetal surveillance plan that is in line with current recommendations.

- Ensure appropriate physician consultation, referral, and transfer of care for any of these conditions that are outside the scope of practice of the primary prenatal care provider.
- Ensure that the fetal surveillance plan is documented in the chart.
- Ensure adequate patient education and consent for tests and documentation of this process. It is especially important that women understand the limitations of the tests.
- Put in place a clear and standardized process to ensure that there is timely review and follow-up of tests.

Summary

Despite the current widespread use of multiple tests of antenatal fetal well-being, there are no established, best-practice guidelines that health-care providers can use to determine who to test, what tests to use, when to begin testing, or how often to test. At this time, there is also not a conclusive answer to the question of whether antenatal fetal testing improves neonatal outcomes. Most guidelines are currently based on observational studies and consensus expert opinions. There is observational evidence that the use of the tests described in this chapter

coupled with immediate delivery when fetal acidemia is suspected can decrease the rates of stillbirth. However, the impact on neonatal mortality and significant morbidity such as cerebral palsy has not been established. Given the risks associated with premature birth, the decision to deliver a fetus prior to term based on the results of antenatal testing should be made with caution especially considering the high rate of false positive results for many of the antenatal tests of fetal well-being. The decision to intervene for fetal indications at term is easier, but the risks to the mother associated with cesarean section for both this and future pregnancies should be taken into consideration.

In the absence of large randomized trials to determine the optimal population, method, and timing for antenatal tests of fetal well-being, health-care providers must create a individualized fetal surveillance plan for each woman taking into account maternal conditions, fetal conditions, obstetric history, and findings during routine prenatal assessments. Consultation, collaboration, or referral may be necessary in certain cases. In addition to providing women with education and instructions on the why, how, when, and where of any recommended fetal testing, health-care providers must also ensure that women understand both the benefits and the limitations of tests of fetal well-being.

Case study

Marjorie is a 26-year-old primigravida at 40 weeks and 3 days EGA who is seen in the office for her routine prenatal care appointment. She knows that many primigravidas are pregnant past their due dates and wants to discuss the plan for the rest of her pregnancy. She would like to avoid induction of labor.

History
Marjorie has had a normal pregnancy thus far. Pregnancy dates were determined by the date of her last normal menstrual period and confirmed by ultrasound at 11 weeks' gestation. She has gained 28 lb at 40 weeks and has remained active throughout her pregnancy. She has no chronic health conditions and does not smoke, drink alcohol, take medication, or use illicit substances. Her family history is negative for chronic disease or inherited disorders. She is in a committed relationship with the father of the baby. They are both excited about this pregnancy and are eager to see their baby.

Physical
Weight: 141, +1 lb in 1 week, B/P = 126/72

Fundal height = 39 cm

Reports regular fetal movement

FHTs are in the 140s with an audible acceleration during listening period. Fetus is active during palpation.

Cervical exam offered and declined.

Plan
Education is provided to Marjorie that placental function starts to decline as gestational age progresses and that this can lead to an increased risk to her baby if her pregnancy continues past 42 weeks of gestation. Assessment of fetal well-being by BPP is scheduled at 41 weeks, and again at 41 weeks and 3 days. Marjorie is pleased to hear that if her testing is normal, an induction of labor for postdate pregnancy will not be considered until 42 weeks' gestation.

Follow-up
Marjorie's antepartum fetal testing at 41 weeks reveals a BPP score of 8/10, which is normal. The day after her test, she goes into spontaneous labor and has a vaginal birth of a healthy baby girl who weighs 3118 g.

References

Alfirevic, Z., & Neilson, J. P. (2000). Biophysical profile for fetal assessment in high risk pregnancies. *Cochrane Database of Systematic Reviews*, (2), CD000038.

American College of Obstetricians and Gynecologists (ACOG). (1999). ACOG practice bulletin. Antepartum fetal surveillance. Number 9, October 1999(replaces Technical Bulletin Number 188, January 1994). Clinical management guidelines for obstetrician-gynecologists. *International Journal of Gynaecology and Obstetrics*, *68*(2), 175–185.

Baskett, T. F., Allen, A. C., Gray, J. H., Young, D. C., & Young, L. M. (1978). Fetal biophysical profile and perinatal death. *Obstetrics & Gynecology*, *70*(3), 357–360.

Brace, R. A. (1997). Physiology of amniotic fluid volume regulation. *Clinical Obstetrics & Gynecology*, *40*(2), 280–289.

Cetrulo, C. L., & Schifrin, B. S. (1976). Fetal heart rate patterns preceding death in utero. *Obstetrics & Gynecology*, *48*(5), 521–527.

Cousens, S., Blencowe, H., Stanton, C., Chou, D., Ahmed, S., Steinhardt, L., & Lawn, J. E. (2011). National, regional, and worldwide estimates of stillbirth rates in 2009 with trends since 1995: A systematic analysis. *Lancet*, *377*, 1319–1330.

East, C. E., Smyth, R., Leader, L. R., Henshall, N. E., Colditz, P. B., & Tan, K. H. (2005). Vibroacoustic stimulation for fetal assessment in labour in the presence of a nonreassuring fetal heart rate trace. *Cochrane Database of Systematic Reviews*, *18*(2), CD004664.

Figueras, F., Martínez, J. M., Puerto, B., Coll, O., Cararach, V., & Vanrell, J. A. (2003). Contraction stress test versus ductus venosus Doppler evaluation for the prediction of adverse perinatal outcome in growth-restricted fetuses with non-reassuring non-stress test. *Ultrasound in Obstetrics & Gynecology*, *21*(3), 250–255.

Flenady, V., Koopmans, L., Middleton, P., Frøen, J. F., Smith, G. C., Gibbons, K., . . . Ezzati, M. (2011). Major risk factors for stillbirth in high-income countries: A systematic review and meta-analysis. *Lancet*, *377*(9774), 1331–1340.

Froen, J. F., Arnestad, M., Frey, K., Vege, A., Saugstad, O. D., & Stray-Pedersen, B. (2001). Risk factors for sudden intrauterine unexplained death: Epidemiologic characteristics of singleton cases in Oslo, Norway, 1986–1995. *American Journal of Obstetrics & Gynecology*, *184*, 694–702.

Giles, W. B., & Bisits, A. M. (1993). Clinical use of Doppler ultrasound in pregnancy: Information from 6 randomized trials. *Fetal Diagnosis and Therapy*, *8*, 247–255.

Grant, A., Valentin, L., Elbourne, D., & Alexander, S. (1989). Routine formal fetal movement counting and risk of antepartum late death in normally formed singletons. *Lancet*, *334*(8659), 345–349.

Grivell, R. M., Alfirevic, Z., Gyte, G. M. L., & Devane, D. (2010). Antenatal cardiotocography for fetal assessment. *Cochrane Database of Systematic Reviews*, (1), CD007863.

Harman, C. R. (2009). Assessment of fetal health. In R. K. Creasy, R. Resnik, J. D. Iams, C. J. Lockwood, & T. R. Moore (Eds.), *Creasy & Resnik's maternal-fetal medicine: Principles and Practice* (6th ed.). Philadelphia: Saunders Elsiever.

Hijazi, Z. R., & East, C. E. (2009). Factors affecting maternal perception of fetal movement. *Obstetrical & Gynecological Survey*, *64*(7), 489–497.

Huang, D. Y., Usher, R. H., Kramer, M. S., Yang, H., Morin, L., & Fretts, R. C. (2000). Determinants of unexplained antepartum fetal deaths. *Obstetrics & Gynecology*, *95*, 215–221.

Khooshideh, M., Izadi, S., Shahriari, A., & Mirteymouri, M. (2009). The predictive value of ultrasound assessment of amniotic fluid index, biophysical profile score, nonstress test and foetal movement chart for meconium-stained amniotic fluid in prolonged pregnancies. *Journal of Pakistan Medical Association*, *59*, 471–474.

Kodama, Y., Sameshima, H., Ikeda, T., & Ikenou, T. (2009). Intrapartum fetal heart rate patterns in infants (≥34 weeks) with poor neurological outcome. *Early Human Development*, *85*, 235–238.

Kontopoulos, E. V., & Vintzileos, A. M. (2004). Condition-specific antepartum fetal testing. *American Journal of Obstetrics & Gynecology*, *191*(5), 1546–1551.

Liston, R. M., Cohen, A. W., Mennuti, M. T., & Gabbe, S. G. (1982). Antepartum fetal evaluation by maternal perception of fetal movement. *Obstetrics & Gynecology*, *60*(4), 424–426.

Low, J. A., Pickersgill, H., Killen, H., & Derrick, E. J. (2001). The prediction and prevention of intrapartum fetal asphyxia in term pregnancies. *American Journal of Obstetrics & Gynecology*, *184*, 724–730.

MacDorman, M. F., & Kirmeyer, S. (2009). Fetal and perinatal mortality, 2005. *National Vital Statistics Reports*, *57*(8), 1–19. Centers for Disease Control and Prevention, National Center for Health Statistics, Division of Vital Statistics.

Macones, G. A., Hankins, G. D., Spong, C. Y., Hauth, J., & Moore, T. (2008). The 2008 National Institute of Child Health and Human Development workshop report on electronic fetal monitoring: Update on definitions, interpretation, and research guidelines. *Journal of Obstetric, Gynecologic, and Neonatal Nursing*, *37*(5), 510–515.

Mangesi, L., Hofmeyr, G. J., & Smith, V. (2007). Fetal movement counting for assessment of fetal well-being. *Cochrane Database of Systematic Reviews*, (1), CD004909.

Manning, F. A. (2009). Antepartum fetal testing: A critical approach. *Current Opinion in Obstetrics and Gynecology*, *21*, 348–352.

Manning, F. A., Morrison, I., & Lange, I. R. (1985). Fetal assessment based on fetal biophysical profile scoring: Experience in 12,620 referred high-risk pregnancies. I. Perinatal mortality by frequency and etiology. *American Journal of Obstetrics & Gynecology*, *151*(3), 343–350.

Manning, F. A., Morrison, I., Lange, I. R., Harman, C. R., & Chamberlain, P. F. (1987). Fetal biophysical profile scoring: Selective use of nonstress test. *American Journal of Obstetrics & Gynecology*, *156*(3), 709–712.

Manning, F. A., Platt, L. D., & Sipos, L. (1980). Antepartum fetal evaluation: Development of a fetal biophysical profile. *American Journal of Obstetrics & Gynecology*, *136*(6), 787–795.

Miller, D. A., Rabello, Y. A., & Paul, R. H. (1996). The modified biophysical profile: Antepartum testing in the 1990s. *American Journal of Obstetrics & Gynecology*, *174*(3), 812–817.

Moore, T. R., & Piacquadio, K. (1989). A prospective evaluation of fetal movement screening to reduce the incidence of antepartum fetal death. *American Journal of Obstetrics and Gynecology*, *160*(5 Pt. 1), 1075–1080.

Neldam, S. (1980). Fetal movements as an indicator of fetal well-being. *Lancet*, *1*(8180), 1222–1224.

Ocak, V., Demirkiran, F., Sen, C., Colgar, U., Ocer, F., Kilavuz, O., & Uras, Y. (1992). The predictive value of fetal heart rate monitoring: A retrospective analysis of 2165 high-risk pregnancies. *European Journal of Obstetrics & Gynecology and Reproductive Biology*, *44*, 53–58.

O'Leary, J., Mendenhall, H., & Andrinopoulos, G. (1980). Comparison of auditory versus electronic assessment and antenatal welfare. *Obstetrics & Gynecology*, *56*(2), 244–246.

O'Sullivan, O., Stephen, G., Martindale, E., & Heazell, A. E. P. (2009). Predicting poor perinatal outcome in women who present with decreased fetal movements. *Journal of Obstetrics and Gynaecology*, *29*(8), 705–710.

Paine, L., Johnson, T. R. B., Turner, M. H., & Payton, R. G. (1986). Auscultated fetal heart rate accelerations part II. An alternative to the nonstress test. *Journal of Nurse-Midwifery, 31*(2), 73–77.

Paine, L., Payton, R. G., & Johnson, T. R. B. (1986). Auscultated fetal heart rate accelerations part I. Accuracy and documentation. *Journal of Nurse-Midwifery, 31*(2), 68–72.

Papageorghiou, A. T., Yu, C. K., Bindra, R., Pandis, G., Nicolaides, K. H., & Fetal Medicine Foundation Second Trimester Screening Group. (2001). Multicenter screening for pre-eclampsia and fetal growth restriction by transvaginal uterine artery Doppler at 23 weeks of gestation. *Ultrasound in Obstetrics & Gynecology, 18*(5), 441–449.

Pearson, J. F., & Weaver, J. B. (1976). Fetal activity and fetal wellbeing: An evaluation. *British Medical Journal, 1*, 1305–1307.

Pillai, M., & James, D. (1990). The development of fetal heart rate patterns during normal pregnancy. *Obstetrics & Gynecology, 76*(5 Pt. 1), 812–816.

Pinette, M. G., Blackstone, J., Wax, J. R., & Cartin, A. (2005). Using fetal acoustic stimulation to shorten the biophysical profile. *Journal of Clinical Ultrasound, 33*(5), 223–225.

Sadovsky, E., & Yaffe, H. (1973). Daily fetal movement recording and fetal prognosis. *Obstetrics & Gynecology, 41*(6), 845–850.

Signore, C., Freeman, R. K., & Spong, C. Y. (2009). Antenatal testing—A reevaluation. *Obstetrics and Gynecology, 113*(3), 687–701. doi:10.1097/AOG.0b013e318197bd8a

Sinha, D., Sharma, A., Nallaswarmy, V., Jayagopal, N., & Bhatti, N. (2007). Obstetric outcome in women complaining of reduced fetal movements. *Journal of Obstetrics and Gynaecology, 27*(1), 41–43.

Stewart, R. D., Bleich, A. T., Lo, J. Y., Alexander, J. M., McIntire, D. D., & Leveno, K. J. (2012). Defining uterine tachysystole: How much is too much? *American Journal of Obstetrics & Gynecology, 207*, 290.e1–290.e6. (Electronic publication ahead of print). doi:10.1016/j.ajog.2012.07.032

Tan, K. H., & Sabapathy, A. (2001). Maternal glucose administration for facilitating tests of fetal wellbeing. *Cochrane Database of Systematic Reviews*, (4), CD003397.

Tveit, J. V. H., Saastad, E., Stray-Pedersen, B., Børdahl, P. E., Flenady, V., Fretts, R., & Frøen, J. F. (2009). Reduction of late stillbirth with the introduction of fetal movement information and guidelines—A clinical quality improvement. *BMC Pregnancy and Childbirth, 9*, 32.

Velazquez, M. D., & Rayburn, W. F. (2002). Antenatal evaluation of the fetus using fetal movement monitoring. *Clinical Obstetrics and Gynecology, 45*(4), 993–1004.

Vintzileos, A. M., Campbell, W. A., Igardia, C. J., & Nochimson, D. J. (1983). The fetal biophysical profile and its predictive value. *Obstetrics & Gynecology, 62*(3), 271–278.

Webster, J., King, H. B., Toomey, L. M., Salisbury, M., Powell, S. M., Craft, B., . . . Salas, E. (2008). Understanding quality and safety problems in the ambulatory environment: Seeking improvement with promising teamwork tools and strategies. In K. Henriksen, J. B. Battles, M. A. Keyes, & M. L. Grady (Eds.), *Advances in Patient Safety: New Directions and Alternative Approaches* (Vol. 3, Performance and Tools). Rockville, MD: Agency for Healthcare Research and Quality.

Willinger, M., Ko, C. W., & Reddy, U. M. (2009). Racial disparities in stillbirth risk across gestation in the United States. *American Journal of Obstetrics & Gynecology, 201*(5), 469.e1–469.e8.

Yudkin, P. L., Wood, L., & Redman, C. W. (1987). Risk of unexplained stillbirth at different gestational ages. *Lancet, 1*, 1192–1194.

11

Common discomforts of pregnancy

Robin G. Jordan

Relevant terms

Anticipatory guidance—the preparation of a patient for an anticipated development and/or situation

Fibroadenomas—common, noncancerous breast lumps of fibrous and glandular tissue

Galactoceles—milk-filled cysts in the breast, common during lactation

Gastroesophageal reflux—a condition where stomach contents leak backward from the stomach to the esophagus

Hirsutism—excess facial and body hair in women

Leukonychia—white spots on nail beds

Leukorrhea—excessive, nonbloody, often white vaginal discharge

Linea nigra—dark vertical line that appears on the abdomen of most women during pregnancy

Lumbar lordosis—a condition in which the curve of the lumbar spine increases

Melasma—an increase in facial pigmentation generally over the cheeks and forehead

Pelvic girdle—also called the bony pelvis, consists of the paired hipbones connected to the symphysis pubis anteriorly and the scarum posteriorly, the ilium, ischium, and scarum; forms the birth canal; transfers the weight of the upper body to the legs

Ptyalism—the excess secretion of saliva in the mouth

Sleep hygiene—the term used to describe the set of behaviors used to control presleep and sleep environments

Striae gravidarum—often referred to as stretch marks, these benign cosmetic changes occur due to tearing in the dermis related to weight gain

Overview

The common discomforts of pregnancy encompass a wide variety of physical and emotional signs and symptoms, occurring at various times throughout pregnancy. Almost all of them are due to the normal anatomical and physiological changes that occur during pregnancy, are self-limiting, and are benign to pregnancy outcome. Antepartum care providers must be well versed in the causes of, timing of, and relief measures for the common discomforts of pregnancy, as pregnant women commonly report pregnancy symptoms that require knowledgeable discussion and appropriate advice.

Some health-care professionals may refer to the common discomforts of pregnancy as temporary minor physical or emotional changes; however, they are often not minor to the woman who is experiencing them. While some physiological changes may induce symptoms that are easily managed, others changes may cause symptoms that create profound discomfort and require alterations in lifestyle and, as a result, can be quite distressing. Women with numerous pregnancy-related physical symptoms and those experiencing significant effects on life quality can develop depressive symptoms and low self-esteem (Kamysheva, Werthmeim, Skouteris, Paxton, & Milgrom, 2009). Also, some physical symptoms can be a somatic manifestation of psychological or emotional concerns.

When a woman reports a pregnancy-related symptom, it is important to ascertain that this symptom is indeed

Prenatal and Postnatal Care: A Woman-Centered Approach, First Edition. Edited by Robin G. Jordan, Janet L. Engstrom, Julie A. Marfell, and Cindy L. Farley.
© 2014 John Wiley & Sons, Inc. Published 2014 by John Wiley & Sons, Inc.

due to pregnancy and not pathology, and is within the limits of normal for the symptom. While each symptom requires different questions, some symptoms share subjective data gathering components. Questions of onset, frequency/duration of the symptom, anything that has made it worse or better, are questions essential to almost all pregnancy discomforts that can quickly distinguish between normal and abnormal. The onset of a symptom can be an important diagnostic clue in determining whether the symptom falls into the category of a common discomfort or a pathology. Additionally, multiple symptoms can represent changes in a single body system or changes in more than one body system. The data obtained from a thorough symptom review guide which aspects of a physical examination are indicated.

OLD CART: a mnemonic for symptom review

O: onset
L: location
D: duration
C: character
A: aggravating/alleviating factors
R: radiation
T: timing

The manner in which these common pregnancy symptoms are viewed and presented to women is an important consideration when providing prenatal care. Most women report their symptoms to their health-care provider and look for advice and information, but they also look for empathetic acknowledgment and active listening to their concerns. Traditional medical vernacular typically uses the title "Common Complaints of Pregnancy" and designates symptom reporting as "complaints." Rather than writing "complained of . . .," the more respectful term, "reports symptoms of . . ." can be used when charting. Complaining implies whining, a negative behavior, and does not provide an accurate perspective on a woman's report of common changes experienced during pregnancy. Changing how these symptoms are viewed and communicated from common discomfort complaints to common discomfort symptoms can also allow women to feel more comfortable sharing their symptoms and seeking help from health-care providers.

During prenatal care visits, it is essential to educate women about the normal changes occurring in their bodies. Pregnant women may perceive normal and benign symptoms as abnormal, promoting a reliance on medical care to interpret and resolve the discomfort.

Prenatal anticipatory guidance, teaching, and reassurance of normalcy for pregnancy discomforts can normalize a woman's perception of her body changes and promote self-knowledge of her body and her pregnancy experience. All pregnant women reporting common discomforts should be advised of the physiological basis for their symptom(s), when she can expect relief, self-help measures to help ameliorate her discomfort(s), and signs and symptoms to be alert for indicating a condition outside of the broad scope of normal when applicable.

Anticipatory guidance for the pregnant woman concerning common pregnancy discomforts and normal body changes requires a solid knowledge base of the normal maternal adaptations to pregnancy and recognition of the limits of normalcy. While most of the discomforts of pregnancy remain within the realm of normal, symptom characteristics that delineate normal from pathology should be considered.

This chapter is organized by topic alphabetically with sections on data gathering and relief measures included for each symptom. Many of the common discomforts of pregnancy can be alleviated with commonsense measures and "tincture of time"; others may require more intervention. A variety of relief measures, including more traditional or alternative remedies that women have used over time are presented. For many pregnancy symptoms, reassurance of normal brings a measure of relief and ability to cope.

Back pain and pelvic girdle pain

Back pain in pregnancy develops under the influence of progesterone and relaxin that soften the ligaments and joints, as well as the shift in a woman's center of gravity as pregnancy progresses. The incidence of back pain during pregnancy is estimated to be 50–70% (Mogran & Pohjanen, 2005). Lower backache is attributed to the lumbar lordosis required to counterbalance the weight of the growing uterus. Upper backache is caused by increasing weight of the breasts, postural factors, and employment requiring extended sitting.

Factors that increase incidence of back pain are older age, higher parity, and occupations with heavy lifting or constant standing. Back pain generally increases as pregnancy advances, and it can interfere with daily activities like carrying, cleaning, sitting, and walking, and can prevent women from going to work and sometimes disturbs sleep.

Some women experience pelvic girdle pain that may or may not be associated with lower back pain. This is sometimes referred to as sacroiliac joint pain. It can be misdiagnosed as sciatica; however, only 1% of pregnant women actually have true sciatica (Richens, Smith, &

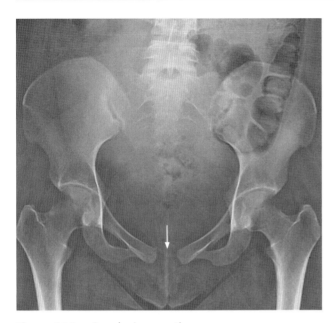

Figure 11.1.   Symphysis separation.

Leddington, 2010). The etiology of pelvic girdle pain is thought to be the same as lower back pain; however, presentation is different: The pain can radiate across the hip joints and the thigh bones, or close to the sacroiliac joints extending to the gluteal area (Kanakaris, Roberts, & Giannoudis, 2011). The pain can be described as shooting, pulsating, or burning. Women will often report shooting pain into the symphysis pubis, and pain on movement, especially walking or anytime up unilateral weight bearing. Women may report a clicking, snapping sound heard or griding sensation felt within the symphysis pubis (Howell, 2012). A waddling gait with short steps may develop to limit hip motion and avoid pain.

The symphysis pubis of the anterior portion of the pelvis widens prenatally under hormonal influence in preparation for birth. The cartilage connecting the two halves of the pelvis at the symphysis pubis widens in all women, and in some, a separation of the bone from the cartilage occurs, creating a diastasis. Symphysis pubis diastasis is more common after birth; however, it can occur prenatally (Fig. 11.1). Pain from symphysis separation can be significant and severely restrict capacity for sitting, standing, and walking.

Assessment

Subjective data gathering

The following information should be obtained: the onset, location and description of symptoms, history of back problems before pregnancy or in prior pregnancies, associated activity, relief measures tried and efficacy, presence of associated signs like contractions, pelvic pressure, symptoms of urinary tract infection (UTI), and history of any recent trauma.

Objective data gathering

Observation of posture, palpation of area for tenderness or signs of trauma, and additional assessment to rule out preterm labor or UTI as indicated should be performed. To diagnose symphysis separation, the active straight leg test is employed. The patient lies supine with straight legs and feet shoulder width apart. Ask the woman to raise one leg, then the other several feet off the table. Women with symptomatic separation feel pain upon this maneuver (Vleeming, Hanne, Ostgaard, Sturesson, & Stuge, 2007).

Relief and preventative measures

Pelvic floor and pelvic tilt exercises can help strengthen core body muscles and improve trunk stability, which can reduce back pain (Borg-Stein & Dugan, 2007). Pelvic floor and pelvic tilting exercises involve the musculature that stabilizes the core and trunk (Table 11.1).

Swimming or aquatic therapy relieves joint and muscle pressure by providing a weightless environment and has been effective in relieving and reducing pregnancy-related back pain (Granath, Hellgren, & Gunnarsson, 2006). Some women report relief of low back pain from chiropractic manipulation (Lisi, 2006). It is common for prenatal care providers to recommend

Table 11.1   Instructions for Pelvic Floor and Pelvic Tilt Exercises

Pelvic floor exercises (Kegels)	Pelvic tilt exercises
• Squeeze the muscles of the pelvic floor. If this is difficult, imagine you are trying to stop yourself from urinating or passing gas. • Hold these muscles in contraction for 10 seconds. • Relax the muscles slowly. Repeat. • Aim for 10 or more repetitions throughout the day. • Do not use muscles like the thighs or buttocks.	• In the standing position: Lean against a wall with knees gently bent. Flatten the lower back against the wall as the abdominal muscles are contracted. • Repeat 5–10 times. • Aim for five or more repetitions throughout the day. • Continue to breathe during the movement. • In the hands/knees position: Keeping the head aligned with the body, straighten the back like a plank. Make the lower back hollowed out and curved. Return to the flat position.

acetaminophen for pain relief during pregnancy. While not associated with teratogenicity, recent data suggest a modest but consistent association of acetaminophen use in pregnancy with asthma in later childhood (Henderson & Shaheen, 2013). More studies are needed to determine causation. Acetaminophen remains the analgesia of choice during pregnancy as needed, yet as with all medications during pregnancy, should be used only when necessary. The following additional remedies can be advised and include relief for symphysis separation pain.

Relief measures for pelvic girdle pain

- Be aware of posture and stand straight with hips pulled forward.
- Avoid standing for long periods of time.
- Place one foot on a low stool if prolonged standing is unavoidable.
- Use proper body mechanics when lifting.
- Sleep on a mattress that offers support.
- Sleep on the side with pillows propped under the uterus and between the knees.
- Wear low-heeled shoes; avoid high heels as they strain the lower back muscles.
- Pelvic tilt exercises help keep the back muscles stretched.
- Acupuncture can effectively relieve pregnancy-related pelvic and back pain (Ee, Manheimer, Pirotta, & White, 2008).
- Supportive maternity belts, binders, or garments such as the BellyBra® provide support to abdominal muscles and improve low back pain (Kalus, Kornman, & Quinlivan, 2008).
- Massage.
- Warm pack to the affected area.
- Apply a sacroiliac belt that fits around the hips to reduce symphysis pubis movement.
- Short term use of acetaminophen can be used in all trimesters of pregnancy. Typical doses are 325–650 mg po q 4–6 h prn up to a maximum of 3000 mg/day.

A pregnancy supporter belt provides compression of the bony pelvis and lifts up the lower segment of the uterus, providing support and some pain relief (Howell, 2012). Women with severe back pain or possible separation or the symphysis pubis may need to stop working for the remainder of the pregnancy to achieve relief. Women with significant back pain or pain unrelieved by common measures can benefit from physical therapy evaluation or a referral to a physiatrist.

Bleeding gums

The effects of estrogen increase blood flow to the mouth and gums and cause swelling of the gingival tissue. This is called gingivitis of pregnancy. The increase in small fragile blood vessels, hyperplasia, and edema can cause minor bleeding to occur while brushing or flossing teeth or when eating certain abrasive or rough foods. Approximately one in two pregnant women will experience bleeding gums during pregnancy (American Academy of Periodontology, 2004). The increase in progesterone changes the saliva to promote bacterial growth in the mouth, enhancing a woman's susceptibility to gingivitis in pregnancy (Gürsoy et al., 2010).

Assessment

Subjective data gathering

The onset, nature and characteristics, predisposing or aggravating factors, oral hygiene practices, and prior history of dental disease should be obtained. Objective data gathering is an oral examination as indicated.

Relief and preventative measures

Women experiencing bleeding gums should be reassured that this is a common and normal event in pregnancy because of estrogen effects and increased blood flow to the area. Women should be advised to continue regular flossing and brushing routines with a softer bristled brush, and acknowledge that these dental hygiene activities can stimulate minor and intermittent bleeding that is not of any significance. Routine dental care and most dental procedures can and should be done during pregnancy. Women with preexisting gingivitis often experience a worsening of gingivitis symptoms in pregnancy. If women experience regular bleeding, oral examination for signs and symptoms of severe gingivitis and referral to a dentist is warranted. Periodontal disease can cause systemic infection processes that are linked with an increase in preterm birth, preeclampsia, and low birth weight (Xiong, Buekens, Vastardis, & Yu, 2007).

Breast tenderness

Breast tenderness is an almost universal symptom in pregnancy and can be one of the first physical signs alerting a woman that she may be pregnant. Initial acute breast tenderness typically begins in weeks 4–6 after the last menstrual period (LMP). The body increases its levels of estrogen and progesterone, enabling the milk ducts and milk-producing cells to form in preparation for breastfeeding. Additional blood flow circulates in the breasts during this time, causing the swelling and tenderness typical of the first trimester. Layers of fat are deposited within the breasts, adding to the change in size and discomfort. Benign breast lumps such as cysts, galactoceles, and fibroadenomas normally enlarge in pregnancy under the influence of estrogen (Graham, 2007). Breast changes continue to occur throughout pregnancy; however, most women experience relief from acute tenderness late first to midsecond trimester. Colostrum starts to form after 20 weeks' gestation, producing nipple discharge in some women in the latter half of pregnancy. Primigravidas are more likely to experience more intense breast tenderness than multigravidas since the breast tissue is expanding in a new way. It is common for many women to experience some relief from breast tenderness when they enter the second trimester.

Normal pregnancy breast symptoms

- Increase in breast size by up to two cup sizes
- Increase in areola size and darkening of the areola
- Breast veins more prominent and visible
- Highly sensitive nipples
- Burning, tingling, or throbbing breast pain
- Sensation of breast heaviness
- Itchy breast skin and nipples
- Throbbing or tingling breasts during sexual activity
- Striae develop on the breasts

Assessment

Subjective data gathering

The onset and characteristics of breast tenderness, prior history of breast problems, current lactation status, any nipple discharge, and its qualities should be obtained.

Objective data gathering

Inspection and palpation of the breast for infection, irritation, and masses are done as indicated. Color of any discharge should be noted.

Relief and preventative measures

Women should be reassured that this is a normal pregnancy symptom and informed of the physiology behind this symptom. Linking the changes to physiological preparation for lactation may help women cope with the discomfort (Johnson & Strube, 2011). Adequate support from garments that limit breast movement is key to reducing the discomfort of breast tenderness.

Relief measures for pregnancy breast discomfort

- Wear a well-fitting bra with adequate support and no underwire.
- Choose cotton bras to help dissipate moisture.
- Wear a sports bra that minimizes breast movement when exercising.
- Apply cool cloth to the breasts.
- Avoid breast stimulation during sexual activity.
- Pat breasts dry after bathing, no rubbing or stimulation.
- Sleep in a bra if the breasts are tender at night.

Carpal tunnel syndrome (CTS)

CTS is a frequently reported common discomfort of pregnancy, affecting an estimated 11–62% of pregnant women (Ablove & Ablove, 2009; Baumann et al., 2007), typically during the third trimester (Pazzaglia et al., 2005). CTS is caused by anything that compresses the median nerve, which runs from the forearm into the palm and the tendons in the carpal tunnel. The pathophysiology of CTS in pregnancy is primarily attributed to increased body fluid volume causing compression of the median nerve. Median nerve compression occurs to some degree in all pregnant women; however, many remain asymptomatic. Common symptoms include numbness and/or tingling in the thumb, index finger, and middle fingers; wrist pain; and loss of grip strength and dexterity. It can occur in one or both hands, and impairment and discomfort can range from mild to severe. Symptoms are more pronounced after a period of rest or after a period of repetitive hand motions like typing. CTS symptoms are common during sleep when the wrist may be in a flexed position, and can wake women contributing to disordered sleep and fatigue. Factors associated with increased incidence of CTS are primigravida status, older age, preeclampsia, excessive weight gain, and edema (Padua et al., 2010).

Though CTS in pregnancy is most often a limited and benign discomfort, severe cases if left untreated can lead to permanent disability. Women developing CTS during the first and second trimesters of pregnancy are more likely to have more severe symptoms and disability.

Diagnosis is made on the basis of clinical symptom history and physical exam.

Assessment

Subjective data gathering

The onset, nature, characteristic and location of sensation, presence of pain, and degree of disability are obtained.

Objective data gathering

Carpal tunnel compression tests are specific and easy to perform in the office. A commonly use test consists of the examiner applying direct thumb pressure over the median nerve at the carpal tunnel and holding for 30 seconds. A positive test consists of paresthesias elicited within this period. Another test consists of flexing the wrist downward while holding the elbow straight; paresthesias elicited within 60 seconds of passive wrist flexion is positive for CTS. Diagnostic nerve conduction studies are often not necessary in pregnancy.

Relief and preventative measures

Treatment for most women during pregnancy is conservative as this condition often improves dramatically within the first 2 weeks postpartum, when the body is losing the excessive pregnancy fluid.

Relief measures for CTS

- Hand splint in neutral position worn at night and/or during the day as needed
- Avoidance of extreme flexion or extension of the wrist
- Decreased use of vibrating tools like lawn mowers
- Decreased repetitive hand and wrist motions
- Massage and gentle stretching of the fingers and wrist
- Acetaminophen 325–650 mg po q 4–6 h prn for pain relief up to a maximum of 3000 mg/day

---

Symptoms can persist after 1 year in more than 50% of pregnant women (Padua et al., 2010). If CTS was present during pregnancy, assessment should be done at the postpartum checkup. Women with persistent CTS symptoms several months after birth should be referred to a hand specialist physician.

Cervical pain

"Cervical zinger" is a term informally coined by some pregnant women used to describe the sensation of sharp shooting pains felt within the cervix. The pain is typically very sudden and brief yet quite uncomfortable. The onset is typically in the third trimester. Women may report an isolated episode every so often, or several episodes a day. It is likely due to the increased pressure of the presenting part of the cervix irritating particular nerve endings. Because of the nature and location of the pain, some women may be concerned that this pain could signal a problem. Women should be reassured that this episodic shooting pain experienced by many women during later gestation is likely due to fetal pressure on the cervix, and is not known to be associated with any complications.

Constipation

Constipation is defined as difficult and infrequent bowel movements, the passage of hard stools, and abdominal discomfort or pain (Vazquez, 2008). It is estimated that between 11% and 40% of pregnant women experience constipation during some point in pregnancy (Bradley, Kennedy, Turcea, Roa, & Nygaard, 2007; Longo, Moore, Canzoneri, & Robichaux, 2010). Pregnancy constipation is likely due to the rise in progesterone and delayed gastric motility. Diets low in fiber and lack of physical activity are also contributing factors. Risk factors for constipation include taking iron supplementation or a prior history of constipation (Vazquez, 2008). In fact, many women will discontinue iron or prenatal vitamins with iron due to constipation. Women who have chronic or episodic constipation prior to conception can find their symptoms worsen during pregnancy. Potential problems due to constipation are development of hemorrhoids or anal fissures, both of which may cause pain and bleeding (Jewell & Young, 2001). Constipation can also induce abdominal pain, nausea, and poor appetite.

Assessment

Subjective data gathering

Areas to evaluate include the onset, usual bowel habits and current pattern, description of a typical stool, diet and fluid intake habits, exercise patterns, medication history, self-help measures including over-the-counter (OTC) medication used to relieve constipation, and presence of abdominal pain or cramping.

Objective data gathering

The abdomen should be palpated for masses and bloating. A rectal exam may be appropriate in some situations. Stool can also be felt through the posterior vaginal wall during a pelvic exam.

Relief and preventative measures

The majority of cases are simple constipation that occurs due to a combination of hormonal, dietary, and mechanical factors affecting normal gastrointestinal (GI) function. Pregnant women with simple constipation can usually find relief with an explanation of the physiological basis, reassurance of normalcy, and self-treatment measures.

Prevention and relief measures for constipation

- *Eat a high-fiber diet*—Approximately 25–30 g/day of dietary fiber is needed to prevent constipation. High-fiber foods include fruits, vegetables, breakfast cereals, whole grain breads, prunes, and bran.
- *Ensure adequate hydration*—Eight to twelve cups of liquid daily in combination with a high-fiber diet can provide enough bulk to promote regular bowel movement.
- *Exercise routinely*—Regular walking, swimming and other moderate exercises can help stimulate bowel activity.
- *Decrease, change, or eliminate iron supplements*— Taking iron every third day can increase hematocrit and hemoglobin and reduce side effects. Changing iron supplement to vegetable-based preparation like Floradix can reduce constipation.
- *Defecate after meals*—Bowel activity is increased at this time.
- *Avoid Valsalva straining during bowel movement to prevent hemorrhoid formation.*

Resources for high-fiber foods should be provided. If dietary and lifestyle changes do not produce relief from constipation, adding a bulking agent like 2–4 tbs of bran or psyllium may be all that is needed. It takes 2–3 days to feel the effects of bulk laxatives. Once desired results are achieved, the amount of supplementation should be titrated to provide constipation prevention. Osmotic and stimulant laxatives are second-line measures if diet and bulk-forming laxatives are ineffective. They have the benefit of quicker relief; however, side effects may limit repeated use. Self-administration of a Fleet-type enema can also be offered as a safe and effective means of constipation relief (Table 11.2).

Dizziness/Syncope

It is estimated that approximately 28% of women experience dizziness during pregnancy, with almost 5% of women going on to have an episode of syncope, or fainting (Gibson, Powrie, & Peipert, 2001). The normal physiological changes predisposing women to syncope include increased vascular resistance and vasodilation and venous pooling in the legs. This leads to a drop in cardiac output and a drop in blood pressure, reducing cerebral blood flow and causing the sensation of dizziness. It is common to hear women report dizziness or fainting while standing and waiting for periods of time during routine activities like waiting in the grocery checkout line or in the post office. Postural hypotension caused by a rapidly changing position from lying down to an upright position can also bring on dizziness. Hypoglycemic episodes in pregnancy can also lead to dizziness

Table 11.2 Remedies for Constipation

Laxative types and examples	Mechanism of action	Side effects
Bulk-forming laxatives • Fiber supplements with oat bran, or wheat fiber in pill, powder, liquid, or chewable form. • Citrucel, Metamucil, FiberCon, Benefiber	Increases stool transit time and frequency of bowel activity Must be taken with liquids to be effective	Bloating, cramping
Stool softeners/ osmotic laxatives • Miralax, Colace, Surfak, and pharmacy or store-branded products containing docusate	Prevents hardening of the feces by adding moisture	Bloating, cramping
Stimulant laxatives • Oral stimulant = Senekot • Rectal stimulant = bisacodyl • Castor oil contraindicated in pregnancy	Causes intestinal contraction to expel stool	Abdominal pain, diarrhea, rectal irritation, electrolyte imbalance, colic Used with caution in pregnancy

Adapted from Tharpe, Farley, and Jordan (2012).

or syncope; a diet history can be done to determine if this is a factor.

Assessment

Subjective data gathering

This includes the onset, nature and characteristic of symptoms, description of activity just prior to episode of dizziness or syncope, most recent food or fluid intake, environmental factors such as heated or unventilated room, associated factors such as palpitations, headache or vomiting, and any significant medical history such as seizure disorder.

Objective data gathering

Observation for any signs of injury, blood pressure, and pulse should be done and heart auscultation performed as indicated.

Relief and preventative measures

Education on the physiology behind this symptom and reassurance of normalcy important elements of care. For dizziness due to postural hypotension, women should be advised to arise from bed slowly and to sit at the side of the bed for several moments.

Prevention measures for pregnancy syncope

- Arise from bed slowly.
- Avoid extended periods of standing when possible.
- Walk in place to promote venous return during those times when standing is unavoidable.
- Eat small meals or snacks every few hours during the day.
- Maintain adequate hydration.
- Consider compression stockings for women in an occupation requiring prolonged standing.
- Avoid overheating.
- Avoid closed-in areas with limited ventilation.

Women who experience dizziness associated with chest pain or significant shortness of breath, or loss of consciousness resulting in possible injury should be evaluated further. Maternal cardiac disease complicates 1% of pregnancies (Pieper, 2008) and is a significant contributor to maternal mortality. It is often undiagnosed until pregnancy and is difficult to differentiate from common symptoms of pregnancy. For this reason, dizziness associated with chest pain or significant shortness of breath, or loss of consciousness should be thoroughly explored. Carefully consider consultation or referral to a specialist care for these women.

Edema

Total body fluids increase by 6–8 L in pregnancy, most of which is extracellular. Several liters of this fluid are found in interstitial space, or the space surrounding the body cells. When excessive fluid accumulates in the interstitial space, edema develops. This is a normal physiological development in pregnancy. Dependent edema, the most common form of edema in pregnancy, affects approximately 75% of women (Davison, 1997). It is most noticeable in the legs in later pregnancy when the weight of the growing uterus interferes with venous return from the lower extremities. Edema of the hands is common in the morning and is likely postural. Edema can also be generalized over the body; this will present most notably as facial edema. Edema can produce symptoms of heaviness in the legs, discomfort, or pain, and can limit mobility. It can also produce inconveniences such as tight or stuck rings and difficulty fitting into regular shoes. Assess the severity of edema with a method such as the four-point scale (+1, slight, to +4, very marked); note its pitting or nonpitting quality, and note the height of the edema in the case of lower extremity edema.

Assessment

Subjective data gathering consists of onset, location of edema, symptom description, and typical diet, noting water and salt intake.

Objective data gathering consists of observation and inspection of edema, noting location, severity, presence of pitting, blood pressure, urine dip for protein, and weight gain pattern.

Relief and preventative measures

Water immersion provides a uniform compression and produces a natural pressure gradient and has been shown to effectively reduce peripheral edema in over 80% of women (Irion & Irion, 2011). Immersion should last at least 20 minutes and should be at least chest deep.

Relief measures for normal edema of pregnancy

- Water immersion for at least 20 minutes
- Exercise such as brisk walking or swimming improves venous return from the legs and reduces edema.
- Apply compression stockings when first arising in the morning before dependent edema worsens.
- Avoid constrictive clothing such as knee-high socks.
- Elevate the legs periodically throughout the day.
- Drink plenty of fluids, especially water.
- Avoid heavily salted foods.

Women with rapid onset edema or signs and symptoms such as blurry vision, hypertension, and/or proteinuria require further evaluation for preeclampsia.

Emotional changes

Pregnant women experience a range of emotions throughout the prenatal course from joy and excitement to ambivalence, fear, and anxiety, sometimes all on the same day (see Chapter 16, "Psychosocial Adaptations in Pregnancy"). The physical changes and pregnancy discomforts and the tremendous hormonal influences play a role in a pregnant woman's emotions. The very nature of creating a new life opens a woman to loss and vulnerability in ways she has not known before, and can manifest itself in anxieties about potential bodily harm to herself and her baby. Pregnant women often report having detailed and vivid dreams that often reflect anxieties and concerns about pregnancy or parenting. These emotional changes are normal and universal across cultures in pregnant women (Thorpe, Dragonas, & Golding, 1992). Most women cope well with their emotional changes and take them in stride.

Assessment

Subjective data gathering

The onset, description of feelings and emotions, family member's reactions, sleep patterns, and usual diet are determined.

Objective data gathering

The woman's general affect and indicators of distress should be noted.

Relief and preventative measures

Active listening is the most helpful strategy a provider can implement in response to emotional issues. Reassurance that emotional changes are normal and expected can go a long way to help a woman cope with this symptom. Encourage the woman to talk with her partner and family members about how she is feeling to help her feel supported and safe. Ensuring adequate sleep and a nutritious diet can help maximize her ability to cope.

Normal emotional changes in pregnancy can sometimes mask the presence of depression, anxiety disorders, or chronic stress. Women who exhibit symptoms consistent with mood disorders, or those who are under severe and long-lasting stress, require additional screening and treatment options as indicated.

Fatigue

Fatigue in the first trimester is one of the most common pregnancy symptoms and is due to the increase in progesterone. It is important to differentiate this fatigue from fatigue due to pathology, such as anemia or depression, both of which are common in women of childbearing age. An efficient determination of normalcy of this symptom can be done with a few questions and a quick visual exam of the woman.

The most common symptom of anemia is fatigue and or weakness. Other signs and symptoms of anemia include shortness of breath, dizziness, headache, coldness in the hands and feet, and pale skin. Common signs and symptoms of depression are very similar to early pregnancy symptoms (see Chapter 42, "Psychological Disorders"). These include a decrease of energy and/or motivation, insomnia, excessive sleeping, irritability, inability to concentrate or make decisions, and a feeling of sadness, heaviness, or apathy. While anemia and depression are fairly common in women of childbearing age, the most likely reason for fatigue in the first trimester is still the normal physiological changes of pregnancy. Fatigue onset corresponding to 5–7 weeks' gestation is the most significant clue as to the normal common discomfort of pregnancy or pathology.

Assessment

Subjective data gathering

The onset and characteristics of fatigue, description of relief measures used, sleep habits, exercise habits, and prior history of anemia or depression are obtained.

Objective data gathering

The woman's affect is observed, and clinical assessment for anemia or depression is done as warranted.

Relief and preventative measures

Women should be reassured that this is a normal and time-limited symptom. Most women will experience relief around 12 weeks' gestation. It is especially important to encourage the woman to enlist help from her family and friends at this time, even writing a "prescription" for increased rest to show her family. Thirty minutes of walking or other aerobic exercise daily can help increase a woman's energy level (Tella, Sokunbi, Akinlami, & Afolabi, 2011). Other strategies for dealing with early pregnancy fatigue are generally commonsense measures.

Relief measures for pregnancy fatigue

- Take a daytime nap or rest if the schedule allows.
- Get adequate night-time sleep.
- Delegate household chores and modify a busy schedule.
- Engage in 30 minutes of daily exercise.
- Eat a diet adequate in protein and iron to maintain adequate iron stores.
- Eat every few hours to keep blood glucose even.

Flatulence

Flatulence is common in pregnancy and can occur during any trimester due to hormonal influence on the GI tract. The increase in progesterone and slowing of GI transit time allows for more gas formation in the gut. During the third trimester, the expanding uterus places increasing pressure on the intestines, slowing digestion further, and pressure on the rectum, decreasing muscle control and leading to increased flatulence. This is an embarrassing pregnancy discomfort that women are often reluctant to discuss; therefore, it is prudent to ask about this discomfort so women can be informed about relief measures.

Assessment

Subjective data gathering

Information on the onset, amount, history of lactose intolerance or bowel disorders, usual diet habits, and level of distress over this symptom are obtained.

Objective data gathering

The abdomen is palpated for distention.

Relief and preventative measures

The pregnancy-induced GI changes should be explained. Emphasis should be placed on preventative measures.

Prevention and relief of flatulence

- Eat six smaller meals per day to avoid digestive system overload.
- Avoid gas-producing foods such as cabbage, beans, fried foods, onions.
- Avoid artificial sweeteners like sorbitol (common in diet soda) as they increase gas formation.
- Keep a food diary to identify patterns.
- Eat slowly to reduce air swallowing.
- Avoid using a straw or drinking from a bottle, which increases air swallowing and gas formation.
- Chew food thoroughly.
- Lightly steaming vegetables can make them more easily digested than raw foods.
- Take time to relax before eating as tension can alter digestion.
- Take a probiotic to balance bowel flora.
- Fresh ginger, carrot, celery, and apple juice will help calm the digestive tract.
- Massage the abdomen in a clockwise rotation.
- Side lying position, knee–chest position, elevating hips above the head (hot air rises)
- Yoga postures promote intestinal circulation.
- Brisk walking or exercise helps mobilize gas and provide relief.
- OTC gas relief medication, such as Bean-o, Di-Gel, or Gas-X

Some women who are especially distressed by this symptom may find relief with and OTC antiflatulence remedy. Those containing simethicone (e.g., Di-Gel) are safe in pregnancy. Activated charcoal tablets should be avoided.

Headache

The most common cause of headache during pregnancy is muscle tension. Most women with a history of migraine headaches may experience decreased frequency and severity of migraines during pregnancy (Sances et al., 2003), while a small percentage of women can experience an increase in headaches in the second or third trimester (Silberstein, 2004). Pregnant women who abruptly eliminate caffeine can experience an increase in headaches for a period of time. Women who have a history of migraine headaches often find that they improve during pregnancy. The vast majority of headaches in pregnancy are tension headaches, which respond readily to common relief measures. Other benign causes include sinus congestion, allergies, low blood sugar, or mild dehydration.

Assessment

Subjective data gathering

The onset, duration of headache, presence of aura, any associated symptoms, precipitating factors, occupational and activities of daily living (ADL) history, prior headache history, pattern of caffeine intake, diet and fluid intake, and relief measures used and efficacy are assessed.

Objective data gathering

The woman's general appearance, blood pressure, weight, assessment of skin, and mucosa for hydration are evaluated. Palpation of periorbital sinus is done as indicated.

Relief and preventative measures

If not associated with hypertension or other obvious medical issues, reassurance that most headaches in pregnancy are benign is appropriate. Keeping a headache diary with food consumed in the 24-hour period preceding the onset of a migraine can help determine food triggers. Exercise such as 30 minutes of brisk walking has been found effective in reducing headache (Marcus, 2007). Acetaminophen within established dose ranges may be used when needed in all trimesters of pregnancy (Office of Teratology Information Specialists (OTIS), 2011).

Relief and prevention measures for headache in pregnancy

- Acetaminophen 325–650 mg po q 4–6 h prn up to 3000 mg daily
- Massage of the head, neck, and back
- Acupuncture
- Warm compress at the base of the head, neck, and forehead
- Relaxation exercises
- Increased rest
- Regular exercise like walking
- Avoid environmental headache triggers (smoke, strong fragrances, skipping meals, stress, glaring lights, excessive heat or cold).
- Avoid food headache triggers (nitrates found in bacon, hot dogs, sulfites found in dried fruits and used as a preservative in packaged salads, artificial sweeteners, chocolate, aged cheeses)

Women with sinus headache or additional symptoms of pharyngitis or fever will need further evaluation for appropriate pharmacological treatment. Specialty care should be sought for severe headache that does not respond to comfort measures and analgesia, new onset headache with neurological symptoms, headache with sudden onset that is severe (see Chapter 38, "Neurological Disorders"), or if the headache is accompanied by an increase in blood pressure, proteinuria, or papilledema (see Chapter 22, "Hypertensive Disorders in Pregnancy").

Heartburn

Heartburn, also called gastroesophageal reflux disease (GERD), is very common during pregnancy. Heartburn occurs when digested food from the stomach is pushed back upward into the esophagus, causing a burning sensation that starts in the stomach and seems to rise up into the lower throat. This can be mildly uncomfortable to extremely debilitating. Heartburn is estimated to occur in 40–80% of women at some point during pregnancy (Keller, Frederking, & Layer, 2008). The prevalence of heartburn increases during pregnancy: approximately 22% of women during the first trimester, 39% in the second trimester, and 72% in the third trimester (Richter, 2003).

There are several causes of heartburn in pregnancy. The two key factors thought to be responsible for heartburn are pregnancy hormones and uterine growth. First, increased levels of estrogen and progesterone in pregnancy cause the lower esophageal sphincter (LES) to relax, which allows acid from the stomach to flow back up, causing burning and pain. In the second and third trimesters, LES pressure that keep the esophagus closed gradually falls to approximately 30–50% of baseline values, reaching a nadir at 36 weeks' gestation (VanThiel et al., 1977). Second, as the uterus grows, it crowds the stomach and intestines, which causes the stomach and acid to back up into the esophagus. Contributors to heartburn are greasy or fatty foods, coffee and other drinks containing caffeine, onion, garlic or spicy foods, certain medications, overfilling the stomach, eating too quickly, and lying down after eating.

Assessment

Subjective data gathering

The onset, description of symptoms, severity, frequency, associated symptoms, foods associated with heartburn, and relief measures used and efficacy should be determined.

Relief and preventative measures

A stepwise approach should be followed, starting with reassurance of normalcy in pregnancy. Lifestyle and dietary modifications can help alleviate heartburn during pregnancy. Women should be encouraged to avoid foods that are known to cause heartburn.

Heartburn preventative measures

- Encourage smaller meals. Eat five to six meals to facilitate digestion avoid overloading the stomach at one time.
- Avoid drinking large amounts of fluids with meals; drink fluids between meals instead.
- Avoid spicy, greasy, and fatty foods. Fats delay gastric emptying.
- Choose low fat or skim milk.
- Avoid a large meal before bedtime.
- Avoid caffeine.
- Avoid lying down right after eating.
- Gain appropriate pregnancy weight for body mass index (BMI). Excess weight exerts extra pressure on the abdomen, increasing potential for heartburn.
- Wear nonrestrictive clothing around the abdomen.
- Elevate the upper body on pillows when lying down.

OTC or prescription medications are used for those women who do not respond adequately to lifestyle modifications. Antacids containing magnesium hydroxide or magnesium trisilicate (Maalox, Mylanta) or sucralfate (a local cytoprotective agent) are commonly used in pregnancy to effectively treat heartburn. Antacids with sodium carbonate like Alka-Seltzer should be avoided as they can cause maternal or fetal metabolic alkalosis. Antacids should not be taken with iron supplements or prenatal vitamins with iron because gastric acid facilitates iron absorption. If symptoms persist, histamine 2-receptor antagonists like ranitidine (Zantac) are Food and Drug Administration (FDA)-approved category B drugs and are effective in treating heartburn.

Women should be advised to report the following:

- heartburn that returns as soon as the antacid wears off
- heartburn that disrupts sleep
- difficulty swallowing
- weight loss
- spitting up blood
- black stools.

Serious reflux complications are uncommon in pregnancy. Women who have evidence of GI bleeding or significant dysphagia require further evaluation for pharmacological or medical treatment.

Heart palpitations

Women may report occasional heart palpitations, or a sensation of the heart fluttering during pregnancy. This is usually normal and is due to the increase in blood volume and heart rate experienced during pregnancy. Palpitations are most commonly seen between 28 and 32 weeks' gestation, when the heart stroke volume peaks (Adamson & Nelson-Piercy, 2007). Sinus tachycardia is seen in the third trimester due to the physiological increase in heart rate. Nonpathological ectopic beats or nonsustained arrhythmias are seen in the majority of women who undergo electrocardiogram (EKG) for a report of palpitations in pregnancy (Adamson & Nelson-Piercy, 2007). Heart palpitations can be perceived as a "flip-flop" sort of feeling, an extra heartbeat, or as a pause in the regular heartbeat, followed by rapid palpitations. This symptom is often very concerning for the woman experiencing this.

Assessment
Subjective data gathering

The onset, nature and characteristics of symptom, precipitating events, associated symptoms, caffeine intake, medication history, and prior history of anxiety or depressive disorders are assessed.

Objective data gathering

The woman's general affect are noted and heart sounds auscultated.

Relief and preventative measures

Explanation of the physiological basis and reassurance of normalcy is the most appropriate course of action. If the perception of palpitations is accompanied by dizziness, shortness of breath, or the woman has a history of cardiac problems, it is appropriate to have her come into the office and be seen by your consultant immediately.

Hemorrhoids

Hemorrhoids are swollen blood vessels in the lower rectum. They are clusters of vascular tissue and connective tissue beneath the normal epithelium of the anal canal that swell and often lead to itching, burning, and bleeding with the passage of stool. The incidence of hemorrhoids in pregnancy is not known; however, it is higher in pregnant women than in nonpregnant women and are more commonly seen in the third trimester (Vazquez, 2008). Etiologies in pregnancy include decreased venous

return, pressure of the enlarging uterus, increased progesterone causing decreased GI motility, and increased Valsalva pressure during defecation (Longo et al., 2010). Symptoms include mild to severe pruritus, protrusion of vein through the anus, and rectal bleeding. Most hemorrhoids resolve spontaneously or with conservative medical therapy alone. However, complications can include thrombosis, secondary infection, ulceration, abscess, and fecal incontinence.

Assessment
Subjective data gathering

Evaluation consists of the quantity, color, amount and timing of any rectal bleeding, usual diet, elimination habits, description of stool consistency, and prior history of constipation or inflammatory bowel disease.

Objective data gathering

A visual inspection of the rectum and a rectal digital exam are done if indicated.

Relief and preventative measures

First-line therapies are conservative measures to treat constipation and facilitate easier passage of stool with less strain. These include increased dietary fiber, and the use of bulk and osmotic laxatives as needed (see the section "Constipation").

Relief measures for hemorrhoids in pregnancy

- Increased dietary fiber
- Avoid prolonged toilet sitting.
- Practice proper anal cleansing after bowel movement.
- Use OTC pain relief preparations after bowel movement as directed (Preparation H or Anusol).
- Use topical hydrocortisone cream or rectal suppositories as directed.
- Kegel exercise to promote pelvic blood flow and muscle tone

---

Women with no relief from conservative measures may benefit from further evaluation for possible hemorrhoid band ligation or injection sclerotherapy.

Increased warmth and perspiration

The increased blood flow through the skin during pregnancy makes most pregnant women feel warmer than usual. Blood volume starts to increase at about 6 weeks, and, by about 32 weeks, it can be as much as 50% more than what it would normally be. This increased blood flow combines with the relaxing effects of progesterone on cell walls to increase capillary vasodilatation, making the pregnant woman feel warmer. The increase in basal metabolic rate during pregnancy increases by about 20%, contributing to increased body and skin temperature. An explanation of the physiological basis and simple measures can help women cope with this symptom.

Relief measures for increased warmth and perspiration

- Wear light or layered clothing.
- Ensure adequate hydration.
- Lower the environmental temperature when possible.
- Bathe or shower as often as needed for comfort.

Leukorrhea

Leukorrhea is the term used for the nonirritating vaginal discharge that starts in the first trimester of pregnancy. This is caused by the increase in pelvic blood flow. The secretions are clear to white in color, have a mild but not offensive odor, and can be thin and watery or more viscous. Estrogen causes the secretions to be more acidic in pregnancy, thereby providing some protection to the mother and fetus against infections.

Assessment

Subjective data gathering

The onset, nature and characteristics of discharge, associated symptoms, sexual history, and condom use are evaluated.

Objective data gathering

If indicated by symptom presentation, a speculum exam and wet prep may be done.

Relief and preventative measures

An explanation of the physiological basis for the increase in vaginal discharge should be provided. Once the possibility of a sexually transmitted infection or vaginitis has been ruled out, women should be advised that this is not a sign of infection, to avoid self-treatment with OTC medications, and to avoid douching. Other advice includes wearing absorbent cotton underwear, changing underwear several times daily, practicing daily perineal hygiene, and using nonscented panty liners as desired. Women with vaginal discharge accompanied by itching, foul odor, or pain require further evaluation for appropriate treatment.

Leg cramps

Cramping of the calf and or foot muscles is common in pregnancy. These cramps often occur at night after a period of inactivity and are more common during the second and third trimesters. The exact cause of leg cramps during pregnancy is unknown. However, some research suggests a connection between leg cramps and the buildup of lactic and pyruvic acids (by-products of metabolizing dietary sugars and starches) that occurs as a result of impaired blood flow in the legs in pregnancy (Jansen, Lecluse, & Verbeek, 1999).

Assessment

Subjective data gathering

The onset, description of symptoms, occupational and ADL history, exercise patterns, and relief measures used and efficacy are evaluated.

Objective data gathering

A visual inspection of the area is done along with palpation of lower extremities for edema, varicosities, and injury as indicated.

Relief and preventative measures

When a leg cramp strikes, standing up and stretching the affected leg, and dorsiflexing the foot can ease the cramp (Fig. 11.2). Women should be advised that these cramps are normal in pregnancy.

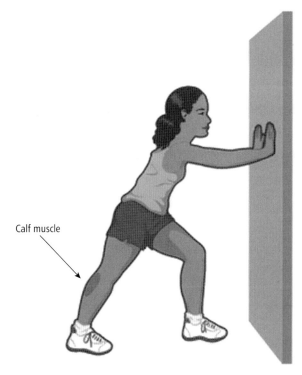

Calf muscle

Figure 11.2.   Stretching calf muscles to prevent leg cramps.

Methods to prevent pregnancy leg cramps

- Exercise like walking promotes circulation of metabolic by-products that can cause cramping and keeps leg muscles stretched and pliant.
- Adequate hydration to avoid dehydration
- Stretching the calf muscles before bed can help reduce legs cramps (see Fig. 11.2, exercise to prevent leg cramps).
- Avoid sitting or standing for prolonged periods of time.
- Warm bath before bed

Some health-care providers have advocated taking magnesium supplements to reduce leg cramps in pregnancy; however, research has not been supportive of this measure. Theoretical physiological explanations for prenatal leg cramps include low levels of vitamin B and disturbances in calcium–phorphorus–magnesium balance. A double-blind randomized controlled trial has demonstrated no effect of magnesium supplements on the frequency of leg cramps in pregnancy (Nygaard, Valbø, Pethick, & Bøhmer, 2008).

Nasal congestion and epistaxis

Local nasal mucosa tissues swell and small vessel vasculature proliferates under the influence of higher estrogen levels in pregnancy. The increased swelling and blood flow exert additional pressure on nasal mucosa, causing nasal congestion and predisposing the vessels to more easily erupt and bleed.

Nasal congestion

Nasal congestion or pregnancy-induced rhinitis is a common discomfort experienced by 20–30% of pregnant women (Namazy & Schatz, 2011). While estrogen-induced hyperemia is considered a primary etiology, the placental growth hormone may play a role. It has been suggested that the presence of pregnancy rhinitis signals a well-functioning placenta, as one study found that women with this symptom had higher levels of placental growth hormone (Ellegard et al., 1998). Women with pregnancy-induced rhinitis will typically report persistent nasal congestion, possibly accompanied by clear nasal secretion, with no additional symptoms of a cold or seasonal allergy. Pregnancy rhinitis typically can last more than 6 weeks and is resolved by 2 weeks postpartum.

Assessment

Subjective data gathering. The onset, nature, characteristics of symptom, signs and symptoms of upper respiratory infection, and the methods used for relief and efficacy are queried.

Objective data gathering. Palpation of nasal sinuses and lymph nodes, inspection of nares as indicated, noting the presence of secretions, noting respirations, and auscultation and percussion of lung fields may be done.

Relief and preventative measures

An explanation of the physiological basis for this symptom should be provided.

Relief of nasal congestion of pregnancy

- Increased humidification and use of saline nasal drops or spray can help relieve symptoms.
- Drinking hot beverages can liquefy secretions and provide temporary symptomatic relief.
- Avoid medicated OTC nasal sprays.

Pregnant women should be advised to avoid the use of OTC nasal decongestant sprays or cold remedies as the rebound congestion that occurs once these are discontinued is often more severe than the original congestion. This often prompts an increase in dose in an effort to obtain relief, thereby entering a cycle of rebound congestion and higher dosing. Pregnant women with symptoms suggestive of allergic rhinitis or bacterial infection such as cough, green nasal discharge, sinus headache, and pain warrant additional evaluation and treatment. For women with severe pregnancy rhinitis, oral decongestants such as pseudoephedrine can be considered in normotensive women after the first trimester (Namazy & Schatz, 2011).

Epistaxis

Approximately 20% of pregnancy women will experience one or more episodes of nosebleed or epistaxis during pregnancy (Namazy & Schatz, 2011). Women with a history of seasonal allergies and epistaxis before pregnancy have an increased risk of epistaxis during pregnancy (Dugan-Kim, Connell, Stika, Wong, & Gossett, 2009). Pregnant women with a history of epistaxis have an increased risk of postpartum hemorrhage, possibly due to factors related to clotting ability or abnormalities in vessel integrity that predispose women to both conditions (Dugan-Kim et al., 2009).

Often, bleeding occurs without warning; however, some symptoms that might precede an episode of epistaxis are itchy nose, dry nose, nasal congestion, sinus headache, or excessive sneezing or nose blowing. Inquire about typical nasal hygiene practices. Women should be reassured that this is a common pregnancy symptom that is typically harmless.

Measures to prevent pregnancy epistaxis

- Use saline nose drops to keep the nasal mucosa moist.
- Increase room humidification, especially when sleeping.
- Avoid vigorous nose blowing or nose picking.
- Eat a nutritious diet to promote healthy tissue.

Measures to stop a nosebleed during pregnancy

- Sit down and lean forward, pinching the nose firmly just under the bridge.
- Maintain pressure for at least 10 minutes continuously.
- Place an ice bag over the nose.
- Avoid nose blowing for at least 12 hours.

Consultation for further evaluation is appropriate for women with frequent and prolonged episodes of epistaxis.

Nausea and/or vomiting during pregnancy

Nausea with or without vomiting is estimated to occur in 70–90% of all pregnant women, with vomiting occurring in approximately 45% of these women (Ismail & Kenny, 2007). The etiology of nausea and vomiting of pregnancy (NVP) is commonly attributed to endocrine factors such as human chorionic gonadotropin and estrogen. Increased levels of progesterone causing delayed gastric emptying also contribute to NVP. The presence of *Helicobacter pylori* has been implicated in worsening this common pregnancy symptom (Goldberg, Szilagy, & Graves, 2007). A familial component is theorized as female relatives of affected women have more NVP than women whose female relatives do not experience NVP. Symptoms vary greatly from one woman to the next and from one pregnancy to the next. NVP typically starts around the sixth week of gestation, peaks at 9–11 weeks' gestation, and tends to subside by 12–14 weeks' gestation. It is absent by 20 weeks' gestation for the vast majority of women.

The term "morning sickness" can be misleading as many women report these symptoms throughout the day. Women who experience NVP suffer fewer miscarriages, with embryonic loss the lowest among those with frequent from vomiting rather than nausea alone (Flaxman & Sherman, 2000). Women with NVP also have lower rates of preterm birth and low birth weight,

infants with congenital anomaly, and stillbirth (Czeizel, Puhó, Ács, & Bánhidy, 2006; Weigel & Weigel, 1989). These positive outcomes can be reassuring and provide a positive perspective on this unpleasant symptom. It is theorized that the purpose of this pregnancy nausea and vomiting may be to protect the embryo by encouraging the mother to avoid potentially harmful foods.

While nausea and vomiting are common early pregnancy symptoms, they may cause significant dehydration and contribute to poor nutrition. About 35% of women who experience NVP experience loss of time at work and negative impact on family relationships (Niebyl, 2010).

Assessment

Subjective data gathering

Evaluation begins with determining the onset, frequency, symptom characteristics, precipitating and aggravating factors, ability to carry out ADL and go to work, appetite, ability to keep food and liquids down, and relief measures tried and efficacy. Assessing the severity of NVP can be done by a relatively simple method known as the Pregnancy-Unique Quantification of Emesis (PUQE) Scale (Table 11.3). This validated scale allows prenatal care providers to efficiently evaluate NVP severity to aid in determining appropriate intervention. Higher scores on the scale are significantly associated with increased hospitalization, emergency room visits, and quality of life measures (Koren et al., 2005).

While most reports of NVP are found to be within normal limits, it is appropriate to gather subjective information from the woman and to observe pertinent physical features, such as weight and skin turgor, to make sure she has not crossed the line to pathology. Though this is an uncommon condition, 1–2% of women experience hyperemesis (see Chapter 24). Pertinent questions such as presence of ptyalism, frequency of vomiting, ability to function normally in her daily routine as well as physical symptoms of dehydration, weight loss, and ketosis are important pieces of data gathering for women with nausea and vomiting in pregnancy to initially decide if she is still within the realm of normal or not.

Objective data gathering

The woman's weight is obtained (noting gain or loss), and general appearance, skin tugor, mucosa, presence of ketonuria, presence of ptyalism, and signs of dehydration are evaluated.

Relief and preventative measures

For normal NVP that has minimal to moderate interference on ADL, relief measures should be instituted from

Table 11.3   PUQE Scale

Pregnancy-Unique Quantification of Emesis and Nausea (PUQE)* scoring system					
How many hours in the past 24 hours had you felt nauseated/sick to stomach?	(1)	(2)	(3)	(4)	(5)
How many times in the past 24 hours did you vomit?	7 or more (5)	5–6 (4)	3–4 (3)	1–2 (2)	None (1)
How many times in the past 24 hours did you experience gagging, retching, or dry heaves?	None (1)	1–2 (2)	3–4 (3)	5–6 (4)	7 or more (5)

PUQE score: _____
How many hours have you slept out of 24 hours? Why? _____
On a scale of 0–10, how would you rate your well-being? _____
0 (worst possible) 10 (the best you felt before pregnancy)
Can you tell me what causes you to feel that way? _____

The total score is the sum of points, noted in parentheses, awarded to each of the three questions.
Nausea score: mild NVP = ≤6; moderate NVP = 7–12; severe NVP ≥ 13.
Source: Ebrahimi, Maltepe, Bournissen, and Koren (2009); used with permission.

least to most systemic. Lifestyle and OTC measures should be advised to all women with NVP so they can try various methods. What is effective varies from one woman to the next and from one pregnancy to the next. For many women, lifestyle and OTC measures are enough to provide adequate relief. Table 11.4 describes measures to help women obtain relief from nausea and vomiting (Fig. 11.3).

OTC remedies are used for women who do not find relief with lifestyle and diet measures and for those presenting with moderate NVP. Prescription pharmacological measures should be instituted for women who report more severe or disabling NVP. Serum ketone and electrolyte levels should be evaluated.

Women should be advised of the physiology and the time-limited nature of NVP, and to eat whatever they can during the duration of this symptom. Instruction should be provided on reporting signs and symptoms of dehydration, unrelieved NVP, or inability to keep any food down for >24 hours. Consultation, IV fluid rehydration, and possible hospitalization are warranted for women with severe and unrelenting NVP.

Table 11.4   Relief Measures for Nausea and Vomiting of Pregnancy

Lifestyle measures	Rationale
Small frequent meals	Keep something in the stomach.
Increase periods of rest.	NVP worse with fatigue
Sip clear carbonated or sour liquids.	Reduces saliva
Sip small amounts of fluids through the day.	Avoid expanding the stomach.
Delay prenatal vitamins until nausea resolves.	Iron increases nausea; take 800 mcg folic acid alone.
Decrease dietary fat.	Fat is digested more slowly.
Avoid strong-smelling foods.	Can be a nausea trigger
Avoid highly spiced foods.	Reduces gastric secretions
Increase intake of high-protein foods.	Reduces gastric secretions
Increase intake of bland foods.	Reduces gastric secretions
Eat something right before bed and upon rising.	Keep something in the stomach.
Brush teeth between meals, not right after.	Can be a nausea trigger
Eat whatever seems appealing.	Short-term nutrient imbalance not harmful

Table 11.4   (*Continued*)

Over-the-counter remedies	Administration	Comments
Acupressure at P6 of the Neiguan point	Seabands or self-administer	More effective for nausea See Figure 11.3—for P6 acupressure point
Ginger 1 g via capsule, tea, candy, soda	250 mg QID; ½ tsp grated rhizome in 1 cup tea X4; 1 × 1 in. pieces crystallized ginger × 2	Various forms to try; up to 1 g daily
Vitamin B$_6$ supplement	25 mg TID or QID; 50 mg BID	More effective for nausea
Vitamin B$_6$ plus doxylamine	25 mg vitamin B$_6$ TID and ½ Unisom tablet (equals 12.5 mg) up to TID	Significant N&V relief Safety is well established. No adverse fetal effects Initiate doxylamine at hs as it causes drowsiness

Pharmacological measures	Administration	Comments
Antihistamines and anticholinergics		
• Doxylamine succinate and pyridoxine hydrochloride (Diclegis)	2 tablets at bedtime	Pregnancy category A
• Diphenhydramine (Benadryl)	25–50 mg po q 4–8 h	Pregnancy category B
• Dimenhydrinate (Dramamine)	50–100 mg po q 4–6 h	Most widely studied for NVP
• Meclizine (Antivert)	25 mg po q 4–6 h	
Antiemetics		
• Ondansetron (Zofran)	8 mg po bid	Pregnancy category B
• Promethazine (Phenergan)	12.5–25 mg po q4–6	Pregnancy category C

Adapted from Botehlo, Emeis, & Brucker, 2011; King & Murphy, 2009; Niebyl, 2010.

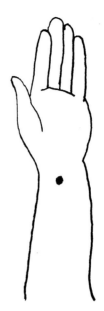

Figure 11.3.   P6 acupressure point for relief of nausea. P6 point is 3 of the woman's fingerbreadths from the wrist.

Ptyalism

Ptyalism is the excess secretion of saliva in the mouth. It is an unusual pregnancy discomfort; however, it is more often seen in women with significant nausea with or without vomiting, particularly women who have difficulty swallowing their saliva. More than 50% of women diagnosed with hyperemesis of pregnancy have associated ptyalism (Godsey & Newman, 1991). For those women experiencing ptyalism associated with normal NVP, it tends to subside by 12–14 weeks' gestation. The etiology is unknown; however, it is theorized that it may be a combination of decreased swallowing in women with NVP, an increase in saliva production, and pregnancy hormonal influences.

Nausea tends to increase salivary gland activity. Saliva is known to be more viscous in the first trimester, which may contribute to less swallowing, perpetuating a cycle of nausea and increased saliva production. Presenting symptoms may be a report of excessive saliva that is bitter tasting and/or a difficulty in swallowing the saliva. Women with ptyalism will often carry tissues with them to spit into and report a decrease in appetite and food intake. Ptyalism can be a significant symptom for some women as sleep is disturbed and work activities and social encounters are limited (van Dinter, 1991). Historical accounts of ptyalism indicate that several cups to several quarts of fluid can be lost in a 24-hour period.

Comfort measures for ptyalism

- Carry a spitting cup.
- Place a towel under the face at night or while resting.
- Lay in a side lying position to facilitate flow of saliva.
- Use soft flannel cloths to wipe the mouth to reduce skin chafing.
- Rinse with mouthwash frequently to reduce the bitter taste.
- Sour candies may improve a woman's ability to swallow.

Assessment

Subjective data gathering

This consists of the onset, description of the amount and characteristics of saliva, and the presence of associated symptoms such as nausea.

Objective data gathering

An inspection of the oral cavity, observation of wiping the mouth frequently, and evaluation for signs and symptoms of dehydration may be done.

Relief and preventative measures

Relief measures for nausea and vomiting can also relieve ptyalism for some women.

Ptyalism in pregnancy can cause psychological distress and interfere with normal daily activities. Women experiencing unrelenting ptyalism leading to dehydration require further evaluation for care.

Restless leg syndrome (RLS)

RLS is a neurological and sensory motor disorder characterized by a strong urge to move the legs and typically occurs during the night during periods of inactivity. It is estimated that 30% of pregnant women experience RLS at some point in pregnancy, though it is widely considered to be underdiagnosed (Balendran, Champion, Jaaniste, & Welsh, 2011). RLS is more common in the third trimester and is a major contributor to poor sleep quality. Risk factors for RLS include a history of growing pains during childhood, a family history of RLS, multiparity, and anemia in pregnancy (Tuğba, Karadağ, Doğulu, & Inan, 2007). The majority of RLS diagnosed in pregnancy will be related to the pregnancy itself or to anemia.

Assessment

Subjective data gathering

Diagnosis is made via four criteria experienced with RSL (Table 11.5). Women will often use the words "creeping," "itching," "crawling," or "gnawing" to refer to the sensation of RSL. Additional history includes onset,

Table 11.5   RSL Diagnostic Criteria

Diagnostic criteria for RLS

These five features must be present for a diagnosis of restless legs syndrome:
1. There is an urge to move the legs, usually accompanied by or caused by uncomfortable and unpleasant sensations in the legs.
2. The urge to move the legs and any accompanying unpleasant sensations begin or worsen during periods of rest or inactivity such as lying or sitting.
3. The urge to move the legs and any accompanying unpleasant sensations are partially or totally relieved by movement, such as walking or stretching, at least as long as the activity continues.
4. The urge to move the legs and any accompanying or unpleasant sensations are worse in the evening or night than during the day or only occur in the evening or night.
5. The urge to move the legs and any accompanying unpleasant sensations are not solely accounted for by another condition, such as leg cramps, positional discomfort, leg swelling, or arthritis.

Adapted from: Restless Leg Foundation http://www.rls.org/Page.aspx?pid=477.

description of symptoms, symptoms prior to pregnancy, history of anemia, typical sleep patterns, history of insomnia, occupational and ADL history, and exercise patterns. Medication history is important.

Objective data gathering

An inspection of the legs for lesions or varicosities is done, and a complete blood count (CBC) with serum ferretin may be obtained as indicated.

Relief and preventative measures

Treatment of anemia decreases the symptoms of RSL. Women with serum ferritin levels < 45 µg/L tend to respond well to iron replacement therapy (Djokanovic, Garcia-Bournissen, & Koren, 2008). Dopamine antagonists such as Benadryl, Reglan, and Zoloft can make RSL worse, so avoiding these drugs if possible can relieve symptoms (Hensley, 2009).

Relief measures for RLS in pregnancy

- Treat underlying anemia.
- Ensure adequate sleep hygiene with the same sleep and arising patterns, quiet room.
- Discontinue strenuous activities after 4 pm.
- Eliminate chocolate and caffeine-containing products.

While there are no FDA-approved drugs for use in pregnancy, opioids such as oxycodone and tramadol currently have the best safety record for the treatment of severe RSL during pregnancy (Djokanovic et al., 2008). Gabapentin (Neurontin) has been shown to be effective and is considered safe in pregnancy. Folic acid supplementation must be given to women taking gabapentin (Balendran et al., 2011; Djokanovic et al., 2008). Comanagement for severe RSL requiring off-label use of these medications is appropriate.

Round ligament pain

This pregnancy symptom is commonly seen in the late first trimester into the second trimester. The round ligaments suspend the uterus within the body. As the uterus expands in size and increases in weight, these ligaments are stretched like rubber bands. Nerve fibers that run next to the ligaments stretch along with them and can cause pain. This stretching can also produce a spasm of the round ligament that can result in sharp and sudden pain. Common symptoms are shooting pain after a sudden movement or sharp, knifelike pain in the lower abdomen or on one side, typically the right side, extending into the groin area. It can last a few seconds to a several minutes. Round ligament pain is often brought on by sudden movement, such as rising from a seated position or arising from bed first thing in the morning. Sometimes, women are awakened during the night by the pain when they turn in bed. Round ligament pain can be quite uncomfortable and worrisome for women, though it is normal and benign (Fig. 11.4).

Assessment

Subjective data gathering

The onset, location of pain, presence of other associated symptoms, and relief measures used and efficacy are evaluated.

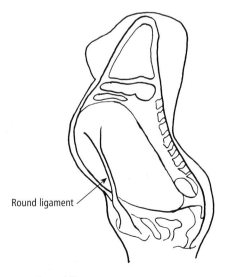

Round ligament

Figure 11.4. Round ligaments.

Objective data gathering

Abdominal palpation for tenderness, rebound tenderness or masses, should be done, and a pelvic examination to rule out ectopic pregnancy or preterm labor done as indicated.

Relief and preventative measures

Explanation of the physiology of round ligament pain using a uterus model and reassurance of normalcy will help women understand what is going on and cope with the pain. Women should be informed on methods to prevent and relieve round ligament pain.

Methods to prevent and relieve round ligament pain

- Avoid sudden movement from sitting to standing.
- Arise slowly from bed in the morning.
- Support the uterus with a pillow under the abdomen and between the knees when side lying.
- Wear an abdominal support garment or sling.
- Apply a warm compress to the area.
- During an episode of round ligament pain, sitting and flexing the knees to the abdomen shortens the ligaments and can provide relief.

Round ligament pain can mimic symptoms of ectopic pregnancy, preterm labor, threatened abortion, and appendicitis. Careful history and additional exam will differentiate pathology from normal round ligament pain. Further evaluation should be done for women with increasing and unrelieved pain or additional symptoms indicative of possible pathology.

Shortness of breath

Feeling short of breath is a common pregnancy discomfort of the first and third trimesters. The increase in progesterone starting in the first trimester causes an increase in respiratory capacity, tidal volume, and respiratory rate (Hill & Pickinpaugh, 2008). This can result in feeling short of breath. In the late third trimester, the uterus compresses the diaphragm, mechanically decreasing capacity of the lungs to fully expand. This can increase shallow breathing, leading to a sensation of being short of breath. Once the fetus engages into the pelvis in late third trimester, the sensation of shortness of breath often decreases. Although lung function is more efficient during pregnancy, the sensation of feeling short of breath can escalate to a feeling of panic for some women.

Subjective data gathering

The onset, nature and characteristics, predisposing or aggravating factors, and history of asthma or other respiratory illness are evaluated.

Objective data gathering

Observation of respirations at rest should be done, and auscultation and percussion of the lung fields done as indicated by additional symptoms.

Relief and preventative measures

Reassurance that this is normal with explanation of physiological basis goes a long way to improving this sensation. Relief strategies for this symptom include measures to expand lung capacity, such as good posture, lifting the arms over the head when shortness of breath occurs, and sleeping in a more upright position with pillow support.

Warning signs accompanying a feeling of shortness of breath include constant coughing, heart palpitations, chest pain, fever or chills, and faintness or dizziness. Women with asthma may experienced heighted shortness of breath and need further assessment when presenting with this symptom.

Skin changes

Skin changes are universal during pregnancy. Physiological skin changes are numerous and include hypermelanosis or darkening of the skin, changes in the size and/or color of moles or nevi, development of spider angioma, and the appearance of striae. The increased production of estrogen, human placental growth factors, and melatonin during pregnancy is primarily responsible for most of the physiological skin changes. Many of the changes in the integumentary system start in the second trimester and progress in the third trimester. Skin changes in pregnancy that may indicate underlying pathology are covered in Chapter 39, Dermatologic Disorders.

Hyperpigmentation

A very mild darkening of all the skin area usually occurs with pregnancy. The anatomical areas most impacted include the areola, nipples, and genitalia. The axilla, inner thighs, and periumbilical areas also have a higher incidence of involvement. These pigmentation changes generally begin early in pregnancy and increase as the pregnancy advances. Even though hyperpigmentation tends to decrease after birth, the nipples, areola, and genital areas do not return to their prepregnant pigmentation (Nussbaum & Benedetto, 2006).

Melasma, also known as the mask of pregnancy or cholasma, is estimated to affect 50–70% of pregnant women to some degree (Gupta, Gover, Nouri, & Taylor, 2006). A genetic component, along with rising levels of

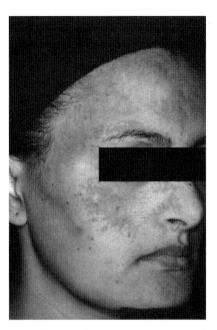

Figure 11.5. Melasma of pregnancy. Permission obtained from Springer.

hormones, may contribute to this condition. Melasma presents as tan or brownish uneven patches of darker skin on the forehead, temples, and cheeks and is more common in women with darker hair and pale skin. Melasma gradually fades and clears spontaneously over time after giving birth, though it is likely to recur in subsequent pregnancies (Fig. 11.5).

Linea nigra begins to appear in the second trimester as a thin vertical line that bisects the navel. Linea nigra appears in women of all skin colors. The vast majority will see a gradual fading and disappearance of this line within a few months after giving birth, though it can take longer in women with darker skin color.

Breast skin changes are seen on the areola with the development of a line of pigmentation surrounding the areola. This is called the secondary areola and is less dark in color with its border merging with the surrounding skin. Small oil-producing glands called Montgomery's tubercles become prominent around the edges of the areola. They make a protective secretion that keeps the nipple and areola supple and moist during breastfeeding.

Striae gravidarum develops on the abdomen, hips, thighs and/or breasts in approximately 80–90% of pregnant women (Kroumpouzos & Cohen, 2001). Onset is usually in the mid to late second trimester and presents as pink and red with a shiny appearance (Fig. 11.6).

The cause of striae gravidarum remains unknown, but both mechanical stretching of the skin and hormonal factors are likely involved. Striae may form due to structural connective tissue and collagen fiber changes. Lower

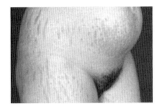

Figure 11.6. Striae gravidarum.

levels of serum relaxin, which decreases the elasticity of connective tissues, are associated with a higher occurrence of striae gravidarum (Lurie, Matas, Fux, Golan, & Sadan, 2011). Although striae gravidarum tends to occur in body areas experiencing extreme skin stretching, there is no correlation between degree of striae formation and extent of body enlargement in pregnancy, which supports hormonal involvement as an etiology. Caucasian women are more likely to develop striae than Asian or African American women, and there appears to be a strong familial tendency (Kumari, Jaisankar, & Thappa, 2007). Also, younger women, particularly teens, and those who gain more than recommended for BMI, are more likely to develop striae gravidarum (Osman, Rubeiz, Tamin, & Nassar, 2007).

Skin tags are harmless small pieces of soft hanging skin that can appear in pregnancy due to pregnancy hormones. They often develop near the neck, under the armpits, or under the breasts near the bra line, but can occur anywhere on the body. Thy commonly fall off during the first 2 months postpartum.

Vascular changes

Changing levels of estrogen and an increase in intravascular pressure account for vascular changes during pregnancy. These factors promote vasodilation and increase the development of spider angioma, palmar erythema, purpura and gingival edema, and hyperemia. Spider angiomas are tiny dilated blood vessels that present as small bright red spots on the trunk, extremities, and occasionally on the face. There can be a central red dot with small radiating vessels on the periphery. Spider angiomas usually appear between 8 and 20 weeks of gestation. White women are much more likely to develop these (67%) than are black women (11%) (Nussbaum & Benedetto, 2006). These fade or disappear after giving birth. Palmar erythema presents as either diffuse or mottling over the entire palm or mottling that is more concentrated over the thenar or hypothenar areas of the hand. Purpura appear as scattered petechia over the lower legs. Gingival edema and hyperemia are common findings in pregnant women and first appear in the first trimester and increase as the pregnancy progresses. Most vascular changes resolve without treatment following birth.

Hair and nail changes

Body hair changes during pregnancy as well. Because the estrogen-induced increase in the hair resting phase delays normal hair loss, many women notice an increase in hair thickness during pregnancy. Mild hirsutism is also commonly seen in pregnancy, especially on the face, with women reporting the development of "peach fuzz" on the jawline and cheeks. Women may also notice fingernails and toenails growing faster than usual, and they may become brittle or soft. Other normal nail changes can include the development of transverse grooves, leukonychia or white spots on nail, and thickening under the nail bed (Muallem & Rubeiz, 2006).

Assessment

Subjective data gathering

The onset, location, sunscreen use habits, history of prior skin conditions, characteristics of symptoms, presence of other associated symptoms such as pruritis or rash, spreading pattern, relief measures used and efficacy, and presence of existing skin conditions are evaluated. If hair loss is reported, amount should be assessed.

Objective data gathering

A visual inspection of skin and hair patterns is done, and palpation or culture of skin lesions are performed as indicated.

Relief and preventative measures

While benign in nature, striae may become cosmetic problems for some women. The cosmetic industry has sought to capitalize on this by marketing treatments claiming to prevent striae; however, their efficacy has not been proven since the development of straie is not totally dependent on external skin stretching. Treatments such olive oil, seaweed wraps, castor oil, glycolic acid, and zinc sulfate have been marketed. There is no evidence to support any products that claim to prevent striae gravidarum (Salter & Kimball, 2006). Emollient creams are useful to decrease itching and dryness and can make the skin feel more pliable. Women should be informed that "stretch mark creams," regardless of marketing claim, are not likely to prevent striae development.

All pregnant women should be advised to use sunscreen as a method to prevent or reduce melasma of pregnancy. Women who develop melasma during pregnancy should be advised to avoid sun exposure and to use sunscreen consistently. If melasma persists postpartum, creams containing a combination of tretinoin and glycolic acids and/or hydroquinone are often successful treatments (Gupta et al., 2006).

The majority of skin, nail, and hair changes regress postpartum. Women should be reassured that facial hair will gradually be lost, skin color will return to normal, and skin tags generally will fall off sometime postpartum. Moles that continue to grow larger, darken, or change should have further evaluation. Women will also notice an increase in hair loss postpartum as the stages of hair growth and loss return to their normal patterns. Striae do not completely disappear, though they fade into less noticeable smaller silvery white lines. While there is no physical discomfort associated with most of these skin, nail, and hair conditions, women may regard them as conditions of concern. Understanding these normal skin changes provides the basis for client education and reassurance.

Sleep disturbances

Sleep disturbance is a common report during pregnancy regardless of parity. Numerous factors contribute to poor sleep quality during pregnancy. Normal pregnancy physiological changes such as increased uterine size and physical discomforts, and increasing progesterone levels contribute to poor sleep quality. Obesity is associated with disturbed sleep in both pregnant and nonpregnant women (Facco, Kramer, Ho, Zee, & Grobman, 2010). Snoring and restless legs increase in the third trimester and can interfere with sleep (Facco et al., 2010). Women with high levels of childbirth fear (tocophobia) can experience an increase in sleep deprivation and fatigue (Hall et al., 2009). Pregnant women with depression have less total sleep time and increased sleep disturbance. Interestingly, women taking selective serotonin reuptake inhibitors (SSRIs) during pregnancy have poorer sleep quality and decreased sleep time than depressed women not taking SSRIs (Okun, Kiewraet al., 2011).

There are two general indicators of sleep quality. Total sleep time is the actual time spent in sleep during the night, and wake after sleep onset (WASO) is the amount of time spent awake during the night after falling asleep. As pregnancy advances, WASO increases and become significant in the weeks prior to labor (Beebe & Lee, 2007).

Excessive fatigue from lack of sleep can affect ability to work and perform daily living activities. In addition, disturbed sleep appears to play a role in adverse pregnancy outcomes.. Excessive sleep debt can interfere with labor progress. Sleep time less than 6 hours per night is associated with longer labors and higher Cesarean rates (Lee & Gay, 2004). Fatigue and poor quality sleep prior to labor can increase pain perception (Beebe & Lee, 2007) and may contribute to decreased coping abilities during labor. One study found that poor sleep quality is associated with an increased risk of preterm birth (Okun,

Schetter, & Glynn, 2011). An underlying mechanism for preterm birth is higher levels of proinflammatory serum cytokines found in women who have poor sleep quality (Chang, Pien, Duntley, & Macones, 2010). Women who are sleep deprived during pregnancy are also more likely to develop postpartum depression (Beebe & Lee, 2007; Lee & Gay, 2004).

Women often hold multiple roles in today's society, with many employed full time while managing the majority of household and family responsibilities. Women should be advised that sleep disturbances are more common in the last 4 weeks of pregnancy and should be helped to strategize ways to obtain adequate sleep during this time.

Assessment

Subjective data gathering

Inquiry regarding sleep quality should be made of all pregnant women at the first visit and periodically during pregnancy. The onset, sleep patterns, sleep hygiene and routine, prior history of insomnia, presence of excessive anxiety or stress, and prior history of depression should be evaluated. A depression inventory is administered as indicated.

Objective data gathering

The woman should be observed for signs of sleep deprivation, such as lethargy and flat affect.

Relief and preventative measures

Education for women and their families about the importance of adequate rest during the prenatal period is essential to reduce poor outcomes associated with lack of sleep. Strategies to increase rest should be encouraged and supported. Acupuncture has been shown to improve sleep quality in pregnant women (da Silva, Nakamura, Corderio, & Kulay, 2005).

Relief measures for prenatal sleep disturbance

- Sleep hygiene instructions include regular bedtime, no working or computer several hours prior to bed, using the bed only for resting and sleeping.
- Delegate chores and responsibilities.
- Diet modifications prior to bedtime include avoiding heavy meals, spicy foods (heartburn), and drinking excessive liquids.
- Use positioning aids to support the gravid uterus.
- Relaxation aids can help, such as relaxation exercises, visualization, music, aromatherapy, and warm bath.
- Prepare the sleep environment—darken the room and lower the room temperature by a few degrees.
- Acupuncture

Sleep quality should be a routine assessment in all pregnant women at various points in gestation. Lack of sleep can cause significant distress in pregnant women. A sympathetic listening ear is essential. It is also appropriate to initiate maternity leave from work in the last 1–2 weeks of pregnancy or sooner if indicated to ensure that women have adequate rest prior to labor.

Supine hypotension syndrome (SHS)

When a pregnant woman is in the supine position, the gravid uterus can compress the inferior vena cava, which returns blood back to the heart from the lower half of the body. This compression decreases blood pressure resulting in symptoms of intense dizziness, tachycardia, pallor, nausea, and sweating. In some women, loss of consciousness can occur. This is called vena cava syndrome or supine hypotension syndrome (SHS) and can occur in the second and third trimesters as the uterus grows. SHS is primarily seen in the third trimester, occurring in up to 15% of women at term since the uterus is at its largest (Chestnut, 2004). Changing position to the side quickly results in alleviation of symptoms.

Traditional advice during pregnancy has been not to exercise in the supine position after the first trimester; however, this advice has come under question. Since most women do not experience SHS, and the rhythmic movement of the legs during exercise increases blood flow to the heart, it is likely that most women can safely exercise on their backs for short periods of time at least until the beginning of the third trimester and perhaps longer. Women may have some misapprehension about the supine position for sleep; however, women should be reassured that there is no evidence to indicate fetal or maternal harm. Importantly, women who become dizzy from SHS will naturally change position to alleviate symptoms.

Assessment

Subjective data gathering

The onset, frequency, description of symptoms, and associated symptoms should be ascertained.

Objective data gathering

Since this only occurs when women are in the supine position, the observations are made during office visits or in labor if the woman is required to be in this position. Observe the woman for signs of discomfort, anxiety, and restlessness.

Relief and preventative measures

Explanation and reassurance of normalcy are essential as this symptom can be frightening. SHS is immediately relieved by turning to the side lying or sitting position. A flat supine position for prenatal care examinations should not be used for prenatal examinations. The head of the examination table should be elevated and the woman can tilt her hips laterally to avoid compression of the vena cava, especially in the third trimester.

Urinary frequency

During the first 12 weeks of pregnancy, the uterus is a pelvic organ. As the uterus grows, it may press on the bladder causing a sensation of bladder fullness and the urge to urinate. This often improves after the 12 weeks' gestation of pregnancy as the uterus rises out of the pelvis and becomes an abdominal organ. In the later weeks of pregnancy when the fetal head descends into the pelvis, urinary frequency may occur again for the same reason. Resting in the lateral recumbent position facilitates venous return and increased urine output, resulting in nocturia, especially in the third trimester. It is important to differentiate normal urinary frequency from urinary tract infection (UTI).

Assessment

Subjective data gathering

This includes determining the onset, presence of dysuria, urgency, voiding small amounts, blood in urine, fluid intake habits, and prior history of UTIs.

Objective data gathering

Palpation of the suprapubic area for pain or tenderness, urine dip for nitrites, and/or urinalysis can be done. Culture and sensitivity tests are done as indicated by other findings.

Relief and preventative measures

Liquids that are known bladder irritants such as caffeine or carbonated beverages can be eliminated to avoid exacerbating this normal discomfort. It is appropriate to advise women to keep the bladder empty. Suggestions include

- voiding soon after feeling the urge
- voiding at scheduled intervals, every 2–3 hours
- urinating before and after intercourse
- reducing fluid intake in the later evening hours.

Women should be informed of the physiological basis for this symptom and that it tends to recur in the third trimester. Instructions on the warning signs of UTI should be given. If frequency is accompanied by other signs of infection, further investigation is warranted to rule out UTI (see Chapter 34, "Urinary Tract Disorders").

Urinary incontinence

The same hormonal and anatomical changes contributing to urinary frequency can lead to involuntary loss of urine, or urinary incontinence, during pregnancy. Increased pressure on the levator ani muscles from the gravid uterus and changes in the ureterovesical angles where the value controlling urine flow from the bladder is located also contribute to involuntary loss of urine in pregnancy. Incontinence can range from the more common mild loss of urine, several drops of urine while sneezing, laughing, or coughing to loss of copious amounts of urine requiring a change of clothing. It is estimated that approximately 27% of pregnant woman may experience some degree of urinary incontinence during pregnancy, typically a small amount of leakage occurring during the third trimester (Kocaöz, Talas, & Atabekoğlu, 2010). This is sometimes mistaken for rupture of membranes by the pregnant woman. Multigravidas, older age, a prior history of incontinence in pregnancy, and those whose mother or sister reports incontinence in pregnancy are more likely to experience this symptom.

Assessment

Subjective data gathering

The onset of the symptom, frequency, predisposing events, characteristics of incontinence; description of the amount of urine lost; and affect on ADL should be evaluated.

Objective data gathering

Visual inspection of the peripad for the amount of urine and whiff test for the odor of urine can be done if needed.

Relief and preventative measures

Urinary incontinence is a disturbing symptom for women who experience it. An explanation of the basis for this symptom during pregnancy and reassurance that tone will be regained postpartum are essential. A referral to a physical therapist knowledgeable in pelvic physiotherapy can be done at this time or postpartum to help women learn how to strengthen the pelvic floor musculature.

Relief measures for mild pregnancy urinary incontinence

- Reassurance of normalcy and explanation of the physiological basis
- Emptying the bladder frequently
- Wearing panty liners as needed
- Kegel exercises to increase muscle tone—approximately 75–100/day.

Most women with small amounts of infrequent incontinence assess the impact of this symptom on their quality of life as minimal. While less common, significant urinary incontinence during pregnancy can cause distress and can negatively impact the quality of life. Incontinence lasting longer than 6 weeks postpartum should prompt a referral for further urogynecological evaluation.

Varicosities (legs/vulva)

Varicose veins, or varices, are abnormally enlarged superficial veins and are usually seen in the thigh and leg and ankles. The veins in the legs are most commonly affected as they are working against gravity. The relaxing effect of progesterone on vessel walls and valves makes them more pliable and is a major factor in the development of varicose veins during pregnancy. The compression of the gravid uterine on pelvic vessels leads to vein engorgement and is also a contributing factor. Conditions that can predispose women to varicosities and/or exacerbate existing varicosities are increased age, family history of varicose veins, obesity, prolonged standing, and existing leg trauma. For women prone to varicosities of the leg or vulva, the varicosities will often worsen in size, shape, and symptoms with subsequent pregnancies.

Leg varicosities

Common symptoms include pain, night cramps, numbness, or tingling in the area of the varicosities; the legs may feel heavy, achy, and may itch. As pregnancy progresses, the varicose veins are more engorged with blood and symptoms increase. The majority of women who develop varicosity of the leg veins will retain these varicosities after pregnancy, though they may decrease in size. For most women, these large superficial veins are a cosmetic nuisance. Complications are not common; however, varicose veins in the legs can cause

- constant itching
- pigmentation around the ankles
- ulcers at the ankles
- mild swelling of the feet
- infection of the vein.

If started early in pregnancy, varicose veins may be prevented. The major preventive measure is to exercise. Instituting a program of regular walking before or at the onset of pregnancy and continuing throughout pregnancy can reduce the incidence of varicose veins (U.S. Department of Health and Human Services, Office on Woman's Health, 2010).

Assessment

Subjective data gathering. This includes the onset, presence of symptoms, occupational and ADL history, exercise patterns, and relief measures used and efficacy; and history of varicosities and history of thrombophilias.

Objective data gathering. This includes a review of prepregnant BMI, current weight, inspection of location, number and size of varicosities, redness, skin color, and palpation for areas of hardness, tenderness, and warmth.

Relief and preventative measures

While there is no cure for varicose veins, measures can reduce symptoms and possibly delay the worsening of existing varicose veins.

Relief measures for varicose veins in pregnancy

- Elevation of the legs at any opportunity
- Lying on the left side with the legs elevated on a pillow. This prevents the fetus from pressing on the vena cava, which is on the right side of the body and decreases the chance of developing varicosities.
- Avoid standing for prolonged periods.
- Avoid crossing the legs when sitting down.
- Walk or exercise daily as this stimulates the muscles that promote venous return in the legs.
- Gain and appropriate amount of pregnancy weight for BMI.
- When lying down, keep the legs elevated.
- Slightly heighten the foot of the bed with bricks or thick books to elevate the legs at night.
- Avoid tight knee-high socks or stockings.
- Wear elastic compression stockings with pressure gradient.

Elastic stocking should have a gradient pressure, with the strongest pressure at the ankle and less pressure at more proximal points of the lower extremity. Compression hosiery is classified according to the pressure level applied at the ankle in three classes: class I = 20–30 mmHg; class II = 30–40 mmHg; and class III = 40–50 mmHg. There is no consensus on the class of compression needed for effective management of varicose veins. These garments should be put on first getting up in the morning before any swelling of the feet and legs occurs. They can be difficult to put on and feel tight and hot when on; thus, it is common for women to discontinue use (Palfreyman & Michaels, 2009).

Vulvar varicosities

Women also can develop varicosities in the vulva. Clinically, vulvar varices may present as small isolated protrusions, mainly in the labia majora, or as large masses, involving the vulvar area. Varicose veins in the vulvar and perivulvar area are estimated to occur in approximately 4% of women (Bell, Kane, Liang, Conway, & Tornos, 2007), though out of embarrassment, women may not mention vulvar veins so it is likely underreported. Vulvar varicosities typically develop after 24 weeks' gestation and are more common in multigravidas. Most of them regress spontaneously after pregnancy. Vulvar varicosities can also open up varicose veins down the inner of back part of the thigh. The risk of vulvar varicosities increases with the number of pregnancies (Van Cleef, 2011). If a woman has varicose veins of the vulva during pregnancy, she will almost always have varicosities of the legs at the same time.

The classical presentation of symptoms includes vulvovaginal swelling, a sensation of heaviness and pressure, and pain with prolonged standing (Gearhart, Levin, & Schimpf, 2011). Pruritus, dyspareunia, and discomfort during walking may also be present. It is common for many women with vulvar varicosities to be asymptomatic. Thrombosis and bleeding are rare but can occur (Van Cleef, 2011). Vulvar varicosities typically do not interfere with normal vaginal birth. Unlike leg varicosities, vulvar varicosities disappear spontaneously by 4 weeks postpartum for most women (Fig. 11.7).

Assessment

Subjective data gathering. The onset, presence of symptoms, occupational and ADL history, exercise patterns, and relief measures used and efficacy should be determined.

Objective data gathering. A visual inspection of the perineal areas affected, size, locations, and the approximate number of varicose veins should be done. Ideally,

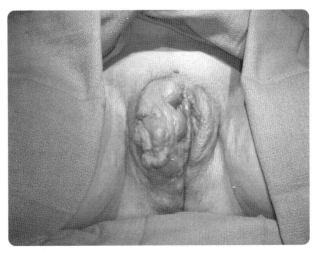

Figure 11.7.   Vulvar varicosities. Permission obtained from Elsevier.

the woman is in the standing position to determine the extent of venous pooling; however, assessment can also be made while in the lithotomy position.

Relief and preventative measures

The treatment of choice of vulvar varicosities during pregnancy is conservative and symptomatic. An explanation of the physiological basis for these symptoms and reassurance they will resolve postpartum can help women cope with symptoms.

Women with leg varicosities should be advised of signs and symptoms of venous thrombosis. While rare, vulvar varicosities presenting in the first trimester in a primigravida requires referral for possible Doppler studies. Persistent vulvar varicosities after pregnancy also should prompt referral for evaluation and potential treatment with surgery or sclerotherapy.

Relief measures for vulvar varicosities

- Avoid prolonged periods of standing.
- Elevate the lower legs when sitting or lying down.
- Use a support device similar in appearance to a male athletic supporter but is contoured to provide compressive support for the vulva, thus preventing the pooling of blood in the labial veins.
- Support garments such as bicycle shorts worn with peripads can put gentle counterpressure on vulvar varicosities.
- Support garments that lift the pregnant abdomen can reduce pressure on lower extremities.

Case study: Nausea and vomiting during pregnancy

Julia, a 31-year-old G1, was presenting to the office for her second prenatal visit at 9 weeks' gestation. She called to schedule her prenatal appointment 1 week earlier because of a significant increase in nausea and vomiting. Julia's medical and family histories are unremarkable. She had no prior history of insomnia, depression, or anxiety disorders.

Today, her weight is 145 lb. Her weight at her first visit 2 weeks ago was 143 lb.

SUBJECTIVE DATA GATHERING: Julia states her nausea and vomiting started about 10 days ago and has progressively gotten worse. She is vomiting one to three times per day. She is able to eat and drink liquids better in the morning and afternoon; by later afternoon, she is too nauseated to eat. She reports that the smells of cooking food make her feel sick. Diet history is obtained. She is able to eat bagels, V-8 vegetable juice, cereal without milk, some fruits and bland vegetables, and chicken; however, it does not always stay down. She indicates she often feels sick enough to leave work in the afternoon. Julia reports using measures such as eating dry carboyhydrates like crackers in the morning, not brushing her teeth right after meals, and sipping small amounts of liquid throughout the day. She is also been trying various forms of ginger every day for the last 5 days, such as ginger tea and ginger candies. She feels all of these measures have been somewhat helpful in the first part of the day, but she still feels has nausea and vomiting in the evening, and is unable to eat much during this time the day.

OBJECTIVE DATA GATHERING: The PUQE scale was administered and her score was 8. An evaluation of skin turgor appears normal, oral mucus membranes are somewhat dry, and urine dip for ketones is +1. Her general affect is pleasant and she is not in acute distress.

PLAN: Julia was advised that a majority of women experience nausea and vomiting in early pregnancy due to the increase in pregnancy hormones, that this is considered a sign of a healthy pregnancy, and that most women experience significant relief by 12–14 weeks' gestation. Positive feedback for using ginger was given with information on making fresh grated ginger tea to increase fluid intake. Julie was advised to continue her current relief measures and a prescription for Diclegis with administration instruction was provided. Education included information that this medication has been studied extensively and is considered safe and effective in pregnancy, and that it will make her sleepy. Avoiding triggers such as the odors of cooking food and discontinuing her prenatal vitamins was advised. She was also shown how to use acupressure at P6 in an effort to reduce her nausea. Julia was comfortable with this plan. A recheck appointment was scheduled for another week for a weight check and to evaluate her progress. She was advised to call with vomiting >24 hours or if she felt her symptoms were not improved with these relief measures.

Visual changes

The physiological increase in third space fluids during pregnancy can result in ocular changes that may be noticeable to a woman. The increase in body fluids can cause an increase in corneal thickness or a change in the corneal curvature. She may report contact lens intolerance or that her lenses or glasses are not providing the same degree of correction. Since these changes are temporary, it is wise to wait several weeks postpartum before changing eye refraction prescriptions.

Subjective data gathering

The onset, description of character of change in vision, history of diabetes, and associated symptoms should be evaluated.

Assessment

Objective data gathering

This consists of obtaining the blood pressure and performing an opthalmoscopic eye exam as indicated. If needed, a visual assessment using a Snellen eye chart can be done.

Case study: Heartburn and sleep deprivation

Rhonda, a 27-year-old G2P1001 at 37 weeks' gestation, was being seen for her routine prenatal visit. She reports a 2-week history of significant substernal pain within an hour after eating that is unrelieved by Tums. The pain lasts for 30 minutes to 2 hours and varies in intensity. She has tried eating food without spices and eliminating fatty foods, but neither strategy has been effective. She also reports being unable to sleep at night for the last 10 days. She states she is very tired when she goes to bed, but her "mind is racing," and when she does fall asleep, she wakes up several times to empty her bladder, leaving her feeling sleep deprived and exhausted during the day. She states she is so tired at work that she often naps for 20 minutes during lunchtime, but that it is difficult to get quality sleep. Her medical and obstetrical histories are normal.

Evaluation was done to rule out preeclampsia as a cause of the substernal pain. Blood pressure was 128/72, reflexes normal, urine dip negative for proteinuria, and she denied visual changes. The assessment of heartburn (pyrosis) was made.

An assessment was done of Rhonda's daily activities, sleep routines, and her emotional status. Rhonda works from 7 am to 3 pm as a nurse in a medical surgical unit and is on her feet most of the day. After work, she picks up her daughter from day care, plays and care for her daughter, prepares dinner, then participates with her husband in their evening ritual of her daughter's bath and story time before bed. She arises at 5:50 am 5 days/week to prepare for work, maintains a regular bedtime of 9:30 pm, reads for 15 minutes before bed, and sleeps in a dark room. She estimated that she is sleeping 5–6 hours per 24 hours right now. A depression inventory was administered

and was negative. She indicates waking up thinking about how she will be able to work full time and care for a newborn and her 2-year-old. She is also feeling worried about going into labor so exhausted.

Rhonda was counseled on the physiological basis for heartburn in pregnancy, and that this is common in later pregnancy. She was advised to institute lifestyle measures such as eating six smaller meals daily to reduce stomach expansion and reflux, avoid food 2 hours before meals, to remain upright after eating, and to continue to avoid highly spiced or fatty foods. The use of liquid antacids and H_2-receptor antagonists was discussed. Liquid antacids are often more effective than chewable tablets as they coat the upper GI tract and neutralize stomach acid. Zantac is more effective as it acts by suppressing stomach acid and is considered safe in pregnancy. Rhonda chose to first try liquid Mylanta 2–4 tsp four times daily and would use OTC Zantac tablets as directed if that was not effective. Rhonda was advised not to use Alka-Seltzer or sodium bicarbonate preparations.

Rhonda's insomnia and lack of sleep were discussed. Rhonda was counseled on the importance of sleep in late gestation. A medical leave from work was provided to enable Rhonda to sleep during the day as needed and to reduce worries about going into labor already exhausted. Measures such as soothing music at bedtime, warm bath prior to bed, relaxation exercises and visualization were advised. She was also counseled to avoid heavy food and excessive fluid intake prior to bedtime. Rhonda felt relieved that she would be off work and have the time to obtain adequate rest and prepare for labor. A revisit was scheduled for 1 week, with instructions to call before then if her symptoms were not improved.

Relief and preventative measures

Women should be informed of the physiological basis and reassured that this symptom is temporary. Women reporting blurry vision after 20 weeks' gestation need immediate evaluation to rule out preeclampsia. Pregnant women with preexisting diabetes reporting eye changes should be referred for further evaluation, as diabetes-related retinopathy can progress during pregnancy (Dinn, Harris, & Marcus, 2003).

Resources for health-care providers and women and their families

American College of Nurse Midwives Share-with-Women—Back Pain during Pregnancy: http://www.midwife.org/Share-With-Women

American College of Nurse Midwives Share-with-Women—Nausea & Vomiting during Pregnancy: http://www.midwife.org/Share-With-Women

American College of Obstetricians and Gynecologists—Frequently Asked Questions: Easing Back Pain during Pregnancy: http://www.acog.org/~/media/For%20Patients/faq100.pdf?dmc=1&ts=20120626T0844442480

American College of Obstetricians and Gynecologists—Frequently Asked Questions: Morning Sickness: http://www.acog.org/~/media/For%20Patients/faq126.pdf?dmc=1&ts=20120626T0846451201

American College of Obstetricians and Gynecologists—Frequently Asked Questions: Skin Conditions during Pregnancy: http://www.acog.org/~/media/For%20Patients/faq169.pdf?dmc=1&ts=20120626T0841117285

Motherisk Nausea & Vomiting of Pregnancy Forum: http://www.motherisk.org/women/forum.jspb

SOS Morning Sickness: http://sosmorningsickness.org/en/

References

Ablove, R., & Ablove, T. (2009). Prevalence of carpal tunnel syndrome in pregnant women. *Wisconsin Medical Journal, 108*(4), 194–196.

Adamson, D., & Nelson-Piercy, C. (2007). Managing palpitations and arrhythmias during pregnancy. *Heart (British Cardiac Society), 93*, 1630–1036. doi:10.1136/hrt.2006.098822

American Academy of Periodontology. (2004). Periodontal management of the pregnant patient. Academy Report.

Balendran, J., Champion, D., Jaaniste, T., & Welsh, A. (2011). A common sleep disorder in pregnancy: Restless leg syndrome and its predictors. *Australian and New Zealand Journal of Obstetrics and Gynaecology, 512*, 262–264.

Baumann, G., Karlikaya, G., Yujsel, G., Citci, B., Kose, G., & Tireli, H. (2007). The subclinical incidence of CTS in pregnancy: Assessment of median nerve impairment in asymptomatic pregnant women. *Neurology, Neurophysiology, and Neuroscience, 3*, 1–9.

Beebe, K., & Lee, K. A. (2007). Sleep disturbance in late pregnancy and early labor. *Journal of Perinatal and Neonatal Nursing, 23*(2), 103–108.

Bell, D., Kane, P., Liang, S., Conway, C., & Tornos, C. (2007). Vulvar varices: An uncommon entity in surgical pathology. *International Journal of Gynecological Pathology, 26*(1), 99–101.

Borg-Stein, J., & Dugan, S. A. (2007). Musculoskeletal disorders of pregnancy, delivery and postpartum. *Physical Medicine and Rehabilitation Clinics of North America, 18*(3), 459–476.

Botehlo, N., Emeis, C., & Brucker, M. C. (2011). Gastrointestinal conditions. In M. Brucker & T. King (Eds.), *Pharmacology for women's health practitioners.* Sudbury, MA: Jones and Bartlett.

Bradley, C., Kennedy, C., Turcea, S., Roa, A., & Nygaard, I. (2007). Constipation in pregnancy: Prevalence symptoms and risk factors. *Obstetrics and Gynecology, 110*(6), 1351–1358.

Chang, J. J., Pien, G. W., Duntley, S. P., & Macones, G. A. (2010). Sleep deprivation during pregnancy and maternal and fetal outcomes: Is there a relationship? *Sleep Medicine Reviews, 14*(2), 107–114. doi:10.1016/j.smrv.2009.05.001

Chestnut, D. H. (2004). *Obstetric anesthesia: Principles and practice* (3rd ed.). Philadelphia: Mosby.

Czeizel, A., Puhó, E., Ács, N., & Bánhidy, F. (2006). Inverse association between severe nausea and vomiting in pregnancy and some congenital anomalies. *American Journal of Medical Genetics, 140A*(5), 453–462.

da Silva, G., Nakamura, M., Corderio, J., & Kulay, L. K. (2005). Acupuncture for insomnia in pregnancy: A prospective quasi-randomized, controlled study. *Acupuncture in Medicine, 23*(2), 47–51.

Davison, J. M. (1997). Edema in pregnancy. *Kidney International. Supplement, 59*, S90–S96.

Dinn, R. B., Harris, A., & Marcus, P. (2003). Ocular changes in pregnancy. *Obstetrical and Gynecological Survey, 58*(2), 137–144.

Djokanovic, N., Garcia-Bournissen, F., & Koren, G. (2008). Medications for restless leg syndrome in pregnancy. *Journal of Obstetrics and Gynaecology Canada, 30*(6), 505–507.

Dugan-Kim, M., Connell, S., Stika, C., Wong, C., & Gossett, D. (2009). Epistaxis of pregnancy associated with postpartum hemorrhage. *Obstetrics and Gynecology, 114*, 1322–1325.

Ebrahimi, N., Maltepe, C., Bournissen, F. G., & Koren, G. (2009). Nausea and vomiting of pregnancy: Using the 24-hour Pregnancy-Unique Quantification of Emesis (PUQE-24) scale. *Journal of Obstetrics and Gynaecology Canada, 31*(9), 803–807.

Ee, C. C., Manheimer, E., Pirotta, M. V., & White, A. R. (2008). Acupuncture for pelvic and back pain in pregnancy: A systematic review. *American Journal of Obstetrics and Gynecology, 198*(3), 254–259.

Ellegard, E., Oscarsson, J., Bougoussa, M., Igout, A., Hennen, G., Edén, S., & Karlsson, G. (1998). Serum level of placental growth hormone is raised in pregnancy rhinitis. *Archives of Otolaryngology–Head and Neck Surgery, 124*(4), 439–443.

Facco, F., Kramer, J., Ho, K., Zee, P., & Grobman, W. (2010). Sleep disturbances in pregnancy. *Obstetrics and Gynecology, 115*(1), 77–83.

Flaxman, S. M., & Sherman, P. W. (2000). Morning sickness: A mechanism for protecting mother and embryo. *Quarterly Review of Biology, 113*–148.

Gearhart, P., Levin, P., & Schimpf, M. (2011). Expanding on earlier findings: A vulvar varicosity grows larger with each pregnancy. *American Journal of Obstetrics and Gynecology, 204*(89), e1–e2.

Gibson, P. S., Powrie, R., & Peipert, J. (2001). Prevalence of syncope and recurrent presyncope during pregnancy. *Obstetrics and Gynecology, 97*(4), 1S–2S.

Godsey, R. K., & Newman, R. B. (1991). Hyperemesis gravidarum. A comparison of single and multiple admissions. *The Journal of Reproductive Medicine, 36*(4), 287–290.

Goldberg, D., Szilagy, A., & Graves, L. (2007). Hyperemesis gravidarum and *Helicobacter pylori* infection: A systemic review. *Obstetrics and Gynecology, 110*, 695–703.

Graham, H. (2007). Breast health and pregnancy. *British Journal of Midwifery, 15*(3), 137–142.

Granath, A. B., Hellgren, M. S., & Gunnarsson, R. K. (2006). Water aerobics reduces sick leave due to low back pain during pregnancy. *Journal of Obstetric, Gynecologic, and Neonatal Nursing, 35*, 465–471. doi:10.1111/j.1552-6909.2006.00066.x

Gupta, A., Gover, M., Nouri, K., & Taylor, S. (2006). The treatment of melasma: A review of clinical trials. *Journal of the American Academy of Dermatology, 55*(6), 1048–1065.

Gürsoy, M., Könönen, E., Tervahartiala, T., Gürsoy, U. K., Pakukanta, R., & Sorsa, T. (2010). Longitudinal study of salivary proteinases during pregnancy and postpartum. *Journal of Periodontal Research, 45*, 496–503.

Hall, W. A., Hauck, Y. L., Carty, E. M., Hutton, E. K., Fenwick, J., & Stoll, K. (2009). Childbirth fear, anxiety, fatigue and sleep deprivation in pregnant women. *Journal of Obstetric, Gynecologic, and Neonatal Nursing, 38*(5), 567–576. doi:10.1111/j.1552-6909.2009.01054.x

Henderson, A. J., & Shaheen, S. O. (2013). Acetaminophen and asthma. *Paediatric Respiratory Reviews, 14*(1), 9–16.

Hensley, J. G. (2009). Leg cramps and restless leg syndrome during pregnancy. *Journal of Midwifery and Women's Health, 54*(3), 211–218. doi:10.1016/j.jmwh.2009.01.003

Hill, C., & Pickinpaugh, J. (2008). Physiologic changes in pregnancy. *Surgical Clinics of North America, 88*(2), 391–401.

Howell, E. R. (2012). Pregnancy-related symphysis pubis dysfunctions management and postpartum rehabilitation: Two case reports. *Journal of the Canadian Chiropractic Association, 56*(2), 102–111.

Irion, J., & Irion, G. (2011). Water immersion to reduce peripheral edema in pregnancy. *Journal of Women's Health Physical Therapy, 35*(2), 46–49.

Ismail, S. K., & Kenny, L. (2007). Review of hyperemesis gravidarum. *Best Practice and Research. Clinical Gastroenterology, 21*(5), 755–769.

Jansen, P. H. P., Lecluse, R. G. M., & Verbeek, A. L. M. (1999). Past and current understanding of the pathophysiology of muscle cramps: Why treatment of varicose veins does not relieve leg cramps. *Journal of the European Academy of Dermatology and Venereology, 12*, 222–229. doi:10.1111/j.1468-3083.1999.tb01032.x

Jewell, D., & Young, G. (2001). Interventions for treating constipation in pregnancy. *Cochrane Database of Systematic Reviews,* (2), CD001142. doi:10.1002/14651858.CD001142

Johnson, T., & Strube, K. (2011). Breast care during pregnancy. *Journal of Obstetric, Gynecologic, and Neonatal Nursing, 40*(2), 144–148.

Kalus, S., Kornman, L., & Quinlivan, J. (2008). Managing back pain in pregnancy using a support garment: A randomized trial. *BJOG: An International Journal of Obstetrics and Gynaecology, 115*, 68–75. doi:10.1111/j.1471-0528.2007.01538.x

Kamysheva, E., Werthmeim, E., Skouteris, H., Paxton, S., & Milgrom, J. (2009). Frequency, severity, and effect on life of physical symptoms experienced during pregnancy. *Journal of Midwifery and Women's Health, 54*(1), 43–49.

Kanakaris, N. K., Roberts, C. S., & Giannoudis, P. V. (2011). Pregnancy-related pelvic girdle pain: An update. *BMC Medicine, 9*(1), 15. Retrieved from http://www.biomedcentral.com/1741-7015/9/15

Keller, J., Frederking, D., & Layer, P. (2008). The spectrum and treatment of gastrointestinal disorders during pregnancy. *Nature Clinical Practice. Gastroenterology and Hepatology, 5*(8), 430–444. doi:10.1038/ncpgasthep1197

King, T., & Murphy, P. (2009). Evidence-based approaches to management of nausea and vomiting of pregnancy. *Journal of Midwifery and Women's Health, 54*(6), 1–8.

Kocaöz, S., Talas, M., & Atabekoğlu, C. (2010). Urinary incontinence in pregnancy women and their quality of life. *Journal of Clinical Nursing, 19*, 3314–3323. doi:10.1111/j.1365-2702.2010.03421.x

Koren, G., Piwko, C., Ahn, E., Boskovic, R., Maltepe, C., Einarson, A., . . . Ungar, W. (2005). Validation studies of the Pregnancy Unique Quantification of Emesis (PUQE) scores. *Journal of Obstetrics and Gynaecology, 25*(3), 241–244.

Kroumpouzos, G., & Cohen, L. (2001). Dermatoses of pregnancy. *Journal of the American Academy of Dermatology, 45*, 1–19.

Kumari, R., Jaisankar, T., & Thappa, D. (2007). A clinical study of skin changes in pregnancy. *Indian Journal of Dermatology, Venereology and Leprology, 73*, 141.

Lee, K. A., & Gay, C. L. (2004). Sleep in late pregnancy predicts length of labor and type of delivery. *American Journal of Obstetrics and Gynecology, 191*, 2041–2046.

Lisi, A. (2006). Chiropractic spinal manipulation for low back pain of pregnancy: A retrospective case series. *Journal of Midwifery and Women's Health, 51*(1), e7–e10.

Longo, S., Moore, R., Canzoneri, B., & Robichaux, A. (2010). Gastrointestinal conditions during pregnancy. *Clinics in Colon and Rectal Surgery, 23*, 80–89.

Lurie, S., Matas, Z., Fux, A., Golan, A., & Sadan, O. (2011). Association of serum relaxin with striae gravidarum in pregnant women. *Archives of Gynecology and Obstetrics, 283*, 219–222.

Marcus, D. (2007). Headache in pregnancy. *Current Treatment Options in Neurology, 9*(1), 23–30. doi:10.1007/s11940-007-0027-0

Mogran, I., & Pohjanen, A. I. (2005). Low back pain and pelvic pain during pregnancy: Prevalence and risk factors. *Spine, 30*(8), 9830991.

Muallem, M. M., & Rubeiz, N. G. (2006). Physiological and biological skin changes in pregnancy. *Clinics in Dermatology, 24*(2), 80–83.

Namazy, J. A., & Schatz, M. (2011). Asthma and rhinitis during pregnancy. *Mount Sinai Journal of Medicine, New York, 78*, 661–670.

Niebyl, J. (2010). Nausea and vomiting in pregnancy. *New England Journal of Medicine, 363*(16), 1544.

Nussbaum, R., & Benedetto, A. V. (2006). Cosmetic aspects of pregnancy. *Clinics in Dermatology, 24*(2), 133–141.

Nygaard, I. H., Valbø, A., Pethick, S. V., & Bøhmer, T. (2008). Does oral magnesium substitution relieve pregnancy-induced leg cramps? *European Journal of Obstetrics, Gynecology, and Reproductive Biology, 141*(1), 23–26. doi:10.1016/j.ejogrb.2008.07.005

Office of Teratology Information Specialists (OTIS). (2011). Acetaminophen and Pregnancy. Retrieved from http://www.otispregnancy.org/files/acetaminophen.pdf

Okun, M. L., Kiewra, K., Luther, J. F., Wisnewski, S. R., & Wisner, K. L. (2011). Sleep disturbance in depressed and non depressed pregnant women. *Depression and Anxiety, 28*, 676–685.

Okun, M. L., Schetter, C. D., & Glynn, L. M. (2011). Poor sleep quality is associated with preterm birth. *Sleep, 34*, 1493–1498.

Osman, H., Rubeiz, N., Tamin, H., & Nassar, A. (2007). Risk factors for the development of striae gravidarum. *American Journal of Obstetrics and Gynecology, 196*(1), 62e1–62 e5.

Padua, L., Pasquale, A., Pazzaglia, C., Liotta, G., Librante, A., & Mondelli, M. (2010). Systematic review of pregnancy-related carpal tunnel syndrome. *Muscle and Nerve, 42*(5), 697–702.

Palfreyman, S., & Michaels, J. (2009). A systematic review of compression hosiery for uncomplicated varicose veins. *Phlebology, 24*(S1), 13–33.

Pazzaglia, C., Caliandro, P., Aprile, I., Mondelli, M., Foschini, M., Tonali, P. A., . . . Italian, C. T. S. (2005). Multicenter study on carpal tunnel syndrome and pregnancy incidence and natural course. *Acta Neurochirurgica, 92*(Suppl.), 35.

Pieper, P. G. (2008). Expected and unexpected cardiac problems during pregnancy. *Netherlands Heart Journal, 16*(12), 403–405.

Richens, Y., Smith, K., & Leddington, S. (2010). Lower back pain during pregnancy: Advice and exercises for women. *British Journal of Midwifery, 18*(9), 562–566.

Richter, J. E. (2003). Gastroesphogeal reflux disease during pregnancy. *Gastroenterology Clinics of North America, 31*(1), 235–261.

Salter, S. A., & Kimball, A. B. (2006). Striae gravidarum. *Clinics in Dermatology, 24*, 97–100.

Sances, G., Granella, F., Nappi, R. E., Fignon, A., Ghiotto, N., Polatti, F., & Nappi, G. (2003). Course of migraine during pregnancy and postpartum: A prospective study. *Cephalalgia, 23*(3), 197.

Silberstein, S. D. (2004). Headaches in pregnancy. *Neurologic Clinics, 22*(4), 727.

Tella, B., Sokunbi, O., Akinlami, O., & Afolabi, B. (2011). Effects of aerobic exercise n the level of insomnia and fatigue in pregnant women. *International Journal of Gynecology and Obstetrics, 15*(1), 1.

Tharpe, N., Farley, C., & Jordan, R. (2012). *Clinical practice guidelines for midwifery and women's health* (4th ed.). Sudbury, MA: Jones & Bartlett.

Thorpe, K., Dragonas, T., & Golding, J. (1992). The effects of psychological factors on the emotional well being of women during pregnancy: A cross cultural study of Britain and Greece. *Journal of Reproductive and Infant Psychology, 10*(4), 205–217.

Tuğba, T., Karadağ, Y., Doğulu, F., & Inan, L. (2007). Predisposing factors to restless leg syndrome in pregnancy. *Movement Disorders, 22*(5), 627–631.

U.S. Department of Health and Human Services, Office on Woman's Health. (2010). Varicose veins and spider veins. Retrieved from http://www.womenshealth.gov/publications/our-publications/fact-sheet/varicose-spider-veins.pdf

Van Cleef, J. (2011). Treatment of vulvar and perineal varicose veins. *Phlebolymphology, 18*(1), 38–44.

van Dinter, M. C. (1991). Ptyalism in pregnant women. *Journal of Obstetric, Gynecologic, and Neonatal Nursing, 20*, 206.

VanThiel, D. H., Gavaler, J. J., Joshi, S. N., et al. (1977). Heartburn of pregnancy. *Gastroenterology, 72*, 668–678.

Vazquez, J. C. (2008). Constipation, haemorrhoids, and heartburn in pregnancy. *Clinical Evidence (Online), 2008*.

Vleeming, A., Hanne, B., Ostgaard, H., Sturesson, B., & Stuge, B. (2007). European guidelines for the diagnosis and treatment of pelvic girdle pain. Retrieved from http://www.backpaineurope.org/web/files/586_2008_602_OnlinePDF.pdf

Weigel, R. M., & Weigel, M. (1989). Nausea and vomiting of early pregnancy and pregnancy outcome. A meta–analytical review. *BJOG: An International Journal of Obstetrics & Gynaecology, 96*(11), 1312–1318.

Xiong, X., Buekens, P., Vastardis, S., & Yu, S. (2007). Periodontal disease and pregnancy outcomes: State of the science. *Obstetrical and Gynecological Survey, 62*(9), 605–615.

12

Medication use during pregnancy

Mary C. Brucker and Tekoa L. King

Relevant terms

Adverse drug reaction—response to a drug that is noxious and unintended and which occurs at doses normally used for prophylaxis, diagnosis, or therapy of disease or for the modification of physiological function

Background risk—risk that is unavoidable; in pregnancy, the background risk of a congenital anomaly is estimated at approximately 3–4%

Behind-the-counter (BTC) drug—a subtype of over-the-counter drugs, behind-the-counter drugs are nonprescription but are not on open shelving due to potential for abuse after modification; the prototype is pseudoephedrine, which can be made into a type of amphetamine

Bioequivalent—a term used to denote that the pharmacokinetics between two agents are essentially the same and the results of administration are anticipated to be the same when administered under similar circumstances

Black box warning—a method that the FDA uses to identify unusual harm associated with an agent; often it is added to package inserts after postmarketing studies to identify unexpected risks

Botanical—a plant, in whole or part, that is used for medicinal purposes

Brand name—a trademarked name assigned to a drug by the manufacturer; some brand names are similar to the generic name (e.g., pseudoephedrine/Sudafed®); others suggest their indications for use (e.g., Tamiflu®)

Clinical trials—controlled studies to ascertain the effectiveness and safety of proposed drugs

Controlled substance—pharmaceuticals listed in schedules found in U.S. Law 21 U.S.C. §802(32)(A); these agents include both opiates as well as nonopiates, and generally have a high risk of addiction, often without valid medicinal use; examples include heroin

Cytochrome P450—the name of a large family of enzymes involved with metabolism, especially of lipids, steroidal hormones, toxins, and various drugs; genetic variations

within the subgroups of the family are often the etiology of drug–drug or drug–other agent interactions

Drug resistance—inability of a drug, usually an anti-infective, to be therapeutic due to changes in the targeted microorganism; in the majority of cases, after initial exposure to the drug or a similar agent, the microorganism evolves so it no longer is sensitive to the agent.

Food and Drug Administration (FDA)—a federal agency whose charges include protecting and promoting public health through regulation of prescription and over-the-counter drugs; other areas under their purview include vaccines, blood transfusions, medical devices, electromagnetic radiation, and food safety

Herbal—a medication that is a subtype of botanicals and is composed of edible plants

Over-the-counter (OTC) drug—Nonprescription drug available directly to consumers

Polypharmacy—the practice of treating individuals using multidrug regimens; this term generally is accepted to mean administration of five or more drugs

Prescriptive authority—legal ability to prescribe drugs, medical devices, and so on

Prescriptive drugs—agents that have been approved by the FDA in the United States and are available by prescription only through a health professional with prescriptive authority

Side effect—physiological responses unrelated to the desired drug effects that occur with therapeutic doses of the medication; side effects may be beneficial or harmful

Teratogen—from the Greek for *monster*, a teratogen is an agent (drug, virus, disease, or other) that causes a permanent congenital anomaly when taken during a critical period in embryonic or fetal development

Therapeutic window—also known as the pharmaceutical window; plasma drug concentration should be between the minimum effective concentration (MEC) in the plasma for obtaining the desired drug action and the mean toxic concentration (MTC)

Prenatal and Postnatal Care: A Woman-Centered Approach, First Edition. Edited by Robin G. Jordan, Janet L. Engstrom, Julie A. Marfell, and Cindy L. Farley.
© 2014 John Wiley & Sons, Inc. Published 2014 by John Wiley & Sons, Inc.

Introduction

Health-care providers must have good diagnostic skills and a broad knowledge of effective therapeutic interventions including nutrition, physical exercise, emotional support, and nonpharmacologic agents. Today, more than ever, health-care providers must also be knowledgeable about pharmacologic interventions.

Clinically relevant pharmacologic information that is applicable to women can be difficult to obtain because data about the pharmacologic effects of drugs on women are limited. Drug trials often have a lower percentage of women enrolled than men, and when women are included in drug trials, gender-specific analysis may not be conducted or published (Franconi, Brunelleschi, Steardo, & Cuomo, 2007). The data are even sparser with regard to pregnant and lactating women. Few rigorous studies have been conducted concerning the use of drugs for pregnant, postpartum, or lactating women secondary to ethical dilemmas, potential fetal risks, or possible litigation years after use. However, as approximately 4 million pregnant women give birth in the United States every year (Martin et al., 2011), pharmacologic principles that apply to this population are an essential body of knowledge. This chapter reviews basic principles of prescribing and presents an overview of pregnancy-specific pharmacologic topics.

Pharmacologic terms

Pharmacology has a language that can be confusing. For example, opioids are rarely termed "narcotics" when used in a therapeutic context, but the term narcotics is widely used when discussing opioids as agents of abuse. The "Relevant terms" at the start of this chapter summarizes some of the more common pharmacologic terms in an effort to facilitate clarity.

Types of pharmaceutical agents

Pharmaceutical agents include all chemical substances used for the prevention, treatment, or cure of diseases. The majority of pharmaceutical agents are referred to as drugs or medications. Nonprescription agents, which include over-the-counter (OTC) medicines and nutritional supplements or botanicals, may be obtained directly without a prescription from a health-care provider. Prescription drugs can only be dispensed to the public if the medication is prescribed by a properly authorized health-care provider.

In addition to nonprescription and prescription drugs, individuals may be exposed to pharmaceuticals in other ways. For example, hormones and antimicrobials fed to animals may enter into the food chain. An analysis of water in the Great Lakes conducted in 2010 found that almost 35% of surface water contained traces of various pharmaceuticals (Klecka, Persoon, & Currie, 2010). Environmental pollutants and metabolites can also have pharmacologic effects that result in endocrine disruptions, including abnormalities in a woman's menstrual pattern. Years ago, people were advised to discard out-of-date medications by flushing them down a toilet or washing them through the kitchen garbage disposal. These practices are no longer recommended due to concerns about environmental contamination. The current recommendation is to take unused medications to a local pharmacy or government agency that offers disposal of pharmaceuticals.

Pharmaceutical agents are used extensively by pregnant women. More than 50% of pregnant women have reported using an herbal remedy, usually ginger, cranberry, or raspberry leaves in an attempt to treat a common discomfort of pregnancy (Dennehy, 2011; Holst, Wright, Haavik, & Nordeng, 2009). Although the number of drugs used by individuals today is alarming to some, there are some nutritional supplements that have great value for women, which, ironically, are underused. All women of reproductive age are encouraged to take folic acid, a B vitamin that decreases the risk of a neonate being born with an open neural tube defect if taken preconceptionally and during the first few weeks of pregnancy. Yet when the National Health and Nutrition Examination researchers analyzed surveys in 2009, they discovered that more than 70% of women 15–44 years of age did not consume folic acid supplements regularly (Tinker, Cogswell, Devine, & Berry, 2010).

The use of OTC drugs is commonplace in the United States. In a survey of more than 650 adults, the most frequently cited reasons for using such agents were familiarity with the agents as well as accessibility and the costs saved by avoiding an ambulatory visit with a health-care professional (National Council on Patient Information and Education (NCPIE), 2008). Among all prescription and nonprescription agents, the one most commonly used by pregnant women is acetaminophen (Tylenol®), either alone or in combination with other analgesics or cough/cold remedies. More than 60% of pregnant women have reported using this drug (Werler, Mitchell, Hernandez-Diaz, & Honein, 2005).

Prescriptive authority

Historically, physicians have had the broadest authority to prescribe drugs and medical devices. Prescriptive authority is governed by state statute and today, a variety of other providers also have various degrees of prescriptive authority, including dentists, nurse-midwives, nurse practitioners, podiatrists, psychologists, physician assistants, and veterinarians (Osborne, 2011; Plank, 2011). The type of prescriptive authority possessed by these health-care providers often varies according to jurisdiction of the state or territory, and may be limited by the discipline's professional scope of practice.

Governmental oversight of pharmaceutical agents

Several different federal agencies are involved in the regulation of pharmaceutical agents. The Food and Drug Administration (FDA) has authority to approve, monitor, and withdraw prescription and nonprescription agents, including monitoring of drug advertising. An important exception concerns nutritional supplements and botanical agents. These OTC products are not classified as drugs and are therefore not regulated by the FDA. They can, however, have important pharmacologic effects, including interactions with other prescribed drugs.

Other organizations that regulate pharmaceuticals include the Federal Trade Commission (FTC), which is authorized to monitor direct-to-consumer advertising of OTC medications. The Drug Enforcement Administration (DEA) regulates drugs that have significant risks of addiction. These agents commonly are known as "controlled substances" and are subdivided into five categories ranked from highest to lowest potential for addiction (Table 12.1). Agents in the first category (schedule I) include drugs rarely if ever prescribed for therapeutic reasons such as heroin and cocaine. Agents in the last category (schedule V) include cough suppressants that contain codeine (United States Department of Justice, 2012). The DEA issues specific DEA prescriber numbers to health-care providers who are approved to write prescriptions for controlled substances and monitors those prescriptions. In some jurisdictions, the prescriptive authority of providers other than physicians may be limited on the basis of the controlled substance categories.

When a pharmaceutical company seeks FDA approval to market a drug for the treatment of a specific condition, they conduct preapproval studies that are designed to demonstrate the drug's efficacy and safety. Clinical trials with human subjects occur in three phases. Phase I trials study healthy individuals to determine the pharmacokinetics and pharmacodynamics of an agent. Phase II trials enroll small numbers of persons with the disorder of interest to determine the initial efficacy of a medication. Phase III trials enroll larger numbers of individuals to see if the initial efficacy is statistically and clinically significant. The FDA's Center for Drug

Evaluation and Research (CDER) evaluates the results of these clinical trials and recommends or denies approval of the medication. It is important to note that a drug can be prescribed to treat a disorder that the drug is not specifically approved to treat. This is called "off-label" use. An example of off-label prescribing is the use of misoprostol (Cytotec®), a drug the FDA has approved for treating ulcers that is also used for cervical ripening prior to induction of labor.

The prescription: Essential components

Historically, prescriptions have been written on a paper pad of preprinted blanks and given to a consumer who took the prescription to a pharmacy where the medication was dispensed. These prescription pads have important components essential for security and prevention of fraud such as anticopy watermarks, ink that turns a copy black upon photocopying, colored backgrounds to prevent erasures, unique batch numbers, and even UV fibers similar to U.S. currency may be embedded in the paper on which the prescription is written. Electronic methods of prescribing (e-prescribing) provide additional protections from fraud and have the additional advantage of minimizing medical errors.

When handwritten prescriptions are used, it is expected that the text will be printed (not written in cursive), legible, and contain a number of essential required components. These include the name, address, and phone number of the provider. If a provider is in a group practice with a listing of all members printed at the top of the prescription, the individual prescriber should circle her/his name. Prescription pads also usually include dedicated lines for the consumer's name, age, address, and current date; generic name of medication, dose, amount to be dispensed, and number of times the medication can be refilled; the letters RX or R/ to signify the "recipe" and to verify that this is a drug prescription; and the provider's signature, license number, and DEA number. The DEA number is a unique number created using a standardized coding method that identifies the type of provider through a letter prefix. Although the DEA is charged with monitoring the prescription of controlled substances only, a DEA number is increasingly being required of all prescribers for all prescriptions.

The use of the generic name for a particular medication on the prescription allows the pharmacist to dispense a less expensive formulation if one is available. Some prescribers will choose to request a particular brand name and indicate in writing that no substitution should be undertaken. Some medications have variable biologic effects in different formulations. When this is the case, a specific brand name may be necessary to

Table 12.1   Schedules for Controlled Substances

Schedule	Definition/examples
I	Substances in this schedule have a high potential for abuse, have no currently accepted medical use for treatment in the United States, and there is a lack of accepted safety for use of the drug or other substance under medical supervision. Some examples of substances listed in schedule I are heroin, lysergic acid diethylamide (LSD), peyote, methaqualone, and 3,4-methylenedioxymethamphetamine ("ecstasy").
II	Substances in this schedule have a high potential for abuse, which may lead to severe psychological or physical dependence. Examples of single entity schedule II narcotics include morphine and opium. Other schedule II narcotic substances and their common name brand products include hydromorphone (Dilaudid®), methadone (Dolophine®), meperidine (Demerol®), oxycodone (OxyContin®), and fentanyl (Sublimaze® or Duragesic®). Examples of schedule II stimulants include amphetamines (Dexedrine®, Adderall®), methamphetamine (Desoxyn®), and methylphenidate (Ritalin®). Other schedule II substances include cocaine, amobarbital, glutethimide, and pentobarbital.
III	Substances in this schedule have a potential for abuse less than substances in schedules I or II, and abuse may lead to moderate or low physical dependence or high psychological dependence. Examples of schedule III narcotics include combination products containing less than 15 milligrams of hydrocodone per dosage unit (Vicodin®) and products containing not more than 90 mg of codeine per dosage unit (Tylenol with Codeine®). Also included are buprenorphine products (Suboxone® and Subutex®) used to treat opioid addiction. Examples of schedule III non-narcotics include benzphetamine (Didrex®), phendimetrazine, ketamine, and anabolic steroids such as oxandrolone (Oxandrin®).
IV	Substances in this schedule have a low potential for abuse relative to substances in schedule III. An example of a schedule IV narcotic is propoxyphene (Darvon® and Darvocet-N 100®). Other schedule IV substances include alprazolam (Xanax®), clonazepam (Klonopin®), clorazepate (Tranxene®), diazepam (Valium®), lorazepam (Ativan®), midazolam (Versed®), temazepam (Restoril®), and triazolam (Halcion®).
V	Substances in this schedule have a low potential for abuse relative to substances listed in schedule IV and consist primarily of preparations containing limited quantities of certain narcotics. These are generally used for antitussive, antidiarrheal, and analgesic purposes. Examples include cough preparations containing not more than 200 mg of codeine per 100 mL or per 100 g (Robitussin AC® and Phenergan with Codeine®).

Adapted from: United States Department of Justice. (2012). Controlled Substance Schedules. Retrieved from http://www.deadiversion. usdoj.gov/schedules/#define.

ensure a consistent effect. In those unusual situations, a note clarifying why the brand is medically indicated should be placed in the woman's health record.

The clinical indication for which the drug is being prescribed also should be prominent (e.g., "metronidazole for trichomonas"). Prescriptions also include dose of the drug; how many doses should be taken at one time (e.g., two tablets); route of administration; number of times per day or hour intervals at which the agent should be taken; any specifics regarding timing of administration, such as "with food"; and amount to be dispensed (e.g., 30 tablets) and the number of refills. When a drug has a dosage that is less than one unit such as 0.25 mcg, it should be written with a zero before the decimal point in order to minimize confusion. Similarly, trailing zeros should not be used. A medication that is available in 250 mg tablets should not be written as 250.0 mg. Prescriptions must be dated and signed by a legal prescriber.

Abbreviations should not be used, even those thought to be in common usage.

Figure 12.1 illustrates a prescription in a common format. Since prescriptive authority differs somewhat based on the legal jurisdiction, minor changes may be found among prescriptions.

Drugs and pregnancy

Today, women are counseled to avoid drugs during pregnancy if possible. However, more than 60% of pregnant women take one or more drugs during pregnancy, excluding vitamins or mineral supplements (Andrade et al., 2004). A major concern about the use of medications during pregnancy is fetal risk, which is often unknown. For the woman and her provider, this is can be a complex challenge as they weigh the risks versus benefits of pharmacologic treatment (Koren, 2011). For example, a

N. E. Physician, MD
C. Smith, FNP-BC
M. Breckenridge, CNM
J. Johnson, PA
123 Any Street
Oakland, CA 94602
(510) 123-4567

Name: <u>Amy Jones</u>   Date: <u>12/1/2014</u>
Address: <u>987 Main Street, Oakland CA</u>

Rx

Nitrofurantoin 100 mg
Disp: 10 tablets
Sig: 1 tablet at bedtime for 10 days
Dx: Asymptomatic bacteruria

Brand Necessary
(May substitute generic)

Refill <u>0 times</u>

_____
Signature

Figure 12.1. Sample prescription.

woman with a seizure disorder may risk experiencing status epilepticus complete with significant oxygen deprivation for herself and her fetus or, if treated with an anticonvulsant, an increased risk of a specific birth defect for her fetus. Some agents, such as folic acid, are therapeutic for the embryo/fetus and provide no benefit to the woman. Identification of the fetal risk associated with individual drugs is difficult because few clinical trials have included pregnant women. In addition, identification of fetal harm may take several years to become apparent.

Teratology

Drugs used by a pregnant woman can cause harm to the fetus in two ways: teratogenosis and fetotoxicity. Drugs that are teratogens cause a permanent change in structure, function, or growth. Most of the well-known teratogenic drugs interfere with organogenesis during the embryonic period, which results in birth defects such as a cleft palate, cardiac anomaly, facial abnormality, or another dysmorphic effect. The other mechanism by which drugs affect the fetus is fetotoxicity. Fetotoxic agents, such as tobacco, exert effects on growth or fetal development in the second and third trimesters.

The first teratogen discovered was not of pharmaceutical origin, but was a virus—rubella. Congenital rubella syndrome was identified in the early 1940s by an Australian ophthalmologist, Norman Gregg, who noticed that there was an increase in neonatal cataracts after an outbreak of rubella some months before (Dunn, 2007). Gregg's discovery was counter to the then prevailing theory that the placenta provided a barrier that protected the fetus and, therefore, any birth defect must be solely inheritable. This observation changed the understanding about the risk to the fetus from environmental exposures.

The American public became aware of the risk of drugs in pregnancy when the mass media widely publicized the dangers of thalidomide. In the late 1950s, thalidomide, produced in Germany, was prescribed as a sedative and antiemetic and marketed as a treatment for women with nausea and vomiting of pregnancy. Data regarding teratogenic effects emerged in Europe while the FDA was scrutinizing the agent for approval in the United States. The data revealed that thalidomide interrupts limb formation such that exposed fetuses are born with various limb deformities. Although the drug was never FDA approved for use in pregnancy, it was estimated that several thousand pregnant women residing in the United States took thalidomide via the samples provided to physicians in anticipation of FDA approval. After the thalidomide tragedy was recognized, the FDA imposed stricter regulations for the approval of new

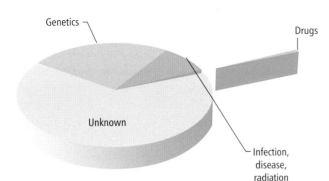

Genetics

Drugs

Unknown

Infection,
disease,
radiation

Figure 12.2. Causes of birth defects. Adapted from: Jacobs
et al. (1974) and Koren (2011).

Table 12.2	Wilson's Six Principles of Teratology
Principle 1	Susceptibility to teratogenesis depends on the genotype of the conceptus and the manner in which this interacts with environmental factors.
Principle 2	Susceptibility to teratogenic agents varies with the developmental stage at the time of exposure.
Principle 3	Teratogenic agents act in specific ways (mechanisms) on developing cells and tissues to initiate abnormal embryogenesis (pathogenesis).
Principle 4	The final manifestations of abnormal development are death, malformation, growth retardation, and functional disorder.
Principle 5	The access of adverse environmental influences to developing tissues depends on the nature of the influences (agent).
Principle 6	Manifestations of deviant development increase in degree as dosage increases from no-effect to a totally lethal level.

drugs. Another result was a general shift to the public belief that all drugs are potential teratogens until disproven, and the misconception that drugs are the most common etiology for birth effects.

Etiology of birth defects

Congenital anomalies secondary to unknown causes occur in approximately 3–4% of all births. This statistic often is referred to as the background risk. Sixty-five to seventy percent of birth defects are idiopathic with no known etiology (Jacobs, Melville, Ratcliffe, Keay, & Syme, 1974; Koren, 2011). Approximately 25% of birth anomalies are identified as having a genetic cause. As illustrated in Figure 12.2, drugs and chemicals account for about 1% of all identified birth defects. The other causes of birth defects are maternal diseases, infections, radiation, chemicals, and various environmental insults. Although the number of medications prescribed during pregnancy has increased greatly during recent years, the number of known teratogenic drugs has remained remarkably small with only a few new discoveries in recent decades. In addition, even though the number of birth defects due to pharmaceutical agents is relatively small, the emphasis on teratogenic drugs remains important because any drug associated birth defect can potentially be avoided entirely if the drug is not taken (Fig. 12.2).

Mechanisms of teratogenic drugs

Contemporary to the thalidomide event, embryologist Jim Wilson identified six principles of teratology that continue to be relevant today (Friedman, 2010; Wilson, 1959, 1977) (see Table 12.2). In the first principle, Wilson noted the importance of host susceptibility, which explains why not all fetuses have the same reaction to a specific teratogen.

The second principle provides credence to the concept of the critical period. When critical periods are discussed, publications often report pregnancy in weeks

Adapted from: Wilson, J. (1977). Current status of teratology: general principles and mechanisms derived from animal studies. In J. Wilson & F. Fraser (Eds.), *Handbook of teratology* (4 vols, 47–74). New York: Plenum Press. Springer.

after fertilization as opposed to gestational weeks that are calculated from the date of the last normal menses. Embryologists describe gestational age using the date of conception as the starting point for calculating the age of the conceptus (postconception dating). In contrast, health-care providers usually calculate the number of gestational weeks from the first day of the last menstrual period (menstrual age or gestational age). Thus, in the area of teratology, it is important to know which type of dating is in use in order to identify critical periods.

For the purposes of teratogenicity, pregnancy can be subdivided into three time periods: pre-embryonic (between fertilization and implantation), embryonic (between implantation and 9 postconception weeks), and the fetal period (after 9 postconception weeks). Exposure to a teratogen during the pre-embryonic period usually results in an "all or none" effect. Since the tissue is undifferentiated, either there is a pregnancy loss or there is no teratogenic effect of exposure to a teratogen during this period of pregnancy. The latter phenomenon also has been illustrated with the technique of preimplantation genetic diagnosis. This type of early embryo assessment used with *in vitro* fertilization consists of removing a few cells with the knowledge that the remaining cells will compensate.

During the embryonic period, organogenesis can be adversely affected by a teratogen. In general, this is the period of greatest concern for use of pharmaceuticals. The fetal period is the time when the fetus is most susceptible to growth restriction and developmental or behavioral abnormalities (Moore & Persaud, 2007). Figure 12.3 is a classic illustration of the critical periods in human development from the viewpoint of an embryologist using postconceptional dating. Some organ systems are susceptible for a few days, whereas the central nervous system may be affected over a period of months.

Wilson's third principle addresses the mechanisms of teratology. A review of drugs in pregnancy identified the mechanisms of most teratogens to be one of folate antagonism, neural crest cell disruption, endocrine disruption of sex hormones, oxidative stress, vascular disruption, or specific receptor- or enzyme-mediated reactions (van Gelder et al., 2010). The newer research regarding mechanisms eventually may result in some changes in the design of the drugs to prevent teratogenic effects or possibly create antidotes.

The last two principles proposed by Wilson reflect the potency and type of teratogen. High doses of a potent teratogen logically would have the potential for causing a more severe effect than lower doses of a less potent drug.

Identification of a teratogen

Unlike a laboratory diagnosis of a condition like diabetes mellitus or a bacterial infection, identification of a teratogen is quite difficult. Most teratogenic drugs are not identified as such before they are approved by the FDA. The randomized clinical trialss (RCTs) conducted to test safety and efficacy prior to FDA approval for marketing are not able to identify rare harms for three reasons: First, they do not have enough participants; second, these trials usually exclude women (pregnant or not), persons who take other medications, or those have comorbid conditions that might interfere with the drug's effects. Thus, the effects are not generalizable to a larger population. Third, the RCTs only document immediate effects as they do not follow participants for long periods after the exposure. Preapproval drug trial RCTs may prove helpful to determine drug benefits but are poor at detecting potential harms (Vandenbroucke & Psaty, 2008).

Unfortunately, teratogens, like other rare adverse drug effects, are a post hoc phenomenon and are revealed only after children are affected. Among the factors for consideration when a drug is being evaluated as a teratogen include an increase in the frequency of the birth defect in the exposed group of women compared to general population. The likelihood of teratogenicity is strengthened if the congenital anomaly is rare and if a similar finding is apparent in animal models. The presence of

two specific effects, namely, dose response and threshold, also serve to validate the probability of a teratogen (Friedman & Polifka, 1994).

Although teratogens are occasionally first identified as such after years of use in the general marketplace, an agent also may be mislabeled as a teratogen by the public without scientific foundation. The ease at which information is placed on the Internet and shared on social media sites may cause unfounded opinions to become accepted as fact. Women may question agents that have little or no scientific data about teratogenicity. An example of this would be the multiple web sites that "link" the artificial sweetener aspartame to birth defects, lupus, multiple sclerosis, cancers, and other conditions in spite of scientific research to the contrary.

As more knowledge of genetics and pharmacogenomics emerge, it is hoped that there may be better predictors of teratogens in the future (Mitchell, 2011). Unfortunately, most teratogens continue to be revealed after children are born with life-changing birth defects (Augustine-Rauch, 2008).

FDA categories for drugs in pregnancy

In 1979, the FDA published a pregnancy-specific categorization of drugs in an attempt to facilitate recognition of teratogenic drugs so the agents could be avoided or at least used judiciously (United States Food and Drug Administration, 1979). The five categories are named after letters of the Latin alphabet, A, B, C, D and X, and are listed in Table 12.3. Few drugs are able to meet the rigor required to be a category A drug; however, a large number of agents such as vitamins, acetaminophen, anti-infectives, and pharmaceuticals used to treat common gastrointestinal ailments are listed in category B.

Drugs assigned to categories D and X are known teratogens, but the two categories are divided on the basis of whether or not the clinical indication for the drug outweighs the risk of using it. For example, some commonly used anticonvulsants are classified as category D because the risk of teratogenicity is not absolute and maternal need for the drug is significant. In contrast, isotretinoin (Accutane) is a category X agent because there are no known situations in which the treatment of acne outweighs the potential teratogenic risk.

FDA category C contains the most complex array of medications and because of this, it is the most confusing. Category C drugs include drugs that cause teratogenic effects in animals but no apparent untoward effects in humans. The prototypical drug for this class is a corticosteroid that is linked to birth defects in rabbits but has not been linked to abnormalities in humans. Additionally, drugs for which no data on safety during pregnancy

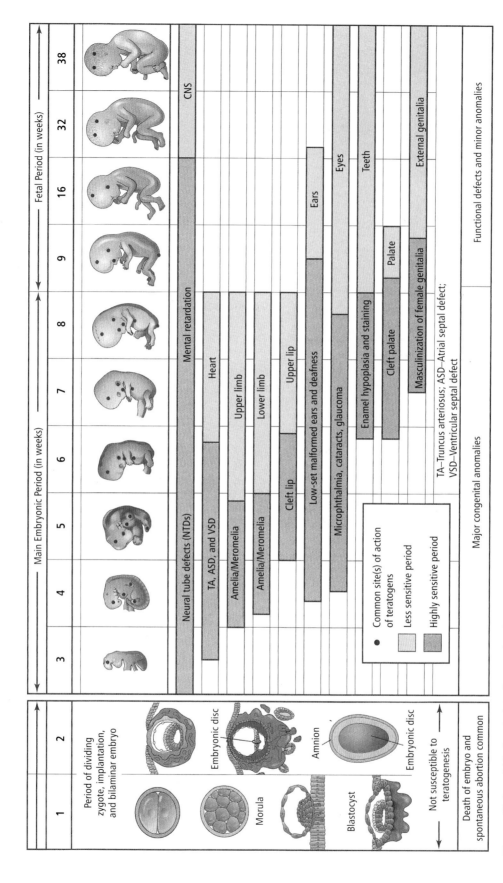

Figure 12.3.   Critical periods in human development according to postconceptional weeks. Adapted from: Moore et al. (2007).

Table 12.3 U.S. FDA Pregnancy Categories

United States FDA pregnancy categories	
Pregnancy category A	Adequate and well-controlled human studies have failed to demonstrate a risk to the fetus in the first trimester of pregnancy (and there is no evidence of risk in later trimesters).
Pregnancy category B	Animal reproduction studies have failed to demonstrate a risk to the fetus, and there are no adequate and well-controlled studies in pregnant women, or animal studies have shown an adverse effect, but adequate and well-controlled studies in pregnant women have failed to demonstrate a risk to the fetus in any trimester.
Pregnancy category C	Animal reproduction studies have shown an adverse effect on the fetus and there are no adequate and well-controlled studies in humans, but potential benefits may warrant use of the drug in pregnant women despite potential risks.
Pregnancy category D	There is positive evidence of human fetal risk based on adverse reaction data from investigational or marketing experience or studies in humans, but potential benefits may warrant use of the drug in pregnant women despite potential risks.
Pregnancy category X	Studies in animals or humans have demonstrated fetal abnormalities and/or there is positive evidence of human fetal risk based on adverse reaction data from investigational or marketing experience, and the risks involved in the use of the drug in pregnant women clearly outweigh potential benefits.

Adapted from: U. S. Food and Drug Administration. (1979). Specific requirements on content and format of labeling for human prescription drugs. Federal Register 44:37434–67.

exist are assigned to category C. Most pharmaceutical agents fall into this subcategory of the larger category C.

The FDA developed and published the categorization method, but drug manufacturers are responsible for assigning a drug to a specific category. In some cases, researchers have differed with the manufacturer based on their analysis of the clinical trial and other data (Briggs, Freeman, & Yaffe, 2011). In an attempt to provide more information for consumers and providers, a revised method has been proposed (United States Food and Drug Administration, 2008). The revision proposes a move from categorizing by letters to one that uses a descriptive format for drugs in pregnancy and lactation.

Each drug would include a summary of data about fetal risk and clinical considerations for use. For example, a drug might be noted to be associated with anomalies of the newborn and will include additional text that specifies the type of abnormalities and the incidence of the birth defects. The section on clinical considerations is proposed to include pragmatic information regarding the risks of nontreatment, dosing variations, and complications. The studies on which the summary information was based also would be included so that it becomes apparent if all relevant research has been considered when assigning the classification. (Frederiksen, 2011). The FDA has not yet approved this proposed change in pregnancy categories.

Selected teratogens

A major difficulty with determining harm from drugs used during pregnancy is that any neonate may be unexpectedly born with a congenital anomaly of unknown etiology. Older drug studies, in particular, have been contaminated with issues such as polypharmacy used by the infant's mother during pregnancy, not recognizing adverse fetal effects of a nontreated disorder, and use of questionable methodologies. Table 12.4 is a list of selected teratogens or common agents proposed to have teratogenic effects (Buhimschi & Weiner, 2009a; Koren, 2011; Shehata & Nelson-Piercy, 2001; Webster & Freeman, 2001). The majority of teratogens have been known for decades. The most recent additions to the list are some of the newer antidepressants, although it seems likely they are weak teratogens.

Lack of evidence of teratology does not indicate that an agent is safe. For example, the daughters of women who took diethylstilbesterol (DES) during their pregnancy did not demonstrate reproductive system cancers until they were postpubescent (Hoover et al., 2011). However, many drugs have been used extensively in a wide array of populations for decades and there is no compelling reason to prohibit their use, assuming that a need for the medication exists. Table 12.5 lists several of the most commonly used pharmaceuticals that have minimal or no known teratogenicity.

Pharmacokinetics in pregnancy

Pharmacokinetics reflects how the body acts on drugs. The normal physiological changes of pregnancy directly influence pharmacokinetic changes. For example, because plasma volume expands approximately 50%, higher doses of antibiotics are necessary to achieve the optimal plasma levels needed to obtain a therapeutic effect. Thus, higher doses of antibiotics are needed for pregnant women. Table 12.6 provides an overview of the

Table 12.4   Selected Teratogens

Teratogen	Time of exposure	Effects
Angiotensin converting enzyme inhibitors (ACEI) and angiotensin II antagonists	Questionable in first trimester Most apparent in late pregnancy due to hemodynamic effects	*Possible* cardiovascular, central nervous system (CNS) defects, intrauterine renal insufficiency, oligohydramnios with complications (e.g., limb contractures, lung hypoplasia), prematurity, fetal death, neonatal hypotension)
Antidepressants (e.g., fluoxetine, sertraline, paroxetine) Note: If severe depression is untreated, it is likely to result in low birth weight, malnutrition, and other poor outcomes.	First trimester (although several studies contradictory in findings)	If teratogenic, considered low potency; linked in some studies (especially paroxetine, with cardiac defects)
Antineoplastic agents	First-trimester exposure	Significant increase in birth defects in general and spontaneous pregnancy loss
Antithyroid drugs (propylthiouracil, methimazole) If untreated, increased risk of congenital anomalies, preterm birth, and intrauterine restriction may result	Less risk with propylthiouracil in first trimester, but higher risk of liver disease First-trimester exposure	Propylthiouracil associated with fetal hypothyroidism and, rarely, aplasia cutis Methimazole associated with cretinism in a dose-dependent fashion and is commonly associated with fetal anomalies such as aplasia cutis, esophageal atresia, and choanal atresia
Benzodiazepines (e.g., diazepam [Valium])	First trimester exposure	No link with significant teratogenic effects; some studies associated with cleft palate, but not with other studies; long term use, especially high doses, associated with floppy newborn, poor sucking, and so on
Carbamazepine (anticonvulsant/mood stabilizer)	First-trimester exposure	1% risk for open neural tube defect (10X baseline), increased risk of cardiovascular defects, syndrome similar to that with hydantoin reported
Cocaine ("agent of abuse")	Methodological issues make interpretation of findings difficult. Data often confounded by various factors such as polypharmacy (including alcohol) and malnutrition	Linked with placental abruptions, prematurity, fetal loss, low birth weight, microcephaly, limb defects, urinary malformations, and behavioral issues
Corticosteroids	*Possibly* first trimester	Cleft palate
Coumarin (anticoagulant, warfarin [Coumadin])	First trimester (4–7 postconceptional weeks) Some defects are found in half of pregnancies when coumarin derivative is given during any trimester. Second and third trimester	Fetal warfarin syndrome (nasal hypoplasia and epiphyseal defects); also associated with intrauterine growth restriction, CNS delays, ophthalmic issues and hearing loss, pregnancy loss Risk of CNS damage due to hemorrhage after the first trimester
Diethylstilbestrol (DES) (synthetic nonsteroidal estrogen) *No longer marketed in United States*	Exposure prior to 16 postconceptional weeks	Increased risk of pregnancy loss and preterm birth (ironically the indication for which it was initially administered); first discovered as a teratogen when "DES daughters" were found to have a high rate of vaginal clear cell carcinoma; questionable influence on children of the DES daughters also; often used as example of an agent in use for decades before teratogenicity was discovered

Table 12.4 (*Continued*)

Teratogen	Time of exposure	Effects
Ethanol/alcohol	Throughout pregnancy; some indication of dose relationship (eight drinks per day), although threshold remains unclear	Fetal alcohol syndrome that includes growth restriction, facial changes, cleft palate, cardiac defects, and developmental delays
Folic acid antagonists (e.g., aminopterin and methotrexate—both antichemotherapeutics)	First trimester (most likely 6–8 postconceptional weeks)	Fetal aminopterin-methotrexate syndrome: growth restriction, CNS defects, cranial/facial defects, cardiovascular abnormalities, mental deficiency
Hormones (especially sex hormones such as estrogen, progesterone, androgens)	First trimester *potential*	No strong evidence of teratogenic effects; *possible* association between progesterone and male virilization of female genitalia; *possible* association of hypospadias and pseudohermaphrodism with androgens; association, although not strong, between combined oral contraceptives and vertebral, anal, cardiac, tracheoesophageal, renal, and limb defects
Hydantoins (phenytoin [Dilantin]—anticonvulsant and antiarrhythmic)	First trimester	Fetal hydantoin syndrome that includes craniofacial abnormalities, hypoplasia of distal phalanges and nails, intrauterine growth restriction, mental deficiency, and cardiac defects
Lithium (mood stabilizer)	First trimester	Cardiac defects, especially Epstein's anomaly, although absolute numbers are small
Misoprostol (prostaglandin)	First trimester	Mobius syndrome (facial paralysis) and limb defects; may have pregnancy loss with large doses
Retinoids (e.g., isotretinoin [Accutane], megadoses of vitamin A)	Appears to be primarily first trimester; consumer education mandates two forms of contraception for at least 1 month prior to starting method and 2 months after discontinuing; also instructs women not to donate blood while on drug	Potent teratogen with structural and behavioral risks; retinoic acid embryopathy that includes craniofacial dysmorphology, cardiac defects, abnormalities of thymus, and alterations in CNS development; estimated 40% risk of pregnancy loss
Tetracyclines (anti-infective)	After 17 weeks postconception/19 weeks' gestation Late third trimester	Discoloration of teeth Risk of staining of permanent teeth
Thalidomide (primarily listed as sedative, limited availability in the United States)	34–50 days after LMP	Predilection for mesodermal tissue, resulting in limb reduction, and defects of gut, ears, and cardiovascular systems The prototype for all teratogenic drugs
Valproic acid (mood stabilizer and anticonvulsant [Depakene])	First trimester	Neural tube defects (including meningomyelocele), lumbar disorders, cardiovascular malformations, and hypospadias; fetal valproate syndrome: craniofacial defects, cardiovascular defects, long digits, abnormal fingernails and cleft lip, in some studies; neurobehavioral changes

Adapted from: Buhimschi and Weiner (2009a), Koren (2011), Shehata and Nelson-Piercy (2001), Webster and Freeman (2001).

Table 12.5   Selected Drugs with Minimal or No Evidence of Teratogenesis or Contraindication to Breastfeeding*

Analgesics
Acetaminophen (Tylenol®)
Codeine (Tylenol #3 and #4®)
Morphine

Antacids
Cimetidine (Tagamet®)
Cisapride (Propulsid®)

Antifungals
Ketoconazole (Nizoral®)
Miconazole (Monistat®)

Antiinfectives
Acyclovir (Zovirax®)
Amoxicillin (Amoxil®)
Azithromycin (Zithromax®)
Cefazolin (Ancef®, Kefzol®)
Ciprofloxacin (Cipro®)
Clindamycin (Cleocin®)
Erythromycin (E-mycin®)
Metronidazole (Flagyl®)
Nitrofurantoin (Macrodantin®, Macrobid®)
Penicillin G

Antihypertensives
Hydralazine (Apresoline®)
Labetalol (Trandate®)
Methyldopa (Aldomet®)
Propanolol (Inderal®)

Antinausea
Diphenhydramine (Benadryl®)
Doxylamine (Unisom®)
Metoclopramide (Reglan®)
Prochlorperazine (Compazine®)
Promethazine (Phenergan®)

Antivirals
Acyclovir (Zovirax®)

Corticosteroids
Betamethasone
Dexamethasone
Prednisone

*This list is not comprehensive. Most drugs are safe for use in pregnancy. This list is provided to give the reader a general overview of the categories most often used by pregnant women.
Adapted from: Buhimschi and Weiner (2009b).

most common pharmacokinetic differences that occur during pregnancy.

Fortunately, most commonly used drugs in pregnancy have wide therapeutic indices. Thus, little customization in route, dosing, or administration is needed. However, as newer sophisticated drugs emerge, the possibility exists that in the future, accommodations will be made to adjust medications for the changes in pharmacokinetics during pregnancy.

Rational use of drugs in pregnancy

No specific guidelines exist to aid the health-care provider when choosing a medication for a pregnant woman in order to avoid fetal risk. However, there are some general strategies that can be used, including choosing drugs listed in Table 12.5 when possible. Additionally, a medication that is older and well known should be used rather than one that is new. When considering dosing, the initial choice should be one in the lowest therapeutic range even though altered pharmacokinetics during pregnancy suggest that higher doses may be necessary to achieve a therapeutic effect. Drugs should be avoided during the first trimester whenever possible because of the potential impact during the period of organogenesis. The use of a single agent is preferred over a combination of drugs to avoid polypharmacy and potential drug–drug interactions. Lastly, women should be counseled that OTC, herbs, nutritional supplements, and botanicals should be regarded as drugs and discussed with a health-care professional before self-administration. The one exception of these rules is prenatal vitamins, which have a combination of vitamins in one pill, although even among such pharmaceuticals, the ingredients such as calcium or iron can cause drug–drug interactions. The common ingredients in prenatal vitamins are listed in Table 12.7.

Summary

Health-care providers are challenged to stay current with advances in pharmacology, especially for the pregnant woman and her offspring. Clinicians should not hesitate to recommend or prescribe agents when they are needed, but also should do so with knowledge about pharmacokinetic changes in pregnancy and how an individual medication works. Drugs used in pregnancy must be scrutinized as to effects (including therapeutic, side, and adverse) as well as risks to the unborn. Issues such as cost, accessibility, and pharmacogenomics also are important considerations. Perhaps most importantly, new information about existing drugs and new medications is emerging at a rapid rate, emphasizing the importance of being current in practice.

Table 12.6 Pregnancy and Pharmacokinetics with Clinical Implications

Pharmacokinetics and pregnancy	Clinical implications
Changes in absorption	
Intestinal motility increased Gestational nausea and vomiting	Delayed or absent drug response/changes in absorption Drug absorption delayed because of decreased time in GI system
Gastric pH increased (by second trimester)	Changes in absorption in stomach of oral drugs
Gastric emptying increased	Potential delay in onset of therapeutic responses
Respiratory minute volume increases approximately 50%	Absorption of inhaled drugs increased through lungs resulting in potential therapeutic effects at lower dosage
Skin perfusion, skin hydration, and perfusion to muscles increased	Intramuscular absorption of drugs increased Transcutaneous absorption of lipophilic and hydrophilic drugs increased
Routine simultaneous use of certain oral agents	Inactivation of absorption (e.g., calcium and iron in some prenatal combination multivitamins and minerals)
Changes in distribution	
Plasma volume increased by approximately 50%	Potential need to increase dosage of hydrophilic drugs because of decreased concentration in plasma (dilutional effect)
Body fat stores increased by 3–4 kg	Long-term use of lipophilic drugs increased accumulation in body fat.
Plasma albumin concentrations decreased (dilutional effect with increased plasma volume), resulting in less protein bound drugs	Increased incidence of free drugs if agents are highly protein bound. Drugs that are highly protein bound will have more pharmacologic activity in a pregnant woman.
Changes in metabolism	
Cytochrome P450 enzyme activity changes due to increased estrogen and progesterone levels (e.g., decreased CYP1A2; increased CYP 3A4 and CYP2C9)	Profound changes in metabolism of some drugs including tripling of half-life of caffeine and increased half-life of other agents such as sertraline (Zoloft®)
Changes in elimination	
Glomerular filtration rate increased throughout pregnancy by 50% at term	Decreased effect of renal drugs because of rapid clearance of such agents
Addition of fetal compartment	
Unique addition of fetal compartment that influences pharmacokinetics, especially in area of distribution	Drugs that are highly lipophilic, low molecular weight and low protein binding can accumulate in fetal compartment Majority of drugs in the fetal compartment are approximately 50–100% maternal concentration
Fetal circulation is more acidic than maternal circulation	Drugs that are of basic pH can concentrate in fetal compartment because of ion trapping
Fetal albumin plasma concentration increases throughout pregnancy until at term approximately 20% higher than maternal concentrations	Drugs highly bound to albumin accumulate in the term fetus and can promote displacement or lack of binding of bilirubin, resulting in neonatal jaundice/kernicterus

Adapted from: Manns-James (2011).

13

Substance use during pregnancy

Daisy J. Goodman, Alane B. O'Connor, and Kelley A. Bowden

Relevant terms

Binge drinking—consumption of alcohol that brings blood alcohol concentration to about 0.08% or above (Centers for Disease Control and Prevention (CDC), 2012)

Motivational interviewing—nonjudgmental, neutral questioning technique to promote dialogue

Neonatal abstinence syndrome (NAS)—the constellation of signs and symptoms displayed by a neonate exposed to prenatal opiates

Standard drink—a standardized serving of an alcoholic beverage contains 15.0 mL of pure ethanol; regular beer (5%) = 12 oz, wine (12%) = 5 oz, cocktail of a 80% spirit = 1.5-oz glass (44.4 mL)

Substance abuse—pattern of harmful use of substances; also termed "substance use disorders"

Substance dependence—persistent use despite problems related to use of the substance; increased tolerance of its effects and presence of withdrawal symptoms upon abrupt cessation; often used interchangeably with "addiction"

Risks of perinatal substance abuse

Perinatal substance abuse is a persistent and expanding public health problem. In the United States, the most commonly abused substances during pregnancy include marijuana, prescription analgesics and anxiolytics, heroin, and amphetamines. Exposure to harmful substances during pregnancy is not limited to illicit drug use. Despite public education campaigns and product labeling about the risks of prenatal smoking and alcohol use, the prevalence of antepartum tobacco use in the United States is approximately 16%, and 12–20% of pregnant women drink at least some alcohol during pregnancy (National Institute for Drug Abuse (NIDA), 2009; U.S. Centers for Disease Control and Prevention (CDC), 2008).

The use of alcohol, tobacco, and drugs during pregnancy places both a woman and her developing fetus at risk through a variety of mechanisms (American Society of Addiction Medicine (ASAM), 2011b; Mengel, Searight & Cook, 2006; National Task Force on Fetal Alcohol Syndrome and Fetal Alcohol Effects, 2009). The type of substance used, the timing of use during embryogenesis and fetal development, and the duration and amount of substance used all contribute to the impact on a woman's pregnancy and to the fetal and neonatal effects. For example, first-trimester methamphetamine and alcohol use are associated with miscarriage, embryopathy, and visible physical defects. Less obvious fetal effects such as developmental, cognitive, and behavioral disabilities are associated with later-trimester exposures and are frequently *not* linked to maternal substance use at the time they are diagnosed in childhood (American College of Obstetricians and Gynecologists (ACOG), 2011b). Perinatal substance abuse is also associated with pregnancy complications, in large part due to a decrease in the ability of the placenta to transfer adequate oxygen and nutrients to the fetus. Dependence on opioids is linked to poor fetal growth, premature birth, and low birth weight. Prenatal exposure to stimulants and acute drug withdrawal cause vasoconstriction of the uteroplacental circulation, increasing the risks of miscarriage, placental abruption, and progressive uterine contractions. Repeated cycles of intoxication and withdrawal associated with dependence on illicit drugs are thought to cause microvascular changes in the placental circulation, which

---

Prenatal and Postnatal Care: A Woman-Centered Approach, First Edition. Edited by Robin G. Jordan, Janet L. Engstrom, Julie A. Marfell, and Cindy L. Farley.

have been observed in the placentas of women exposed to heroin (Binder & Vavrinková, 2008).

The worst perinatal outcomes appear to be associated with pregnancies exposed to multiple substances (Binder & Vavrinková, 2008). However, it is difficult to distinguish the impact of substance abuse from other factors impacting the health and safety of a pregnant woman who is abusing multiple substances. Social and economic stress, homelessness, poor nutritional status, comorbid psychiatric conditions, and domestic abuse all contribute to an environment of chronic stress which adversely affects the pregnancy (Shannon, King, & Kennedy, 2006).

Prevalence of prenatal substance abuse

According to the U.S. Department of Health and Human Services (DHHS) (2010), 4.4% of pregnant women aged 15–44 were current illicit drug users during 2009 and 2010. This was lower than the rate among women of the same age group who were not pregnant (10.9%). Pregnant women of a younger age were at a much greater risk of using illicit drugs than older pregnant women. Drug use rates among pregnant women 15–17 years of age were as high as 16.2%. In other studies, rates of abuse of illicit substances during pregnancy have been as high as 27%, particularly among vulnerable populations (Bolnick & Rayburn, 2003).

The illicit drug use problem among women of childbearing age may be worsening as the use and misuse of prescription medications are significantly increasing in the United States. Among women, emergency department visits for suicide attempts involving medications used to treat anxiety and insomnia increased 56% from 2005 to 2009 (U.S. Substance Abuse and Mental Health Services Administration (SAMHSA), Center for Behavioral Health Statistics and Quality, 2011). Similarly, emergency department visits for suicide attempts involving hydrocodone and oxycodone, two commonly prescribed narcotic analgesics, increased 67% and 210%, respectively, among women during the same time period (U.S. SAMHSA, 2011).

Trends among women at risk for alcohol abuse often look quite different from illicit substance use with older, more educated, and employed women at greater risk than younger women with less education (U.S. DHHS, 2009). For example, 17.7% of pregnant women aged 35–44 reported alcohol use compared to 8.6% of pregnant women aged 18–24. Pregnant women with a college degree (14.4%) or at least some college education (11.2%) were more likely to report alcohol use than pregnant women with a high school diploma or less (8.5%). A greater percentage of employed pregnant women (13.7%) reported alcohol use than those that were unemployed (8.3%). In addition, employed pregnant women were more likely to report binge drinking (2.3%) than unemployed pregnant women (1.3%).

Nicotine is a highly addictive substance and is the most common form of chemical dependence in the United States (ASAM, 1998). The use of nicotine is particularly prevalent among those abusing alcohol and illicit substances. More than 22% of women report smoking in the 3 months before pregnancy, during pregnancy, or after birth (U.S. CDC, 2009). Compared with nonsmokers, women who smoke are more likely to be younger than 25 years of age, unmarried, Caucasian, have fewer than 12 years of education, have an annual income of less than $15,000, be underweight, and have an unintended pregnancy (U.S. CDC, 2009).

Among the broader population, rates of illicit substance use tend to vary by ethnicity with the highest rates among American Indians (12.5%), Alaska Natives (12.1%), and blacks (10.7%). Among whites, the rate was 9.1% followed by Hispanics (8.1%) and Asians (3.5%) (U.S. DHHS, 2010). Rates of illicit substance use tended to be highest among persons living in large metropolitan counties (9.4%) and lowest in completely rural counties (3.7%), and were greater in the West (11.0%) and Northeast (9.4%) than in the Midwest (8.2%) and South (7.8%) (U.S. DHHS, 2010).

Definitions

Terminology within the field of addiction is often confusing. The *Diagnostic and Statistical Manual of Mental Disorders, Fourth Edition* (DSM-IV) has two broad categories, substance abuse and substance dependence. Substance dependence includes the continuing and compulsive use of substances despite physiological, physical, and social harm (Rastegar & Fingerhood, 2005). Physical dependence on a substance is defined as the increased tolerance of its effects as well as the presence of withdrawal symptoms upon abrupt cessation, and is an element of substance dependence. However, physical dependence on its own does not meet the criteria for substance dependence (Rastegar & Fingerhood, 2005). For example, an individual who is prescribed opioids for chronic pain would likely be physically dependent but would only meet the criteria for substance dependence if also engaging in maladaptive behaviors.

The term substance abuse refers to a situation in which an individual uses substances in a harmful and/or dangerous manner but does not necessarily meet the criteria for substance dependence. For example, an individual who uses substances recreationally but does not seem to be escalating her/his behavior and/or is not physically dependent would meet the criteria for substance abuse but not substance dependence.

The term addiction, rather than substance dependence, is most commonly used by the general public (Rastegar & Fingerhood, 2005).

ASAM definition of addiction

"Addiction is a primary, chronic disease of brain reward, motivation, memory and related circuitry. Dysfunction in these circuits leads to characteristic biological, psychological, social and spiritual manifestations. This is reflected in an individual pathologically pursuing reward and/or relief by substance use and other behaviors. Addiction is characterized by inability to consistently abstain, impairment in behavioral control, craving, diminished recognition of significant problems with one's behaviors and interpersonal relationships, and a dysfunctional emotional response. Like other chronic diseases, addiction often involves cycles of relapse and remission. Without treatment or engagement in recovery activities, addiction is progressive and can result in disability or premature death." (ASAM, 2011a)

Practically speaking, the distinction between substance abuse and dependence is a critical one for prenatal health-care providers to understand in assessing and referring patients to an appropriate level of care. Problematic substance use can be described using the general term "substance use disorder."

Historical approaches to maternal substance use

Historically, pregnant women with substance use disorders have been victims of significant stigma and punitive actions on the part of health-care providers and the criminal justice system. Criminal prosecution of pregnant women caught using drugs was justified by a perceived irresolvable conflict between fetal "rights" to be free of exposure to substances *in utero* and the maternal right to privacy and bodily integrity (Wolff, 2011). In many areas of the country, pregnant women were routinely arrested and prosecuted for drug use under a variety of statutes, including distribution of drugs to a minor and child abuse and neglect. During the 1980s, concerns about an epidemic of "crack babies" led to nonconsensual drug testing and the illegal release of patient information to law enforcement (Wolff, 2011). Between 1980 and 2000, over 200 women in 30 states were arrested and charged for alleged drug use and related actions

during pregnancy. Some cases were successfully argued in favor of the defendants as violating the fourteenth amendment's guarantee of freedom from unreasonable search; in others, women served long sentences and lost custody of their children (Flavin, 2002).

While there is some variability in the prevalence of substance use by race and ethnicity, selective drug testing of vulnerable populations, particularly poor women and women of color, has been widely reported (Wolff, 2011). During the 1980s, arrest and incarceration was 10 times more likely in South Carolina for African American women than for white women who used cocaine (Wolff, 2011). The result of these discriminatory drug screening policies was to foster avoidance of the health-care system by poor women and women of color, and to further decrease access to prenatal care.

Harm reduction approach to prenatal substance use

The approach just described illustrates the perceived antagonism between the actions of a pregnant, substance-using woman and the safety and well-being of her fetus. An alternate model strives to reduce harm to both mother and fetus through the reduction of risk factors affecting pregnancy outcomes. Behavior is perceived as a continuum from extreme to minimal risk, with the mother and the fetus being one unit to be protected as they move along that continuum. Complete abstinence from substance use during pregnancy is a goal that may or may not be attainable; however, every step toward abstinence should be recognized as positive (Boyd & Marcellus, 2007). The "harm reduction" framework promotes collaboration between women and their prenatal care providers toward this mutual goal. Success, no matter how subtle, is built upon the recognition that harmful exposures are being decreased incrementally (Flavin, 2002). This model also helps reduce provider burnout among providers caring for this population.

Position statements on prenatal substance use

The American College of Nurse-Midwives (ACNM), the American Society of Addiction Medicine (ASAM), and the American Congress of Obstetricians and Gynecologists (ACOG) have published position statements regarding the care of pregnant women with substance use disorders. All three organizations promote a comprehensive, treatment-centered approach consistent with a harm reduction model (ACOG, 2011a, 2011b; American College of Nurse-Midwives (ACNM), 2004; ASAM, 2011b).

Key features of professional position statements on prenatal substance use

- Universal screening using validated screening instruments
- A nonpunitive, multidisciplinary approach to prenatal substance use
- Support of legislation that protects women with addiction from criminal prosecution when seeking health care
- High-quality substance abuse treatment for pregnant women
- Screening and prevention programs targeting all women of childbearing age
- Preconception education on substance use
- Professional education for health-care providers in the identification, intervention, referral, and treatment of pregnant women

Comorbid conditions and prenatal substance use

Psychiatric disease

Pregnant women with substance use disorders have a high prevalence of anxiety disorders and depression. There is also a strong correlation with current and past physical and sexual trauma (Horrigan, Schroeder, & Schaffer, 2000). In one study, high scores on the Patient Health Questionnaire (PHQ-9) depression scale doubled the rate of continued alcohol use during pregnancy (Harrison & Sidebottom, 2009). Untreated psychiatric disorders and post-traumatic stress symptoms place a woman at additional risk for relapse.

Untreated psychiatric disorders are particularly associated with a dependence on opioids, with a prevalence rate over 50% in most studies. The majority of opioid-dependent pregnant women report post-traumatic stress symptoms rooted in histories of sexual and physical abuse as children and adults (Hans, 1999; Helmbrecht & Thiagarajah, 2008; Horrigan et al., 2000; Jessup & Brindis, 2005; Kearney, 1998; Maine OSA, 2009; Merikangas, et al. 1998; Moylan, Jones, Haug, Kissim, & Svikis, 2001; Velez et al., 2006). Current intimate partner violence may further complicate a woman's ability to seek and continue in treatment, especially when the partner is substance dependent (Velez et al., 2006).

Pregnant women using substances frequently express guilt and require significant reassurance regarding the progress of their pregnancies (Jessup & Brindis, 2005; Kearney, 1998). Regular participation in substance abuse counseling is a necessary component of addiction treatment; however, it is difficult to track participation if counseling is provided separately from medical treat-

ment and from prenatal care (Brady & Ashley, 2005). This is further complicated logistically when a woman needs both psychiatric care and addiction treatment. Thus, prenatal health-care providers should request a woman to give written consent to communicate with her psychiatric provider and substance abuse counselor so that all providers can communicate regarding her treatment plan, determine whether appointments are being kept, and assess the risk for relapse.

Medical risks

Perinatal substance use is associated with significant medical risk. Intranasal and intravenous drug use potentially exposes women to hepatitis B and C and HIV. These risks are exacerbated by unsafe sexual practices, prostitution, and the need to trade sex for drugs. Pregnant women with substance abuse disorders have an increased risk for repeated occurrence of sexually transmitted infection (Horrigan et al., 2000). Incarceration increases risk of exposure to multidrug-resistant organisms and tuberculosis.

Thrombophlebitis and deep vein thrombosis are frequent sequelae of intravenous drug use (Winklbaur et al., 2008). Nonsterile injection technique leads to needle-site abscess and, potentially, endocarditis. Maternal and fetal death can occur from accidental or intentional drug overdose.

Risks associated with the social environment surrounding many pregnant women with substance dependence are difficult to separate from medical risk factors. These may include malnutrition, risk for traumatic injury related to homelessness and domestic abuse, prostitution, and incarceration.

Commonly abused substances and pregnancy implications

It is often difficult for the health-care provider to quantify the amount of fetal exposure to an illicit substance. Self-reported data can be unreliable as women are generally motivated to underreport illicit substance use. The use of one illicit substance during pregnancy places a woman at greater risk of polysubstance abuse, and it is nearly impossible to distinguish the potential fetal effects of one substance from the effects of another substance. In addition, substance use often occurs in tandem with poor prenatal care and poverty, which, even without a substance use disorder, places the maternal–fetal dyad at risk for poor outcomes.

Alcohol

Alcohol use during pregnancy is the leading known preventable cause of intellectual disabilities and birth defects in the United States. Alcohol is a teratogen, associated with a range of disorders grouped together as fetal alcohol spectrum disorders (FASDs). Central nervous system (CNS) damage is the primary feature of any FASD diagnosis. The identifiable conditions associated with prenatal alcohol exposure under the FASD umbrella are fetal alcohol syndrome (FAS), partial fetal alcohol syndrome (PFAS), alcohol-related neurodevelopmental disorder (ARND), and alcohol-related birth defects (ARBDs). Of these, FAS is the most severe, associated with damage to multiple structures in the brain and lifelong disabilities. Impairments are in three categories: (1) growth deficiency, (2) CNS dysfunction with developmental disability or brain damage, and (3) characteristic facial dysmorphology. Prenatal alcohol use is associated with multiple perinatal complications.

Pregnant women who are alcohol dependent require medically assisted withdrawal ("detoxification"), which should be managed in the inpatient setting.

Maternal child risks associated with prenatal alcohol use

Pregnancy-related risks
Spontaneous abortion
Preterm birth
Stillbirth

Neonatal/childhood risks
Decreased muscle tone and poor coordination
Heart defects (ventricular septal defect, atrial septal defect)
CNS damage
Visual impairment
Failure to thrive
Growth disorders
Facial dysmorphism, including
- narrow, small eyes with large epicanthal folds
- small head
- small upper jaw
- smooth groove in the upper lip
- smooth and thin upper lip
Delayed psychomotor development
Cognitive impairment and learning disabilities
Behavioral and social disorders

Source: National Organization on Fetal Alcohol Syndrome (NOFAS) http://www.nofas.org/living-with-fasd/

FASD is 100% preventable. Women should avoid consuming alcohol when trying to conceive and during pregnancy as no amount of alcohol consumption is considered safe. Alcohol consumption can damage the fetus at any stage of pregnancy even in the earliest weeks before a woman knows she is pregnant (U.S. CDC, 2010). However, according to ACOG (2011a), low-level alcohol consumption during early pregnancy is not an indication for pregnancy termination. Women who are drinking during pregnancy should be advised to quit and offered support at each prenatal visit. Duration of alcohol exposure, especially into the third trimester, is positively associated with cognitive-behavioral problems in childhood (ACOG, 2011a). Unfortunately, approximately 12% of pregnant women continue to drink alcohol during pregnancy, and 2% continue binge drinking (U.S. CDC, 2009).

All women of childbearing age should be screened for alcohol use and misuse. The highest rate of late-trimester alcohol consumption is found among white, college-educated women over age 35. This group of women is also screened with the least frequency by health-care providers (ACOG, 2011a; Chang et al., 2011).

Nicotine

Cigarette use in women of childbearing age is associated with reduced fertility and an increased risk of ectopic pregnancy (Briggs, Freeman, & Yaffe, 2011). The use of cigarettes during pregnancy is associated with multiple complications including spontaneous abortion, placental abruption and preterm birth, fetal growth restriction, and low birth weight (Briggs et al., 2011). The Centers for Disease Control estimate that "20% or more of low birth weight births could be prevented by eliminating smoking during pregnancy" (U.S. CDC, 2008, p. 168). Chronic *in utero* exposure to nicotine leads to neonatal withdrawal, potentially intensifying symptoms associated with withdrawal from other drugs such as opioids (Choo, Huestis, Schroeder, Shin, & Jones, 2004). Exposure to maternal cigarette use has been associated with a higher prevalence of sudden infant death syndrome (SIDS), asthma, other respiratory disorders, and cognitive, emotional, and behavioral problems during childhood (U.S. CDC, 2008). Nicotine has a direct inhibitory effect on lung tissue maturation and reduces the infant's ability to respond during episodes of hypoxia. This likely contributes to the higher incidence of SIDS (U.S. CDC, 2008). Infants exposed to secondhand smoke also show an increased prevalence of upper respiratory problems. Harm from maternal smoking appears to be the result of a combination of neurotoxic effects of nicotine and of carbon monoxide in smoke, as well as vasoconstriction, which compromises placental function. Rapid placental transfer of carbon monoxide also inhibits fetal oxygenation.

Maternal–child risks associated with prenatal smoking

Pregnancy risks
Ectopic pregnancy
Early pregnancy loss
Fetal growth restriction
Preterm birth
Low birth weight
Stillbirth
Placental abruption
Placenta previa
Preterm premature rupture of membranes (PPROM)

Neonatal/childhood risks
Cleft lip and palate
Musculoskeletal defects (clubfoot, craniosynostosis)
Gastrointestinal defects (gastroschisis, hernia)
Asthma and other atopic diseases
Middle ear infections
Neurological development deficits
SIDS
Reduced head circumference
Altered brainstem development
Altered lung structure
Cerebral palsy

Adapted from: Anderka et al. (2010), Hackshaw, Rodeck, and Boniface (2011), U.S. CDC (2008), Wehby et al. (2011).

Cocaine

A powerful stimulant drug, either in its pure powder form or in the less expensive form, "crack," cocaine is highly addictive and produces intense physiological cravings. Long-term use causes depletion of dopamine receptors in the brain, decreasing sensitivity to natural reward systems and motivational factors.

The use of cocaine during pregnancy is associated with lower gestational age at delivery, an increased risk of preterm labor and delivery, lower birth weight, and delivery of small-for-gestational-age infants (MacGregor et al., 1987). The use of cocaine during pregnancy decreases blood flow to the uterus, thereby inducing uterine contractions (Briggs et al., 2011). In addition to the increased risk of fetal demise, significant morbidity is also associated with *in utero* cerebrovascular accidents. The fetus exposed to cocaine is also at risk for a number of congenital abnormalities in the heart, genitourinary tract, limbs, and face, as well as atresia of the bowel (Briggs et al., 2011). Neurobehavioral abnormalities and an increased risk of SIDS may be seen after birth.

Women who chronically abuse cocaine are at high risk for unsafe sexual practices, exchanging sex for drugs, and the transmission of blood-borne diseases (NIDA, 2011).

Cognitive-behavioral therapies are currently the only evidence-based treatment for cocaine addiction, although research to identify pharmacological agents that can reduce cravings or block the drug's pleasurable effects is ongoing. Clonidine and baclofen have been used off-label with some success in small studies, but further research is needed. Pregnant women dependent on cocaine should be offered residential treatment as abstaining from the drug entirely is the safest alternative during pregnancy.

Opioids

The complications associated with the misuse of opioids during pregnancy appear to be largely related to the recurrent intoxication and withdrawal experienced by both the mother and the fetus. This is true of both the commonly abused opioid analgesics such as oxycodone and hydrocodone as well as heroin. Clinicians should be particularly concerned about maternal use of heroin during pregnancy as it is often adulterated with other substances including amphetamines, strychnine, and lidocaine and may also contain bacteria. The maternal–fetal effects of opioid dependence during pregnancy are variable, ranging from minimal effects to intrauterine growth restriction, placental insufficiency, preeclampsia, preterm rupture of membranes, premature delivery, and perinatal mortality (Bolnick & Rayburn, 2003; Kaltenbach, Berghella, & Finnegan, 1998). Withdrawal from opioids during pregnancy is particularly associated with adverse pregnancy outcomes. The majority of newborns exposed to opioids prenatally undergo a neonatal abstinence syndrome (NAS) after birth, which may require prolonged hospitalization (Jansson, Velez, & Harrow, 2009; Winklbaur et al., 2008).

Benzodiazepines

Benzodiazepines (diazepam, alproazolam, lorazepam, clonazepam) are among the most commonly abused prescription drugs. Prescribed for the short-term management of severe anxiety, this class of CNS depressants produces high tolerance and physical dependence. Abrupt discontinuation after chronic use causes severe anxiety and may precipitate seizure activity similar to withdrawal from alcohol. When used concurrently with opioids or alcohol, benzodiazepines enhance respiratory depression and can be fatal.

Benzodiazepines freely cross the placenta and can impact the fetus, although specific data about the implications of benzodiazepine use and misuse during pregnancy are variable. Some studies show an increase in congenital malformations while other studies have not confirmed these findings (Briggs et al., 2011). Regular use during pregnancy has been associated with fetal dependence and consequently a withdrawal syndrome in infants. There is also concern that *in utero* exposure may impact infant neurobehavioral outcomes (Briggs et al., 2011).

Pregnant women who are dependent on benzodiazepines require medically assisted withdrawal in order to minimize harm to themselves and the developing fetus. Referral for inpatient management is strongly recommended.

Marijuana

Cannabis is the most commonly used illicit drug among pregnant women, with an estimated prevalence of 10–15% (Garry et al., 2009; Tennes et al., 1985). Data about the potential effects of marijuana use during pregnancy are variable. Some studies have shown an association between marijuana use and congenital defects, neurobehavioral changes in the infant, as well as a possible association to leukemia among children exposed to marijuana *in utero* (Astley & Little, 1990; Briggs et al., 2011). Further studies have not always reproduced these findings and research is often limited by the difficulty quantifying exact exposure levels. Women abusing marijuana during pregnancy are at greater risk of also using nicotine, alcohol, and other illicit substances.

Amphetamines/Methamphetamines

Amphetamines are among the most common drugs of abuse in North America. Both the amphetamines commonly prescribed for the treatment of attention deficit/hyperactivity disorder, such as dextroamphetamine, and methamphetamine, an illicit substance manufactured in drug labs, are abused during pregnancy. The appropriate use of prescribed amphetamines during pregnancy appears to be low risk for the fetus (Briggs et al., 2011). Because of the vasoconstriction effects of amphetamines, fetal growth in exposed pregnancies should be monitored. Illicit amphetamine use during pregnancy, however, increases an infant's risk of being low birth weight and may put the infant at risk for neurodevelopmental problems in the future (ACOG, 2011b). Since the abuse of amphetamines is associated with significant toxicity, clinicians may want to avoid prescribing amphetamines during pregnancy.

Among pregnant women, methamphetamine abuse accounted for 24% of all admissions to federally funded treatment centers, and increased from 8% in 1994 (Derauf et al., 2007). The vast majority of these admissions were to facilities in the western United States (NIDA, 2012). Nationally, pregnant methamphetamine users are more likely to be white, young, and unmarried and substance dependent rather than casual users. Perinatal use of the drug is associated with homelessness, police involvement, psychiatric comorbidities, single parent status, intimate partner violence, and loss of custody of previous children. Infants born to mothers using methamphetamine have lower Apgar scores, higher neonatal mortality and neonatal intensive care unit (NICU) admissions, although it is difficult to determine the exact causation due to the high prevalence of polysubstance exposure. Children with antenatal methamphetamine exposure also score lower on tests of antenatal, visual-motor integration and memory (ACOG, 2011b; Derauf et al., 2007; Oei, Abdel-Latif, Clark, Craig, & Lui, 2010).

Women who continue to use methamphetamine during pregnancy should be referred for comprehensive substance abuse treatment. Given the significant risk posed to pregnancy, health-care providers should seriously consider referral to a residential program as a harm reduction strategy, to separate a woman from her environment of use, and to provide physical safety during her pregnancy. Repeat testing for sexually transmitted infection in the third trimester is advised, as well as nutritional counseling and dental care. Because of the high risk for placental insufficiency among methamphetamine users, monthly ultrasounds should be performed to assess fetal growth (ACOG, 2011b).

Designer drugs

New, potentially addictive substances are continuously being developed, primarily in illicit drug labs, marketed, and sold throughout the United States. For example, during 2011, synthetic stimulants containing mephedrone, methylenedioxypyrovalerone, and/or methylone—commonly called either "bath salts" or "plant food"—became available in large quantities in many parts of the United States. Common symptoms associated with bath salt ingestion include agitation, hallucinations, paranoia, chest pain, and suicidal ideations. The effects of bath salts and other designer drugs on pregnancy are unknown, but pregnant women should be discouraged from inhaling or ingesting any unknown substance.

Screening for prenatal substance abuse

Pregnancy is a time of high motivation for self-care and presents a unique opportunity for promoting behavioral change (Jessup & Brindis, 2005). National data on substance use patterns reveal that alcohol use among women of childbearing age was highest for those who were not pregnant or raising children at home (63%). Rates were much lower in the first trimester of pregnancy (19%) and further decreased in the second and third trimesters (7.8% and 6.2%). Similar patterns are reported for marijuana and cigarette use (National Institute for Drug Addiction, 2009).

Early screening enables clinicians to provide timely intervention and referral to treatment for women at risk for prenatal substance use, and to maximize potential harm reduction. Even in the case of known teratogens such as alcohol exposure, outcomes may be improved with cessation of use as pregnancy progresses.

Motivational interviewing techniques can help facilitate conversation and information gathering on substance use in pregnancy. The following are examples of statements that can promote effective engagement: (1) "I want to ask you a series of questions today about your lifestyle. I ask all women these questions because it helps me get a better understanding of your daily life and will help me provide better care to you," and (2) "I ask all women these questions because it's important to their health and the health of their babies. In a typical week, on how many occasions did you have something to drink?" Unless otherwise reported, assume use of alcohol by all women.

The use of a validated instrument specifically designed to screen pregnant women has been shown to significantly increase the number of women with potentially harmful substance use who receive treatment (Chang et al., 2011; Chasnoff, Wells, McGourty, & Bailey, 2007). Integrating substance abuse screening and intervention into routine prenatal care is associated with a decrease in pregnancy complications including preterm delivery, placental abruption, and intrauterine fetal demise (Goler, Armstrong, Taillac, & Osejo, 2008).

Universal screening of pregnant women for drug and alcohol use should be done during the first prenatal visit, ideally in the first trimester, and at least once more during pregnancy. The earlier the screening and referral for treatment occurs, the greater the potential to reduce harm to both mother and fetus.

Ideally, women of childbearing age should be screened preconceptionally and provided with education and intervention to minimize the risks of continued substance use during pregnancy. Unfortunately, many women who use alcohol and drugs do not present for care until they are already pregnant.

Screening tools

Universal screening for substance abuse allows the health-care provider to discuss the risks of alcohol, drug, and tobacco use with *every* pregnant woman, eliminating provider bias in determining who is screened. Screening can be performed using interview-based or self-administered questionnaires. Using a validated instrument increases the chance that prenatal substance

Table 13.1 T-ACE Screening Tool for Alcohol Use

T-ACE screening tool questions and scoring
- **T**olerance: "How many drinks does it take to make you feel high?" (more than 2 drinks = 2 points)
- **A**nnoyed: "Have people annoyed you by criticizing your drinking?" (positive response = 1 point)
- **C**ut down: "Have you ever felt that you ought to cut down on your drinking?" (positive response = 1 point)
- **E**ye opener: "Have you ever had a drink first thing in the morning to steady your nerves or get rid of a hangover?" (positive response = 1 point)

Scoring = any score of 2 total points or higher on the T-ACE survey indicates a positive screen for at-risk drinking.
Adapted from: Sokol, R. J., Martier, S. S., & Ager, J. W. (1989). The T-ACE questions: Practical prenatal detection of risk-drinking. *American Journal of Obstetrics and Gynecology, 160,* 863–871.

abuse will be identified, addressed, and potentially reduced (Chasnoff et al., 2005).

A number of instruments have been developed and tested for use with pregnant women. These include the T-ACE, TWEAK, and AUDIT C, which screen solely for alcohol use, and the 4Ps Plus and CRAFFT, which screen more generally for substance use (Burns, Gray, & Smith, 2010; Chang et al., 2011; Gavin, Ross, & Skinner, 1989; Humeniuk et al., 2008; Yonkers et al., 2010). In two large studies of disadvantaged, minority, pregnant women, the T-ACE and TWEAK screening tools were superior in identifying risk drinking during pregnancy (Hankin & Sokol, 1995; Russell et al., 1996). The T-ACE tool identifies lower levels of alcohol consumption than the TWEAK tool and is the preferred tool for use in pregnancy (ACOG, 2011a) (Table 13.1). Any alcohol consumption during pregnancy increases the risk of continued drinking during pregnancy (Chang, Wilkins-Haug, Berman, & Goetz, 1999). Structured screening using a validated tool and brief intervention services for at-risk drinking are billable services (ACOG, 2011a).

Some health-care providers advocate universal urine drug testing during pregnancy. Although urine toxicology is a useful follow-up test when a woman is at risk for drug or alcohol use, or to monitor success during substance abuse treatment, there are many drawbacks to using urine testing as a screening tool. Standard urine drug screens have limited ability to detect intermittent use, may not include all drugs in use in a particular community, do not routinely include testing for the metabolites of alcohol, and add significant cost to prenatal care. Accurate urine drug screening requires an observed collection and is not recommended as a screening method for pregnant women (ACOG, 2008).

Brief intervention and treatment

Although substance abuse screening can identify a patient *at risk* for alcohol or drug use, it does not differentiate between intermittent and habitual use, or diagnose drug or alcohol dependence. Intervention is essential with a positive screen to explore the extent of her substance use, her willingness to address this as an issue, and her options for treatment. The pattern of use as well as the woman's social environment, and the presence or absence of symptoms suggestive of physiological dependence should be further evaluated. Outcomes appear to be improved for drug-affected pregnancies when substance abuse screening and treatment are closely linked with prenatal care (Goler et al., 2008).

The initial intervention should consist of accurate and factual information about the maternal and fetal potential problems associated with the substance use. Appropriate options for treatment based on the type of substance(s) used should be provided. For example, the 5 A's are commonly used for pregnant women who smoke cigarettes (Table 13.2). Concern should be conveyed that the woman is at risk for alcohol or drug use during her pregnancy, take a nonjudgmental approach, and support her ability to change. The health-care provider should affirm a mutual goal of achieving a healthy pregnancy and ensuring safety for the mother, the fetus, and the newborn.

Smoking cessation during pregnancy

Optimally, tobacco cessation should occur prior to conception; however, many women are still actively smoking when they become pregnant. Individual psychosocial interventions are essential due to the gravity of harm potentially caused by maternal tobacco use and should be repeated at several points prenatally. Fortunately, counseling to decrease smoking during pregnancy has some documented success. Provider advice to quit accompanied by self-help materials has been shown to increase abstinence from tobacco almost twofold (OR 1.9, CI 95%). A cognitive-behavioral approach appears to be the most effective (U.S. CDC, 2008).

The 5 A's and the 5 R's model of smoking cessation

A brief, five-step intervention program, referred to as the "5 A's" model, is recommended in clinical practice to help pregnant women quit smoking (ACOG, 2010; Fiore et al., 2008) (Table 13.2). Each of these steps may take 1–5 minutes. Although damage from tobacco use begins in the first trimester, harm can be reduced by decreasing the dose and/or smoking cessation at any point during the pregnancy. Screening, intervention, and encouragement should be performed at every prenatal visit. A similar five-step process is outlined by the CDC (U.S. CDC, 2008).

Bupropion (Zyban®, Wellbutrin®)

Most of the data pertaining to the use of bupropion during pregnancy suggest that it is low risk. Although some early studies have shown an increased risk of heart defects, further research has not supported this finding. Limited data suggest that the use of bupropion during pregnancy is associated with an increased risk of attention deficit/hyperactivity disorder; however, maternal cigarette use may have contributed to this finding (Briggs et al., 2011). If a woman requires the use of bupropion during pregnancy to successfully quit smoking, she should be informed of these potential risks, but the medication should not be withheld if medically indicated.

Nicotine replacement therapy

The risks of cigarette smoking during pregnancy are well established. While nonpharmacological interventions are likely the safest option for both the mother and the fetus, nicotine replacement therapy is a reasonable option if these approaches fail. While the nicotine contained in replacement therapies continues to present a risk of fetal harm, the risk of exposure to pure nicotine is considered smaller than exposure to tobacco products as these contain both nicotine and a variety of other substances including carbon monoxide and ammonia. If the woman continues to smoke while using the replacement therapies, the benefits of using nicotine replacement therapy may outweigh the risks (Briggs et al., 2011).

Varenicline (Chantix®)

There is no information on the safety of varenicline use in pregnancy. Significant concerns about the safety of this medication have been raised for nonpregnant patients. Documented adverse effects of the medication include mood changes, depression, and suicide. The National Institutes of Health is currently sponsoring clinical trials of varenicline during pregnancy (National Institutes of Health, 2012). Varenicline is classified as pregnancy category C drug. However, given that the serious potential risks of smoking during pregnancy are well documented, the clinician may weigh the benefits and risks of the use of varenicline during pregnancy if both nonpharmacological and other available pharmacological interventions have been ineffective (Briggs et al., 2011).

General principles of prescribing drugs during pregnancy should be followed when using pharmaceutical

Table 13.2   The 5 A's and the 5 R's Model of Smoking Cessation

The 5 A's—initial smoking counseling and intervention

Ask—Ask the woman about her tobacco use at the first prenatal visit, document it as a vital sign, and track smoking status at every visit.

Advise—Advise smoking cessation, focusing on the positive benefits of smoking cessation.

Assess—Assess the woman's willingness to quit smoking. For women who indicate that they want to quit and are committed to trying within the specified time frame, the clinician should move on to the fourth A. For women who indicate that they are not yet ready to quit or commit to trying to quit within the time frame, the clinician should use techniques designed to increase the patient's motivation to quit smoking.

Assist—Assist with a cessation plan by providing support, self-help materials, and problem-solving techniques, and by helping to identify other sources of support. Examples of assistance are setting a quit date, providing techniques to cope with cravings and social situations when others are smoking, avoiding smoking triggers, and using substitute behaviors like walking or gum chewing.

Arrange—Arrange follow-up to monitor smoking status and provide support, encouragement, and positive reinforcement for their efforts to help maintain motivation.

The 5 R's—subsequent smoking counseling and intervention

Relevance—Ask the woman to identify why quitting might be personally relevant, such as children in her home, money saved by quitting, and a history of smoking related illness.

Risks—Ask the woman to identify her own negative consequences from smoking. Additional risks to bring up in the discussion are the following:
* Acute risks—shortness of breath, exacerbation of asthma, impotence, infertility
* Long-term risks—heart attacks, strokes, lung and other cancers, chronic obstructive pulmonary disease (COPD)
* Environmental risks—increased risk of lung cancer in spouse and children; higher rates of smoking by children; increased risk for sudden infant death syndrome (SIDS), asthma, middle ear disease and respiratory infection in children.

Rewards—Ask the woman to identify
* positive benefits they currently derive from smoking; discuss alternative methods for filling the potential void after cessation
* the potential rewards of smoking cessation including improved health, improved sense of smell and taste, money saved, healthier children, freedom from addiction, more physically fit, and reduced wrinkling and aging of skin.

Roadblocks—Ask the woman to identify barriers to quitting smoking. As she self-identifies barriers, each should be addressed and reassurance provided that assistance and encouragement are available. She needs to know that roadblocks can be overcome.

Repetition—Repeat the above strategies every time an unmotivated patient has a visit.

Source: http://www.ahrq.gov/professionals/clinicians-providers/guidelines-recommendations/tobacco/clinicians/reference/index.html.

agents for smoking cessation. These include using the lowest dose necessary to achieve success in order to minimize fetal exposure and delaying therapy until the second trimester in order to avoid the period of embryogenesis when the fetus is most sensitive to teratogens. Consultation and or collaboration with an obstetrician or perinatogist may be considered when using pharmaceutical smoking cessation strategies for pregnant women.

Care of pregnant women with substance use disorders

Those who provide services for pregnant, drug-using women must recognize that care of women with social problems that affect pregnancy outcomes should be approached in the same way as care of all women with medical problems that potentially impact fetal well-being. The overall goal of treatment for drug dependence during pregnancy is to improve outcomes for both mother and baby by minimizing perinatal risk, increasing maternal participation in prenatal care, and assisting the mother to transition to a safe and stable lifestyle. Opioid maintenance therapy, in conjunction with a comprehensive prenatal care program, enables a pregnant woman to access the services needed for this transition. Harm reduction should be the guiding principle for the prenatal care of women with substance use disorders. A collaborative model provides the most comprehensive care for the pregnant woman.

Antepartum assessment

Pregnancy dating

Accurate pregnancy dating is a critical component of managing substance exposed pregnancies for a variety of reasons. Physiological stress leading to anovulation frequently causes amenorrhea or oligomenorrhea in women who are substance dependent and contributes to both late entry to care and uncertainty determining the timing of conception. An ultrasound for pregnancy dating should be performed shortly after a woman presents for prenatal care. As much precision as possible in determining gestational age is essential due to the increased risk for preterm labor and the potential need to accelerate delivery in the case of intrauterine growth restriction or other pregnancy complications.

Prenatal laboratory testing

In addition to routine prenatal labs and HIV testing, women with substance use disorders should be screened for hepatitis C antibodies, hepatic function, and tuberculosis. HIV, hepatitis C virus (HCV), hepatitis B, and gonorrhea and chlamydia testing should be repeated in the third trimester as indicated (American Academy of Pediatrics, 2009). Routine antepartum urine drug testing should be performed only with patient consent and when test results would influence the course of prenatal care.

Screening for medical comorbidities

Viral blood-borne disease should be managed collaboratively with the consulting obstetrician, family medicine, and/or infectious disease specialist. Exposure to tuberculosis is most likely when there is a history of immigration from an area where the disease is endemic or a history of incarceration. Colonization with multidrug-resistant organisms such as methicillin-resistant *Staphylococcus aureus* (MRSA) is frequent among women with substance abuse disorders. Pregnant women with substance dependence are at higher risk for viral transmission through risky sexual practices. Patient education about transmission prevention is essential.

Psychosocial assessment

Pregnant women with substance use disorders are more likely to have inadequately treated psychiatric diseases. Conversely, untreated psychiatric problems are a risk factor for continued substance use (Hans, 1999). Assessment for depression and anxiety disorders is an essential part of supporting women's recovery.

Screening for depression and domestic violence should be included in the initial assessment of all pregnant women and should be intensified when caring for women at risk for substance abuse (Horrigan et al., 2000). Patients with complex psychiatric disorders or severe depression and anxiety should be referred to psychiatry or other mental health specialists. Anxiety disorders, post-traumatic stress, and mild to moderate depression may be managed collaboratively when within the knowledge base and scope of practice of the prenatal provider.

All pregnant women screening positive for substance use should be offered weekly substance abuse counseling. An intensive outpatient treatment program that meets daily is also an excellent option, if available. When comorbid psychiatric disease is identified, patients should be referred for dual-diagnosis counseling as well as medication management when indicated. First-line pharmacological agents used for the treatment of depression and anxiety in pregnancy should be considered.

The possibility of drug–drug interaction is important to consider for women on opioid maintenance therapy who are also receiving psychiatric medications. Metabolism of buprenorphine and methadone may be altered by medications that inhibit or induce cytochrome p450 3A4 activity, such as selective serotonin reuptake inhibitors (SSRIs). Concurrent treatment with fluoxetine (Prozac®) has been found to increase serum concentrations of methadone due to inhibition of opioid metabolism, although this has not been demonstrated to date with buprenorphine. Sertraline (Zoloft®) inhibits cytochrome p450 3A4 activity and may result in higher buprenorphine levels (Jones et al., 2010; U.S. Center for Substance Abuse Treatment, 2004).

Certain substance interactions can be lethal, for example, when those on opioid maintenance therapy self-medicate with benzodiazepines or drink alcohol. Reported cases of lethal buprenorphine overdose have primarily been attributed to polysubstance use (Johnson, Strain, & Amass, 2003; Walsh & Eissenberg, 2003). Interaction with benzodiazepines significantly augments the respiratory depressant effects of opioids and can overcome the protective ceiling effect of buprenorphine. Concern has also been expressed about the additive effects of withdrawal from psychiatric medications and opioids on the newborn after birth (O'Connor, Monroe, & Alto, 2012). Concurrent withdrawal from nicotine also appears to worsen neonatal abstinence symptoms.

Social risks

Women with a positive screen for drug use need screening for domestic violence and referral for domestic violence services as indicated. Women should be asked about additional barriers to care, including lack of transportation, childcare, and access to essential resources such as food and shelter. Special consideration should be given to placement in residential treatment programs or in shelters when women who are dependent on drugs are at risk for homelessness and/or domestic violence. Because of these social risks, clinicians need to be tolerant of missed appointments and may even consider offering drop-in appointments as their clinic schedule allows.

Fetal assessment

Little data are available on which to base protocols for fetal assessment for substance exposed pregnancies. A targeted anatomy scan around 18–20 weeks is recommended for all substance exposed pregnancies. A plan for fetal monitoring during the second half of pregnancy should be individualized based on an estimate of each patient's risk for poor pregnancy outcomes. A limited early third-trimester ultrasound may be helpful to determine fetal growth and amniotic fluid volume as indicators of placental function. Factors to consider in planning follow-up include whether a woman is stable in treatment, whether she is using illicit drugs, the severity of concurrent social risk factors, and the amount of tobacco consumption. Monthly growth ultrasounds are often justified to follow fetal growth and placental function, depending on the level of substance use. Scheduled fetal nonstress testing should be avoided for the first few hours after methadone dosing, as peak methadone levels alter fetal heart rate variability and can reduce fetal breathing motion on biophysical profile (Jansson, DiPietro, & Elko, 2005).

Anticipatory guidance

Pregnant women who are substance dependent often experience significant guilt and anxiety regarding impending hospitalization for labor and birth. Anticipatory guidance in the antepartum period is essential. Whenever possible, information should be given in writing to ensure accurate recall. Education should include options for management of labor pain, and hospital policies including routine drug screening, continuation of opioid maintenance therapy, protection of patient confidentiality, and smoking. Women and their families must be provided with accurate information about surveillance for and treatment of NAS during the antepartum period. Written institutional policies regarding breastfeeding for women with substance dependence should be made available. State rules regarding mandatory reporting to child protective services should be openly discussed. A woman may attempt to avoid being reported by changing prenatal care providers late in the course of pregnancy unless institutional policies are discussed in an open and supportive manner.

Referral to treatment

There are a number of barriers to the treatment of substance use disorders during pregnancy. The significant social stigma, shame, and guilt associated with ongoing addiction during pregnancy may cause a woman to attempt to quit using substances on her own. Women often fear that the disclosure of a substance abuse disorder during pregnancy will result in mandated reporting and unwanted attention from a variety of social service agencies. In addition, low levels of self-esteem and education in addition to past and continuing legal problems may interfere with self-reporting and seeking assistance.

The treatment plan for pregnant women with substance use disorders needs to be comprehensive, collaborative, and individualized to the woman's specific needs. The benefits of treatment as well as the risks of continuing illicit substance use during pregnancy should be discussed and a referral to a substance abuse treatment facility should be provided (Johnston, Mandell, & Meyer, 2010). If a woman is unwilling to seek treatment, the woman should be given the opportunity to take any resources with her in case she decides to seek treatment. It is important for the clinician to schedule additional appointments to continue to engage the woman in discussions related to recovery as well as to monitor for the potential effects of illicit substance use on her pregnancy. Facilitating access to treatment for any psychological comorbidities that may exist is an important component of care (Johnston et al., 2010). A readily accessible and up-to-date list of treatment resources should be maintained. Pregnant women should expect to gain priority access to most substance abuse treatment facilities. Ideally, treatment should be made available on the same day as diagnosis of drug abuse.

Nonadherence to treatment is a common obstacle in the care of pregnant women abusing substances. Together with the treatment team, the prenatal care provider needs to evaluate whether the outpatient care treatment approach meets the needs of the woman. A more structured treatment environment such as inpatient treatment and/or bringing in additional treatment specialists may be needed for successful intervention. The clinician should always be assessing the patient's position on the recovery spectrum. Sometimes, treatment nonadherence is related to external factors such as existing childcare demands and/or transportation problems. Additional referrals to social service agencies might reduce some of these barriers.

Opioid replacement therapy in pregnancy

Acute opioid withdrawal is associated with a variety of potential maternal–fetal complications including tachycardia, hypertension, gastrointestinal distress, as well as an increased risk of mortality for the fetus. Medication-assisted treatment is recommended to reduce these complications as well as to stabilize the maternal social situation, reduce the risk of drug overdose, and reduce the potential risk of blood-borne infections that may accompany intravenous drug use. Medically supervised opioid withdrawal has also been tried, but long-term abstinence in these situations is typically low. Methadone (category C) is the standard of care treatment option for opioid-dependent pregnant women and it has been shown to improve prenatal care, reduce illicit drug use, and reduce the risk of fetal withdrawal *in utero* (Johnston et al., 2010). Office-based treatment and/or outpatient treatment options as well as those that are residential should both be considered for the treatment of opioid-dependent pregnant women. The patient, the mental health/addiction treatment specialists, as well as the prenatal care providers should all participate in decisions pertaining to substance abuse treatment options.

Methadone

Methadone is a highly effective, evidence-based treatment of opioid dependence. It is a full agonist for the mu-opioid receptor and has a long half-life, which allows for daily dosing. It is dispensed through federally licensed methadone treatment centers that often provide substance abuse counseling, and in some cases medical care, in addition to the medication. Pregnant women should expect priority admission to methadone treatment centers. The clinician should have the patient sign appropriate consent forms to coordinate care with the methadone treatment providers. This may require specialized forms due to the federal regulations regarding the confidentiality of substance abuse treatment services.

Relatively high doses of methadone, often greater than 100 mg daily, are often required during pregnancy. The dose may need to be split into twice daily dosing, particularly later in pregnancy, due to increased excretion of the drug. Higher maintenance dosing of methadone is not associated with an increased frequency or severity of NAS or other adverse perinatal outcomes. Therefore, concerns about NAS should not restrict methadone dosing during pregnancy (Pizarro et al., 2011).

Buprenorphine

Buprenorphine is a partial agonist for the mu-opioid receptor and is also Food and Drug Administration (FDA) approved for the treatment of opioid dependence (but not in pregnancy). Although less data are available about its use during pregnancy, a growing body of evidence suggests that maternal–infant outcomes are similar

and in some cases improved when women are maintained on buprenorphine during pregnancy (Alto & O'Connor, 2011; Binder & Vavrinková, 2008; Johnson et al., 2001; Johnson, Jones & Fisher, 2003; Jones et al., 2010; Kahila et al., 2007; Kakko, Heilig, & Sarman, 2008). Buprenorphine can be dispensed in the context of an office visit, thereby reducing some of the barriers to treatment associated with methadone, particularly the daily dosing schedule, which requires transportation to the methadone clinic. If methadone treatment is refused or unavailable, the clinician should consider opioid-substitution therapy with buprenorphine after informed consent is obtained and the risk of inadequate experience during pregnancy is clearly documented in the patient's record. Outpatient treatment with buprenorphine should occur in tandem with substance abuse counseling.

The Drug Addiction Treatment Act of 2000 limits the outpatient prescriptive authority of buprenorphine to specially trained and federally waivered physicians (O'Connor, 2011). In the inpatient setting, providers with prescriptive authority for Drug Enforcement Administration (DEA) schedule III medications can prescribe buprenorphine to prevent acute opioid withdrawal. The prenatal care provider should work in close collaboration with the buprenorphine prescriber and the remainder of the substance abuse treatment team. Buprenorphine monotherapy should be used during pregnancy as it avoids the potential fetal risk of acute withdrawal if the buprenorphine/naloxone combination therapy (Suboxone®) is misused. The average dose of buprenorphine at the end of pregnancy is 16 mg (Johnston et al., 2010). Many women maintained on buprenorphine during pregnancy will often require dose increases during the course of the pregnancy, usually ranging from 3 to 6 mg (Fischer et al., 2006; Jones et al., 2005; O'Connor et al., 2011).

Treatment with methadone vs. buprenorphine

The decision between methadone and buprenorphine requires careful consideration and is often accomplished within an interdisciplinary care team. If the woman has been stabilized on either medication prior to pregnancy, it is reasonable to continue with the same medication. Methadone and/or inpatient residential treatment may be considered for women with polysubstance use, unstable living situations, and those who require more intensive levels of care, or have previously abused buprenorphine (Johnston et al., 2010). Appropriate candidates for office-based treatment with buprenorphine may include women who are willing to seek substance abuse treatment and prenatal care, those in a more stable social situation, and those that are only abusing opioids. It is possible to initiate buprenorphine treatment in an inpatient facility and then transfer to an outpatient treatment facility when she is stabilized on the medication. While outpatient treatment offers many benefits, it is harder to verify that the patient is taking her full dose daily, and some clinics are moving toward observed daily dosing during pregnancy.

While the buprenorphine or methadone provider will likely be managing most aspects of the medication-assisted treatment, the prenatal care provider should be aware of the importance of maintaining close contact with pregnant women in recovery including frequent assessments of opioid craving and/or potential opioid withdrawal symptoms, which can include anxiety, agitation, muscle aches, insomnia, gastrointestinal distress, and dilated pupils. Pregnant women in treatment with buprenorphine require frequent pill counts and urine drug screens to assure that the medication is being taken properly and to monitor for potential illicit substance use.

Whether the pregnant woman is maintained on methadone or buprenorphine, many of the prenatal care issues are the same. Between 24 and 32 weeks, a consultation or referral should be made to the pediatric provider who will monitor the infant for NAS (Johnston et al., 2010). An anesthesia consult can also be beneficial as it can reduce some of the maternal anxiety associated with pain management during birth.

Pain management during birth can be a complex issue. The pregnant woman with a substance abuse disorder often requires more frequent and higher doses of analgesics and, in these cases, it should not be assumed that she is exhibiting drug seeking behavior. Opioid analgesics can be safely used, often in tandem with buprenorphine or methadone, though caution is advised if using combination products with acetaminophen due to the potential risks of liver toxicity if acetaminophen dosing exceeds 4 g daily. Epidurals are often the ideal pain management option. Nalbuphine and butorphanol are contraindicated during birth as they can precipitate acute opioid withdrawal.

Throughout the pregnancy, issues pertaining to NAS, potential referrals to child welfare agencies (as required by individual states), as well as breastfeeding issues in women receiving medication-assisted treatment should be regularly discussed. NAS tends to be longer and more severe in women using multiple addictive substances, including nicotine. Knowledge of this may motivate a pregnant woman to reduce her exposure of these substances.

Laws pertaining to mandated reporting of substance use during pregnancy and/or infants affected by exposure to substances *in utero* vary by state. Clinicians should be aware of these laws in the state(s) in which they practice. None of the states have laws explicitly stating that substance use during pregnancy is a criminal act of child abuse. However, several states have laws requiring health-care providers to test and/or report prenatal drug exposure and, in some cases, this can be grounds for termination of parental rights.

Breastfeeding and medication-assisted treatment counseling

The decision to encourage breastfeeding should be made in conjunction with the newborn's health-care provider. Breastfeeding is generally encouraged in women receiving medication-assisted treatment with either methadone or buprenorphine unless other contraindications exist. Women maintained on methadone during pregnancy can continue on methadone while breastfeeding (McCarthy & Posey, 2000). Women maintained on buprenorphine monotherapy during pregnancy should be switched to the combination buprenorphine/naloxone therapy unless the breastfeeding infant is being treated for NAS with an opioid medication (Grimm, Pauly, Poschl, Linderkamp, & Skopp, 2005; Johnston et al., 2010). In these cases, the mother should continue on buprenorphine monotherapy until either the infant no longer needs treatment with an opioid medication or the mother decides to stop breastfeeding (Johnston et al., 2010; Lindemalm, Nydert, Svensson, Stahle, & Sarman, 2009).

Communication and coordination of care

Comprehensive and well-coordinated care by a multidisciplinary team provides optimal support for pregnant women with substance use disorders. Providing screening and intervention services for alcohol, tobacco, and drug use within the context of prenatal care has been shown to improve not only perinatal outcomes but also related costs (Goler et al., 2008, 2012). However, in rural practice, the elements of a comprehensive plan of care may need to be coordinated between a team of providers in disparate locations. The pregnant woman should be asked to provide written consent for communication between her pregnancy, addiction medicine, psychiatric, and pediatric health-care providers. Once appropriate consent is obtained, regular communication between members of the team is essential.

Federal and state laws regarding the confidentiality of records pertaining to substance abuse treatment are appropriately restrictive. Consultation with an institutional risk management team is recommended to ensure that patient privacy is protected without jeopardizing the providers' ability to share information essential for optimal patient care and safety.

Neonatal abstinence syndrome

The term NAS refers to the constellation of signs and symptoms displayed by a neonate exposed to opiates *in utero*. These signs and symptoms may also occur iatrogenically after administration of opioids for the purpose of treating pain or sedating the newborn (Weiner & Finnegan, 2011). Opiate withdrawal symptoms are generally categorized by CNS and gastrointestinal dysfunction (American Academy of Pediatrics (AAP), 1998). The timing of NAS may vary, but in most babies, symptoms appear within 72 hours. Signs and symptoms that may persist for several weeks include restlessness, tremors, high-pitched cry, increased muscle tone, irritability, and exaggerated Moro reflex. Seizures occur rarely. Sleep pattern disturbance, irritability, and hypertonia may last for 4–6 months (Weiner & Finnegan, 2011).

The severity of symptoms in the newborn is not predicted by maternal opiate dose (Seligman et al., 2010; Thajam, Atkinson, Sibley &, Lavender, 2010). It is important to recognize that prenatal tobacco exposure does impact newborn neurobehavior and this is likely to affect the severity of symptoms (Choo et al., 2004; Law et al., 2003). Mothers should be counseled to reduce or eliminate cigarette smoking to reduce the severity of NAS.

NAS may mimic other illnesses and, in situations where providers are unaware of a mother's opiate use, the infant will require testing to rule out other illnesses. Differential diagnoses include hypoglycemia, hypocalcemia, hypomagnesemia, hyperthyroidism, CNS hemorrhage, anoxia, and sepsis (AAP, 1998).

Assessment and treatment of neonatal abstinence syndrome

Several scoring tools exist to objectively assess an infant's symptoms of NAS and the progression or alleviation of those symptoms. Parents should anticipate that scoring begins in the first few hours after birth and will continue every 3–4 hours throughout hospitalization.

When a newborn requires treatment of NAS, the goals of therapy are to promote weight gain, sleep, and periods of time when the infant may interact and bond with the family. Treatment may begin with nonpharmacological measures, which may include swaddling, decreasing exposure to light and noise, pacifiers, and frequent small feedings, which may consist of hypercaloric formula because of the increased caloric requirements (AAP, 1998). The decision to treat NAS with pharmacological agents should be individualized and based on prenatal exposure(s). A drug from the same class as that causing withdrawal is preferable (AAP, 1998). Length of stay for infants with NAS will vary by prenatal exposures and need for pharmacological treatment. The length of stay for infants not requiring pharmacological treatment may be as short as 4 days. Those requiring treatment may anticipate a hospital stay of several weeks.

Breastfeeding and neonatal abstinence syndrome

Breastfeeding is encouraged for infants exposed prenatally to opioids and may reduce the severity of NAS. Maternal barriers to breastfeeding may include lack of education, psychiatric comorbidity, depression, polysubstance use, low self-esteem, and a history of physical and/or sexual abuse. Infant barriers to breastfeeding include irritability, hypertonicity, difficulty coordinating suck and swallow, nasal stuffiness, and hypersensitivity to minor stimuli (Jansson, Velez &, Harrow, 2004). Coordinating services with lactation consultant prenatally may be useful to promote successful breastfeeding.

Long-term implications of neonatal abstinence syndrome

When babies have a particularly difficult NAS course that is associated with polysubstance exposure and/or requires a combination of therapeutic agents, parents should be counseled that the risk of SIDS is 5–10 times higher than that of the general population. This increased risk may be related to several issues such as decreased lung maturity, sleep pattern disturbances, and/or vomiting and loose stools leading to dehydration and electrolyte imbalance (Weiner & Finnegan, 2011). Parents should be encouraged to utilize safe sleep practices including putting their baby on his/her back to sleep, in their own crib on a firm mattress without toys. Babies should not sleep with adults or siblings. Newborn sleeping arrangements should be discussed during the prenatal period (AAP, 2011).

Long-term outcomes for newborns with NAS continue to be studied. In 2003, the Keeping Children and Families Safe Act (PL 108-36) reauthorized the Child Abuse Prevention and Treatment Act (CAPTA) and is the first federal legislation to direct states to established policies and procedures to address the safety and well-being of infants affected by prenatal drug exposure. The Act requires that health-care providers notify child protective services in the event an infant is born affected by illegal substances or with withdrawal symptoms due to *in utero* exposures and that a plan of care is developed for the affected infant. The overall goal is that notification of the substance exposure will lead to greater identification of children at risk for poor developmental outcomes, and therefore greater access to early intervention services (National Abandoned Infants Assistance Resource Center, 2006). Parents should anticipate and be encouraged to accept referrals to support services such as public health nurses and child development services.

Postpartum care

Relapse prevention is a primary goal of postpartum care. Postpartum resumption of substance use is common and generally occurs within the first few months, as women often identify the fetus as the primary motivating factor for recovery during pregnancy (Jessup & Brindis, 2005; NIDA, 2009). Women with at-risk drinking patterns rapidly resume use after giving birth (NIDA, 2009). Opioid maintenance therapy should be continued for patients who require treatment. Women with substance use disorders are at high risk for postpartum depression and should be followed closely, treated aggressively, and/or referred. Referral to Public Health Nursing and other home visiting services are recommended. When antidepressant therapy is indicated, potential drug–drug interactions should be considered. Substance abuse counseling and/or dual-diagnosis therapy should be continued.

Repeat pregnancy prevention is also an important consideration in postpartum care for women with substance use disorders. Providing information on and access to reliable contraception is essential.

Breastfeeding and substance use

Advising a woman with a substance use disorder about breastfeeding is often a controversial area in clinical practice. It is important for institutions to have a written policy to assure consistency across the health-care team and to limit the potential impact of clinician bias. As a general rule, the benefits and risks of breastfeeding should be weighed. This would include the benefit of the medication to the mother (as in the case of opioid replacement therapy), the benefits of breast milk to the infant, and the enhanced maternal–infant bonding that occurs with breastfeeding. Risks would include potential exposure to both prescribed and illicit substances in the breast milk as well as issues associated with abrupt discontinuation of breastfeeding. While maternal HIV is a contraindication to breastfeeding, maternal hepatitis B and C are not contraindications to breastfeeding as long as the mother does not have cracked or bleeding nipples.

Transfer of medications and/or illicit substances from maternal serum into breast milk depends on a variety of factors including lipid solubility, molecular weight, and half-life. It is important to remember that pregnancy risk is not necessarily the same as breastfeeding risk. Historically, women with substance abuse disorders exhibit low rates of breastfeeding. It is difficult to determine to what extent this is related to individual choice

or clinician recommendation. In addition, limited evidence is available about the risks of exposure to illicit substances in breast milk often due to the ethical considerations of administering these substances to nursing mothers. If polysubstance use is a concern, particular emphasis should be placed on monitoring the infant for drowsiness, adequate weight gain, and developmental milestones.

In response to the limited research available about breastfeeding and substance use, the Academy of Breastfeeding Medicine (ABM) (2009) developed guidelines for breastfeeding in drug-dependent women. Unless other contraindications (e.g., maternal HIV) exist, women engaged in substance abuse treatment, who have received consistent prenatal care and who have abstained from illicit substance use in the 90 days prior to delivery should be encouraged to breastfeed (ABM, 2009). Women who are not currently or planning to engage in substance abuse treatment as well as those who have abused substances in the 30 days prior to delivery should be discouraged from breastfeeding. The ABM suggests a careful evaluation of women who have relapsed in the 30–90 days prior to birth, those who have only recently entered treatment, as well as those who have maintained sobriety only in an inpatient setting (Table 13.3).

Infants born to mothers who are using cigarettes are at risk of exposure through breast milk and in their environment.

> If a breastfeeding mother is actively smoking, she should be advised to
>
> - smoke away from the baby, preferably outdoors
> - smoke right after nursing sessions
> - smoke as few cigarettes as possible; infant risks increase with smoking more than 20 cigarettes a day
> - be aware that reduction in milk supply, inhibition of the let-down reflex, and physical symptoms in the baby, such as nausea, abdominal cramps, vomiting, and diarrhea, may occur.

There are no reports pertaining to the use of nicotine replacement therapies during breastfeeding. While smoking cessation is generally encouraged during lactation, no professional organizations have recommended the use of nicotine replacement therapies, probably due to insufficient data regarding risks. Similarly, there is little data about the use of bupropion or varenicline during breastfeeding.

Bupropion is found in low levels in breast milk. If a nursing mother requires bupropion, it is not a reason to discontinue breastfeeding (National Library of Medicine, 2011c). However, adequacy of milk supply and

Table 13.3 Specific Substances and Breastfeeding

Substance	Comments
Alcohol	• The daily use of small amounts of alcohol, such as one glass of wine or beer, is not likely to cause problems for the breastfeeding infant (National Library of Medicine [Alcohol], 2011b). • Mothers should be advised to wait at least two hours after a drink to breastfeed as peak alcohol levels in breast milk occurs shortly after ingestion. • Daily use of larger amounts of alcohol can decrease milk production, may be associated with impaired infant growth and motor function, and may interfere with parenting skills.
Amphetamines	• In regularly prescribed doses, breastfeeding does not appear to be contraindicated. Breastfeeding is discouraged in women actively abusing methamphetamines (ACOG Com. Op. No. 479, 2011).
Benzodiazepines	• Breastfeeding is not explicitly contraindicated if the medications are taken as prescribed. Breastfeeding is not recommended for women who are abusing benzodiazepines (Hale, 2010). • These medications and their metabolites pass freely into breast milk and cause sedation, breastfeeding difficulty, and poor weight gain (National Library of Medicine, 2011a).
Buprenorphine	• Breastfeeding is not contraindicated; very limited safety data are available (U.S. DHHS, 2011).
Cocaine	• Breastfeeding is discouraged if a woman is actively abusing cocaine (Sarkar, Djulus, & Koren, 2005). • Infants may be exposed to significant amounts of cocaine through breast milk (Winecker et al., 2001). • Serious adverse reactions include vomiting, diarrhea, and seizures (Chasnoff, Lewis, & Squires, 1987).
Illicit opioids	• When used in excess by the breastfeeding mother, infants can experience increased lethargy and breathing difficulties.
Marijuana	• Breastfeeding is discouraged in women regularly using cannabis (ABM, 2009; AAP, 2005). • Tetrahydrocannabinol (THC) transfers readily into breast milk and may be present in higher concentrations than in maternal serum due to its high lipophilicity (Hale, 2010).
Methadone	• Women who received methadone maintenance during pregnancy and are stable in treatment should be encouraged to breastfeed their infants (AAP, 2001). • Women in treatment with methadone should be cautioned against abrupt cessation as the sudden termination of breastfeeding in infants exposed to methadone in breast milk has been associated with acute withdrawal symptoms (Isemann, Meinzen-Derr, & Akinbi, 2011; Malpas & Darlow, 1999).
Nicotine	• Breastfeeding is not contraindicated. • Cigarette smoking reduces maternal milk yield. • Nicotine and other cigarette chemicals pass into breast milk.

neonatal and infant behavior should be carefully monitored.

Varenicline's molecular weight and long half-life suggest that it will likely be present in breast milk. The actual risk of exposure in breast milk is unknown. An infant exposed to varenicline during breastfeeding should be monitored for the common side effects experienced by adults, including nausea, vomiting, constipation, and sleep disturbances (Briggs et al., 2011).

Cultural considerations

Nationwide, women of childbearing age are significantly less likely to use substances when pregnant than either prior to pregnancy or postpartum (National Institute for Drug Addiction, 2009). Non-Hispanic white women report the highest rates of substance use during preg-

nancy, followed by Hispanics and non-Hispanic African Americans (Muhuri & Gfroerer, 2009). Postpregnancy, all women are at risk for resuming substance use within the first few months after birth (NIDA, 2009).

Women reporting illicit drug use are more likely to have lower levels of education, a household income below $20,000 annually, or be unemployed (van Gelder, et al., 2010). The choice of primary substance used varies both geographically and economically, and is dependent on availability and price. Historically, privately insured women are less likely to be screened for substance abuse during pregnancy than women who are on public assistance (Wolff, 2011). Treatment success is heavily dependent on the acceptability of a given program (Kearney, 1998), as well as its accessibility. Health-care providers should be familiar with available local and regional addiction treatment resources.

Case study: Washington County, Maine

Never doubt that a small group of thoughtful, committed citizens can change the world.
Indeed, it is the only thing that ever has.
~Margaret Mead~

BACKGROUND: "Down East" Maine is an entirely rural area with a natural resource and service based economy. This area consists of 47 widely dispersed towns, ranging in population from 10 to 4000. The heavily wooded region encompasses 2569 square miles roughly twice the size of Rhode Island. Severe winters, poor road conditions, and a lack of public transportation add to the geographic isolation of the area. The extreme poverty, poor economic environment, and low educational attainment contribute to a social climate characterized by high stress, broken families, poor preventative health care, and an increased risk for substance abuse.

PROBLEM: In 1999, Maine's Office of the U.S. Attorney noted that law enforcement seizures and arrests for illegal possession of prescription narcotics had jumped ninefold. Arrests for illegal possession had quadrupled in less than four years and substance abuse admissions for narcotic abuse had increased by 500%. On the very day that the U.S. Attorney traveled to Down East Maine to declare that narcotic abuse was the most serious criminal and social problem facing Maine, I was approached by a 19-year-old pregnant woman who was desperate to find help for her 4-year history of opiate addiction. After hours of phone calls, I found that there were no treatment options in Down East Maine. Eventually, because of her pregnancy, she was accepted into a "detox" program that was 4 hours away. Had she not been pregnant, the waiting list at this facility was at least 6 months long. Three months later, I found myself caring for 10 opiate-addicted pregnant women. I began seeing unusual preterm labor patterns that I now recognize as acute opiate withdrawal in the third trimester. Many of these women abused prescription drugs because they thought they were "safe" and would not harm their unborn babies. As abuse of narcotics grew, hepatitis C and HIV became significant public health risk factors in our community. The drug problem was contributing to the breakup of families, and an estimated 50% of child protective and custody cases involved prescription drug abuse within the family.

ACTION: Neighbors Against Drug Abuse (NADA) is a group of citizens who came together in response to the overwhelming substance abuse problem in Down East Maine. Initially, we acted as a fact-finding group. We quickly determined that we needed to inform as many organizations and public officials as possible about the drug problem. I represented NADA in Washington, DC, by testifying before the U.S. Senate Committee on Health and Education at the invitation of one of our State Senators. This testimony provided us with federal recognition, acknowledgment of the problem, and national and state support.

To address the crisis, we were then able to develop a coordinated program with three areas of focus: prevention/education, treatment, and law enforcement.

RESULTS: Community awareness of the scope of the substance abuse problem promoted further progress in increasing resources. Educational workshops, counselor training, collaboration with federal agencies, and grants for treatment and prevention grants were obtained.

A local treatment center was established. This center provided methadone maintenance, medical examinations, short-term detoxification, counseling services, relapse prevention and support groups, addiction education, HIV counseling, job training and placement assistance, educational assistance, nutritional counseling, and after care. The Maine Adult Drug Court was instituted. This is a specialized court given the responsibility to handle cases involving drug offenders through comprehensive supervision, drug testing, treatment services, and immediate sanctions/incentives.

Several pregnancy-related coalitions and services were formed from these efforts. The infant–family support specialist focuses on women with substance abuse disorders who are receiving prenatal care. The Bridging program connects pregnant women with substance abuse disorders with specially trained, intensive case management providers who offer additional support in the home during pregnancy and for the first 6 months after birth until they are transitioned into local services. The Bridging program addressed critical needs, specifically getting the family through the infant hospitalization for NAS, following-up with child development services and other agencies, and helping the family connect with the new baby.

Nancy Green, CNM

Personal and family considerations

The prenatal care of women with substance abuse disorders can be complex and requires a comprehensive approach. Treatment must be accessible and many women may require assistance with transportation. The clinician also needs to consider other potential barriers to care such as the need for childcare during appointments. A woman may be at risk of violence within the home when she seeks treatment, particularly if she was the primary source of prescription opioids prior to entering recovery. If her partner is unable to access treatment at the same time, he or she might also demand access to medications prescribed to treat substance dependence. This places both the mother and the fetus at risk for poor outcomes. Some programs will not provide a pregnant woman with buprenorphine if her partner is actively abusing opioids.

Scope of practice considerations

A woman struggling with substance abuse and addiction during pregnancy is at high risk both socially and physically. The likelihood that she will achieve a sustained recovery is increased compared to when she is not pregnant *if* she receives appropriate support (Boyd & Marcellus, 2007; Jessup & Brindis, 2005). A holistic, woman-centered approach is essential. Because midwives and other advanced practice nurses are trained to provide care for women in the context of family and community, they are well prepared to coordinate a comprehensive treatment approach addressing both pregnancy and social needs. Prenatal care should be delivered in collaboration with a consulting obstetrician, an addiction medicine specialist or a family practice physician, a licensed substance abuse counselor, and if indicated, a psychiatric provider. Social services and public health nursing services should be involved whenever possible. Referral to specialties such as infectious disease is necessary if comorbidities such as hepatitis or HIV are present.

Summary

Substance abuse during pregnancy continues to present a major public health concern. Early identification of at risk maternal–fetal dyads improves outcomes as it reduces potential complications associated with recurrent intoxication and withdrawal and limits exposure to infectious diseases as well as the medical problems associated with intravenous drug use. Multidisciplinary medical and behavioral health care is cost-effective as it reduces the potential financial burden of extended hospital stays for undertreated maternal–fetal dyads. Substance abuse

often occurs in tandem with other mental health comorbidities including depression, anxiety, and post-traumatic stress disorder that may be the result of a previous history of violence and abuse. Prenatal clinicians are ideally positioned to care for pregnant women with substance abuse disorders due to their ongoing care over time. Clinicians have an ethical responsibility to provide evidence-based and nonjudgmental care to this highly vulnerable patient population.

Resources for health-care providers

Interactive Web-based program designed for health-care professionals to hone their skills in assisting pregnant women to quit smoking: http://www.smokingcessationandpregnancy.org/

Methamphetamine abuse and addiction—NIDA research report: http://www.drugabuse.gov/publications/research-reports/methamphetamine-abuse-addiction

Motivational interviewing techniques: http://www.ncbi.nlm.nih.gov/books/NBK26158/

National Drug Threat Assessment 2011: http://www.justice.gov/ndic/pubs44/44849/44849p.pdf

National Library of Medicine's LactMed, a searchable evidence-based database of the compatibility of medications/substances with breastfeeding: http://toxnet.nlm.nih.gov/cgi-bin/sis/htmlgen?LACT

NIDA report: Cocaine-NIDA report: http://www.drugabuse.gov/sites/default/files/rrcocaine.pdf

NIDA-linked training program: http://www.sbirttraining.com/sbirtcore

Patient information on alcohol and pregnancy, English and Spanish text available: English: http://www.niaaa.nih.gov/publications; Spanish: http://www.niaaa.nih.gov/publications/publicaciones-en-espanol

Reducing alcohol-exposed pregnancies: http://www.cdc.gov/ncbddd/fasd/documents/redalcohpreg.pdf

Resources for women and their families

Information and resources on quitting smoking targeted at women: http://women.smokefree.gov/Default.aspx

Web site dedicated to helping smokers quit: http://www.smokefree.gov/

Web site from the NOFAS provides information and resources on FASDs and the risk of drinking alcohol during pregnancy: http://www.nofas.org/

References

Academy of Breastfeeding Medicine (ABM). (2009). ABM Clinical Protocol #21: Guidelines for breastfeeding and the drug-dependent woman. *Breastfeeding Medicine*, 4(4), 225–228.

Alto, W. A., & O'Connor, A. B. (2011). Management of women treated with buprenorphine during pregnancy. *American Journal of Obstetrics and Gynecology, 205*(4), 302–308.

American Academy of Pediatrics (AAP). (1998, June). *Neonatal Drug Withdrawal.* Retrieved from http://aappolicy.aappublications.org/cgi/reprint/pediatrics;101/6/1079.pdf

American Academy of Pediatrics. (2001). The transfer of drugs and other chemicals into human milk. *Pediatrics, 108*(3), 776–789.

American Academy of Pediatrics. (2005). Breastfeeding and the use of human milk. *Pediatrics, 115*(2), 496–506.

American Academy of Pediatrics. (2009). *Hepatitis C.* Retrieved from http://aapredbook.aappublications.org

American Academy of Pediatrics. (2011). SIDS and other sleep-related infant deaths: Expansion of recommendations for a safe infant sleeping environment (policy statement). *Pediatrics, 128*(5), 1030–1039.

American College of Nurse-Midwives (ACNM). (2004). *Position statement: Addiction in pregnancy.*

American College of Obstetricians and Gynecologists (ACOG). (2008). At-risk drinking and illicit drug use: Ethical issues in obstetric and gynecologic practice. ACOG Committee Opinion No. 422. *Obstetrics & Gynecology, 112*, 1449–1460.

American College of Obstetricians and Gynecologists (ACOG). (2010). Smoking cessation during pregnancy. Committee Opinion No. 471. *Obstetrics & Gynecology, 116*, 1241–1244.

American College of Obstetricians and Gynecologists (ACOG). (2011a). American Congress of Obstetricians and Gynecologists Committee Opinion No. 496. *At-risk drinking and alcohol dependence: Obstetric and gynecologic implications.* Retrieved from http://www.acog.org/~/media/Committee%20Opinions/Committee%20on%20Health%20Care%20for%20Underserved%20Women/co496.ashx?dmc=1&ts=20111220T0654563639

American College of Obstetricians and Gynecologists (ACOG). (2011b). American Congress of Obstetricians and Gynecologists Committee Opinion No. 497. *Methamphetamine abuse in women of reproductive age.* Retrieved from http://www.acog.org/~/media/Committee%20Opinions/Committee%20on%20Health%20Care%20for%20Underserved%20Women/co479.ashx?dmc=1&ts=20111212T0858208959

American Society of Addiction Medicine. (1998). *Public policy statement on nicotine addiction and tobacco.* Retrieved from http://www.dshs.wa.gov/pdf/dbhr/ASAM%20Position%20Paper%20on%20Nicotine%20Addiction.pdf

American Society of Addiction Medicine (ASAM). (2011a). *Definition of addiction.* Retrieved from http://www.asam.org/for-the-public/definition-of-addiction

American Society of Addiction Medicine (ASAM). (2011b). Public policy statement on women, alcohol and other drugs, and pregnancy. Retrieved from http://www.asam.org/advocacy/find-a-policy-statement/view-policy-statement/public-policy-statements/2011/12/15/women-alcohol-and-other-drugs-and-pregnancy

Anderka, M., Romitti, P. A., Sun, L., Druschel, C., Carmichael, S., & Shaw, G. (2010). Patterns of tobacco exposure before and during pregnancy. *Acta Obstetricia et Gynecologica Scandinavica, 89*(4), 505–514.

Astley, S. J., & Little, R. E. (1990). Maternal marijuana use during lactation and infant development at one year. *Neurotoxicology and Teratology, 12*, 161–168.

Binder, T., & Vavrinková, B. (2008). Prospective randomized comparative study of the effect of buprenorphine, methadone and heroin on the course of pregnancy, birth weight of newborns, early postpartum adaption and course of the neonatal abstinence syndrome

(NAS) in women followed up in the outpatient department. *Neuroendocrinology Letters, 29*, 80–86.

Bolnick, J. M., & Rayburn, W. F. (2003). Substance use disorders in women: Special considerations during pregnancy. *Obstetrics and Gynecology Clinics of North America, 30*, 545–558.

Boyd, S., & Marcellus, L. (2007). *With child: Substance use during pregnancy: A woman-centred approach.* Nova Scotia: Fernwood.

Brady, T. M., & Ashley, O. S. (Eds.). (2005). *Women in substance abuse treatment: Results from the Alcohol and Drug Services Study (ADSS) (DHHS Publication No. SMA 04-3968, Analytic Series A-26).* Rockville, MD: Substance Abuse and Mental Health Services Administration, Office of Applied Studies.

Briggs, G. G., Freeman, R. K., & Yaffe, S. J. (2011). *Drugs in pregnancy and lactation.* Philadelphia: Lippincott, Williams & Wilkins.

Burns, E., Gray, R., & Smith, L. (2010). Brief screening questionnaires to identify problem drinking during pregnancy: A systematic review. *Addiction (Abingdon, England), 105*, 601–614.

Centers for Disease Control and Prevention (CDC). (2012). Alcohol and public health. Retrieved from http://www.cdc.gov/alcohol/factsheets/binge-drinking.htm

Chang, G., Orav, E., Jones, J., Buynitsky, T., Gonzalez, S., & Wilkins-Haug, L. (2011). Self reported alcohol and drug use in pregnant young women. *Journal of Addiction Medicine, 5*(3), 221–226.

Chang, G., Wilkins-Haug, L., Berman, S., & Goetz, M. (1999). A brief intervention for alcohol use in pregnancy: A randomized trial. *Addiction, 94*, 1499–1508.

Chasnoff, I., McGourty, R., Bailey, G., Hutchins, E., Lightfoot, S., & Pawson, L. (2005). The 4Ps Plus Screen for substance use in pregnancy. *Journal of Perinatology, 25*, 368–374.

Chasnoff, I., Wells, A., McGourty, R., & Bailey, L. (2007). Validation of the 4Ps Plus screen for substance use in pregnancy. *Journal of Perinatology, 27*, 744–748.

Chasnoff, I. J., Lewis, D. E., & Squires, L. (1987). Cocaine intoxication in a breast-fed infant. *Pediatrics, 80*, 836–838.

Choo, R. E., Huestis, M. A., Schroeder, J. R., Shin, A. S., & Jones, H. E. (2004). Neonatal abstinence syndrome in methadone-exposed infants is altered by level of prenatal tobacco exposure. *Drug and Alcohol Dependence, 75*, 253–260.

Derauf, C., LaGasse, L. L., Smith, L. M., Grant, P., Shah, R., Arria, A., . . . Lester, B. M. (2007). Demographic and psychosocial characteristics of mothers using methamphetamine during pregnancy. *The American Journal of Drug and Alcohol Abuse, 3*.

Fiore, M. C., Jaen, C. R., Baker, T. B., Bailey, W. C., Benowitz, N., & Curry, S. J. (2008). Treating tobacco use and dependence: 2008 update US Public Health Service Clinical Practice Guideline executive summary. *Respiratory Care, 53*(9), 1217–1222.

Fischer, G., Ortner, R., Rohrmeister, K., Jagsch, R., Baewert, A., Langer, M., & Aschauer, H. (2006). Methadone versus buprenorphine in pregnant addicts: A double-blind, double-dummy comparison study. *Addiction (Abingdon, England), 101*, 275–281.

Flavin, J. (2002). A glass half full? Harm reduction among pregnant women who use cocaine. *Journal of Drug Issues, 32*(3), 973–998. doi:10.1177/002204260203200315

Garry, A., Rigourd, V., Amirouche, A., Faurous, V., Aubry, S., & Serreau, R. (2009). Cannabis and breastfeeding. *Journal of Toxicology.*

Gavin, D., Ross, H., & Skinner, H. (1989). Diagnostic validity of the drug abuse screening test in the assessment of DSM-III drug disorders. *British Journal of Addiction, 84*, 301–307.

Goler, N., Armstrong, M., Caughey, A., Haimowits, M., Hung, Y., & Osejo, V. (2012). Early Start, a cost-beneficial perinatal substance abuse program. *Obstetrics and Gynecology, 19*(1), 102–110.

Goler, N., Armstrong, M., Taillac, C., & Osejo, V. (2008). Substance abuse treatment linked with prenatal visits improves perinatal outcomes: A new standard. *Journal of Perinatology, 28*, 597–603.

Grimm, D., Pauly, E., Poschl, J., Linderkamp, O., & Skopp, G. (2005). Buprenorphine and norbuprenorphine concentrations in human breast milk samples determined by liquid chromatography-tandem mass spectrometry. *Therapeutic Drug Monitoring, 27*, 526–530.

Hackshaw, A., Rodeck, C., & Boniface, S. (2011). Maternal smoking in pregnancy and birth defects: A systematic review based on 173 687 malformed cases and 11.7 million controls. *Human Reproduction Update, 17*(5), 589.

Hale, T. (2010). *Medications and mothers' milk.* Amarillo, Texas: Hale Publishing.

Hankin, J., & Sokol, R. J. (1995). Identification and care of problems associated with alcohol ingestion in pregnancy. *Seminars in Perinatology, 19*, 286–292.

Hans, S. L. (1999). Chapter 3: Parenting and parent-child relationships in families affected by substance abuse. In H. E. Fitzgerald, B. M. Lester, & B. S. Zuckerman (Eds.), *Children of addiction: Research, health and public policy issues.* New York: RoutledgeFalmer.

Harrison, P., & Sidebottom, A. (2009). Alcohol and drug use before and during pregnancy: An examination of use patterns and predictors of cessation. *Maternal and Child Health Journal, 13*, 386–394.

Helmbrecht, G. D. & Thiagarajah, S. (2008). Management of addiction disorders in pregnancy. *Journal of Addiction Medicine, 2*(1), 1–16.

Horrigan, T., Schroeder, A., & Schaffer, R. (2000). The triad of substance abuse, violence and depression are interrelated in pregnancy. *Journal of Substance Abuse Treatment, 18*, 55–58.

Humeniuk, R., Ali, R., Babor, T. F., Farrell, M., Formigoni, M. L., Jittiwutikarn, J., . . . Simon, S. (2008). *Validation of the alcohol, smoking and substance involvement screening test (ASSIST).* Geneva, Switzerland: World Health Organization.

Isemann, B., Meinzen-Derr, J., & Akinbi, H. (2011). Maternal and neonatal factors impacting response to methadone therapy in infants treated for neonatal abstinence syndrome. *Journal of Perinatology, 31*, 25–29.

Jansson, L., DiPietro, J., & Elko, A. (2005). Fetal response to maternal methadone administration. *American Journal of Obstetrics and Gynecology, 193*, 611–617.

Jansson, L., Velez, M., & Harrow, C. (2009). The opioid-exposed newborn: Assessment and pharmacological management. *Journal of Opioid Management, 5*(1), 47–55.

Jansson, L. M., Velez, M., & Harrow, C. (2004). Methadone maintenance and lactation: A review of the literature and current management guidelines. *Journal of Human Lactation, 20*(1), 62–70.

Jessup, M., & Brindis, C. (2005). Issues in reproductive health and empowerment in perinatal women with substance use disorders. *Journal of Addictions Nursing, 16*, 97–105.

Johnson, R., Jones, H., & Fischer, G. (2003). Use of buprenorphine in pregnancy: Patient management and effects on the neonate. *Drug and Alcohol Dependence, 70*, S87–S101.

Johnson, R. E., Jones, H. E., Jasinski, D. R., Svikis, D. S., Haug, N. A., Jansson, L. M., . . . Lester, B. M. (2001). Buprenorphine treatment of pregnant opioid-dependent women: Maternal and neonatal outcomes. *Drug and Alcohol Dependence, 63*, 97–103.

Johnson, R. E., Strain, E. C., & Amass, L. (2003). Buprenorphine: How to use it right. *Drug and Alcohol Dependence, 70*, S59–S77.

Johnston, A., Mandell, T. W., & Meyer, M. (2010). *Treatment of opioid dependence in pregnancy: Vermont guidelines.* Retrieved from https://www.med.uvm.edu/VCHIP/downloads/VCHIP_1%20 NEONATAL_GUIDELINES_FINAL.pdf

Jones, H. E., Johnson, R. E., Jasinski, D. R., O'Grady, K. E., Chisholm, C. A., Choo, R. E., . . . Milio, L. (2005). Buprenorphine versus methadone in the treatment of pregnant opioid-dependent patients: Effects on the neonatal abstinence syndrome. *Drug and Alcohol Dependence, 79*, 1–10.

Jones, H. E., Kaltenbach, K., Heil, S.H., Stine, S. M., Coyle, M.G., Arria, A. M., . . . Fischer, G. (2010). Neonatal abstinence syndrome after methadone or buprenorphine exposure. *The New England Journal of Medicine, 363*, 2320–2331.

Kahila, H., Saisto, T., Kivitie-Kallio, S., Haukkamaa, M., & Halmesmaki, E. (2007). A prospective study on buprenorphine use in pregnancy: Effects on maternal and neonatal outcome. *Acta Obstetricia et Gynecologica Scandinavica, 86*, 185–190.

Kakko, J., Heilig, M., & Sarman, I. (2008). Buprenorphine and methadone treatment of opiate dependence during pregnancy: Comparison of fetal growth and neonatal outcomes in two consecutive case series. *Drug and Alcohol Dependence, 96*, 69–78.

Kaltenbach, K., Berghella, V., & Finnegan, L. (1998). Opioid dependence during pregnancy. *Obstetrics and Gynecology Clinics of North America, 25*, 139–151.

Kearney, M. (1998). Truthful self-nurturing: A grounded formal theory of women's addiction recovery. *Qualitative Health Research, 8*(4), 495–512.

Law, K. L., Stroud, L. R., LaGasse, L. L., Niaura, R., Liu, J., & Lester, B. M. (2003). Smoking during pregnancy and newborn neurobehavior. *Pediatrics, 111*(6), 1318–1323.

Lindemalm, S., Nydert, P., Svensson, J.-O., Stahle, L., & Sarman, I. (2009). Transfer of buprenorphine into breast milk and calculation of infant drug dose. *Journal of Human Lactation, 25*, 199–205.

MacGregor, S. N., Keith, L. G., Chasnoff, I. J., Rosner, M. A., Chisum, G. M., Shaw, P., & Minogue, J. P. (1987). Cocaine use during pregnancy: Adverse perinatal outcome. *American Journal of Obstetrics and Gynecology, 157*(3), 686–690.

Malpas, T. J., & Darlow, B. A. (1999). Neonatal abstinence syndrome following abrupt cessation of breastfeeding. *The New Zealand Medical Journal, 112*, 12–13.

McCarthy, J., & Posey, B. (2000). Methadone levels in human milk. *Journal of Human Lactation, 16*, 115–120.

Mengel, M., Searight, R., & Cook, K. (2006). Preventing Alcohol-exposed pregnancies. *Journal of the American Board of Family Medicine, 19*, 494–505.

Merikangas, K. R., Mehta, R. L., Molnar, B. E., Walters, E. E., Swendsen, J. D., Aguilar-Gaziola, S., . . . Vega, W. A. (1998). Comorbidity of substance use disorders with mood and anxiety disorders: Results of the international consortium in psychiatric epidemiology. *Addictive Behaviors, 23*(6), 893–907. doi.org/10.1016/S0306-4603(98)00076-8

Moylan, P. L., Jones, H. E., Haug, N. A., Kissim, W. B., & Svikis, D. S. (2001). Clinical and psychosocial characteristics of substance-dependent pregnant women with and without PTSD. *Addictive Behaviors, 26*(3), 469–474.

Muhuri, P., & Gfroerer, J. (2009). Substance use among women: Association with pregnancy, parenting and race/ethnicity. *Maternal and Child Health Journal, 13*(3), 376–385. doi:10.1007/s10995-008-0375-8

National Abandoned Infants Assistance Resource Center. (2006, September). *Substance exposed infants: Noteworthy policies and practices.* Retrieved from http://aia.berkeley.edu/information_resources/substance_exposed_newborns.php

National Institute for Drug Addiction (NIDA). (2009). Substance use among women during pregnancy and following childbirth. National Survey on Drug Use and Health, NSDUH report. Rockville, MD:

Office of Applied Studies, Substance Abuse and Mental Health Services Administration (SAMHSA).

National Institute for Drug Addiction (NIDA). (2011). Cocaine. Retrieved from http://www.drugabuse.gov/drugs-abuse/cocaine

National Institute for Drug Addiction (NIDA). (2012). Methamphetamine. Retrieved from http://www.drugabuse.gov/drugs-abuse/methamphetamine

National Institutes of Health. (2012). Varenicline Pregnancy Cohort Study. Retrieved from http://clinicaltrials.gov/ct2/show/NCT01290445

National Library of Medicine. (2011a). *Clonazepam.* Retrieved from http://www.nlm.nih.gov/medlineplus/druginfo/meds/a682279.html

National Library of Medicine. (2011b). *Alcohol.* Retrieved from http://www.nlm.nih.gov/medlineplus/alcohol.html

National Library of Medicine. (2011c). *Bupropion.* Retrieved from http://www.nlm.nih.gov/medlineplus/druginfo/meds/a695033.html

National Task Force on Fetal Alcohol Syndrome and Fetal Alcohol Effects. (2009). Preventing Alcohol-exposed pregnancies. U.S. Department of Health and Human Services, Washington, DC.

O'Connor, A., Alto, W., Musgrave, K., Gibbons, D., Llanto, L., Holden, S., & Karnes, J. (2011). Observational study of buprenorphine treatment of opioid-dependent pregnant women in a family medicine residency: Reports on maternal and infant outcomes. *Journal of the American Board of Family Medicine, 24,* 194–201.

O'Connor, A., Monroe, R., & Alto, W. (2012). *Concurrent in utero exposure to antidepressants and buprenorphine delays the resolution of neonatal abstinence syndrome in infants born to opioid dependent pregnant women.* Unpublished manuscript.

O'Connor, A. B. (2011). Nurse practitioners' inability to prescribe buprenorphine: Limitations of the Drug Addiction Treatment Act of 2000. *Journal of the American Academy of Nurse Practitioners, 23*(10), 542–545.

Oei, J., Abdel-Latif, M., Clark, R., Craig, F., & Lui, K. (2010). Short-term outcomes of mothers and infants exposed to methamphetamine. *Archives of Disease in Childhood. Fetal and Neonatal Edition, 95*(1), 36–41.

Oei, J., & Lui, K. (2007). Management of the newborn affected by maternal opiates and other drugs of dependency. *Journal of Paediatrics and Child Health, 43,* 9–18.

Pizarro, D., Habli, M., Grier, M., Bombrys, A., Sibai, B., & Livingston, J. (2011). Higher maternal doses of methadone does not increase neonatal abstinence syndrome. *Journal of Substance Abuse Treatment, 40*(3), 295–298.

Rastegar, D. A., & Fingerhood, M. I. (2005). *Addiction medicine: An evidence-based handbook.* Philadelphia: Lippincott Williams & Wilkins.

Russell, M., Martier, S. S., Sokol, R. J., Mudar, P., Jacobson, S., & Jacobson, J. (1996). Detecting risk drinking during pregnancy: A comparison of four screening questionnaires. *American Journal of Public Health, 86*(10), 1435–1439. doi:10.2105/AJPH.86.10.1435

Sarkar, M., Djulus, J., & Koren, G. (2005). When a cocaine-using mother wishes to breastfeed: Proposed guidelines. *Therapeutic Drug Monitoring, 27,* 1–2.

Seligman, N. S., Almario, C. V., Hayes, E. J., Dysart, K. C., Berghella, V., & Baxter, J. K. (2010). Relationship between maternal methadone dose at delivery and neonatal abstinence syndrome. *The Journal of Pediatrics, 157*(3), 428–433.

Shannon, M., King, T., & Kennedy, H. (2006). Allostasis: A theoretical framework for understanding and evaluating perinatal outcomes.

Journal of Obstetric, Gynecologic, and Neonatal Nursing, 36(2), 125–134.

Tennes, K., Avitable, N., Blackard, C., Boyles, C., Hassoun, B., Holmes, L., & Kreye, M. (1985). Marijuana: Prenatal and postnatal exposure in the human. *NIDA Research Monograph, 59,* 48–60.

Thajam, D., Atkinson, D. E., Sibley, C. P., & Lavender, T. (2010). Is neonatal abstinence syndrome related to the amount of opiate used? *Journal of Obstetric, Gynecologic, and Neonatal Nursing, 39*(5), 503–509.

U.S. Center for Substance Abuse Treatment. (2004). *Clinical guidelines for the use of buprenorphine in the treatment of opioid addiction.* Treatment Improvement Protocol (TIP) Series 40. DHHS Publication No. (SMA) 04-3939. Rockville, MD: Substance Abuse and Mental Health Services Administration.

U.S. Centers for Disease Control and Prevention (CDC). (2008). *Treating Tobacco Use and Dependence (2008 Update): Clinical practice guideline.* Retrieved from http://books.google.com/books?hl=en&lr=&id=dUI4JJzIsikC&oi=fnd&pg=PR1&dq=treating+tobacco+use+and+dependence+clinical+practice+guideline&ots=Tpxzaa4tM5&sig=bT6bXDL0Xzqi0GItj1DRfkRUyM0#v=onepage&q&f=false

U.S. Centers for Disease Control and Prevention (CDC). (2009). *Trends in smoking before, during, and after pregnancy—Pregnancy risk assessment monitoring system (PRAMS), United States, 31 Sites, 2000–2005.* Retrieved from http://www.cdc.gov/mmwr/preview/mmwrhtml/ss5804a1.htm

U.S. Centers for Disease Control and Prevention. (2010). *Alcohol use in pregnancy.* Retrieved from http://www.cdc.gov/ncbddd/fasd/alcohol-use.html

U.S. Department of Health and Human Services (DHHS). (2009). *Alcohol use among pregnant and nonpregnant women of childbearing age—United States, 1991–2005.* Retrieved from http://www.cdc.gov/mmwr/preview/mmwrhtml/mm5819a4.htm?s_cid=mm5819a4_e

U.S. Department of Health and Human Services (DHHS). (2010). *Results from the 2010 national survey on drug use and health: Summary of national findings.* Retrieved from http://www.samhsa.gov/data/NSDUH/2k10NSDUH/2k10Results.pdf

U.S. Department of Health and Human Services (DHHS). (2011). *Clinical guidelines for the use of buprenorphine in the treatment of opioid addiction.* Retrieved from http://buprenorphine.samhsa.gov/Bup_Guidelines.pdf

U.S. Substance Abuse and Mental Health Services Administration (SAMHSA), Center for Behavioral Health Statistics and Quality. (May 12, 2011). *Trends in emergency department visits for drug-related suicide attempts among females: 2005 and 2009.* Rockville, MD.

van Gelder, M. M., Reefhuis, J., Caton, A. R., Werler, M. M., Druschel, C. M., & Roeleveld, N. (2010). Characteristics of pregnant illicit drug users and associations between cannabis use and perinatal outcome in a population-based study. *Drug and Alcohol Dependence, 109*(1), 243–247.

Velez, M. L., Montoya, I. D., Jansson, L. M., Walters, V., Svikis, D., Jones, H. E., . . . Campbell, J. (2006). Exposure to violence among substance-dependent pregnant women and their children. *Journal of Substance Abuse Treatment, 30,* 31–38.

Walsh, S. L., & Eissenberg, T. (2003). The clinical pharmacology of buprenorphine: Extrapolating from the laboratory to the clinic. *Drug and Alcohol Dependence, 70*(2), S13–S27.

Wehby, G. L., Prater, K., McCarthy, A. M., Castilla, E. E., & Murray, J. C. (2011). The impact of maternal smoking during pregnancy on early child neurodevelopment. *Journal of Human Capital, 5*(2), 207. doi:10.1086/660885

Weiner, S. M., & Finnegan, L. P. (2011). Drug withdrawal in the neonate. In S. L. Gardner, B. S. Carter, M. Enzman-Hines, & J. A. Hernandez (Eds.), *Handbook of neonatal Intensive care* (7th ed., pp. 201–222). St. Louis, MO: Mosby.

Winecker, R. E., Goldberger, B. A., Tebbett, I. R., Behnke, M., Eyler, F. D., Karlix, J. L., . . . Bertholf, R. L. (2001). Detection of cocaine and its metabolites in breast milk. *Journal of Forensic Sciences, 46*(5), 1221–1223.

Winklbaur, B., Kopf, N., Ebner, N., Jung, E., Thau, K., & Fischer, G. (2008). Treating pregnant women dependent on opioids is not the same as treating pregnancy and opioid dependence: A knowledge synthesis for better treatment for women and neonates. *Addiction (Abingdon, England), 103*, 1429–1440.

Wolff, K. (2011). Panic in the ER: Maternal drug use, the right to bodily integrity, privacy, and informed consent. *Politics and Policy, 39*(5), 679–714.

Yonkers, K., Gotman, N., Kershaw, T., Forray, A., Howell, H., & Rounsaville, B. (2010). Screening for prenatal substance use: Development of the Substance Use Risk Profile-Pregnancy Scale. *Obstetrics and Gynecology, 116*(4), 827–833.

14

Social issues in pregnancy

Nena R. Harris

Relevant terms

Food insecurity—uncertainty about the availability of adequate and safe nutrition

Health disparity—differences in the incidence, prevalence, and burden of disease that exist between a subgroup and the larger population

Intimate partner violence—the action of causing bodily harm or injury by hitting, kicking, slapping, biting, punching, stabbing, raping, or any other use of force, and/or repetitive emotional harm

Near-poverty—characterizes having an annual income between 100% and 200% of the federal poverty threshold, which is based on family size and composition

Poverty—the circumstance of having an annual income less than the federal poverty thresholds, which are based on family size and composition

---

Introduction

Of the many variables that impact pregnancy-related maternal and infant outcomes, social issues are perhaps the most multifaceted and complex. Social issues present challenges that are unlikely to be solved through a one-on-one conversation with a patient in an office setting. Comprehensive, multilevel assessment and intervention that involves a team of professional personnel is usually necessary. This, in turn, increases the investment of time and resources, creating a true burden for the already-busy provider. In this chapter, issues related to poverty, homelessness, abuse, and incarceration will be explored.

Issues such as these contribute to significant health disparities in maternal and infant morbidity and mortality that persist in the United States despite increases in health-care spending and programs to improve access to prenatal care for vulnerable populations (Adams, Gavin, & Benedict, 2005). The impact on a pregnant woman, her family, and her unborn baby should be a concern for all health-care providers with patients experiencing any of these issues.

When thinking about health disparities in the clinical setting, it is important to recognize that many of the contributing factors have no easy, quick solution. In fact, many of them are deep-seated societal and historical factors that are likely impossible for the health-care provider to completely resolve in his or her brief interactions with the patient. So why is there a need to understand them? Health disparities, defined as differences in the incidence, prevalence, or burden of disease in a subgroup when compared to a larger population, are rooted in inequities in access to health care, education, income, and sanitary and safe living and work environments (Carter-Pokras & Baquet, 2002); minority women are more likely to be at a disadvantage in each of these areas of inequity (Adams et al., 2005; Murray-García, 1999; Walker, Mays, & Warren, 2004). It is necessary for health-care providers to understand the life issues that may affect the course of the pregnancy and present risks to the woman and her unborn baby. While resolving all of the factors that might contribute to a woman's risk for poor outcomes will likely not be possible for an individual health-care provider, a team-based approach to assisting the woman to access available resources is a beginning step in optimizing her and her child's health

Prenatal and Postnatal Care: A Woman-Centered Approach, First Edition. Edited by Robin G. Jordan, Janet L. Engstrom, Julie A. Marfell, and Cindy L. Farley.

and in decreasing the nation's health disparities. Having a basic understanding of the issues being faced, knowing what resources are needed, and assisting women to access those resources are key first steps to providing quality, compassionate care for women facing various social issues during pregnancy.

Poverty

Poverty during pregnancy can present challenges that affect the health of the woman and her unborn baby and place them at risk for poor outcomes. Low-income women are likely to experience more stressors and hardship around the time of pregnancy than those with higher incomes; these life stressors can include job loss, homelessness, domestic violence, relationship dissolution, and incarceration (Braveman et al., 2010). Women living in poverty are more likely to have an unplanned pregnancy (Finer & Henshaw, 2006), which impacts their ability and readiness to make the lifestyle adjustments necessary to prepare for a healthy pregnancy, birth, and postpartum experience. Poverty has been noted as a risk factor in preterm birth and low birth weight (Nkansah-Amankra, Dhawain, Hussey, & Luchok, 2010; Weck, Paulose, & Flaws, 2008). Furthermore, children who are born into impoverished environments are exposed to a variety of related stressors and have an increased risk for poor behavioral, emotional, and physical outcomes including malnutrition, chronic disease, developmental delays, and low school performance (Evans & English, 2002).

While poverty likely does not directly lead to poor outcomes for pregnant women, the conditions resulting from poverty create hardships that affect health outcomes. First, a lack of financial resources characteristic of poverty impacts the woman's ability to obtain adequate nutrition, which is a significant factor in maintaining a healthy pregnancy and baby (Cox & Phelan, 2008; Harnisch, Harnisch, & Harnisch, 2012; Kaiser & Allen, 2002). Food insecurity, or concerns about one's ability to obtain adequate and safe nutrition, can lead to women being either underweight or overweight (Sarlio-Lähteenkorva & Lahelma, 2001; Townsend, Peerson, Love, Achterberg, & Murphy, 2001). Inadequate nutrition can be characterized by insufficient intake of calories as well as the presence of deficiencies of vitamins and minerals in spite of adequate caloric intake. The latter often occurs when women purchase foods that are less expensive but have low nutritional value (Sarlio-Lähteenkorva & Lahelma, 2001). These foods often contain high amounts of saturated fats, sodium, and calories but contain very little in the way of vitamins and minerals. Alternatively,

women may experience cycles of food unavailability followed by availability, during which times they overeat or indulge in energy-dense foods (Townsend et al., 2001). Women with this type of eating pattern may be overweight, whereas women with a chronically insufficient caloric intake will likely be underweight or lose weight during pregnancy if the demands of the pregnancy outweigh intake. In both cases, the woman and baby are not provided the nutrients and calories needed for optimal health. Pregnant women should be directed to their local office of Women, Infants, and Children (WIC). The WIC program is federally funded and located in each state. Eligibility requirements are determined based on categorical, residential, financial, and nutritional risks. Women are categorically eligible during pregnancy and up to 6 weeks after birth or at the end of pregnancy. Infants up to 1 year and children up to 5 years of age are also categorically eligible. Residential requirements are that the woman, infant, or child live in the state through which the benefit is administered. There is no requirement for the length of residency. Local offices may be assigned to the individuals for services. Financial eligibility is determined by each state but must be 100% of federal poverty requirements but no more than 185% of the requirements. Nutritional risk is determined either by the WIC office or by a health-care provider. A preapplication assessment is available online to determine eligibility and lists the documentation needed for the appointment as well as the address of the local WIC office (U.S. Department of Agriculture, 2012).

Understanding the health-care implications of poor housing, safe and sanitary housing has long been a goal of public health advocates (Winslow, 1937). Access to safe and comfortable shelter is significantly influenced by poverty, and women living in poverty often have limited options for housing. Increased odds of preterm birth and low birth weight have been identified in women living in low-income neighborhoods (Nkansah-Amankra et al., 2010). Furthermore, housing that is crowded, unsanitary, with poor lighting and aeration, surrounded by violence and drug use, or infested with insects and/ or rodents creates unsafe and stressful conditions that expose the woman and her baby to physical, environmental, and psychological threats to health (Chaudhuri, 2004; Raugh, Landrigan, & Claudio, 2008; Shaw, 2004; Winslow, 1937). In pregnancy, psychological distress caused by stressful living conditions can lead to biophysical changes such as increased cortisol levels that impact fetal intrauterine growth and development (LeWinn et al., 2009; Obel et al., 2005).

Poverty plays a key role in the homelessness of families and individuals since the majority of homeless persons cite the inability to afford housing and/or unemployment as the reasons behind their homelessness (National Alliance to End Homelessness, 2012). Rates of poverty have increased in recent years due to the economic recession, and the national homelessness rate continues to be a national crisis.

The health-care needs of homeless pregnant women can be varied and complex. Homeless women are more likely to have poorly managed chronic illness, communicable diseases, mental illness, and substance abuse (Beal & Redlener, 1995; Little et al., 2005). Unstable housing can result in delays or disruptions in health care for conditions that are easily prevented or managed; concerns about shelter, food, and safety take priority over health-care needs (Broussard, 2010). These concerns, along with barriers such as lack of transportation or childcare for other children, interfere with a woman's ability to obtain consistent prenatal care (Beal & Redlener, 1995; Bloom et al., 2004; Braveman, Marchi, Egerter, Pearl, & Neuhaus, 2000; Richards, Merrill, & Baksh, 2011). These problems are only exacerbated for the pregnant woman since the demands of the growing baby place additional stressors on the mother's body. Consequently, homeless pregnant women are at an increased risk for preterm birth (Beal & Redlener, 1995; Little et al., 2005; Richards et al., 2011). An assessment of a woman's living arrangements should always be conducted during care since many homeless women might be hesitant to disclose their homelessness. Some homeless women have been reported to child protective services and have had their children taken away because of their homelessness (Smid, Bourgois, & Auerswald, 2010). A punitive process such as this should be avoided; rather, women should be assisted in obtaining safe and sanitary living arrangements. Building a trusting and compassionate relationship during prenatal care will increase the likelihood that women will continue their care in an attempt to enhance health outcomes. Although many of these resources will be accessed through the local state's social services departments, the health-care provider can become familiar with the process of obtaining available resources in order to educate women of their options.

Families in poverty are more likely to be headed by single mothers and are more vulnerable to experiencing homelessness. In 2010, 32% of single-mother families in the United States were living in poverty compared to only 6% of two-parent families (DeNavas-Walt, Proctor, & Smith, 2011). Single mothers who are also homeless experience compounded stress at a level higher than dealing with either of the two conditions alone, creating significant concerns for her health and the health of her baby; depression, lack of social support, compromised health, unintended pregnancy, unemployment or underemployment, low parenting satisfaction, and punitive parenting practices are common in single mothers (Broussard, 2010; Crosier, Butterworth, & Rodgers, 2007; Eamon & Wu, 2011; Finer & Henshaw, 2006; Wu & Eamon, 2011; Zhan, 2006). Lack of paternal involvement during pregnancy and birth has been implicated in preterm birth, low birth weight, and small-for-gestational-age (SGA) infants (Alio, Kornosky, Mbah, Marty, & Salihu, 2009).

While financial security does not address all of the challenges that single mothers face, it goes a long way in relieving some of the burden of providing for a family. Single mothers are often forced to rely on government programs for financial assistance. Health-care providers can assist patients experiencing or facing single motherhood to access community and government financial resources. Assisting the woman in obtaining child support from the father of the baby is another possible intervention that might alleviate some of the financial hardships she faces and decrease her need for government assistance (Huang & Han, 2011). The Office of Child Support Enforcement, a division of the U.S. Department of Health and Human Services, exists to assist custodial parents in establishing paternity in cases of uncertainty or contest, determining the amount of support that is owed, and acquiring the support from the noncustodial parent. Women should be directed to their state Child Support Enforcement Office for information on the specific procedure and documentation required to initiate a case in that state. Links to information on collecting child support and contact information to state Child Support Enforcement Offices are located in the "Resources for Women and Their Families" section.

Interdisciplinary care

Pregnant women who are living in poverty will need referrals to a variety of social services to best serve their needs. Coverage for pregnancy care is a priority, so assistance to access Medicaid for Pregnant Women (MPW) for women without health insurance is an ideal starting point. An interdisciplinary approach that includes medical and social as well as legal services will provide the most comprehensive overview of available options. Since the breadth of many services is determined by income levels, it might be helpful for health-care providers to help women locate where they fall in respect to federal poverty thresholds. A basic understanding of how her income will be defined by agencies offering medical, social, and legal assistance might help her to anticipate a decision about her eligibility.

Poverty thresholds by family size and number of adults at home		
Family unit size (includes unborn baby)	One adult	Two adults
2	$15,504	$15,063
3	$18,123	$18,106
4	$22,891	$22,811
5	$26,434	$26,844
6	$29,494	$30,056
7	$32,340	$33,665
8	$36,697	$37,011

Source: U.S. Census Bureau (2012).

Incarceration

Estimates of the number of incarcerated women who are pregnant range from 6% to 10% (Clarke et al., 2006; Harrison & Beck, 2004). Substance abuse is a significant factor for the incarceration of women; other reasons for incarceration include prostitution, theft, and possession of drug paraphernalia (Harrison & Beck, 2004; James, 2004). In many cases, a woman's drug abuse and drug-related activities are precipitated by her relationship with a male partner who is also involved in drugs. Incarcerated women experience disease and mental illness at higher rates than women in the general population (Blitz, Wolff, Pan, & Pogorzelski, 2005; Gunter, 2004; Magee, Hult, Turalba, & McMillan, 2005; Nijhawan, Salloway, Nunn, Poshkus, & Clarke, 2010; Sterk, Theall, & Elifson, 2005). Health-care providers working in jail or prisons provide a vital service to this vulnerable population with complex health-care needs.

Women who have been incarcerated have an increased likelihood of having a history of substance abuse, exposure to sexually transmitted infections (Clarke et al., 2006), and being a victim of intimate partner violence (IPV) (Knudsen et al., 2008; Zust, 2009). Women who have been incarcerated at any point in their pregnancy are also at risk for exposure to communicable diseases that are prevalent in places with close living arrangements, such as influenza and tuberculosis. For these women, prenatal care can be the avenue by which they receive comprehensive assessment and access treatment and interventions. Prenatal care will enable women to receive adequate screening, treatment, education, and referrals for problems that might otherwise go unattended (Dooley & Ringler, 2012). However, prenatal care is likely to be initiated later in the pregnancy with

inconsistent subsequent care; for women at risk for incarceration, their pregnancies likely occurred in the midst of chaotic life circumstances and attention to the pregnancy is not an urgent need compared to all of the other hardships that require immediate attention. Managing stressful life circumstances often presents barriers to obtaining the prenatal care and the benefits that it would offer for this high-risk population. Women with drug-related incarcerations are unlikely to be eligible for federal programs such as Medicaid for Pregnant Women, WIC, or housing assistance, which exacerbates the financial barriers that might interfere with timely and consistent prenatal care.

Substance abuse issues that lead to incarceration for many pregnant women negatively impact fetal and maternal health (see Chapter 13, "Substance Use during Pregnancy"). For women who are using drugs during their pregnancy, the fear of detection and punishment and an altered appreciation of the importance of prenatal care may play a role in a woman's lack of timely and sufficient prenatal care. This prevents possible entry into drug rehabilitation to minimize the exposure of the unborn baby to drugs and alcohol. For any substance abuse, the infant will experience withdrawal symptoms after birth and go on to face developmental, neuropsychological, and behavioral sequelae as a result of the *in utero* exposure to drugs or alcohol. Thus, caring for a woman who has been incarcerated should include a thorough assessment of the reasons for her incarceration, with an understanding that a history of substance abuse is a significant possibility. The health-care provider must be familiar with the laws guiding his or her practice since some states require reporting of cases in which a child is being exposed to illegal substances during the pregnancy or at birth; currently, 14 states require mandatory reporting of suspected prenatal drug abuse (Guttmacher Institute, 2012). For women who will give birth while incarcerated, anticipatory guidance as to the policies that will affect her care during labor is necessary. While organizations such as the American College of Obstetricians and Gynecologists (2011) and the Association of Women's Health, Obstetric and Neonatal Nurses (AWHONN) (2011) have highlighted the risks associated with and have taken a stance opposing the practice of shackling incarcerated women during labor, many state correction agencies still enforce this policy.

Nurse practitioners and other health-care providers not working within a jail or prison system are unlikely to encounter an incarcerated patient; midwives who provide labor and birth services might, on occasion, attend the birth of a woman who is incarcerated. Nonetheless, health-care providers care for women who have a history of incarceration or who are at risk for future incarceration. Those working in a jail or prison system will likely be required to follow strict protocols for prenatal care developed by prison officials. Early prenatal care for women who are at risk for incarceration is essential; the health education and counseling that is a hallmark of quality prenatal care has the potential to influence women to make positive health-related changes (Dooley & Ringler, 2012; Hotelling, 2008).

Guidelines to consider for incarcerated pregnant women

1. Recognize that a woman's effort to attain prenatal care is a step toward caring for herself and her baby and that she has likely overcome significant barriers to attend the appointment. Praise her for her efforts to prioritize her and her baby's health.
2. Understand the characteristics of women with histories of incarceration and develop a plan for assessment based on common risk factors.
3. Assess for the following:
   - reasons for incarceration
   - nature of life circumstances leading up to and following the period of incarceration
   - history of childhood and adult exposure to violence, including sexual, physical, and IPV
   - thoughts about the pregnancy, including circumstances surrounding pregnancy, whether the pregnancy was planned or unplanned, plans for pregnancy and child placement, involvement of the father of the baby, involvement of family members, concerns about life after the birth, and structure of family and living arrangements
   - depression and emotional distress
   - all possible sexually transmitted infections, including HIV; provide treatment as needed according to practice guidelines (see Chapter 41)
   - substance abuse, including last use, drugs used, and attempts at rehabilitation; refer to an obstetrician or perinatologist for initiation of opioid therapy for opioid-dependent women (see Chapter 13).
4. Obtain permission to access any medical records for previous prenatal visits at other clinics.
5. Encourage timely follow-up and assist with removing any identified barriers to attending appointments, such as lack of transportation, lack of childcare (for other children), and lack of insurance.
6. Provide anticipatory education on the circumstances of labor and birth while incarcerated. Advocate for nonuse of shackles to ensure freedom of movement during labor and birth (AWHONN, 2011).

Sources: American College of Obstetricians and Gynecologists (ACOG) (2011), AWHONN (2011), Clarke and Adashi (2011), National Commission on Correctional Health Care (NCCHC) (2005).

Intimate partner violence during pregnancy

IPV is defined as physical injury caused by someone with whom the woman has an intimate relationship and can consist of pushing, slapping, pushing, hitting, kicking, biting, and punching as well as rape. The perpetrator can use verbal threats or physical force to overcome the woman and commit the act of abuse. Physical abuse in childhood and during pregnancy is a national concern. According to the Center for Disease Control and Prevention (CDC) (2010), one of every four women will experience physical abuse by a man at some point in her life. Prevalence rates of IPV during pregnancy range from approximately 4% to 10% (Chu, Goodwin, & D'Angelo, 2010). However, these are likely low estimates due to underreporting by women (Gunter, 2007). Furthermore, a preexisting pattern of IPV might escalate in episodes and severity during pregnancy (Anderson, Marshak, & Hebbeler, 2002). In light of this information, healthcare providers encounter many women who are or have been victims of abuse but are not aware of it. IPV can affect a woman throughout her life and certainly can impact maternal child health and her perception of the pregnancy.

Women experiencing IPV have poor quality of life and are more likely to experience depression, post-traumatic stress disorder, anxiety, sexually transmitted infections, and unplanned pregnancy (Humphreys, 2011; Lapierre, 2010; McMahon, Huang, Boxer, & Postmus, 2011; Zlotnick, Capezza, & Parker, 2011). During pregnancy, IPV poses a threat to both the mother and her unborn baby (Zlotnick et al., 2011); pregnant victims of IPV have increased rates of delayed prenatal care, miscarriage, second- and third-trimester bleeding, placental abruption, preterm labor and birth, neonatal death, and other adverse outcomes (Boy & Salihu, 2004; El-Mohandes, Kiely, Gantz, & El-Khorazaty, 2011; Leone et al., 2010; Sarkar, 2008). Adolescents are especially vulnerable to IPV and require targeted intervention since experiencing IPV during adolescence is a risk factor for victimization in adulthood (ACOG, 2012). Children born into abusive home environments are at risk for experiencing various forms of abuse and are more likely to have difficult temperaments, poor health outcomes, poor school performance, and experience anxiety and depression (Chambliss, 2008; McMahon et al., 2011). Some states require mandatory reporting of IPV that occurs in homes with children, regardless of whether it is known that a child is or is not being directly abused. See "Resources for Health-Care Providers" for resources summarizing specific state laws.

IPV usually takes on a cycle of building tension, battering, and attempts at reconciliation (Gunter, 2007).

Arguments, verbal threats, and low-level assaults such as pushing characterize the tension-building phase. The abuse victim tends to appease the abuser in an effort to avoid escalating the abuse. The explosive battering phase is manifested with serious acts of abuse and control like slapping, punching, or rape. The next phase tends to immediately follow the overtly violent actions and is commonly referred to as the "honeymoon stage." This phase is characterized by the abuser's display of overly affectionate, remorseful, and apologetic behavior (Gunter, 2007). This attempt to convince the woman that the behavior will change so that she will not leave the relationship is often effective and women can remain in abusive relationships for months and even years. Poverty and lack of immediate housing in the event of her departure also play a significant role in a woman's decision to remain in an abusive relationship (Gunter, 2007). Further, threats of severe physical harm or death from her abuser create an overwhelming fear that leads women to choose injury over possible death by staying in the relationship. Homicide is a leading cause of death for women of childbearing age (Murphy, Xu, & Kochanek, 2012). In 2010, almost 38% of female homicide victims were murdered by a husband or boyfriend (Federal Bureau of Investigation, 2012). For a woman in an abusive relationship, the most dangerous time is when she leaves. However, many women are able to leave abusive relationships and lead productive lives if given the appropriate support. Understanding the context of a woman's choice to remain in or leave an abusive relationship will counteract judgmental reactions to a choice with which the provider disagrees. Empathy for the enormity of the decision at hand will produce compassion and minimize judgment.

Research demonstrating that a woman's legal action—in the form of a court order of protection—against her abuser will result in a decrease in abuse is strong; however, some studies have found that incidences of IPV increased after a court order of protection (McFarlane et al., 2004). Furthermore, there is evidence that temporary court orders for protection might increase psychological abuse, while permanent court orders are more effective in decreasing physical abuse (Holt, Kernic, Lumley, Wolf, & Rivara, 2002; Kratochvil, 2010). In light of these inconsistent findings and the inherent limitations in such studies, women should be educated about the potential for such action to exacerbate her abuser's rage and assisted in taking the steps necessary to ensure her safety and the safety of her children. The health-care provider should never force a woman to take such action if she is not ready or comfortable with the potential consequences. Instead, steps to enhance her sense of safety, self-worth, and empowerment may provide her with the resolve to take legal action should she feel ready to do so in the future.

In order to initiate effective interventions, assessment of IPV must occur at regular intervals throughout prenatal care; women who are being abused might find it hard to disclose the abuse until they have developed a trusting relationship with the health-care provider (American College of Nurse Midwives (ACNM), 2002; Anderson et al., 2002). Table 14.1 contains some general principles to follow when assessing for IPV and planning interventions to assist women in accessing appropriate resources.

Pregnancy and a history of childhood sexual abuse

The incidence of childhood sexual abuse (CSA) is estimated at between 18% and 25% of U.S. women (Sperlich & Seng, 2008). Pregnancy can be a trigger for a return of the feeling of terror and shame for many women due to the changes in the pregnant body, the feelings of vulnerability that pregnancy naturally brings, and the office procedures like vaginal exams. This can take the form of flashbacks of previously repressed memories, nightmares, increased anxiety, and behavior changes. For some women, pregnancy is the event that causes repressed memories of CSA to resurface for the first time in many years, especially among those abused at younger ages. Women who have survived CSA have an increase in perinatal complications such as hyperemesis, preterm labor, cervical insufficiency, and increase in hospitalizations during pregnancy (Leeners, Stiller, Block, Görres, & Rath, 2010). These complications may be related to higher levels of catecholamines and stress hormones found in women with prior CSA (DeBellis, Lefter, Trickett, & Putnam, 1994). CSA is also associated with a significant increase in the risk for adolescent pregnancy (Noll, Shenk, & Putnam, 2009), extreme fear of childbirth (Lukasse et al., 2010), labor dysfunction, and postpartum depressive disorders (Kendall-Tackett, 2007).

Assessing for childhood sexual abuse

All pregnant women should be asked about a prior history of CSA during the prenatal intake interview. While some pregnant women may share their history of CSA, many will not. For women who have not disclosed prior abuse, they may not disclose until they have been asked numerous times or until they can judge that the provider "gets it" and is competent at addressing these issues (Sperlich & Seng, 2008). The health-care provider must be alert to physical, psychological, and behavioral clues that may indicate CSA (Table 14.2).

Table 14.1 Intimate Partner Violence: Assessment and Planning

1. Assess for IPV using a formal screening tool or informal questions. Preface with a statement that normalizes universal screening for all women. Assess for the following:
   - emotional abuse, humiliation, intimidation, use of threats
   - physical abuse, including hitting, biting, kicking, slapping, pushing, punching
   - sexual abuse or rape.
   All women should be assessed for IPV at the initial prenatal visit and regularly throughout the remainder of the pregnancy, at least once per trimester.

2. Assess frequency of abuse and history of injuries and trips to the ER. If she has current injuries, document them in the record with specific descriptions and drawings. Photograph them if a camera is available.

3. Assess her perception of imminent danger. Ask about guns or other weapons in the home. Inquire about suicidal ideations from her and/or her partner.

4. Ask about her perceptions of the future of the relationship. Avoid judgment if she has no intentions of ending the relationship. Ask sensitive questions to understand the factors that are preventing her from leaving.

5. If there are suspicions of abuse and a woman's partner is always with her, use strategies to separate them such as asking for a urine sample and following her to the bathroom.

5. Assess her support network, including sources of financial help, housing, and transportation.

6. Provide contact information for local shelters for battered women and local social services for housing, financial, and medical assistance. Place posters and flyers in the women's bathrooms. Advise her on places to keep the numbers hidden, such as under the insert of her shoe or inside the lining of a purse.

7. If she wants to obtain a court order of protection, provide information for local agencies that are equipped to provide women with legal assistance. Do not call agencies or law enforcement on her behalf without her permission.

8. Validate the woman's experience, choices, and fears and reinforce her self-worth. Withhold judgment and engage in active listening. Refrain from humiliating her because of her choices and adding to the feelings of victimization that she feels from her abuser.

Sources: ACNM (2002), ACOG (2012), Anderson et al. (2002), Gunter (2007).

Table 14.2 Possible Signs and Symptoms of Prior CSA

Physical signs and symptoms	Psychological signs and symptoms	Behavioral signs and symptoms
Prior history of multiple somatic illnesses: • dizziness and fainting • chronic pain and fatigue • morbid obesity • gastrointestinal (GI) disorders • migraine headaches Obstetric/gynecologic symptoms: • sexual dysfunction • breast disease • chronic menstrual problems • chronic urinary tract infection (UTI) • premenstrual syndrome • history of multiple sexually transmitted infections (STIs) • multiple unplanned pregnancies Scars from self-mutilation	Post-traumatic stress disorder Compulsive disorders Dissociative disorders Panic attacks Low self-esteem Depression Negative reaction to pregnancy Denial of pregnancy	Promiscuity Anorexia or bulimia Substance abuse Seeks female health-care providers Little or no prenatal care Frequent health-care visits for somatic symptoms

Providing care

The acute need for control motivates behavior that may be exhibited by women who have experienced CSA. Certain behaviors may help her manage feelings of extreme anxiety and fear that emerge during pregnancy. Some women may seek to learn everything about pregnancy and birth in order to prepare for every possible scenario that might happen to them. This may be manifested as attending multiple childbirth preparation class series, gathering multiple accounts of women's childbirth experiences, reading many books, and researching childbirth on the Internet (Hobbins, 2004). Some women may develop very detailed and lengthy birth plans in an effort to control events covering a variety of birth scenarios. This overload of information may contribute to confusion and further anxiety. Some women may exhibit hypervigilance in interpreting their body changes and sensations during pregnancy. This may be manifested as frequent telephone contacts with health-care providers and multiple office visits with problems and many questions (Hobbins, 2004). A history of CSA is associated with an increased reporting of common discomforts and symptoms of pregnancy during the antepartum period (Lukasse, Schei, Vangen, & Øian, 2009). Women may also increase visits to health-care providers for various somatic symptoms in the hopes of obtaining help or relief from her abusive situation (Sperlich & Seng, 2008).

Some women may actively avoid discussions related to her body and childbearing, such as breastfeeding, perineal preparation for birth, and pain or sexuality during pregnancy. These discussions may cause visible anxiety and discomfort, and the woman may appear to be noncommunicative, sarcastic, indifferent, or fearful.

Health-care providers should knock on the door prior to entering the examination space and provide self-introduction by name and occupation (midwife, nurse practitioner, etc). The initial interview and history should be conducted before the woman has changed into an examination gown. Since many women have an unknown history of CSA, these should all be routine practice habits. When abuse is disclosed, a calm, nonjudgmental, and empathetic response is essential.

It is of the utmost importance to avoid the use of traumatizing or paternalistic language when providing care to all women, but most particularly to women with a history of CSA. Some things that may be commonly stated during the course of prenatal care but should be avoided are things like "just open your legs a little bit wider," "lift your bottom up for me," "good girl—just hold still for a minute," and the like. Not only are these phrases infantilizing to women, they can also reintroduce traumatizing memories and cause extreme anxiety to CSA survivors (Squire, 2009).

When providing prenatal care, it is essential to understand that a woman with a history of CSA is likely to have strong need for a safe, trusting relationship with her health-care provider in addition to control over what happens to her body. While developing trust is a vital aspect of obtaining quality prenatal care, this can be a difficult task for CSA survivors. To facilitate this process, recognizing and verbalizing understanding of the concerns she may be facing is important. For example, "I know it may take some time to feel that I am trustworthy. So here are some things about me you can count on. I will keep your confidentiality. I'll try to remember to ask permission to touch you, and I will keep you informed of your condition" (Sperlich & Seng, 2008, p. 68).

Almost half of CSA survivors experience memories of their abuse when undergoing a medical vaginal exam (Leeners, 2007). They need to be in control of when the exams are done and when they can be stopped for any reason, without penalty. For those women who have disclosed CSA (and women showing distress during a pelvic exam with no disclosure of abuse), it is appropriate to say, "I see that this is stressful for you. I am going to stop now. Are you okay? Let me know if I may continue." Throughout the perinatal period, vaginal examinations should only be done when absolutely indicated and the woman should be informed of her plan of care. Any procedure or examination should be explained prior to being done, and again during every step of the process. This will help the woman anticipate what is being done and gives her the opportunity to accept or decline. Women with a prior history of CSA need to have control of when examinations are allowed. Having control over what happens to their bodies is important in reducing retraumatization of women during pregnancy care.

Women with a history of CSA have babies of lower birth weight and shorter gestation (Seng, Low, Sperlich, Ronis, & Liberzon, 2011). CSA linked post-traumatic stress syndrome (PTSD) may contribute to these adverse perinatal outcomes. Close attention should be paid to maternal diet, weight gain, fundal height, and other signs of adequate fetal growth.

Summary

The social circumstances in which women live their lives exert significant influence on prenatal health and pregnancy outcomes. Health-care providers should be prepared to invest the time required to assist women who are experiencing poverty, homelessness, single motherhood, IPV, or a history of CSA during pregnancy. Realizing that these issues are key contributors to health disparities in maternal and infant morbidity and mortality, it is imperative that they be addressed in a compassionate and expedient manner. In many cases, the health-care provider must operate as a case manager in the beginning stages of the relationship until other professionals with expertise in social services can take over. A familiarity with local community, state, and federal agencies that exist to provide aid to individuals in vulnerable circumstances is essential.

Case study

Brenda is a 27-year-old woman pregnant with her third child. This is her second prenatal visit and her first at your clinic; her first prenatal visit was 1 month ago in the neighboring town where she lived up until 3 weeks ago. She is now 25 weeks pregnant and has moved to live closer to her sister after leaving her boyfriend who was abusive to her and her children; he is not the father of her other two children. The abuse had escalated since she became pregnant. Although her sister does not have room in her apartment for her and her children, she wanted to move closer so that she could have help with childcare when she finds a new job. Her last job was over a year ago, but she is hoping to find something soon so that she can save up money for a deposit on her own apartment before the baby comes. Right now, she is living at the local homeless shelter. It is not ideal, but she was able to get a small private room with two beds for herself and her children. Her children are 5 and 10 years old; the 5-year-old will start kindergarten in the fall.

Upon reviewing her intake forms, you note that Brenda is 5'7" and weighs 120 lb. She thinks that she weighed around 132 lb before she got pregnant. She had moderate nausea with occasional vomiting during her early pregnancy; her appetite was very low during that time, which she reports was a good thing since money was very tight anyway. She does not have her records from her first prenatal visit and does not know any of the labs that were drawn or their results. She reports being in good health; her only history is two episodes of gonorrhea in her early 20s and a recent treatment for trichomoniasis, which she suspects she got from her boyfriend.

Case study response

Since Brenda was seen at another clinic, her medical records were requested. She filled out the necessary permissions for you to obtain her records. You reviewed what was done at that visit and then completed the care that she needed at this point in her pregnancy, including a complete physical exam, prenatal labs, and STD testing. After a thorough assessment of her last menstrual period, it was determined that her dates were uncertain. Brenda stated that she did not have an ultrasound at the last clinic. You advised that she have an ultrasound to date her pregnancy, and the indications, procedures, and safety where discussed with her.

Her nausea and vomiting were assessed and education was provided on minimizing symptoms.

Her body mass index (BMI) was calculated. Education was provided about nutrition and healthy weight gain in pregnancy. You discussed the importance of adequate nutrition and how to select healthy, nutrient-dense food options. Having WIC will give her access to nutritious foods while she is pregnant and after the birth. Her children will also qualify for nutrition assistance.

You assessed her sense of danger regarding her abusive boyfriend. Leaving the relationship can be a very dangerous time for abused women. You helped her to formulate a safety plan that includes limiting knowledge of her whereabouts and access to a cell phone for emergencies. If she felt that she was in danger, you would have developed a plan to involve law enforcement. You checked for shelters for battered women in your area where there are more safeguards in place than a typical homeless shelter.

Brenda was referred to local social services offices for assistance with housing, nutrition, MPW, job training, childcare, and child support. She can have assistance with finding affordable housing and will likely qualify for WIC and MPW, which will cover her pregnancy care retroactively. You advised her to provide the office where she was previously seen her coverage information to avoid being billed. Job training will increase her chances of securing gainful employment. Identifying childcare options will allow her children to receive quality care while she is looking for a job and working or returning to school. You explored whether she is comfortable with filing for child support. She might prefer to not initiate a case against her boyfriend, but the State might do so on her behalf if she applies for certain types of assistance.

A list of potential problems was created to include in Brenda's record. This list prompted providers to assess Brenda for issues that might influence her physical and mental well-being during the pregnancy and postpartum period.

Resources for health-care providers

American College of Obstetricians and Gynecologists—Committee opinion on health-care for pregnant and postpartum incarcerated women and adolescents: http://www.acog.org/Resources_And_Publications/Committee_Opinions/Committee_on_Health_Care_for_Underserved_Women/Health_Care_for_Pregnant_and_Postpartum_Incarcerated_Women_and_Adolescent_Females

American College of Obstetricians and Gynecologists—Committee opinion on intimate partner violence: http://www.acog.org/Resources_And_Publications/Committee_Opinions/Committee_on_Health_Care_for_Underserved_Women/Intimate_Partner_Violence

American College of Obstetricians and Gynecologists—Committee opinion on health-care for homeless women: http://www.acog.org/Resources_And_Publications/Committee_Opinions/Committee_on_Health_Care_for_Underserved_Women/Health_Care_for_Homeless_Women

Guttmacher Institute—State policies on substance abuse during pregnancy: http://www.guttmacher.org/statecenter/spibs/spib_SADP.pdf

Health care and multiple diagnosis issues of homeless people: http://hivinsite.ucsf.edu/insite?page=pr-06-03-01

Homeless and pregnant—*Healing Hands*, a publication of the Health Care for the Homeless Clinicians' Network, National Health Care for the Homeless Council: http://www.nhchc.org/wp-content/uploads/2012/02/August2001HealingHands.pdf

Improving screening of women for violence—Basic guidelines for health-care providers, including "How to Make Your Office Survivor-Friendly": http://www.medscape.org/viewprogram/2777

National Commission on Correctional Health Care—Women's Health Care in Correctional Settings (Position Statement): http://www.ncchc.org/resources/statements/womenshealth2005.html

National Health Care for the Homeless Council—Provides clinical guidelines adapted for use with homeless populations; it consists of organizations and individual who seek to improve health care, housing, and income for the homeless: http://www.nhchc.org/resources/clinical/adapted-clinical-guidelines/

National Coalition for the Homeless—A network of individuals committed to preventing and ending homelessness; their efforts are centered around advocacy, public education, and grassroots organization to address civil rights and housing, health care, and economic justice: http://www.nationalhomeless.org/index.html

World Health Organization—Report about IPV during pregnancy around the world: http://whqlibdoc.who.int/hq/2011/WHO_RHR_11.35_eng.pdf

U.S. Department of Health and Human Services, Child Welfare Information Gateway—A summary of state laws mandating reporting of child abuse and neglect: http://www.childwelfare.gov/systemwide/laws_policies/statutes/manda.pdf

Women's Prison Association—A summary of jail and prison nursery programs: http://wpaonline.org/pdf/Mothers%20Infants%20and%20Imprisonment%202009.pdf

Resources for women and their families

How to obtain child support: Child support enforcement steps: http://www.acf.hhs.gov/programs/cse/fct/fct2.htm

Local food pantries—Assist women in locating local food banks or pantries using the link: http://feedingamerica.org/foodbank-results.aspx. Women may obtain food items as well as common household items from some pantries.

Medicaid for Pregnant Women—provides medical insurance for women during pregnancy and up to 60 days postpartum. This program is available in all 50 states and allows low-income women to access adequate prenatal care. Women may even receive retroactive coverage (defined as "presumptive eligibility") so that they can begin prenatal care before their approval is final. For eligibility and application information, women should contact their state's Department of Human Services. For more information, visit: http://www.medicaid.gov/Medicaid-CHIP-Program-Information/By-Population/Pregnant-Women/Pregnant-Women.html

State Child Support Enforcement Offices: http://www.acf.hhs.gov/programs/css

Temporary Assistance for Needy Families (TANF)—a program that helps families transition from public assistance to work by providing financial support, work opportunities, and childcare assistance. For details about the program and eligibility, visit: http://www.acf.hhs.gov/programs/ofa/programs/tanf

The National Association of Child Care Resource & Referral Agencies—provides information about state Child Care Resource offices, which provide assistance with locating and paying for quality childcare: http://www.naccrra.org/

The National Association of Free Clinics—organization for clinics providing free health care for uninsured or underinsured individuals across the country. To find a free clinic in your area, visit: http://www.nafcclinics.org

The Office of Child Support Enforcement—provides assistance in obtaining child support for custodial parents.

The Special Supplemental Nutrition Program for WIC—the U.S. Department of Agriculture provides supplemental nutrition and nutritional education for low-income pregnant, postpartum, and nursing women and children up to age 5 years old with identified nutritional risks. The program exists in all 50 states and the District of Columbia, 34 Indian tribal organizations, and other U.S. territories. For details about the program and eligibility, visit: http://www.fns.usda.gov/wic/

U.S. Department of Housing and Urban Development—public housing assistance is offered in the form of public housing or housing choice vouchers (section 8). Women should contact their local Public Housing Agency (PHA) for assistance. Assistance for finding affordable local housing or help with utility bills is also available. For more information, visit: http://portal.hud.gov/hudportal/HUD?src=/topics/rental_assistance

References

Adams, E. K., Gavin, N. I., & Benedict, M. B. (2005). Access for pregnant women on Medicaid: Variation by race and ethnicity. *Journal of Health Care for the Poor and Underserved, 16*, 74–95.

Alio, A. P., Kornosky, J. L., Mbah, A. K., Marty, P. J., & Salihu, H. M. (2009). The impact of paternal involvement of feto-infant morbidity among Whites, Blacks, and Hispanics. *Maternal and Child Health Journal, 14*, 735–741. doi:10.1007/s10995-009-0482-1

American College of Nurse Midwives (ACNM). (2002). Assessment for intimate partner violence in clinical practice. *Journal of Midwifery & Women's Health, 47*(5), 386–390.

American College of Obstetricians and Gynecologists (ACOG). (2011). Health care for pregnant and postpartum incarcerated women and adolescent females (Committee Opinion No. 511). *Obstetrics and Gynecology, 118*, 1198–1202.

American College of Obstetricians and Gynecologists (ACOG). (2012). Intimate partner violence (Committee Opinion No. 518). *Obstetrics and Gynecology, 119*, 412–417.

Anderson, B. A., Marshak, H. H., & Hebbeler, D. L. (2002). Identifying intimate partner violence at entry to prenatal care: Clustering routine clinical information. *Journal of Midwifery & Women's Health, 47*, 353–359.

Association of Women's Health, Obstetric and Neonatal Nurses (AWHONN). (2011). Shackling incarcerated women (position statement). *Journal of Obstetric, Gynecologic, and Neonatal Nursing, 40*, 817–818. doi:10.1111/j.1552-6909.2011.01300.x

Beal, A. C., & Redlener, I. (1995). Enhancing perinatal outcomes in homeless women: The challenge of providing comprehensive health care. *Seminars in Perinatology, 19*(4), 307–313.

Blitz, C. L., Wolff, N., Pan, K., & Pogorzelski, W. (2005). Gender-specific behavior health and community release patterns among New Jersey prison inmates: Implications for treatment and community reentry. *American Journal of Public Health, 95*(10), 1741–1746.

Bloom, K. C., Bednarzyk, M. S., Devitt, D. L., Renault, R. A., Teaman, V., & Van Loock, D. M. (2004). Barriers to prenatal care for homeless pregnant women. *Journal of Obstetric, Gynecologic, and Neonatal Nursing, 33*, 428–435. doi:10.1177/ 0884217504266775

Boy, A., & Salihu, H. M. (2004). Intimate partner violence and birth outcomes: A systematic review. *International Journal of Fertility and Women's Medicine, 49*(4), 159–164.

Braveman, P., Marchi, K., Egerter, S., Kim, S., Metzler, M., Stancil, T., & Libet, M. (2010). Poverty, near-poverty, and hardship around the time of pregnancy. *Maternal and Child Health Journal, 14*, 20–35.

Braveman, P., Marchi, K., Egerter, S., Pearl, M., & Neuhaus, J. (2000). Barriers to timely prenatal care among women with insurance: The importance of prepregnancy factors. *Obstetrics and Gynecology, 95*, 874–880.

Broussard, C. A. (2010). Research regarding low-income single mothers' mental and physical health: A decade in review. *Journal of Poverty, 14*, 443–451.

Carter-Pokras, O., & Baquet, C. (2002). What is a "health disparity"? *Public Health Reports, 117*, 426–434.

Center for Disease Control and Prevention (CDC). (2010). National intimate partner and sexual violence survey: 2010 summary report. Retrieved from http://www.cdc.gov/ViolencePrevention/pdf/ NISVS_Report2010-a.pdf

Chambliss, L. R. (2008). Intimate partner violence and its implication for pregnancy. *Clinical Obstetrics and Gynecology, 51*(2), 385–397.

Chaudhuri, N. (2004). Interventions to improve children's health by improving the housing environment. *Reviews on Environmental Health, 19*, 197–222.

Chu, S. Y., Goodwin, M. M., & D'Angelo, D. V. (2010). Physical violence against U.S. women around the time of pregnancy, 2004–2007. *American Journal of Preventive Medicine, 38*, 317–322. doi:10.1016/j.amepre.2009.11.013

Clarke, J., & Adashi, E. (2011). Perinatal care for incarcerated patients: A 25-year-old woman pregnant in jail. *Journal of the American Medical Association, 305*(9), 923–929.

Clarke, J. G., Hebert, M. R., Rosengard, C., Rose, J. S., DaSilva, K. M., & Stein, M. D. (2006). Reproductive health care and family planning needs among incarcerated women. *American Journal of Public Health, 96*(5), 834–839.

Cox, J. T., & Phelan, S. T. (2008). Nutrition during pregnancy. *Obstetrics and Gynecology Clinics of North America, 35*, 369–383.

Crosier, T., Butterworth, P., & Rodgers, B. (2007). Mental health problems among single and partnered mothers: The role of financial hardship and social support. *Social Psychiatry and Psychiatric Epidemiology, 42*, 6–13. doi:10.1007/s00127-006-0125-4

DeBellis, M., Lefter, L., Trickett, P. K., & Putnam, F. W. (1994). Urinary catecholamine excretion in sexually abused girls. *Journal of the American Academy of Child and Adolescent Psychiatry, 33*(3), 320–327.

DeNavas-Walt, C., Proctor, B. D., & Smith, J. C. (2011). *Income, poverty, and health insurance coverage in the United States: 2010.* U.S. Census Bureau, Current Population Reports. Washington, DC: U.S. Government Printing Office.

Dooley, E. K., & Ringler, R. L. (2012). Prenatal care: Touching the future. *Primary Care, 39*, 17–37.

Eamon, M. K., & Wu, C.-F. (2011). Effects of unemployment and underemployment on material hardship in single-mother families. *Children and Youth Services Review, 33*, 233–241.

El-Mohandes, A., Kiely, M., Gantz, M. G., & El-Khorazaty, N. (2011). Very preterm birth is reduced in women receiving an integrated behavioral intervention: A randomized controlled trial. *Maternal and Child Health Journal, 15*, 19–28. doi:10.1007/s10995-009-0557-z

Evans, G. W., & English, K. (2002). The environment of poverty: Multiple stressor exposure, psychophysiological stress, and socioemotional adjustment. *Child Development*, 73(4), 1238–1248. doi:10.1111/1467-8624.00469

Federal Bureau of Investigation. (2012). Crime in the United States, 2010: Murder circumstances by relationship. Retrieved from http://www.fbi.gov/about-us/cjis/ucr/crime-in-the-u.s/2010/crime-in-the-u.s.-2010/tables/10shrtbl10.xls

Finer, L. B., & Henshaw, S. K. (2006). Disparities in rates of unintended pregnancy in the United States, 1994 and 2001. *Perspectives on Sexual and Reproductive Health*, 38(2), 90–96.

Gunter, J. (2007). Intimate partner violence. *Obstetrics and Gynecology Clinics of North America*, 34, 367–388.

Gunter, T. D. (2004). Incarcerated women and depression: A primer for the primary care provider. *Journal of the American Medical Women's Association*, 59(2), 107–112.

Guttmacher Institute. (2012). Substance abuse during pregnancy. Retrieved from: http://www.guttmacher.org/statecenter/spibs/spib_SADP.pdf

Harnisch, J. M., Harnisch, P. H., & Harnisch, D. R. (2012). Family medicine obstetrics: Pregnancy and nutrition. *Primary Care*, 39, 39–5.

Harrison, P. M., & Beck, A. J. (2004). Prisoners in 2003. U.S. Department of Justice, Bureau of Justice Statistics (NCJ205335). Retrieved from http://bjs.ojp.usdoj.gov/content/pub/pdf/p03.pdf

Hobbins, D. (2004). Survivors of childhood sexual abuse: Implications for perinatal nursing care. *Journal of Obstetric, Gynecologic, and Neonatal Nursing*, 33(4), 485–497.

Holt, V. L., Kernic, M. A., Lumley, T., Wolf, M. E., & Rivara, F. P. (2002). Civil protection order and risk of subsequent police-reported violence. *JAMA: The Journal of the American Medical Association*, 288(5), 589–594.

Hotelling, B. A. (2008). Perinatal needs of pregnant, incarcerated women. *The Journal of Perinatal Education*, 17(2), 37–44. doi:10.1624/105812408X298372

Huang, C.-C., & Han, K.-Q. (2011). Child support enforcement in the United States: Has policy made a difference? *Children and Youth Services Review*, 34, 622–627.

Humphreys, J. (2011). Sexually transmitted infections, pregnancy, and intimate partner violence. *Health Care for Women International*, 32, 23–38. doi:10.1080/07399332.2010.529211

James, D. J. (2004). Profile of jail inmates, 2002. U.S. Department of Justice, Bureau of Justice Statistics (NCJ201932). Retrieved from http://bjs.ojp.usdoj.gov/content/pub/pdf/pji02.pdf

Kaiser, L. L., & Allen, L. (2002). Position of the American Dietetic Association: Nutrition and lifestyle for a health pregnancy outcome. *Journal of the American Dietetic Association*, 102(10), 1479–1490.

Kendall-Tackett, K. (2007). Violence against women and perinatal period: The impact of lifetime violence and abuse on pregnancy postpartum and breastfeeding. *Trauma, Violence and Abuse*, 8(3), 344–353.

Knudsen, H. K., Leukfeld, C., Havens, J. R., Duvall, J. L., Oser, C. B., Staton-Tindall, M. . . . Inciardi, J. A. (2008). Partner relationships and HIV risk behaviors among women offenders. *Journal of Psychoactive Drugs*, 40(4), 471–481.

Kratochvil, R. (2010). Intimate partner violence during pregnancy: Exploring the efficacy of a mandatory reporting statute. *Houston Journal of Health Law and Policy*, 10, 63–113.

Lapierre, S. (2010). Striving to be "good" mothers: Abused women's experiences of mothering. *Child Abuse Review*, 19, 342–357. doi:10.1002/car.1113

Leeners, B. (2007). Effect of childhood sexual abuse on gynecological care as an adult. *Psychosomatics*, 48, 385–393.

Leeners, B., Stiller, R., Block, E., Görres, G., & Rath, W. (2010). Pregnancy complications in women with childhood sexual abuse experiences. *Journal of Psychosomatic Research*, 69(5), 503–510.

Leone, J. M., Lane, S. D., Koumans, E. H., DeMott, K., Wojtowycz, M. A., Jensen, J., & Aubry, R. H. (2010). Effects of intimate partner violence on pregnancy trauma and placental abruption. *Journal of Women's Health (2002)*, 19(8), 1501–1509. doi:10.1089/jwh.2009.1716

LeWinn, K. Z., Stroud, L. R., Molnar, B. E., Ware, J. H., Koenen, K. C., & Buka, S. L. (2009). Elevated maternal cortisol levels during pregnancy are associated with reduced childhood IQ. *International Journal of Epidemiology*, 38(6), 1700–1710. doi:10.1093/ije/dyp200

Little, M., Shah, R., Vermeulen, M. J., Gorman, A., Dzendoletas, D., & Ray, J. G. (2005). Adverse perinatal outcomes associated with homelessness and substance use in pregnancy. *Canadian Medical Association Journal*, 173(6), 615–618.

Lukasse, M., Schei, B., Vangen, S., & Øian, P. (2009). Childhood abuse and common complaints in pregnancy. *Birth (Berkeley, Calif.)*, 36, 190–199. doi:10.1111/j.1523-536X.2009.00323.x

Lukasse, M., Vangen, S., Øian, P., Kumle, M., Ryding, E. L., Schei, B., & on behalf of the Bidens Study Group. (2010). Childhood abuse and fear of childbirth-a population-based study. *Birth (Berkeley, Calif.)*, 37, 267–274. doi:10.1111/j.1523-536X.2010.00420.x

Magee, C. G., Hult, J. R., Turalba, R., & McMillan, S. (2005). Public health consequences of imprisonment preventive care for women in prison: A qualitative community health assessment of the Papanicolaou test and follow- up treatment at a California state women's prison. *American Journal of Public Health*, 95(10), 1712–1717.

McFarlane, J., Malecha, A., Gist, J., Watson, K., Batten, E., Hall, I., & Smith, S. (2004). Protection orders and intimate partner violence: An 18-month study of 150 Black, Hispanic, and White women. *American Journal of Public Health*, 94(4), 613–618.

McMahon, S., Huang, C.-C., Boxer, P., & Postmus, J. L. (2011). The impact of emotional and physical violence during pregnancy on maternal and child health at one year postpartum. *Children and Youth Services Review*, 33, 2103–2111. doi:10.1016/j.childyouth.2011.06.001

Murphy, S. L., Xu, J., & Kochanek, K. D. (2012). Deaths: preliminary data for 2010. *National Vital Statistics Reports*, 60(4), Retrieved from http://www.cdc.gov/nchs/data/nvsr/nvsr60/nvsr60_04.pdf

Murray-García, J. (1999). The public's health, its national identity, and the continuing dilemma of minority status. *Journal of Health Care for the Poor and Underserved*, 10, 397–408.

National Alliance to End Homelessness. (2012). The state of homelessness in America, 2012. Retrieved from http://www.endhomelessness.org/files/4361_file_FINAL_The_State_of_Homelessness_in_America_2012.pdf

National Commission on Correctional Health Care (NCCHC). (2005). Women's health care in correctional settings (position statement). Retrieved from http://www.ncchc.org/resources/statements/womenshealth2005.html

Nijhawan, A. E., Salloway, R., Nunn, A. S., Poshkus, M., & Clarke, J. G. (2010). Preventive healthcare for underserved women: Results of a prison survey. *Journal of Women's Health (2002)*, 19(1), 17–22.

Nkansah-Amankra, S., Dhawain, A., Hussey, J. R., & Luchok, K. J. (2010). Maternal social support and neighborhood income inequality as predictors of low birth weight and preterm birth outcome disparities: Analysis of South Carolina Pregnancy Risk Assessment and Monitoring Survey, 2000–2003. *Maternal and Child Health Journal*, 14, 774–785.

Noll, J., Shenk, C., & Putnam, K. (2009). Childhood sexual abuse and adolescent pregnancy: A meta-analytic update. *Journal of Pediatric Psychology, 34*(4), 366–378.

Obel, C., Hedegaard, M., Henriksen, T. B., Secher, N. J., Olsen, J., & Levine, S. (2005). Stress and salivary cortisol during pregnancy. *Psychoneuroendocrinology, 30,* 647–656. doi:10.1016/j.psyneuen.2004.11.006

Raugh, V. A., Landrigan, P. J., & Claudio, L. (2008). Housing and health: Intersection of poverty and environmental exposures. *Annals of the New York Academy of Sciences, 1136,* 276–288.

Richards, R., Merrill, R. M., & Baksh, L. (2011). Health behaviors and infant health outcomes in homeless pregnant women in the United States. *Pediatrics, 128,* 438–446. doi:10.1542/peds.2010-3491

Sarkar, N. N. (2008). The impact of intimate partner violence on women's reproductive health and pregnancy outcome. *Journal of Obstetrics and Gynaecology, 28*(3), 266–271. doi:10.1080/01443610802042415

Sarlio-Lähteenkorva, S., & Lahelma, E. (2001). Food insecurity is associated with past and present economic disadvantage and body mass index. *The Journal of Nutrition, 131,* 2880–2884.

Seng, J., Low, L., Sperlich, M., Ronis, D., & Liberzon, I. (2011). Post-traumatic stress disorder, child abuse history, birthweight and gestational age: A prospective cohort study. *BJOG: An International Journal of Obstetrics and Gynaecology, 118,* 1329–1339. doi:10.1111/j.1471-0528.2011.03071.x

Shaw, M. (2004). Housing and public health. *Annual Review of Public Health, 25,* 397–418. doi:10.1146/annurev.publhealth.25.101802.123036

Smid, M., Bourgois, P., & Auerswald, C. L. (2010). The challenge of pregnancy among homeless youth reclaiming a lost opportunity. *Journal of Health Care for the Poor and Underserved, 21,* 140–156.

Sperlich, M., & Seng, J. (2008). *Survivor moms: Womens' stories of birthing, mothering and healing after sexual abuse.* Eugene, OR: Motherbaby Press.

Squire, C. (2009). Childbirth and sexual abuse during childhood. In C. Squire (Ed.), *The social context of birth.* Abingdon, United Kingdom: Radcliffe.

Sterk, C. E., Theall, K. P., & Elifson, K. W. (2005). African-American female drug users and HIV risk reduction: Challenges with criminal involvement. *Journal of Health Care for the Poor and Underserved, 16*(4), 89–107.

Townsend, M. S., Peerson, J., Love, B., Achterberg, C., & Murphy, S. P. (2001). Food insecurity is positively related to overweight in women. *The Journal of Nutrition, 131,* 1738–1745.

U.S. Census Bureau. (2012). Poverty: Poverty thresholds by size of family and number of children, 2011. Social, Economic, and Housing Statistics Division. Retrieved from http://www.census.gov/hhes/www/poverty/data/threshld/index.html

U.S. Department of Agriculture (2012). Food and Nutritional Service: Women, Children and Infants. Retrieved from http://www.fns.usda.gov/wic/

Walker, B., Mays, V. M., & Warren, R. (2004). The changing landscape for the elimination of racial/ethnic health status disparities. *Journal of Health Care for the Poor and Underserved, 15,* 506–521.

Weck, R. L., Paulose, T., & Flaws, J. A. (2008). Impact of environmental factors and poverty on pregnancy outcomes. *Clinical Obstetrics and Gynecology, 51*(2), 349–359.

Winslow, C.-E. A. (1937). Housing as a public health problem. *American Journal of Public Health, 27,* 56–61.

Wu, C.-F., & Eamon, M. K. (2011). Patterns and correlates of involuntary unemployment and underemployment in single-mother families. *Children and Youth Services Review, 33*(6), 820–828. doi:10.1016/j.childyouth.2010.12.003

Zhan, M. (2006). Economic mobility of single mothers: The role of assets and human capital development. *Journal of Sociology and Social Welfare, 33*(4), 127–150.

Zlotnick, C., Capezza, N. M., & Parker, D. (2011). An interpersonally based intervention for low-income pregnant women with intimate partner violence: A pilot study. *Archives of Women's Mental Health, 14,* 55–65. doi:0.1007/s00737-010-0195-x

Zust, B. L. (2009). Partner violence, depression, and recidivism: The case of incarcerated women and why we need programs designed for them. *Issues in Mental Health Nursing, 30,* 246–251.

15

Exercise, recreational and occupational issues, and intimate relationships in pregnancy

Meghan Garland

Relevant terms

Endocrine disruptors—chemicals that either mimic or antagonize the effects of endogenous hormones in the endocrine system

Interval training—a series of low- to high-intensity exercise workouts interspersed with brief rest or relief periods

Pedometer—a device that counts each step a person takes by detecting hip motion

Shift work—an employment practice of providing service over a 24-hour period, requiring workers to cover various segments of time of work; the term also includes both regular night shifts and work schedules in which employees change or rotate shifts

Transtheoretical model of stages of change—a strategy to assess an individual's readiness to act on a new healthier behavior; it also provides processes of change to guide the individual through the stages of change

---

Exercise in pregnancy

Traditional recommendations for exercise in pregnancy have been based more on cultural and social practices than on scientific evidence (Barakat, Pelaez, Montejo, Luaces, & Zakynthinaki, 2011). Healthy pregnant women should engage in 30 or more minutes of moderate-intensity exercise most, if not all, days of the week (American College of Obstetricians and Gynecologists (ACOG), 2002). These guidelines are consistent with the American College of Sports Medicine and American Heart Association guidelines for healthy adults between the ages of 18 and 65 years old. These updated exercise recommendations include definitions of "moderate" and "vigorous" exercises to reflect current data on the amount

of energy expenditure needed to improve health outcomes. The benefits of regular exercise during pregnancy are immensely greater than any risk for the vast majority of pregnant women.

Physiological changes during pregnancy and exercise

Pregnancy has effects on maternal systems that are directly affected during exercise including cardiovascular, respiratory, musculoskeletal, and thermoregulatory systems. Numerous cardiovascular changes are associated with pregnancy including an overall increased cardiac workload. Physiological responses to exercise during pregnancy include increased oxygen consumption, redistribution of blood flow away from the viscera and myometrium into the skin and skeletal muscle. Reduced uterine blood flow would have to exceed 50% to induce fetal hypoxia, a rare occurrence associated only with prolonged, strenuous exercise in a healthy pregnant woman (Blackburn, 2013). Several compensatory mechanisms preserve fetal oxygen availability during exercise. The decrease in blood flow to the placenta is much lower than the decrease to the myometrium due to selective distribution mechanisms. Additionally, sustained exercise during pregnancy is associated with increased placental villous size and volume. Maternal hematocrit rises during exercise, thus increasing maternal oxygen carrying capacity (Blackburn, 2013). Uterine oxygen uptake also increases during exercise.

The normal changes in maternal respiratory function in pregnancy are the same as those during mild to moderate exercise in the nonpregnant state. Respiratory rate during mild exercise is greater than that of nonpregnant women, but this difference ceases during moderate

---

Prenatal and Postnatal Care: A Woman-Centered Approach, First Edition. Edited by Robin G. Jordan, Janet L. Engstrom, Julie A. Marfell, and Cindy L. Farley.
© 2014 John Wiley & Sons, Inc. Published 2014 by John Wiley & Sons, Inc.

exercise. Gas exchange is not altered by pregnancy and exercise-induced acid–base balance is similar to non-pregnant women.

Exercise is associated with increased heat production and body temperature and may alter fetal heat dissipation. However, most women can tolerate moderate exercise with no change in core body temperature. The ability of pregnant women to dissipate heat generated during exercise increases as pregnancy progresses. The pregnancy-induced lordosis, increase in joint laxity, changes in joint kinetics, and decreased abdominal muscle strength may increase the risk of injury during exercise.

Benefits of exercise in pregnancy

Entering pregnancy with a habit of engaging in regular physical activity and exercise during pregnancy may be one of the most effective ways to ameliorate a wide range of pregnancy discomforts and may reduce potential for complications. One of the strongest benefits of physical activity is a dramatic reduction in rates of gestational diabetes (GDM). Women with the highest levels of physical activity prepregnancy have a 55% lower risk of developing GDM than women with the lowest rates (Zavorsky & Longo, 2011b). Increasing weekly energy expenditure through physical activity decreases metabolic syndrome, systemic inflammation, coronary heart disease, and cardiovascular disease while delaying aging and disability in all populations. Women who continue to exercise during pregnancy gain less weight, deposit less fat, have increased fitness, and have lower cardiovascular risk profiles in the perimenopausal period of life than women who stop exercise during pregnancy. Additionally, women who are cardiovascularly fit during pregnancy have significantly shorter first- and second-stage labors (Zavorsky & Longo, 2011b; Smith & Michel, 2006).

Women who engaged in regular physical activity during pregnancy are less likely to be diagnosed with hypertensive disorders in pregnancy (Martin & Brunner Huber, 2010). A dose–response relationship suggests that women who engage in the most physical activity prior to and during pregnancy have the lowest risk of developing hypertensive disorders. The development of hypertensive disorders in pregnancy is associated with endothelial dysfunction, which may produce vasoconstriction. Exercise improves vascular health and placental growth in addition to reversing endothelial dysfunction. Randomized controlled trials among sedentary obese pregnant women who take up exercise during pregnancy demonstrate significant benefits (Evenson & Wen, 2011; Foxcroft, Rowlands, Byrne, McIntyre, & Callaway, 2011).

Regular participation in exercise programs is associated with numerous psychosocial benefits, and improved muscular strength is beneficial in preventing low-back pain and improving balance (Barakat et al., 2011). Specifically, women who engage in 3 hours a week of vigorous exercise in pregnancy report greater satisfaction

---

Benefits of exercise during pregnancy

- Reduced risk of preeclampsia
- Reduced risk of GDM
- Reduced risk of preterm birth
- Improved pain tolerance
- Lower total weight gain
- Less fat mass gain
- Improved self-image
- Shorter first and second stages of labor
- Fewer pregnancy discomforts such as low-back pain
- Higher newborn Apgar scores
- Decreased rates of operative birth

Sources: Forouhari, Yazdanpanahi, Parsanezhad, and Ragain-Shirazi (2009), Martin and Brunner Huber (2010), Penney (2008).

Absolute and Relative Contraindications to Exercise

Relative contraindications	Absolute contraindications
- Severe anemia - Unevaluated maternal cardiac arrhythmia - Chronic bronchitis - Poorly controlled type I diabetes - Extreme morbid obesity - Extreme underweight (body mass index [BMI] < 12) - History of extremely sedentary lifestyle - Intrauterine growth restriction in current pregnancy - Poorly controlled hypertension - Orthopedic limitations - Poorly controlled seizure disorder - Heavy smoker	- Hemodynamically significant heart disease - Restrictive lung disease - Cerclage/cervical insufficiency - Multiple gestation at risk for preterm labor - Persistent second- or third-trimester bleeding - Placenta previa after 20 weeks of gestation - Premature labor during current pregnancy - Ruptured membranes - Preeclampsia in current pregnancy

Source: Zavorsky and Longo (2011b).

with their stamina, energy levels, appearance, and general health than sedentary pregnant women. Exercise also has positive effects on the neonate with moderate-intensity physical activity being associated with normal fetal growth. Exercise during pregnancy plays an important role in preventing obesity and excessive weight gain and in controlling weight in women who are already obese (Barakat et al., 2011). Women should be informed about the potential benefits of exercise for themselves and the fetus and that there is a lack of evidence for any harmful effects. This may be a change of thinking from previous generations of pregnant women. Some pregnant women with preexisting medical or pregnancy conditions should not exercise or have a greatly reduced level of activity, and these women should be appropriately counseled on the rationale for limited activity.

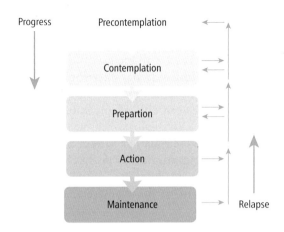

Figure 15.1.   Transtheoretical stages of change. http://en.wikipedia.org/wiki/File:Stages-of-change.png.

Motivating women to exercise in pregnancy

Despite all these benefits, pregnant women spend less time exercising than their nonpregnant counterparts. Most pregnant women do not meet the minimum recommendations for physical activity set forth by the American College of Obstetricians and Gynecologists and, contrary to best practices, have low activity or sedentary lifestyles (Evenson & Wen, 2011; Olson & Blackwell, 2011). A recent review of pregnancy and exercise studies shows that as pregnancy progresses, rates of exercise decrease, but the factors that influence exercise patterns are numerous and complex (Gaston & Cramp, 2011). Less than 16% of pregnant women meet recommended activity guidelines in pregnancy compared to 26.1% of nonpregnant women (Gaston & Cramp, 2011), though the reasons are unknown.

"Teachable moments occur during significant life transitions that motivate people to adopt risk-reducing health behaviors" (Olson & Blackwell, 2011, p. 401). Each pregnancy is a period of life transition, and the moment should be seized to instruct and reinforce adoption of regular physical exercise as one of the best methods of reducing maternal and neonatal risk and improving quality of life not only during pregnancy but across the life span. There is a strong correlation between engaging in physical activity prior to pregnancy and continuing exercise during pregnancy. Exercise interventions should be targeted at inactive women prior to conception with the hope of improving exercise rates during pregnancy; given the positive physical and mental health outcomes associated with regular exercise in pregnancy, promotion of exercise should be a crucial health promotion objective for prenatal care providers.

Various counseling approaches have been initiated in an attempt to promote adoption of regular exercise habits during pregnancy. Outcomes including psychosocial measures (increased sense of well-being and positive self-image) and gestational weight gain have been used to gauge success (Lewis, Martinson, Sherwood, & Avery, 2011; Olson & Blackwell, 2011; Phelan et al., 2011; Smith & Michel, 2006). Many trials have based intervention on the transtheoretical model of stages of change (TTM SOC) (Lewis et al., 2011; Olson & Blackwell, 2011; Phelan et al., 2011; Smith & Michel, 2006). Interventions have included phone-based, mail-based, and face-to-face counseling based on TTM SOC principles, but no method or technique has been shown to be superior to another (Fig. 15.1).

TTM SOC was developed in the 1970s from naturalistic studies of smokers as they struggled to quit (Prochaska, 2008). TTM SOC is especially helpful for people in early stages of change that may be labeled as "unmotivated" or "noncompliant." Persons in the initial stage of precontemplation may lack information or may be demoralized after repeated attempts and failures to modify a given behavior. These individuals will not be receptive to change advice but may benefit from information about the disadvantages of their current behavior. It is not until a move is made into the preparation stage and plan to take action in the immediate future, that the cons of continuing a behavior outweigh the pros of no change, will specific advice about behavior modification be welcomed.

A systematic review of TTM SOC based dietary and exercise modification programs for overweight and obese adults revealed that the combination of TTM SOC with diet and exercise modification tended to produce limited but significant positive effects on weight gain (Tuah et al., 2011).

Exercise activities

Pedometers may be a useful measure of activity intensity and can help women assess their baseline activity level. Most women move during their daily lives far less than they estimate. An established pedometer-based guideline is that 30 minutes of moderate-intensity exercise would translate into 3000–4000 steps. Pedometers have the advantage of being used in any setting with any type of land-based physical activity. For a woman not engaged in any regular exercise, walking daily or 4–5 days/week is an easy exercise to initiate. The woman should start with 10-minute walks and gradually work up to 30 minutes. Walking, low-impact aerobic activity (70% of maximal heart rate), and group fitness classes are good options. Jumping or jerky movements and activities that could result in blunt force abdominal trauma should be avoided. Alternatives to land-based physical activity include swimming or water aerobics. There may be several advantages to aquatic exercise during pregnancy. Immersion to chest level increases buoyancy and the sensation of physical comfort, improves mobility, and utilizes both the flexor and extensor portions of muscle groups; and hydrostatic pressure changes increase venous blood return, thus decreasing dependent edema. Water-based exercise is also associated with decreased physical discomforts such as low-back pain and leg cramps and decreased psychological stress (Smith & Michel, 2006). The advantages of aquatic exercise might be greatest later in pregnancy when discomforts are most pronounced and the feelings of buoyancy are most welcomed.

Exercise guidelines

Zavorsky and Longo (2011a, 2011b) suggest guidelines for exercise intensity, addition of strength training, and caloric expenditure guidelines to current exercise recommendations for pregnant women. They suggest that interspersing periods of vigorous-intensity exercise near aerobic maximum throughout lower-intensity activity (commonly referred to as interval training) and including light weight training activity in the second and third trimester may further optimize maternal and fetal health beyond those achievable under the current recommendations without any negative impact of newborn size, weight, or health. Higher-intensity exercise may be most important for obese and overweight pregnant women who are at greater risk of maternal and fetal complications. The Borg rating of perceived exertion (RPE) is used to measure total exertion, overall exertion, and fatigue level of exercise (Fig. 15.2). Physical exertion

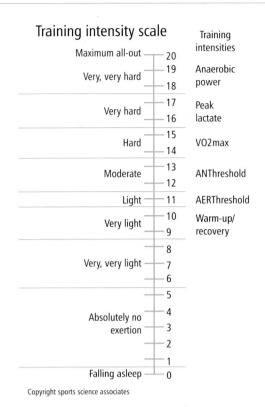

Figure 15.2.   Borg RPE. http://coachsci.sdsu.edu/csa/vol45/rushall.htm (permission received from Brent S. Rushall).

during pregnancy should be between 12–14 (somewhat hard or moderate activity) and 15–16 (hard or vigorous activity). The more vigorous the activity, the shorter the amount of time needed to achieve recommended weekly physical activity expenditure goals. Vigorous exercise reduces total exercise time by 60% compared to light exercise. Exercising at higher intensity for shorter periods of time is more beneficial than exercising at lower-intensity levels for long periods of time. This is especially true for overweight and obese women.

Interval-type exercise

For busy women who are often caring for other children, increased vigor traded for decreased total time may increase rates of achieving metabolic expenditure goals on a regular basis. In studies of exercise toleration, pregnant women who exercise vigorously have lower serum lactate levels and a decrease in postexercise oxygen consumption, which appears to aid in maintaining fetal well-being (Penney, 2008). Additionally, pregnancy does not affect a woman's capacity for prolonged exercise (Penney, 2008). While there appear to be advantages of vigorous exercise in pregnancy, there is a lack of randomized control trials with large enough study populations and special populations such as overweight and obese pregnant women. There are no established guidelines on vigorous exercise in pregnancy set forth by professional organizations. However, studies of interval training in older and health compromised populations have demonstrated efficacy and safety (Zavorsky & Longo, 2011a), suggesting no adverse risks for pregnant women.

Strength exercises

Adding light resistance strength training three times weekly for 35–40 minutes as part of total metabolic expenditure does not negatively affect newborn weight, and those who engage in strength training gained less weight in a randomized controlled trial of 160 pregnant women (Zavorsky & Longo, 2011a). Light strength training is defined as using 3 kg or smaller weights or resistance bands and no more than 10–12 repetitions per set. Although strength training has not been added specifically to exercise recommendations for pregnant women in the United States, Canadian guidelines recommend a combination of strength and aerobic

---

Guidelines for safe strength training in pregnancy

For pregnant women aged 18–45 years old, 8–10 muscle strength exercises can be performed over one to two sessions per week (nonconsecutive days). One aerobic training session can be replaced by a muscle strength training session in the weight room or at home.

Use Lighter Weights and More Repetitions
- Heavy weights may overload joints already loosened during pregnancy. Use lighter weights and do more repetitions instead. For example, if one usually performs leg presses with 10-lb weights for 8–12 reps, try 6 or 7 lb for 15–20 reps.

Use Resistance Bands, Not Free Weights
- Resistance bands are a safer alternative as free weights may hit the abdomen.

Avoid the Supine Position after 16–20 Weeks of Gestation
- An easy modification is to use an inclined bench rather than a flat bench.

Avoid the Valsalva maneuver
- Valsalva means forcefully exhaling without actually releasing air. This can result in a rapid increase in blood pressure and decrease blood flow to the fetus.

Avoid Walking Lunges
- These may increase the risk of pelvic and groin ligament strain.

Listen to Your Body
- If you feel muscle strain or extreme fatigue, modify your activity or decrease the frequency of the workouts. Pregnancy is not a time for heavy weight lifting.

Adapted from: Zavorsky and Longo (2011a).

---

training with the advice that adverse maternal and neonatal outcomes are not increased for women who exercise (Penny, 2009).

Women who engage in strenuous exercise and strength training should be advised to increase caloric intake more than the additional 300 kcal needed to cover increased metabolic needs in pregnancy. The additional amount of kilocalories will depend on the individual woman, her recommended weight gain for gestation, and her individual patterns of exercise.

General advice for exercising in pregnancy

Many women have concerns about the level of exertion that is safe while exercising. This concern can be exacerbated by the slight dyspnea related to normal physiological changes of pregnancy in the respiratory system, but they should not perceive substantial differences in exertion when exercising. Women can use several methods to assess cardiorespiratory exertion. The "talk test" is an easy method to employ. Women should be able to talk while exercising if they are exercising at an appropriate level. If carrying on a conversation while exercising is difficult due to fatigue and "losing their breath," the intensity is considered too high. They should trust how they feel and adjust accordingly. Recent research suggests a target heart rate of 145–160 beats per minute (bpm) for fit pregnant women between ages 20 and 29, and 140–156 bpm for women aged 30–39 (Avery, Jennings, Sherwood, Martinson, & Crane, 2008). Women at lower fitness levels can use a heart rate range of 129–144 bpm between ages 20 and 29, and 128–144 bpm for those aged 30–39. This correlates to 60–80% of aerobic capacity. Women can manually check their heart rate during exercise or use a heart rate monitor. Another guide to appropriate intensity is the Borg RPE scale, a rating scale from 6 to 20, with 6–7 being "very, very light" and 19–20 being "very, very hard." Exercising at 12–14 represents a "somewhat hard" level, which is a safe level of exertion for most pregnant women. Exercising above a Borg rating of 14 would typically be considered too high for pregnant women.

Strength training should be assessed individually. It is acceptable during pregnancy to use moderate resistance and multiple repetitions. It is suggested that exercise in the supine position be limited after 16–20 weeks' gestation to reduce the possibility of potential supine hypotension related to vena caval compression by the gravid uterus. Most women develop sufficient collateral circulation to prevent symptomatic hypotension. Abdominal exercises can be modified to prevent vena caval compression, but they should be discontinued if significant rectus diastasis develops. Exercises that may lead to

General advice for exercising in pregnancy

- Healthy pregnant women should exercise for 30 or more minutes at moderate-intensity exercise most days of the week.
- Women can anticipate feeling slightly short of breath during mild exercise related to normal respiratory changes during pregnancy.
- Use the "talk test" to monitor intensity. Women should be able to talk while exercising. If carrying on a conversation while exercising is difficult due to fatigue and "losing their breath," the intensity is considered too high.
- Exercise at 12–14 on the Borg RPE: Exercising above a Borg rating of 14 would typically be considered too high for pregnant women.
- Exercise at 60–80% of aerobic capacity: a target heart rate of 145–160 bpm for physically fit pregnant women between ages 20 and 29, and 140–156 bpm for women aged 30–39. Women at lower fitness levels can use a heart rate range of 129–144 bpm between ages 20 and 29, and 128–144 bpm for those aged 30–39.
- Prepregnancy exercise routines can be modified to adhere to the "somewhat hard" level by reducing frequency/intensity/duration.
- Women who do not regularly engage in exercise prior to pregnancy should begin walking 10 minutes four to five times weekly and gradually increase duration to 30 minutes at moderate exertion four or more times weekly.
- Avoid exercising in the fasting state and in very high heat and humid conditions.
- Adequate hydration during exercise is important. Check urine color and maintain light yellow or straw color to monitor hydration.
- Exercise in loose, comfortable clothing that allows heat dissipation and evaporation of sweat.
- Strength training using moderate resistance and multiple repetitions is acceptable during pregnancy for most women.
- Abdominal exercises should be discontinued if significant diastasis rectus develops.
- Exercise in the supine position should be limited after 16–20 weeks' gestation to reduce possible vena caval compression by the gravid uterus.
- Avoid exercise that may lead to falls, musculoskeletal injury, or abdominal trauma. Scuba diving is not recommended.
- Women should consume a healthy diet to maintain a normal rate and amount of weight gain during pregnancy.

Warning signs to stop exercising while pregnant

- Vaginal bleeding
- Dyspnea prior to exertion
- Dizziness
- Headache
- Chest pain
- Muscle weakness
- Calf pain or swelling of unknown origin
- Preterm labor
- Decreased fetal movement
- Ruptured membranes

Adapted from: Zavorsky and Longo (2011b).

Summary

Exercise before and after pregnancy is an essential tool to ameliorate pregnancy discomforts and to reduce the risks of serious obstetric complication such as GDM and hypertensive disorders. Ideally, women would enter pregnancy physically fit and maintain adequate physical activity throughout gestation. Although high prepregnancy BMI tends to blunt the reduction of risk, overweight and obese women may benefit the most from vigorous exercise. The addition of weight training may further enhance metabolic changes that promote energy utilization and discourage fat deposition. Although there is not one clearly superior method of counseling to promote adoption of healthy behaviors, the principles of TTM SOC provide a framework for clinicians to begin a conversation about exercise during pregnancy. Above all, reassure women that moderate exercise during normal pregnancy is safe, is healthy for her and her fetus, and encourage women to take a commonsense approach to exercise.

Environmental exposures in pregnancy

Since the industrial revolution, humans have been exposed to an increasing number of chemical and environmental substances, and most of the time, the exposure is unknown to us. Pregnancy is an especially vulnerable time with regard to toxic exposure. A growing fetus is very sensitive to drugs and chemicals, especially in the first trimester. All persons are exposed to a variety of chemical exposures on a daily basis in the home, workplace, and neighborhoods. For many toxicants, there is little empirical human data to demonstrate safety or adverse effects (Grason & Misra, 2009). Heavy metals such as lead and mercury, organic solvents, alcohol, and ionizing radiation are confirmed environmental teratogens, and exposure could contribute to pregnancy loss (Jain & Parviainen, 2012). All of these

musculoskeletal injury or abdominal trauma such as horseback riding and downhill skiing should be discontinued. Scuba diving is also not recommended. Women should be advised of symptoms or conditions in which exercise should be stopped.

substances are readily found in our environment, homes, food sources, and workplaces. Environmental toxins have been implicated in contributing to poor reproductive outcomes.

All employees face some workplace risks to their health. Pregnant women (including those who do not realize they are pregnant) are, however, at an even greater risk of harm not only to themselves, but also to their unborn child. Certain occupations and exposures are linked to specific adverse pregnancy outcomes. Efforts should be made to identify, eliminate, or reduce the risks associated with each pregnant employee's duties. The changing nature of employment has caused new workplace hazards for reproductive age women. While there are numerous workplace reproductive hazards, only a few apply to each individual employee. Thus, care should be taken not to raise undue fear or worry about the risks associated with work.

Toxins now pervade the ecosystem and it is impossible to eliminate all exposure. However, further data gathering, topic research, and client education are always essential when caring for a woman with substance exposure. Before definitive conclusions can be drawn regarding the teratogenicity of environmental exposures, several clinical factors need to be considered. These include gestational age at the time of exposure, the amount of toxin reaching the developing embryo/fetus, the duration of exposure, the impact of other factors or substances to which the mother or her fetus is simultaneously exposed, and the overall health of the mother and fetus.

Although there are methodological challenges to studying exposures and birth outcomes, evidence exists that air pollution, heavy metals, and pesticides may increase risks of low birth weight, intrauterine growth restriction, preterm birth, and birth defects. There is growing literature about the ubiquitous nature of endocrine disruptors including bisphenol A (BPA), phalates, and perchlorates (Grason & Misra, 2009). The poor, racial, and ethnic minorities are disproportionally exposed to air pollution such as lead-based paints indoors and particulate air pollution from living near busy highways or industrial facilities (Morello-Frosch, Zuk, Jerrett, Shamasunder, & Kyle, 2011). Living near a hazardous industrial waste site increases the risk of poor perinatal outcomes including low birth weight, spontaneous abortion, and prematurity (Morello-Frosch et al., 2011). However, the threshold for harm is often unknown (Grason & Misra, 2009). Some workplaces have special concerns such as hospitals, where ionizing radiation and exposure to chemotherapeutics pose special risks to health-care personnel (Alex, 2011; Chalupka & Chalupka, 2010; McDiarmid & Gehle, 2006).

Health-care providers are not well versed in the subject of environmental exposures (Grason & Misra, 2009; McDiarmid & Gehle, 2006). Moving from a strategy of risk awareness to implementing strategies to reduce maternal–fetal risk will provide actual benefit. Many environmental toxicants remain in tissues for some period of time after exposure (such as heavy metals stored in teeth and bones), making the preconception period the best time to identify toxicant exposures and to implement strategies to reduce exposure. The earliest weeks of pregnancy is when the fetus is most vulnerable to toxicant effects. The blood–brain barrier is not fully formed until about 6 months after birth, making the fetal brain especially vulnerable (Chalupka & Chalupka, 2010).

Making an environmental exposure assessment

Specific information about employment including tasks performed, chemicals in the environment (including metals and solvents), as well as other potential exposures should be obtained preconceptionally or at the first prenatal visit (Chalupka & Chalupka, 2010). The Environmental and Occupational Health History Profile can be used during the preconception period or at the first prenatal visit (Table 15.1). If substance exposure is noted, then further detailed history on route, timing, and duration of exposure is essential. Use of protective equipment such as gloves or masks should be noted. Many women may not know the names of chemicals used in their workplace. The Occupational Health and Safety Administration (OSHA) mandates that the names and health effects of all chemicals be available to workers on site via the material safety data sheet (MSDS). Women should be informed of their right to access MSDSs about any potential workplace toxicants and to access their employer's occupational health nurse about personal protective equipment and other environmental controls to reduce or eliminate exposures (Chalupka & Chalupka, 2010).

Metals and metalloids

Lead, cadmium, mercury, and arsenic are associated with adverse pregnancy outcomes. Exposures to heavy metals generally occur in industrial workplaces, but contaminated soil, air, and water can lead to environmental exposure as well (Red, Richards, Torres, & Adair, 2011). Animal studies have demonstrated that such metals cross the placenta, are terotogenic, and can cause fetal death. It is likely that similar effects can be observed in humans (Red et al., 2011).

Lead occurs naturally in the environment and has many industrial uses. Lead exposure occurs commonly

Table 15.1. Environmental and Occupational Health History

Please help us understand your home and work environment so we can provide better reproductive care to you. Please check the appropriate boxes below.

Present work
Please tell us where you work:

- Agriculture
- Beauty salon/nail salon
- Construction
- Dry cleaning
- Metal work
- Mining

- Education
- Health care
- Hospitality (hotel/restaurant)
- Hazardous waste
- Office/clerical
- Printing

- Pharmaceuticals
- Public safety
- Veterinary care
Other:
_____

Please explain your job to us:
_____

Potential workplace exposures
In your work, are you exposed to any of the following:

Biological agents
- Animal dander
- Bacteria
- Enzymes/proteins
- Endotoxin
- Fungi
- Protozoa
- Viruses
Other (specify): _____

Physical/psychological conditions
- High demand/low pay
- Prolonged standing/lifting
- Rotating shift work
- Strenuous work/musculoskeletal strain
- Other (specify): _____

Physical agents
- Cold
- Heat
- Ionizing radiation (X-rays)
- Lasers
- Loud noises
- Nonionizing radiation
- RF radiation/microwave
- Infrared radiation
- UV radiation
- Vibration
- Other:_____

Chemical agents
- Chemotherapeutics/pharmaceuticals
- Inorganic chemicals
- Metals
- Arsenic
- Lead
- Mercury
- Cadmium
- Beryllium
- Chromium
- Other (specify):_____

Environmental history

Home
- When was your home built?
- What type of heating do you have in your home?
- What chemicals are stored on your property?
- Where does your drinking water come from?
- If you have well water, is it tested annually? If so, for what?

Neighborhood
- Do you have any environmental concerns in your neighborhood?
- What type of industry or farm is near your home?
- Do you live near a hazardous waste site?

Hobbies/activities
- What are your hobbies?
- Do you garden?
- Do you burn, smelt, or solder any products?
- Do you eat what you catch and grow?
- Do you use alternative healing or healing practices involving lead or mercury?

Instructions for use: All questions answered in the affirmative should be followed up with questions to elicit specific information to quantify exposure. Quantitative information should include route of exposure (inhalation, dermal, ingestion), timing (relation of exposure to critical time windows), duration (of exposure, hours in work shift), and frequency (of exposures per shift/per week).

Adapted from: figure 1, "Environmental and Occupational Health History Profile," in Chalupka and Chalupka (2010).

in work environments that involve lead smelting, soldering, mining, welding, brass foundries, stained glass manufacture, construction and demolition, battery storage, printing, painting, shipping, and automobile manufacture (Red et al., 2011). Hobbies such as stained glass and ceramics involve lead. The most common route of exposure is through inhalation of lead dust. Environmental exposure can also occur through ingestion of contaminated foods or water. Lead poisoning is less common since leaded gasoline was banned in 1996. Lead paint remains a possible exposure source as does lead pipes in older homes (Morello-Frosch et al., 2011).

In high enough doses, prenatal exposure to lead is toxic to every organ system. Prenatal exposure can cause delayed development, reduced intelligence, and behavioral problems. Lead is stored in teeth and bones. It is theorized that mobilization of maternal calcium stores during pregnancy may increase lead levels in the blood. Prenatal lead exposure has been implicated in still birth, neonatal death, spontaneous abortion, and preterm birth.

Mercury is also a naturally occurring metal found in the air, water, and soil. Several occupations involve mercury exposure, including dentistry and manufacture of mercury containing lamps, lights, batteries, electrical equipment, catalysts, thermometers, thermostats, paints, and jewelry (Red et al., 2011). Individuals may also be exposed through use of skin-lightening creams produced in Mexico, and typically used by Hispanic women (Centers for Disease Control and Prevention (CDC), 2012a). Power plants are the largest industrial source of environmental mercury. Mercury emitted from power plant stacks falls in rain and snow onto the land and into water bodies around the power plants, thus contaminating fish. The most common route of human mercury is through ingestion of high-mercury fish such as shark, swordfish, and tilefish. Methylmercury crosses the placenta and can have adverse effects including mental deficit, blindness, deafness, cerebral palsy and language deficits (Red et al., 2011). High levels of exposure can cause maternal brain, heart, liver, and kidney damage.

Arsenic is a naturally occurring metalloid that combines oxygen, sulfur, and chlorine to form inorganic arsenic compounds. Occupations such as copper or lead smelting, wood treatment, and pesticide application can lead to exposure (Red et al., 2011). Additionally arsenic compounds are used extensively in poultry and swine feed for meat pigmentation, disease prevention, and growth promotion (Sutton et al., 2011). Arsenic crosses the placenta and cause fetal toxicity. Prenatal arsenic exposure at high levels is linked to fetal growth restriction, spontaneous abortion, still birth, and neonatal death (Red et al., 2011). Emerging data also suggest that early life exposure to arsenic in drinking water is associated with liver, lung, and kidney cancer in adults (Sutton et al., 2011).

Preventing exposure is the primary method of preventing heavy metal. Pregnant women and children should not be present in housing built before 1978 that is undergoing renovation. They should not participate in activities that disturb old paint or in cleaning up paint debris after work is completed. Women living in homes with lead pipes should be advised to only use cold water from the tap for cooking and drinking (CDC, 2012b). Lead is found in hot water heaters and municipal water lines. Women should be advised to let tap water run for 1 minute before using it if the water has not been turned on for more than 6 hours (Chalupka & Chalupka, 2010). Women should be cautioned not to expose themselves to mercury. If mercury is spilled in the home, another household member should clean it up. Mercury should never be vacuumed because it aerosolizes easily. Women who are pregnant or plan to become pregnant should eat fish for optimal fetal health, yet should be aware of local fishery advisories regarding mercury contamination and avoid eating tilefish, shark, king mackerel, and swordfish (see Chapter 6, "Nutrition during Pregnancy"). Women who live in areas with high arsenic concentrations in the water supply should be encouraged to use alternate water supplies or a reverse osmosis filter (CDC, 2010).

Heavy metal poisoning can be treated with chelating agents that prevent or reverse binding of heavy metals and enhance excretion, though fetal outcomes and safety have not been established in pregnancy (Red et al., 2011).

Organic solvents

Organic solvents such as benzene, toluene, hydrogen sulfide, carbon tetrachloride, aliphatic hydrocarbons, phenols, and phthalates are carbon-containing liquids that can dissolve or disperse other substances (Red et al., 2011). Organic solvents are found in some paints, varnishes, glues, and cleaning/degreasing agents, and in the production of dyes, printer inks, plastics, textiles, and agricultural products. Pregnant women may be more susceptible to organic solvents due to increased respiratory rate and oxygen consumption. Organic solvent exposure in the first 2 weeks after conception is linked to increased risk of spontaneous abortion (Red et al., 2011). Toluene is an organic solvent of special concern because of its potential to be used as a substance of abuse (Red et al., 2011). Women who abuse toluene-containing products such as paints, varnishes, lacquers, glues, and enamels have increased risks of preterm birth, perinatal death, and intrauterine growth restriction (Red et al., 2011).

Pesticides

Our industrialized food system is largely dependent on the application of petroleum-based pesticides and fertilizers (Sutton et al., 2011). Pesticide is a broad term that includes insecticides, fungicides, herbicides, rodenticides, and fumigants (Red et al., 2011). Many classes of compounds are used as pesticides. Examples include endocrine modulators, such as DDT, and organic synthetic compounds. Pesticides can spread beyond crops into the wider environment where they contaminate the air, water, and soil, and this exposure is ubiquitous among pregnant women. Exposure can come from home or commercial pesticide use, use on pets, and from residue on home or commercially grown produce. Review studies suggest an increased risk of fetal harm associated with pesticides in general and with maternal employment in agricultural industries (Jain & Parviainen, 2012). Exposure to pesticides in pregnancy has been shown to increase risk of poor prenatal growth, birth defects, leukemia, and impaired neurodevelopment. Pesticides act on the central nervous system and could affect a developing fetus. Forty percent of U.S. children have enough cumulative exposure to pesticides to potentially impact their brains and nervous systems (Sutton et al., 2011). Research documents that when children's diet change from conventional to organic food, pesticide levels decrease, thus indicating that a primary source of exposure is in the food supply (Sutton et al., 2011).

Organophosphates, such as parathion, malathion, and diazinon—all commonly found in home pesticides—are cholinesterase inhibitors. Malathion is a common organophosphate that is used to kill insects in agriculture, household gardens as well as lice, flea, and mosquito control. Malathion exposure among agricultural workers is associated with shortened gestation especially with increasing exposure late in pregnancy (Red et al., 2011). Animal studies show decreased fertility, increased miscarriage rates, and fetotoxicity (Morello-Frosch et al., 2011; Sutton et al., 2011). Carbamates, such as the popular home pesticide Sevin, are widely used insecticides that inhibit cholinesterases. At high doses, noted effects in animal studies included omphalocele, ventricular septal, and other structural anomalies. Women who work in agricultural industries and who garden should be advised to reduce exposure to pesticides, herbicides, and other agricultural chemicals.

Endocrine-disrupting chemicals

Endocrine-disrupting chemicals (EDCs) are defined as chemicals that either mimic or antagonize the effects of endogenous hormones in the endocrine system and consequently can cause adverse health effects that can be passed on to future generations (United States Environmental Protection Agency (EPA), 2011). EDCs include BPA and phthalates are commonly found in food containers. These chemicals can mimic or block the effects of naturally occurring hormones in the body. In some cases, the adverse health effects can be passed on to future generations. Prenatal exposure to phthalates is associated with changes in male reproductive anatomy and behavioral changes in young girls (Vandenberg, Hauser, Marcus, Olea, & Welshons, 2007). Animal studies suggest prenatal exposure to BPA is associated with obesity, reproductive abnormalities, and neurodevelopmental abnormalities in offspring. To reduce exposure, decrease consumption of processed and canned foods. Avoid the food- or drink-related use of plastics with recycling codes #3, #4, and #7.

Reducing exposures

A comprehensive approach is needed to meaningfully reduce perinatal exposure to environmental toxicants (Grason & Misra, 2009). The first step is to identify toxicants and their sources. Information on potential local toxicants present in communities should be used to help women and health-care providers learn about environmental hazards at work and at home. Many environmental toxicants are found in work settings. MSDSs are by law available for employees to review regarding workplace toxicants. Surprisingly, reproductive health information may not be included even for substances known to impact reproduction (Grason & Misra, 2009). The second step is to inform women about toxicant exposure and how to reduce exposure. Exposure reduction strategies depend on the toxicant and route of exposure. Some occupational exposures can be reduced with the use of personal protective equipment such as gloves and respirators. Other toxicants may require total avoidance as best as possible.

Quantifying the amount of an exposure is a much greater challenge than simple identification of an exposure. Consultation with an occupational medicine specialist is advised for those women who may have significant exposure. Women with acute exposures to toxic substances are best served by referral to the emergency department. All prenatal health-care providers need to be familiar with online toxicology resources to be able to quickly and accurately inform pregnant women about potential risks and to provide appropriate counsel to reduce risk during pregnancy. Sensitivity to the emotional issues raised in the inadvertent or unintentional exposure to potentially fetotoxic substances is essential. Keep in mind that much of the time, a known exposure may be brief—often,

Reducing adverse environmental exposures

- Follow Environmental Protection Agency (EPA) Guidelines on fish conception in pregnancy.
- Do not use skin-lightening creams or home remedies that might contain mercury.
- Recycle all mercury-containing thermometers.
- Wash fruits and vegetables with water and a brush when applicable. Soap is not needed.
- Remove outer leaves of leafy vegetables and discarded before washing.
- Choose organic fruits and vegetables when possible.
- Do not eat nonfood items such as dirt or clay.
- Avoid jobs or hobbies that may involve lead exposure.
- Avoid alternative cosmetics, food additives, and medicines imported from overseas.
- Avoid exposure to deteriorated lead-based paint in older homes.
- Have water tested if you suspect lead contamination from wells or solder in pipes.
- Use cold tap water instead of hot for drinking or cooking.
- Avoid the use of plastics with the recycling codes (often found on the outside bottom of containers) #3, #4, and #7 because they can contain phthalates and/or BPA.
- Eat more fresh food instead of canned or processed foods.
- Avoid rooms when removing old carpet because the padding may contain polybrominated diethyl ethers.

reassurance is an appropriate part of an appropriate plan of care.

Summary

The number of potential toxicants in the environment continues to grow. A disturbing body of research indicates that an increasing number of these toxicants can profoundly affect fetal growth and development. Assessment of possible exposures in the home and workplace during prenatal care is required to evaluate potential risks. Women need adequate information on potential exposures so they are able to avoid and reduce unnecessary exposures that can increase health risk.

Sexuality in pregnancy

Pregnancy is a time of profound and complex psychosocial examination and change. Sexual feelings and function are impacted by physical changes, hormonal changes, shifting roles, and relationships. The majority of research about patterns of sexual behavior during pregnancy demonstrates a decrease in frequency of

intercourse and sexual desire as pregnancy progresses (Bartellas, Crane, Daley, Bennett, & Hutchens, 2000; De Judicibus & McCabe, 2002; Foux, 2008; Fox, Gelber, & Chasen, 2008; Johnson, 2011; Trutnovsky, Haas, Lang, & Petru, 2006). Yet the topic of sexuality is not routinely addressed during antepartum care. Often when the subject is broached during prenatal care, it is to advise women to refrain from sexual activity (Murtagh, 2010). Health-care providers frequently cite lack of time and lack of confidence in dealing with issues of sexual health as reasons why they do not address it routinely in practice (Foux, 2008; Murtagh, 2010). Many women do not bring up questions about sexual health with providers because of embarrassment or fear of being judged. However, both men and women express a desire to be able to discuss these issues with their providers (Foux, 2008). Patterns of sexual behavior vary tremendously from woman to woman; thus, any evaluation of sexual dysfunction must take into account normal patterns for an individual woman. Sexual behavior changes may not need intervention unless it is accompanied by distress on the part of the woman: That which bothers only her partner is not considered a female sexual dysfunction (Murtagh, 2010).

Pregnancy influences on sexuality

Patterns of sexual behavior are profoundly influenced by physical symptoms of pregnancy. Sexual activity often declines during the first trimester due to the normal pregnancy symptoms of fatigue, sore breasts, emotional lability, and nausea. Fears of miscarriage can also decrease sexual desire. During the second trimester, women may find an increase in sexual desire as first-trimester discomforts cease, although this can be quite variable (Johnson, 2011). Women may report feeling more erotic and energetic, and fears of miscarriage may subside (Murtagh, 2010). Increased genital blood flow and lubrication may make orgasm easier to achieve (Foux, 2008; Murtagh, 2010). However, there is research that indicates the opposite as well and women may suffer from diminished clitoral sensation and inability to achieve orgasm (Johnson, 2011). During the third trimester, physical discomforts and the gravid abdomen may make traditional sex acts less appealing.

Regardless of the stage of pregnancy, most women report a decrease in sexual activity compared to patterns prior to pregnancy with the most pronounced decrease occurring in the third trimester. However, women report an increase in relationship satisfaction during pregnancy compared to prepregnancy. Few women report a complete loss of sexual desire or completely avoid sexual intercourse in the third trimester (De Judicibus & McCabe, 2002). Male partners may also experience sexual dysfunction during pregnancy including loss of libido, erectile dysfunction, and premature ejaculation (Johnson, 2011). Men also express reluctance to share fears about sex during pregnancy with their partners either out of shame for expressing vulnerability or not wanting to burden their partner during a vulnerable time (Foux, 2008). Although desire to engage in sexual acts may decrease, the desire for tenderness and nongenital physical contact remains unchanged or may increase.

Fear of fetal harm or pregnancy complications such as bleeding, ruptured membranes, and preterm labor likely plays a role in decreased sexual activity. However, research does not support an association between sexual activity and preterm birth (Yost et al., 2006). It is important for providers to dispel myths and to reassure women and their partners that the vast majority of couples can engage in sexual activity without fear of somehow harming the pregnancy. Few complications are contraindications to sexual activity. A pregnancy perceived as "at risk" can cause emotional distance in a relationship (Foux, 2008). For those women who do have contraindications to sex, advising that sex is not safe without providing education about alternatives to vaginal intercourse and ways to maintain intimacy can lead to sexual frustration (Faux).

Contraindications to sexual intercourse during pregnancy

Absolute contraindications	Relative contraindications
• Unexplained vaginal bleeding • Placenta previa • Premature cervical dilation • Premature rupture of membranes	• History of preterm birth • Multiple gestation

---

Sexual activities during pregnancy

Some types of sexual activity decrease during pregnancy, although kissing, fondling, and vaginal intercourse tend to remain stable (Johnson, 2011). Breast stimulation, cunnilingus, and self-stimulation decline. The decline in cunnilingus may be due to a fear of air embolism following oral-genital stimulation (Johnson, 2011). Positioning for sexual intercourse also changes over the course of pregnancy with face-to-face and man-on-top positions declining as gestation advances. Woman on top, side by side, on all fours, and rear entry are used more frequently and can be suggested to relieve discomfort and facilitate coitus (Johnson, 2011; Murtagh, 2010). Mutual masturbation may be an alternative to genital-to-genital contact as well.

Sexual history

Taking a sexual history can be brief or extensive. It can be accomplished while taking a review of systems or in a general health history (Murtagh, 2010). Important information to obtain includes assessment of the relationship (sexually and otherwise), her support network, whether the pregnancy was planned, outcomes of previous pregnancies, previous births (assess for physical or psychological trauma), health of living children, and contraceptive history (Johnson, 2011). Physical data may be needed for a complete picture of a woman's sexual practices. A trusting and comfortable environment as well as maintaining an attitude that normalizes sexual behavior and conveys a nonjudgmental attitude will facilitate disclosure. Women may disclose personal and sometimes traumatic experiences, and the provider must be prepared to handle disclosures of childhood sex abuse, rape, and domestic violence. Depending upon the issues uncovered, a referral to a specialist may be warranted.

Counseling

Adequate communication between women and their providers about sexual health is often lacking (Murtagh, 2010). Couples are often unaware of the changes in sexual function common in pregnancy, and they may not receive adequate anticipatory guidance or information from their health-care providers (see "Assessment of Prenatal Sexual Health and Prenatal Counseling"). Women may rely more on the advice and experiences of female friends (Johnson, 2011). Couples especially need

---

Assessment of prenatal sexual health and prenatal counseling

Initial assessment
- Assessment of current/past sexual relationship
- Explore woman/couple's support network
- Ascertain if the pregnancy was planned
- Outcomes of previous pregnancies
- Previous births (route, presence of trauma)
- Current children's health
- Contraception use (past and future)

Antepartum counseling
- Range of sexual changes that may be experienced during pregnancy
- Incorporation of safe sex practices, if appropriate
- Reassurance of the normalcy of a wide range of sexual expressions during pregnancy
- Exploration of different sexual positions and noncoital contact

to be aware of the reduction in sexual activity common in the third trimester and it should be communicated as a normal part of pregnancy and not pathology. Awareness of the normal decline in libido, desire, and orgasm frequency and intensity should also be discussed. Couples should be reassured that these changes will gradually recover over time postpartum. Alternatives to vaginal intercourse should be discussed and the importance of maintaining intimacy acknowledged. Nongenital contact can reinforce emotional intimacy, reinforce sexual health, and may help couples to explore new and satisfying ways of expressing sexuality (Johnson, 2011).

Summary

Prenatal health-care providers should include periodic assessment of sexual function and satisfaction into routine care practices. Many cultural myths surround sexuality in pregnancy. Women and couples should be encouraged to ask questions and discuss how normal pregnancy-related changes impact sexual relationships.

Working during pregnancy

Nearly three-quarters of pregnant women in the United States will continue to work outside the home until the last month of pregnancy (Pompeii, Savitz, Evenson, Rogers, & McMahon, 2005). Employment in general is associated with better pregnancy outcomes, but some components of work may pose potential risks for the mother and the fetus.

The effect of specific work tasks on pregnancy outcomes is a difficult phenomenon to study. Many occupational activities involve multidimensional mental and physical tasks rather than an isolated metric such as only standing or only lifting. It has also been noted that tasks such as standing and lifting have no standard definition making meta-analysis difficult. However, some conclusions can be made about the effects of specific work situations on pregnancy outcomes.

Shift work

There is a statistical association between adverse pregnancy outcomes and shift work, especially rotating shifts and working the night shift. Shift work has been implicated in suboptimal pregnancy outcomes including preterm birth and low birth weight (Alex, 2011; Croteau, Marcoux, & Brisson, 2007). Risks of preeclampsia may also increase with shift work, but the evidence is conflicting and few high-quality studies have examined it (Bonzini et al., 2011). The mechanisms that may contribute to poor pregnancy outcomes related to shift work are not completely understood. Disruption of the circadian rhythm, psychosocial stress, and disturbed sleep have been proposed (Bonzini et al., 2011). Shift work has a negative effect on several physiological pathways including neuroendocrine (disruptions in melatonin production), behavioral (stress response), immune, and vascular mechanisms (Bonzini et al., 2011).

Most studies to date do not indicate more than moderate risk of shift work alone as a contributing factor to small-for-gestational-age babies, but when combined with other environmental risks, the effects are compounded (Bonzini et al., 2011). There appears to be a small risk for preterm birth associated with shift work and it appears to be more pronounced for women's work schedules that do not change over the course of pregnancy (Bonzini et al., 2011). Significant associations for preterm birth associated with shift work are found in countries with restrictive prenatal leave policies and with few measures to protect pregnant workers rights (Bonzini, Coggon & Palmer, 2007; Vrijkotte, van der Wahl, Eijsden, & Bonsel, 2009). It is prudent to make reasonable workplace accommodation regarding reasonable workloads, opportunities to rest when fatigued, and reduced exposure to shift and night work.

Heavy lifting and long work hours

As an isolated risk factor, heavy lifting (defined as heavy or repetitive load carrying, lifting, manual labor, or significant exertion) is not a risk factor for growth restriction or preterm birth (Magann et al., 2005). Bending, squatting, and raising the arms above shoulder level for >3 h/day especially combined with moderate or poor social support is associated with preterm birth (Croteau et al., 2007).

Prolonged standing at work has been linked to an increased risk for preterm birth in some studies but not in others. A meta-analysis on long working hours (more than 40 hours weekly) demonstrated a modest to null association with small-for-gestational-age or preterm birth (Bonzini et al., 2007). Currently, uncertainty in the evidence does not make a compelling case for mandatory occupational restrictions in pregnancy. However, no benefit has been found by engaging in long working hours, heavy lifting, or prolonged standing. It is prudent to advise pregnant women to limit engagement in such activities especially in late pregnancy when fatigue is increased and joint laxity is more pronounced.

Fatigue associated with work outside the home as a potential cause of adverse perinatal outcome has also been examined. Little is known about the affects of fatigue associated with work inside the home. Fatigue has been linked to adverse health outcomes such as cardiovascular disease, metabolic syndrome, and depression in other populations (Okun et al., 2012). However, fatigue and sleep disturbances are common concerns during pregnancy and determining causality from a single variable is challenging. Many tools used to evaluate workplace fatigue have not been validated in pregnancy. Many items on these questionnaires are commonly experienced by pregnant women (e.g., backache and headache) or are symptomatic of other conditions like depression (body aches, anxiety, and inability to concentrate) (Chien & Ko, 2003).

There does appear to be evidence that lack of sleep or severely disturbed sleep may contribute to poor obstetric outcomes such as preterm birth and prolonged labor (Lee & Gay, 2004, Okun et al., 2012). Pregnant women should routinely be asked about their sleep habits, especially women reporting excessive fatigue. Sleeplessness is a risk factor for developing depression as well as a symptom of depression. Women who experience a lack of sleep (less than 7 hours nightly) or who are experiencing severe sleep disturbances (sleeping 6 or fewer total hours three or more times weekly resulting in impaired daytime functioning) should be screened for depression with a tool validated for pregnant women. Pregnant women should be advised to maintain good sleep practices to enhance rest. Women should be encouraged to sleep for 7 or 8 hours nightly. Women who wake up frequently should be encouraged to stay in bed and rest rather than get out of bed. Adjusting bed and wake times to facilitate adequate rest may also be suggested (Lee & Gay, 2004).

Noise exposure

Excessive noise exposure in the general population has been linked to hearing impairment, hypertension, heart disease, adverse work performance, and aggressive behavior (Magann et al., 2005). Noise exposure has been implicated with poor pregnancy outcomes especially when combined with shift work (Magann et al., 2005). Other investigators have found no link between excessive noise and poor pregnancy outcome (Magann et al., 2005). Except in the most extreme circumstances, it is highly unlikely that fetal hearing loss will occur *in utero* due to occupational noise exposure (Thurston & Roberts, 1991).

Psychosocial stress

Psychosocial stress has been thought to contribute to poor pregnancy outcomes such as preterm birth and low birth weight through several proposed mechanisms. Based on animal studies, it is thought to affect neuroendrocrine pathways and impair cellular immunity (Mutambudzi, Meyer, Warren, & Reisine, 2011). Additionally, women who experience psychosocial stress may be more likely to engage in unhealthy activities like drinking alcohol, smoking, skipping meals, entering care late in pregnancy, or attending prenatal care infrequently.

Research examining the relationship between stress and perinatal outcomes has been inconsistent due to how stress is defined and assessed.

A meta-analysis assessing 31,323 women found a small but significant association between psychosocial stress during pregnancy and lower birth weight (Littleton, Bye, Buck, & Amacker, 2010). A greater negative perinatal affect from major life stressors such as death or divorce was found than with other types of stress and women of ethnic minorities experience a greater negative affect from major life stressors, demonstrating a stronger correlation between stress and negative perinatal outcomes than white women. Life stress and emotional symptoms such as anxiety are associated with a shorter length of gestation (Tegethoff, Greene, Olsen, Meyer, & Meinlschmidt, 2010). Psychosocial stress as a lone risk factor has a negligible impact on pregnancy and it likely needs to be of severe intensity to affect perinatal outcomes.

Although there are no strong correlations between workplace stress and poor birth outcomes, several associated factors seem to compound workplace stress and to increase the risk of poor pregnancy outcomes. Poor social support and a perception of little control in the work environment are both associated with preterm birth and low birth weight. High-demand work alone does not pose a risk in pregnancy and workplace stress shows only a moderate impact on pregnancy outcomes. However, much more quality research needs to be done before any firm conclusions can be made.

Pregnancy discrimination in the workplace

In 1978, the Pregnancy Discrimination Act was enacted to protect pregnant women who have increasingly chosen to work while pregnant. Pregnancy discrimination in the form of layoff, firing, or denial of time off has continued and discrimination charges have increased despite legislation (Equal Employment Opportunity Commission, 2013). When discussing work during pregnancy, the woman's plan for continued employment during and after pregnancy and her plans for time off with her newborn should be evaluated. This can provide an opportunity to facilitate information about her rights regarding pregnancy and the workplace and maternity leave.

Data gathering and counseling

During an occupational assessment at the first prenatal visit, the types of activities performed and the number of hours worked should be determined. Her feelings about her work should be assessed. Does she have adequate social support to engage in work outside the home (transportation, childcare, etc.)? Does she see herself as a valued and autonomous employee? Does she have control over her work environment? Women with low social support can be directed to community services to help with transportation and childcare. Many employers also have employee stress reduction and assistance programs as well. Women in extremely physically demanding jobs should be encouraged to modify their work as pregnancy progresses. In many cases, it may be prudent for health-care providers to provide a pregnancy disability for women who perform certain tasks or to modify working hours. Examples would be restricting the work week to 40 hours and shift length to 8 hours as well as avoiding repetitive motions if musculoskeletal overuse injury is a concern. Using validated antenatal depression tools such as the Edinburgh Postpartum Depression Scale in women with low levels of control in their work environments or who present with psychosomatic complaints such as disturbed sleep may also be useful to identify women at risk for poor obstetric outcomes.

Summary

Occupational activities can affect a woman's health during pregnancy and should be evaluated at the first prenatal visit. A complete assessment is essential to determine perinatal risk in the workplace. Work responsibilities should be modified to accommodate a woman's changing physical abilities as needed and to promote adequate rest during the last part of pregnancy. Women should be encouraged to avoid extreme and ongoing fatigue during pregnancy. Measures to address work-related stress should be explored as indicated. Women should be aware of their employer policies regarding maternity and disability leaves and also be familiar with federal laws on pregnant women and work.

Resources on pregnancy and environmental exposure for women

American College of Obstetricians and Gynecologists Basic information about common exposures, particularly in the workplace. The Web site includes message boards and blogs for women to post and respond to questions: http://www.acog.org/For%20Patients.aspx

March of Dimes Birth Defects Foundation provides fact sheets, brochures, and an exposure screening checklist: http://www.marchofdimes.com/pnhec/159.asp

National Institute of Environmental Health Sciences (NIEHS), HHS, maintains ToxTown, a Web site with an interactive tool for the general public to learn about toxic chemical and environmental health risks. Some information included about risks to pregnant women is available: http://www.toxtown.nlm.nih.gov

National Institute of Occupational Safety and Health (NIOSH) conducts research and makes recommendations on preventing work-related injury and illness. Specific information about reproductive health and work for pregnant women is available: http://www.cdc.gov/niosh

National Institutes of Health (NIH) provides a Household Product Database: http://www.hpd.nlm.nih.gov

Women's Voices for the Earth is a grassroots environmental health and justice organization. Reports and fact sheets with specific information on risks of household products and exposures are available: http://www.womenandenvironment.org

Resources on pregnancy and environmental exposure for health-care providers

Food and Drug Administration, Health and Human Services (HHS), provides fact sheets on pregnancy and medicines, infections, and food safety. The Web site allows users to research the safety and effectiveness of medications that might be used during pregnancy: http://www.fda.gov/womens/healthinformation/pregnancy.html

Motherisk provides a telephone helpline to answer questions about pregnancy exposures. Links to peer-reviewed articles about environmental exposures and child health are available: http://www.motherisk.org

National Library of Medicine TOXNET provides information on many toxic substances: http://www.toxnet.nlm.nih.gov

NIEHS provides Links to NIEHS studies regarding reproductive health: http://www.niehs.nih.gov/oc/factsheets/pregnant/home.htm

Organization of Teratology Information Specialists (OTIS) provides fact sheets in English and Spanish on a variety of common exposures: http://www.otispregnancy.org

Resource on work during pregnancy for women

The U.S. Equal Employment Opportunity Commission (EEOC) provides information to pregnant women and employers on nondiscrimination during pregnancy: http://www.eeoc.gov/laws/types/pregnancy.cfm

References

Alex, M. (2011). Occupational hazards for pregnant nurses: Finding a balance between service and safety. *The American Journal of Nursing, 111*(1), 28–37.

American College of Obstetricians and Gynecologists (ACOG). (2002). Exercise during pregnancy and the postpartum period. ACOG committee opinion no. 267. *Obstetrics and Gynecology, 99,* 171–173.

Avery, M., Jennings, E., Sherwood, N., Martinson, B., & Crane, L. (2008). Effects of exercise during pregnancy on maternal outcomes: Implications for practice. *American Journal of Lifestyle Medicine, 2*(5), 441–455. Retrieved from http://www.medscape.com/viewarticle/580466

Barakat, R., Pelaez, M., Montejo, R., Luaces, M., & Zakynthinaki, M. (2011). Exercise during pregnancy improves maternal health perception: A randomized control trial. *American Journal of Obstetrics and Gynecology, 204*(402), e1–e7. doi:10.1016/j.ajog.2011.01.043

Bartellas, E., Crane, J., Daley, M., Bennett, K., & Hutchens, D. (2000). Sexuality and sexual activity in pregnancy. *BJOG: An International Journal of Obstetrics and Gynaecology, 107,* 964–968.

Blackburn, S. (2013). *Maternal, fetal and neonatal physiology: A clinical perspective.* Maryland Height, MO: Elsevier.

Bonzini, M., Coggon, D., & Palmer, K. (2007). Risk of prematurity, low birth weight and pre-eclampsia in relation to work hours and physical activities: A systematic review. *Occupational and Environmental Medicine, 64,* 228–243. doi:10.1136/oem.2006.026872

Bonzini, M., Palmer, K., Coggon, D., Carungo, M., Cromi, A., & Ferrario, M. (2011). Shift work and pregnancy outcomes: A systematic review with meta-analysis of currently available epidemiological studies. *BJOG: An International Journal of Obstetrics and Gynaecology, 118,* 1429–1437. doi:10.1111/j.1471-0528.2011.03066.x

Centers for Disease Control and Prevention (CDC). (2012a). Mercury exposure among household users and nonusers of skin-lightening creams produced in Mexico—California and Virginia, 2010. *Morbidity and Mortality Weekly Report (MMWR), 61*(02), 33–36, January 20, 2012. Retrieved from http://www.cdc.gov/mmwr/preview/mmwrhtml/mm6102a3.htm

Centers for Disease Control and Prevention (CDC). (2012b). Basic information about lead in drinking water. Retrieved from http://water.epa.gov/drink/contaminants/basicinformation/lead.cfm

Chalupka, S., & Chalupka, A. (2010). The impact of environmental and occupational exposures on reproductive health. *Journal of Obstetric, Gynecologic, and Neonatal Nursing, 39,* 84–102. doi:10.1111/j.1552-6909.2009.01091.x

Chien, L., & Ko, Y. (2003). Fatigue during pregnancy predicts cesarean deliveries. *Journal of Advanced Nursing, 45*(5), 487–494.

Croteau, A., Marcoux, S., & Brisson, C. (2007). Work activity in pregnancy, preventive measures, and the risk of preterm delivery. *American Journal of Epidemiology, 166*(8), 951–965. doi:10.1093/aje/kwm171

De Judicibus, M., & McCabe, M. (2002). Psychological factors and the sexuality of pregnant and postpartum women. *Journal of Sex Research, 39*(2), 94–103.

Equal Employment Opportunity Commission. (2013). Pregnancy discrimination charges: EEOC & FEPAs combined: FY 1997-FY 2011. Retrieved from http://www.eeoc.gov/eeoc/statistics/enforcement/pregnancy.cfm

Evenson, K., & Wen, F. (2011). Prevalence and correlates of objectively measured physical activity and sedentary behavior among U.S. pregnant women. *Preventive Medicine, 53,* 39–43. doi:10.1016/j.ypmed.2011.04.014

Forouhari, S., Yazdanpanahi, Z., Parsanezhad, M., & Ragain-Shirazi, M. (2009). The effects of regular exercise on pregnancy outcomes. *Irainan Red Crescent Medical Journal, 12*(1), 57–60.

Foux, R. (2008). Sex education in pregnancy: Does it exist? A literature review. *Sexual and Relationship Therapy, 23*(3), 271–277. doi:10.1080/14681990802226133

Fox, N., Gelber, S., & Chasen, S. (2008). Physical and sexual activity during pregnancy and near delivery. *Journal of Women's Health, 17*(9), 1431–1435. doi:10.1089/jwh.2007.0730

Foxcroft, K. F., Rowlands, I. J., Byrne, N. M., McIntyre, H. D., & Callaway, L. K. (2011). Exercise in obese pregnant women: The role of social factors, lifestyle and pregnancy symptoms. *BMC Pregnancy and Childbirth, 11*(1), 4.

Gaston, A., & Cramp, A. (2011). Exercise during pregnancy: A review of patterns and determinants. *Journal of Science and Medicine in Sport, 14,* 299–305. doi:10.1016/j.jsams.2011.02.006

Grason, H., & Misra, D. (2009). Reducing exposure to environmental toxicants before birth: Moving from risk perception to risk reduction. *Public Health Reports, 124,* 629–641.

Jain, V., & Parviainen, E. K. (2012) Psychosocial and environmental pregnancy risks. eMedicine from WebMD. Updated July 2, 2012. Retrieved from http://emedicine.medscape.com/article/259346-overview

Johnson, C. (2011). Sexual health during pregnancy and the postpartum. *The Journal of Sexual Medicine, 8,* 1267–1284. doi:10.1111/j.1743-6109.2011.02223.x

Lee, K., & Gay, C. (2004). Sleep in late pregnancy predicts length of labor and type of delivery. *American Journal of Obstetrics and Gynecology, 191,* 2041–2046. doi:10.1016/j.acog.2004.05.086

Lewis, B., Martinson, B., Sherwood, N., & Avery, M. (2011). A pilot study evaluating a telephone-based exercise intervention for pregnant and postpartum women. *Journal of Midwifery and Women's Health, 56,* 127–131. doi:10.1111/j.1542-2011.2010.00016.x

Littleton, H., Bye, K., Buck, K., & Amacker, A. (2010). Psychosocial stress during pregnancy and pregnancy outcomes: A meta-analytic review. *Journal of Psychosomatic Obstetrics and Gynaecology, 31*(4), 219–228. doi:10.3109/0167482X

Magann, E., Evans, S., Chauhan, S., Nolan, T., Henderson, J., Klausen, J., . . . Morrison, J. (2005). The effects of standing, lifting and noise exposure on preterm birth, growth restriction, and perinatal death in healthy low-risk working military women. *The Journal of Maternal-Fetal and Neonatal Medicine, 18*(3), 155–162. doi:10.1080/14767050500224810

Martin, C. L., & Brunner Huber, L. R. (2010). Physical activity and hypertensive complications during pregnancy: Findings from 2004 to 2006 North Carolina Pregnancy Risk Assessment Monitoring System. *Birth, 37*(3), 202–210.

McDiarmid, M., & Gehle, K. (2006). Preconception brief: Occupational/environmental exposures. *Maternal and Child Health Journal, 10,* S123–S128. doi:10.1007/s10995-006-0089-8

Morello-Frosch, R., Zuk, M., Jerrett, M., Shamasunder, B., & Kyle, A. (2011). Understanding the cumulative impacts of inequalities in environmental health: Implications for policy. *Health Affairs, 30*(5), 879–887. doi:10.1377/hlthaff.2011.0153

Murtagh, J. (2010). Female sexual function, dysfunction and pregnancy: Implications for practice. *Journal of Midwifery and Women's Health, 55*(5), 438–466. doi:10.1016/j.jmwh.2009.12.006

Mutambudzi, M., Meyer, J., Warren, N., & Reisine, S. (2011). Effects of psychosocial characteristics of work on pregnancy outcomes: A critical review. *Women and Health, 51,* 279–297. doi:10.1080/03630242.2011.560242

Okun, M., Luther, J., Wisniewski, S., Sit, D., Prairie, B., & Wisner, K. (2012). Disturbed sleep, a novel risk factor for preterm birth? *Journal of Women's Health, 21*(1), 54–60. doi:10.1089/jwh.2010.2670

Olson, G., & Blackwell, S. (2011). Optimization of gestational weight gain in the obese gravida: A review. *Obstetrics and Gynecology Clinics of North America, 38,* 397–407. doi:10.1016/j.ogc.2011.03.003

Penney, D. (2008). The effect of vigorous exercise during pregnancy. *Journal of Midwifery and Women's Health, 53*, 155–159. doi:10.1016/j.jmwh.2007.12.003

Phelan, S., Phipps, M., Abrams, B., Darroch, F., Schaffner, A., & Wing, R. (2011). Randomized trial of a behavioral intervention to prevent excessive gestational weight gain: The fit for delivery study. *The American Journal of Clinical Nutrition, 93*, 772–779. doi:10.3945/ajcn.110.005306

Pompeii, L., Savitz, D., Evenson, K., Rogers, B., & McMahon, M. (2005). Physical exertion at work and the risk of preterm birth and small for gestational age birth. *Obstetrics and Gynecology, 106*(6), 1279–1288.

Prochaska, J. (2008). Decision making in the transtheoretical model of behavior change. *Medical Decision Making, 28*, 845–849. doi:10.1177/0272989X08327068

Red, B., Richards, S., Torres, C., & Adair, C. (2011). Environmental toxicant exposure during pregnancy. *Obstetrical and Gynecological Survey, 66*(3), 159–169. Retrieved from http://www.obgynsurvey.com

Smith, M., & Michel, Y. (2006). A pilot study on the effects of aquatic exercises on discomforts of pregnancy. *Journal of Obstetric, Gynecologic, and Neonatal Nursing, 35*, 315–323. doi:10.1111/j.1552-6909.2006.00045x

Sutton, P., Wallinga, D., Perron, J., Gottlieb, M., Sayre, L., & Woodruff, T. (2011). Reproductive health and the industrialized food system: A point of intervention for health policy. *Health Affairs, 30*(5), 888–897. doi:10.1377/hlthaff.2010.1255

Tegethoff, M., Greene, N., Olsen, J., Meyer, A. H., & Meinlschmidt, G. (2010). Maternal psychosocial adversity during pregnancy is associated with length of gestation and offspring size at birth: Evidence from a population-based cohort study. *Psychosomatic Medicine, 72*(4), 419–426.

Thurston, F., & Roberts, S. (1991). Environmental noise and fetal hearing. *Journal of the Tennessee Medical Association, 84*(1), 9–12.

Trutnovsky, G., Haas, J., Lang, U., & Petru, E. (2006). Woman's perception of sexuality during pregnancy and after birth. *The Australian and New Zealand Journal of Obstetrics and Gynaecology, 46*, 282–287. doi:10.1111/j.1479-828X.2006.00592.x

Tuah, N., Amiel, C., Qureshi, S., Car, J., Kaur, B., & Majeed, A. (2011). Transtheoretical model for dietary and physical exercise modification in weight loss management for overweight and obese adults. *Cochrane Database of Systematic Reviews, 10*. doi:10.1002/14651858.CD008066.pub2

United States Environmental Protection Agency (EPA). (2011). What are endocrine disruptors? Retrieved from http://www.epa.gov/endo/pubs/edspoverview/whatare.htm

U.S. Centers for Disease Control and Prevention (CDC). (2010). Arsenic and drinking water from private wells. Retrieved from http://www.cdc.gov/healthywater/drinking/private/wells/disease/arsenic.html

Vandenberg, L. N., Hauser, R., Marcus, M., Olea, N., & Welshons, W. V. (2007). Human exposure to bisphenol A (BPA). *Reproductive Toxicology (Elmsford, N.Y.), 24*(2), 139–177.

Vrijkotte, T., van der Wahl, M., Eijsden, M., & Bonsel, G. (2009). First trimester working conditions and birthweight: A prospective cohort study. *American Journal of Public Health, 99*(8), 1409–1416.

Yost, N., Owen, J., Berghella, V., Thom, E., Swain, M., Dildy, G., . . . Langer, O. (2006). Effect of coitus on preterm birth. *Obstetrics and Gynecology, 107*(4), 793–796.

Zavorsky, G., & Longo, L. (2011a). Adding strength training, exercise intensity, and caloric expenditure to exercise guidelines in pregnancy. *Obstetrics and Gynecology, 117*(6), 1399–1402. doi:10.1097/AOG.0b013e31821b1f5a

Zavorsky, G., & Longo, L. (2011b). Exercise guidelines in pregnancy. *Sports Medicine (Auckland, N.Z.), 41*(51), 345–360. doi:0112-1642/11/0005.1045/s49.95/0

16

Psychosocial adaptations in pregnancy

Cindy L. Farley

Relevant terms

Adaptation—the process of making necessary accommodations to changing circumstances while maintaining a coherent identity

Affective state—a range of feeling conditions that includes motives, attitudes, moods, and emotions

Anxiety—a state of uneasiness and apprehension about a real or imagined threat

Attachment—a lasting psychological connectedness between human beings (Bowlby, 1978)

Attitude—a relatively enduring organization of beliefs, feelings, and behavioral tendencies toward socially significant objects, groups, events, or symbols (Hogg & Vaughan, 2009)

Body Image—a subjective awareness and attitude toward one's body and its parts that may or may not correspond to objective measures

Cognition—processes of knowing, including attending, remembering, and reasoning; also the content of the processes, such as schemas, concepts, and memories (Gerrig & Zimbardo, 2002)

Coping—the process of dealing with internal or external demands that are perceived to be threatening or overwhelming (Gerrig & Zimbardo, 2002)

Culture—the sum total of ideas, beliefs, values, material goods and tools, and nonmaterial aspects that individuals make as members of a society

Emotion—a perception of a stimulus that results in a physiological reaction interpreted by the individual as a particular feeling or affective state (Cacioppo, Tassinary, & Berntson, 2007)

Expectation—a strong belief that something will happen or be the case in the future

Family—a social group traditionally composed of two parents and their biological children with the primary function of raising children to the age of maturity; variations of this definition are emerging in contemporary society

Fear—a psychophysiological response to a perceived threat that is consciously recognized as danger

Pain—a complex and subjective interaction of multiple physiological and psychological factors on an individual's interpretation of noxious stimuli

Perception—cognitive processes that organize sensory information and interpret its meaning

Psychophysiology—the study of cognitive, emotional, and behavioral phenomenon as related to and revealed through physiological processes and events (Cacioppo et al., 2007)

Role—a pattern of expected behaviors associated with a particular position or status in a social system

Self-efficacy (confidence)—a dynamic cognitive process involving an individual's beliefs regarding personal capabilities to undertake and successfully complete a stressful task (Bandura, 1977)

Self-esteem—a person's overall evaluation or appraisal of self-worth

Sexuality—how people experience and express themselves as sexual beings

Social systems—two or more individuals interacting within a structured situation with a common focus or foci

Stress—an adverse reaction an individual has to perceived pressure, demands, or challenging tasks

---

Prenatal and Postnatal Care: A Woman-Centered Approach, First Edition. Edited by Robin G. Jordan, Janet L. Engstrom, Julie A. Marfell, and Cindy L. Farley.

Introduction

Pregnancy, labor, and birth are psychophysiological processes embedded in a sociocultural context. Many profound changes occur within the individual woman and within her family structure during the childbearing year. These changes call for an approach to care that is concerned with more than just screening for pathology. These changes call for an approach to care that is based on a relationship of trust and mutual respect between care providers and the women they serve, and a provision of services that address psychological, social, and spiritual needs in addition to biological needs.

Prenatal care offers a unique opportunity to get to know a woman and her family over time. Beyond meeting the woman's physical needs, the health-care provider will work in the context of a developing relationship to support the pregnant woman to "achieve her own goals and hopes for her pregnancy, birth, and baby, and for her role as mother" (Rooks, 1997, p. 2). In addition to assessing the growth of the fundus and the development of the fetus at each visit, assessment of the changes and development in maternal and family psychosocial attachment and adaptation processes must occur as well. Providers of prenatal care seek not only safe passage through pregnancy, labor, and birth for mother and baby, but also the promotion of psychological health and resiliency that will assist the woman in facing the challenges of the long process of raising her newborn child to maturity.

Time spent in relating is an essential element of the development of a relationship. While rapport (an affinity or sympathetic understanding) with a woman can be developed in the early minutes of a first meeting, developing a therapeutic relationship of mutuality and trust takes time—time to listen to and honor a woman's life stories, time to respond with support and acceptance, and time to reconvene, reconnect, and follow up on previous conversations.

In order to actualize relationship-based care, it is important to deliberately structure generous amounts of time for initial and return prenatal visits and to provide continuity of care with the same clinician or set of clinicians to foster the development of a therapeutic relationship. It is an ongoing struggle to allow for unhurried client encounters in an era of productivity measures applied to health care. Productivity tends to be defined as seeing a certain number of clients in a truncated amount of time. Effective, high-quality, humanistic prenatal care requires focus and engagement in the moment with the woman who is in front of you now.

Maternal attachment and adaptation

The attachments we form with a small circle of family and friends give meaning and direction to our lives. Joys, sorrows, triumphs, and challenges are shared; information and tangible aids are given and received through these important social relationships. Mental and physical health processes and outcomes are mediated by psychosocial connections. Perhaps no single relationship in a life is as important as the bond between mother and child in setting the stage for later life. Maternal–infant bonding has its roots in the mother's early life experiences and circumstances surrounding the current pregnancy. Attachment to the fetus and adaptation of the woman, her partner, and her family during pregnancy are processes that can be evaluated by the prenatal care provider. Interventions, education, support, and referrals can be made to ameliorate problems and to promote psychosocial health.

Maternal adaptation to the pregnancy and attachment to the fetus are critical to the survival of the newly born baby and to the ongoing health of the mother. Healthy maternal adaptation and attachment are evidenced by the mother's physical caretaking and emotional attentiveness to her baby's needs (Scharfe, 2012); this is enacted during pregnancy as self-care measures, such as avoiding alcohol and eating a nutritious diet. Emotional attentiveness may manifest in other behaviors, such as giving the fetus a nickname, talking to the fetus, and playing music for the fetus. Failure to adapt and attach can lead to a variety of disorders after birth; for the mother, these can include postpartum depression, detached parenting, abusive parenting, social isolation, and deterioration of self-care practices; for the baby, these can include failure to thrive without organic cause, battering, and the inability to form social bonds with others (O'Connor & Zeanah, 2003).

Pregnancy as a transitional event in the life of the woman and her family has been conceptualized from two overarching psychosocial perspectives: (1) pregnancy as a crisis and (2) pregnancy as a developmental life phase (Sherwen, 1987). Each perspective informs theoretical relationships and care strategies. Paradoxically, both perspectives may operate jointly or alternately in the individual woman's experience of pregnancy. For the prenatal care provider, conceptual frameworks, philosophical tenets, and approaches to care logically follow from each perspective. Therefore, each perspective will be considered here.

The word crisis derives from the Greek and literally translates "to decide" (Merriam Webster Online Dictionary, 2012). While the word typically is used to express more negative connotations of disaster or the likelihood of a poor outcome, it has also been interpreted as a turning point or opportunity. A crisis is said to occur whenever an event or circumstance disrupts normal functioning or perspectives. The individual enters a state of disequilibrium and must find new methods of problem solving in order to reach an altered yet effective state of functioning. Pregnancy can be considered a crisis as it necessitates physical and psychosocial adjustments in functioning and perspectives by the woman and her family. Whether a crisis is resolved in a positive or negative manner depends on such factors as the meaning of the crisis to the individual, the experience and resources available to deal with the crisis, and the resiliency of the individual and the individual's support systems.

Pregnancy has also been conceptualized as a developmental phase or challenge (Lederman, 1984, 1996; Lederman & Weis, 2009). In this world view, pregnancy is seen as a maturational stage that most women will experience in their lives. It is estimated that 80% of adult American women will become biological mothers, while 10% will voluntarily choose childlessness and the remaining 10% will struggle with infertility (Livingston & Cohn, 2010). The changes inherent in this developmental phase are tasks that must be mastered in order to move to a new level of functioning. A developmental phase can lead to growth or decline in individual or family functioning. Importantly, in either paradigm of pregnancy, the woman and her family are open to the services and ministrations of a professional to assist them in this process of transition and change.

Bowlby and Ainsworth

A number of theoreticians have contributed to modern understandings of maternal psychosocial attachment and adaptation in the childbearing year and will be mentioned here (Bowlby, 1978; Brazelton, 1973; Kennell & Klaus, 1976; Lederman, 1984; Rubin, 1984). John Bowlby, a British psychoanalyst, described attachment theory from his observations working with maladapted adolescents (Bowlby, 1978). He noted that the presence of the mother or a primary caretaker was a key variable in healthy personality development for an individual. His premise is that the mother and the infant are biologically preprogrammed to form a strong attachment relationship, but their roles are different. The baby's role is to lead the relationship through behavioral cues and the mother's role is to respond to these cues in a timely and sensitive manner. Infant behavior, such as cooing and crying, is designed to attain and maintain proximity to the mother.

Mary Ainsworth was a protégé and colleague of John Bowlby. She created a psychological tool to explore infant attachment called the strange situation. A mother and her infant were brought into a room with a stranger. After several minutes, the mother unobtrusively exited the room. The infant's behavior upon recognition of the absence of the mother was observed and was considered a reflection of the degree of attachment. This test is still used in research in the area of attachment psychology. Bowlby and his associates focused more on delineating infant behaviors; their work served as a foundation for Kennell and Klaus in their development of a theory of maternal–infant bonding that revolutionized thinking about prenatal and birth practices in America in the 1970s and beyond (Kennell & Klaus, 1976; Kennell, Klaus, & Klaus, 1995).

Kennell and Klaus

Marshall Kennell and John Klaus, physicians in neonatal intensive care units, noted that premature babies who spent extended periods of separation from their mothers from birth would graduate from the nursery to the home environment, presumably healthy and growing (Kennell & Klaus, 1976; Kennell et al., 1995). And yet a disproportionate number of these children would return to the emergency department, victims of abuse or nonorganic failure to thrive. Upon further investigation by these physicians, it was found that the mothers were emotionally detached from these fragile infants due to fear that they would die. In the early days of neonatal intensive care nurseries, limited to no contact was afforded to mothers. Upon discharge, these mothers harbored feelings that their babies did not belong to them and were not long for the world. The mothers also had no authentic skills in handling or providing care for their babies and therefore had no confidence that they could nurture their babies. Their lack of mothering skills and emotional stamina during this transition led to conditions under which their infants did not grow and develop properly.

Kennell and Klaus (1976) began to examine neonatal intensive care practices that exacerbated this emotional disconnect for mothers, which led to investigation of birth practices for both preterm and term infants. These investigations were foundational in adding to our knowledge of the bonding process from the perspective of the mother's behaviors toward the infant. Kennell and Klaus observed births in Guatemala in environments where the laboring woman was continuously attended by a female support person and where the baby was never separated from its mother. They found that both the mother and the baby are in a special sensitive period immediately postbirth in which postpartum physiology and prolonged physical contact lead to profound connections between the mother and the neonate.

Mothers follow a specific and universal pattern of behavior in becoming acquainted with their newborn (Kennell & Klaus, 1976). Mothers tend to touch with fingertips first starting at the face, followed by gentle rubbing motion using the palms. They will align their face with their baby's face in the en face position to establish eye contact and for full visual exploration of their newborn. A high-pitched voice is used as they softly speak to their newborn. Maternal behavior such as this tends to elicit satisfying responses from the baby, which in turn stimulates release of oxytocin and prolactin in the mother and affirms her mothering skills, leading to beneficial health effects for postpartum recovery. Postbirth bonding processes are important to review in the prenatal period with the mother as some birth routines persist that do not honor the reciprocal interaction of the mother and the baby (Mercer, 1985).

Prenatal preparation for postbirth bonding

1. Obtain the services of providers whose labor and birth practices are woman-centered and baby friendly.
2. Attend childbirth education classes.
3. Articulate preferences for the conduct of labor, birth, and immediate postpartum in a written birth plan.
4. Arrange for continuous labor support with sensitive family, friends, a doula or a midwife.
5. Have baby placed skin to skin with mother immediately postbirth and leave undisturbed for a prolonged period of time.
6. Delay nonurgent procedures, such as cord clamping, newborn measurements, and eye prophylaxis.
7. Allow generous amounts of time for the baby to breastfeed and interact with the family.

Brazelton

The contribution of newborn behavior to the establishment of the early mother–infant bond was not acknowledged until the past few decades (Brazelton, 1973). T. Berry Brazelton is a pediatrician who led the way in this work by calling attention to the remarkable behaviors and resiliency of the newly born baby. Prior to this, the neonate was considered a "tabula rasa" or a blank slate that was primarily a product of her/his environment and therefore did not evolve a personality until after birth. As neonatal behaviors, such as crying, rooting, and gazing, that call forth maternal responses, such as singing, nursing, and comforting, became appreciated by modern science, it became apparent that the amazing newborn emerged from the amazing preborn (Verny & Kelly, 1981). A Native American cultural sentiment is that at birth, a baby is already 9 months old. Science is now catching up with this idea as genetically determined

temperaments evidenced by fetal activity patterns are being discerned (DiPietro, 2010). A critical concept for prenatal care practice is that as fetal sensorimotor capabilities develop, the fetus is acting, reacting, and learning in his/her intrauterine environment. Sharing the developing wonder of what the fetus is capable of and experiencing at various gestational weeks are important teaching points during prenatal care and can support the development of maternal–fetal attachment (Alhusen, 2008) Additionally, preparing the pregnant woman for the range of normal early newborn activities, including the various newborn states, such as sleep, drowsiness, quiet alert, activeness, excitability, and crying, and her ability to console the baby as well as the baby's ability to self-soothe in certain states will give her tools for beginning her role as mother with her neonate.

Prenatal teaching regarding fetal growth and development

1. Share the average weight and length of the fetus for gestational age at each visit, easily available on gestational wheels or apps.
2. Motor capabilities develop in the late embryonic phase at 6–8 weeks' gestation and change in quality and pattern as nerves and muscles mature.
3. Fetal sensitivity to touch and pressure begins early, at 10–12 weeks' estimated gestational age (EGA).
4. Fetal hearing develops at 23–24 weeks; the fetus will respond to sound.
5. Fetal vision is the last sense to develop; eyes unfuse at 24–26 weeks and sight matures over time.

Source: Blackburn (2013).

Rubin

The theories of Reva Rubin, a nurse researcher, have been seminal in the area of maternal role attainment and maternal attachment (Mercer, 1995, 2010; Rubin, 1984; Sherwen, 1987). She conceptualized a series of maternal tasks that were achieved through specific cognitive processes. Her work has been extended, revised and critiqued over time by herself and by other researchers (Mercer, 1995, 2010; Parratt & Fahy, 2010; Rubin, 1984; Sleutel, 2003). Rubin's four tasks of maternal role attainment arise from a lifetime of social learning that becomes internalized within the individual mother. These tasks include (1) safe passage, (2) acceptance by others, (3) binding in to the child, and (4) giving of oneself. Indicators of positive or impaired development of maternal role attainment are listed as follows (Flagler & Nicholl, 1990).

Indicators for maternal role development

Positive development	Impaired development
1. Robust fantasies about baby and motherhood	1. Persistent unrealistic or negative fantasies
2. Can identify maternal role models	2. No positive maternal role models in her life
3. Aware of fetal/newborn capabilities	3. Knowledge deficit regarding fetal/newborn capabilities
4. Wearing clothes that accommodate the pregnant body	4. Wearing clothes that constrict the pregnant body
5. Acceptance of bodily changes of pregnancy	5. Negative response to bodily changes of pregnancy
6. Seeking care, support, and advice from professionals and family	6. Dismissing care, support, and advice by professionals and family
7. Engaging in health-promoting practices	7. Engaging in practices that are harmful to health
8. Enriching and empathetic social environment	8. Impoverished or abusive social environment

The maternal task of "safe passage" is defined as seeking the means to assure a secure and healthy pregnancy and childbirth for herself and her fetus/newborn. Early in pregnancy, the woman is self-aware and has not yet differentiated the fetus as an individual. She experiences early bodily changes and pregnancy discomforts, such as breast tenderness and enlargement, and nausea and vomiting; her concerns for safety are primarily involved with her own health. However, severe nausea and vomiting will raise concerns about the fetus getting enough nourishment, and vaginal spotting will raise concerns about the possibility of spontaneous abortion or miscarriage; in such instances, safety concerns expand to include embryonic/fetal health and well-being. As the fetus becomes psychologically differentiated as an individual for the pregnant woman, usually through quickening but sometimes earlier with the advent of early ultrasound images of the baby, she becomes aware of the intertwined fates of herself and her baby. Danger for one constitutes danger for the other. Labor and birth are seen as particularly risky events to navigate. Successful attainment of this task is achieved through acquiring knowledge and skills to help her successfully manage pregnancy and childbirth and through arrangement of tangible aid and social support by family, friends, and professionals.

Pregnancy signals impending changes in the nature of social relationships for the mother and her child. This requires some letting go of old ways of being to make way for the newer ways, particularly by the woman herself. To achieve the task of "acceptance by others" for herself as a mother and for her baby-to-be as a new family member, the pregnant woman reflects on her current life, on her past relationships, and role models with respect to parenting and on her current relationships and aspirations for mothering. She will need to give up certain behaviors of her prechild lifestyle and will want acknowledgment for these behaviors. If this is a second or more baby, acceptance of the new baby by the siblings will be an important milestone. The ages and developmental stages of the siblings will dictate how she will approach them in gaining this acceptance for her new baby. Her success in navigating this task will largely depend on the quality of her relationships with her partner, her mother, and other important members of her kinship and friendship networks.

The task of "binding-in to the child" is one of establishing a direct form of experience between the mother and her fetus/infant. This entails moving the abstraction of the baby-to-be into a real relationship. An awareness of a separate being, not just a pregnancy, is facilitated by ultrasound images, listening to the fetal heartbeat, and recognizing its separate rhythm from her own, and the sine qua non in differentiating the idea of the baby into its own reality—quickening. The sensation of fetal movement begins an internal awareness of the fetus and its activity patterns for the pregnant woman. The mother can begin to ascribe certain attributes to the fetus. If the gender of the baby is known, social sex role assumptions begin in the womb. For example, some women will predict that their male baby will become a soccer player after a period of intense activity, while the female fetus will have a future envisioned as a prima ballerina. This is a sociocultural phenomenon that sets up expectations related to gender rather than individual characteristics and proclivities; for this reason, one couple took the extreme measure of not revealing their child's gender until that child's fourth birthday (Pappas, 2011).

Early fetal movements are felt only by the mother and as such are a very special period in gestation. Later in gestation, fetal movements can be felt externally by partners and professionals. Mothers-to-be will engage in conversations with their babies about their movements as pregnancy goes along. A dimension of relatedness to the fetus is added to the pregnancy and marks the onset of maternal–infant attachment.

The fourth task of maternal role attainment is "giving of oneself" and is felt by Rubin to be the most complex and demanding task of childbearing. Physical, emotional, and social changes of pregnancy progressively require more and more modifications in the woman's lifestyle and choices. And yet she must embrace these changes willingly and see their purpose in giving to her child for the child's benefit and well-being. This state of "giving-to" creates a sense of vulnerability, dependence, and a need to be "given-to" in return. "Mothering the mother" is a phrase that symbolizes ways in which family and professionals can support the pregnant woman by assuring her she will have tangible aid and emotional support that will see her through her more vulnerable moments.

Rubin articulated three cognitive processes through which the four tasks of maternal role attainment are achieved. The first process is *replication*. Replication is the active search by the woman for elements of the maternal role that she wishes to incorporate into her interpretation of becoming mother and that she believes are valued by society. Mimicry is a replicative behavior that is an imitation of simple behaviors or practices she has seen other mothers execute. Current trends and recommendations of childbearing and childrearing experts are also tried on through mimicry. For example, the pregnant woman may have to purchase a certain stroller that she has seen others use or prepare homemade baby food in the manner of her own mother. Role playing is an interactive form of replication and requires a partner in the role-play situation. Examples of this type of replication may include interaction with a friend's or relative's infant or discussions with her partner on parenting issues. The woman will closely observe signals from the role-playing partner to see if she is receiving positive or negative feedback from her early mothering behaviors or ideas. She will evolve her role accordingly. Rubin refers to this as "binding-in" to a maternal identity.

Fantasy is an essential cognitive component of maternal role taking. It is not to be confused with a stream of consciousness daydream, but is rather a series of mental operations that help the pregnant woman accept the pregnancy and the baby and deal with the hopes and fears she has for her new life ahead. *Introjection* is the pregnant woman's identification of someone who copes well with the pending situation and incorporation of that behavior into her fantasy work. *Projection* is done as the woman contemplates future imagery of herself and her baby. She imagines a fantasy child in various situations and inserts herself into the picture. *Rejection* is the identification of behaviors that will not be incorporated, although they may be assumed by the woman in her fantasy work. An example of these operations is the observation of a good friend who is successfully breast-feeding her child. The pregnant woman will imagine herself and her baby-to-be in a similar behavior pattern and yet may reject the openness with which her friend

breastfeeds in public and imagines a more modest display of breastfeeding. *Grief work* is another aspect of fantasy work that refers to the gradual disengagement with aspects of the pregnant woman's prior life no longer useful in the new imagined life. Moving through the grief work allows her to accept her new maternal role.

Dedifferentiation is the third cognitive process by which a woman assumes the maternal role. This is an exploration of the goodness of fit of prior fantasy work with the woman's current self-image. The determination of congruence of the fantasized behaviors, attitudes, and interactions examined in replication and fantasy work are then assimilated into the woman's formulation of the maternal role.

What can prenatal care providers incorporate into their care practices from Rubin's theory of maternal role development? Providers should inquire about

---

Assessment of maternal attachment and adaptation

1. How do you feel about being pregnant?
2. Was this a planned pregnancy or was it unintended?
3. How was pregnancy achieved? Easily? With difficulty? Through reproductive technologies?
4. How do others in your life feel about your pregnancy? Your partner? Your children? Your mother? Your friends?
5. Do you have tangible and emotional support from your partner, family, and friends during pregnancy and beyond?
6. What was your relationship with your mother like? What were her birth experiences like?
7. How has your relationship with your partner changed during the pregnancy?
8. What bodily changes are you experiencing? How do you feel about these changes?
9. Are you having any dreams or fantasies about the baby or about your transition to motherhood? Please describe these for me.
10. What are you doing differently now that you are pregnant to avoid harm and maintain your health and your baby's health? Changes in habits, such as diet, exercise, rest? Avoidance of smoking, alcohol, drugs?
11. What are you doing to prepare for the baby? Car seat? A room or sleeping space? Clothing, diapers, and other items?
12. Do you talk to your baby *in utero*? Have a name or nickname for the baby?
13. Are you aware of the baby's movements and position? How would you describe your baby's activities?
14. Are you planning to breastfeed your baby?
15. What are your plans and preferences for labor and birth?

relationships and behaviors important to the woman's attachment to the fetus and her attainment of the maternal role. Clear communication can be encouraged within her primary affiliative relationships and can be role-modeled by the prenatal provider. Descriptions of the wide range of normal social and emotional changes she faces can be reassuring to the pregnant woman. Asking about fantasy work and dreams are a chance to engage in discussions that can lead to exploration of her hopes and fears regarding impending childbirth and motherhood. Providing information to enhance the woman's knowledge of her changing needs throughout the course of pregnancy and early postpartum, and of newborn characteristics and behaviors is an essential service. For women who are struggling with serious relationship issues, strategies to assist her include clarifying the problem situation, reviewing steps to conflict resolution, and providing her with appropriate referrals for her psychosocial issues.

Lederman

Another important theorist in psychosocial concerns in pregnancy is Regina Lederman (1984, 1996; Lederman & Weis, 2009), a nurse researcher, who described seven dimensions of maternal development for women from her work examining psychophysiological correlates among pregnancy and childbirth variables, such as maternal anxiety, coping and safety, labor progress indices, and biochemical markers of stress—epinephrine, norepinephrine, and cortisol. Her seven dimensions of psychosocial adaptation include the following areas: (1) acceptance of pregnancy, (2) identification with a motherhood role, (3) relationship with the mother, (4) relationship with the partner, (5) preparation for labor, (6) fear of loss of control in labor, and (7) fear of loss of self-esteem in labor (Lederman, 1984, 1996). Her work offers additional important insights to the development of the maternal role, is compatible with Rubin's theories, and will be discussed here.

"Acceptance of pregnancy" is the adaptive response by the woman to the pregnancy and all that it means in her life. A common feature as a woman works through to accept her pregnancy is ambivalence toward being pregnant. Ambivalence is holding opposing positive and negative thoughts, attitudes, and emotions simultaneously for the same event. Ambivalence is expected to occur in women with an unintended pregnancy as they take in the fact that they are pregnant and consider the implications and choices they have ahead, but it also occurs in women who have planned to be pregnant. The feeling of ambivalence is considered a normal reaction and may be largely resolved in the early months of pregnancy, but it may recur as the enormity

of the life changes are felt by the woman. In Lederman's seminal research (1984), acceptance of the pregnancy was found to be related to a woman's identification with a motherhood role, her relationship with her own mother, and her level of preparation for labor. Additional factors found to be important were the woman's reaction to her bodily changes and whether these manifested in any discomforts of pregnancy. While there are anatomical and physiological explanations for the multitude of common discomforts of pregnancy, the astute care provider will also consider whether these discomforts are a psychosomatic expression of ambivalence, anxiety, stress, or personality issues (Kuo, Wang, Tseng, Jian, & Chou, 2007).

The transition from woman-without-child to woman-mother is a process that when navigated successfully will end with the "identification with a motherhood role" (Lederman, 1984). The extent to which a woman is identifying with a motherhood role can be assessed by exploring the motivation and preparation she has for such a life event. The motivations leading to pregnancy are as varied as are the life stories of the women we serve. And while about one-third (37%) of pregnancies are categorized as unintended (Mosher, Jones, & Abma, 2012), there is a school of thought in psychology that contends there is no such thing as an accidental pregnancy. The pregnant woman herself may not recognize the diverse psychosocial influences and meanings that led to her pregnancy. Some variants on the circumstances surrounding a pregnancy and its meaning can include a planned pregnancy accomplished without difficulty in a committed couple relationship, pregnancy achieved with the use of artificial reproductive technologies amid financial concerns, complicated therapeutic procedures and side effects, a pregnancy in a single woman with several casual sexual partners in the time frame of conception, and an urban adolescent who feels social pressure to become pregnant for confirmation that she is desirable and healthy. In some cultures, pregnancy will tie a man to a woman in a provider role while the baby is young. This is particularly true in areas of desperate poverty, such as Haiti, where outsiders view pregnancy as detrimental to the woman's circumstance, and yet her reality is that a pregnancy and the new baby keep the baby's father in a provider role and will help her feed herself and her children for the next several years.

The desire to be pregnant can be separate from the desire to bear and raise a child. Concerns are raised if the mother-to-be is not preparing for the eventual baby through gathering of supplies and cognitive preparation. Congruent with Rubin's theories, Lederman (1984; 1996; Lederman & Weis, 2009) found that fantasizing and dreaming were important mental strategies in trying on various maternal behaviors and styles of parenting. These mental operations allowed the woman to envision herself as a mother with characteristics that she desires to develop in that role and to anticipate future life changes as a result of becoming a mother. Her own childhood is reconsidered from a new perspective, including mothering behaviors she experienced that she plans to incorporate or eliminate in her repertoire of mothering behaviors. Role conflicts are anticipated, including the common concerns of job or career conflicts, childcare arrangements, and concomitant financial implications. Positive identification with the motherhood role involves clarification of the woman's self-image as mother and progressive development of confidence in her abilities to successfully complete the tasks of mothering. Women who struggle with low self-esteem, excessive narcissism, lack of good role models, and excessive career/motherhood conflicts can experience extreme anxiety that impedes their ability to move forward in identifying with a motherhood role. Lederman (1984) found that the psychophysiological influences of these conflicts played out in prolonged labors and difficult births for a disproportionate number of these women.

The pregnant woman's "relationship with her own mother" is an important line of inquiry for the prenatal clinician to discuss. Intergenerational parenting patterns, while not destiny, are foundations that serve as reference for the development of the maternal role. The love and support present or lacking in her own childhood will shape the pregnant woman's approach to mothering. Gently ask about the pregnant woman's own mother or mother figure. Given the nature of blended and alternative families today, it is not a certainty that the mother figure will be her own biological mother. Ascertain the past and current availability of the pregnant woman's mother to her. This can give rise to discussions about her experiences of being mothered. The grandmother's reaction to the pregnancy and acknowledgment of her daughter as a mother are influential. Typically, the grandmother-to-be enjoys sharing memories and reminiscing about her childbearing and child-rearing experiences with her pregnant daughter. Their relationship takes on new dimensions as the pregnant woman empathizes with her mother from a new perspective and the grandmother sees her daughter as a mature autonomous adult.

A common practical and social postpartum arrangement is for the grandparent(s) to come spend a week or so after the baby is born to help with meals and household chores, to care for the new mother, and to meet and bond with the new baby. Even with geographic distances, new avenues of connecting via social networking systems allow visual and audio connection among grandparents and the growing family. Mother–daughter relationships fraught with conflict can adversely affect the gravida's adjustment to motherhood and, in Lederman's research (1984), was also significantly related to prolonged labor and its negative sequelae. The mind–body relationship is real and powerful and can reflect social stressors as the pregnant woman makes her physical and psychic transition to mother.

The "relationship with the woman's partner" is a vital element in her adjustment to the mother role. The relationship from the pregnant woman's point of view will be examined here; the perspective of the male or lesbian partner will be considered under "Partner Adaptation and Attachment." How the pregnant woman perceives the response of her partner to the pregnancy is key and consists of the partner's empathy toward her, the ability to cooperate under changing conditions, availability for communication and sharing, and reliability in being present to her in both a physical and emotional sense.

The pregnant woman will typically have concerns about the partner's adjustment to the parenting role; this is something the prenatal care provider can inquire about and provide suggestions and support as appropriate. The nature of the relationship will be important to understand—an interdependent relationship with give and take by both parties sets the stage for success for both parents in assuming their impending parental duties. Mutual care-taking activities during pregnancy are positive signs for the partners' relationship and support for each other as parents. Pregnancy enhances dependency needs in both partners as they face the restructuring of life as they know it; however, excessive dependency is counterproductive and associated with low autonomy and low self-esteem (Lederman, 1984).

Intimate relations will change over the course of pregnancy and early parenting; this can be characterized as a normal evolution of this life phase for the couple and strategies for fostering ongoing closeness and intimacy, such as designating daily time for communication, affection, and connection, can be suggested. Role conflicts that are common can be presented for discussion and consideration. For example, if both partners work, childcare issues are something to begin to sort out during the pregnancy. Who will arrange childcare, transport the child, pack the diaper bag, and so forth? Some places of employment offer parental leaves that support either or both partners during their transition to parenthood; these work policies are important to investigate during the pregnancy. The partner relationship contributes significantly to the adaptation of the woman to pregnancy and motherhood, and will undergo changes that provide the framework for family patterns that extend far into the future.

"Preparation for labor" is a dimension of psychosocial adaption to pregnancy that has elements of practical preparation and imagined rehearsal. An important standardized method of practical preparation for childbirth and early parenting is attendance at childbirth education classes. The second-wave feminist movement of the 1960–1970s raised the consciousness of childbearing women through childbirth classes. Interest in unmedicated or "natural" childbirth, taking back control of the childbirth process and placing it in women's hands led to the development of independent childbirth classes. These classes were part of a movement passionate to reform the childbirth practices of the day that did not allow family or friends to observe or participate in the birth and that did not allow choice in labor and birth procedures. These classes were so successful that they established a niche in the health-care system and were incorporated into the programming offered by hospitals to pregnant women and their families, or professionalized into organizations requiring training and certification to teach. However, such recognition has come at a cost—the relinquishment of independence and the ability to critique and reform the system. Third-wave feminism and the green movement have stimulated a reemergence of independent and alternative classes (see Resources for Health-Care Providers for Web sites of selected childbirth education groups). The important point is to know the types of childbirth education classes that are available in your area and to consider the influence that the classes chosen and taken will have on the pregnant woman's knowledge and attitudes toward the childbirth interventions and processes and how this will shape her expectations and hopes for her own childbirth.

Language as a reflection and construction of social realities

"Natural" childbirth is an unfortunate term still in common use. Implied is its polar opposite, "unnatural" childbirth—any birth where medical interventions are used. Examples of other problematic terms in common parlance in the childbearing field are such phrases as "You have an 'adequate' pelvis"; "I 'delivered' her baby"; and "You have an 'incompetent' cervix." Note the subtle but pervasive message that is negative and disempowering to women. Even the term "obstetric care" refers to the physician providing care, not the woman receiving care. We prefer the terms "maternity care," "prenatal care," or "antepartum care." Challenge questions: What other common phrases used in prenatal care have a negative or disempowering connotation? What are better terms to use in their place?

Another preparatory activity for the maternal role is the gathering of supplies for the baby. A rite of passage for pregnant women commonly observed in American society today is the baby shower, typically a party hosted by a friend or family member at which gifts for the honored mother and baby are an expected contribution for attendance. This is usually a gathering of women only. This ritual has the practical aspect of providing material goods necessary for the new baby, such as diapers, clothing, and toys, but it should also be understood from a social perspective. Rituals function as a means of delineating and defining social roles and communicating the scope of the new role (Engelhardt, 2012). Rituals link the past to the future by sharing structured symbolic activities imbued with meaning. Activities at a baby shower center around games that create positive memories, festive food and drink, and wisdom and advice from the circle of females present. It should be noted that ethnically diverse cultures vary in prenatal preparatory practices and rituals (Ahern & Ruland, 2003). The sensitive care provider will recognize cultural variation in the meaning and expectations ascribed to preparatory activities during pregnancy and will consider maternal behavior in this context.

Maternal detachment as a protective mechanism

Women who live with conditions of chronic scarcity and daily struggles to survive, as is seen in impoverished or remote areas of the world, often delay forming attachments to their infants. Maternal attachment is muted and protectively distanced when one's frame of reference is a high fertility rate combined with a high infant mortality rate (Scheper-Hughes, 1985), as is seen in areas such as Haiti, Ethiopia, South Sudan, and remote rural Brazil. Clinicians serving immigrant women from areas of abject poverty or clinicians traveling to provide prenatal care in these areas may note maternal indifference that is in marked contrast to American expectations. Such flat affect is often a reflection of the difficult life path and history of losses experienced in the woman's own precarious efforts to survive. The delay in attachment does not preclude the eventual formation of a secure attachment between mother and child and should be understood in its cultural context.

Much of a woman's preparatory activity and therefore knowledge about labor and birth today is gained through secondary sources, such as friends and family's oral histories, books, Internet sources, and television, video, and movie depictions. The Internet is becoming a more important source of information and influence for women's birth decisions, especially as women who have grown up with the ubiquitous Internet are reaching adulthood (Khanna, 2008; Lagan, Sinclair, & Kernohan, 2010). Symbolic depictions of others' birth experiences, such as stories of friends' births and television portrayals of labor and birth, are pervasive and almost unavoidable in American culture today. Direct observation of another's birth experience presents a unique learning opportunity. Under the liberal visiting policies in hospitals today, more people have attended the birth of a friend or a family member (Klaidman et al., 1999). One study examining the influence of witnessing birth on childbirth confidence or self-efficacy reported that about one-fourth of the nulliparous pregnant women ($n = 159$) had actually witnessed birth prior to giving birth themselves (Farley, 1999); this number has presumably grown since this study was conducted. Birth has its own special sights, sounds, smells, and sensations, thus creating a multisensory barrage of information for those present. Birth is not experienced directly, but vicariously and within a particular social context. From her perceptions of the witnessed birth, the female observer gives meaning to this witnessed event, its relevance to her own life experience, and incorporates these perceptions into her feelings and beliefs about her own abilities to labor and give birth.

Logic would dictate that preparation for an unknowable labor and birth is tentative at best. And yet planning for labor and birth is done by women and encouraged by clinicians (Carty & Tier, 1989). The problem with planning for birth is that there are not simply two contingencies—normal or abnormal—vaginal or cesarean birth. Rather, there are multiple possibilities of unforeseen situations that may alter birth plans slightly or drastically, calling into play one or many of the labor and birth procedures that had previously been chosen or rejected. The unknowable can be frightening. How does one make plans under conditions of uncertainty? Clearly, uncertainty is part and parcel of the anticipation and the experience of labor and birth. Women turn to approaches that have helped them in the past: seeking information, checking with credible authorities, garnering social support, reflecting on previous successful coping strategies, and using cognitive strategies, such as positive self-talk, to plan for their unknowable labor and birth. Mental rehearsals, fantasy work, and dreams are important methods of working through these uncertainties and developing strategies for dealing with various contingencies. Some women will avoid thinking about the upcoming labor and birth. This may represent a dysfunctional state or a coping strategy for the woman and should be investigated further.

From a psychological perspective, preparing for labor is also preparing for separation from the fetus. This separation begins with the onset of labor. Contractions and pain in labor are a phenomenon toward which much thought and anticipation are invested on the part of the pregnant woman. The concept of contractions can be difficult for some women to imagine, particularly nulliparous pregnant women who have not experienced contractions. On the other hand, multigravida women may have increased fear because they have authentic experience to inform their expectations. However, multiparous women need to understand that each labor and birth has the potential to be different than previous experiences. A sense of the work, pain, risks, and benefits of labor that are balanced and based on a healthy sense of realistic possibilities is the best place from which to anticipate labor for the pregnant woman.

Lederman's (1984) final two tasks are related to dealing with significant fears for many childbearing women: "fear of loss of control in labor" and the "fear of loss of self-esteem in labor." Fear is a powerful emotion with psychological and physical components. These fears are largely centered on the anticipated pain of childbirth and the ability to handle it. The concept of control explored by Lederman was not an internal versus external locus of control, but rather a woman's sense that she could maintain control over her physical reactions and emotional responses while in labor.

In addition to control of self in labor, there were concerns of maintaining social control in terms of interpersonal interactions of respect and mutuality with the staff in the birth setting. The ability to trust the medical/nursing staff and her support people to help the pregnant woman maintain control will contribute to her level of fear. While the relationship between the prenatal care provider and the pregnant woman has typically had several months to develop, the relationship between professional caregivers and support people present at birth may just be established with the onset of labor. Expectations, beliefs, and preferences may coincide or may be discordant with the woman's choices and unfolding events. The caregivers' priorities at this time are related to the provision of care and related professional tasks, while support people vary from passive observers to active advocates for the laboring woman. Established functional or dysfunctional patterns of relating among the laboring woman and her supportive others and how they interact with staff can set the stage for a positive experience or one fraught with misunderstandings. It is important to discuss with the pregnant woman who will be at her birth and what role they will play. Encourage the woman to consider inviting only those individuals she can rely on for authentic support.

What is an emotion?

What is an emotion? The primary components of this multidimensional, dynamic phenomenon include a physiological arousal state and the psychological processes of perception and cognition. Emotion is also a deeply social phenomenon that is influenced by cultural expectations and by interpersonal relationships. It is here that the mind–body connection is evident.

Acute emotional events in life can have powerful but time-limited effects on an individual's psychophysiology. Just as interesting are the chronic emotional influences on mental and physical health. For example, what are the effects of a chronic anxiety or dread of the upcoming labor and birth on maternal health and birth outcomes? (Or the dread of an upcoming exam on the immune system of a student?) Be observant in the clinical setting for cues of psychological distress—much anxiety during pregnancy can be relieved by timely and responsive care.

The fear of loss of self-esteem in labor is related to how well the woman feels she is able to maintain the level of control she has set for herself. However, a woman's underlying general sense of self-esteem is important here as well. In Lederman's analysis (1984, 1996; Lederman & Weis, 2009), childbearing women who held themselves in high self-esteem were tolerant with their own imperfections, persistent in working toward their goals, and were able to set boundaries with others who did not value their goals. Women with low self-esteem struggled with a pessimistic attitude toward events in their lives and were less likely to assert their abilities to influence the process and outcomes of their labor and birth experiences.

Fear is a feature of the complex and dynamic emotional response women have to the childbearing experience. For most women, this fear is moderated by psychological defense mechanisms, such as rationalization and denial, as well as cognitive processes, such as self-esteem and self-efficacy. However, severe fear in childbirth is an issue that is often undetected and therefore unexplored in clinical practice (Saisto & Halmesmäki, 2003). The most common fears are related to the health of the baby and the experience of pain (Geissbuehler & Eberhard, 2002). Fears of interventions and of being at the mercy of health-care personnel are also common. Fear of dying in childbirth is rarely stated but is considered by women. For female immigrants from other countries, such as Haiti, Nepal, or Ethiopia, the fear of dying in childbirth is a real fear born of their life experiences, not a hypothetical construct. Extreme levels of childbirth fear are estimated to affect 6–10% of

women (Areskog, Kjessler, & Uddenberg, 1982; Saisto & Halmesmäki, 2003). A request for an elective cesarean section should trigger a discussion about fears and self-esteem, not simply risks and benefits of the procedure. Such Swedish and Finnish women who received counseling during pregnancy withdrew their initial request for a surgical birth and went on to have successful vaginal births (Saisto & Halmesmäki, 2003). Predisposing variables to extreme childbirth fear include prior traumatizing birth or medical experiences, low self-esteem, high numbers of daily stressors, and lack of social support. Depression, anxiety, and other psychological stressors also play a role in the development of childbirth fear.

In later updates to Lederman's work (1996; Lederman & Weis, 2009), she explored differences in psychosocial adaptation in pregnancy of multigravidas in a longitudinal study similar to her original research. Consistently over the last several years, 40% of childbearing women in the United States are first-time mothers, while 60% are having repeat pregnancies. This has implications for the woman's expectations, psychological concerns, and family structure adjustments. Multigravidas have an authentic reference point from which to anticipate their impending labor, and while this is highly predictive, it also not a given. Some women will have to be encouraged to open their expectations to other possible trajectories for their labors. The maternal role has been attained to varying degrees of success in multigravida women; now it is expanded to include another child. Concerns of multiparas are practical and range from the financial concerns of an additional child to the work of a newborn added to the care and needs of older children. Additionally, reactions from her partner and extended family will help or hinder her adjustment to becoming mother again.

Sibling adaptation and attachment

Preparation of siblings for the birth of a new baby is part of the work of the multigravida pregnant woman. Sometimes, siblings accompany their mother to prenatal visits and can be asked about their feelings and expectations for the new baby directly in an age-appropriate manner. If her children do not accompany the pregnant multigravida woman, selected questions can be asked of the pregnant woman in regard to her other children. Sibling relationships are a dynamic force within the family; children and their parents exert mutual influence on each other in their interactions. While the arrival of a new baby may lead to some regressive behaviors in a young sibling for a short period of time, often the new baby is an object of great interest to younger and older siblings alike. An estimated 80% of children will grow up with siblings, so this is a common adjustment in family structure. Much sibling research tends to focus on birth order, with particular emphasis on primogeniture, in other words, the influence of other children on the firstborn child. However, for the prenatal care provider, the most appropriate focus is in assessment, education, and support of the mother and her other children as she adjusts her maternal role to include another child. It should not be assumed that a mother knows everything about pregnancy, labor, and birth simply by virtue of having given birth previously. Knowledge must be assessed, verified, and either reinforced or re-explained for the multigravida.

Assessment of sibling attachment and adaptation

1. What are the ages of the siblings?
2. What have they been told about the pregnancy? How have they responded?
3. What is their understanding of pregnancy, birth, and becoming a big sister or brother?
4. What is their understanding of the needs of newborn babies? Of the new demands on their mother's time and energy?
5. What are their expressed feelings about the pregnancy and baby? Are there any notable changes in sibling behavior that coincide with the news of the pregnancy?
6. How are siblings to be included in prenatal visits? In labor and birth?
7. What is the nature of the maternal relationship with each sibling? Paternal/partner relationship with each sibling? The sibling-to-sibling relationship? Grandparent relationships with each sibling? Relationship of each sibling with friends or other family?
8. Are the basic needs of the siblings—food, shelter, clothing, developmentally appropriate activities, positive emotional climate, and appropriate supervision and guidance of behavior—provided for by responsible adults? Are there plans in place for the additional resources needed for the new baby?

The theories presented in this section give the prenatal care provider a structure for exploring a variety of psychosocial issues important to healthy adaptation, attachment, and maternal role attainment in the pregnant woman. These issues are best explored over several visits and in the context of a developing relationship of mutual

dialogue and trust. The prenatal visit offers opportunity for casual but concentrated conversation in which to hear the pregnant woman's stories while examining the pregnant abdomen. The prenatal care provider can encourage disclosure of important information by using active listening; liberal use of affirmations and probes; and maintaining a warm, caring, and nonjudgmental attitude. While prenatal care providers are not psychological therapists per se, much of the information, counseling, and support provided during prenatal care will prove reassuring and therapeutic to the pregnant woman.

Partner adaptation and attachment

With changing lifestyles and emerging new configurations of family structures, it is not a given that pregnant women today will have partners in a committed social and legal relationship. The standard marital relationship between a mother and a father is becoming less common. More babies today are born to unmarried women than in years past (Copen, Daniels, Vespa, & Mosher, 2012) (Table 16.1). More lesbian couples are choosing to have babies through a pregnancy of one of the partners. Women carrying surrogate pregnancies for gay and infertile couples, while not common, are encountered from time to time in prenatal care. Some women chose to proceed with pregnancy without a partner, availing themselves of artificial means of reproduction to achieve pregnancy. Other women are abandoned by their partners with the onset of an unplanned pregnancy; other women are not certain of paternity, interjecting an element of discord into these relationships. A partner relationship must not be assumed, it must be assessed.

Pregnant women feel the weight of responsibility for the growing fetus; this leads to heightened vulnerability and dependency needs that will influence all relationships, but most particularly their relationship with their partner. New roles are forged as the pregnancy progresses in anticipation of the baby. Emotional support and tangible assistance between the pregnant woman and her partner are critical elements for positive parental and partner role development requiring clear communication and ongoing effort at this time. Sound information and sensitive guidance by the prenatal care provider can facilitate these changes.

Table 16.1 Trends in the Marital or Cohabitation Status of Women Aged 15–44 (Copen et al., 2012)

Years	Number of women	Married (%)	Cohabiting (%)	Not cohabiting (%)
Total, 2002	21,018,000	64.4	14.3	21.3
Total, 2006–2010	21,161,000	59.7	23.4	16.9

Assessment of partner attachment and adaptation

1. What is the nature of the partner relationship with the pregnant woman?
2. Was this a planned pregnancy with partner involvement?
3. What is partner perception of the pregnancy—positive, negative?
4. Does the partner have other children?
5. What past and current experience with parenting does the partner have?
6. Does the partner exhibit bonding behaviors toward the fetus, such as talking to the fetus, patting the pregnant abdomen, protective behavior toward the pregnant woman?
7. Is the partner involved in the provision of food, shelter, clothing, and positive emotional climate for the pregnant woman? Are there plans in place for the additional resources needed for the new baby?

Male partners

The experience of becoming a father is an important milestone in male adult development. Traditionally, the father has been characterized as a remote figure, busy with the work involved in maintaining financial security for the family. However, men today are rejecting exaggerated definitions of masculinity and are redefining their father roles to include hands-on involvement and a nurturing component in their relationship with their partner and their children (Draper, 2002).

Tradition has delegated to the father rather minor roles in the childbearing experience, although this is changing. From colonial times, when childbearing was largely a social function of a group of midwives and women gathered to support the mother and the infant, to recent times when childbirth has been under the domain of medical science and technology, and hospital rules and regulations, the father has been an obscure figure. Hospitals have relaxed their policies for support people attending the laboring woman from exclusion of all family and friends prior to the 1970s, to inclusion of only married men who attended formal childbirth classes in the 1970s–1980s, to liberal visiting policies emerging in the 1990s and beyond that may only specify a number of support people allowed in the room at one time. Access to labor and birth areas has allowed male partners to play a greater role in providing labor comfort and support measures to the laboring woman. At the birth, some couples want the father to catch the baby or to cut the umbilical cord in an effort to create powerful emotional bonds and family legacy memories.

Couvade, a French verb meaning to brood or to hatch, is a term applied to fatherhood rituals across various historical eras and cultural groups. These rituals serve several purposes for the father and the new family, including warding off evil spirits, publicly acknowledging the new baby as his own, and strengthening the emotional bond between father and child (Dunham et al., 1991). Examples of these archaic rituals for men are avoidance of certain foods or use of knives during pregnancy and labor, adornment with the pregnant woman's clothing, and confinement to a hut for the length of his mate's labor and birth. While ritual couvade is practiced only in primitive cultures today, the couvade syndrome is a common condition in which the male partner of a pregnant woman experiences physical and emotional symptoms of pregnancy. Estimates of the occurrence of couvade syndrome range from 11% to 80% of male partners, although symptoms may not be recognized as a psychogenic manifestation of the partner's pregnancy (Lipkin & Lamb, 1982). Expectant fathers may have one or more signs and symptoms of pregnancy, including nausea, vomiting, weight gain, breast tenderness, food cravings, headaches, abdominal cramps, and sleep disturbances. The couvade syndrome is thought to be a psychosomatic manifestation of the changes in social roles, a reflection of either an overidentification with or an envy reaction to his partner's pregnancy. It is not considered a mental health disorder. Most men will appreciate a simple explanation of the couvade syndrome along with the reassurance that this common male experience will abate with time.

While paternal attachment appears to go through processes similar to maternal attachment, the timing is different. The pregnancy and the baby remain abstractions for the man during early pregnancy; for the woman, the reality of the pregnancy is evident in physical changes. For the man, the changes in his pregnant partner inform his experience and elicit his response and involvement in the pregnancy. His experience of the pregnancy is through those embodied experiences of his partner that can be shared. Notable events include procuring a home pregnancy test kit, sharing the results, announcing the pregnancy to family and friends, feeling the baby's movements, viewing the ultrasound, supporting the pregnant woman through her bodily changes, and participating in childbirth classes, prenatal visits, labor, and birth.

The partner relationship is altered by the woman's experiences of pregnancy. For example, sexual relations may become less frequent in the first trimester due to fatigue, malaise, and nausea experienced by the pregnant woman, or in the third trimester due to the aches and pains of the enlarging uterus. At times, it is the male partner who is reluctant to engage in sexual relations for fear of hurting the baby. The perspective here is not the sexual act per se but rather the meaning of sexual intimacy to the relationship. The couple can be reassured that a new normal will be reestablished as they move through a period of fluctuating needs and desires for sexual intimacy.

The male partner can be encouraged to develop his nurturing father skills with the woman throughout pregnancy. He can play a role in buffering some of the stress that the mother undergoes in her transitions. However, this depends on the context of the partner relationship. Committed partners, whether married, cohabiting, or dating, are found to be a positive influence for the mother's role enactment and stress (Nomaguchi, Brown, & Leyman, 2012). For mothers no longer linked romantically with the baby's father, the status of relationship with a current partner is the crucial element. Mother–father relationships are varied and complex in contemporary society.

Men have their own psychological processes in their transition to the fatherhood role. The pregnancy can raise psychological issues of sexual identity in the man. The Freudian concept of "penis envy" has its counterpart in "parturition envy"—an envy of the creative force that grows and brings forth new life. The pregnancy and birth cycle are the most distinctive female capacities that men do not possess. And in their early formative years, the central figure for most men is their own mother—a powerful female. Consciously or not, men will explore where they fit on the masculine–feminine continuum. The father role contains aspects that reflect the range of this spectrum, such as breadwinner-provider, nurturer, teacher, and caregiver. Role stress and conflict can occur as men adjust their self-image to include the role of father and as they incorporate this new facet of their development into their current social roles and obligations.

Today, a man is expected to be more actively involved with his pregnant partner and their children. Participation in pregnancy, labor, and birth are interesting and rewarding experiences for men. The role of the male partner/father includes expressive and nurturant aspects. Direct physical care of very young children and continued open, warm emotional support of his partner and children are among the expectations of the continuous process of learning to negotiate the challenges of fatherhood. Changing societal expectations are based on several assumptions gaining widespread acceptance: (1) The burdens of childrearing are too great to be under the exclusive domain of mothers; (2) the joys of childrearing are too great to be under the exclusive domain of mothers; and (3) children are the responsibility of both parents.

Lesbian partners

Lesbian women are estimated to comprise 2–12% of the female population (Markus, Weingarten, Duplessi, & Jones, 2010). Thirty years ago, lesbian women typically had children in the context of a prior heterosexual relationship, but today, more lesbian women are choosing to become pregnant and parent in the context of an ongoing lesbian relationship. Lesbian partners are given special consideration here as many assumptions made by prenatal care providers do not hold true for lesbian couples. Indeed, if heterosexual assumptions form the basis of early encounters with a pregnant lesbian client, she may feel a sense of discrimination that can lead to defensiveness or withholding of important health and psychosocial information. In order to avoid this situation, a thorough social and sexual history should be taken before prenatal education or advice is rendered. Additionally, an honest self-assessment of your own cultural sensitivity to lesbian and bisexual women and an audit of language and practices used in the office are important quality improvement procedures to complete (GLBT Health Access Project, n.d.; Planned Parenthood, 2009). For example, the option of "partnered" should be available on the health history form.

The term lesbian is broader than a sexual or romantic attraction between two women; it encompasses issues of identity, sexual experimentation, sexual orientation, sexual preference, gender presentation, and lifestyle. While lesbianism has been covertly practiced in human societies since ancient times, it has only recently made its way into mainstream American culture via positive media portrayals and the willingness of popular celebrities to share their personal stories. This has led to more women feeling comfortable to self-identify as lesbian or bisexual, although it also leaves them open to the backlash of criticism, discrimination, bullying, and hate crimes. Of great relevance here is how lesbian, bisexual, and transgendered women and their partners are treated in health care and specifically in prenatal care. First and foremost, be sensitive to the woman before you as a pregnant woman with unique and universal needs and inquire about her partner's role in the pregnancy and parenting.

Caring for the pregnant woman in a lesbian relationship

1. Use inclusive language on office forms and in conversation.
2. Inquire about the partner relationship.
3. Welcome and include all members of her family.
4. Inquire about the method of conception to determine health risks, if any.
5. Discuss potential legal concerns regarding partner rights; know relevant state laws.
6. Focus on her needs as a pregnant woman and as an individual.

A unique feature for lesbian couples is that either partner has the biological capability to become pregnant. How the couple negotiated which partner becomes pregnant and by what method are issues to explore early in prenatal care (Pelka, 2009). Equality in a relationship is highly valued among lesbian couples; unequal biological ties to the baby can be a source of discord during pregnancy and beyond. Only one partner will carry the baby *in utero*; typically only one will breastfeed. Some lesbian couples are accessing artificial reproductive technologies through the health-care system, using *in vitro* fertilization to biologically comother by using the egg of one partner and the womb of the other. More common conception strategies are using frozen sperm from a known or unknown donor. Using sperm from an unknown donor can be costly, and the donor has been screened for a variety of health-related issues (Markus et al., 2010). Those couples unable or unwilling to go this route can use fresh sperm from a known donor with home insemination techniques. This choice carries a higher risk of inadvertently acquiring a sexually transmitted infection.

Just as heterosexual couples vary in psychosocial roles, relationships, and dynamics, so do lesbian couples. Lesbian couples may turn to peers for social support more often than family members, although this is highly dependent on how the lesbian relationship and partner have been accepted into each partner's extended family network. This, in turn, affects how well the new baby will be accepted into the family. Rejection or begrudging acceptance of the lesbian relationship can complicate the developmental tasks in pregnancy of gaining acceptance of the new baby by others and reviewing the pregnant woman's relationship with her own mother (Wismont & Reame, 1989).

Lesbian parents are creating autonomous family units that do not fit into neat predetermined societal categories. Even language is negotiated as the partners establish their roles. Positive terminology in use today for the lesbian partner are the terms "coparent," "comother," or "social mother." Later, there is the negotiation of what the child will call each of them. Children raised in lesbian and gay families fare as well as children raised in heterosexual families on a variety of indices, such as psychosocial health and educational attainment, in spite of a background of discrimination against such family structures (Amato, 2012).

Legal issues are another unique concern for lesbian couples and vary by state (Zeidenstein, 2004). Parental rights are not assured for the lesbian partner, even in the few states where gay marriage is legal. Second parent adoption is a process to ensure equal rights to the child, but the legality of this option varies by state as well. Legal rights and obligations of the sperm donor are additional considerations that the prenatal clinician will want to call to the couple's attention.

Lesbian couples' experiences of prenatal care are positive when the provider focuses more on pregnancy and parenting issues than on sexual orientation, involves the partner, and uses inclusive, neutral language in interviewing and counseling (Röndahl, Bruhner, & Lindhe, 2009).

Body image

We are embodied spirit; we experience life and interact with our environments through our physical bodies. Most women have a love–hate relationship with aspects of their body and this varies over time. Pregnancy is a time in life when rapid body changes are normal, early postpartum even more so. At no other time of life can a woman lose 10–15 lb (of baby, placenta, fluid, and blood) in the course of a few minutes. Body image is an important psychological concept that influences other psychological processes internal to the individual, as well as behaviors and social relationships. Satisfaction with one's body in pregnancy has been linked to eating behaviors, weight gain, depressive symptoms, and exercise behaviors (Rauff & Downs, 2011).

Body image is a subjective awareness and attitude toward one's body and its parts that may or may not correspond to objective measures. There is an element of individual assessment that is dynamic and varies over time, but there is also an element of social comparison; that is, how do I compare in relation to a particular reference group? This is largely culturally based. Ideals of youthful slender bodies in contemporary culture in America are not achievable by most women but are internalized nonetheless. In fact, nearly half of all women in United States are overweight or obese, and this percentage is projected to increase unless a cultural shift in eating and exercise patterns occurs (Mamun et al., 2010; Mehta, Siega-Riz, & Herring, 2010). More than 40% of pregnant women today are either overweight or obese; of these women, 8% are in the extremely obese category with a body mass index (BMI) of 40 or higher (Gunatilake & Perlow, 2011).

The simple routine measure of obtaining weight during prenatal care has an emotionally charged meaning to many pregnant women. A woman's weight factors in to her body image. This single numeric objective measure can elicit an emotional response for many women and is typically done at each client visit. It is not uncommon to have a pregnant woman step on the scales for her routine weight and burst into tears. Women who enter pregnancy already dissatisfied with their body are more likely to gain outside the recommended weight gain guidelines

(Bagheri et al., 2012; Mehta et al., 2010). Beyond the physical health consequences of weight, weight has a powerful link to a woman's body image and self-worth that the insightful prenatal care provider will recognize.

Body awareness in pregnancy focuses on the obvious areas of breast and abdominal growth. Other aspects of a woman's body may also enter into this increased self-surveillance and awareness, for example, skin coloration changes, such as the linea nigra or areolas, and redistribution of body fat and fluid, such as in the face or feet. Some of these changes are received positively; others cause dismay. The prenatal care provider can help by providing anticipatory guidance and explanation of the physical changes that can occur. The pregnant body has been celebrated in art since ancient times and is considered beautiful by many people. This fact can be shared with the pregnant woman as inspiration and positive affirmation.

The pregnant body is perceived as a protective container for the baby. For women who accept and embrace the pregnancy, the body changes are tangible evidence that she and the baby are healthy and growing well. Until the very end of pregnancy, most women do extremely well adapting their body image to incorporate the anatomic changes of pregnancy. The last weeks of pregnancy bring about a change. Eager anticipation of the baby's arrival coupled with the physical discomforts of late pregnancy lead to a readiness for birth and a return to the prepregnant body. However, most women are unprepared for the body changes in early postpartum and the time it can take to return to a nonpregnant body shape. Very few women regain their prepregnant body shape, although many will approximate it within a few weeks postpartum. This is an area of anticipatory guidance by the prenatal care provider for education, healthy lifestyle promotion, and support.

Clothing can be an extension of the body image. Besides the practical nature of clothing for skin protection and temperature regulation, a woman's choice of clothing can communicate identity and project a statement or an image. The change from regular clothing to pregnancy clothes usually occurs of necessity by the twentieth week for nulliparous pregnant women and by the sixteenth to eighteenth week for multiparous women. Some women will want to camouflage their pregnancies and others will want to flaunt their pregnancies.

By paying attention to her body, the pregnant woman has a unique knowledge of her body processes and the life of the fetus (Young, 1990). She feels the movements of the fetus and the contractions of her uterus, with an immediacy and certainty that nothing can replicate. Technologies in prenatal care, such as ultrasound imaging, fetal heart rate monitors, and screening tests for Down syndrome are often given more credence in our technologically dependent society. The prenatal care provider needs to honor the information provided by the woman and to carefully balance the information obtained by machine. Although machine-generated information is typically considered more objective than human-generated information, it can result in creating as much uncertainty as it reduces (Haninger & Farley, 2001; Sandelowski, 1993). The illusion of certainty (and sometimes blatant uncertainty) that machine-generated information creates leads to further technological measures to validate the uncertain technologically generated information. The outcome of technology dependency (uncertain results and information) is the creation of an increased requirement for and further dependency upon technology (Lawson & Turriff-Janasson, 2006). Still another effect of dependence on technology as the only, the best, or most promising solution to health problems is the masking of the existence of other viable solutions in the prevention and treatment domains. Additionally, medically controlled information creates a distance between the woman and her organic experience of pregnancy. Just as we encourage women to listen to their bodies, so too are we obligated to listen and respond to women's accounts of their body awareness and body knowledge.

Childbirth confidence

Enhancement of childbirth confidence in the pregnant woman is a facet of the art of prenatal care. Prenatal care providers need to assess a woman's expectations for her labor and birth experience and her beliefs in her own abilities. Interventions to enhance childbirth confidence, when indicated, are provided through the vehicle of an ongoing therapeutic relationship during prenatal care. It is important to assist the pregnant woman in understanding that a wide range of responses to varying circumstances in childbirth can be considered a successful mastery experience. The belief in her own abilities and her body's intrinsic power to work properly to bring forth a child are ideas to be explored and facilitated with the pregnant woman. Confidence for childbirth can be modified. Confidence for childbirth is best understood as the psychological concept of self-efficacy (Farley, 1999; Lowe, 1991).

Self-efficacy and childbirth

Self-efficacy is a dynamic cognitive process that is an individual's evaluation of her own capabilities to cope with a stressful situation and to perform required behaviors (Bandura, 1977). There are four sources of information that affect an individual's self-efficacy beliefs. The first and most potent source of self-efficacy information is *performance accomplishment*. Simply put, if a person has performed a task successfully in the past, she is more likely to believe that she can do it again. Therefore, a woman's previous experiences with childbirth have a powerful influence on her beliefs that she can do it again. Performance accomplishments are the most reliable sources of self-efficacy expectancies because they are based on the individual's own personal experiences of mastery or failure for the given task. A positive prior experience can lead to a positive outlook for the current pregnancy, whereas a traumatic prior birth experience can require psychological healing work.

The second source of self-efficacy information is *vicarious experience*. If a person is exposed to others' successful achievements of a particular task, then she is more likely to think "I can do it too," particularly if she identifies with the model. Vicarious experiences can be categorized into live modeling versus symbolic modeling. Live modeling experiences are those experiences in which the individual is a direct observer, that is, physically present at the model's performance of the task. Being present at a live birth is less common than symbolic modeling experiences but is available to enough women today that it is worth inquiring about and discussing the influence of this event with the pregnant woman (Farley, 1999).

Symbolic modeling experiences are representations of the task in symbolic form, in this case labor and birth. Examples of symbolic modeling experiences in our culture today include the oral or written accounts, photographs, drawings, and videos delivered in person or via books, magazines, and media. Because symbolic modeling vicarious experiences are plentiful in our culture today, they can be assumed to have a pervasive effect on American women and their beliefs about their birth capabilities. Unlike drugs or physical interventions, symbolic representations do not contribute directly to the physiology of labor and birth, but they can exert an indirect influence. Symbolic vicarious modeling experiences mediate their effects through elicitation of images in the parturient's mind, interpreted through the shared meanings and associations of the symbolically enacted task. These meanings and associations, when invoked, promote certain behaviors or emotional states that may affect the physiology of labor and birth.

Playing with dolls as young girls, sharing dreams about becoming a mother, hearing other women's birth stories, reading books and posts, attending childbirth classes, and watching birth videos are all examples of symbolic modeling experiences. Ubiquitous in our society are condensed, highly edited, and often overly dramatized birth depictions, such as those found in 5-minute YouTube videos or a 30-minute television show such as "A Baby's Story." The laboring woman is shown as fine in one moment, screaming and writhing in agony the next moments, and has a baby in her arms in the next moment. These depictions are far from the truth for the vast majority of women and can impart an erroneous view of the work of birth and, as such, are a disservice to women. Prenatal care providers can provide corrective information to their clients, but should appreciate the power of popular cultural influences on the way that pregnancy, labor, and birth are perceived in America.

Verbal persuasion is the third source of self-efficacy information. This is the encouragement or discouragement for the task at hand received from others related to the individual's ability to perform the task at hand. A well-timed "Yes, you can do it!" can positively influence a woman's perception of her abilities to give birth. Self-efficacy beliefs based on verbal persuasion are likely to be short-lived and weak because these beliefs are created without an authentic experiential base to support them (Bandura, 1977). Effective verbal persuasion can be provided by those who make the commitment to be "with woman" throughout her labor, as signs of discouragement must be recognized and addressed as they occur. The short-lived positive effects of verbal persuasion—"You can do this! You are doing this!"—may need to be repeated a number of times to combat the undermining physical sensations of labor.

The fourth and final source of self-efficacy information is *visceral arousal*. Visceral arousal is the physiological response produced by autonomic arousal that can occur while anticipating or experiencing a stressful situation. These internal cues are often interpreted by the individual as signs of impending failure. As such, this arousal state may be detrimental to performance. Common discomforts during pregnancy can include musculoskeletal aches and pains, shortness of breath, intermittent feelings of fear and panic, swelling, fatigue, and nausea. Some of these discomforts can be viewed by the woman as her body not dealing well with the pregnancy, and this can skew her perception of her ability to labor effectively. Additionally, common signs and symptoms of labor, such as pain, pressure, flushing, and rapid heart rate, can also serve to undermine confidence and therefore performance. Prenatal care providers can assist the pregnant woman by reinterpreting these discouraging signs and symptoms as falling within the range of normal or indicating encouraging signs of progress.

Self-efficacy is a major determinant of the amount of effort and degree of persistence an individual will apply to a difficult situation (Bandura, 1982). Self-efficacy has been related to a number of phenomena of interest to professionals caring for childbearing women, such as exercise during pregnancy and postpartum (Downs &

Hausenblas, 2004), amount of pain reported in labor (Lowe, 1991, 1996), persistence in laboring without analgesia or anesthesia versus use of epidural anesthesia during labor (Hodnett, 2002), and initiation and maintenance of breastfeeding (Blyth et al., 2002).

Labor and birth represent unique applications of self-efficacy theory. Unlike many other stressful events, labor cannot be avoided or stopped once it has begun. The course of labor for any given woman is essentially an unknown (Lowe, 1993, 2000), and there is no one single externally defined right way to give birth. Successful performance will be judged by the woman herself against her own expectations of her ideal performance during labor and birth. Prenatal care providers can assist by offering a view of a wide range of options and conditions for success and by using strategies to enhance childbirth confidence to support the woman's belief in her own strength and capabilities.

Practical strategies to enhance childbirth confidence (self-efficacy) in pregnant women

Performance accomplishment
- Review and build on prior positive childbirth experiences.
- Address and discuss prior negative childbirth experiences:
  - Listen to her stories.
  - Acknowledge her fears.
  - Point out differences between then and now.
  - Reframe the story for learning value.
- Explore emotional issues related to early pregnancy losses, whether spontaneous or elective.

Vicarious Experience
- Review prior attendance at a live birth and the emotions elicited.
- Inquire about what reading, viewing, listening about birth she is exposed to and
  - review her feelings about these
  - correct any misinformation
  - describe probabilities as well as possibilities.

Verbal Persuasion
- Inquire about others' messages to her regarding her plans for birth and her capabilities and help her frame them in a positive manner.
- Plant positive seeds using your own verbal persuasion skills regarding your faith in her ability to do well.

Visceral Arousal
- Review her health status and prenatal growth; point out the body's inherent ability to grow and to heal.
- Review prior pain experiences for coping strategies.
- Deal with emotional responses; do not dismiss them.
- Prepare her to deal with signs and symptoms of labor as positive progress.

Summary

The prenatal care provider is privileged to see pregnant women over time and at a key transitional point in their lives. The relationship between a woman and her prenatal care provider begins with a conversation starter as simple as "Tell me about yourself." The process of assessing a woman's psychosocial adaptation to pregnancy brings to consciousness and dialogue important concerns for women that cover a broad range of life experiences, social circumstances, and personality characteristics.

In dealing with psychosocial issues in pregnancy, the primary therapeutic strategy for the prenatal care provider is active and empathetic listening. Psychosocial adaptation is not something that is "cured" by the clinician. Information, support, and affirmations are provided to assist the woman in gaining insight to her situation. Pregnancy adds another dimension to a woman's life that can enhance or overwhelm her ability to cope and function. When a woman's coping mechanisms are overwhelmed or mental health concerns are raised, the care provider will turn to local social service agencies and mental health professionals for assistance in meeting her needs (Tharpe, Farley, & Jordan, 2013).

Psychosocial and physiological health outcomes for the mother and the baby are linked to prenatal processes. Attending to the psychosocial adaptations of the woman and her family throughout pregnancy is a preventive aspect of prenatal care and includes assessments and interventions to enhance psychosocial wellness and to reduce psychosocial risk. It is important to appreciate the psychosocial milieu of the pregnant woman in order to best serve her needs and to assist her in achieving her goals and optimum health outcomes.

Resources for women and their families

American Pregnancy Association. Promoting pregnancy wellness: http://www.americanpregnancy.org/index.htm

Body Image and Pregnancy: http://www.womenshealth.gov/body-image/pregnancy/

Childbirth Connection. Evidence based childbirth practice to empower childbearing women: http://www.childbirthconnection.org/

Family Equality Council: http://www.familyequality.org/

University of Michigan Health System. (2012). New baby sibling: Helping your older child (or children) adjust: http://www.med.umich.edu/yourchild/topics/newbaby.htm

Case study

A 25-year-old G1P0 woman presents for her initial prenatal visit at 10 weeks' EGA by certain last menstrual period (LMP). She is single, has had some college education, and works in the banking industry as a teller. She lives in an apartment with two girlfriends from college. She is involved with the baby's father, who is her supervisor at work. This pregnancy was unintended.

SUBJECTIVE: She and the father of her baby were initially shaken by the news of the pregnancy but are planning to continue the pregnancy. They are making plans to move in together. This client describes her own relationship with her mother as generally positive but rocky at times. Her mother has bipolar disorder and initially reacted poorly to the news of this pregnancy, but came around quickly to be supportive. This client's parents are divorced; she has been estranged from her father for 2 years. However, she called him to announce the pregnancy and resume relations with him. He was grateful for the chance to reconnect and offered his support of her and the baby. She is excited about becoming a mother and wants to have a birth with as little intervention as possible.

OBJECTIVE: Her vital signs and physical exam are within normal limits. Her bimanual exam reveals an anteverted uterus consistent with 10 weeks' size.

ASSESSMENT:

1. Intrauterine pregnancy at 10 weeks by dates and size; 2. Normal attachment and adaptation to pregnancy, including resolving expressed ambivalence, seeking acceptance for her baby from family members, connecting with her own mother, reconnecting with her father, and strengthening her relationship with her partner.

PLAN:

1. Affirm and support her continued growth and development into the maternal role.
2. Reassess her progress at the next scheduled visit.
3. Continue prenatal care and psychosocial support per routine and per individual needs.

Resources for health-care providers

Birthing from within. (2012). Philosophy: http://www.birthingfromwithin.com/philosophy

Bradley method. (2012). Why take Bradley classes? http://www.bradleybirth.com/WhyBradley.aspx

Childbirth Connection. For professionals: http://www.childbirthconnection.org/home.asp?Visitor=Professional

ChildStats.gov. (2011). America's children: Key national indicators of well-being: http://childstats.gov/americaschildren/

GLBT Health Access Project. (n.d.). Community Standards of Practice for the Provision of Quality Health Care Services to Lesbian, Gay, Bisexual, and Transgender Clients: http://www.glbthealth.org/CommunityStandardsofPractice.htm

Hypnobirthing. (2011). Taking the birthing world by calm: http://www.hypnobirthing.com/howitworks.htm

International Childbirth Education Association. (2012). Mission & Philosophy: http://www.icea.org/content/mission

Lamaze International. (2012). About Lamaze International: http://www.lamaze.org/CoreValues

Planned Parenthood. (2009). Out for health: http://www.outforhealth.org/for-providers.html

References

Ahern, N. R., & Ruland, J. P. (2003). Maternal-fetal attachment in African-American and Hispanic-American women. *The Journal of Perinatal Education, 12*(40), 27–35. doi:10.1624/105812403X107044

Alhusen, J. L. (2008). A literature update on maternal-fetal attachment. *Journal of Obstetric, Gynecologic, & Neonatal Nursing, 37*(3), 315–328. doi:10.1111/j.1552-6909.2008.00241.x

Amato, P. (2012). The well-being of children with gay and lesbian parents. *Social Science Research, 41*, 771–774.

Areskog, B., Kjessler, B., & Uddenberg, N. (1982). Identification of women with significant fear of childbirth during late pregnancy. *Gynecologic and Obstetric Investigation, 13*, 98–107.

Bagheri, M., Dorosty, A., Sadrzadeh-Yegneh, H., Eshraghian, M., Amirir, E., & Khamoush-Cheshm, N. (2012). Pre-pregnancy body size dissatisfaction and excessive gestational weight gain. *Maternal and Child Health Journal, 17*(4), 1–9. doi:10.1007/s10995-012-1051-6

Bandura, A. (1977). Self-efficacy: Toward a unifying theory of behavioral change. *Psychological Review, 84*, 191–215.

Bandura, A. (1982). Self-efficacy mechanism in human agency. *American Psychologist, 37*(2), 122–147. doi:10.1037/0003-066X.37.2.122

Blackburn, S. T. (2013). *Maternal, fetal and neonatal physiology* (4th ed.). St. Louis, MO: Saunders Elsevier.

Blyth, R., Creedy, D. K., Dennis, C., Moyle, W., Pratt, J., & De Vries, S. M. (2002). Effect of maternal confidence on breastfeeding duration: An application of breastfeeding self-efficacy theory. *Birth (Berkeley, Calif.), 29*(4), 278–284. doi:10.1046/j.1523-536X.2002.00202

Bowlby, J. (1978). *A secure base: Clinical applications of attachment theory*. London: Routledge.

Brazelton, T. B. (1973). *Neonatal behavioral assessment scale*. Philadelphia: J. B. Lippincott Co.

Cacioppo, J. T., Tassinary, L. G., & Berntson, G. G. (2007). *Handbook of psychophysiology* (3rd ed.). New York: Cambridge University Press.

Carty, E. M., & Tier, D. T. (1989). Birth planning: A reality based script for building confidence. *Journal of Nurse-Midwifery, 34*(3), 111–114.

Copen, C. E., Daniels, K., Vespa, J., & Mosher, W. D. (2012). *First marriages in the United States: Data from the 2006–2010 National Survey of Family.* National Health Statistics Reports, No. 49. Hyattsville, MD: National Center for Health Statistics.

DiPietro, J. A. (2010). Psychological and psychophysiological considerations regarding the maternal–fetal relationship. *Infant and Child Development, 19,* 27–38. doi:10.1002/icd.651

Downs, D. S., & Hausenblas, H. A. (2004). Women's exercise beliefs and behaviors during their pregnancy and postpartum. *Journal of Midwifery & Women's Health, 49*(2), 138–144. doi:10.1016/j.jmwh.2003.11.009

Draper, J. (2002). It's the first scientific evidence: Men's experience of pregnancy confirmation—Some findings from a longitudinal ethnographic study of transition to fatherhood. *Journal of Advanced Nursing, 39*(6), 563–570.

Dunham, C., Myers, F., Barnden, N., McDougall, A., Kelly, T. L., & Aria, B. (1991). *Mamatoto: A celebration of birth.* New York: Viking Penguin Press.

Engelhardt, H. T. (2012). Ritual, virtue and human flourishing: Rites as bearers of meaning. *Ritual and the Moral Life: Philosophical Studies in Contemporary Culture, 21*(1), 29–51. doi:10.1007/978-94-007-2756

Farley, C. (1999). *Vicarious experience: A source of self-efficacy for birth.* Retrieved from http://www.nursinglibrary.org/vhl/handle/10755/172803

Flagler, S., & Nicholl, L. (1990). A framework for the psychological aspects of pregnancy. *NAACOG's Clinical Issues in Perinatal and Women's Health Nursing, 1*(3), 267–278.

Geissbuehler, V., & Eberhard, G. (2002). Fear of childbirth during pregnancy: A study of more than 8000 pregnant women. *Journal of Psychosomatic Obstetrics and Gynaecology, 23*(4), 229–235. doi:10.3109/01674820209074677

Gerrig, R., & Zimbardo, P. G. (2002). Glossary of psychological terms. Retrieved from http://www.apa.org/research/action/glossary.aspx

GLBT Health Access Project. (n.d.). Community standards of practice for the provision of quality health care services to lesbian, gay, bisexual, and transgender clients. Retrieved from http://www.glbthealth.org/CommunityStandardsofPractice.htm

Gunatilake, R. P., & Perlow, J. H. (2011). Obesity and pregnancy: Clinical management of the obese gravida. *American Journal of Obstetrics and Gynecology, 204*(2), 106–119.

Haninger, N. C., & Farley, C. L. (2001). Screening for hypoglycemia in healthy term neonates: Effects on breastfeeding. *Journal of Midwifery & Women's Health, 46*(5), doi:10.1016/S1526-9523

Hodnett, E. D. (2002). Pain and women's satisfaction with the experience of childbirth: A systematic review. *American Journal of Obstetrics and Gynecology, 186,* S160–S172.

Hogg, M., & Vaughan, G. (2009). *Essentials of social psychology.* Boston: Pearson Education, Ltd.

Kennell, M. H., & Klaus, J. H. (1976). *Maternal-infant bonding.* St. Louis, MO: The C. V. Mosby Company.

Kennell, M. H., Klaus, J. H., & Klaus, P. (1995). *Bonding: Building the foundations of secure attachment and independence.* Boston: Addison Wesley.

Khanna, P. M. (2008). Icyou: How social media is the new resource for online health information. Retrieved from http://www.ncbi.nlm.nih.gov/pmc/articles/PMC2438491/

Klaidman, D., Hosenball, M., Gideonse, T., Howard, L., O'Donnell, P., & Stevenson, S. (1999). Bear down, push, and smile for the camera. *Newsweek,* May 24, 1999, p. 8.

Kuo, S.-H., Wang, R.-H., Tseng, H.-C., Jian, S.-Y., & Chou, F.-H. (2007). A comparison of different severities of nausea and vomiting during pregnancy relative to stress, social support, and maternal adaptation. *Journal of Midwifery & Women's Health, 52*(1), e1–e7. doi:10.1016/j.jmwh.2006.10.002

Lagan, B. M., Sinclair, M., & Kernohan, W. G. (2010). Internet use in pregnancy informs women's decision making: A web-based survey. *Birth (Berkeley, Calif.), 37,* 106–115. doi:10.1111/j.1523-536X.2010.00390.x

Lawson, K. L., & Turriff-Janasson, S. I. (2006). Maternal serum screening and psychosocial attachment to pregnancy. *Journal of Psychosomatic Research, 60,* 371–378.

Lederman, R. P. (1984). *Psychosocial adaptation in pregnancy.* New York: Springer Publishing Company.

Lederman, R. P. (1996). *Psychosocial adaptation in pregnancy* (2nd ed.). New York: Springer Publishing Company.

Lederman, R. P., & Weis, K. (2009). *Psychosocial adaptation in pregnancy* (3rd ed.). New York: Springer Publishing Company.

Lipkin, M., Jr., & Lamb, G. S. (1982). The couvade syndrome: An epidemiologic study. *Annals of Internal Medicine, 96*(4), 509–511.

Livingston, G., & Cohn, D. (2010). Childlessness up among all women; Down among women with advanced degrees. Retrieved from http://www.pewsocialtrends.org/2010/06/25/childlessness-up-among-all-women-down-among-women-with-advanced-degrees/1/

Lowe, N. K. (1991). Maternal confidence in coping with labor: A self-efficacy concept. *Journal of Obstetric, Gynecologic, and Neonatal Nursing, 20,* 457–463.

Lowe, N. K. (1993). Maternal confidence for labor: Development of the childbirth self-efficacy inventory. *Research in Nursing & Health, 16,* 141–149.

Lowe, N. K. (1996). The pain and discomfort of labor and birth. *Journal of Obstetric, Gynecologic, and Neonatal Nursing, 25,* 82–92.

Lowe, N. K. (2000). Self-efficacy for labor and childbirth fears in nulliparous pregnant women. *Journal of Psychosomatic Obstetrics and Gynaecology, 21,* 219–224.

Mamun, A. A., Kinarivala, M., O'Callaghan, M. J., Williams, G. M., Najman, J. M., & Callaway, L. K. (2010). Associations of excess weight gain during pregnancy with long-term maternal overweight and obesity: Evidence from 21 y postpartum follow-up. *The American Journal of Clinical Nutrition, 91*(5), 133.

Markus, E., Weingarten, A., Duplessi, Y., & Jones, J. (2010). Lesbian couples seeking pregnancy with donor insemination. *Journal of Midwifery & Women's Health, 55,* 124–132. doi:10.1016/j.jmwh.2009.09.014

Mehta, U. J., Siega-Riz, A. M., & Herring, A. H. (2010). Effect of body image on pregnancy weight gain. *Maternal and Child Health Journal, 15*(3), 324–332. doi:10.1007/s10995-010-0578-7

Mercer, R. T. (1985). Relationship of the birth experience to later mothering behaviors. *Journal of Nurse-Midwifery, 30*(4), 204–211. doi:10.1016/0091-2182

Mercer, R. T. (1995). A tribute to Reva Rubin. *MCN. The American Journal of Maternal Child Nursing, 20*(4), 184.

Mercer, R. T. (2010). Becoming a mother versus maternal role attainment. In A. I. Meleis (Ed.), *Transitions theory: Middle-range and situation-specific theories in nursing research and practice.* New York: Springer Publishing Company.

Merriam Webster Online Dictionary. (2012). Etymology of the word crisis. Retrieved from http://www.merriam-webster.com/dictionary/crisis

Mosher, W. D., Jones, J., & Abma, J. C. (2012). *Intended and unintended births in the United States: 1982–2010*. National health statistics reports; no 55. Hyattsville, MD: National Center for Health Statistics.

Nomaguchi, K. M., Brown, S. L., & Leyman, T. M. (2012). Father involvement and mothers' parenting stress: The role of relationship status. Retrieved from http://papers.ccpr.ucla.edu/papers/PWP -BGSU-2012-033/PWP-BGSU-2012-033.pdf

O'Connor, T. G., & Zeanah, C. H. (2003). Attachment disorders: Assessment strategies and treatment approaches. *Attachment & Human Development, 5*(3), 223–244. doi:10.1080/14616730310001 593974

Pappas, S. (2011). The truth about genderless babies. Retrieved from http://www.livescience.com/14323-genderless-baby-gender -anxiety.html

Parratt, J. A., & Fahy, K. M. (2010). A feminist critique of foundational nursing research and theory on transition to motherhood. *Midwifery, 27*(4), 445–451.

Pelka, S. (2009). Sharing motherhood: Maternal jealousy among lesbian co-mothers. *Journal of Homosexuality, 56*(2), 195–217.

Planned Parenthood. (2009). Out for health. Retrieved from http:// www.outforhealth.org/for-providers.html

Rauff, E. L., & Downs, S. D. (2011). Mediating effects of body image satisfaction on exercise behavior, depressive symptoms, and gestational weight gain in pregnancy. *Annals of Behavioral Medicine, 42*(3), 381–390. doi:10.1007/s12160-011-9300-2

Röndahl, G., Bruhner, E., & Lindhe, J. (2009). Heteronormative communication with lesbian families in antenatal care, childbirth and postnatal care. *Journal of Advanced Nursing, 65*, 1–11. http://dx.doi .org/10.1111/j.1365-2648.2009.05092.x

Rooks, J. P. (1997). *Midwifery and childbirth in America*. Philadelphia: Temple Press.

Rubin, R. (1984). *Maternal identity and the maternal experience*. New York: Springer Publishing Co.

Saisto, T., & Halmesmäki, E. (2003). Fear of childbirth: A neglected dilemma. *Acta Obstetricia et Gynecologica Scandinavica, 82*, 201–208. doi:10.1034/j.1600-0412.2003.00114.x

Sandelowski, M. (1993). Toward a theory of technology dependency. *Nursing Outlook, 41*(1), 36–42.

Scharfe, E. (2012). Maternal attachment representations and initiation and duration of breastfeeding. *Journal of Human Lactation, 28*(2), 218–225.

Scheper-Hughes, N. (1985). Culture, scarcity and maternal thinking: Maternal detachment and infant survival in a Brazilian shantytown. *Ethos (Berkeley, Calif.), 13*(4), 291–317.

Sherwen, L. N. (1987). *Psychosocial dimensions of the pregnant family*. New York: Springer Publishing Company.

Sleutel, M. R. (2003). Intrapartum nursing: Integrating Rubin's framework with social support theory. *Journal of Obstetric, Gynecologic, & Neonatal Nursing, 32*(1), 76–82.

Tharpe, N. L., Farley, C. L., & Jordan, R. G. (2013). *Clinical practice guidelines for midwifery & women's health* (4th ed.). Sudbury, MA: Jones & Bartlett Publishers.

Verny, T., & Kelly, J. (1981). *The secret life of the unborn child*. New York: Dell Publishing.

Wismont, J. M., & Reame, N. E. (1989). The lesbian childbearing experience: Assessing developmental tasks. *Journal of Nursing Scholarship, 21*, 137–141. doi:10.1111/j.1547-5069.1989.tb00118.x

Young, I. M. (1990). *Throwing like a girl and other essays in feminist philosophy and social theory*. Bloomington, IN: Indiana University Press.

Zeidenstein, L. (2004). Health issues of lesbian and bisexual women. In H. Varney, J. Kriebs, & C. Gegor (Eds.), *Varney's midwifery* (4th ed., pp. 299–311). Sudbury, MA: Jones and Bartlett.

17

Health education during pregnancy

Lisa Hanson, Leona VandeVusse, and Kathryn Shisler Harrod

Relevant terms

Birth plan—a written plan that guides birth attendants as to what the birthing family would like for the labor and birth

Childbirth education—childbirth education teaches a woman and her significant others about childbearing

Health literacy—an individual's ability to read, understand, and use health-care information to make decisions and follow instructions for treatment

Internatal care—a system of care that begins with the birth of the first child and extends through the birth of the next

Literacy—the ability to read for knowledge, to write coherently, and to think critically about the written word

---

Introduction

Pregnancy is an ideal time for a woman to learn how to improve her health and that of her developing fetus. Indeed, pregnancy is an optimal time to provide health information since most women are particularly receptive to learning and using new health information during pregnancy. Research has demonstrated that the provision of health information to a pregnant woman positively impacts the health of her entire family (Lu et al., 2006). Well-planned health education interactions during pregnancy also provide opportunities for health-care providers to establish an ongoing health-care relationship that forms the foundation for continued, comprehensive care after pregnancy (Lu et al., 2006).

Educational interactions during women's routine health-care visits during internatal care (the time from the birth of one child that extends through the birth of the next child) can be used to maximize positive health benefits (Lu et al., 2006). Thus, health-care professionals should take advantage of each health-care encounter during and between pregnancies to improve the health of the woman, her family, and future children.

Since all systems of prenatal care involve multiple visits with a health-care provider, health education during pregnancy can be strategically planned to optimize its impact on the health of women and their families. This chapter summarizes the specific components of health education that should be addressed during pregnancy and suggests the optimal timing for when specific topics should be addressed. Also included in this chapter are several broad topics related to prenatal education such as the quality of health information, cultural influences, health disparities, and the learner's developmental level, literacy level, and health literacy level. Specific aspects of prenatal education addressed in this chapter include prenatal care guidelines, the recommended timing of topics, scope of practice considerations, and documentation of the education provided.

Sources and quality of consumer childbirth education

Surprisingly, high-quality scientific evidence is lacking for both individual and group prenatal health education, according to the authors of a Cochrane Review of nine

Prenatal and Postnatal Care: A Woman-Centered Approach, First Edition. Edited by Robin G. Jordan, Janet L. Engstrom, Julie A. Marfell, and Cindy L. Farley.

studies on the topic (Gagnon & Sandall, 2007). Gagnon and Sandall (2007) criticized the published research for underrepresentation of economically, educationally, and socially disadvantaged participants in prenatal education studies. Another criticism was that the existing research was based on educators' priorities versus attendees' stated or unstated educational needs. The authors' conclusion was that the effects of prenatal education are not yet known.

In the past, it was commonplace for women and their partners to attend formal childbirth education classes beginning at approximately 28 weeks of gestation. The purpose of these classes is to educate women and their support people about labor and birth, and to prepare them with coping strategies such as breathing, relaxation, and massage as well as how to prepare for unexpected emergencies. The theoretical foundation for childbirth education is the proposition that knowledge lessens fear, which leads to less tension and, consequently, less pain (Dick-Read, 2006). Although individual studies show a positive impact on outcomes, overall, the evidence for effectiveness of childbirth education is inconclusive (Koehn, 2002). This may be because childbirth education is viewed as a "single uniform intervention" (Nolan, 2000) rather than from within the context of the broader influences on the participants, such as self-care, health promotion, quality of life, and outcomes beyond childbirth (Humenick, 2000).

The two most common forms of childbirth education available in use today are the Bradley Method® (American Academy of Husband-Coached Childbirth, 2012) and Lamaze (Lamaze International, 2013). Both of these contemporary childbirth education methods have a unique philosophy that provides the basis for the structure and content of classes.

Hypnobirthing is another method of preparing for childbirth that utilizes mental preparation and relaxation and has gained recognition in recent years. This method is based on the prior work of Dr. Grantly Dick-Read, an English obstetrician who was first to propose the concept of reducing pain through eliminating fear and anxiety and thereby reducing stress hormones that increase pain.

Another alternative available to women is attending hospital-based classes. However, these hospital-based classes have frequently been criticized for teaching in a manner that is biased toward interventions and/or practices that are commonplace at the particular facility (Walker, Visger, & Rossie, 2009). In spite of these critiques, some couples favor these classes because they are convenient and provide reassurance and familiarity with the birth setting. Prenatal health-care providers should be knowledgeable about the different types of

Childbirth education: comparison of the Bradley and Lamaze approaches

	Bradley	Lamaze
Philosophy	The Bradley Method teaches families how to have natural births. Techniques are based on how the human body works in labor.	Lamaze was originally based on the Pavlovian theory of conditioned behavioral responses through preparation and training (in dogs). Contemporary Lamaze is based on six natural, healthy birth practices that are supported by research about maternity care practices.
Foci	What to expect and how to avoid pain in labor, focusing on a healthy pregnancy and the relationships of the pregnant woman and her support people	The six healthy birth practices: • Let labor begin on its own. • Move around and change positions. • Have continuous support. • Avoid interventions. • Avoid being on your back. • Keep mother and baby together.
Number of classes	12 classes that follow a workbook with a certified instructor	6 weeks of classes taught by a Lamaze Certified Childbirth Educator

childbirth education classes available to women in their local area, and the cost and time commitment required of each. Further, health-care providers with knowledge of the types of classes and educators available can help women with special considerations, such as women from diverse cultures, single women, and lesbian couples select childbirth classes that meet their individual needs.

The findings of the Listening to Mothers II survey demonstrated that only about 25% of pregnant women participate in formal education childbirth classes and fewer than 10% identified the classes as their most important source of information about pregnancy and childbirth (Declercq, Sakala, Corry, & Applebaum, 2006). Instead, women reported that their most important sources of information were books, friends and relatives, and the Internet (Armstrong & Pooley, 2005; DeClercq et al., 2006). Women with higher education levels and incomes are more likely to have searched for health information on the Internet. However, most women do not discuss their Internet search findings with their health-care providers (Diaz et al., 2002). Health-care providers' knowledge of Web resources could facilitate open discussions and educational exchanges with patients during health-care visit interactions.

Recently, reality television shows have become a common, yet controversial, source of information for pregnant women and their families. For example, a content analysis of 85 American reality-based television shows that portrayed 123 births revealed that the shows emphasized the use of medical intervention during birth (Morris & McInerney, 2010). The television shows also underrepresented the diversity of women and their family structures (Morris & McInerney, 2010).

Unfortunately, consumers do not have safeguards and assurances concerning the accuracy and currency of health resources. Therefore, it is imperative for prenatal care providers to develop a list of recommended resources that they check regularly for the content contained. Internet sources of information can be evaluated using established criteria such as the MedlinePlus Guide to Healthy Web Surfing (U.S. National Library of Medicine National Institutes of Health, 2010). The link to this guide is located in the Resources for Health-Care Providers and Women at the end of this chapter. Health-care professionals may want to follow these guidelines to find appropriate Web sites for their clients' use.

Public libraries continue to be good sources of free reading material. Since digital readers have become more common, some pregnancy books are available for use in digital formats for loan through libraries or for purchase through online bookstores. The ever-expanding options of free or low-cost sources of Internet accessible materials add both opportunity and complexity for women and their families. Prenatal care providers can help direct women to the most optimal sources for reading materials by keeping current with the materials that are available. A list of Web resources is provided at the end of this chapter to assist health-care providers and the women for whom they provide care.

Health-care professionals providing prenatal care are encouraged to develop a recommended reading list or a lending library, based on the principles outlined in this chapter. The reading list can be individualized to the philosophy of normal physiological birth, as well as the culture, language, and age of the population served. Books chosen for inclusion need to be carefully reviewed for content, accuracy, and currency.

Prenatal visit approach to individual childbirth education

Historically, a major component of prenatal education has taken place during individual prenatal visits and formal prenatal classes. Since fewer women are attending prenatal classes, there needs to be an increased emphasis on education during prenatal visits and also independently by the woman and her family. During individual prenatal visits, there is variable time devoted specifically to education. In a classic study, Lehrman (1981) demonstrated that certified nurse-midwives (CNMs) spent an average of 24 minutes for each prenatal visit and devoted at least some of that time to prenatal education. As health-care providers are increasingly pressured to see higher volumes of prenatal clients, efficient use of time during prenatal visits is essential.

Class education and group prenatal care

Group prenatal care (introduced in Chapter 5) is a system of care that allows more time to be spent on health education. Group prenatal care includes women of similar gestational ages who share concerns and questions with each other while receiving prenatal care. At least one group member is a health professional who contributes to and facilitates the discussions. The most well-known form of group prenatal care is the version called CenteringPregnancy™ that involves following a specific curriculum plan so that information covered is comprehensive and relevant (Centering Healthcare Institute, 2011). Group prenatal care involves multiple directions of information exchange, with the group participants viewed as equals and important sources of information and experience.

Developmental considerations in prenatal health education

Adolescents

Cognition impacts both teaching and learning in adults (Long, McCrary, & Ackerman, 1979). While the rate of adolescent pregnancy and births has recently declined (Guttmacher Institute, 2012), teen clients require special consideration regarding prenatal health education because their cognitive abilities are not fully developed. The cognitive features of early, middle, and late adolescence are summarized in the following textbox. The completion of adolescence is independent of age and is characterized by the person's ability to solve abstract problems and compare plausible explanations for phenomena (Friedman, 2006). Because pregnancy has been associated with regression to earlier cognitive states, assessing the predominant cognitive features of individual adolescents can aid in developing, implementing, and evaluating an appropriate plan of prenatal health education (Friedman, 2006; Maehr & Felice, 2006a, 2006b). Strategies for optimal communication with adolescents include the following: Be succinct; use questions that are nonthreatening, open-ended, and do not ask "why"; listen in a nonjudgmental manner and listen more than you speak; reflect the adolescent's mood during interactions (except when it is hostile); model rational decision making; and raise multiple perspectives (American Psychological Association (APA), 2002).

Adult education principles

Knowles (1970, 1980) outlined the principles of adult education and key principles are summarized in the following textbox (Ozuah, 2005) with examples of how they can be incorporated into prenatal education. Adult learners share a goal: to enrich their knowledge. Applying the principles of adult education creates an environment of mutual exchange of information that is viewed as relevant by the pregnant woman and her family. Adult learning principles include respecting the knowledge the adult already has and building beyond it. Women enter pregnancy with preconceived thoughts, feelings and motivation to change while learning more about bodily changes, pregnancy, breastfeeding, and childcare.

Adolescent cognitive development

Time frame	Cognitive features
Early teen 11–14 years	• Concrete thinking predominates • Mainly present oriented • Planning is vague, unrealistic • Limited ability to be introspective and to reason abstractly • Commonly reasons by trial and error • Learns and retains information but sometimes unable to apply it • Often exclusive identification of a "best friend" • Concerns about conformity to peers
Middle teen 15–17 years	• Egocentric • Rebellious • Mostly reason by trial and error • Abstract reasoning and introspection becoming more common • Present oriented with limited future planning abilities • Magical thinking leads to "risk taking" and "impulsive" behavior • Short-term relationships may become sexual
Late teen 18–20 years	• Identity developed, along with "other orientation" • Can apply and use information • Engages in abstract reasoning • Sexual relationships become more interpersonal • Able to plan for the future • Sets goals and takes steps to meet them • Transitioning into adult roles in society (work and family)

Principles of adult education as applied to prenatal education

Principle	Example of incorporation into prenatal education
Autonomous and self-directed	"What would you like to talk about today?"
Need to connect new learning to prior knowledge	"Tell me what you have learned about the discomforts of pregnancy."
Goal and relevancy oriented	"You are in your third trimester, let's talk about some things that you may experience in the coming weeks."
Practical	"Since you are 36 weeks today, it would be a good idea to finalize your birth plan and discuss the signs and symptoms of labor."
Treat with respect in order to learn effectively	"Good afternoon Ms. Jones. My name is Lisa and I will be your nurse-midwife. Would it be acceptable to you if I bring a student to your first prenatal visit today?"

Issues integral to prenatal education

Women's experiences of prenatal care have been examined in an integrative review of 36 studies (Novick, 2009). The described components of prenatal care included three subthemes: continuity, comprehensiveness, and control. While women preferred a single prenatal provider, they will accept a substitute with notification. Although women highly valued counseling, education, and support groups as a part of prenatal education, these were not made readily available to them. In terms of decision making, women valued providers who were good listeners and involved them in decision making. This last finding is aligned with Quality and Safety Education for Nurses (QSEN) (2012) recommendations for patient-centered care as an essential component of nursing education and practice, to "Recognize the patient or designee as the source of control and full partner in providing compassionate and coordinated care based on respect for patient's preferences, values, and needs." Therefore women's preferences in prenatal education and counseling (patient-centered care) are clearly linked to safety.

Literacy, health literacy, written materials, and reading level

Literacy includes the ability to read, gain knowledge, write coherently, and think critically about what the individual has read. However, even highly literate and educated people may not be "health literate." Health literacy is defined by the U.S. Department of Health and Human Services Health Resources & Services Administration (n.d.) as "the degree to which individuals have the capacity to obtain, process and understand basic health information needed to make appropriate health decisions regarding services needed to prevent or treat illness." However, in one study of two U.S. hospitals, up to two-thirds of patients could not understand basic health information, medication directions, or an informed consent document (Williams et al., 1995). Since health literacy is linked to patient safety, the Partnership for Clear Health Communication at the National Patient Safety Foundation (n.d.) has launched the "Ask me 3" program. This program promotes three simple questions that all patients are encouraged to ask of their providers at every health-care interaction: "(1) What is my main problem? (2) What do I need to do? [and] (3) Why is it important for me to do this?" Health-care providers should use these questions to frame prenatal education in a clear and understandable manner, especially if the woman develops a complication during pregnancy.

It is recommended that written health information be presented at a fourth to sixth grade reading level (U.S. National Library of Medicine National Institutes of Health, 2011), and various tools are available to assess the reading level of a document. For example, the Flesch reading ease test formula is available online and uses the number of words, sentences, and syllables to determine a reading level estimate of inserted text (Edit Central, 2011). It is recommended that written patient education materials be subjected to a reading level test before they are introduced to patients for use. Presenting complex information in simple and understandable terms in written materials will improve their utility and impact. Additionally, selective use of graphics may convey important information using fewer words in a more memorable manner for some learners. The goal of health literacy stated in the *Healthy People 2020* document (U.S. Department of Health and Human Services, 2010) is that "everyone [be able] . . . to make good health decisions . . . [using the internet and] printed materials, media campaigns, community outreach, and interpersonal communication."

Prenatal health education guidelines

Recently, five major guidelines for prenatal care were reviewed and critiqued (Hanson, VandeVusse, Roberts, & Forristal, 2009). Seven themes were identified across the guidelines that organized the critique and are relevant for this discussion: "(1) the direction of communication between patient and provider, (2) a predominant focus on [the woman's] physical versus psychological needs, (3) the increasing attentiveness to risk, (4) additive expectations for prenatal care [with decreasing time to provide it], (5) lack of a broad health promotion focus, (6) inconsistent endorsement of component parts of prenatal care, and (7) lack of attention to prenatal education." This last major criticism of the published guidelines for prenatal care demonstrates the need for prenatal care providers to fill this gap (Hanson et al., 2009).

This critical analysis of published antenatal care guidelines also demonstrated significant gaps in prenatal health education (Hanson et al., 2009). Specifically, there were inconsistencies between guidelines regarding which prenatal and general health education topics were included. Evidence for or against the inclusion of topics was lacking. Further, the timing of introduction of prenatal education topics varied among guidelines. Therefore, health professionals are encouraged to develop a comprehensive approach for prenatal health education that can be individualized to meet the needs and priorities of their clients.

Prioritizing prenatal education needs

Roberts (1976) identified four priorities in prenatal education in her classic work. In order of importance, these were (1) responding to a woman's specific questions; (2) addressing essential health and safety issues; (3) providing anticipatory guidance about pregnancy changes, birth, and infant care; and finally (4) adding detailed explanations on any topics or policies that were beyond the woman's self-identified needs at the visit. Roberts (1976) organized the information by gestation and recommended that the prenatal education plan be refined as pregnancy progressed. This approach is consistent with principles of adult learning, specifically the desire for practical information that is relevant and meets women's needs. Each of these priorities is discussed in detail in the following sections and can be adapted for individual and group prenatal care.

Responding to questions

Responding to questions of a woman and her partner may seem like a simple task. However, in a busy prenatal clinic, the challenge becomes immediately apparent. Prenatal visits are often scheduled for a brief and even overbooked in relatively short time frames. While women can ask questions during a prenatal visit at any time, some may be unable to remember their questions if they perceive that the provider is rushing. Taking time to sit and talk to each woman (and her significant other) before or at the end of the appointment will provide the opportunity to answer questions and provide needed education.

Discussing health and safety issues

Issues of safety include environmental health; diet, supplements, and food safety; psychosocial and physical assessments; laboratory testing; and plans to modify risk factors. A careful chart review either before entering the room or with the woman will assure that vital signs and laboratory findings are carefully addressed. A substantial amount of prenatal health education time is devoted to discussing and reviewing the ever-increasing number of laboratory and diagnostic tests incorporated into the accepted standard of prenatal care. At the same time, as more prenatal tests are added, the expectations for productivity are also increasing (Hanson et al., 2009); however, attention to other important aspects of education may help refocus prenatal visits on wellness.

Anticipatory guidance

Anticipatory guidance is the third priority and refers to a specific form of health education in which health-care providers prepare women for likely pregnancy experiences including physical and emotional symptoms, events, and sensations. The woman is growing and developing as a mother during pregnancy. She is experiencing a unique connection between her mind and her body. The emotional and physiological changes that are occurring may be viewed as welcome and exciting, frightening and strange, or for some women, they may even be ignored. Discussions about what she can expect can help reframe the normal discomforts of pregnancy and target education to her developing needs.

A clear understanding of women's experiences during each trimester will help guide the development of a plan of anticipatory guidance. For example, during the first trimester, women focus on their profound physiological changes including nausea, fatigue, urinary frequency, and breast tenderness. Education aimed at coping with these changes will be more effective than attempting to address issues further from her physical and emotional experience. It is important to maintain a balance between the time spent on the many genetic tests that are offered during early pregnancy and the woman's needs to know about the physical and emotional changes occurring.

During the second trimester, relative comfort is accompanied by quickening and a greater awareness of the individuality of the fetus. Therefore, prenatal educational topics can be broadened during this time to include issues of breastfeeding, infant care, and parenting.

During the final trimester, women become increasingly ready to discuss and ultimately experience the process of labor and birth. While all women want optimal outcomes for themselves and their babies, tapping into this emotional readiness allows for meaningful dialogues about labor and birth, including fears and hopes for the experience.

Providing anticipatory guidance

Providing information about other topics or policies beyond the woman's immediate needs is the final priority the provider can address. An example is the development of a written birth plan for the last trimester. A pragmatic approach to begin a birth plan discussion is sharing features of the birth environment and the processes of care with the woman and her family. This will allow her to develop a birth plan that is realistic and useful to guide her care during labor and birth.

Trimester-based approaches to prenatal education

Depending on the structure of the prenatal care environment (individual versus group), women may experience up to a dozen or more prenatal visits. Considering the priorities of prenatal education and the relative predictability of the emotional and physical changes of pregnancy, education can be efficiently structured by trimester. Table 17.1 contains teaching timing on specific prenatal education topics such as laboratory testing, labor preparation, and physiological changes and discomforts of pregnancy and is based on the priorities for prenatal education (Roberts, 1976). Additional recommendations based on gestational age and an analysis of existing prenatal care guidelines are provided (Hanson et al., 2009). No plan for prenatal health education is complete without making sure it is individualized for each woman. Careful planning of education topics may help to avoid information overload at any single prenatal visit. Prenatal providers are encouraged to adapt the teaching plans presented to the needs of their clients and the ever-changing components of prenatal care.

Table 17.1. Prenatal Care Health Education Topics and Suggested Timing

Prenatal health education topics	Gestational weeks*				
	0†–12	12–24	24–32	32–36	36-term
Cervical examination			X		X
Depression screening	X	X	X		X
EDB calculation compared to uterine size	X	X	X	X	X
Fetal growth and status	X	X	X	X	X
Fetal heart tones	X	X	X	X	X
Fetal movement/quickening		X	X	X	X
Fetal presentation			X	X	X
Fundal height measurement	X	X	X	X	X
Hypertensive disorder screening	X	X	X	X	X
Intimate partner violence	X		X	X	
NST, BPP, Doppler flow if indicated			X	X	X
RhoGAM/antepartum			X		
Risk identification/assessment	X	X	X	X	X
Tuberculosis testing	X				
Vaccines					
• Diphtheria	X				
• Hepatitis B	X				
• Influenza	X	X	X	X	X
• TDaP status	X				
Weight gain	X	X	X	X	X
Birth setting information/tour	X				X
Cessation of harmful substances†					
• Alcohol	X				
• Drugs	X				
• Teratogens	X				
• Tobacco	X				
Circumcision decision making					X
Dental care	X				
Employment or school plans	X	X	X		X
Exercise/activity	X	X	X	X	X
Family planning/postpartum				X	X
Genetics counseling as needed	X				
Hot tub/sauna use	X				
Infant feeding method					
• Breastfeeding education	X	X	X	X	X
• Formula feeding education					X
Labor and birth preparation					
• Analgesia and anesthesia				X	X
• Birth planning/preparation				X	X

Table 17.1. (*Continued*)

Prenatal health education topics	Gestational weeks*				
	0†–12	12–24	24–32	32–36	36-term
• Childbirth class attendance		X		X	X
• Involvement of significant other		X			X
• Labor signs/symptoms/when to call provider				X	X
• Plan for care of other children				X	
• Relaxation and comfort techniques			X	X	X
Musculoskeletal discomforts					
• Back pain		X	X	X	
• Leg ache/cramping/varicosities		X	X	X	
• Round ligament pain		X	X	X	
• Sciatica				X	
Nausea and vomiting	X				
Nutrition					
• Balanced diet counseling	X	X			
• Body mass index calculation	X				
• Folic acid	X				
• Food safety	X				
Orientation to provider/practice/prenatal care processes	X				
Over-the-counter medications	X				
Pediatric provider selection			X		X
Personal hygiene					
• Body mechanics			X	X	
• Breast care and supportive bra		X	X		
• Comfortable clothing		X	X		
Physiological changes/pregnancy discomforts					
• Breast fullness/tenderness	X				
• Constipation		X		X	
• Contractions (Braxton Hicks)			X	X	
• Dyspnea/shortness of breath		X	X	X	
• Emotional changes/fears			X		X
• Fatigue	X				X
• Heartburn			X	X	X
• Hemorrhoids			X		X
Postdate management					X
Preparation for baby:			X	X	X
• Household assistance			X		
• Supplies			X		X
Preterm labor education		X	X	X	
Rest	X				X

(*Continued*)

Table 17.1. *(Continued)*

Prenatal health education topics	Gestational weeks*				
	0†–12	12–24	24–32	32–36	36-term
Review laboratory results with woman	X	X	X	X	X
Safety/seatbelts	X				
Sexuality	X		X		X
Supine hypotension		X			
Travel	X	X		X	
Tubal ligation authorization			X		
Urinary frequency	X				
Vaginal discharge		X		X	X
VBAC informed consent	X		X		
Genetic testing options					
• Disease specific	X				
• Nuchal translucency screen	X				
• Maternal serum screening	X	X			
• Ultrasound anatomy screen		X			
Routine lab testing:					
• Antibody screen	X		X		
• Blood type and Rh	X				
• Chlamydia (at risk in the third trimester)	X				X
• Complete blood count	X				
• Gonorrhea	X				
• Group B strep				X	X
• Hemoglobinopathies	X				
• Hepatitis B surface antigen	X				
• HIV	X				
• Papanicolau smear	X				
• Rubella	X				
• Syphilis	X				
• Urinalysis/urine culture	X	X			
• Varicella	X				
Selective testing as indicated					
• Hepatitis C testing	X				
• Gestational diabetes serum screen	X	X	X		

Note: Adapted from "A critical appraisal of guidelines for antenatal care: Components of care and priorities in prenatal education," by L. Hanson, L. VandeVusse, J. Roberts, & A. Forristal, 2009, *Journal of Midwifery & Women's Health, 54*, pp. 466–468. Copyright 2009 by the American College of Nurse-Midwives.
*Several prenatal visits can occur within each time frame specified, allowing multiple opportunities and chances to revisit topics as needed; †zero weeks refers to possible preconception care topics; ‡follow-up positive results with discussion at each subsequent visit including cessation plan.
BPP, biophysical profile; EDB, estimated date of birth; NST, nonstress test; VBAC, vaginal birth after cesarean.

Cultural considerations

Each woman's cultural background affects the manner in which she prepares for and perceives childbirth (Greene, 2007). Prenatal health-care providers need to consider cultural background when preparing the education plan for an individual woman. Written prenatal educational materials should be culturally relevant whenever possible. Fortunately, educational materials depicting women from the diverse cultures are available at no cost from several government-sponsored Web sites, and many of these materials are available in several languages. These Web sites are highlighted in the Web resource list at the end of this chapter. The predominantly government-sponsored Web sites are intended to better serve diverse communities as well as conserve health-care resources for translation of health information. Several of these Web sites also contain portals to government and community resources for the care of women who are refugees.

The importance of culturally relevant health education was demonstrated in a study of 59 minority women, 76.3% of whom were Spanish speakers and 93.2% were foreign-born (Berman, 2006). Of the women, 80% indicated that attending childbirth education classes was important, preferably with instructors from similar cultural backgrounds. The topics in which they were primarily interested varied by gestational age, with discomforts (57.6%), nutrition (50.8%), and emotional changes (45.8%) taking precedence in early pregnancy; in late pregnancy, they wanted to learn the most about postpartum self-care (55.9%) and reducing labor pain (54.2%). The women identified the top three barriers to attending classes as transportation (42.4%), childcare (35.6%), and cost (27.1%). These findings indicate that prenatal education should incorporate cultural practices as well as informational topics that are relevant to the population and offering childcare in an accessible site.

Health disparities and vulnerable populations

Health disparities are associated with poorer perinatal outcomes in vulnerable populations. Health-care providers can positively impact the health of women and families in vulnerable populations by consistently incorporating information on health promotion during health-care visits (Lu et al., 2006; McDorman & Mathews, 2008). Vonderheid, Norr, and Handler (2007) demonstrated an association between prenatal education and positive health behaviors in a study of 159 low-risk African American and Mexican prenatal clinic attendees. The average participant was exposed to 17 of the 22 "health-promoting" prenatal education topics during the course of pregnancy. Improved health behaviors were associated with patients having discussed a higher number of health promotion topics with health-care providers. These findings suggest that health education positively impacts women's health behaviors.

Documentation of teaching

Prenatal health education needs to be carefully documented in the prenatal record to assure that all relevant and needed topics are covered. Documenting that the appropriate topics have been covered and that the woman responded in a manner that indicates understanding of the material facilitates continuity, especially when different health-care providers are involved the woman's care. Although many of the standardized prenatal health records include a minimal checklist for such documentation, prenatal health education should also be documented in progress notes. Some electronic health record systems include triggers or reminders for health education and timing of laboratory testing. In the absence of these reminders, health-care providers need to carefully attend to both the timing and documentation of prenatal health and safety information. It is recommended that documentation of teaching include statements that the woman verbalized understanding of the health education, and that she indicates that she knows how and when to contact the health-care provider, and also that she denied further questions. Such documentation is especially important for topics such as the danger signs of pregnancy complications and the onset of labor. The effectiveness of health teaching can be evaluated at the subsequent visit when the woman is asked if she has any questions or concerns about what was discussed at her last visit.

Summary

Prenatal care visits provide opportunities for education that can impact the health of the woman, her unborn fetus, and her entire family. Special consideration of the woman's culture, her chronological age, cognitive skills, her access and use of health resources, and her health literacy all impact the delivery and receipt of prenatal education. Education incorporated into prenatal visits by prioritizing the woman's learning needs allows for individualization of information and opportunities to present the information when women are best able to comprehend, remember, and use the information. A well-planned approach with careful documentation of individual and group education is essential to meet the extensive informational needs of pregnant women. Prenatal health-care providers play an essential role in providing evidence-based and patient-centered health education throughout the prenatal period.

Case study

Gloria is a G1 P0 who presents as a transfer to care at 16 weeks of gestation from a reproductive endocrinologist. She achieved pregnancy with the help of assisted reproductive technologies. She is currently 32 weeks of gestation at this visit and her baby has been in breech position since 28 weeks.

SUBJECTIVE: "I really want a vaginal birth, is there anything I can do to change this baby's position? I have been reading a number of books and Internet sites and they seem to say that it can be done. There was so much intervention at the beginning of the pregnancy, I was hoping to have less intervention at birth. It seems like there is a trend in doctors and midwives doing breech births these days. That is what they were saying in my childbirth classes. Plus they are saying there are lots of alternatives to try that are often successful. What do you think?"

OBJECTIVE: Gloria presents her questions in an emotional manner, tearing up when she says she wants a vaginal birth.

ASSESSMENT: Gloria needs specific education regarding the various techniques and their probabilities of success for strategies to turn a breech baby. She also needs emotional support in the hope that her baby will turn on its own and in the event that her desired birth is not able to be accomplished.

PLAN: A discussion regarding what Gloria has read and heard should be undertaken in a calm and unhurried manner. Simply waiting to see whether the baby turns without intervention is the best strategy at this point in time, so provide reassurance that the fetal position can change and is in fact very likely to do so. The important point regarding the formal and informal prenatal education she has had to date is to respectfully acknowledge what she has learned from the various sources she has explored and to add the evidence base, or lack thereof, for the procedures she has encountered. Conflicting information from various sources can lead to confusion for women as to what is the best plan of care. If she brings up procedures or alternative therapies that are unfamiliar, such as the Webster chiropractic procedure or moxibustion, welcome the information she brings and make a point to investigate the current literature and bring this information to her at her next visit. The commitment of the health-care provider is not to know everything but to follow up and learn as new ideas are brought forward. The health-care provider is viewed as a source of credible information for women; with this comes with the responsibility to be a lifelong learner.

Resources for health-care providers and women

Selected government Web sites

Agency	Topics	Web site
Centers for Disease Control and Prevention (CDC)	Pregnancy	http://www.cdc.gov/ncbddd/pregnancy_gateway/during.html
Department of Health and Human Services (DHHS): Multicultural Resources for Health Information	• Cultural competency • Dictionaries • Glossaries • Online translation tools • Health literacy • Health resources in multiple languages • Limited English proficiency • Multicultural research • Organizations and portals • Refugee health portals	http://sis.nlm.nih.gov/outreach/multicultural.html
DHHS: Office of Women's Health	Pregnancy	http://www.womenshealth.gov/pregnancy/
Food and Drug Administration (FDA)	Food safety for pregnant women	http://www.fda.gov/food/resourcesforyou/healtheducators/ucm081785.htm

Selected government Web sites

Agency	Topics	Web site
National Institutes of Health (NIH)	Downloadable patient education handouts (some in Spanish)	http://health.nih.gov/topic/Pregnancy (pregnancy) http://health.nih.gov/ (general topics by alphabetical listing)
National Library of Medicine (NLM)	MedlinePlus Guide to Healthy Web Surfing How to write easy to read health materials	http://www.nlm.nih.gov/medlineplus/ healthywebsurfing.html http://www.nlm.nih.gov/medlineplus/etr.html
Refugee Health Information Network (RHIN)	Multilingual downloadable health information sheets for refugees and providers	http://rhin.org/default.aspx

Resources for women and their families

Selected nongovernment Web sites

Agency	Content	Web site
American College of Nurse-Midwives (ACNM)	Downloadable health information sheets called "Share with Women" on many topics, some in Spanish	http://www.midwife.org/
American Congress of Obstetricians and Gynecologists (ACOG)	Information pamphlets for purchase, some in Spanish. A FAQ page for consumers	http://www.acog.org/
March of Dimes (MOD)	Many consumer-friendly resources on various pregnancy topics	http://www.marchofdimes.com/
Childbirth Connections	Consumer and professional information on evidence-based care practices for pregnancy and birth	http://www.childbirthconnection.org/
Lamaze Method	To learn about Lamaze and find a Lamaze certified childbirth instructor	http://www.lamaze.org/p/cm/ld/fid=1
Bradley Method	To learn about the Bradley Method and find a Bradley certified childbirth instructor	http://www.bradleybirth.com/
Hypnobirthing method	To learn about hypnobirthing and find a certified hypnobirthing instructor	http://www.hypnobirthing.com/

References

American Academy of Husband-Coached Childbirth. (2012). *The Bradley Method of husband-coached natural childbirth.* Retrieved from http://www.bradleybirth.com/

American Psychological Association. (2002). *Developing adolescents: A reference for professionals.* Washington, DC: Author. Retrieved from http://www.apa.org/pi/cyf/develop.pdf

Armstrong, T. M., & Pooley, J. A. (2005). Being pregnant: A qualitative study of women's lived experience of pregnancy. *Journal of Prenatal and Perinatal Psychological and Health, 20*(1), 4–24.

Berman, R. O. (2006). Perceived learning needs of minority expectant women and barriers to prenatal education. *The Journal of Perinatal Education, 15*(2), 36–42.

Centering Healthcare Institute. (2011). *Centering model overview: Group healthcare model.* Retrieved from https://www.centering healthcare.org/pages/centering-model/pregnancy-overview.php

Declercq, E. R., Sakala, C., Corry, M. P., & Applebaum, S. (2006). *Listening to Mothers II: Report of the second national U.S. survey of women's childbearing experiences.* New York: Childbirth Connection.

Diaz, J. A., Griffith, R. A., Ng, J. J., Reinert, S. E., Friedmann, P. D., & Moulton, A. W. (2002). Patients' use of the internet for medical information. *Journal of General Internal Medicine, 17*(3), 180–185. doi:10.1046/j.1525-1497.2002.10603.x

Dick-Read, G. (2006). *Childbirth without fear.* London: Pollinger. (Original work published 1942).

Edit Central. (2011). *Flesch reading ease test.* Retrieved from http://www.editcentral.com/gwt1/EditCentral.html

Friedman, L. S. (2006). Seventeen to twenty-one years: Transition to adulthood. In S. D. Dixon & M. T. Stein (Eds.), *Encounters with children: Pediatric behavior and development* (4th ed., pp. 601–620). Philadelphia: Mosby Elsevier.

Gagnon, A. J., & Sandall, J. (2007). Individual or group antenatal education for childbirth or parenthood, or both. *Cochrane Database of Systematic Reviews*, (3), CD002869. doi:10.1002/14651858.CD002869.pub2

Greene, M. J. (2007). Strategies for incorporating cultural competence into childbirth education curriculum. *Journal of Perinatal Education*, *16*(2), 33–37. doi:10.1624/105812407X191489

Guttmacher Institute. (2012). *Facts on American Teens' Sexual and Reproductive Health*. Retrieved from http://www.guttmacher.org/pubs/FB-ATSRH.html

Hanson, L., VandeVusse, L., Roberts, J., & Forristal, A. (2009). A critical appraisal of guidelines for antenatal care: Components of care and priorities in prenatal education. *Journal of Midwifery & Women's Health*, *54*, 458–468.

Humenick, S. S. (2000). Program evaluation. In F. H. Nichols & S. S. Humenick (Eds.), *Childbirth education: Practice, research, and theory* (2nd ed., pp. 593–608). Philadelphia: W.B. Saunders.

Knowles, M. S. (1970). *The modern practice of adult education: Andragogy vs. pedagogy*. New York: Association Press.

Knowles, M. S. (1980). *The modern practice of adult education: From pedagogy to andragogy*. Englewood Cliffs, NJ: Cambridge.

Koehn, M. L. (2002). Childbirth education outcomes: An integrative review of the literature. *Journal of Perinatal Education*, *11*(3), 10–19. doi:10.1624/105812402X88795

Lamaze International. (2013). *Healthy birth practices*. Retrieved from http://www.lamaze.org/HealthyBirthPractices

Lehrman, E. J. (1981). Nurse-midwifery practice: A descriptive study of prenatal care. *Journal of Midwifery and Women's Health*, *26*(3), 27–41. doi:10.1016/0091-2182(81)90057-4

Long, H. B., McCrary, K., & Ackerman, S. (1979). Adult cognition: Piagetian based research findings. *Adult Education*, *30*(1), 3–18. doi:10.1177/074171367903000101

Lu, M. C., Kotelchuck, M., Culhane, J. F., Hobel, C. J., Klerman, L. V., & Thorp, J. M. (2006). Preconception care between pregnancies: The content of internatal care. *Maternal and Child Health Journal*, *10*(5 Suppl.), S107–S122.

Maehr, J., & Felice, M. E. (2006a). Eleven to fourteen years: Early adolescence—Age of rapid changes. In S. D. Dixon & M. T. Stein (Eds.), *Encounters with children: Pediatric behavior and development* (4th ed., pp. 535–562). Philadelphia: Mosby Elsevier.

Maehr, J., & Felice, M. E. (2006b). Fifteen to seventeen years: Mid-adolescence—Redefining self. In S. D. Dixon & M. T. Stein (Eds.), *Encounters with children: Pediatric behavior and development* (4th ed., pp. 565–598). Philadelphia: Mosby Elsevier.

McDorman, M. F., & Mathews, T. J. (2008). *Recent trends in infant mortality in the US NCHS Data Brief, no. 9*. Hyattsville, MD: National Center for Center for Health Statistics.

Morris, T., & McInerney, K. (2010). Media representations of pregnancy and childbirth: An analysis of reality television programs in the United States. *Birth (Berkeley, Calif.)*, *37*(2), 134–140.

National Patient Safety Foundation. (n.d.). *Ask Me 3™*. Retrieved from http://www.npsf.org/askme3/

Nolan, M. (2000). The influence of antenatal classes on pain relief in labour: A review of the literature. *The Practising Midwife*, *3*(5), 23–26.

Novick, G. (2009). Women's experience of prenatal care: An integrative review. *Journal of Midwifery and Women's Health*, *54*, 226–237.

Ozuah, P. O. (2005). First, there was pedagogy and then came andragogy. *Einstein Journal of Biology & Medicine*, *21*, 83–87.

Quality and Safety Education for Nurses (QSEN). (2012). *Patient-Centered Care*. Retrieved from http://www.qsen.org/definition.php?id=1

Roberts, J. E. (1976). Priorities in prenatal education. *JOGN Nursing; Journal of Obstetric, Gynecologic, and Neonatal Nursing*, *5*(3), 17–20.

U.S. Department of Health and Human Services. (2010). *Healthy People 2020*. Retrieved from http://www.healthypeople.gov/2020/default.aspx

U.S. Department of Health and Human Services Health Resources & Services Administration. (n.d.). *About health literacy*. Retrieved from http://www.hrsa.gov/publichealth/healthliteracy/healthlitabout.html

U.S. National Library of Medicine National Institutes of Health. (2010). *MedlinePlus: Guide to healthy web surfing*. Retrieved from http://www.nlm.nih.gov/medlineplus/healthywebsurfing.html

U.S. National Library of Medicine National Institutes of Health. (2011). *MedlinePlus: How to write easy-to-read health materials*. Retrieved from http://www.nlm.nih.gov/medlineplus/etr.html

Vonderheid, S. C., Norr, K. F., & Handler, A. S. (2007). Prenatal health promotion content and behaviors. *Western Journal of Nursing Research*, *3*, 258–276.

Walker, D. S., Visger, J. M., & Rossie, D. (2009). Contemporary childbirth education models. *Journal of Midwifery and Women's Health*, *54*(6), 469–476.

Williams, M. V., Parker, R. M., Baker, D. W., Parikh, N. S., Pitkin, K., Coates, W. C., & Nurss, J. R. (1995). Inadequate functional health literacy among patients at two public hospitals. *Journal of the American Medical Association*, *274*(21), 677–682. doi:10.1001/jama.274.21.1677

18

Assessment and care at the onset of labor

Amy Marowitz

Relevant terms

Active labor—the phase of labor during which contractions are strong and regular and rapid cervical dilation occurs

Braxton Hicks contractions—the uterine activity of pregnancy, perceived as painless by many women, so named after John Braxton Hicks, who wrote about this phenomenon in 1871

Continuous labor support—the presence of a supportive companion throughout the labor process

Contractions—periodic tightening and relaxing of the uterine muscle (myometrium)

Dilation—the diameter of the opening of the cervix, measured in centimeters

Early labor—the preparatory phase of labor during which time contractions become more regular and stronger, and the cervix slowly effaces and dilates; different terms are used to denote this part of labor, for example, latent labor, prelabor and prodromal labor

Effacement—the thinning out of the cervix that occurs during labor, measured as a percentage

Ketonuria—the presence of ketones in the urine resulting from inadequate caloric intake

Labor—a function of the female by which the infant is expelled from the uterus through the vagina into the outside world

Labor dystocia—difficult labor, or labor judged to be progressing more slowly than normal

Multipara—a woman who has given birth two or more times

Nullipara—a woman who has never given birth

Oxytocin—a hormone that stimulates contractions of the smooth muscle of uterus

Primipara—a woman who has given birth once

Prostaglandins—a group of hormones that stimulate contractions of the smooth muscle of the uterus and aid in cervical ripening, in part by causing collagen breakdown

Station—the location of the presenting part of the fetus relative to the ischial spines of the maternal pelvis, measured in centimeters above or below the spines; presenting part at the spines is zero station.

Therapeutic rest—administration of medication to relieve discomfort so a woman can sleep during the early part of labor.

Introduction

Although the onset of labor is often portrayed in popular media as an abrupt and dramatic event, the signs and symptoms of early labor are often subtle or indistinguishable from uterine activity and other discomforts associated with late pregnancy. The elusive nature of labor onset can make this a challenging time for women and families as well as their health-care providers. This chapter reviews issues related to diagnosing labor onset, teaching and anticipatory guidance regarding the onset of labor, components of an evaluation for labor, and ways to support women during the early phases of labor.

Determining the onset of labor

It has long been recognized that uterine activity in the form of contractions occurs throughout much of pregnancy (Reynolds, 1968). Studies utilizing uterine monitoring to quantify uterine activity objectively document

---

Prenatal and Postnatal Care: A Woman-Centered Approach, First Edition. Edited by Robin G. Jordan, Janet L. Engstrom, Julie A. Marfell, and Cindy L. Farley.
© 2014 John Wiley & Sons, Inc. Published 2014 by John Wiley & Sons, Inc.

a gradual increase in the strength and frequency of contractions that builds over the course of pregnancy and finally results in labor (Nageotte, Dorchester, Porto, Keegan, & Freeman, 1988). The hormonal milieu to initiate and support labor evolves during this time as well. Increasing secretion of prostaglandins, estrogen, and oxytocin causes remodeling of the connective tissue of the cervix and gradually more coordinated and frequent uterine contractions (Liao, Buhimschi, & Norwitz, 2005).

The continuous remodeling of the connective tissue and the ongoing contractions throughout pregnancy explain why it can be difficult to precisely define when labor begins. Adding to the uncertain nature of diagnosing labor onset is the significant variation in how women experience the uterine activity leading up to established labor. Some women are unaware of these contractions, whereas other women find them to be very mild and have little difficulty continuing their activities of daily living when they occur. In contrast, some women experience considerable discomfort for hours, days, or longer, resulting in life disruption, lost sleep, and several trips to the health-care provider for evaluation. In addition, some women experience periods of regular, painful contractions that appear to be labor but then stop for hours, days, or weeks.

There is no consensus among clinicians and researchers on how to define the onset of labor. Various criteria are used in different combinations including cervical change; bloody show; ruptured membranes and characteristics of the contractions such as regularity, frequency, and strength (Friedman, 1978; O'Driscoll, Stronge, & Minogue, 1973; Simkin & Ancheta, 2011). Women themselves may define it differently, noting not only contractions, bloody show, and leaking fluid but also emotional changes, sleep alterations, and gastrointestinal symptoms as heralding the onset of labor (Gross, Haunschild, Stoexen, Methner, & Guenter, 2003).

Timing of admission to the birth setting

One of the most challenging decisions for women and their health-care providers is when to seek admission to the planned birth site. It is generally accepted that it is best to delay admission until the woman has reached the period of relatively rapid cervical dilation commonly known as active labor. This recommendation is based on three considerations. First, a number of studies have found that rates of cesarean section and other interventions such as the use of epidural analgesia and oxytocin augmentation are higher in women admitted prior to the active phase of labor (Bailit, Dierker, Blanchard, & Mercer, 2005; Holmes, Oppenheimer, & Wen, 2001;

McGiven, Williams, Hodnett, Kaufman, & Hannah, 1998). A systematic review found that women admitted to the labor unit in active labor have shorter labor unit stays, feel in more control of their experience and use fewer drugs to progress labor or for pain relief (Lauzon & Hodnett, 2009). Second, caring for women in the hospital or birth center prior to active labor increases the cost of health care by requiring more staffing, equipment, and space. Finally, there is a long-standing assumption that women will more comfortable at home during this early part of labor.

Recently, the assumption that women are more comfortable at home has been challenged by a research on the experience of women in early labor. This research demonstrates tension between clinicians trying to delay admission and women who want to be admitted to the birth setting (Barnett, Hundley, Cheyne, & Kane, 2008; Beebe & Humphreys, 2006; Carlsson, Hallberg, & Pettersson, 2009; Cheyne et al., 2007; Eri, Blystad, Gjengedal, & Blaaka, 2010; Low & Moffat, 2006; Nolan & Smith, 2010). These studies were done in several different countries and included women cared for by midwives and physicians in both hospital and birth centers. This research has demonstrated that women perceive incongruence between what they are told and what they experience. Other important findings include that women are uncertain about when to seek care, and are worried about erroneously seeking care too early. Women also report that they feel unsupported by care providers who did not appreciate the difficulty of this part of labor. Another important finding was that family members were uncomfortable with the responsibility of caring for the woman, and both women and families wanted to "hand over" responsibility to health-care professionals.

What is "false labor"?

When a woman experiences what she believes to be labor contractions that later stops, this may be referred to as "false" labor. True labor contractions are said to steadily increase in strength and frequency, and increase with activity. False labor contractions are said to be irregular, do not increase in strength or frequency, and stop or decrease with activity. Although these distinctions between true and false labor are widely accepted, they are not evidence based. Quantified uterine activity in late gestation and uterine activity in early labor are similar in pattern and intensity, indicating there may be no difference in the contractions of so-called false versus true labor (Nageotte et al., 1988).

Periods of contractions that appear to be labor but then stop are very common. While this can be disappointing for women anxiously awaiting the onset of labor, reassurance should be given that these contractions help prepare the cervix for labor. It can be argued that the term "false labor" is problematic and inappropriate. In addition to its questionable physiological accuracy, the phrase false labor invalidates women's experiences of this phenomenon. A better choice of terminology is "prelabor." Exchanging the term prelabor for false labor acknowledges that the contractions experienced are real and serve a necessary preparatory purpose. Numerous studies have documented the negative impact on women when they are sent home after a labor evaluation during which they are told they are experiencing false labor and have come to the birth setting too soon (Barnett et al., 2008; Eri et al., 2010). Women in this situation report feeling anxious, confused, and unsupported and uncertain about how to recognize "true" labor. Providing anticipatory guidance during prenatal visits regarding the normalcy of periods of contractions before the onset of labor, emphasizing the purpose of these contractions in preparing the cervix for labor, and validating women's experience may help the woman be better prepared for the experience of prelabor.

Determining active labor

Just as definitions of the onset of labor vary, so do definitions of active labor. It is common practice to utilize a simple definition of regular contractions and a cervical dilation of 3 or 4 cm. However, recent research indicates this may not be an accurate way to define the onset of active labor (Neal & Lowe, 2012; Neal, Lowe, Patrick, Cabbage, & Corwin, 2010). Some women are in active labor before the cervix is dilated 3 or 4 cm, whereas other women are not in active labor until a more advanced cervical dilation. This distinction is important because once a woman is thought to be in active labor, there are often specific cultural and institutional expectations regarding labor progression. If a woman is mistakenly diagnosed as being in active labor when she is not, interventions such as oxytocin augmentation and cesarean sections for labor dystocia may be used unnecessarily (Gifford, 2000; Neal & Lowe, 2012; Neal et al., 2010).

An alternative definition for the onset of active labor is the time when the rate of cervical dilation sharply increases (Friedman, 1978). This definition is considered the most accurate but can be difficult to recognize in real time. A useful approach is to avoid strict criteria and to consider multiple factors including cervical effacement and dilation, contraction frequency, intensity and pattern development over time, and the woman's affect and behavior during contractions. Diagnostic accuracy increases if several factors point to active labor.

Anticipatory guidance during the prenatal period

Anticipatory guidance during the prenatal period can help women prepare more effectively for the onset of labor. Adequate time should be spent during late pregnancy prenatal visits to provide information on the process of labor onset and self-care in early labor. Specific instructions on when and how to contact the health-care provider should be given.

Anticipatory guidance should emphasize that labor onset is a gradual process and it is often difficult to distinguish from the contractions and common discomforts of late pregnancy. The variability in women's experience of labor onset should be explained. The normalcy of a lengthy preparatory phase and common experience of contractions that stop and start over days and weeks should also be discussed. Finally, anticipatory guidance should include an explanation of the reasons to delay admission to the birth site until active labor begins.

Commonly, women are told to contact their health-care provider or go to the planned birth site when they have contractions that are 5 minutes apart or closer and painful for at least 1 hour, if they think their membranes have ruptured membranes, or if they have heavy bleeding. These are reasonable guidelines, but it is essential to explain that not all women are in active labor when these events occur, and that returning home may be suggested if active labor has not yet started at the time of the evaluation. An acknowledgment of the challenging nature of determining the onset of active labor for both the woman and health-care provider may decrease a woman's negative feelings about going home following a labor evaluation. Finally, women should be encouraged to contact the health-care provider with any questions or if she experiences difficulty coping with early labor.

Other important topics to cover during prenatal teaching about labor are the importance of adequate food, fluids, and rest. Coping strategies and comfort measures for early labor should also be addressed. The benefits of continuous support during early labor should be emphasized. Women should be encouraged to identify support people before labor begins, seeking those who are knowledgeable about birth and who can provide a calming presence. Including support people during prenatal visits is a good way to make sure these individuals are prepared to provide support and comfort measures during early labor.

Data collection

An encounter with a woman regarding the possible onset of labor may occur by telephone or in person. Any such encounter must begin with the necessary collection of data. This includes information on the mother, the fetus, and the labor. Questions should be tailored to the woman and the circumstances.

General

What is the time of day and the weather? How far away from the birth site does the woman live? Does she have transportation problems? Is home a quiet place she can rest if needed?

What is her affect? If the contact is by telephone, how does she sound? Does she stop talking during contractions? Does she sound anxious, relaxed, energetic, exhausted? If this is a face-to-face visit, what is her general appearance? How does she seem to be coping? How does she feel she is coping? What has she been doing?

Uterine contractions

The presence of contractions may or may not be the primary symptom leading the woman to contact you. If she is having contractions, when did they start? What has the contraction pattern been since starting? What are the current frequency, length, and strength of the contractions? Does she need to stop what she is doing when they occur, or can she continue her activities? Can she sleep through them? Where does she feel them? What is she doing to cope with contractions? Does she have any other pain? If the visit is face to face, palpate the strength and interval of the contractions. Observation of a woman's behavior and affect during contractions can be very helpful in making a diagnosis as many women exhibit a characteristic inward focus during contractions of active labor.

Other signs and symptoms of possible labor

Is there any vaginal bleeding or spotting, or leaking fluid?

Fatigue

Recent sleep history: If it is night, has she slept? If it is day, how much sleep did she have last night?

Recent history regarding rest and activity: Her degree of fatigue will be different if she has been walking for hours trying to get labor going or working with all day, as compared to relaxing. How tired does she feel? How is her energy? If it is night, does she feel like she could sleep?

Hydration/nutrition

Has she been eating and drinking normally? What is her recent food/fluid intake? How is her appetite? Does she have any nausea or vomiting? Is she urinating with usual frequency and a normal amount? Is her urine a light yellow color or dark and concentrated in appearance? If this is a face-to-face visit, perform a urinalysis by dipstick for ketonuria and assess urine specific gravity as needed.

Fetal status

Is fetal movement normal? If this is a face-to-face visit, evaluate the fetal heart rate.

Support

Who is with her? Are they providing adequate support? What is their comfort level with the situation?

Other information

Assess for any signs or symptoms of a urinary tract infection such as burning or pain with urination or increased frequency of urine. Urinary tract infections can stimulate contractions.

Has she had recent sexual intercourse or a recent digital vaginal examination? Both of these can stimulate contractions and a small amount of bleeding or spotting.

Additional Information for a Face-to-Face Visit:

- Vital signs
- Urine dipstick for proteinuria
- Leopold's maneuvers to determine fetal lie, presentation, and position

Digital vaginal exam for cervical dilation, effacement, position, and consistency; fetal station; confirm presentation should be performed by a health-care provider skilled in this type of assessment. If there is a possibility of ruptured membranes, this exam should be deferred. Assessment of cervical effacement is an important aspect of the evaluation since the cervix usually effaces considerably before more rapid dilation can occur, particularly in nulliparous women. Thus, a cervix that is 2 cm dilated and 100% effaced may be more indicative of active labor than one that is 5 cm dilated and 25% effaced. It is important to note that often some cervical effacement and dilation occurs prior to the onset of labor. For this reason, one digital vaginal exam may not be definitive in determining if a woman is in labor. Serial cervical examinations with cervical change noted are a more accurate indication of labor.

Plan of care

At the onset of an encounter with a woman for labor evaluation, the need for immediate admission to the planned birth site must be determined. Reasons for immediate admission include but are not limited to active labor, vaginal bleeding heavier than normal bloody show, or concerns about the fetal status. Institutional policies and individual health-care provider practices regarding timing of admission vary greatly for women with ruptured membranes in the absence of labor. If immediate admission is necessary, assessment by phone or in the office is limited and the woman is directed to the planned birth site. In this situation, the health-care provider will usually notify the birth setting that the woman should arrive in the birth unit shortly.

If there is no indication of a need for immediate admission and early labor is occurring, the plan of care should be tailored to meet the woman's needs. Thus, it is essential to include the woman in the decision making. For example, if the encounter is by telephone, it is helpful to ask the woman if she wants to be evaluated in person. If the woman is comfortable remaining at home, management is centered on self-care, coping strategies, social support, and timing of admission.

The following discussion on self-care and coping should be read with the understanding that little to no research has been conducted on optimal strategies for early labor. Common recommendations come from conventional wisdom, empirical data, and general nursing and midwifery principles.

Self-care

Self-care in early labor primarily involves hydration, nutrition, and rest. Close attention to these issues is needed when longer periods of early labor occur. There are several reasons why women may not keep themselves hydrated and nourished in early labor. Some women believe that they should not eat or drink once labor begins. This misconception should be corrected and the importance of continued intake of fluids and calories in early labor should be emphasized during prenatal education about labor. Most women do not feel well if they are dehydrated, and dehydration may make the uterus irritable, resulting in increased discomfort and inefficient contractions. Once significant dehydration occurs, it can be difficult to correct with oral fluids. Thus, many clinicians recommend the consumption of at least 8 oz of fluid per hour when awake. Women can easily monitor their own hydration status by observing the color of their urine, which should be light yellow. Continued caloric intake is also important during early labor. The goal is for the woman to remain well nourished with adequate caloric reserves for the physical exertion of labor. Eating normally during early labor is ideal, although frequent light snacks and caloric beverages can be an adequate source of nutrition and calories.

Some women experience nausea and/or vomiting in early labor, making it more difficult to stay adequately hydrated and nourished. With mild nausea, it is often possible for the woman to continue to sip fluids and eat small amounts of easily digestible food such as refined carbohydrates or fruits. With significant nausea or vomiting, admission for intravenous fluids and possibly antiemetic medication may be needed.

Sleep and rest

Sufficient rest and sleep are important with long periods of early labor. Coping with early labor and subsequent active labor is much more difficult with significant sleep deprivation and fatigue. As with hydration and nourishment, adequate rest and sleep help a woman manage the physical exertion of active labor. There are several reasons why women may experience fatigue in early labor. Many women have difficulty sleeping in advanced pregnancy, and may start labor with a sleep deficit. For some women, the excitement and/or anxiety experienced with the onset of labor makes it difficult to sleep. Some women believe they should be physically active once early labor begins in order to speed labor progress. Finally, some women cannot sleep due to the pain of early labor contractions.

Advising women on the importance of adequate rest and sleep in early labor should start during prenatal visits and be emphasized during any encounter related to possible labor. Suggestions for preventing fatigue include napping frequently in the last weeks of gestation, trying to sleep between the contractions if it is night, and conserving energy by alternating periods of rest and activity during the day. If the woman cannot sleep through contractions, dozing in between may be helpful. Various relaxation measures may also help the woman sleep. Examples include a warm bath, massage, guided imagery or meditation and listening to relaxing music. A small amount of alcohol to promote sleep, such as a half glass of wine, has been a time-honored recommendation to promote rest in early labor. Alcohol also inhibits contractions, and in fact was used as a tocolytic in the 1960s. Though some consider any alcohol consumption in pregnancy to be inappropriate, it can be argued that it has the same fetal effects as opioids, a class of drug often used to promote rest in early labor (Greulich & Tarrant, 2007).

When a woman cannot sleep during a lengthy preparatory phase of labor and becomes fatigued or exhausted, medication may be a useful tool. Medications that can be given to the woman to take at home include antihistamines such as Benadryl® (diphenhydramine) and Vistaril® (hydroxyzine), and nonbenzodiazepine sedative-hypnotics such as Ambien® (zolpidem). Barbiturate sedative-hypnotics such as Seconal® (secobarbital) were commonly used in this circumstance in the past. However, these drugs have prolonged depressant effects in the newborn and are now considered contraindicated for use in early labor by many clinicians (Greulich & Tarrant, 2007; King & Brucker, 2011). Importantly, none of the sedative-hypnotics have analgesic properties and are not helpful in promoting rest when painful contractions prevent sleep. If a woman is extremely fatigued and cannot sleep due to painful contractions, admission to the planned birth site for therapeutic rest with an opioid analgesic such as morphine sulfate should be considered.

Coping strategies and comfort measures for early labor

One strategy for coping in early labor is distraction. Distracting activities help pass the time and may decrease the woman's focus on her contractions. Suggestions include continuing a normal routine as much as possible or engaging in diverting activities such as watching a movie, playing cards, preparing food, or working on a project.

The degree of discomfort experienced in early labor varies greatly. Generally, recommendations for comfort and nonpharmacological pain relief in early labor are similar to those suggested for active labor. Measures such as water immersion, superficial application of heat and cold, position changes and other movements, touch, and massage are effective in active labor (Simkin & Bolding, 2004) and may be helpful in managing the discomforts of early labor.

Continuous support during labor has well-established benefits (Hodnett, Gates, Hofmeyr, Sakala, & Weston, 2011), and there is some evidence of its benefits in early stages of labor (Simkin & Bolding, 2004). The evidence shows the greatest benefit when support is provided by a person who is experienced and trained and is not part of the woman's social network (Hodnett et al., 2011); however, it is most commonly provided by a partner, family member, or friend in early labor. The support women receive at this time impacts their experience and ability to cope and sets the stage for improved coping in later labor.

Ambulation in early labor

Unrestricted movement in active labor is associated with greater satisfaction with the birth experience, decreased pain, and possibly shorter labor (Carlson et al., 1986; Rossi & Lindell, 1986). Though no studies have examined the benefits of unrestricted movement in early labor, common sense dictates that women should be encouraged to move around as desired during this time. Some women and clinicians believe that ambulation hastens the transition from early to active labor. Women may be told by health-care providers that continued walking helps determine if their contractions are "real" labor because of the belief that activity diminishes the contractions of false labor and stimulates the contractions of true labor. Neither of these rationales is evidence based. The common practice of instructing women in early labor to walk for an hour or two to assess the effect on the contraction pattern should be critically evaluated. This practice contributes to fatigue and is unlikely to be beneficial. Women should be advised to move about and rest during early labor as comfort dictates.

Summary

Progression from late pregnancy to established labor is a process that, for many women, unfolds over days or weeks. Identifying the onset of labor and coping with the early phases of labor can be challenging. An understanding of the physiological nature of these events is needed to provide appropriate teaching to women and to support them during this unique period of time.

Case study

Savannah is a 31-year-old gravida 1 para 0 at 39 weeks and 5 days of gestation. She has received care from your midwifery group practice since her pregnancy was diagnosed at 6 weeks of gestation. She does not have a history of any medical conditions and has never had surgery or been hospitalized. Her pregnancy has been uncomplicated. She calls the midwife at 11 pm to report regular contractions for the past 6 hours.

The following information is obtained: There is no vaginal bleeding or leaking fluid. Fetal movement is normal. The contractions are occurring every 5–10 minutes and are about 45 seconds long. Savannah has a contraction during the phone conversation and is able to continue talking without difficulty. She reports that the contractions are slightly painful and feel different from the Braxton Hicks contractions she has been having for weeks. She worked today at her office job, her last day of work before beginning her maternity leave. She slept well last night and is feeling quite tired now. She thinks she may be able to sleep through these contractions. She has consumed her usual amount of food and fluids today, and has been sipping on water all evening and is urinating normal amounts of light yellow urine. Her husband is with her and is supportive.

After speaking with Savannah through two more contractions that were 8 minutes apart, the midwife discusses the uncertainty of knowing if the contractions she is experiencing will develop into labor. After reviewing information on the characteristics of early labor and the benefits of delayed admission to the birth setting, the midwife and Savannah formulate the following plan: Savannah will have a snack and something nonalcoholic and decaffeinated to drink, take a warm bath, then go to bed and try to sleep.

Since Savannah has a prenatal appointment scheduled for tomorrow afternoon, the midwife plans to see her at that appointment if her condition does not change before then. However, the midwife encourages Savannah to call again if the contractions continue to come regularly, every few minutes apart and painful for an hour, or if she begins to leak fluid or bleed heavily, or is having difficulty coping.

The midwife sees Savannah for her prenatal visit the next afternoon. She reports that her contractions slowed down and more or less stopped following a warm bath, and she slept all night. She requests a digital vaginal exam, which reveals that the cervix is 1–2 cm dilated and 50% effaced. The midwife reassures Savannah about the normalcy of a period of regular contractions that stop and discusses the role these contractions play in preparing the cervix for labor. Guidelines for when to contact the health-care provider are reviewed, as well as suggestions for self-care and coping at home. She is scheduled for a prenatal visit for 1 week in the event that labor does not begin before then.

One week later, Savannah returns for her prenatal visit at 10 am. She says she began having regular contractions last night at about 11 pm. The contractions have gradually gotten closer and stronger and are now every 4–7 minutes and painful. She appears to be relaxed, in good spirits, and coping well. She stops talking several times during the conversation to focus on her contractions. She is not bleeding or leaking fluid. Fetal movement is normal. She slept for a couple of hours early in the night, and then dozed off and on until early morning. She has been sipping fluids through the night, urinating a normal amount, and has eaten a light breakfast before coming to her appointment. Her husband and friend are with her and are supportive. Vital signs and fetal heart rate are normal. A digital vaginal exam reveals that the cervix is 2 cm dilated and 75% effaced.

The midwife meets with Savannah and her support people and explains the difficulty with making a definitive diagnosis of labor at this time. The evolution of the contraction pattern and the change in her cervix since last week suggest that labor may be starting. The options of hospital admission, going home, or staying close to the hospital for a couple of hours are discussed, and Savannah's preferences are explored. Savannah lives an hour away from the hospital and prefers not to drive home, so she decides to walk around a nearby shopping mall. Guidelines for self-care and when to return are reviewed, and the normalcy of her experience emphasized.

Savannah goes to the hospital maternity unit 3 hours later. At that time, her contractions are every 3–4 minutes and stronger. A digital vaginal exam is performed and her cervix is found to be 5 cm dilated and 100% effaced. She is admitted in active labor and gives birth later that night to a healthy baby boy.

References

Bailit, J. L., Dierker, L., Blanchard, M. H., & Mercer, B. M. (2005). Outcomes of women presenting in active versus latent phase of spontaneous labor. *Obstetrics & Gynecology, 105*, 77–79.

Barnett, C., Hundley, V., Cheyne, H., & Kane, F. (2008). "Not in labour": Impact of sending women home in the latent phase. *British Journal of Midwifery, 16*, 144–153.

Beebe, K. R., & Humphreys, J. (2006). Expectations, perceptions, and management of labor in nulliparas prior to hospitalization. *Journal of Midwifery & Women's Health, 51*, 347–353.

Carlson, J., Diehl, J., Sachtleben-Murray, M., McRae, M., Fenwick, L., & Friedman, E. (1986). Maternal position during parturition in normal labor. *Obstetrics & Gynecology, 68*, 443–447.

Carlsson, I., Hallberg, L. R., & Pettersson, K. O. (2009). Swedish women's experiences of seeking care and being admitted during the latent phase of labour: A grounded theory study. *Midwifery, 25*, 172–180.

Cheyne, H., Terry, R., Niven, C., Dowding, D., Hundley, V., & McNamee, P. (2007). "Should I come in now?": A study of women's early labour experiences. *British Journal of Midwifery, 15*, 604–609.

Eri, T. S., Blystad, A., Gjengedal, E., & Blaaka, G. (2010). Negotiating credibility: First time mothers' experiences of contact with the labour ward before hospitalisation. *Midwifery, 26*, e25–e30.

Friedman, E. (1978). *Labor: Clinical evaluation and management* (2nd ed.). New York: Appleton.

Gifford, D. (2000). Lack of progress in labor as a reason for cesarean. *Obstetrics & Gynecology, 94*, 589–595.

Greulich, B., & Tarrant, B. (2007). The latent phase of labor: Diagnosis and management. *Journal of Midwifery and Women's Health, 52*, 190–198.

Gross, M. M., Haunschild, T., Stoexen, T., Methner, V., & Guenter, H. (2003). Women's recognition of the spontaneous onset of labor. *Birth (Berkeley, Calif.), 30*, 267–271.

Hodnett, E. D., Gates, S., Hofmeyr, G. J., Sakala, C., & Weston, J. (2011). Continuous support for women during childbirth. *Cochrane Database of Systematic Reviews*, (2), CD003766.

Holmes, P., Oppenheimer, L. W., & Wen, S. W. (2001). The relationship between cervical dilatation at initial presentation in labour and subsequent intervention. *BJOG: An International Journal of Obstetrics and Gynaecology, 108*, 1120–1124.

King, T. L., & Brucker, M. C. (2011). *Pharmacology for women's health.* Boston: Jones and Bartlett.

Lauzon, L., & Hodnett, E. D. (2009) Labour assessment programs to delay admission to labour wards (Cochrane Review). *Cochrane Database of Systematic Reviews*, (1), CD000936. Oxford: Update Software.

Liao, J. B., Buhimschi, C. S., & Norwitz, E. R. (2005). Normal labor: Mechanism and duration. *Obstetrics and Gynecology Clinics of North America, 32*, 145–164.

Low, L. K., & Moffat, A. (2006). Every labor is unique, but "call when your contractions are 3 minutes apart." *MCN. The American Journal of Maternal Child Nursing, 31*, 307–312.

McGiven, P. S., Williams, J. I., Hodnett, E., Kaufman, K., & Hannah, M. E. (1998). An early labor assessment program: A randomized, controlled trial. *Birth (Berkeley, Calif.), 25*, 5–7.

Nageotte, M. P., Dorchester, W., Porto, M., Keegan, K. A., & Freeman, R. K. (1988). Quantification of uterine of uterine activity preceding preterm, term, and post term labor. *American Journal of Obstetrics and Gynecology, 6*, 1254–1259.

Neal, J., Lowe, N. K., Patrick, T. E., Cabbage, L. A., & Corwin, E. J. (2010). What is the slowest-yet-normal cervical dilation rate among nulliparous women with spontaneous labor onset? *Journal of Obstetric, Gynecologic, and Neonatal Nursing, 39*, 361–369.

Neal, J. L., & Lowe, N. K. (2012). Physiologic partograph to improve birth safety and outcomes among low-risk, nulliparous women with spontaneous labor onset. *Medical Hypotheses, 78*, 319–325.

Nolan, M., & Smith, J. (2010). Women's experience of following advice to stay at home in early labour. *British Journal of Midwifery, 18*, 286–291.

O'Driscoll, K., Stronge, J. M., & Minogue, M. (1973). Active management of labour. *British Medical Journal, 3*, 135–137.

Reynolds, S. R. (1968). The uses of Braxton Hicks contractions. *Obstetrics and Gynecology, 32*, 134–140.

Rossi, M. A., & Lindell, S. G. (1986). Maternal positions and pushing techniques in a non-prescriptive environment. *Journal of Obstetric, Gynecologic, and Neonatal Nursing, 15*, 203–208.

Simkin, P., & Ancheta, R. (2011). *The labor progress handbook: Early interventions to prevent and treat dystocia.* John Wiley & Sons.

Simkin, P., & Bolding, A. (2004). Update on nonpharmocologic approaches to relieve labor pain and prevent suffering. *Journal of Midwifery and Women's Health, 49*, 489–504.

Part III
Common complications of pregnancy

19

Bleeding during pregnancy

Robin G. Jordan

Relevant terms

Cervical motion tenderness (CMT)—done during the bimanual exam by grasping the cervix between the gloved examining fingers and moving the cervix side to side; CMT can be a sign of ectopic pregnancy

Couvelaire uterus—a condition in which blood invades the uterine musculature; can occur with placental abruption

Ectopic pregnancy—a fertilized ovum implanting outside of the uterine endometrium

Kleihauer–Betke test—a maternal blood test that measures the amount of fetal hemoglobin transferred from the fetus to the maternal bloodstream and is a standard measure to quantify fetal–maternal hemorrhage

Leiomyoma—benign uterine tumors, also known as fibroids

Pelvic rest—a general term denoting no intercourse, no use of tampons, and no orgasm

Placental abruption—premature separation of the placenta from the uterine wall prior to birth

Placenta previa—the placenta implants at the margin of or over the cervical os

Recurrent pregnancy loss—three or more consecutive pregnancy losses prior to 20 weeks' gestation or less

Spontaneous pregnancy loss—pregnancy loss before 20 weeks' gestation or with a fetal weight of <500 g

Subchorionic hemorrhage—separation of the chorion from uterine lining resulting in a collection of blood between the uterine wall and the chorionic membrane

Tocolysis—inhibition of uterine contractions typically done by pharmaceutical methods

Vasa previa—a placental condition where the fetal vessels run through the membranes over the cervix unprotected by the umbilical cord or placental tissue

Introduction

Vaginal bleeding occurs in approximately 10–20% of women during pregnancy (Yang et al., 2009). It is not always an easy task to pinpoint the etiology of vaginal bleeding; however, the source of bleeding is almost always maternal rather than fetal. Causes vary depending on gestational age. While most women who experience vaginal bleeding in early pregnancy go on to have a normal pregnancy, first-trimester bleeding is associated with an increased risk for preterm birth (Edwards et al., 2012; Lykke et al. 2010). Vaginal bleeding in the second half of pregnancy is often of a greater magnitude and is linked to increased perinatal morbidity and mortality. This section of the chapter organizes pregnancy bleeding by those etiologies in the first half of pregnancy and by causes more common to the second half of pregnancy.

Bleeding during the first half of pregnancy

The etiology of bleeding during the first half of pregnancy is often unknown and the diagnostic process is one of exclusion. Timing and the amount of vaginal bleeding and visualization of the cervix are essential data to discriminate between normal and abnormal etiology. Bleeding without cramping that occurs after intercourse or around the time of the first missed menses can usually be attributed normal causes and woman can be reassured. Additionally, light bleeding episodes, especially those without pain and lasting only a day or two, do not increase the risk of miscarriage above the baseline

Prenatal and Postnatal Care: A Woman-Centered Approach, First Edition. Edited by Robin G. Jordan, Janet L. Engstrom, Julie A. Marfell, and Cindy L. Farley.
© 2014 John Wiley & Sons, Inc. Published 2014 by John Wiley & Sons, Inc.

Table 19.1   Benign Causes of Bleeding in Pregnancy

Etiology	Physiology	Comments
Implantation spotting	Blastocyst implants into the endometrium 6–11 days after conception	Lasts one episode to several days, small amount, bright red to darker in color
Cervical polyps	Benign tumor on the surface of the cervical canal, bleeding caused by inflammation or vasocongestion	More common in parous women, dark or birth red color. Often intermittent spotting
Vaginal or cervical infection	Infection causes cervicitis with local inflammation and increased cervical friability	Common infections include *Chlamydia trachomatis*, human papilloma virus, *Neisseria gonorrhoeae*
Postcoital spotting	Increase in pelvic blood flow causes cervix to become engorged and friable or can be attributed to infection	Bleeding may also occur after pelvic exam or Pap smear

risk for all women (Hasan et al., 2009). There are several common and benign causes of bleeding in the first half of pregnancy (Table 19.1). The bleeding from non-pathological etiologies is typically of small volume and subsides within hours. Patient history and speculum examination often will confirm a benign etiology or have negative findings.

Some women experience significant bleeding in early pregnancy. The primary pathological considerations for bleeding in the first half of pregnancy are spontaneous pregnancy loss and ectopic pregnancy.

Evaluation

Because bleeding in pregnant women may signal a severe condition, health-care providers need to obtain the menstrual, maternal, and gynecologic history while performing the initial steps of assessment and management. It is essential to recognize an early ectopic pregnancy in women presenting with vaginal bleeding before tubal rupture occurs. A systematic approach to evaluating the woman with vaginal bleeding in pregnancy allows for the development of an appropriate and efficient management plans.

During this history and examination of a woman presenting with early pregnancy vaginal bleeding, the following questions must be answered:

- Is the patient hemodynamically stable?
- Is fever present?
- Is the bleeding intrauterine or extrauterine?
- Is the pregnancy intrauterine or ectopic?
- Is the pregnancy viable?

Problem-focused history

A detailed history is key in evaluating women presenting with vaginal bleeding during pregnancy. The date of the last known menstrual period is ascertained to estimate gestational age along with any ultrasounds done for pregnancy dating. Bleeding severity, amount, location, and severity of pain or cramping are determined to assess the acuity of the woman's situation. The woman may be able to quantify the number of pads used over a specified time and the amount that each pad is soaked. This estimate can be helpful as soaking a pad in less than an hour suggests significant amounts of bleeding that require prompt attention. The presence of clots can indicate heavy bleeding. The woman should be asked about the presence of associated symptoms such as shoulder pain, feeling faint, and vomiting. History is reviewed for risk factors for various etiologies of pregnancy bleeding such as previous ectopic, prior early pregnancy loss, history of uterine fibroids, or current use of an intrauterine device.

The present pregnancy history should be obtained. The woman should be queried on the presence and onset of early pregnancy signs such as breast tenderness, date of pregnancy diagnosis, any illness, fever, or substance exposures since pregnancy. When inquiring about personal habits, sexual history, medication use, and environmental exposures, providers must proceed with great sensitivity. Most women experiencing a spontaneous pregnancy loss search their past actions diligently to find an explanation for the loss and may experience needless guilt over causing a pregnancy loss.

Physical exam

Vital signs including blood pressure, pulse, and temperature are obtained. The abdomen is palpated for adnexal masses or tenderness and assessment of uterine size if possible. Auscultation of fetal heart sounds by Doppler is attempted if the last normal menses was at least 10 weeks prior. During the speculum examination, external tissues are observed for nonobstetrical causes of bleeding such as trauma, infection, and nonvaginal bleeding from external or internal hemorrhoids. The cervix should be examined for signs of infection, discharge, polyps, active bleeding, tissue at the os, and dilation. Any tissue found in the vaginal vault or removed from the cervical os can be sent to pathology to determine the presence of chorionic villi, which verifies that the pregnancy was intrauterine. Bimanual pelvic examination is done to assess uterine size, shape, and cervical motion tenderness. Pain during this procedure can be significant in women with an ectopic pregnancy. Assessment of the adnexa is made for masses and tenderness.

Laboratory evaluation

The determination of serial beta-human chorionic gonadotropin (β-hCG) can aid the provider with interpretation of ultrasound findings and differentiating between normal and abnormal pregnancy conditions. Serial β-hCG should be obtained in women suspected of having an ectopic pregnancy or if viability of the fetus is in question. The level of β-hCG doubles every 2–3 days from the time of blastocyst formation, peaks at 8–10 weeks, then declines starting at 10–12 weeks' gestation to a nadir at 16 weeks' gestation (Table 19.2). For women who are experiencing more than minimal bleeding, a complete blood count (CBC) with differential blood type and screen with possible crossmatch should also be done.

Diagnostic testing

The rapid availability of ultrasonography has allowed for a more individualized management of women experiencing first-trimester bleeding. A combination of transabdominal and transvaginal ultrasound may be used.

Subchorionic hemorrhage or hematoma

Subchorionic hemorrhage is defined as bleeding due to separation of the chorion from the uterine lining. This results in a collection of blood between the uterine wall and the chorionic membrane. Painless spotting or bleeding is a common sign of subchorionic hemorrhage; however, many are detected as an incidental finding during a routine ultrasound without any signs or symptoms noted by the woman.

In those women whose ultrasound shows a subchorionic hematoma, the outcome depends on the size of the hematoma and the fetal gestational age. Pregnancy outcomes are typically good for those women experiencing bleeding earlier in gestation as the hematomas are often small in size and typically regress. Most clots resolve on their own by 20 weeks of gestation by reabsorption. Poorer prognoses are seen in women experiencing late first- or early second-trimester bleeding as the amount of bleeding and the size of the clot is generally larger. Women with subchorionic hemorrhage may experience intermittent bleeding periodically throughout pregnancy. The typical management of subchorionic hemorrhage is pelvic rest for several weeks, and reassurance that this condition often resolves spontaneously.

Leiomyomas

Leiomyomas, commonly called uterine fibroids, are benign smooth muscle tumors that are found in approximately 2% of all pregnant women. They can be a cause of vaginal bleeding during pregnancy. They are more common in African American women and with increasing maternal age. Leiomyomas can grow under the influence of pregnancy hormones, or they may decrease in size or remain unchanged. There are several types of fibroids, classified by location within the myometrium (Fig. 19.1) Most pregnant women with fibroids will be asymptomatic; however, bleeding can occur when an intramural fibroid twists on its stalk or the placenta implants over a fibroid. Pregnant women with uterine fibroids have twice the rate of spontaneous pregnancy loss compared to women without fibroids (Benson, Chow, Chang-Lee, Hill, & Doubilet, 2001).

Spontaneous pregnancy loss

The period of pregnancy prior to fetal viability outside of the uterus is considered early pregnancy. Most consider early pregnancy to end at 20 weeks' gestation or

Table 19.2 Discriminatory Levels for Beta-Human Chorionic Gonadotropin (β-hCG)

Parameter	Ultrasound detection (approximate weeks' gestation)	Quantitative β-hCG (mIU/mL)
Gestational sac detection	Detectable at 4.5 weeks when mean diameter is 2–3 mm	Detectable on TVUS at 1,000 mIU/mL, detectable on abdominal ultrasound at 1,800 mIU/mL
Yolk sac identification	5 weeks at 5–6 mm	1,000–7,200
Fetal pole identification	5–7 weeks	7,200–10,800
Cardiac activity detection	6–7 weeks	>10,800

Source: Snell, B. J. (2009), Assessment and management of bleeding in the first trimester of pregnancy. *Journal of Midwifery and Women's Health*, *54*(6), 483–491.
TVUS: transvaginal ultrasound.

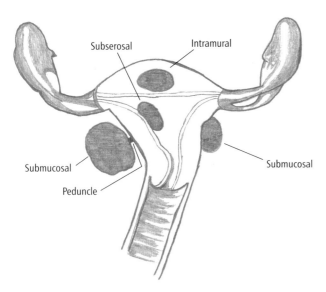

Figure 19.1. Intramural—most common, develop within the uterine wall; subserosal—develop on the outside wall of the uterus and grow outward; submucosal—least common, develop on the inside wall of the uterine cavity and grow inward. Source: http://www.nichd.nih.gov/health/topics/uterine/conditioninfo/Pages/default.aspx, National Institute of Child Health and Development.

Table 19.3   Classification of First-Trimester Pregnancy Loss

Diagnosis	Characteristics and presentation
Complete pregnancy loss (complete abortion)	Women report a history of heavy cramping, bleeding, and passage of clots and/or tissue follow by an abrupt decrease in pain and bleeding.
	Complete passage of products of conception
	Cervix closed
	Uterus small
	May see blood in vaginal vault
Incomplete pregnancy loss (threatened abortion, inevitable abortion)	Cramping may be intense; bleeding may be heavy.
	Partial passage of products of conception
	Cervix open or closed
Delayed pregnancy loss (missed abortion or blighted ovum)	Cervix closed
	The uterus may be small or appropriate for gestational age.
	Amenorrhea many be the only symptom often found during routine office visits when fetal heartbeat is not heard at the appropriate time.
Septic pregnancy loss (septic abortion)	Loss accompanied by uterine infection and possible sepsis
	Is very rare

Sources: Jauniaux et al. (2005), Snell (2009).

when the fetus weighs 500 g. Spontaneous pregnancy loss is defined as pregnancy loss before 20 weeks' gestation or with a fetal weight of <500 g. Several terms are commonly used to describe early spontaneous pregnancy loss. Miscarriage is the lay term to describe early pregnancy loss. Spontaneous abortion is the technically correct term and a common medical term used; however, it is not the ideal term to use in patient discussions as the word "abortion" can be emotionally charged for some people. The term spontaneous pregnancy loss is considered to be more suitable for use in describing the unplanned loss of a pregnancy, regardless of cause. Spontaneous pregnancy loss has been traditionally been categorized according to presentation with the categories forming a continuum of spontaneous loss progression. Simplification of the terms to describe spontaneous pregnancy loss characterizes the loss according to this stage of the process the woman is in at the time of presentation to the health-care provider (Jauniaux, Johns, & Burton, 2005). Both sets of terms are presented in Table 19.3.

Spontaneous pregnancy loss is the most common early pregnancy complication. Determining precise incidence is challenging as many women will miscarry before being aware of the pregnancy. However, it is estimated that 20% of all documented pregnancies and more than half of all conceptions end in loss prior to 14 weeks' gestation (Allison, Sherwood, & Schust, 2011). Approximately 42% of women who experience early

pregnancy bleeding go on to miscarry (Davari-Tanha, Shariat, Kaveh, Ebrahimi, & Jalalvand, 2008). The peak timing of early pregnancy loss is between 5 and 8 weeks' gestation (Hasan et al., 2009), and the vast majority of losses are due to chromosomal abnormalities.

Although the etiologies of first-trimester loss are multifactorial and often remain unknown, certain risk factors increase the likelihood of pregnancy loss (Table 19.4). Advanced maternal age and the number of prior early pregnancy losses are two independent risk factors for spontaneous early pregnancy loss. The rate of spontaneous pregnancy loss increases with advancing maternal age due to aging oocytes (Table 19.5).

Differential diagnosis

Ectopic pregnancy is the most concerning cause of early pregnancy bleeding and must be considered as a differential diagnosis. Nonpathological causes of early pregnancy bleeding may also present early in pregnancy.

Table 19.4 Risk Factors for Early Pregnancy Loss

Prior history of early spontaneous pregnancy loss

Advanced maternal age

Advanced paternal age

Uterine abnormalities
Leiomyomas
Bicorunate, unicornuate, septate, or didelphic uterus

Medication use in early pregnancy
Isotretinoin (Accutane)
Nonsteroidal anti-inflammatory drugs (NSAIDs)

Endocrine disorders
Diabetes mellitus
Progesterone deficiency and leuteal phase defects

Smoking

Alcohol use

Coffee intake of 200 mg/day or more

Malnutrition

Chronic diseases such as factor V Leiden coagulation defect, kidney or cardiac disease

Autoimmune disorders such as systemic lupus erythematosis (SLE) or antiphospholipid antibody syndrome (APS).

Adapted from: American College of Obstetricians and Gynecologists (ACOG) (2001), Nakhai-Pour, Broy, Sheehy, and Bérard (2011), RCOG (2011).

Table 19.5 Age and Early Pregnancy Loss Rate

Age	Early pregnancy loss rate (%)
<35	15
35–39	25–25
40–42	35
>42	50

Source: American Society for Reproductive Medicine (ASRM). (2003). *Age and fertility: A guide for patients.* Birmingham, AL: ASRM.

An empty uterus found on ultrasound examination may signal a completed spontaneous abortion, but the diagnosis is not definitive until ectopic pregnancy is excluded (Table 19.6).

Diagnosis and management

No single parameter is highly sensitive for predicting an impending loss, although certain clinical and ultrasound findings are suggestive of pregnancies that will not reach viability. Vaginal and or abdominal ultrasound will identify an absent or slowing fetal heart rate, an empty yolk sac, and retained products of conception

Table 19.6 Signs, Symptoms, and Differential Diagnosis of Spontaneous Pregnancy Loss

Sign and symptoms
Bleeding that progresses from light to heavy
Cramps that continue until tissue is passed
Abdominal pain
Weakness
Vomiting
Back pain

Differential diagnosis
Nonpathological causes of vaginal bleeding (see Table 20.1)
Ectopic pregnancy
Uterine fibroids
Molar pregnancy
Subchorionic hemorrhage
Vaginal trauma

(POCs), hematoma, or other abnormalities. The most reassuring marker of a healthy pregnancy is the presence of cardiac activity, which should be evident after 5 weeks of gestation or once the embryo reaches 2 mm in length. If cardiac activity is present, the risk of spontaneous loss declines to 3–6% (Juliano, Dabulis, & Heffner, 2008). β-hCG levels in conjunction with ultrasound findings guide diagnosis.

There are no effective therapies for women experiencing threatened or inevitable early pregnancy loss. Most first-trimester spontaneous abortions occur completely without further need for intervention. Women who are experiencing a spontaneous loss should be counseled to expect bleeding and cramping until the uterus has emptied. Over-the-counter analgesia such as acetaminophen can be suggested. Although infection and hemorrhage are rare, women should be advised of signs and symptoms of both and instructed to report them. A follow-up visit should be established to assess for any retained POCs, review contraceptive needs, and assess emotional aspects of the woman's experience.

For those women with missed or incomplete early pregnancy loss, additional management options include expectant, medical, and surgical management, and selection is guided by clinical presentation, maternal hemodynamic stability, the presence of infection, and most importantly, the woman's preference. In a nonviable pregnancy without complications, the woman's preference should be a primary consideration in management.

Expectant management

Expectant management is often the initial treatment choice for women experiencing a spontaneous pregnancy loss. If a woman is unable to make an immediate decision because of her distress about the pregnancy loss, it is appropriate to allow her time to consider her options as long as her condition remains stable. However, women who choose this option should be counseled that complete expulsion may take up to 1 month (Allison et al., 2011). The likelihood of spontaneous expulsion declines rapidly after 1 week of expectant management. Women with an incomplete loss generally respond well to expectant management (85% completion) compared to women with a delayed pregnancy loss (33% completion) (Bagratee et al., 2004).

Medical management

The use of oral or vaginal misopristol in hemodynamically stable women with an incomplete pregnancy loss and a uterus less than 12 weeks' gestation has been shown to be an effective and safe alternative to surgical management (American College of Obstetricians and Gynecologists (ACOG), 2009). Pregnancy expulsion with misoprostol occurs in approximately 66–99% of women with incomplete or delayed pregnancy loss in the first trimester (Allison et al., 2011). The common protocol for medical management of women with an incomplete pregnancy loss and a uterus less than 12 weeks in size is misoprostol, 600 μg orally or 400 μg sublingually. Misoprostol can be increased to 800 μg vaginally or 600 μg sublingually for those women with a delayed pregnancy loss (ACOG, 2009). Doses can be repeated every 3 hours for up to three total doses if needed; however, this frequency results in more pronounced gastrointestinal (GI) side effects, and 6- to 12-hour spacing is often more tolerable for women. Misopristol usually takes 4–16 hours to evacuate uterine content.

Counseling women on what to expect with medical management is an important component of care. GI distress such as nausea and vomiting is the most frequently reported side effect, and some women can experience fever or chills. Women need to be informed that bleeding will become heavier with visible clots likely, and cramping will increase. Once the gestational tissue is passed, cramping dramatically improves. The bleeding pattern experienced with tissue passage is typically described as heavier than the usual menstrual flow and lasts approximately 3 or 4 days. This is followed by a transition to vaginal spotting that may last for a week or longer. Prescription strength analgesia such as hydrocodone for pain management should be provided. Women choosing medical management of early pregnancy loss report a high degree of satisfaction with this method (Bagratee et al., 2004).

Surgical management

Immediate surgical management of first-trimester pregnancy loss can be done by electric vacuum aspiration, manual vacuum aspiration, or sharp curette. Cervical ripening agents are often used first to facilitate the evacuation procedure. Surgical management is indicated for women with severe hemorrhage, signs of infection, significant pain, and failure of medical management. Surgical management is also appropriate if a woman chooses this path as her preferred option.

Early pregnancy loss follow-up care

Any woman with vaginal bleeding who is Rh negative and is nonsensitized should receive anti-D immuinoglobulin (RhoGAM) within 48–72 hours of onset of bleeding, regardless of whether the pregnancy ends in a loss or continues. Before 12 weeks' gestation, the dose of RhoGAM is 50 μg; after 12 weeks' gestation, the dose is 300 μg.

The utility and timing of follow-up serum β-hCG levels after a spontaneous pregnancy loss are not clear (Allison et al., 2011). Some health-care providers routinely monitor the β-hCG level until it has dropped to below the detectable level (usually <5 mIU/mL) to ensure complete expulsion of the pregnancy and absence of gestational trophoblastic disease (GTD). The average time for serum c to reach this level varies depending on the initial β-hCG value at the time of pregnancy loss and the mode of management.

It is common practice to advise 1–2 weeks of pelvic rest for women who have experienced a pregnancy loss. Ovulation may resume as early as day 21 after pregnancy loss, so a return visit should be scheduled within this time frame for discussion and initiation of contraception as needed. Menses typically returns by approximately 6 weeks after the spontaneous loss. Women who have experienced an early spontaneous pregnancy loss often ask about the optimal timing for attempting the next pregnancy. There is no physiological reason to wait.

Early pregnancy loss and family considerations

Pregnancy loss is often a deeply felt event for women and couples. Emotional attachment to the pregnancy and the developing fetus typically begins early in the first trimester, and feelings of loss and grief are often more intense than women expect. Emotional healing takes longer than physical healing. More than half of women (55%) experiencing first-trimester pregnancy loss presented with significant psychological distress immediately, 25% at 3 months, 18% at 6 months, and 11% at 1 year (Lok, Yip, Lee, Sahota, & Chung, 2010). Women's responses stem from loss of future plans, dreams, and hopes for her family. It is also common for a woman experiencing pregnancy loss to feel guilt if the pregnancy was unwanted or if she felt any actions on her part contributed to the loss.

The way in which we communicate news of a nonviable loss is important. The use of sensitive, caring language is imperative during communication with the woman and her family. Inadvertent use of terms such as "pregnancy failures" or "incompetent cervix" can increase a woman's sense of guilt and insecurity. Reassurance about the commonplace nature of pregnancy loss and what does *not* cause early loss to reduce self-blame is important in providing care. Women's experiences vary, but for many, it is a difficult and vulnerable time and grief reactions should be evaluated. While grief reaction and depression are not the same, providers should be alert for depression, as up to 30% of women develop clinical depression after pregnancy loss (Mann, McKeown, Bacon, Vesselinov, & Bush, 2008). See Chapter 25, "Perinatal Loss and Grief," for information on emotional care of women and couples after a pregnancy loss.

A follow-up visit is typically scheduled about 2 weeks after a pregnancy loss. The physical exam is focused on confirming uterine involution and resolution of pregnancy symptoms. Women should be advised that it is safe to resume intercourse after bleeding stops, which is typically 1–2 weeks after a loss.

Women who have experienced an early spontaneous pregnancy loss often ask about the optimal timing for attempting the next pregnancy. There is no physiological reason to wait. All conceptions following the pregnancy loss are more likely to result in a subsequent loss regardless of the interval between pregnancies; however, the vast majority of women will go on to have a subsequent healthy pregnancy (DaVanzo et al., 2007). The ideal interconceptual time frame is unknown. The World Health Organization guidelines recommend waiting at least 6 months before trying to become pregnant after early pregnancy loss, while other studies indicate there is no increase in adverse outcome when conception occurs immediately after pregnancy loss (Love, Bhattacharya, Smith, & Bhattacharya, 2010). One study found that an interval of 27–50 months resulted in a significantly lower repeat loss rate than intervals of less than 6 months (DaVanzo et al., 2007). Subsequent pregnancy timing must be weighed against maternal age and other personal factors. It is common practice to advise most women that it is safe to try for conception when they feel emotionally and physically ready. Most women go on to experience a successful pregnancy after a spontaneous loss, regardless of the interpregnancy interval. An informed balance among increased risk and patient preference must be discussed with women in considering a future pregnancy.

Recurrent pregnancy loss

Recurrent pregnancy loss (RPL), also termed habitual abortion, is defined as three or more consecutive pregnancy losses prior to 20 weeks' gestation or less, and affects up to 2% of couples trying to establish a family (Duckett & Qureshi, 2008). The likelihood of a repeat early pregnancy loss increases after each successive loss, reaching approximately 40% after three consecutive early pregnancy losses (Royal College of Obstetricians and Gynaecologists (RCOG), 2011). The causes of recurrent pregnancy loss include genetic chromosomal abnormalities; uterine structural abnormalities like bicornuate uterus; immunologic factors; thrombophelias; endocrine problems like hypothyroidism, polycystic ovarian syndrome (PCOS), diabetes mellitus, and progesterone deficiency; and infectious causes and environmental factors such as excessive alcohol or caffeine intake. Women experiencing recurrent early spontaneous pregnancy loss should be offered genetic counseling and be referred to a specialist for further evaluation and management. Because the risk of subsequent miscarriages is similar among women that have had two versus three miscarriages, and the probability of finding a treatable etiology is similar among the two groups, most experts agree that there is a role for evaluation after two losses (Ford & Schust, 2009).

Potential problems of unexplained early pregnancy bleeding

Recent investigations report an association between early pregnancy bleeding and adverse pregnancy outcomes. Women with threatened miscarriage are at higher risk for placenta previa, placental abruption, premature rupture of membranes, fetal growth restriction, and antepartum hemorrhage of unknown origin (Saraswat, Bhattacharya, Maheshwari, & Bhattacharya, 2010). While these associations are poorly understood, it is theorized that impaired placentation and placental development play a role in later pregnancy complications. However, since the risk of adverse outcomes is relatively modest and there are no specific interventions to prevent these adverse events, increased fetal and maternal surveillance is not warranted (Saraswat et al., 2010).

Ectopic pregnancy

An ectopic pregnancy occurs when a fertilized ovum implants outside of the uterine cavity. Approximately

Table 19.7   Risk Factors for Ectopic Pregnancy

High risk factors

- Tubal ligation
- Tubal pathology/surgery
- Prior ectopic pregnancy
- IUD—especially Mirena

Moderate risk factors

- Infertility
- Assisted reproduction technology
- Prior history of genital tract infection
- Multiple sex partners secondary to increased risk for PID
- Smoking—risk is dose dependent
- African American race

Lower risk factors

- Prior cesarean
- Douching

Source: Creanga et al. (2011), Cunningham et al. (2010), Hoover et al. (2010).

Table 19.8   Signs and Symptoms of Ectopic Pregnancy

Abdominal pain

Amenorrhea, positive pregnancy test

Bleeding often brownish in color

May have breast tenderness, nausea, and other pregnancy signs

Physical exam
Adnexal mass
Acute pain on cervical motion

Signs of rupture include
Hypotension
Nausea
Pallor
Shoulder pain (blood irritating diaphragm)
Urge to defecate (blood pooling in cul de sac)

1–2% of all documented pregnancies are ectopic (Chang et al., 2003). Ectopic pregnancy is the leading cause of maternal death in the first trimester and accounts for 9% of all maternal mortality in the United States (Chang et al., 2003). Ectopic pregnancy can result in loss of a fallopian tube and reduce fertility. Ruptured ectopic pregnancy can be a life-threatening emergency.

The incidence of ectopic pregnancy increased significantly since the early 1970s; however, has become stable in the last decade. This increase is attributed to the rise of risk factors associated with ectopic pregnancy such as smoking and pelvic inflammatory disease (PID) among reproductive age women, the growing use of assisted reproductive technology (ART), and improvement in detection and diagnosis of ectopic pregnancy (Sivalingam, Duncan, Kirk, Shephard, & Horne, 2011). Risk factors can be categorized by strength of association with occurrence of ectopic pregnancy (Table 19.7); however, 50% of all ectopic pregnancies occur in women without risk factors (Creanga et al., 2011).

Ectopic pregnancy commonly occurs in the fallopian tubes. More rarely, ectopic pregnancy occurs in the ovary, the cervical canal, or the peritoneum.

Clinical presentation

Ectopic pregnancy may develop enough to produce symptoms such as bleeding or lower quadrant pain commonly between 6 and 8 weeks. Many women are asymptomatic when attending the first prenatal visit. Since β-hCG is produced, women may have early pregnancy

symptoms such as breast tenderness and nausea (Table 19.8).

Diagnosis and management

Ectopic pregnancy may be subacute in early stages; however, it can quickly become an obstetric emergency. Early diagnosis is critical to reducing maternal morbidity and mortality and outcomes preserving tubal function and fertility. Ectopic pregnancy should be suspected in all reproductive age women presenting with vaginal bleeding and a positive pregnancy test in the first trimester. Diagnosis of an unruptured ectopic pregnancy is accomplished by serum β-hCG measurements and transvaginal ultrasound. Serial measurement of serum β-hCG values can help to distinguish among a potentially viable intrauterine gestation, a resolving spontaneous abortion, and an ectopic pregnancy. Approximately 50% of women with an ectopic pregnancy present with increasing β-hCG levels, and 50% present with decreasing β-hCG values (Silva et al., 2006). However, the majority of women who have an ectopic pregnancy have serial serum β-hCG values that increase more slowly than would be expected with a viable intrauterine pregnancy or decrease more slowly than would be expected with a miscarriage. Ultrasound findings are correlated with β-hCG levels to determine the most appropriate management.

Treatment of an ectopic pregnancy can be expectant, surgical, or medical, depending on a woman's presentation and preferences (Table 19.9). When β-hCG values decrease at a rate that is at least as high as that expected in a spontaneous pregnancy loss, continued outpatient surveillance and expectant management is warranted until levels are undetectable.

Table 19.9   Criteria for Managing Ectopic Pregnancy

Expectant management
No evidence of tubal rupture
Minimal pain or bleeding
Patient reliable for follow-up
Starting β-hCG level less than 1000 mIU/mL (1000 IU/L) and falling
Ectopic or adnexal mass less than 3 cm or not detected
No embryonic heartbeat

Medical management with methotrexate
Stable vital signs
No medical contraindication for methotrexate therapy
Unruptured ectopic pregnancy
Absence of embryonic cardiac activity
Ectopic mass of 3.5 cm or less
Starting β-hCG levels less than 5000 mIU/mL (5000 IU/L)
Dosage: single intramuscular dose of 1 mg/kg or 50 mg/m²
Follow-up: β-hCG on the fourth and seventh posttreatment days, then weekly until undetectable, which usually takes several weeks
Expected β-hCG changes: initial slight increase, then 15% decrease between days 4 and 7; if not, repeat dosage or move to surgery
Special consideration: prompt availability of surgery if patient does not respond to treatment

Surgical management
Unstable vital signs or signs indicating rupture
Advanced ectopic pregnancy (high β-hCG levels, large mass, cardiac activity)
Patient unreliable for follow-up
Contraindications to expectant management or methotrexate

Source: Deutchman, Tubay, and Turok (2009).

Medical management of ectopic pregnancy with administration of methotrexate, a folic acid antagonist, is a common and safe alternative to surgery. A single-dose intramuscular administration regimen is most common (Barnhart, 2009). Surgical treatment may involve removing the affected fallopian tube (salpingectomy) or dissecting the ectopic pregnancy with conservation of the tube.

The risk of recurrence is approximately 10% among women with one previous ectopic pregnancy and at least 25% among women with two or more previous ectopic pregnancies (Kårhus, Egerup, Skovlund, & Lidegaard 2013; Seeber & Barnhart, 2006). Most women who experience ectopic pregnancy can go on to have a healthy pregnancy. It should be remembered that the woman is still experiencing loss of a pregnancy, even though it was not viable, and is likely to experience grieving similar to women with any other early pregnancy loss.

Gestational trophoblastic disease

GTD encompasses several types of pregnancy-related tumors that originate in the placenta. GTD is divided into molar and nonmolar tumors and can be benign or malignant. Hydatidiform mole is a benign neoplastic disease where a normally fertilized ovum implants into the uterus, but the chorionic villi do not develop properly. The pregnancy is not viable, and the normal pregnancy process turns into a benign tumor. There are two subtypes of hydatidiform mole: complete hydatidiform mole and partial hydatidiform mole (Table 19.10). Genetic markers have shown that the vast majority of hydatidiform moles are derived entirely from paternal

Table 19.10   Types of Gestational Trophoblastic Disease

Type	Physiology	Physical findings
Hydatidiform mole		
Partial hydatidiform mole	Some fetal tissue present Result from one set of maternal haploid genes and two sets of paternal haploid genes	Vaginal bleeding Absence of fetal heart tones Signs and symptoms consistent with an incomplete or missed abortion Uterus may be smaller for gestational age
Complete hydatidiform mole	No fetal tissue present Results from duplication of the haploid sperm after fertilization of an empty ovum Has greater potential for malignancy	Vaginal bleeding Absence of fetal heart tones Uterus may be greater than expected for gestational age
Gestational trophoblastic neoplasm		
Invasive mole	Trophoblastic invasion confined to the myometrium	Continued bleeding after any type of pregnancy Uterine subinvolution
Gestational choriocarcinoma	Rapidly growing trophoblastic cells invade the myometrium and blood vessels Extremely malignant	Continued bleeding after any type of pregnancy Uterine subinvolution

Sources: Berkowitz and Goldstein (2009), Secki et al. (2010).

Table 19.11   Risk Factors for Gestational Trophoblastic Disease

Maternal age >35
Teens
Prior molar pregnancy
Oral contraceptive use
Smoking

genes. This can happen when the sperm penetrates an ovum that has no nucleus.

A hydatidiform mole is considered malignant if metastases or invasion of the myometrium occurs, or when the serum β-hCG levels plateau or rise during the postpartum period in the absence of a subsequent pregnancy. Partial moles are rarely followed by malignant changes, where as this may occur in approximately 10–15% of complete moles (Secki, Sebire, & Berkowitz, 2010).

Hydatidiform moles occur in approximately 1 in 1200 pregnancies in the United States (Atrash, Hogue, & Grimes, 1986) and are more common at the extremes of reproductive age. Women older than 35 years have a twofold increase in risk. Women older than 40 years experience a 5- to 10-fold increase in risk compared to younger women (Table 19.11).

Potential problems

A major potential problem with hydatidiform mole is the development of a malignancy in the molar tissue. This typically occurs within 6 months of molar evacuation (Berkowitz & Goldstein, 2009).

Presentation

The most common classic symptom of a complete mole is vaginal bleeding, occurring in over 50% of women. Molar tissue separates from the decidua, causing bleeding that can vary from spotting to heavy bleeding. The bleeding can persist intermittently for weeks. Uterine growth is often more rapid than is expected for gestational age. No fetal heartbeat is present. Due to extremely high levels of human chorionic gonadotropin (hCG), women may report severe nausea and vomiting. Signs and symptoms of hyperthyroidism can be present due to stimulation of the thyroid gland by the high levels of circulating hCG or by a thyroid-stimulating substance produced by the trophoblasts.

Diagnosis and management

Most molar pregnancies are diagnosed in the first trimester prior to the onset of the classic signs and symptoms due to the widespread availability of pelvic ultrasonography. A quantitative serum β-hCG is also important to diagnosis. Levels greater than 100,000 mIU/mL indicate trophoblastic growth and raise suspicion for a molar pregnancy. However, a molar pregnancy may have a normal hCG level. Complete blood cell count with platelets should be obtained as anemia could be present and coagulopathy could occur. Although women with molar pregnancies are usually clinically euthyroid, plasma thyroxine can be markedly elevated.

Some women present with early spontaneous passage of molar tissue. After the expulsion of tissue, it is essential to determine whether a miscarriage is complete. A physical examination and, in some cases, evaluation with ultrasound or serial β-hCG levels are necessary shortly after or, if the woman's symptoms are stable, within a few days of expulsion. For those who do not pass molar tissue spontaneously, treatment is always surgical by dilation and curettage. Pelvic rest is recommended for 2–4 weeks after evacuation of the uterus, and the woman is instructed not to become pregnant for 6 months. Some women who have completed childbearing or who have higher risk for malignancy may be offered hysterectomy.

Because of the small but real potential for development of malignant disease and because these malignancies are absolutely curable, the importance of consistent follow-up care must be emphasized. Once a molar pregnancy is diagnosed, a baseline chest X-ray is often done as the lungs are a primary site of metastasis for malignant trophoblastic tumors. Serial β-hCG levels are commonly monitored weekly until they are within normal limits for 3–4 weeks, then monthly for 6 months to 1 year (Berkowitz & Goldstein, 2009). This is to identify the rare patient who develops malignant disease. Levels should consistently drop and should never increase. Normal levels are usually reached within 8–12 weeks after evacuation of the hydatidiform mole. As long as the hCG levels are falling, intervention is not needed. To avoid any confusion about the development of malignant disease, the woman must avoid pregnancy during the period of follow-up described earlier. Effective contraception should be used. If a pregnancy does occur, the elevation in β-hCG would be confused with development of malignant disease.

The risk of recurrence of hydatidiform mole is 1–2% (Berkowitz & Goldstein, 2009). Women with a prior history of GTD should undergo early ultrasound evaluation to rule out molar gestation.

Early pregnancy bleeding and scope of practice considerations

Obstetrical consultation is appropriate for women in stable condition and the cause of bleeding is

Table 19.12 Suggested Indications for Physician Consultation, Collaboration, or Referral (May Not Be Inclusive)*

Severe pain: lower abdominal, unilateral or bilateral, shoulder pain

Excessive blood loss or severe bleeding

Signs/symptoms of infection

Adnexal mass, tenderness, or other abnormal clinical findings; hCG levels, 1500 IU/L, that increase more slowly than expected

Presumed diagnosis of, strong suspicion for, or abnormal sonographic findings suggesting ectopic pregnancy

Curettage chosen or clinically indicated before or after trial of expectant management

Incomplete miscarriage with significant bleeding and/or pain

Amount of time to complete expulsion interferes with physical/emotional well-being

Woman desires to wait for spontaneous passage of tissue over 4 weeks after diagnosis of nonviable pregnancy

Serum hCG levels do not decline normally after miscarriage or curettage clinically thought to be complete

Fetal (not embryonic) demise

Suspected or diagnosed gestational trophoblastic disease (*gynecologic oncologist suggested*)

Request of woman/couple

Reproductive endocrinologist suggested
   3 or more miscarriages
   2 or more miscarriages in woman who is in mid-thirties or older, has contributory medical condition, or has significant anxiety about future miscarriage
   Infertility history or previous pregnancy conceived with assisted reproductive technology

Psychiatric provider suggested
   Current depression, anxiety disorder, or other psychiatric disorder
   Symptoms of complicated grief reaction: persistent symptoms of grief, depression, or anxiety; somatic complaints without physical cause; inability to perform daily activities; disproportionate concerns or grievances; unrealistic idealization of the pregnancy or baby

*The guidelines differentiating among consultation, collaboration, and referral vary among practices.
Source: Thorstensen (2000).

undetermined. Women experiencing an uncomplicated early intrauterine pregnancy loss can be managed independently. Referral for management options is appropriate for any pregnancy bleeding event that is potentially life threatening. Table 19.12 provides a guideline for interprofessional evaluation and management of women experiencing first-trimester bleeding.

Bleeding during the second half of pregnancy

Bleeding during the later second or third trimester of pregnancy is almost always abnormal. The bleeding can range from very mild to extremely brisk, and may or may not be accompanied by abdominal pain. The role of the health-care provider is to move toward diagnosis and to determine the need for direct care and the need for referral or consultation. Additionally, reassurance as appropriate, and/or comfort, especially if the bleeding results in a poor pregnancy outcome, is an important component of competent care. Common etiologies of second- and third-trimester bleeding include preterm labor, cervical insufficiency, placenta previa, and placental abruption.

Placenta previa

Placenta previa is a condition where the placenta is implanted very close to or over the cervical os. Normally, the placenta implants in the muscular upper uterine segment. In placenta previa, the placenta is totally or partially implanted in the lower uterine segment, which is thinner and less vascular. Placenta previa is classified according to the location of the placenta relative to the cervix (Fig. 19.2).

A low-lying placenta is a common finding on second-trimester ultrasonography; however, it is not necessarily pathologic. It is estimated that over 90% of low-lying placentas seen on ultrasound at 20 weeks' gestation will move away from the cervix and out of the lower uterine segment (Oleyese, 2009). This movement, called trophotropism, occurs as the placenta naturally grows toward the more highly vascularized uterine fundus. The majority of women with a placenta previa seen on ultrasound in the second trimester will no longer have a placenta previa in the third trimester.

Placenta previa in the third trimester occurs in approximately 2–4 per 1000 singleton pregnancies (Yang et al., 2009). The incidence of placenta previa is rising in correlation with the increase in cesarean section in the United States. Cesarean birth in any pregnancy is associated with an increased risk for placenta previa in the subsequent pregnancy with the risk increasing with each cesarean birth (Getahun, Oyelese, Salihu, & Ananth, 2006). Additional risk factors for placenta previa are noted in Table 19.13.

Potential problems

Placenta previa is associated with an increase in preterm birth and an increase in perinatal morbidity and

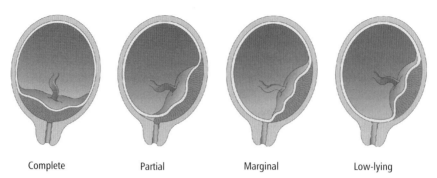

| Complete | Partial | Marginal | Low-lying |

Figure 19.2. Types of placenta previa.

Table 19.13 Risk Factors for Placenta Previa

Advanced maternal age >35
Multiparity
Prior cesarean section
Infertility treatments
Smoking
Unexplained elevated alpha-fetoprotein (AFP)
Multiple gestation
Short interpregnancy interval
Prior uterine curettage

mortality. Women with placenta previa are more likely to experience cesarean section and thus are exposed to surgical potential problems. Women with placenta previa may suffer considerable emotional distress due to recurrent bleeding, hospitalizations, feelings of helplessness, and acute concern for maternal and fetal health.

Presentation

The classic clinical presentation of placenta previa includes painless vaginal bleeding in the late second or early third trimester of pregnancy. The first episode of bleeding often stops after a few hours. Subsequent episodes of bleeding tend to become worse due to increased development of the lower uterine segment and further detachment of the placenta. The painless bleeding occurs due to stretching of the lower uterine segment and detachment at the placenta. Some women may experience associated pain and cramping due to uterine irritability caused by bleeding.

Differential diagnoses

Cervical bleeding from conditions like cervicitis, cervical ectropion, or polyps should be considered. Spotting after intercourse or a digital vaginal examination due to cervical friability is common at any gestation in pregnancy. Also, a woman may experience a small amount of bleeding during cervical dilation during the normal course of labor. Placental abruption should be considered with any late pregnancy bleeding.

Placental abruption

Placental abruption is defined as antepartal decidual hemorrhage leading to the premature separation of the placenta. The immediate cause of the premature placental separation is often the rupture of maternal vessels in the decidua basalis, where it comes into contact with the anchoring villi of the placenta. Since the separation lies within the maternal deciduas, the bleeding is almost always maternal in origin.

Placental abruption occurs in approximately 1% of all pregnancies (Oyelese & Ananth, 2006). One of the most common conditions associated with placental abruption is hypertension. The presence of hypertension during pregnancy, whether from chronic hypertension or a hypertensive disease in pregnancy, approximately doubles the risk of placental abruption (Ananth, Peltier, Kinzler, Smulian, & Vintzileos, 2007), as does interpregnancy interval of less than 1 year (Oyelese & Ananth, 2006). The underlying pathophysiological mechanism may be ischemic placental disease, characterized by chronic reduced blood flow to some degree. Preterm prelabor rupture of membranes is associated with a threefold increase in placental abruption, possibly due to infection and inflammatory processes (Oyelese & Ananth, 2006). Cesarean birth is known to cause lasting damage to the myometrium and endometrium. A cesarean birth is associated with an increased risk of placental abruption in subsequent pregnancies, with a 30–50% increase in the risk of abruption in the third birth among women with a cesarean second birth (Oyelese & Ananth, 2006). Smoking is a risk factor with a dose–response relationship between the number of cigarettes smoked and the risk of placental abruption (Table 19.14).

Potential problems

Women with placental abruption are more at risk for shock, consumptive coagulopathy, and renal failure and death, all of which are associated with significant blood loss during pregnancy. Couvelaire uterus, a condition describing blood seeping into the uterine musculature, is more common with placental abruption. Women who experience placental abruption have a high recurrence rate in subsequent pregnancies. Fetal complications include decreased oxygenation causing cerebral compromise and stillbirth.

Presentation

The signs and symptoms of placental abruption can vary markedly making timely diagnosis difficult. In its early stages, there may be no signs or symptoms clinically evident. A concealed abruption occurs when a midsection of placenta has separated from the uterine wall within the margins of placenta that remains attached. The only symptoms may be cramping, contractions, and or uterine tenderness. A placental separation at the margins often produces visible bleeding (Figure 19.3). The clinical hallmarks of placental abruption are vaginal

Table 19.14 Risk Factors for Placental Abruption

Prior placenta abruption
Hypertension (chronic hypertension, preeclampsia, gestational hypertension)
Increased maternal age
Premature prelabor rupture of membranes
Smoking
Prior cesarean birth
Short interpregnancy interval
Cocaine use
African American and Caucasian races
Polyhydramnios
Multiple gestation
Uterine decompression
Thrombophelias
Uterine leiomyoma
Maternal trauma such as car accident, assault, or fall
Unexplained abnormally elevated maternal serum AFP

Adapted from: Ananth et al. (2005); Oyelese and Ananth (2006).

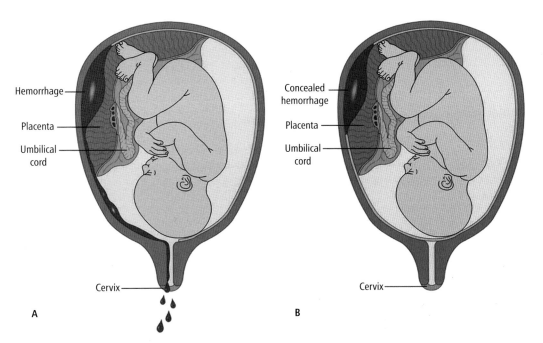

Figure 19.3. Visible and concealed bleeding in placental abruption. Types of abruption: (A) With revealed abruption, blood tracks between the membranes and escapes through the vagina and cervix; (B) with concealed abruption, blood collects behind the placenta, with no evidence of vaginal bleeding. Reprinted with permission from Oyelese, Y., & Anathe, C. (2006). Placental abruption. *Obstetrics & Gynecology, 108*(4), 1005–1016. Illustration by John Yanson.

bleeding with abdominal pain. These classic symptoms are often accompanied by uterine hypertonicity and tenderness. Maternal tachycardia and a nonreassuring fetal heart rate pattern may be present. In a woman whose placenta is located in the posterior wall of the uterus, back pain may accompany uterine abruption.

Diagnosis and management of bleeding in the second half of pregnancy

The amount, color, and characteristics of the bleeding as well as any associated symptoms should be ascertained. Chart review should be done for blood type and Rh, risk factors, and placenta location noted with any prior ultrasound examination. Abdominal palpation for uterine tone and tenderness and vital sign assessment should be performed. A digital pelvic examination in women experiencing second- or third-trimester bleeding should never be performed until placental location is identified. Even a gentle digital exam can precipitate severe prenatal hemorrhage in the presence of placenta previa.

Sonographic evaluation is required to determine placental location. Transvaginal ultrasound is superior to abdominal ultrasound in diagnosing placenta previa (Society of Obstetricians and Gynaecologists of Canada (SCOG), 2007). Transvaginal ultrasound allows for visualization of the internal cervical os and the lower placental edge. In addition, the fetal head does not obscure visualization of the placental edge when using transvaginal ultrasound. Ultrasound may reveal retroplacental clotting indicating possible placental abruption; however, because the placenta and fresh bleeding have similar appearances on sonography images, negative findings on ultrasound do not exclude the possibility of placental abruption. A CBC and type and screen should be done. Coagulation studies may be helpful in women suspected of experiencing placental abruption. Rh-negative women should receive Rh immune globulin within 48–72 hours of the onset of bleeding. A Kleihauer–Betke test should be performed first to determine the appropriate dose of Rh immune globulin.

Hospitalization is appropriate for women with placenta previa during an acute bleeding episode or in the presence of uterine contractions. Conservative expectant management is appropriate for women whose bleeding from documented placenta previa subsides so that birth can occur as close to term is possible. Outpatient management of placenta previa may be appropriate for women in stable condition with home support, close proximity to a hospital, and ready access to transportation.

The management for placental abruption varies depending on gestational age and the status of the mother and fetus. Placental abruption can be associated with poor placentation in early pregnancy which can lead to fetal growth restriction. Therefore, women with a history of a prior placental abruption would be candidates for serial ultrasound evaluation of fetal growth.

Scope of practice considerations in later pregnancy bleeding

Since most causes of second- and third-trimester bleeding are abnormal, obstetrical collaboration or referral is warranted. In the case of placenta previa, consultation or referral is done for possible tocolysis, outpatient or inpatient management decisions, and steroid administration. Placental abruption is an obstetrical emergency and obstetrician management is essential.

Family considerations in later pregnancy bleeding

Women with later pregnancy bleeding may suffer considerable emotional distress due to recurrent bleeding, hospitalizations, feelings of helplessness, and acute concern for maternal and fetal health. Family support systems can be crucial to maintaining family function and reducing maternal stress. Women with limited family support may benefit from social and community services.

Summary

Bleeding during pregnancy is a common event and may or may not signal a problem. Any occurrence of vaginal bleeding during pregnancy requires investigation to differentiate between nonsignificant and potentially harmful processes. Vaginal bleeding is more often benign in early pregnancy, though it can be a sign of miscarriage or ectopic pregnancy. Later pregnancy bleeding can indicate more serious problems such as placental abruption or placenta previa, and requires rapid evaluation and consultation and or referral to specialty care.

Resources for women and their families

American College of Obstetricians and Gynecologists— Frequently Asked Questions: Bleeding during Pregnancy: http://www.acog.org/~/media/For%20 Patients/faq038.pdf?dmc=1&ts=20120626T084256 5527

American College of Obstetricians and Gynecologists— Frequently Asked Questions: Repeated Miscarriage: http://www.acog.org/~/media/For%20Patients/faq 100.pdf?dmc=1&ts=20120626T0844442480

Case study 1

TL, a 27-year-old G2P1 1001, called into the office reporting mild vaginal bleeding, changing a pad once this morning, though it did not soak through. She was advised to come in for evaluation. TL had been seen in the office 3 weeks prior to her first prenatal visit. She is now 9 weeks in gestation.

TL was assessed immediately upon her arrival to the office. She stated the bleeding started approximately 2 hours ago and seemed to be decreasing somewhat. During the visit, TL was very anxious and concerned about losing this wanted pregnancy. She was reassured that early pregnancy bleeding does not always lead to miscarriage, and was told that many women do experience early pregnancy bleeding and go on to complete a full-term pregnancy.

TL denied trauma, intercourse in the last 24 hours, signs and symptoms of vaginal infection, and presence of any pain or cramping. Medication history was negative. She reports mild nausea and breast tenderness, and daily fatigue.

Dark red bleeding was noted over approximately one-third of her pad, which was the second pad since the bleeding started. Her blood pressure was 110/72, pulse 76, temperature 36.6°C, and respirations 20 breaths per minute. Urine hCG test pregnancy text was positive.

Abdominal exam revealed soft nontender adnexa and uterus nonpalpable. On speculum exam, a small amount of red blood was noted in the vaginal vault with a scant amount coming from the cervical os mixed with cervical mucus. The cervix was closed with a small amount of ectropy noted; no polyps or signs of infection were noted. Bimanual examination revealed an anteverted uterus compatible with 9 weeks' gestation, a closed cervix, and no cervical motion tenderness or adnexal mass noted. The findings of her exam were within normal limits and TL was again reassured.

A transvaginal ultrasound was done by the in-office ultrasound technologist. A viable pregnancy was seen with a fetal heart tone in 150 s, gestational age 9 weeks 3 days. No sonographic evidence of subchorionic hemorrhage was noted.

Based on the physical findings and the ultrasound examination, it was determined that TL had a normal viable pregnancy and 9 weeks' gestation. Discussion then ensued with TL regarding various causes of early pregnancy bleeding, that etiology remains unknown in more than half of the women presenting with early pregnancy bleeding, and that most women with early pregnancy bleeding go on to have a full-term pregnancy. Pelvic rest was discussed. TL was informed that limited data are available on the efficacy of pelvic rest, however, that she might feel more comfortable if she abstain from intercourse for several days. TL was instructed to call the office if she had further episodes of bleeding, developed pain or fever, or had other concerns. TL had an appointment the next week for her routine prenatal visit, and follow-up was done at that point. TL experienced no further bleeding or pregnancy complications and gave birth to a 6 lb. 12 oz. girl at 38 weeks' gestation.

Case study 2

AC, a 32-year-old Caucasian G3 P1011 at 34 weeks' gestation, called the office with a report of dull aching pain primarily felt in her back over the last 4 hours. She had tried a heating pad and over-the-counter analgesics with no relief, and it seemed to be getting worse, with her abdomen tightening somewhat in conjunction with the back pain. She reported normal fetal movement that morning. On chart review, it was noted that AC smokes approximately one-half to one pack per day. Routine laboratory studies were within normal limits, and her pregnancy had progressed normally. It was initially thought that AC may be experiencing preterm labor, so she was advised to come into the office for evaluation.

Upon arrival to the office, AC noted the back pain and abdominal tightening were now constant. She reported no bleeding, headache, visual disturbances, or epigastric pain. Her blood pressure was 126/80, pulse 82, temperature 98.8, and respirations 22 breaths per minute. She pointed to her left lower sacral area as where she felt the most pain earlier, but noted that the pain had also moved to the front of her abdomen, right above the pubic bone.

The abdominal exam revealed a tense and somewhat firm uterus, leading to difficulty in palpating fetal parts, although it was determined to be a cephalic presentation. AC reported tenderness on abdominal palpation. Fetal heart tones were found in the right lower quadrant at 130 bpm. The bimanual pelvic exam found the cervix closed.

Because of the increasing nature of the pain and hypertonic uterus, obstetrical referral was initiated. AC was transferred to the labor and birth unit for further evaluation, where it was determined that she was experiencing a concealed placental abruption. AC underwent an emergency cesarean section within 2 hours of arriving in the office, and was delivered of a 3 lb. 9 oz. male with Apgars of 4 and 7, who was transferred to the neonatal intensive care unit (NICU).

Case study 3

RG is a 25-year-old married G1P0 at 7 weeks' gestation according to her last menstrual period. This is a planned and welcomed pregnancy. She called the office with reports of bright red bleeding, lighter than a menstrual period but requiring sanitary pad protection. She also reported intermittent cramping. She denied lightheadedness, dizziness, nausea, vomiting, or lower right or left quadrant pain. She reported continued breast tenderness.

On arrival in the office, her vital signs were obtained. Her height was 65 in., weight 142 lb, blood pressure 112/68 mmHg, and pulse 72 bpm. She appeared to be in some discomfort from the cramping, though she was able to answer questions without difficulty. Upon questioning, she denied any trauma, recent intercourse, or changes in discharge preceding the onset of bleeding. Her last Pap smear was done 3 months previously and was normal. Routine cervical cultures at the time were negative for chlamydia and gonorrhea.

The pelvic examination reveals the following:

- *External genitalia*—A small amount of dark red blood is noted at the vaginal introitus. No lesion, trauma, or lacerations are noted.
- *Vagina*—Pink; a small amount of dark red, mucustinged blood is noted in the vaginal vault. No trauma or lacerations are noted.
- *Cervix*—Appears closed, pink without lesion; a small amount of dark blood is noted coming from the cervical os.

The bimanual exam indicated a 7- to 8-week gestation-sized, anteverted uterus, mildly tender to palpation. No adnexal masses were appreciated; the cervix felt closed.

The results of laboratory studies indicated

- blood type: O
- Rh: positive
- antibody screen: negative
- CBC: normal
- B-hCG: 2400 mIU/mL.

An ultrasound examination was performed. An intrauterine pregnancy was seen with fetal cardiac activity of 152 bpm. A normal gestational sac was seen consistent with a pregnancy of 7 weeks, 1 day. No subchorionic hemorrhage was noted.

The differential diagnosis for RG includes

- normal pregnancy
- threatened abortion.

Because RG continued to bleed, a repeat quantitative β-hCG in 48 hours was ordered. The warning signs and symptoms of spontaneous abortion were discussed with RG. She was advised to call with changes in symptoms, including an increase in bleeding saturating more than a pad an hour, passage of clots, severe cramping, lightheadedness, dizziness, fever, chills, or any other concerning symptoms.

Two days later, RG returned to the office with her husband for her repeat β-hCG, which was 1600 mIU/mL. She continued to bleed lightly. She denied fever, chills, or passing clots. Her vital signs remained stable. The pelvic exam was unchanged from the exam done 2 days prior.

RG and her husband were advised that the falling β-hCG levels indicate a pregnancy loss or miscarriage. Definitive diagnosis was made when a repeat ultrasound revealed no fetal cardiac activity and a collapsing gestational sac. A diagnosis of incomplete abortion or abortion in progress was made.

Time was given for RG and her husband to express their grief and ask questions. Information regarding the unknown etiologies of early pregnancy loss was discussed, and RG was reassured that it is highly unlikely that maternal behavior contributed to the loss, that future fertility is not compromised. The options of care were discussed. They were offered the choices of expectant management, medical management, or surgical evacuation of the uterus. RG chose expectant management and was sent home with instructions to call if the bleeding saturated more than a pad an hour or if she developed fever or chills. RG was instructed in nonsteroidal anti-inflammatory drug (NSAID) pain relief measures but was asked to call if additional pain control was needed. Plans were made for a follow-up telephone call later that week, and the couple was encouraged to call with any questions or concerns. A follow-up appointment was scheduled in 2 weeks, at which time β-hCG levels could be measured if indicated, birth control provided, and RG's grief response assessed. RG's bleeding increased, and she passed uterine contents during the night, with immediate relief of cramping and reduction in bleeding.

References

Allison, J. L., Sherwood, R. S., & Schust, D. J. (2011). Management of first trimester pregnancy loss can be safely moved into the office. *Review in Obstetrics & Gynecology, 4*(1), 5–14.

American College of Obstetricians and Gynecologists (ACOG). (2009). ACOG committee opinion No. 427. Misoprostol for postabortion care. *Obstetrics & Gynecology, 113*(2 Pt1), 465–468.

American College of Obstetricians and Gynecologists (ACOG). (2001, reaffirmed 2008). Committee on Practice Bulletins.

Management of recurrent early pregnancy loss. Clinical Management Guidelines for Obstetrician-Gynecologists No. 24. Washington, DC. ACOG.

Ananth, C. V., Olelese, Y., Yoe, L., Pradhan, A., & Vintzileos, A. M. (2005). Placental abruption in the United States, 1979 through 2001: temporal trends and potential determinants. *American Journal of Obstetrics and Gynecology, 192*(1), 191–198.

Ananth, C. V., Peltier, M. R., Kinzler, W. L., Smulian, J. C., & Vintzileos, A. M. (2007). Chronic hypertension and risk of placental abruption: Is the association modified by ischemic placental disease? *American Journal of Obstetrics and Gynecology, 197*(3), 273–e1.

Atrash, H. K., Hogue, C. J., & Grimes, D. A. (1986). Epidemiology of hydatidiform mole during early gestation. *American Journal of Obstetrics & Gynecology, 154*(4), 906–909.

Bagratee, J. S., Khullar, V., Regan, L., Moodley, J., & Kagoro, H. (2004). A randomized controlled trial comparing medical and expectant management of first trimester miscarriage. *Human Reproduction, 19*(2), 266–271.

Barnhart, K. T. (2009). Clinical practice: Ectopic pregnancy. *New England Journal of Medicine, 361*, 379–387.

Benson, C. B., Chow, J. S., Chang-Lee, W., Hill, J. A., 3rd, & Doubilet, P. M. (2001). Outcome of pregnancies in women with uterine leiomyomas identified by sonography in the first trimester. *Journal of Clinical Ultrasound, 29*, 261–264.

Berkowitz, R. S., & Goldstein, D. P. (2009). Molar pregnancy. *The New England Journal of Medicine, 360*(16), 1639.

Chang, J., Elam-Evans, L. D., Berg, C. J., Herndon, J., Flowers, L., Seed, K. A., & Syverson, C. J. (2003). Pregnancy-related mortality surveillance—United States, 1991–1999. *MMWR Surveillance Summary, 52*(2), 1–8.

Creanga, A., Shapiro-Mendoza, C. K., Bish, C. L., Zane, S., Berg, C. J., & Callaghan, W. M. (2011). Trends in ectopic pregnancy mortality in the United States 1980–2007. *Obstetrics & Gynecology, 117*(4), 837–843.

Cunningham, C., Levano, K., Bloom, S., Hauth, J., Rouse, D., & Spong, C. (2010). *Williams Obstetrics* (23rd ed.). New York: McGraw Hill.

DaVanzo, J., Hale, L., Razzaque, A., & Rahman, M. (2007). Effects of interpregnancy interval and outcome of the preceding pregnancy on pregnancy outcomes in Matlab, Bangladesh. *British Journal of Obstetrics and Gynaecology, 114*, 1079–1087.

Davari-Tanha, F., Shariat, M., Kaveh, M., Ebrahimi, M., & Jalalvand, S. (2008). Threatened abortion: A risk factor for poor pregnancy outcome. *Acta Medica Iranica, 46*, 314–320.

Deutchman, M., Tubay, A. T., & Turok, D. (2009). First trimester bleeding. *American Family Physician, 79*(11), 985.

Duckett, K., & Qureshi, A. (2008). Recurrent miscarriage. *American Family Physician, 78*(8), 977–978.

Edwards, D. V., Baird, D. D., Hasan, R., Savitz, D. A., & Hartmann, K. E. (2012). First-trimester bleeding characteristics associate with increased risk of preterm birth: Data from a prospective pregnancy cohort. *Human Reproduction, 27*(1), 54–60.

Ford, H. B., & Schust, D. J. (2009). Recurrent pregnancy loss: Etiology, diagnosis, and therapy. *Reviews in Obstetrics and Gynecology, 2*(2), 76.

Getahun, D., Oyelese, Y., Salihu, H., & Ananth, C. (2006). Previous cesarean delivery and risks of placenta previa and placental abruption. *Obstetrics & Gynecology, 107*(4), 771–778.

Hasan, R., Baird, D. D., Herring, A. H., Olshan, A. F., Funk, M. L. J., & Hartmann, K. E. (2009). Association between first-trimester vaginal bleeding and miscarriage. *Obstetrics and Gynecology, 114*(4), 860.

Hoover, K. W., Tao, G., & Ken, C. K. (2010). Trends in the diagnosis and treatment of ectopic pregnancy in the United States. *Obstetrics & Gynecology, 115*(3), 495–502.

Jauniaux, E., Johns, J., & Burton, G. J. (2005). The role of ultrasound imaging in diagnosing and investigating early pregnancy failure. *Ultrasound in Obstetrics and Gynecology, 25*, 613–624.

Juliano, M., Dabulis, S., & Heffner, A. (2008). Characteristics of women with fetal loss in symptomatic first trimester pregnancies with documented fetal cardiac activity. *Annals of Emergency Medicine, 52*(2), 143–147.

Kårhus, L. L., Egerup, P., Skovlund, C. W., & Lidegaard, Ø. (2013). Long-term reproductive outcomes in women whose first pregnancy is ectopic: A national controlled follow-up study. *Human Reproduction, 28*(1), 241–246.

Lok, I. H., Yip, A. S., Lee, D. T., Sahota, D., & Chung, T. K. (2010). A 1-year longitudinal study of psychological morbidity after miscarriage. *Fertility and Sterility, 93*(6), 1966–1975.

Love, E., Bhattacharya, S., Smith, N. C., & Bhattacharya, S. (2010). Effect of interpregnancy interval on outcomes of pregnancy after miscarriage: Retrospective analysis of hospital episode statistics in Scotland. *British Medical Journal, 341*, c3967. Retrieved from http://www.ncbi.nlm.nih.gov/pmc/articles/PMC2917004/

Lykke, J. A., Dideriksen, K. L., Lidegaard, Ø., & Langhoff-Roos, J. (2010). First trimester vaginal bleeding and complications later in pregnancy. *Obstetrics and Gynecology, 115*(5), 935–944.

Mann, J. R., McKeown, R. E., Bacon, J., Vesselinov, R., & Bush, F. (2008). Predicting depressive symptoms and grief after pregnancy loss. *Journal of Psychosomatic Obstetrics & Gynecology, 29*(4), 274–279.

Nakhai-Pour, H. R., Broy, P., Sheehy, O., & Bérard, A. (2011). Use of nonaspirin nonsteroidal anti-inflammatory drugs during pregnancy and the risk of spontaneous abortion. *Canadian Medical Association Journal, 183*, 1713–1720. Retrieved from http://www.cmaj.ca/content/early/2011/09/06/cmaj.110454.full.pdf

Oleyese, Y. (2009). Placenta previa: The evolving role of ultrasound. *Ultrasound in Obstetrics and Gynecology, 34*, 123–126.

Oyelese, Y., & Ananth, C. (2006). Placental abruption. *Obstetrics & Gynecology, 108*(4), 1005–1016.

Royal College of Obstetricians and Gynaecologists (RCOG) (2011). The investigation and treatment of couples with recurrent first-trimester and second-trimester miscarriage. RCOG Green-top Guideline No. 17. Retrieved from http://www.rcog.org.uk/womens-health/clinical-guidance/investigation-and-treatment-couples-recurrent-miscarriage-green-top-

Saraswat, L., Bhattacharya, S., Maheshwari, A., & Bhattacharya, S. (2010). Maternal and perinatal outcome in women with threatened miscarriage in the first trimester: A systematic review. *British Journal of Obstetrics & Gynecology, 117*, 245–257.

Secki, M. J., Sebire, N. J., & Berkowitz, R. S. (2010). Gestational trophoblastic disease. *The Lancet, 36*(9742), 717–729.

Seeber, B. E., & Barnhart, K. T. (2006). Suspected ectopic pregnancy. *Obstetrics & Gynecology, 107*, 399–343.

Silva, C., Sammel, M. D., Zhou, L., Gracia, C., Hummel, A. C., & Barnhart, K. (2006). Human chorionic gonadotropin profile for women with ectopic pregnancy. *Obstetrics & Gynecology, 107*, 605–610.

Sivalingam, V., Duncan, W. C., Kirk, E., Shephard, L. A., & Horne, A. W. (2011). Diagnosis and management of ectopic pregnancy. *Journal of Family Planning & Reproductive Health Care, 37*(4), 231–240.

Snell, B. J. (2009). Assessment and management of bleeding in the first trimester of pregnancy. *Journal of Midwifery and Women's Health, 54*(6), 483–491.

Society of Obstetricians and Gynaecologists of Canada (SCOG). (2007). Diagnosis and management of placenta previa. *Journal of Obstetrics & Gynaecology of Canada, 29*(3), 261–266.

Thorstensen, K. A. (2000). Midwifery management of first trimester bleeding and early pregnancy loss. *Journal of Midwifery & Women's Health, 45*, 481–497.

Yang, Q., Wen, S., Phillips, K., Oppenheimer, L., Black, D., & Walker, M. (2009). Comparison of maternal risk factors between placental abruption and placenta previa. *American Journal of Perinatology, 26*(4), 279–286.

20

Amniotic fluid and fetal growth disorders

Victoria H. Burslem and Cindy L. Farley

Relevant terms

Amniotic fluid index (AFI)—The largest vertical pocket (LVP) of amniotic fluid visualized by ultrasound without the presence of umbilical cord is measured in centimeters in each of the four maternal abdominal quadrants. The AFI is the sum of those four pockets. An AFI between 5 and 20 cm is considered normal.

Amniotic fluid volume (AFV)—the total amniotic fluid present *in utero*; approximately 800 mL at term, 400 mL by 42 weeks' gestation

Arterial Doppler flow velocity waveforms—a measurement of blood flow in the umbilical arteries, fetal aorta, and middle cerebral artery during the diastolic phase to determine downstream vascular resistance; commonly performed on the umbilical artery; may be referred to as Doppler flow studies or umbilical artery Doppler (Gabbe et al., 2012, p. 719)

Biophysical profile (BPP)—ultrasound assessment of five fetal biophysical activities sensitive to hypoxia, including gross body movements, fetal breathing, fetal tone, amniotic fluid volume, and nonstress test (NST) variables computed as a total score which has a strong correlation to fetal acidemia within 1 week of the test

Doppler velocimetry—a Doppler flow ultrasonic measurement of the arterial and/or venous vascular beds in the fetus to detect normal or abnormal uteroplacental blood flow patterns

Fern test—a microscopic examination of a fluid sample obtained on a cotton-tipped swab from the posterior fornix of the vagina by sterile speculum exam. If present, amniotic fluid will crystallize on the slide due to its high sodium chloride concentration, seen as a fern pattern. Vaginal secretions will not produce a fern pattern.

Idiopathic—arising spontaneously or occurring without a known cause

Individual growth potential curve—methodology for assessing optimal growth potential in both fetal and newborn weight calculated by computer software that is based on a number of variables, which include fetal gender and the maternal characteristics of height, weight in first trimester, parity, and ethnic origin

Intrauterine growth restriction (IUGR)—poor growth of the fetus *in utero*, leading to a failure to attain his/her full growth potential

Large for gestational age (LGA)—newborn weight greater than or equal to the ninetieth percentile for gestational age; one range of a method used to classify neonates into risk categories by weight relative to gestational age

Low birth weight (LBW)—newborn weight <2500 g; one range of a method used to classify neonates into risk categories by weight; not categorized in relation to gestational age

Macrosomia—variously defined as birth weight greater than 4000 or 4500 g. Recent literature has described it as 4000 g in a diabetic mother (of any type, due to increased fetal abdominal circumference) or 4500 g in a nondiabetic mother.

Modified biophysical profile (modified BPP)—the combined results of an NST and amniotic fluid index (AFI), two of the BPP components most associated with correct assessment of current fetal status and acidemia

Nonstress test (NST)—antenatal assessment of the fetal heart rate (FHR) pattern. A reactive FHR pattern in the normal range of 110–160 beats per minute with variability,

---

Prenatal and Postnatal Care: A Woman-Centered Approach, First Edition. Edited by Robin G. Jordan, Janet L. Engstrom, Julie A. Marfell, and Cindy L. Farley.
© 2014 John Wiley & Sons, Inc. Published 2014 by John Wiley & Sons, Inc.

two accelerations, and no decelerations over a 20-minute period has a very low likelihood of adverse perinatal outcome within 1 week following the test.

Oligohydramnios—less than normal amniotic fluid volume (AFV); variously defined as an AFV of ≤200–500 mL, a largest vertical pocket (LVP) of ≤2 cm or an amniotic fluid index (AFI) of ≤5 cm

Polyhydramnios—greater than normal amniotic fluid volume; commonly defined as an amniotic fluid volume of >2100 mL, an AFI of ≥25 cm at any gestational age, or a single measurement of any LVP >8 cm

Ponderal index—the ratio of birth weight to length [(birth weight (g)/crown heel length)³ × 100]

Small for gestational age (SGA)—a weight for gestation below a given threshold; commonly defined as less than or equal to the tenth percentile, less than the third percentile (very small for gestational age [VSGA] > 2 SD below normal) associated with a significantly increased risk of poor outcome

Targeted ultrasound—also known as a level II ultrasound; this ultrasound examination is done by a certified technician to look for specific fetal anomalies

Introduction

The gestational intrauterine environment is influenced by multiple factors, each of which has the ability to significantly impact fetal growth and development, positively or negatively. Placental development and functioning, amniotic fluid production and volume, as well as numerous maternal and fetal conditions, all contribute individually and cumulatively to the environmental factors influencing *in utero* and neonatal outcomes. This chapter provides a review of normal amniotic fluid physiology, normal placentation, and patterns of fetal development, along with maternal, fetal, and placental conditions that contribute to abnormal amniotic fluid and fetal growth patterns.

Amniotic fluid dynamics

The amniotic fluid is a clear, watery fluid that is filtered out of the maternal blood via the amniotic epithelium into the amniotic cavity. The main constituents are water and electrolytes (99%) together with glucose, lipids from the fetal lungs, proteins with bacteriocidal properties, and flaked-off fetal epithelium cells. Amniotic fluid is found within the amniotic cavity by 6 weeks' gestation from the last menstrual period (LMP) date.

Amniotic fluid surrounds the fetus during intrauterine development and is vital to the well-being of the fetus. Amniotic fluid cushions the fetus from maternal abdominal trauma, provides a constant temperature, protects the umbilical cord from compression, and provides the necessary fluid, space, and growth factors to allow normal development of the fetal lungs and musculoskeletal and gastrointestinal systems. Amniotic fluid also contains antibacterial properties that help protect the fetus from infection. Studies of the amniotic fluid through amniocentesis provide fetal genetic karyotyping and information about fetal lung maturity. Given the important functions of amniotic fluid, it is not surprising that abnormalities in amniotic fluid volume (AFV) are associated with increased perinatal morbidity and mortality.

Amniotic fluid maintains a balanced volume by constantly being produced and reabsorbed in a dynamic process, a process that increases with gestational age. Early in pregnancy, most amniotic fluid comes from maternal sources. By the second trimester, the fetus contributes to amniotic fluid volume (AFV) and composition through the production of lung fluid and, predominantly, urination. During the first half of pregnancy, amniotic fluid volume correlates with fetal weight and thus is fairly predictable. At 10 weeks' gestation, the average volume is 30 mL; at 16 weeks, it is 190 mL (Blackburn, 2013).

After 20 weeks' gestation, there is a greater variation in volume of amniotic fluid, with a general increase in total volume up to approximately 33 weeks' gestation. At this time, the amniotic fluid volume plateaus. Near 38 weeks' gestation, volume starts to decline by an estimated 125 mL/week to an average volume of 800 mL by 40 weeks' gestation (Brace & Wolf, 1989) (Fig. 20.1). There is a wide range of normal biological variability to

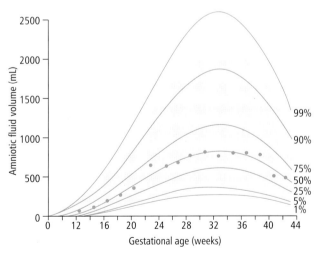

Figure 20.1. Nomogram showing amniotic fluid volume as a function of gestational age. The black dots are the mean for each 2-week interval. From Brace, R. A. & Wolf, E. J. (1989). Normal amniotic fluid volume throughout pregnancy. *American Journal of Obstetrics & Gynecology, 161*, 382.

the volume that fluctuates from day to day within the same woman, influenced by maternal plasma volume and maternal hydration (Blackburn, 2013). After 40 weeks' gestation, amniotic fluid volume declines at a rate of 8% a week (Blackburn, 2013), with an average of 400 mL volume at 42 weeks' gestation (Crowley, O'Herlihy, & Boylan, 1984).

The fetus begins to swallow amniotic fluid at 16–18 weeks' gestation. Near term, a fetus swallows from 200 to 500 mL/day, removing 50% of the amniotic fluid produced through fetal urination (Gabbe et al., 2012, p. 30). This fluid is absorbed through the fetal gastro-intestinal system and is either recycled through the kidneys or is transferred to maternal tissues through the placenta. Near term, the amniotic fluid turns over approximately 1000 mL/day regardless of the total volume present.

Normal placentation and fetal development

Fetal development is largely dependent on proper implantation and function of the placenta, beginning with its formation and secure attachment to the uterine wall by day 10 after fertilization (Blackburn, 2013; Gabbe et al., 2012) (see Fig. 20.2). The cytotrophoblast, the embryo at 7 days after fertilization, forms several types of extravillous trophoblastic tissue, the tissue responsible for the formation of the placenta. By 10–12 weeks' gestation, the trophoblast has eroded the mater-nal spiral arterioles sufficiently so that blood flows into the intervillous space, signaling a properly maturing placenta. A number of pregnancy complications can be related back to this earliest process of trophoblastic invasion. If the invasive process is defective and a failure to properly invade the endometrium results, in a worst case scenario, with only 10% of the spiral arterioles fully penetrated rather than the 96% penetration seen in a normal pregnancy, the placenta will fail to establish proper maternal circulation (Gabbe et al., 2012). This defective process of invasion has been definitively asso-ciated with the development of preeclampsia and intra-uterine growth restriction (IUGR). Conversely, this reduced arteriole invasion may actually be the result of a conceptus that is defective in and of itself, as in the case of chromosomal abnormalities.

Throughout pregnancy, the fetus is in a constant state of rapid growth, in both cellular formation and cellular size. To meet this need, uteroplacental blood flow increases throughout the pregnancy, resulting in greater than 50-fold increase in uterine blood flow as compared to the nonpregnant female. Placental growth and factors contributing to vasodilation of maternal arteries permit the increased uterine blood flow that result from a blood

volume increase of 40% and a doubling of maternal cardiac output (Gabbe et al., 2012). A disruption to either the placental attachment process or the uterine blood flow will impact fetal growth and development; the greater and longer the disruption, the greater the insult.

Amniotic fluid disorders

Oligohydramnios

Oligohydramnios, or less than normal amniotic fluid volume, is diagnosed by ultrasound and defined by varying parameters in the literature, such as an amniotic fluid volume (AFV) of ≤200–500 mL, a largest vertical pocket (LVP) of ≤2 cm, or an amniotic fluid index (AFI) of ≤5 cm. Oligohydramnios, defined as an AFI less than the fifth percentile, may be a better predictor of fetuses at risk for adverse perinatal outcomes compared with using an AFI <5 cm (Shanks, Tuuli, Schaecher, Odibo, & Rampersad, 2011). Figure 20.3 shows AFI values at various points in gestation.

The exact incidence of oligohydramnios is difficult to determine since varying criteria are used to establish a diagnosis, but the generally accepted rate is between 1% and 3% of all pregnancies. However, it is of note that approximately 20% of pregnancies requiring increased antepartum surveillance for a maternal or fetal condi-tion also have oligohydramnios (Blackburn, 2013; Gabbe et al., 2012).

Oligohydramnios is associated with a number of fetal and maternal conditions, including fetal renal abnor-malities, placental insufficiency, and abnormalities of the amnion. It is also true that it may simply be an isolated, idiopathic condition not associated with any underlying pathology. Understanding the timing of gestational onset as well as the causation of oligohydramnios is paramount because implications for neonatal outcome and, therefore, antenatal management of the condition vary significantly (Petrozella, Dasche, McIntire, & Leveno, 2011).

Oligohydramnios that develops in the second trimes-ter is considered early onset and has a high perinatal mortality rate (PMR) due to the etiologies associated with it. Early-onset low amniotic fluid volume (AFV) is commonly caused by fetal anomalies, such as renal agenesis, dysplasia, or obstructive disorders, where there is either a lack of urine production or the inability to pass urine produced due to obstruction. Because amniotic fluid is necessary for fetal lung development, renal anomalies carry a PMR close to 100%. With preterm premature rupture of membranes (PPROM), another etiology for midpregnancy low AFV, the PMR will depend on the fetus's gestational age and

🔒 〰️ The placenta is formed by the chorionic villi of the embryo and the decidua basalis of the endometrium of the mother.

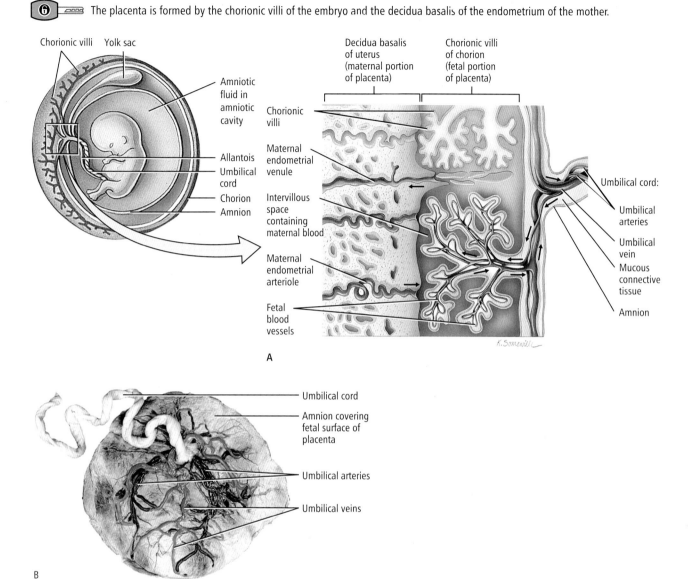

Figure 20.2. Formation of the placenta and umbilical cord. (A) Details of the placenta and the umbilical cord. (B) Fetal surface of the placenta.

other conditions that may result from PPROM, like chorioamnionitis.

In the third trimester, oligohydramnios is more commonly associated with either uteroplacental insufficiency or prolonged pregnancy. Additionally, in the presence of an otherwise normal pregnancy, it is of note that a "significant percentage of third trimester onset oligohydramnios is idiopathic, resolving spontaneously in 3–4 days or in response to maternal hydration" (Gabbe et al., 2012, p. 763). The clinical management dilemma results from oligohydramnios having an association with poor outcome. However, low amniotic fluid volume should not be used as the sole indication in determining the need for an expedited delivery, due to the high rate of

idiopathic oligohydramnios. The clinical condition of the pregnant woman and additional assessment parameters of fetal status must also be taken into account for management decisions. Expectant management is preferred over intervention by induction when the decision is based solely on an isolated low AFI. Neonatal outcomes are similar between the two management options when comparing those with AFIs <5 cm to those with AFIs ≥5 cm because assessment of AFI by ultrasound has been found to have very low sensitivity (Casey et al., 2000; Magann et al., 2000). However, interventions can lead to unwarranted risks for the mother's short- and long-term health. While neonates born to women with low AFIs in one study had lower 5-minute Apgar scores,

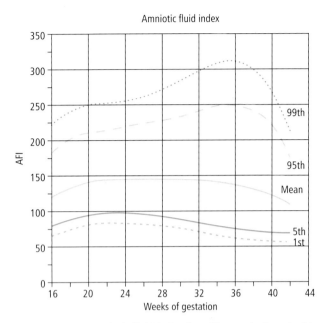

Figure 20.3. Amniotic fluid index (in millimeters) plotted with gestational age (weeks). The solid line denotes the fiftieth percentile; dashed lines, the fifth and ninety-fifth percentiles; and dotted lines, +2 standard deviations (2.5th and 97.5th percentiles). From Moore T.R., & Cayle J.E. (1990) The amniotic fluid index in normal human pregnancy. *American Journal of Obstetrics & Gynecology, 162,* 1168.

no association with neonatal acidosis was found (Figueras & Gardosi, 2011).

The importance of differentiating idiopathic oligohydramnios from that associated with an abnormal maternal or fetal condition is in the recognition of risks inherent to labor induction with an unfavorable cervix. If all other fetal assessment and surveillance parameters are reassuring, the risks of cesarean section due to failed induction must be taken into account in the provider's and the woman's clinical decision-making process.

Fetal and maternal causes of oligohydramnios

Fetal
Renal agenesis
Urinary tract obstruction
Premature spontaneous rupture of the membranes
Abnormal placentation
Elevated maternal serum alpha-fetoprotein (AFP)
Pregnancy at or past 42 weeks' gestation
Severe fetal growth restriction (FGR)

Maternal
Dehydration
Hypertensive disorders
Uteroplacental insufficiency
Antiphospholipid syndrome
Unknown etiology

Oligohydramnios found in association with hypertensive disorders or IUGR carries with it a high risk of poor perinatal outcomes. The low fluid volume is due to decreased fetal kidney perfusion, a result of the vascular constriction that accompanies hypertension of any type or placental insufficiency resulting from poor placentation in early gestation (Blackburn, 2013). While the PMR of later-onset oligohydramnios is not as high as that associated with early onset, nonetheless, it carries with it a strong association with perinatal morbidity and mortality and has been linked to delayed effects of cerebral palsy (CP) and adult-onset disease, such as cardiovascular disease (Figueras & Gardosi, 2011). In this case, the oligohydramnios generally is the result of a maternal condition requiring close observation and prudent decision making for the timing of delivery. An evaluation of the environment that is best for the fetus, *in utero* or extrauterine, is determined by close monitoring with diagnostic tests that assess the fetus's current status.

Prolonged pregnancy is another causative factor in the development of late-onset oligohydramnios. Although AFV has a wide range of normal variations, it is known to decrease from an average of 700–800 mL at term to 400 mL by 42 weeks' gestation. Oligohydramnios in a prolonged pregnancy is associated with an increased risk of meconium-stained amniotic fluid (MSAF), found in approximately one-third of women with oligohydramnios (Gabbe et al., 2012), fetal intolerance of labor, neonatal intensive care unit (NICU) admissions, and poor neonatal outcomes (Casey et al., 2000). Meconium aspiration syndrome, with its risk of chemical pneumonitis and neonatal death, is one of the more serious sequelae associated with MSAF in the presence of oligohydramnios.

Diagnostic assessment and management

Screening, detection, collaborative management, and referral are the focus of primary care management for a woman with suspected oligohydramnios. Accurate pregnancy dating and serial assessment of fundal height are essential to detecting oligohydramnios. If the woman's fundal height is measuring size less than dates, a screening ultrasound should be obtained, if not previously performed, to confirm the expected date of birth (EDB). The status of the amniotic sac should be evaluated by history and physical exam as indicated. If screening ultrasound for dating has been performed and EDB is confirmed, a targeted ultrasound should be scheduled to obtain an anatomy scan and AFV. This will assist in determining if fetal anomalies or signs of aneuploidy are the cause of the oligohydramnios with the provision of genetic counseling and testing made available. If PPROM is suspected, examination by sterile speculum for pooling of amniotic fluid in the posterior vagina, a nitrazine test to assess if vaginal pH has changed from acid to neutral, and a fern test should be done. Serial Doppler blood flow studies will be obtained for a pregnancy confirmed to have oligohydramnios. This noninvasive ultrasound exam assesses placental function by measuring changes in blood flow in the maternal and fetal circulations visualized as Doppler peak velocity waveforms. These studies provide information on current fetal status with data that support either expectant management or the need to intervene and facilitate birth (Blackburn, 2013; Gabbe et al., 2012). Fetal surveillance measures include fetal movement counting, nonstress testing, biophysical profile (BPP), or the modified BPP (Oyelese & Vintzileos, 2011).

Significant debate is found in the professional and lay literature regarding management of pregnancy after 40 weeks' gestation, with various opinions about the value and type of antepartum surveillance, the pros and cons of spontaneous labor versus induction of labor, and the decision about if and when to intervene. This is clearly a multifaceted issue, and any discussion with a pregnant woman should include the findings of current well-designed studies, local provider practice patterns and outcomes, along with the woman's cultural perspective and personal preferences. Current evidence suggests that induction of labor at or after 41 weeks' gestation is not associated with an increase in cesarean section compared to expectant management. This finding is reassuring to health-care providers desiring to minimize the risk of poor neonatal outcomes and to maximize the probability of a vaginal birth. Labor induction at 41 weeks' gestation or beyond may improve perinatal outcome slightly, but if fetal and maternal status are reassuring, either induction or expectant management is a reasonable choice (Gabbe et al., 2012; Gülmezoglu, Crowther, & Middleton, 2012).

The decision to continue expectant management with close monitoring or to schedule an immediate induction is one that is medically determined in collaboration with or referral to a physician colleague, depending on the practice model and setting.

Polyhydramnios

Polyhydramnios, greater than normal amniotic fluid, has been defined as an amniotic fluid volume of >2100 mL or 2.1 L. However, more recent definitions are correlated to the advent of LVP and AFI measurements and include an AFI of ≥25 cm at any gestational age, although some researchers suggest a ≥20 cm cutoff (Magann et al., 2010), or a single measurement of any LVP >8 cm. The overall incidence of polyhydramnios is 1–3% and, as in the case of oligohydramnios, the earlier it develops, the

longer it persists, and the larger the quantity, the greater the perinatal morbidity and mortality. Polyhydramnios can develop gradually or rapidly, with or without a causation identified, and benignly run its course or be associated with poor maternal and/or fetal outcomes.

The most common cause of polyhydramnios is labeled idiopathic in 60% of cases with as much as a 40–50% spontaneous resolution of cases discovered in the second trimester with good outcomes (Hill, Breckle, Thomas & Fries, 1987). Polyhydramnios, however, is also found to be associated with significant fetal and maternal conditions. Congenital anomalies, primarily those of gastrointestinal, cardiac, and neural tube defects, aneuploidy, preterm birth, multiple gestation, macrosomia, fetal intolerance of labor, meconium-stained fluid, emergency cesarean sections, cord pH <7, low 5-minute Apgar scores, and increased NICU admissions all are fetal conditions or outcomes found in conjunction with polyhydramnios. Maternal conditions associated with polyhydramnios are poorly controlled type I or II diabetes and fetal–maternal hemorrhage, in addition to the idiopathic etiology. Placental abruption and postpartum hemorrhage are serious maternal outcomes that can result from polyhydramnios due to uterine overdistension (Magann et al., 2010).

Fetal and maternal causes of polyhydramnios

Fetal
Gastrointestinal disorders: duodenal atresia, gastroschisis, diaphragmatic hernia
Central nervous system abnormalities: anencephaly, other neural tube defects
Cystic hygromas
Nonimmune hydrops
Genetic syndromes: Beckwith–Wiedemann syndrome
Congenital infections: toxoplasmosis, rubella, cytomegalovirus (CMV), herpes simplex, parvovirus B19
Placental abnormalities
Twin gestation

Maternal
Idiopathic
Poorly controlled diabetes mellitus
Maternal–fetal hemorrhage

Assessment and management

Screening, detection, and collaborative management and/or referral are the focus of primary care management for a woman with suspected polyhydramnios. Assessment measures are similar to those employed with suspected oligohydramnios. Accurate pregnancy dating and serial assessment of fundal height are essential to detecting polyhydramnios. The woman's medical and family history for the presence of diabetes and the results of any screening tests for gestational diabetes (GDM) should be reviewed. A repeat GDM screen can be considered if sudden onset polyhydramnios occurs with high-normal prior testing results. Serial Doppler blood flow studies are typically obtained for a pregnancy confirmed to have polyhydramnios. Fetal surveillance measures depend on the etiology of polyhydramnios but include various schedules of NSTs, BPP or modified BPP, and fetal movement counting.

Treatment may include administration of a prostaglandin synthetase inhibitor, such as indomethacin, administered to decrease production of fetal urine, increase fluid reabsorption by the fetal lungs, and increase the amount of intermembranous fluid movement from the fetus to the mother (Blackburn, 2013). Amniotic fluid volume has been noted to decrease within 24 hours of the administration. Prostaglandin synthetase inhibitors as a long-term treatment option are limited due to serious maternal and fetal side effects noted with exposure, particularly if given after 32 weeks' gestation (Gabbe et al., 2012).

Reduction of fluid by serial amniocentesis reductions may be done in women with severe polyhydramnios. This is an effective method of removing from 1 to 5 L of amniotic fluid; however, it must be repeated since the amniotic fluid is regenerated in the body every 48–72 hours. The most common risks to this procedure are rupture of membranes, premature labor, and placental abruption if the fluid is decompressed too rapidly. This management strategy is typically reserved for women suffering from acute cardiopulmonary decompensation due to the polyhydramnios (Gabbe et al., 2012).

The decision to continue expectant management with close monitoring or to schedule an immediate induction is one that is medically determined in collaboration with or referral to a physician colleague, depending on the practice model and setting.

Fetal growth disorders

Determination of growth disorders

Historically, the terms small for gestational age (SGA) and IUGR have been used interchangeably in the professional literature. This practice evolved because, prior to the advent of diagnostic fetal ultrasound assessment, research into fetal growth and development was based solely on neonatal outcomes. Earlier twentieth century observers noted that two parameters were associated with better or worse newborn outcomes, gestational age, and birth weight, with the distinction not yet clear in

how they differed. By the 1960s, newborn birth weight ranges had become standardized, providing an initial frame of reference for weight relative to outcome. These weight classifications are

- extremely low birth weight (ELBW <1000 g)
- very low birth weight (VLBW <1500 g)
- low birth weight (LBW <2500 g)
- macrosomia (>4000 g).

With advancements in the field of neonatology, it was ascertained that a newborn's weight relative to gestational age increased the ability to correctly ascertain a probability of perinatal and neonatal morbidity and mortality. Population-based reference ranges of birth weight relative to gestational age norms were developed, adding significantly to providers' ability to assess risks and to determine management strategies. The classifications are

- very small for gestational age (VSGA less than the third percentile)
- SGA less than the tenth percentile
- appropriate for gestational age (AGA tenth to the ninetieth percentile)
- large for gestational age (LGA greater than the ninetieth percentile) (Fig. 20.4).

While this methodology brought great improvement in the ability to further separate out those infants at greater risk for poor outcomes, it still did not take into account differences inherent to an individual neonate's anthropometric measurements. Therefore, a newborn could fit by weight in the AGA category but be IUGR by characteristics, while an SGA infant by weight could be simply constitutionally small, resulting in false negatives and false positives. In fact, 70% of newborns in the SGA category are normally developed, small newborns who are not at risk for adverse outcome. To address this flaw, the ponderal index was developed, defined as the ratio of birth weight to length (crown to heel). Ponderal index percentiles were derived using North American, subsequently Australian, and later, European populations (Landmann, Reiss, Misselwitz, & Gortner, 2006). This classification was the first methodology that more closely correlated with actual perinatal morbidity and outcomes (Gabbe et al., 2012; Walther & Ramaekers, 1982; Weiner & Robinson, 1989).

Coinciding with the advancements in treatment options available to neonatologists, the field of ultrasound technology was growing in its ability to analyze fetal growth patterns prior to birth. A new avenue of research opened, focused on identification of *in utero* patterns of abnormal growth, while exploring modalities to assess fetal well-being and to improve outcomes by

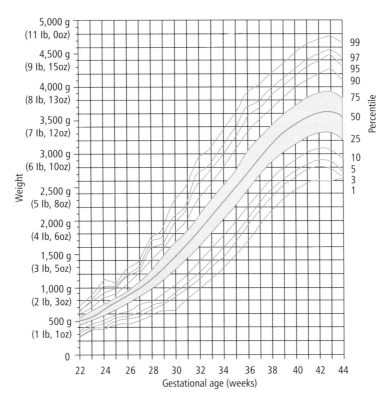

Figure 20.4.   Fetal weight percentiles throughout gestation. Source: Peleg, D., Kennedy, C.M., & Hunter, S.K. (1998). Intrauterine growth restriction: Identification and management. *American Family Physician, 58*(2), 453–460.

antenatal intervention. Concern arose as studies began to show that some neonates diagnosed with IUGR *in utero* were being incorrectly identified, leading to unnecessary intervention and iatrogenic prematurity, adding both cost and morbidity as a result of the false positive IUGR identification.

Recent research has identified yet another improvement in the ability to correctly identify fetal growth and classification of birth weight, a customized growth potential. This model assesses an individual growth potential calculated for each baby in each pregnancy, applying this new standard to fetal weight as well as birth weight. The model takes into account, or is customized, for fetal gender in addition to maternal characteristics of height, weight, parity, and ethnic origin. The optimal birth weight that is calculated is then projected backward for all gestational ages, thus avoiding the standard of preterm neonatal weights, which are skewed by the pathology of many preterm neonates. Research validates that the use of this methodology results in more correct identification of fetuses and newborns previously categorized as SGA by population referencing, as normal size by customized growth potential calculations and not at risk. Additionally, this calculation identifies a substantial number of fetuses greater than the tenth percentile that are actually IUGR and at risk (Figueras & Gardosi, 2011).

For the purposes of this discussion, IUGR will refer to those neonates identified as growth restricted and SGA will refer to those neonates constitutionally small but not growth restricted.

Studies have noted a stronger association of abnormal Doppler studies, fetal intolerance of labor, need for cesarean section, NICU admissions, stillbirths, and neonatal deaths with those infants identified as having true SGA by the customized growth potential model (Gardosi & Francis, 2009). Evidence is mounting that validates this approach in identifying the truly growth-restricted fetus, with the anticipation that growth potential curves will become the standard tool utilized for antenatal identification of a fetus at risk.

Intrauterine growth restriction

IUGR, also known as FGR, is defined as "a fetus that fails to reach his potential growth" (American College of Obstetricians and Gynecologists (ACOG), 2000) or as "the failure of a fetus to achieve its genetic growth potential in utero" (Blackburn, 2013, p. 417). While the various classifications previously discussed focus primarily on establishing neonatal risk status by birth weight, the focus of IUGR is on the impact of the antenatal environment on fetal development, one variable of which is birth weight. IUGR is the second highest cause of perinatal mortality, after prematurity. The IUGR neonate is generally in the SGA category, although not always as was previously described, with those in the VSGA category (less than the third percentile) having a significant association with IUGR. The negative effects of IUGR are well documented: increased perinatal and neonatal morbidity, stillbirth, neonatal mortality, in addition to the delayed effects of CP and adult-onset diseases. IUGR affects 8% of pregnancies. It is associated with 52% of stillbirths and 10% of all perinatal mortality, with 72% of unexplained fetal deaths occurring in those below the tenth percentile of growth (Mandruzzato et al., 2008; Rocha, Bittar, & Zugaib, 2010; Stanojevic, 2008).

The causes of IUGR are multifactorial and can be synergistic. Maternal, placental, and/or fetal factors, in addition to maternal disease, and/or environmental factors are each possible contributors to the development of IUGR. It is detected by a growth pattern found to be slowing on serial ultrasounds. Two types of IUGR are described in the literature: symmetric IUGR, associated with 25% of IUGR, and the more common asymmetric IUGR, accounting for 75% of IUGR.

Symmetric IUGR is due to an early alteration in the process of normal cell division that results in the creation of a smaller number and size of cells, commonly caused by genetic, infectious, or teratogenic insults. It can be apparent even in early second-trimester ultrasounds, with uniform diminishment of fetal organs, length, and weight, resulting in an overall proportionately smaller newborn. Symmetric IUGR is usually caused by chromosomal or congenital anomalies (<10%), infections (<10%) such as CMV and rubella, or exposure to other teratogens, such as smoking, alcohol, cocaine, narcotics, or therapeutic drugs, such as phenytoin or valproate, used in the treatment of seizure disorders (Gabbe et al., 2012). Because the insult has occurred during the period of hyperplasia, it is less amenable to improvement by antenatal interventions. Management decisions are informed by weighing the risk of prematurity against the risk of an adverse *in utero* environment.

Asymmetric IUGR, on the other hand, is usually the result of uteroplacental insufficiency, which causes chronic fetal hypoxemia and malnutrition *in utero*. In this case, the insult occurs during the phase of hypertrophy, causing the fetal cell size to be smaller but normal in number. With this growth pattern, the abdomen and lower body experience a delay with relative sparing of head growth. Asymmetric IUGR is associated with maternal hypertensive disorders, including preeclampsia, malnutrition (with protein and glucose restriction having greater impact than caloric restriction), diabetes,

and other diseases, such as renal disease, affecting vascularity, abnormal placentation, such as circumvallate placenta or placenta previa, multiple gestation, autoimmune disorders, such as systemic lupus erythematosis, and hemoglobinopathies, such as sickle cell anemia. Antenatal interventions, focused on nutrition, hydration, and improvement of uteroplacental blood flow, have shown promise in the ability to impact IUGR progression and perinatal outcome, in addition to strategies aimed at determining optimal timing of delivery.

Assessment and management

Screening, detection, and collaborative management and/or referral are the focus of primary care management for a woman with suspected IUGR.

Precise documentation of gestational age is essential to detecting and diagnosing IUGR. Screening should include identification of those at risk for the development of IUGR (Table 20.1).

The clinical hallmark of IUGR is a fundal height measurement of size less than dates of more than 3 cm in women with certain pregnancy dating. Diagnosis of IUGR is typically done by consecutive ultrasound measurements performed at least 2 weeks apart.

If not previously involved in the screening process, the health-care provider should include his/her collaborative physician in a plan for ongoing management once IUGR has been identified by ultrasound. Due to the variety of practice agreements, locale settings, and distance to facilities with the ability to provide appropriate follow-up, the health-care provider may continue involvement in the provision of prenatal primary care in conjunction with the collaborative physician. However, the woman may need to be referred to a facility equipped to handle the antenatal, perinatal, and neonatal requirements of the pregnancy.

If screening ultrasound for dating has been performed and EDB confirmed, a targeted ultrasound should be scheduled to obtain an anatomy scan and AFV. This will assist in determining if fetal anomalies or signs of aneuploidy are the cause of the IUGR, with the provision of genetic counseling and testing made available (Gabbe et al., 2012). There is no single protocol on optimal methods and timing of fetal surveillance measures for women with a growth-restricted fetus. Care strategies should be individualized in each situation and modified as indicated. Serial fetal growth ultrasounds are commonly performed at 3–4 weeks apart to assess the fetal growth curve (Figueras & Gardosi, 2011). Measurements of the biparietal diameter (BPD), head circumference (HC)/abdominal circumference (AC) ratio, fetal weight, and AFV should be included. The fetal AC provides the best single measurement to screen for poor growth (Gabbe

Table 20.1   Risk Factors for Development of IUGR

Risk Factors for Development of IUGR	
Maternal prepregnancy conditions	• Hypertensive disorders • Diabetes • Renal disease • Collagen vascular disease • Autoimmune disorders • Thrombophilias • Some hemoglobinopathies • Severe anemia • Prepregnancy BMI <20 or ≥30
Present pregnancy conditions	• Multiple gestation • Inadequate weight gain, particularly if associated with low protein intake • Placental abnormalities identified on ultrasound (circumvallate placenta, placenta accreta, single umbilical artery, partial placental infarction, hemangioma, placental abruption, and placenta previa) • Relative hypoglycemia or a "flat response" on a 3-hour glucose tolerance test, reflecting reduced glucose supply to the placenta • Unexplained abnormal biochemical markers on genetic screening
Prior maternity and family history	• Prior history of IUGR infant • Family or personal history of infant with chromosomal abnormalities, congenital malformations, or genetic syndromes
Maternal teratogenic exposures	• Smoking • Substance use • Environmental exposures
Maternal exposure to infection (especially during the first trimester)	• CMV • Rubella • Toxoplasmosis • Herpes simplex • Syphilis

Sources: Figueras and Gardosi (2011), Gabbe et al. (2012).

et al., 2012). Serial arterial Doppler flow studies of the umbilical artery are performed weekly or biweekly to assess for the presence of fetal acidemia. Good evidence exists that demonstrates Doppler flow studies improve perinatal outcomes and reduce perinatal deaths (Figueras & Gardosi, 2011). Serial nonstress tests (NSTs) performed weekly, possibly biweekly, depending on the risk status of the fetus, also provide evidence of fetal acid–base status. The BPP or the modified BPP provides a highly sensitive reflection of chronic hypoxia and is considered an important component of assessment of the fetal status. An estimate of AFV by itself is poorly correlated with fetal acidemia; however, a declining AFI in the presence of IUGR is an indicator of worsening uteroplacental function and warrants a complete BPP, umbilical artery Doppler flow studies, and/or a period of prolonged monitoring (Gabbe et al., 2012). Daily maternal evaluation of fetal movement is an appropriate adjunct to antepartum fetal surveillance.

The decision to continue expectant management with close monitoring or to schedule an immediate induction is one that is medically determined in collaboration with or referral to a physician colleague, depending on the practice model and setting.

Macrosomia

Historically, macrosomia was defined as a birth weight of greater than 5000 g (11 lb). More recently, as studies have evaluated birth weights in relation to a higher risk of perinatal complications, the definition of macrosomia has been modified. It has now been variously defined as a newborn weight of greater than 4000 g (8 lb 13 oz) to 4500 g (9 lb 14 oz), with the latter definition more commonly used. An alternative descriptor of macrosomia is the classification of birth weight relative to gestational age, which defines LGA as birth weight above the ninetieth percentile.

Further differentiation of this definition has been initiated due to the association of diabetes to the development of macrosomia. Because the fetal abdominal diameter (AD) of a diabetic mother tends to be larger relative to the BPD than does the fetal AD of a nondiabetic mother, the risk of vaginal birth complicated by shoulder dystocia in a diabetic mother is increased significantly (Jazayeri, Heffron, Phillips, & Spellacy, 1999). Thus, there is a trend in current literature to consider macrosomia to be greater than 4500 g in a nondiabetic mother, but greater than 4000 g in a diabetic mother, due to the increased risk of shoulder dystocia in a diabetic mother with a fetus of lower weight (Gabbe et al., 2012).

Risk factors for the development of fetal macrosomia

Diabetes (all types, including gestational)
Abnormal 1-hour glucose screen with a normal 3-hour glucose tolerance test
Birth of an infant >4000 g
Maternal prepregnant obesity
Excessive prenatal weight gain
Prolonged pregnancy
Fetal male gender
High paternal birth weight

Assessment and management

While the identification of risk factors is clear, correct antenatal identification of a macrosomic fetus is much more difficult and the various assessment methods available have demonstrated a high rate of inaccuracy. A change in fundal height growth pattern with a measurement >3 cm than expected for gestation, particularly if performed serially by the same examiner, is an initial indicator of possible macrosomia. This gross assessment of fetal size is fraught with inherent variation—multiple provider measurements, changes in fetal station, presentation, or position, maternal obesity, or personal bias. Interestingly, a woman's own perception of fetal size has been found to have as good a correlation to actual birth weight as fetal weight estimation by Leopold's maneuvers and/or sonographic estimated fetal weight (EFW) determination (Ashrafganjooei, Naderi, Eshrati, & Babapoor, 2010; Torloni et al., 2008).

Ultrasound assessment of fetal weight once appeared to hold great promise to detect macrosomia, but evaluation of its ability to prognosticate has found disappointing results. Research confirms that in order to correctly identify that a fetal weight is >4000 g at a 90% confidence level, the ultrasound EFW estimate must be >4600 g. (Gabbe et al., 2012). Others have documented that ultrasound estimation of fetal weight ≥4800 g is associated with only about a 50% chance that the infant's birth weight will be ≥4500 g. An increasing reliance on sonographic determination of an EFW in late pregnancy is due to the increasing reluctance of physicians and midwives to attempt vaginal birth if there is concern about perinatal risks associated with macrosomia. The inaccuracy of ultrasound EFW estimation is resulting in an increased number of early induction of labor or scheduled cesarean sections, only to discover at birth a number of infants <4500 g and not at high risk of shoulder dystocia (Chauhan et al., 2005).

The woman's medical, obstetrical, and family history, as well as current physical examination findings for risk factors associated with the development of macrosomia, should be reviewed. The woman's medical and family history for the presence of diabetes and the results of any screening tests for GDM should be reviewed. A repeat screen can be considered if sudden onset of polyhydramnios occurs with high-normal prior testing results or significant family history.

If an ultrasound for dating has been performed and EDB confirmed, a targeted ultrasound should be scheduled to obtain an anatomy scan and an EFW. This will assist in determining if fetal anomalies or signs of aneuploidy are the cause of the size greater than dates, with the provision of genetic counseling and testing made

available (Gabbe et al., 2012). Serial fetal growth ultrasounds at 3- to 4-week intervals to assess the fetal growth curve should be initiated. Measurements of the BPD, HC/AC ratio, fetal weight, and AFV should be included. A fetal AC of >35 cm identifies more than 90% of macrosomic infants (Jazayeri, et al., 1999).

A prudent course to follow clinically is the combination of EFW estimation clinically with Leopold's maneuvers by an experienced examiner, sonographic findings, and the woman's own perception of fetal size when having any discussion regarding mode of delivery. A question frequently posed by women in this situation is about the possible benefit of labor induction prior to the due date in the hope of avoiding continued fetal growth, an even bigger baby, and concern that waiting longer will increase her risk of needing a cesarean section to give birth. On the contrary, in nondiabetic mothers, studies have documented an increased rate of cesarean section in those women induced prior to 41 weeks, particularly with a low Bishop's score of <6. Awaiting the onset of labor or delaying induction until >41 weeks' gestation is associated with a lower rate of cesarean section, even in the presence of macrosomia (Bailey & Kalu, 2009). Further, when counseling the pregnant client, the healthcare provider should convey the information that obstetrical professional organizations and research findings have not published any definitive statements or recommendations about the advisability of having a scheduled cesarean section for a macrosomic fetus. It is imperative that any conversation is approached with that understanding, and the woman's perspective on management and personal perception of risk is taken into account as an important consideration (Gabbe et al., 2012).

The decision to offer an early elective induction or a scheduled cesarean section for macrosomia is one that is medically determined in collaboration with or referral to a physician colleague, depending on the practice model and setting.

Summary

A careful and systematic approach to the examination of the pregnant abdomen will reveal concerns related to amniotic fluid and fetal growth disturbances to the astute health-care provider. Additionally, listening to the woman as she relates her interval history and her sense of fetal growth and activity will provide clues that assist in the clinical determination of a normal variation versus a condition requiring further testing and treatment. Amniotic fluid and fetal growth disturbances are important contributors to perinatal morbidity and mortality with short-term implications regarding timing and route of birth and long-term implications regarding the health

Case study

Anna, a 22-year-old G1 P0 woman, presents for her routine 30-week prenatal care visit.

CHART REVIEW: She began care at 6 weeks' gestation by LMP and confirmed by ultrasound. Her history is noncontributory. Her prenatal course has been normal except for an episode of minor bleeding at 7 weeks that resolved spontaneously and an episode of preterm contractions at 27 weeks that was managed with oral hydration.

SUBJECTIVE: Anna reports no further contractions, good fetal activity, and no other problems. She says she is eating well and getting enough rest.

OBJECTIVE: Maternal blood pressure is 114/76; FHRs are 150.

Fundal height is 26 cm. The fetus palpates in breech position.

Urinalysis is negative for glucose and protein. Her prior fundal height measurement at 27 weeks' gestation was 25 cm.

ASSESSMENT: Intrauterine pregnancy at 30 weeks by dates and 26 weeks by size; size smaller than dates.

PLAN: Anna was sent for an ultrasound evaluation later that same day in order to determine if that fundal height measurement reflected a problem or if this was within normal limits. Upon ultrasound, the fetus was found to be at less than the tenth percentile in weight; therefore, further ultrasound studies were undertaken. EFW below the tenth percentile defines the fetus as SGA. Diagnosis of IUGR is typically done in consecutive ultrasound measurements performed at least 2 weeks apart. However, ultrasound techniques evaluating various biophysical parameters are useful surveillance tools in determining fetal well-being and timing of intervention, particularly for preterm pregnancies. In this case, fetal blood flow abnormalities were noted upon spectral Doppler blood flow velocimetry; specifically, the middle cerebral artery and the umbilical artery were markedly below normal values. Anna was admitted to the labor and birth unit for administration of steroids for fetal lung maturation. Fetal monitoring, Doppler studies, and BPP testing were done. On day 5 of her hospital stay, the fetal condition deteriorated as noted by BPP testing, so birth was accomplished by cesarean section and a live male infant weighing 690 g (1 lb 8 oz) with an Apgar of 8 at 1 minute was born. Anna had a normal recovery from her surgery; the baby was transferred to the NICU and required ventilation for 4 days. After that, he had a positive progression in his growth and development and was discharged home close to his estimated due date.

and well-being of the mother and baby. Establishment of an accurate due date early in the pregnancy, along with the use of customized fetal growth charts, will assist the health-care provider in identifying the fetus at risk.

Resources for women and their families

Amniotic fluid disorders: http://pregnancy.about.com/cs/amnioticfluid/a/aaafv.htm
Low birth weight: http://www.marchofdimes.com/baby/premature_lowbirthweight.html

Resources for health-care providers

Amniotic fluid disorders: http://www.marchofdimes.com/professionals/25079_4536.asp; http://www.womenshealthsection.com/content/obs/obs027.php3
Fetal macrosomia: http://www.aafp.org/afp/2001/0701/p169.html
Intrauterine fetal growth restriction: http://www.fetal.com/IUGR/treatment.html

References

American College of Obstetricians and Gynecologists (ACOG). (2000). Practice bulletin #12: Intrauterine growth restriction: Clinical management guidelines for obstetrician-gynecologists. Chicago, IL: Author.

Ashrafganjooei, T., Naderi, T., Eshrati, B., & Babapoor, N. (2010). Accuracy of ultrasound, clinical and maternal estimates of birth weight in term women. EMHJ, 16(3).

Bailey, C., & Kalu, E. (2009). Fetal macrosomia in non-diabetic mothers: Antenatal diagnosis and delivery outcome. Journal of Obstetrics & Gynecology, 29(3), 206–208.

Blackburn, S. T. (2013). Maternal, fetal, and neonatal physiology: A clinical perspective (4th ed.). Maryland Heights, MO: Elsevier Saunders.

Brace, R. A., & Wolf, E. J. (1989). Normal amniotic fluid volume changes throughout pregnancy. American Journal of Obstetrics & Gynecology, 161, 382–388.

Casey, B. M., McIntire, D. D., Bloom, S. L., Lucas, M. J., Santos, R., Twickler, D. M., . . . Leveno, K. J. (2000). Pregnancy outcomes after antepartum diagnosis of oligohydramnios at or beyond 34 weeks' gestation. American Journal of Obstetrics & Gynecology, 182(4), 909–912. doi:10.1067/mob.2000.104231

Chauhan, S. P., Grobman, W. A., Gherman, R. A., Chauhan, V. B., Chang, G., Magann, E. F., & Hendrix, N. W. (2005). Suspicion and treatment of the macrosomic fetus: A review. American Journal of Obstetrics & Gynecology, 193(2), 332–346.

Crowley, P., O'Herlihy, C., & Boylan, P. (1984). The value of ultrasound measurement of amniotic fluid volume in management of prolonged pregnancies. *British Journal of Obstetrics and Gynaecology, 91,* 444–448.

Figueras, F., & Gardosi, J. (2011). Intrauterine growth restriction: New concepts in antenatal surveillance, diagnosis, and management. *American Journal of Obstetrics & Gynecology, 204*(4), 288–300. doi:10.1016/j.ajog.2010.08.055

Gabbe, S. G., Niebyl, J. R., Simpson, J. L., Landon, M. B., Galan, H. L., Jauniaux, E. R., & Driscoll, D. A. (Eds.). (2012). *Obstetrics: Normal and problem pregnancies* (6th ed.). Philadelphia: Elsevier Saunders.

Gardosi, J., & Francis, A. (2009). Adverse pregnancy outcome and association with small for gestational age birthweight by customized and population-based percentiles. *American Journal of Obstetrics & Gynecology, 201,* 28.e1–28.e8. doi:10.1016/j.ajog.2009.04.034

Gülmezoglu, A. M., Crowther, C. A., & Middleton, P. (2012). Induction of labour for improving birth outcomes for women at or beyond term. *Cochrane Database of Systematic Reviews,* (4), CD004945, 2006.

Hill, L. M., Breckle, R., Thomas, M. L., & Fries, J. K. (1987). Polyhydramnios: Ultrasonically detected prevalence and neonatal outcome. *Obstetrics and Gynecology, 69*(1), 21–25. PMID:3540761.

Jazayeri, A., Heffron, J. A., Phillips, R., & Spellacy, W. N. (1999). Macrosomia prediction using ultrasound fetal abdominal circumference of 35 centimeters or more. *Obstetrics & Gynecology, 93*(4), 523–526.

Landmann, E., Reiss, I., Misselwitz, B., & Gortner, L. (2006). Ponderal index for discrimination between symmetric and asymmetric growth restriction: Percentiles for neonates from 30 weeks to 43 weeks of gestation. *The Journal of Maternal-Fetal and Neonatal Medicine, 19*(3), 157–160. doi:10.1080/14767050600624786

Magann, E. F., Chauhan, S. P., Barrilleaux, P. S., Whitworth, N. S., & Martin, J. N. (2000). Amniotic fluid index and single deepest pocket: Weak indicators of abnormal fluid volumes. *Obstetrics & Gynecology, 96*(5), 737–740.

Magann, E. F., Doherty, D. A., Lutgendorf, M. A., Magann, M. I., Chauhan, S. P., & Morrison, J. C. (2010). Peripartum outcomes of high-risk pregnancies complicated by oligo- and polyhydramnios: A prospective longitudinal study. *The Journal of Obstetrics and Gynaecology Research, 36*(2), 268–277. doi:10.1111/j.1447-0756.2009.01145.x

Mandruzzato, G., Antsaklis, A., Botet, F. A., Chervenak, F., Figueras, F., Grunebaum, A., . . . Stanojevic, M. (2008). Recommendations and guidelines for perinatal practice—Intrauterine restriction (IUGR). *Journal of Perinatal Medicine, 36,* 277–281. doi:10.1515/jpm.2008.050

Oyelese, Y., & Vintzileos, A. M. (2011). The uses and limitations of the fetal biophysical profile. *Clinical Perinatology, 38,* 47–64.

Petrozella, L., Dasche, J., McIntire, D., & Leveno, K. (2011). Clinical significance of borderline amniotic fluid index and oligohydramnios in preterm pregnancy. *American College of Obstetrics and Gynecology, 117*(2), 338–342.

Rocha, C. O., Bittar, R. E., & Zugaib, M. (2010). Neonatal outcomes of late-preterm birth associated or not with intrauterine growth restriction. *Obstetrics and Gynecology International, V 2010,* 231842. doi:10.1155/2010/231842; 1-5.

Shanks, A., Tuuli, M., Schaecher, C., Odibo, A. O., & Rampersad, R. (2011). Assessing the optimal definition of oligohydramnios associated with adverse neonatal outcomes. *Journal of Ultrasound Medicine, 30*(3), 303–307.

Stanojevic, M. (2008). Recommendations and guidelines for perinatal practice—Intrauterine restriction (IUGR). *Journal of Perinatal Medicine, 36,* 277–281. doi:10.1515/jpm.2008.050

Torloni, M. R., Sass, N., Sato, J. L., Renzi, A. C. P., Fukuyama, M., & Lucca, P. R. D. (2008). Clinical formulas, mother's opinion and ultrasound in predicting birth weight. *Sao Paulo Medical Journal, 126*(3), 145–149.

Walther, F. J., & Ramaekers, L. H. J. (1982). The ponderal index as a measure of the nutritional status at birth and its relation to some aspects of neonatal morbidity. *Journal of Perinatal Medicine, 10,* 42–47.

Weiner, C. P., & Robinson, D. (1989). Sonographic diagnosis of intrauterine growth retardation using the postnatal ponderal index and the crown-heel length as standards of diagnosis. *American Journal of Perinatology, 6*(4), 380–383.

21

Preterm labor and birth

Robin G. Jordan

*To prevent an early birth, wear a lodestone (magnet)
to hold the child within . . .*
(Cotton Mather, 1710, in Wertz & Wertz, 1989)

Relevant terms

Age of viability—occurs sometime between 22 and 26
weeks, usually when fetal weight is greater than 500 g

Cervical cerclage—a minor surgical procedure to stitch the
cervix closed to prevent preterm birth (PTB) in women
with short cervix or cervical insufficiency

Cervical insufficiency—a condition where the cervix is
weakened and tends to begin to dilate early in pregnancy

Late preterm birth rate—the number of births between 34
and 36 weeks gestation

Moderate preterm birth rate—the number of births
between 32 and 33 weeks

Preterm birth rate—the number of births delivered at less
than 37 completed weeks of gestation per 100 total
births

Stress—demands that tax or exceed the adaptive capacity
of an organism and that result in psychological and
biological changes.

Very preterm birth rate—the number of births <32 weeks
gestation

Introduction

Preterm birth (PTB) is defined as a birth after 20 weeks
of gestation and prior to 37 completed weeks' gestation
and is a major cause of neonatal morbidity and mortality worldwide. Gestational age is never rounded up, so
36 weeks and 6 days of gestation is 36 weeks and not 37

weeks of gestation (Institute of Medicine (IOM), 2007).
The prevalence of PTB has increased significantly over
the last several decades with the prevalence approximately 12–13% of all births in the United States. This is
one of the highest PTB rates in the developed world. A
2012 World Health Organization report on PTB ranks
the United States 130 out of 184 in the world for its rate
of PTB (World Health Organization (WHO), 2012).

This increase is occurring despite advancing knowledge of the mechanisms of PTB and medical interventions to reduce the incidence of PTB. Part of this increase
is due to the higher rates of multiple births following the
use of assisted reproduction techniques. Another contributing factor is thought to be the rise in elective induction and operative delivery (Bannerman, Fuchs, Young,
& Hoffman, 2011; Martin, Kirmeyer, Osterman, & Shepherd, 2009) (Fig. 21.1). Prevention of elective early births
for the convenience of the mother or the provider are
the subject of a March of Dimes education campaign and
government initiatives (March of Dimes (MOD), 2012a).
Approximately one-third of all PTBs are intentional or
medically indicated births, and two-thirds are spontaneous births (Hodgson & Lockwood, 2010).

Accurate measures of gestational age are needed to
operationalize the current definition of prematurity.
Most often, prenatal ultrasound is used to provide assessment of gestational age with first trimester measures
of fetal size the most accurate, when there is little individual variation in fetal growth (IOM, 2007). Individual
variations in fetal growth increase as gestation increases.
Use of the date of the last menstrual period (LMP) may
also be used in women with a history of normal cycles
however biological variations in menstrual cycles,

Prenatal and Postnatal Care: A Woman-Centered Approach, First Edition. Edited by Robin G. Jordan, Janet L. Engstrom, Julie A. Marfell,
and Cindy L. Farley.

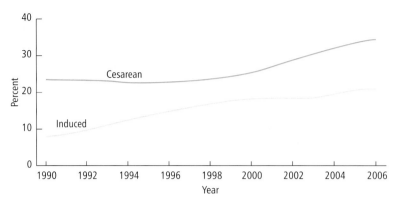

Figure 21.1. Induction of labor and cesarean birth rate among late preterm birth: United States 1990–2006. From U.S. CDC/NCHS National Vital Statistics System.

ovulation, and implantation can contribute to reduced accuracy in gestational age calculation for some women.

Fetal growth and maturation occur along the continuum throughout pregnancy; therefore, categorizations of PTBs based on gestational age are useful in evaluating risks for infant morbidity and mortality.

- **Late preterm**: 34–36 weeks' gestation
- **Moderate preterm**: 32–33 weeks' gestation
- **Very preterm**: 28–31 weeks' gestation
- **Extremely preterm**: <28 weeks' gestation

Social and racial disparities

Disparities in PTB rates by socioeconomic status are well documented in the United States (IOM, 2007). Social factors such as education, employment, housing, and access to quality health care may be implicated in these disparities, not just as individual risk factors but also as environmental and social contextual factors among the population as a whole. For example, socioeconomically disadvantaged women experience more stressful life events and more chronic stress than women who are not socioeconomically disadvantaged (Lu, Lu, & Schetter, 2005). Poverty is one of the strongest predictors of PTB, and socioeconomic disparities in PTB often are closely paralleled by racial and ethnic categories.

The risk of PTB for black women is approximately 1.5 times the rate seen in white women (Center for Disease Control and Prevention (CDC), 2012). The reasons for these disparities remain poorly understood. Possible explanations include differences in access to care and quality of care, social determinants of health including the effects of psychosocial stress, poverty, and living environment; prevalence of comorbidities; and genetic factors (MacDorman, 2011). Even when adjusting for socioeconomic factors, an increased risk of PTB persists among black women (Collins, David, Simon, & Prachand, 2007). Genetic contributions to the etiology of PTB may

include specific factors that increase the risk of preterm premature rupture of membranes and spontaneous PTB among black women. The PTB rate rises at a younger age and at a greater rate for black women compared with white women (Anum, Springel, Shriver, & Strauss, 2008). This differential rise with increasing age may be explained by the weathering hypothesis (Love, David, Rankin, & Collins, 2010). Weathering is the process of deteriorating health with cumulative disadvantage and suggests that the health effects of social inequality compound as individuals age. This increasing gap in health status between black and white women during the reproductive years can negatively impact reproductive outcomes.

Physiology of preterm birth

PTB is not a single entity but an outcome of a multifactorial and complex process that is poorly understood. For PTB to occur, the cervix undergoes considerable change including collagen remodeling and altered cellular content, allowing effacement and dilatation. Despite various contributing factors to PTB, clinical pathways leading to these changes can be categorized by four overall processes (Buhimschi, Schatz, Krikun, Buhimschi, & Lockwood, 2010; Goldenberg, Culhane, Iams, & Romero, 2008):

1. *Premature activation of the maternal or fetal hypothalamus pituitary adrenal axis*—This activation leads to a release of prostaglandins and stimulation of placental estrogens related to myometrium activation and labor.
2. *Pathological uterine distention*—Both multifetal gestation of polyhydramnios and risk factors for PTB of the myometrium increase the formation of gap junctions and oxytocin receptors, which contribute to contractions.
3. *Inflammation*—Both systemic infection and ascending genital tract infections are linked to spontaneous

PTB. The inflammatory response increases prosta-glandin production, which can break down the extra-cellular matrix of the fetal membranes and cervix.

4. *Decidual hemorrhage*—This causes the release of thrombin, which promotes inflammation-associated PTB mechanisms.

Table 21.1   Potential Neonatal Problems of Prematurity

Respiratory distress syndrome
Intraventricular hemorrhage
Feeding difficulties
Hypoglycemia
Difficulty maintaining body temperature
Necrotizing enterocolitis
Apnea
Patent ductus arteriosis
Infection
Jaundice
Hypothermia
Neurobehavioral problems
Retinopathy of prematurity
Anemia
Cerebral palsy
Cognitive and developmental deficits

Complications related to prematurity

Premature infants are at greater risk for short- and long-term complications, including disabilities and impediments in growth and mental development (Table 21.1). With each additional week of prematurity, a newborn is at greater risk for having medical complications.

Risk factors for preterm birth

There are multiple risk factors for PTB (Table 21.2), although 50% of women who give birth prematurely have no clearly delineated risk factor. While most women with a prior history of PTB will go on to have a term birth, a prior PTB is the strongest risk factor for a repeat PTB.

The most significant risk factor is a prior history of a PTB, accounting for up to 42% of PTBs (McManemy, Cooke, Amon, & Leet, 2007). Women who have a low prepregnancy body mass index (BMI) have a decreased blood volume and therefore less uterine blood flow. They also consume less vitamins and minerals, which has been associated with decreased blood flow and increased risk for maternal infection.

Chronic stress has been associated with PTB. Research implicates several of the stress response hormones (e.g., corticotropin releasing hormone, corticotropin, and cortisol) as likely contributors to PTB as well as term birth. While a solid physiological foundation may exist for the

Table 21.2   Risk Factors for Preterm Birth

Prior obstetric/gynecological history
Prior history of PTB
Cervical surgery(cone biopsy, LEEP, etc.)
Multiple cervical dilation and uterine evacuations
Uterine anomalies

Maternal demographics
<17, >35 years of age
Less education (<12 years)
Single marital status
Lower socioeconomic status
Short interpregnancy interval (<18 months)

Nutritional status/physical activity
Prepregnancy BMI <19 or weight <50 kg
Poor nutritional status
Long working hours (>80 h/week)
Hard physical labor (including standing >8 hours)

Current pregnancy characteristics
Assisted reproductive techniques
Multiple gestation
Fetal disease
Congenital malformations
Poly- or oligohydramnios
Maternal medical condition (e.g., hypertension, diabetes, thyroid disease, and asthma)
Maternal abdominal surgery
Psychological factors (e.g., stress, depression)
Substance abuse
  Smoking
  Heavy alcohol consumption
  Cocaine
  Heroin
Infection
  Bacterial vaginosis
  Trichomoniasis
  Chlamydia
  Gonorrhea
  Syphilis
  Urinary tract infection (e.g., asymptomatic bacteria, pyelonephritis)
  Severe viral infection
  Intrauterine infections
Short cervical length between 14 and 28 weeks
Positive fetal fibronectin between 22 and 34 weeks

Adapted from: Goldenberg and McClure (2010).

relationship between stress and PTB, stress has been a difficult concept to uniformly measure and treat (Chen, Grobman, Gollan, & Borders, 2011; Hobel, Goldstein, & Barrett, 2008). Research results are quite consistent in pointing to anxiety as a possible risk factor for PTB (Schetter & Tanner, 2012). Anxiety regarding the pregnancy itself is fairly consistent in predicting gestational age at birth or PTB (IOM, 2007). Psychological counseling during pregnancy (Mamell & PPPB Study Group, 2001), prenatal care in a group setting (Ickovics et al., 2007), and relaxation techniques such as yoga (Narendran, Nagarathna, Narendran, Gunasheela, & Nagendra, 2005) have demonstrated effective in reducing PTB in select groups; however, more study is needed before universal recommendations can be made.

Occupational physical activity and exposures have been implicated in the etiology of PTB. A recent study of the work patterns in over 62,000 childbearing aged women found a dose response relationship between occupational lifting and PTB with the strongest associations for extremely and very PTB (Runge et al., 2013). Several meta-analyses reported a small adverse effect of shift work on the risk of PTB (Bonzini, Coggon, & Palmer, 2007; Mozurkewich, Luke, Avni, & Wolf, 2000). The underlying theories include sleep deprivation or disrupted circadian rhythms resulting in neuroendocrine changes that affect the timing of parturition, although direct links have not yet been established.

Predicting preterm birth

Risk factor based prenatal scoring systems have been developed in an effort to identify women who are most likely going to experience PTB; however, they have failed to achieve that goal. More than half of women who go on to give birth prematurely will not be identified by risk scoring (low sensitivity), and the majority of women who screen positive go on to give birth at term (low predictive value) (Mercer et al., 1996).

Fetal fibronectin (fFN) testing

A method to predict PTB is the use of the biochemical marker fFN. This is a glycoprotein found in high concentrations in the amniotic fluid and in the interface between the decidua and the trophoblast cells, and is thought to play a role in implantation and maintenance of the attachment between the maternal deciduas and fetal chorion during pregnancy. Although normally found in the cervical and vaginal secretions before 16–20 weeks' gestation, its presence in the cervicovaginal secretion after 20 weeks' gestation is abnormal, except as a marker of the imminent onset of labor at term. A positive test is modestly useful in predicting the risk of a PTB occurring within 1–2 weeks (Kiefer & Vintzileous, 2008). A negative fFN result is more strongly predictive of a woman who will *not* have a PTB (>90% negative predictive value). To illustrate, in women with a negative fFN, 99% will be undelivered in 7 days, 95% undelivered at 14 days, and 90% undelivered at 21 days (Peaceman et al., 1997). Using fFN to confirm risk status can help decrease

unnecessary and potentially harmful interventions. The fFN test must be done prior to vaginal ultrasonography and a digital cervical exam. A swab is placed in the posterior fornix of the vagina and rotated for 10 seconds. The test may not be reliable if the woman had a vaginal examination, sexual intercourse, endovaginal ultrasonography, or cervical examination within the previous 24 hours, or if she presents with vaginal bleeding.

Cervical length measurement

Transvaginal ultrasound to determine cervical length measurement is an effective screening tool to predict PTB. Decreasing cervical length is associated with increased risk of PTB. A short cervical length <25 mm in the early or late second trimester has been associated with a marked increased risk of PTB (Domin, Smith, & Terplan, 2010). Cervical length measurement has false positives and has no utility in preventing PTB. Expert groups have not formed a consensus on routine cervical length screening for all pregnant women (The American College of Obstetricians and Gynecologists, 2012; Parry, Sumhan, Elovitz, & Iams, 2012). Many advocate its use for women at risk for PTB such as those with a history of prior cervical procedures like conization and loop electrosurgical excision procedure (LEEP) and for women with uterine abnormalities (Campbell, 2011; Parry et al., 2012; Rafael, 2010). When fFN and cervical length measurement are used together, it increases the predictive power of both tests. The information gained from both of these prediction strategies may be useful in deciding whom to treat for preterm labor with corticosteroids and possibly tocolytics.

Diagnosing preterm labor

Symptoms of PTB that women may report are menstrual-like cramps or regular contractions, low backache, diarrhea, and a sensation of pelvic pressure. Specific clinical signs to make the diagnosis of preterm labor criteria include persistent uterine contractions of four every 20 minutes or eight every 60 minutes with documented cervical change or cervical effacement of at least 80% or cervical dilatation greater than 2 cm (MOD, 2012b). Women who do not meet these criteria are diagnosed with false labor. Many women with suspected preterm labor stop contracting and go on to give birth at term.

Management of women with preterm labor

Although preterm labor is one of the most common reasons for hospitalization of pregnant women, identifying women with preterm contractions who will go on to give birth preterm is an inexact process. More than half of women presenting with reports of preterm labor will go on to give birth at term (McPheeters et al., 2005). Establishment of an institutional practice protocol to evaluate women with signs and symptoms of preterm labor can provide a methodical and complete evaluation strategy that may improve diagnostic accuracy and appropriate treatment.

A thorough history should be done to evaluate symptoms, fetal well-being, and integrity of the membranes and to assess for possible underlying infection. In addition to the initial evaluation, an obstetrical ultrasound may be done to look for maternal and fetal anatomical anomalies and amniotic fluid volume. The decision to admit, discharge, or transport the woman should be made within 4 hours of evaluation (MODb, 2012b).

Initial preterm labor evaluation

Review of prenatal record for historical risk factors

- Verification of pregnancy dates and methods of dating used
- Prior history of urinary tract infection (UTI), bacterial vaginosis (BV), trichomoniasis, gonorrhea, or chlamydia

Subjective history and evaluation of symptoms

- Presence of leaking fluid
- Onset, duration, characteristics, contraction pattern
- Precipitating events, if any

Vital signs
Evaluation of uterine contractions
Examination of the uterus for signs of abruption, tone, fetal size, fetal position
Evaluation of fetal heart rate tracingSpeculum examination for

- Cervical dilation and effacement
- Presence of bleeding
- Status of fetal membranes
- FFN swab obtained in women 35 weeks gestation or less
- Rectovaginal swab for GBS
- Chlamydia and gonorrhea cultures on women with risk factors

Vaginal ultrasound in women 35 weeks gestation or less

- Cervical length
- Placental location

Urine culture to diagnose asymptomatic bacteriuria
Drug screening in women with risk factors for illicit drug use
Digital cervical examination for dilation and effacement *after*

- Membrane status and placental location determined
- Swabs and cultures done

Adapted from: Audibert et al. (2010), Sayres (2010).

Preterm birth prevention

Prevention of PTB is the primary goal of many healthcare organizations and remains a challenge for healthcare providers. Many strategies aimed at prevention have been tried with varying degrees of success. Home uterine monitoring, bed rest, and prenatal treatment of various vaginal infections have not been proven effective in PTB prevention. Some risk factors, however, are modifiable and amenable to change. Risk factors that may predispose a woman to PTB should be identified during the first prenatal visit and risk reduction interventions implemented. PTB prevention strategies that have significant research support as effective in preventing PTB are improved weight and nutrition; reducing infection; avoiding cocaine; smoking cessation, avoiding a short (<18 months) interpregnancy interval; diagnosis and treatment of asymptomatic bacteriuria; improving sleep quality and reducing fatigue; and the use of progesterone and cerclage in women at high risk.

Nutrition

A low prepregnancy BMI is one of strongest predictors of adverse pregnancy outcomes such as PTB and fetal growth restriction. Underweight status before pregnancy nearly doubles the likelihood of delivering preterm (Bloomfield, 2011; Han, Mulla, Beyene, Liao, & McDonald, 2011). A low body mass interacts with other factors such as smoking and stress to increase risk of these outcomes. The association between maternal thinness and adverse pregnancy outcomes may be mediated more by a low plasma volume than by decreased protein or energy status. Maternal micronutrient status may partially influence plasma volume expansion in pregnancy. Therefore, improving maternal micronutrient status may reduce adverse outcomes through this mechanism.

Specific deficiencies in iron, folic acid, zinc, vitamin D, calcium, and magnesium, and imbalances in the appropriate dietary ratio of omega-3 and omega-6 fatty acids have various levels of evidence in playing a role in PTB (Dunlop, Kramer, Hogue, Menon, & Ramakrishan, 2011). Evidence exists regarding the role of adequate calcium, iron, and omega-3 fatty acids in reducing risk for PTB (Imdad & Bhutta, 2012; Mozurkewich & Klemens, 2012).

The burden of nutritional deficiencies is greater among black women compared with white women. A systematic review on the effect of prenatal supplementation on pregnancy outcomes documented a significant improvement in birth weight, but no reduction in the rate of PTB (Shah & Ohlsson, 2009). Iron deficiency during pregnancy increases the risk of PTB and low birth weight. For those women who are anemic during pregnancy, iron supplementation has been shown in some trials to reduce the risk of PTB (Christian, 2010). The role of micronutrients the contribution to PTB is complex, and precise mechanisms of action and optimal requirements are not fully known.

Nutritional interventions to reduce PTB risk

Assist all pregnant women to

- achieve an appropriate prepregnancy weight
- gain an adequate amount of pregnancy weight for BMI
- take 200–300 mg of omega-3 fatty acids daily or eat two fish meals/week
- have a healthy balanced diet
- eat three meal/day plus two snacks and not miss meals
- achieve adequate iron stores.

A multicenter trial examined the association between frequency of eating and preterm birth in more than 200 women (Siega-Riz, 2008). Women who fell short of the current Institute of Medicine guidelines for eating three meals plus two snacks daily had a 30% increase in risk of PTB compared to those with adequate nutrition. The study's author postulates that the body reacts to missed meals as a stressor, and elevated levels of stress hormones have been implicated in the events leading to a PTB. Additional research links missing meals and lack of walking increases risk of PTB in African American women (Hennessy, Volpe, Sammel, & Gennaro, 2010). Working with women to improve diet during pregnancy has the potential to make an important impact on preventing PTB.

Smoking cessation

Smoking cessation is considered one of the most important measures to reduce PTB and other complications of pregnancy. Cigarettes contain numerous compounds such as nicotine and carbon monoxide that cause uteroplacental insufficiency via vasoconstriction (Wickström, 2007). A higher proportion of women stop smoking in pregnancy during any other time in their lives (Lumley et al., 2009). One-to-one counseling using the 5-A's and the 5-R's interventions is an effective method to reduce smoking during pregnancy. Counseling should include education on the specific risk of tobacco use on maternal and fetal health. For further information on smoking cessation during pregnancy, refer to Chapter 13, "Substance Use during Pregnancy."

Interpregnancy interval

A short interpregnancy interval less than 18 months is a risk factor for PTB (Conde-Agudelo, Rosas-Bermúdez, & Kafury-Goeta, 2006). One proposed mechanism of action is maternal micronutrient depletion and insufficient time for maternal nutrient replenishment, particularly folate and iron (Getz, Anderka, Werler, & Case, 2012). Advising women to wait at least 1.5 years between pregnancies and providing reliable birth control options are appropriate interventions in reducing PTB.

Treating infections

Multiple studies have reported an association between PTB and various genitourinary tract infections including group B streptococci, *Chlamydia trachomatis*, BV, *Neisseria gonorrhoeae*, syphilis, and *Trichomonas vaginalis*. However, a causal association for most of these infections has not been proven, making treatment recommendations for PTB prevention challenging. Some areas of infection treatment do show efficacy in PTB prevention.

BV is characterized by an overgrowth of a variety of anaerobic organisms, including *Garderella vaginalis*, *Mycoplasma hominis*, *Mobiluncus* species, *Atopobium vaginae*, and an associated reduction in normal vaginal *Lactobacillus* species. Studies conclude that BV is associated with PTB; however, data supporting universal screening and treatment of BV in reducing the rate of PTB are lacking. Current recommendation is that pregnant women with symptoms should be screened and treated if positive (CDC, 2012; USPSTF, 2008).

Periodontal disease has been associated with a sevenfold increase in PTB (Boggess & Edelstein, 2006) and is considered be a potential risk factor for PTB. The theory behind this association lies in the subclinical systemic infectious process that occurs in periodontal infections. Chronic oral infection is common; it has been estimated that over 50% of the U.S. population has some degree of periodontal disease (Boggess & Edelstein, 2006). Despite this association, studies on treating periodontal infections in pregnancy and reducing PTB have been equivocal. Identification and treatment of periodontal disease prior to pregnancy or an early gestation is considered to be beneficial, especially for women at risk for PTB (Huck, Tenenbaum, & Davideau, 2011).

Asymptomatic bacteriuria has long been associated with PTB. Treatment of asymptomatic bacteriuria decreased the incidence of PTB (Smaill, 2007). Screening for asymptomatic bacteriuria with a midstream clean-catch urine culture between 12 and 16 weeks' gestation should be done for all pregnant women, and treatment initiated for those women who screen positive (USPSTF, 2008). Women at higher risk for asymptomatic bacteriuria such as women with sickle cell trait and a history of recurrent UTI should be screened more frequently.

Disturbed sleep and fatigue

Disturbed sleep appears to play a role in adverse pregnancy outcomes, including PTB (Okun et al., 2012). Poor sleep quality and occupational fatigue have been associated with preterm premature rupture of membranes and preterm labor (Newman et al., 2001). The specific pathways through which disturbed sleep and fatigue contribute to PTB are unknown. It is speculated that fatigue and poor sleep quality contribute to increased risk of PTB independently and in conjunction with other risk factors such as stress. Sleep is a modifiable behavior. Assessing women's sleep quality and habits during pregnancy and implementing behavioral interventions may be a relatively simple option to reduce the risk of PTB for some women.

Improving sleep quality and reducing fatigue

Evaluate sleep habits.
Evaluate sleep quality.
Evaluate the level of fatigue. Measures to improve sleep quality:

- Exercise regularly.
- Avoid large meals close to bedtime.
- Establish a consistent bedtime and waking time.
- Establish a regular relaxing bedtime routine.
- Associate the bed with sleep, avoid watching TV, reading, or using a computer in bed.
- Use comfortable bedding and a cooler room.
- Block out distracting noise.
- Practice relaxation techniques before bedtime.

Some women are exposed to highly demanding occupational physical activities during pregnancy that might represent a threat to the fetus and to their own health. Studies on the relation between occupational activities and PTB have yielded contradictory results. Two specific areas of activity—prolonged standing and working >40 h/week—have stronger links with risk for PTB (Mozurkewich et al., 2000; Saurel-Cubizolles et al., 2004). Currently, no guidelines exist on reducing work and standing hours as a PTB risk reduction strategy. It is common practice to limit pregnant women's work week to 40 hours and to recommend no work in the last 1–2 weeks of pregnancy to promote adequate rest prior to labor onset. It is appropriate to evaluate each woman's employment situation in the context of her total health picture to make individual recommendations.

Progesterone therapy

It is theorized that progesterone maintains uterine quiescence in the latter half of pregnancy by limiting the production of stimulatory prostaglandins and inhibiting the expression of protein genes that develop the uterine muscle ability to contract. The use of 250 mg intramuscular 17-hydroxyprogesterone caproate from weeks 16–20 through term in a singleton pregnancy reduces the incidence of PTB in women with a history of prior PTB before 37 weeks' gestation (Likis et al., 2012). Progesterone suppositories reduce the rate of PTB before 33 weeks in women with a short cervix (Hassan et al., 2011). Vaginal progesterone is recommended for women with no prior spontaneous PTB and with a cervical length of 20 mm or less at 24 weeks' gestation or earlier (The American College of Obstetricians and Gynecologists, 2012). Women qualifying for this type of care benefit from physician comanagement or referral to high risk specialists.

Cerclage

Cervical cerclage is a therapeutic option for women with documented cervical insufficiency. Women with cervical insufficiency may be asymptomatic or may present with mild symptoms such as pelvic pressure, premenstrual-like cramping or backache, and increased vaginal discharge. These symptoms have usually been present over several days or weeks. Cervical cerclage reduces the incidence of PTB in women at risk of recurrent PTB (Alfirevic, Stampalija, Roberts, & Jorgensen, 2012). The optimal timing, method, and selection criteria for cerclage remain controversial, though it is generally performed prior to 24 weeks' gestation. Women with a prior history of cervical trauma such as conization or LEEP procedures, of progressively earlier births, two or more consecutive prior second-trimester pregnancy losses, or three or more early (<34 weeks) PTBs should receive obstetrical evaluation for possible cerclage placement.

Summary

Preventing PTB remains one of the great challenges in maternity care. PTB rates continue to increase. The etiologies are complex and influenced by genetics and environmental factors. During the course of prenatal care, risk factors should be identified and risk reduction interventions initiated. Women with previous PTB are at an increased risk of subsequent PTB and may be candidates for treatment with prenatal progesterone. fFN testing and vaginal ultrasonography for cervical length measurement are useful for triage and subsequent care decisions. For women in preterm labor, only prenatal corticosteroids and birth in a facility with a level III neonatal intensive care unit have been shown to improve outcomes consistently.

Case study

Brianna is a 19-year-old G2P1 African American woman here for her first prenatal visit at 8 weeks' gestation in a planned pregnancy. She had her first child, Caleb, 2 years ago. Caleb was born at 33 weeks' gestation in another state and spent 10 weeks in the hospital before coming home. She states he is now a busy toddler and is followed in a health clinic on a regular basis. Brianna lives with her 21-year-old boyfriend from high school and he is active in parenting Caleb. A complete history was done. Of significance to her prior history of PTB are the following: Her boyfriend and his friends are smokers and smoke in the house; Brianna often skips meals as she works full time; she drinks 3–5 cups of coffee daily; and she and her family eat fast food four to five times per week on average. Brianna does not smoke, drink alcohol, or use drugs. She indicates she and her boyfriend have a very happy relationship and are pleased to be pregnant. Her family support consists of her sisters and her mother who live nearby. Brianna states she thinks she gained about 14–15 lb with her son. Her labor started over a day with low back cramps that she tried to ignore until they started to come more often. Her boyfriend insisted that she go to the hospital, and on arrival, she was found to have contractions every 5 minutes and was dilated "a little." She denied any bleeding or pain other than the back cramps. She said she was given medication to make her labor stop that made her shake, and she got another "shot for the baby's lungs to hurry up." She was in the hospital 2 days and her contractions started up again, and she had the baby after 9–10 hours of labor.

A complete physical exam and cervical cultures were done. Her dental health appeared excellent and her physical findings were within normal, with the uterus enlarged to approximately 8 weeks' size, and her cervix was long, thick, and closed. Her prepregnant BMI is 18.6 and BP 130/74.

In addition to routine pregnancy topics, PTB was discussed. Brianna was advised that since she had one PTB, she was at higher risk to have another one, though she was reassured that a repeat PTB was not "a given." She was further reassured that her physical exam findings were within normal. Brianna expressed great motivation to reduce her risk in any way possible. She was advised to avoid cigarette smoke in her house for her and Caleb's health. Brianna was advised that nutritional status and weight gain during pregnancy have a significant impact on the risk of PTB. She was instructed in the importance of not missing meals, eating nutritious food every few hours during the day, and gaining between 28 and 40 lb. Brianna thought that was a lot of weight and expressed concern about "getting fat." This was discussed at length with the rationale for adequate weight, information about weight gain and fetal needs, and reassurance that she would most likely lose the weight quickly after childbirth. She stated she would "do it if it would help me be able to take the baby home right away." Pregnancy nutritional needs and food sources were reviewed, meal planning was discussed, and a dietary consult initiated. Brianna felt she could make changes in her diet to improve nutrition and weight gain during this pregnancy. She stated she was going to share this information with her mother who would make sure she "did what she was supposed to do."

The use of 250 mg intramuscular 17-hydroxyprogesterone caproate from weeks 16–20 through term was discussed with rationale. Brianna readily agreed to this therapy. The use of transvaginal cervical length measurement in the second trimester was also discussed as a means to detect early cervical change. The midwife indicated she was going to consult with the obstetrician in the office to create a tailored plan schedule for Brianna.

In addition to routine laboratory testing, a screen for BV was done and was negative. A clean-catch midstream urine was done to detect asymptomatic bacteriuria, and cervical cultures were obtained to assess for infection.

A prescription for a prenatal supplement containing 27 mg iron, 800 mcg folic acid, and 300 mg n-3s was given. Brianna was informed about the significance of these specific nutrients in possibly reducing risk of PTB.

Normal pregnancy issues such as fetal growth and development, common discomforts, and starting a 30-minute five times per week walking program were discussed. Brianna was advised that in subsequent visits, the warning signs of preterm labor would be reviewed. An appointment was made with the dietician for 1 week with a revisit with the midwife in 2 weeks. A request was submitted for her prior prenatal and birth records.

Resources for women and health-care providers

Center for Disease Control and Prevention—State-specific data and many consumer and professional resources: http://www.cdc.gov/features/premature birth/

March of Dimes—A global organization with the mission to prevent premature births: http://www.marchofdimes.com/

References

Alfirevic, Z., Stampalija, T., Roberts, D., & Jorgensen, A. L. (2012). Cervical stitch (cerclage) for preventing preterm birth in singleton pregnancy. *Cochrane Database of Systematic Reviews*, (4), CD008991.

Anum, E. A., Springel, E. H., Shriver, M. D., & Strauss, J. F., 3rd. (2008). Genetic contributions to disparities in preterm birth. *Pediatric Research*, 65(1), 1–9.

Audibert, F., Fortin, S., Delvin, E., Djemli, A., Brunet, S., Dubé, J., & Fraser, W. D. (2010). Contingent use of fetal fibronectin testing and cervical length measurement in women with preterm labour. *Journal of Obstetrics and Gynaecology Canada*, 32(4), 307–312.

Bannerman, C. G., Fuchs, K. M., Young, O. M., & Hoffman, M. K. (2011). Non-spontaneous late preterm birth: Etiology and outcomes. *American Journal of Obstetrics and Gynecology*, 205, 456.e1–456.e6.

Bloomfield, F. H. (2011). How is maternal nutrition related to preterm birth? *Annual Review of Nutrition*, 31, 235–261.

Boggess, K. A., & Edelstein, B. L. (2006). Oral health in women during preconception and pregnancy: Implications for birth outcomes and infant oral health. *Maternal and Child Health Journal*, 10(5 Suppl.), S169–S174.

Bonzini, M., Coggon, D., Palmer, K. T. (2007). Risk of prematurity, low birthweight and pre-eclampsia in relation to working hours and physical activities: A systematic review. *Occupational & Environmental Medicine*, 64, 228–243.

Buhimschi, C. S., Schatz, F., Krikun, G., Buhimschi, I. A., & Lockwood, C. J. (2010). Novel insights into molecular mechanisms of abruption-induced preterm birth. *Expert Reviews in Molecular Medicine*, 12, e35.

Campbell, S. (2011). Universal cervical-length screening and vaginal progesterone prevents early preterm births, reduces neonatal morbidity and is cost saving: Doing nothing is no longer an option. *Ultrasound in Obstetrics and Gynecology*, 38(1), 1–9. doi:10.1002/uog.9073

Center for Disease Control and Prevention (CDC). (2012). Preterm birth. Retrieved from http://www.cdc.gov/reproductivehealth/maternalinfanthealth/PretermBirth.htm

Chen, M. J., Grobman, W. A., Gollan, J. K., & Borders, A. E. (2011). The use of psychological stress scales in preterm birth research. *American Journal of Obstetrics and Gynecology*, 205(5), 402–434. Retrieved from http://www.AJOG.org

Christian, P. (2010). Micronutrients, birth weight, and survival. *Annual Review of Nutrition*, 30, 83–104.

Collins, J. W., Jr., David, R. J., Simon, D. M., & Prachand, N. G. (2007). Preterm birth among African American and white women with a lifelong residence in high-income Chicago neighborhoods: An exploratory study. *Ethnicity and Disease*, 17(1), 113–117.

Conde-Agudelo, A., Rosas-Bermúdez, A., & Kafury-Goeta, A. C. (2006). Birth spacing and risk of adverse perinatal outcomes: A meta-analysis. *JAMA: The Journal of the American Medical Association*, 295(15), 1809–1823.

Domin, C. M., Smith, E., & Terplan, M. (2010). Transvaginal ultrasonographic measurement of cervical length as a predictor of preterm birth: A Systematic review with meta-analysis. *Ultrasound Quarterly*, (26).

Dunlop, A. L., Kramer, M. R., Hogue, C. J., Menon, R., & Ramakrishan, U. (2011). Racial disparities in preterm birth: An overview of the potential role of nutrient deficiencies: Nutrient deficiencies and racial disparities in preterm birth. *Acta Obstetricia et Gynecologica Scandinavica*, 90(12), 1332–1341.

Getz, K. D., Anderka, M. T., Werler, M. M., & Case, A. P. (2012). Short interpregnancy interval and gastroschisis risk in the national birth defects prevention study. *Birth Defects Research. Part A, Clinical and Molecular Teratology*, 94, 714–720.

Goldenberg, R. L., Culhane, J. F., Iams, J. D., & Romero, R. (2008). Epidemiology and causes of preterm birth. *Lancet*, 371(9606), 75–84.

Goldenberg, R. L., & McClure, E. M. (2010). The epidemiology of preterm birth. In V. Berghella (Ed.), *Preterm birth: Prevention and management* (pp. 22–38). Oxford, UK: Wiley-Blackwell.

Han, Z., Mulla, S., Beyene, J., Liao, G., & McDonald, S. (2011). Maternal underweight and the risk of preterm birth and low birth weight: A systematic review and meta-analyses. *International Journal of Epidemiology*, 40(1), 65–101.

Hassan, S., Romero, R., Vidyadhari, D., Fusey, S., Baxter, J., et al. (2011). Vaginal progesterone reduces the rate of preterm birth in women with a sonographic short cervix: A multicenter randomized, double blind placebo controlled trial. *Ultrasound in Obstetrics & Gynecology*, 38, 18–21.

Hennessy, M. D., Volpe, S. L., Sammel, M. D., & Gennaro, S. (2010). Skipping meals and less walking among African Americans diagnosed with preterm labor. *Journal of Nursing Scholarship*, 42(2), 147–155. doi:10.1111/j.1547-5069.2010.01345.x

Hobel, C. J., Goldstein, A., & Barrett, E. S. (2008). Psychological stress and pregnancy outcome. *Clinical Obstetrics and Gynecology*, 51, 333–339.

Hodgson, E. J., & Lockwood, C. J. (2010). Preterm birth: A complex disease. In V. Berghella (Ed.), *Preterm birth: Prevention and management* (pp. 8–16). New York: Wiley-Blackwell.

Huck, O., Tenenbaum, H., & Davideau, J. L. (2011). Relationship between periodontal diseases and preterm birth: Recent epidemiological and biological data. *Journal of Pregnancy*, 2011, Article ID 164654. doi:10.1155/2011/164654; 8 pages.

Ickovics, J. R., Kershaw, T. S., Westdahl, C., Magriples, U., Massey, Z., Reynolds, H., & Rising, S. S. (2007). Group prenatal care and perinatal outcomes: A randomized controlled trial. *Obstetrics and Gynecology*, 110(2 Pt 1), 330–339.

Imdad, A., & Bhutta, Z. A. (2012). Effects of calcium supplementation during pregnancy on maternal, fetal and birth outcomes. *Paediatric & Perinatal Epidemiology*, 26, 138–152.

Institute of Medicine (IOM). (2007). Committee on Understanding Premature Birth and Assuring Healthy Outcomes. Behavioral and psychosocial contributors to preterm birth. In R. E. Behrman & A. S. Butler (Eds.), *Preterm birth: Causes, consequences, and prevention*. Washington, DC: National Academies Press (US). Retrieved from http://www.ncbi.nlm.nih.gov/books/NBK11362/

Kiefer, D., & Vintzileous, A. (2008). The utility of fetal fibronectin in the prediction and prevention of preterm birth. *Reviews in Obstetrics and Gynecology*, 1(3), 106–112.

Likis, F. E. L., et al. (2012). Progestogens for preterm birth prevention a systematic review and meta-analysis. *Obstetrics and Gynecology*, 120(4), 987–907.

Love, C., David, R. J., Rankin, K. M., & Collins, J. W., Jr. (2010). Exploring weathering: Effects of lifelong economic environment and maternal age on low birth weight, small for gestational age, and preterm birth in African-American and white women. *American Journal of Epidemiology, 172*(2), 127–134.

Lu, Q., Lu, C., & Schetter, C. D. (2005). Learning from success and failure in psychosocial intervention: An evaluation of low birth weight prevention trials. *Journal of Health Psychology, 10*(2), 185–195.

Lumley, J., Chamberlain, C., Dowswell, T., Oliver, S., Oakley, L., & Watson, L. (2009). Interventions for promoting smoking cessation during pregnancy. *Cochrane Database of Systematic Reviews,* (3), Art. No.: CD001055, doi:10.1002/14651858.CD001055.pub3

MacDorman, M. F. (2011). Race and ethnic disparities in fetal mortality, preterm birth, and infant mortality in the United States: An overview. *Seminars in Perinatology, 35,* 200e8.

Mamelle, N. J., & PPPB Study Group. (2001). Psychological prevention of early pre-term birth: A reliable benefit. *Biology of the Neonate, 79*(3–4), 268–273.

March of Dimes (MOD). (2012a). Healthy Babies are Worth the Wait. Retrieved from http://www.marchofdimes.com/professionals/medicalresources_pprc.html

March of Dimes (MOD). (2012b). Preventing prematurity. Retrieved from https://www.prematurityprevention.org/portal/server.pt

Martin, J. A., Kirmeyer, S., Osterman, M., & Shepherd, R. A. (2009). Born a bit too early: Recent trends in late preterm births. NCHS data brief, no 24. Hyattsville, MD: National Center for Health Statistics.

McManemy, J., Cooke, E., Amon, E., & Leet, T. (2007). Recurrence risk for preterm delivery. *American Journal of Obstetrics and Gynecology, 196*(6), 576–577.

McPheeters, M. L., Miller, W. C., Hartmann, K. E., Savitz, D. A., Kaufman, J. S., Garrett, J. M., & Thorp, J. M. (2005). The epidemiology of threatened preterm labor: A prospective cohort study. *American Journal of Obstetrics and Gynecology, 192*(4), 1325.

Mercer, B. M., Goldenberg, R. L., Das, A., et al. (1996). The preterm prediction study: A clinical risk assessment system. *American Journal of Obstetrics and Gynecology, 174,* 1885–1893.

Mozurkewich, E., & Klemens, C. (2012). Omega-3 fatty acids and pregnancy: Current implications for practice. *Current Opinion In Obstetrics & Gynecology, 24*(2), 72–77.

Mozurkewich, E. L., Luke, B., Avni, M., & Wolf, F. M. (2000). Working conditions and adverse pregnancy outcome: A meta-analysis. *Obstetrics and Gynecology, 95,* 623–635.

Narendran, S., Nagarathna, R., Narendran, V., Gunasheela, S., & Nagendra, H. R. J. (2005). Efficacy of yoga on pregnancy outcome. *Journal of Alternative and Complementary Medicine (New York, N.Y.), 11*(2), 237–244.

Newman, R. B., et al. (2001). Occupational fatigue and preterm premature rupture of membranes. *American Journal of Obstetrics and Gynecology, 184*(3), 438–444.

Okun, M. L., Luther, J. F., Wisniewski, S. R., Sit, D., Prairie, B. A., & Wisner, K. L. (2012). Disturbed sleep, a novel risk factor for preterm birth? *Journal of Women's Health, 21*(1), 54–60.

Parry, S., Sumhan, H., Elovitz, M., & Iams, J. (2012). Universal maternal cervical length screening during the second trimester: Pros and cons of a strategy to identify women at risk of spontaneous preterm delivery. *American Journal of Obstetrics and Gynecology, 207*(2), 101–106.

Peaceman, A. M., et al. (1997). fetal fibronectin as a predictor of preterm birth in patients with symptoms: A multicenter trial. *American Journal of Obstetrics and Gynecology, 177,* 13–18.

Rafael, T. J. (2010). Short cervical length. In V. Berghella (Ed.), *Preterm birth: Prevention and management* (pp. 130–148). New York: Wiley-Blackwell.

Runge, S. B., Pedersen, J. K., Svendsen, S. W., Juhl, M., Bonde, J. P., & Andersen, A. M. N. (2013). Occupational lifting of heavy loads and preterm birth: A study within the Danish National Birth Cohort. *Occupational and Environmental Medicine.*

Saurel-Cubizolles, M. J., Zeitlin, J., Lelong, N., Papiernik, E., Di Renzo, G. C., & Bréart, G.; for the Europop Group. (2004). Employment, working conditions, and preterm birth: Results from the Europop case-control survey. *Journal of Epidemiology and Community Health, 58,* 395–401.

Sayres, W. G., Jr. (2010). Preterm labor. *American Family Physician, 81*(4), 477.

Schetter, C. D., & Tanner, L. (2012). Anxiety, depression and stress in pregnancy: Implications for mothers, children, research, and practice. *Current Opinion in Psychiatry, 25*(2), 141–148.

Shah, P. S., & Ohlsson, A. (2009). Effect of multimicronutrient supplementation on pregnancy outcomes: A meta-analysis. *Canadian Medical Association Journal, 180*(12), e99–e108.

Siega-Riz, A. (2008). Outcomes of maternal weight gain. *American Journal of Epidemiology, 153,* 647–652.

Smaill, F. (2007). Asymtomatic bacteriuria in pregnancy. *Best Practice & Research Clinical Obstetrics and Gynaecology, 21*(3), 439–450.

The American College of Obstetricians and Gynecologists. (2012). Practice bulletin No. 130: Prediction and prevention of preterm birth. *Obstetrics and Gynecology, 120*(4), 964–973.

U.S. Preventive Services Task Force (USPSTF). *Screening for Asymptomatic Bacteriuria in Adults: U.S. Preventive Services Task Force Reaffirmation Recommendation Statement.* AHRQ Publication No. 08-05120-EF-1, July 2008. Retrieved from http://www.uspreventiveservicestaskforce.org/uspstf08/asymptbact/asbactrs.htm

Wertz, R. W., & Wertz, D. C. (1989). *Lying-in: A history of childbirth in America.* New Haven, CT: Yale University Press.

Wickström, R. (2007). Effects of nicotine during pregnancy: Human and experimental evidence. *Current Neuropharmacology, 5*(3), 213.

World Health Organization (WHO). (2012). Born too soon: The global action report on preterm birth. Retrieved from http://www.who.int/pmnch/media/news/2012/201204_borntoosoon-report.pdf

22

Hypertensive disorders in pregnancy

Robin G. Jordan

Relevant terms

Arteriovenous (AV) nicking—a small artery is seen
crossing a small vein on fundoscopic examination; this is
due to compression of the vein with bulging on either
side of the crossing

Disseminated intravascular coagulation (DIC)—
pathological activation of the clotting system that leads
to clot formation in small vessels throughout the body
and can cause multiple organ failure

Papilledema—optic disk swelling that is caused by
increased intracranial pressure

Proteinuria—excess protein in the urine and a diagnostic
marker for hypertensive disorders in pregnancy

Thrombocytopenia—a decrease in platelets that can be
defined as platelet count less than 150,000/mL or platelet
count below the 2.5th percentile for pregnant women
(116,000/µL).

Introduction

Approximately 5–10% of pregnant women have hypertension (Cunningham et al., 2010), making it the most common medical disorder encountered during pregnancy. Most women with hypertensive disorders in pregnancy have mild disease and have outcomes similar to women with normotensive pregnancies. However, pregnant women experiencing more severe disease are at risk for substantial maternal and perinatal morbidities. Hypertensive disorders are responsible for 11% of

maternal deaths in the United States in 2006–2007 (Centers for Disease Control and Prevention, 2012). It is essential for health-care providers to make timely and accurate diagnoses to prevent adverse maternal and perinatal outcomes associated with pregnancy hypertensive disorders. Preeclampsia is the most common hypertensive disorder in pregnancy and is a focus of this chapter.

Classification of hypertensive disorders of pregnancy

The National High Blood Pressure Education Program Working Group (NHBPEP) has set forth a commonly accepted classification of hypertensive disorders in pregnancy (Table 22.1).

Chronic hypertension

When hypertension is first identified in a pregnant woman prior to 20 weeks' gestation, or a pregnant woman is on antihypertensive medication prior to conception, she is diagnosed as having chronic hypertension. Approximately 5% of pregnancies are complicated by chronic hypertension (ACOG, 2012). Most women with chronic hypertension have good pregnancy outcomes; however, risk for pregnancy complications is increased (Table 22.2). The risk of adverse outcome is related to the severity of the hypertension.

Chronic hypertension is further classified into mild and severe categories with BP ≥140/90 (mild), and BP

Prenatal and Postnatal Care: A Woman-Centered Approach, First Edition. Edited by Robin G. Jordan, Janet L. Engstrom, Julie A. Marfell,
and Cindy L. Farley.
© 2014 John Wiley & Sons, Inc. Published 2014 by John Wiley & Sons, Inc.

Table 22.1   Classification and Definitions of Hypertensive Disorders of Pregnancy

Chronic hypertension	BP ≥140/90 mmHg before pregnancy or before the twentieth week of gestation; persists for >12 weeks postpartum
Gestational hypertension	Systolic BP ≥140 or diastolic BP ≥90 on at least two occasions at least 6 hours apart for the first time during pregnancy after 20 weeks' gestation; no proteinuria; BP returns to normal at 12 weeks postpartum; final diagnosis made postpartum
Preeclampsia–eclampsia syndrome	A pregnancy-specific disorder that is a multisystem disease characterized by hypertension ≥140/90 mmHg on ≥2 occasions at least 6 hours apart, and proteinuria ≥300 mg in a 24-hour urine collection after 20 weeks' gestation The convulsive form of preeclampsia is eclampsia.
Preeclampsia superimposed on chronic hypertension	New onset proteinuria ≥300 mg in a 24-hour urine in hypertensive women after 20 weeks' gestation or a sudden increase in proteinuria or blood pressure or platelet count <100,000 μL in women with hypertension and proteinuria before 20 weeks' gestation

Table 22.2   Maternal–Fetal Potential Problems due to Chronic Hypertension

Condition	Estimated incidence or risk*
Preeclampsia	17–25%
Fetal growth restriction	10–20%
Placental abruption	1.6%
Preterm birth	Fivefold increase
Cesarean birth	Threefold increase
Postpartum hemorrhage	Onefold increase
Small for gestational age (SGA)	–
Cardiovascular accident (CVA)	–
Stillbirth	–

*ACOG Practice Bulletin 119 (2012), Sibai (2002).

≥180/110 (severe). Pharmaceutical treatment of mild chronic hypertension is not recommended during pregnancy as it does not benefit the fetus or prevent the development of preeclampsia (Abalos, Duley, Steyn, & Henderson-Smart, 2007), and may even cause excessive lowering of blood pressure (BP) and decreased placental perfusion. Most women with chronic hypertension have a decrease in BP during the second trimester of pregnancy with the rise to prepregnancy values during the third trimester, a pattern similar to that observed in normotensive women.

Women presenting with severe chronic hypertension in pregnancy typically have a history of known hypertension and have been on antihypertensive medications in the past. These women are at risk for increased maternal and fetal morbidities and should have perinatal or obstetrical interprofessional care (Table 22.2).

Women with chronic hypertension are at significant risk for developing superimposed preeclampsia. Another 7–20% of women with chronic hypertension have worsening of hypertension during pregnancy without the development of preeclampsia (Abalos et al., 2007).

Gestational hypertension

This condition previously known as "pregnancy-induced hypertension" is one that describes hypertension reaching 140/90 mmHg for the first time after 20 weeks' gestation but without proteinuria or other features of preeclampsia. BP returns to normal by 12 weeks postpartum. Often, the diagnosis of gestational hypertension is a provisional one and women are eventually diagnosed with preeclampsia, chronic hypertension, or transient hypertension in pregnancy. Of women who initially present with apparent gestational hypertension, approximately 50% are eventually diagnosed with preeclampsia, especially in those women who exhibit gestational hypertension prior to 30 weeks' gestation (Sibai, 2003).

Preeclampsia–eclampsia

Preeclampsia is a multisystem disorder that occurs only during pregnancy and the postpartum period and is typically characterized by hypertension and proteinuria. Preeclampsia is covered in more detail in the next section. Eclampsia is the onset of grand mal seizures that cannot be attributed to other causes in a woman with preeclampsia. Adequate prenatal care has significantly reduced the rate of eclampsia in the United States and is a rare condition. Approximately 0.1% of women with preeclampsia develop eclampsia (Sibai, 2004). Eclamptic seizures typically are preceded by increasingly severe preeclampsia manifestations; however, they may also occur unexpectedly in women with mild BP elevations and minimal or no proteinuria. Since this condition reflects central nervous system (CNS) compromise, typical symptoms include headaches, visual changes, and restlessness. Headache is the most common prodromal symptom (Shamil, Edmonds, Tong, Samarasekera, & Whitehead, 2011); however, it is very difficult to predict who will go on to develop eclampsia. Although part of the formal diagnostic criteria for preeclampsia, it has been demonstrated that up to 20% of women who go on to develop eclampsia do not have significant proteinuria prior to their seizure (Sibai, 1990a). Eclampsia can result in fetal distress, placental abruption, and fetal or maternal death. Eclamptic seizures can occur during the prenatal, intrapartum, and postpartum time frames, with the majority occurring prenatally.

Preeclampsia superimposed on chronic hypertension

Superimposed preeclampsia is the major adverse pregnancy condition associated with chronic hypertension. The diagnostic criteria include the presence of hypertension prior to 20 weeks' gestation and one or more of the following:

- new onset proteinuria ≥300 mg/24 h after 20 weeks' gestation
- thrombocytopenia after 20 weeks' gestation
- worsening of hypertension as pregnancy progresses

This complication can be challenging to diagnose, especially if women present late to prenatal care and demonstrate hypertension at the first visit. The acute onset of proteinuria or a sudden increase over baseline hypertension should prompt a laboratory and physical evaluation for superimposed preeclampsia. Large, randomized, placebo-controlled trials have shown no significant reduction in the risk of preeclampsia associated with the use of low-dose aspirin, calcium supplementation, or antioxidant supplementation (Seely & Ecker, 2011). Women with chronic hypertension and superimposed preeclampsia have additional perinatal risks and should be referred to specialized perinatal care.

Preeclampsia

Preeclampsia is a multisystem disorder typically manifesting as hypertension and proteinuria during pregnancy affecting between 2% and 8% of pregnant women in the United States. The majority of cases occur near term at 36 weeks' gestation and beyond. While giving birth is the only cure for preeclampsia, preeclampsia can also develop during the intrapartum and postpartum periods, though this is less common. Hypertension and proteinuria are the cardinal clinical manifestations used to diagnose and estimate the severity of the disease. Preeclampsia is typically categorized as mild or severe (Table 22.3) and is considered a progressive disease, but is variable in severity and unpredictable. Mild preeclampsia can rapidly progress to severe disease. On the mild end of

Table 22.3 Criteria to Diagnose Mild and Severe Preeclampsia

Mild preeclampsia	Severe preeclampsia
Minimum criteria • Systolic ≥140 mmHg or • Diastolic ≥90 mmHg • On two BP readings at least 6 hours apart • Proteinuria ≥300/mg/24-hour urine or • ≥+1 on dipstick on two specimens (on two samples at least 6 hours apart) • Occurs after 20 weeks' gestation	Minimum criteria • Systolic ≥160 mmHg or • Diastolic ≥110 mmHg • On two BP readings at least 6 hours apart • Proteinuria ≥ 5 g/24-hour urine or • ≥+3 on dipstick (on two samples at least 6 hours apart) • Occurs after 20 weeks' gestation
May see • Elevated reflexes • Elevated hemoglobin due to hemoconcentration • Mild edema	May see • Epigastric pain • Visual disturbances • Headaches • Edema • Clonus • Diminished renal function • Thrombocytopenia • Oliguria <400 mL/24 hours

Source: ACOG Practice Bulletin No. 33 (2002/2008), National High Blood Pressure Education Program Working Group (NHBPEP) (2000).

the continuum, women may present with hypertension and proteinuria, yet feel well and report no symptoms. Women with more severe disease are often symptomatic and at risk for liver failure, renal failure, disseminated intravascular coagulation (DIC), CNS abnormalities, and significant fetal complications. Women who develop early preeclampsia with onset before 34 weeks' gestation have higher rates of adverse maternal and neonatal outcomes than women developing late-onset preeclampsia. Most cases of preeclampsia are late-onset preeclampsia, occurring during the last few weeks of pregnancy and are mild with favorable outcomes.

Pathophysiology of preeclampsia

Various theories have existed regarding the etiology and pathogenesis of preeclampsia. Preeclampsia is currently considered to be primarily a disorder of placental dysfunction that leads to a syndrome of endothelial dysfunction and vasospasm. Preeclampsia develops in stages, with the last being the clinical illness. A three-stage model of the development of preeclampsia has been proposed (Fig. 22.1) (Redman & Sargent, 2010).

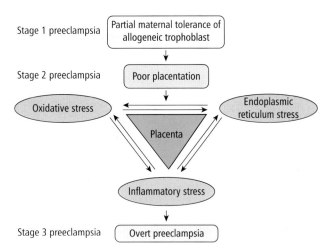

Figure 22.1. Stages of preeclampsia development. Redman & Sargent (2010).

Stage I occurs before conception with the woman developing tolerance to alloantigen in male sperm. The term, "immune priming" has been used to describe this period of time. Immunologic factors are thought to play a role in the development of preeclampsia. It is theorized that a maternal immune response to exposure to paternal antigens in sperm may contribute to alteration of placental implantation. Prior and repeated exposure to partner sperm is thought to decrease this immune response in women. It is well established that a longer exposure time to paternal sperm prior to conception reduces the risk of developing preeclampsia (Saito, Sakai, Sasaki, Nakashima, & Shiozaki, 2007). This may explain the higher incidence of preeclampsia in very young women and in those women who consistently use barrier methods of contraception (Young, Levine, & Karumanchi, 2010). Additionally, a change of partner seems to restore the risk of preeclampsia in multigravidas to that of primiparity, adding further support to the physiological foundation of immune priming prior to conception (Zhang & Patel, 2007).

Stage II is the development of the disease and begins early in the first trimester with placental development, well before maternal signs and symptoms of preeclampsia develop. It has been hypothesized that the abnormal placental development is caused by altered immune responses, genetic factors, or early hypoxic episodes during cell differentiation. At the beginning of a normal pregnancy, the placenta should cause remodeling of the uterine spiral arteries, which allows for the increased blood and oxygen flow required in pregnancy. This remodeling is done as the cytotrophoblast cells of the developing placenta invade the endothelium and the maternal spiral arteries, and change them into large capacity blood vessels with low resistance for maternal fetal exchange. In women with preeclampsia, this remodeling of the spiral arteries is incomplete. There is incomplete penetration into the maternal myometrium resulting in narrow vessels and hypoperfusion.

Stage II is the manifestation of preeclampsia and can be detected by clinical screening. Endothelial cell damage produces several factors that constrict and obstruct vascular beds. This damage, in conjunction with an exaggerated maternal inflammatory response, cause maternal vasospasm, increased capillary permeability, and clotting dysfunction, which negatively affects target organs such as the brain, liver, kidney, and placenta.

It is also theorized that the inflammatory signal processing seen in preeclampsia may depend on fetal genes, whereas the maternal response to the inflammatory signals depends on maternal genes, suggesting that both maternal and fetal genes are involved (Sibai, Dekker, & Kupferminc, 2005).

Insulin resistance is more common in women who develop preeclampsia; however, it is uncertain as to whether the insulin resistance is a component of the pathophysiology or whether it is a preexisting risk factor (Parretti et al., 2006). Pregnant women with gestational diabetes are at higher risk of developing preeclampsia.

Potential problems due to preeclampsia

The potential maternal and fetal problems are related to the gestational age at which preeclampsia develops and the severity of the disease. Increased vascular resistance characteristic of preeclampsia can lead to poor perfusion through the placenta, increasing the risk for potential problems related to uteroplacental insufficiency. These potential problems include

- oligohydramnios
- placental abruption
- fetal growth restriction
- nonreassuring fetal status.

Preeclampsia is one of the leading causes of preterm birth through both spontaneous onset of labor and indicated delivery.

Risk factors for developing preeclampsia

Preeclampsia is more common at the extremes of childbearing age. The increased incidence of chronic hypertension in women older than 35 years may explain the increased incidence of preeclampsia and women of this age group.

Risk factors for developing preeclampsia

Nulliparity
Multifetal gestation
Age extremes: <18 and >35
Black race
Pregestational diabetes
Obesity
Chronic hypertension
Prior history of preeclampsia
In vitro fertilization
Family history of hypertension or preeclampsia in a
  first-degree relative
New paternity partner (limited exposure to partner sperm
  and immunologic factors involved)
Preexisting renal, autoimmune disorders or cardiac disease

Diagnostic evaluation

History

The medical obstetrical history obtained early in pregnancy should be reviewed for risk factors for the development of preeclampsia. During each prenatal visit after 20 weeks' gestation, all pregnant women should be asked about the presence of specific symptoms of preeclampsia. These symptoms include visual disturbances (blurring, double vision, and spots), persistent headaches, right upper quadrant or epigastric pain, and increased edema. The presence of visual disturbances and headaches indicate potential CNS vasospasm, and right upper quadrant pain indicates liver involvement. Both symptoms are more commonly seen with increasingly severe disease. Women should be asked if there is a noticeable increase in edema especially in the face; nondependent edema is more significant in preeclampsia than dependent edema, which is common in most pregnant women in later gestation.

Blood pressure

An accurate BP reading is imperative in women with hypertensive disorders in pregnancy. The cuff size should be appropriate for the woman's size, with cuff length 1.5 times the upper arm circumference or a cuff with a bladder that encircles 80% or more of the arm. BP is best measured after a rest period of 10 minutes or more, with the pregnant woman in an upright position with cuff position at the level of her heart. The woman should not use tobacco or caffeine within 30 minutes of the measurement. Diagnostic criteria require that a repeat BP be done at least 6 hours later to verify the initial high BP measurement. This can be difficult in actual clinical practice. It is common for a repeat BP to be done at the

Table 22.4 Urine Dipstick Proteinuria Thresholds*

Results	Concentration of protein
Negative	0
1+	30–100 mg/dL
2+	100–300 mg/dL
3+	300–1000 mg/dL
4+	>1000 mg/dL

*Multistix®.

conclusion of the office visit, and a working diagnosis made from both readings until confirmation can be made with a later BP reading.

Proteinuria

Assessment of proteinuria can be done in several ways. In the office, assessment is done via dipstick urinalysis on a fresh midstream specimen. A positive dipstick urinalysis reaction (1+) usually occurs once the protein concentration reaches a threshold of 30 mg/dL. It is well established that the dipstick urinalysis method of proteinuria assessment has a high degree of false negative results, thus providing limited utility for clinical decision making. Additionally, observer error in evaluating color change on the dipstick can be problematic. The dipstick urinalysis method does offer a convenient screening test for initial detection and for following proteinuria patterns at home (see Table 22.4). The albumin:creatinine ratio is used in the office setting for a rapid evaluation of proteinuria; however, this test does not always correlate well with the 24-hour urine sample (Wikström, Wikström, Larsson, & Olovsson, 2006). The albumin:creatinine test is commonly done as a rapid screening test while awaiting results of the 24-hour urine. The 24-hour and urine is the gold standard for evaluating proteinuria and should be obtained on all women with hypertension in pregnancy or those with continued proteinuria by dipstick regardless of BP. Providing women with adequate information on the importance of obtaining a complete 24-hour sample is essential.

Edema and weight gain pattern

Observation for new-onset edema in the hands and lower extremities should be done with the degree of pitting noted. While not part of the clinical diagnostic criteria, significant edema can result from protein loss in the urine, which causes fluids to leak out of the blood vessels and into the tissues, causing swelling or edema. A sudden increase in weight could signify fluid retention often associated with preeclampsia.

Physical examination

Additional components of the physical exam include abdominal assessment for epigastric or right upper quadrant tenderness. An ophthalmic exam may reveal changes such as papilledema, vascular spasm, or arteriovenous nicking related to increased edema. Deep tendon reflexes may be hyperactive due to CNS irritability.

Laboratory evaluation

There is no single reliable screening laboratory evaluation. An overall picture of the severity and progression of the disease is obtained from the evaluation of a variety of labs reflecting preeclampsia pathology (Table 22.5). Laboratory evaluation includes

- complete blood count (CBC) including platelets
- liver enzymes (AST, LDH, ALT)
- serum uric acid or a complete renal function panel (creatinine clearance, serum uric acid, BUN, serum creatinine)
- peripheral smear
- coagulation studies if platelets are low (PTT, fibrinogen).

In women with stable and mild preeclampsia, a CBC, and 24-hour urine should be obtained weekly. If progression of preeclampsia is suspected, the test should be repeated more frequently. This baseline lab panel should be done in early pregnancy in women at high risk for preeclampsia.

Management of women with preeclampsia

The optimal management of a woman with preeclampsia depends on gestational age and disease severity. Maternal and fetal surveillance is indicated for all women with gestational hypertension and preeclampsia, with the goal of evaluating for disease progression or the development of organ dysfunction. The NHBPEP (2000) advocates hospitalization for new-onset preeclampsia for initial evaluation and assessment of disease severity and progression, after which outpatient management is instituted. Other health-care providers proceed directly to outpatient management in cases of mild preeclampsia. Regardless of location, all women who present with new-onset hypertension should have symptom screening, a 24-hour urine collection for proteinuria evaluation, accurate weight and BP measurement, and laboratory evaluation. Some experts advocate for a baseline ultrasound to assess fetal growth pattern, depending on gestational age at the time of diagnosis. This is especially important in early-onset preeclampsia.

Maternal and fetal surveillance

Outpatient monitoring recommendations include daily fetal movement counting, maternal monitoring of symptoms, serial fetal testing, regular health-care provider evaluation, and lab assessment. While there is little consensus regarding the types of tests to be used and frequency of testing, the gestational age and the severity of the condition are guiding principles. For women with mild preeclampsia or mild gestational hypertension, it is appropriate to recommend a nonstress test (NST) and a biophysical profile (BPP) at the time of diagnosis and usually twice per week until labor begins (see Chapter 10). Health-care provider symptom assessment, BP measurement, and urine protein check are typically done at 3- to 4-day intervals. Some health-care providers instruct women with preeclampsia and gestational hypertension to regularly monitor their own BP and urine at home (Cunningham et al., 2010).

Lifestyle recommendations

The role of various nutrients in reducing the effects of preeclampsia has been investigated. Most studies have not demonstrated a relationship between specific nutrients in the onset or improvement of hypertensive disorders of pregnancy. It is appropriate to advise women with mild gestational hypertension or mild preeclampsia to consume a diet adequate in all major and micronutrients required for optimal fetal growth such as protein, calcium, folic acid, omega-3 fatty acids, and vitamins. Salt restricted diets are not helpful in preeclampsia and should not be advised.

Reduced daily activity should be encouraged. This can be in the form of periods of rest in the morning, afternoon, and evening. Resting in the left lateral position is preferred as this reduces fetal pressure on the vena cava and increases maternal fetal blood flow. Complete or partial bed rest for the duration of pregnancy has often been recommended for women with mild preeclampsia or mild gestational hypertension; however, there is no evidence that suggests that this improves pregnancy outcomes (Meher & Duley, 2006). Prolonged bed rest can increase the risk of thromboembolism and is often a significant hardship for most women and their families. Women with preeclampsia should be advised to stop working and provided with documentation to this effect as needed.

Medication

Antihypertensive medication in women with mild preeclampsia or gestational hypertension does not improve perinatal outcome and is not recommended. Women considered to have severe disease may be placed on antihypertensive medications, corticosteroids,

Table 22.5 Laboratory Manifestations of Preeclampsia–Eclampsia–HELLP Syndrome

Laboratory indices	Abnormal values and trends		Comments
Renal dysfunction			
24-hour urine	Proteinuria >300 mg/24 hours		Reflects glomerular damage and renal compromise
Blood urea nitrogen (BUN)	increased	⬆	Elevated due to decrease in glomerular filtration rate and renal blood flow
Serum uric acid	>5.6 mg/dL; increasing trend	⬆	Elevated due to decreased intravascular volume, increased uric acid production by poorly perfused tissues and decreased glomerular filtration rate Hyperuricemia is one of the earliest laboratory manifestations of preeclampsia.
Serum creatinine	>1.2 mg/dL	⬆	Normal in mild preeclampsia; may be elevated in severe preeclampsia due to decreased intravascular volume and decreased glomerular filtration rate
Hematologic dysfunction			
Hemoglobin		⬆	Increase reflects reduced plasma volume with redistribution of intravascular volume to the interstitial fluid space due to increased capillary permeability
		⬇	Decrease reflects hemolysis in severe disease and HELLP syndrome; caused by coagulation cascade and fibrin deposits in microvessels that destroy RBCs.
Platelet count	<100,000–150,000/ mL, decreasing t rend	⬇	Reflects platelet consumption during increased thrombus formation and intravascular coagulation; thrombocytopenia is the most common hematologic abnormality in women with preeclampsia
Peripheral smear	Presence of Burr cells and schistocytes		Reflects the presence of microangiopathic hemolysis suggestive of severe disease and HELLP syndrome
Prothrombin time (PT), partial thromboplastin time (PTT)	Elevated	⬆	Measure clotting time, can be increased in preeclampsia
Hepatologic dysfunction			
Aspartate transaminase (AST)	>70 U/L	⬆	An enzyme associated with liver parenchymal cells, reflects hepatocellular injury
Alanine transaminase (ALT)	>70 U/L	⬆	An enzyme present in hepatocytes, increased serum levels reflect liver damage
Lactic acid dehydrogenase (LDH)	>600 U/L	⬆	LDH is present in erythrocytes in high concentration. An increase may be a sign of hemolysis.

Sources: NHBPEP (2000), Sibai (2005).

or magnesium sulfate and are often medically managed within the hospital.

Education

Providing adequate information to women with pre-eclampsia about their condition is an especially important component of care. Women should be advised in understandable terms what preeclampsia is, appropriate management options, and symptoms to report. Women with mild preeclampsia should be reassured that they will most likely have a normal birth and birth outcome.

Education includes emphasis on her need to report:

- persistent headache
- visual disturbances such as spots or blurry vision
- epigastric pain
- feeling of general malaise
- sudden weight gain or facial edema.

The only cure for preeclampsia is giving birth. Induction is a reasonable option for women with mild pre-eclampsia at term with favorable cervix or with worsening preeclampsia. Discussions about birth plans and choices should be initiated once the stability of the disease has been established, and reviewed at subsequent visits.

HELLP syndrome

HELLP syndrome is a serious complication of pregnancy characterized by hemolysis (H), elevated liver enzymes (EL), and low platelet count (LP). This syndrome can be considered a variant of severe preeclampsia; however, the pathophysiology includes a more acute inflammatory process targeting the liver and a greater activation of the coagulation system. HELLP syndrome occurs in approximately 4–12% of all women with preeclampsia, especially those with severe preeclampsia, but the precise incidence is difficult to establish due to a lack of consensus on diagnostic criteria and missed diagnoses. About 70% of the cases develop during the prenatal period with the majority occurring in the third trimester between 27 and 37 weeks' gestation (Haram, Svendsen, & Abildgaard, 2009). Women who develop HELLP syndrome tend to be older, white, and multiparous compared with other women with preeclampsia. The onset and progression from early symptoms to seizure can be rapid. This condition always calls for immediate referral. HELLP syndrome increases a woman's risk for severe complications including renal failure, pulmonary edema, DIC, placental abruption, adult respiratory distress syndrome (ARDS), and liver hematoma.

The physical symptoms of HELLP syndrome vary and can be mistaken for normal pregnancy symptoms, or other conditions such as gastritis, flu, acute hepatitis, gallbladder disease or acute fatty liver of pregnancy (AFLP). Clinically, malaise, fatigue, and nonspecific physical symptoms are experienced in 90% of women with HELLP syndrome shortly before seeking medical attention (Sibai, 1990b). Nausea and vomiting, headache, and abdominal pain are very prevalent. BP is severely elevated in the majority of women experiencing this disease. Common presentation includes a report of general malaise or feeling like the case of the flu is starting. Additional typical symptoms include nausea and vomiting, right upper quadrant pain, and other signs and symptoms of preeclampsia.

Because of the tendency to present with vague symptoms, delay in making the correct diagnosis of HELLP syndrome can occur. A report of malaise or feeling unwell, or of indigestion or heartburn (both symptoms common in many pregnant women) should be further investigated in those women with preeclampsia. While the majority of women with HELLP syndrome have hypertension and proteinuria, the presence and degree of both manifestations can vary. Hypertension may be severe, mild, or normal. Proteinuria may be significant or absent. Reflexes should be examined and maybe brisk, reflecting increased CNS excitability.

The laboratory screening should be done in any woman suspected of HELLP syndrome as the diagnosis is based on laboratory evidence of hemolytic anemia, hepatic damage, and thrombocytopenia in women suspected to have preeclampsia. The basic laboratory screening for women suspected of HELLP syndrome varies in practice and generally includes a CBC with platelets, coagulation studies if platelet count is less than 100,000, urinalysis, serum creatinine, liver function tests, uric acid, indirect and total bilirubin levels, and peripheral smear.

Women suspected of developing HELLP syndrome require immediate specialist attention for further evaluation and management. Women with a diagnosis of HELLP syndrome have a significant increase in the risk for recurrence of hypertension in some form in a subsequent pregnancy (Leeners et al., 2011).

Atypical presentation preeclampsia

Data in the last decade suggest that some women with preeclampsia will not have the classic presentation of the disease. Women with atypical cases are those that have some of the signs and symptoms of preeclampsia without the usual hypertension or proteinuria and that develop at less than 20 weeks' gestation or greater than 48 hours after giving birth. Some women with preeclampsia may not have the hallmark sign of proteinuria, and yet their disease may more severe than women with proteinuria

Table 22.6 Signs and Symptoms of Atypical Presentation Preeclampsia

Gestational hypertension plus one of the following items:

Symptoms of preeclampsia (headache, dizziness, visual changes, epigastric pain)

Hemolysis

Thrombocytopenia (<100,000/mm³)

Elevated liver enzymes

or

Gestational proteinuria plus one of the following items:

Symptoms of preeclampsia (headache, dizziness, visual changes, epigastric pain)

Hemolysis

Thrombocytopenia

Elevated liver enzymes

or

Early signs and symptoms of preeclampsia–eclampsia at <20 weeks of gestation

Late postpartum preeclampsia–eclampsia (48 hours after birth)

Adapted from: Sibai and Stella (2009).

(Thornton, Makris, Ogle, Tooher, & Hennessy, 2010). Although hypertension is an important characteristic of preeclampsia because of the underlying pathophysiology, hypertension does not necessarily precede other symptoms or laboratory abnormalities characteristic of preeclampsia (Sibai & Stella, 2009). The physical symptoms of preeclampsia such as headache or visual changes may present prior to the onset of hypertension or proteinuria (Table 22.6). Women reporting these physical symptoms in the latter part of pregnancy should be evaluated by further history or laboratory testing.

Prediction of preeclampsia

Women with hypertensive disorders have a 50% chance of recurrence in a subsequent pregnancy (van Oostwaard et al., 2012). The earlier the disease manifests during a prior pregnancy, the higher the chance of recurrence rises. If preeclampsia presented clinically before 30 weeks' gestation, the chance of recurrence in a subsequent pregnancy may be as high as 40% (Sibai, Mercer, & Sarinoglu, 1991).

Serum markers of endothelial dysfunction and use of Doppler velocimetry are being investigated as biomarkers for predicting who will go on to develop symptomatic preeclampsia, allowing for earlier diagnosis and opportunities for optimizing pregnancy outcome. However, neither method has yet been found useful in predicting who will develop preeclampsia (Repke, 2013).

Prevention of preeclampsia

Prevention of preeclampsia has been a topic that has generated much research in the last decade. Strategies to prevent preeclampsia have been focused on attempts to correct theoretical abnormalities in preeclampsia and are limited by the lack of a complete understanding of the pathophysiological process. Unfortunately, many therapies have been either disproved or have shown only minimal benefit. Researchers concluded that calcium supplementation of 1.5–2.0 g daily during pregnancy appears to be beneficial for women at high risk for preeclampsia and for women with low calcium intake (Sibai & Cunningham, 2009; World Health Organization (WHO), 2011). However, these supplements do not prevent preeclampsia in women not at risk for the disease. Calcium supplements are not recommended for all pregnant women as a preventative measure.

Aspirin has been proposed to prevent preeclampsia by inhibiting the production of thromboxane, a vasoconstrictor and platelet aggregator. Research and recommendations on aspirin therapy have been inconsistent. Aspirin therapy may provide some benefit and is recommended for women at high risk for developing preeclampsia (Duley, Henderson-Smart, Meher, & King, 2007; WHO, 2011). The use of low-dose aspirin therapy (75 mg) to prevent preeclampsia should be done on an individual basis.

Antioxidants have been investigated with the idea that oxidative stress may cause the endothelial dysfunction associated with preeclampsia. None of the randomized controlled trials evaluating vitamin C and E supplementation have demonstrated benefit, and several reported an increase in adverse perinatal events with vitamin C and E supplementation (Roberts, 2008). The majority of evidence on supplementation with omega-3 fatty acids via fish oil does not support routine use for preeclampsia prevention or preventing disease progression after diagnosis.

Long-term sequelae of preeclampsia

Preeclampsia is becoming a disease of interest to internists as emerging evidence links preeclampsia with disease in later life. Strong associations between preeclampsia and cardiovascular disease have been established. Women diagnosed with preeclampsia have a fourfold risk of later hypertension and a twofold risk of heart disease, thromboembolism, and stroke (Bellamy,

Casas, Hingorani, & Williams, 2007; Valdiviezo, Garovic, & Ouyang, 2012). These associations are even stronger in women who have experienced preeclampsia in several pregnancies. Preeclampsia may be a risk factor for permanent cerebrovascular changes. Women with pre-eclampsia have a higher rate of white matter brain lesions than controls (Aukes et al., 2012), which may explain deficits in visual function (Wiegman et al., 2012) and memory (Workman, Barha, & Galea, 2012) found in women with a prior history of preeclampsia. A prior history of preeclampsia is also strongly associated with an increased risk of diabetes later in life (Feig et al., 2013; Wang et al., 2012). These findings support the importance of counseling during routine health visits on disease prevention measures such as appropriate diet, weight management and exercise habits to reduce risk.

Risk management issues in the office setting

Because preeclampsia/eclampsia is the third leading cause of death in pregnant women, appropriate recognition, treatment, and referral are clearly important issues for those providing prenatal care. Common diagnostic and treatment mistakes that can occur in the maternity triage setting include the following: (Kelly, 1999).

- ignoring a BP elevation
- not following up on proteinuria
- misinterpreting the cause of visual changes, nausea, vomiting, malaise, or epigastric pain
- sending a patient with preeclampsia home before verification of maternal and fetal well-being
- failure to follow up on milder symptoms of disease with more frequent ambulatory visits
- failure to reflect/implement collaborative or medical management when it is appropriate.

Interprofessional practice issues

Many prenatal health-care providers, especially midwives, who provide prenatal care regularly as part of their specialty responsibilities manage the care of women with mild preeclampsia, depending on the setting. Pregnant women with severe preeclampsia, chronic hypertension, and women with chronic hypertension who develop superimposed preeclampsia require medical consultation, interprofessional care, or referral. Women who develop early-onset preeclampsia are best managed in a tertiary care setting with appropriate maternal–fetal medicine specialists. In practices where optimal specialty care collaboration is not possible, women are referred for management as the risk of complications is significant in this subgroup of women. Providing emotional and supportive care as appropriate to the practice setting may still be a responsibility of the nurse practitioner or midwife.

Summary

Hypertensive disorders represent the most common medical complication of pregnancy and are a major cause of maternal and fetal morbidity and mortality in the United States and worldwide. Management depends upon the woman's gestational age, symptom constellation and presentation, and fetal status. Most women with mild to moderate hypertension or preeclamspia are at low risk for perinatal complications. The risk of complications is increased in women with severe hypertension or severe preeclampsia. Hypertensive disorders in pregnancy are an important risk factor for cardiovascular disease in women. Therefore, lifestyle modifications, regular BP control, and control of metabolic factors are recommended after birth, to avoid complications in subsequent pregnancies and to reduce maternal cardiovascular risk in the future.

Resources for women and their families

The Preeclampsia Foundation offers consumer material and information on the diagnosis and management of preeclampsia: http://www.preeclampsia.org/

The U.S. National Library of Medicine offers consumer information on multiple health topics, including preeclampsia: http://www.ncbi.nlm.nih.gov/pubmed health/PMH0001900/

The March of Dimes provides an overview of preeclampsia with additional resources for women: http://www .marchofdimes.com/pregnancy/complications_ preeclampsia.html

Resources for health-care providers

U.S. Department of Health and Human Services: Agency for Healthcare Quality and Research (AHRQ): Guideline summary on prediction, prevention, and prognosis of preeclampsia. In *Diagnosis, evaluation and management of the hypertensive disorders of pregnancy*: http://sogc.org/guidelines/diagnosis-evaluation-and -management-of-the-hypertensive-disorders-of-pre gnancy/

Case study

Mindy is a 26-year-old G1 P0 married Caucasian woman at 35 weeks' estimated gestational age (EGA), accompanied by her husband. She is receiving care from a local certified professional midwife (CPM) and had planned to have a home birth. She has been referred to you by a CPM for evaluation of her BP.

SUBJECTIVE: Mindy is very passionate about a noninterventionist birth and plans to give birth at home. She is currently pursuing her master's degree in art history. She and her husband have done quite a bit of research on birth options. She is here to see you reluctantly and has a wary attitude. She feels fine and thinks her CPM is being overly cautious.

Mindy reports she has not had any recent headache, dizziness, or visual changes. She indicates that she cannot wear her rings anymore due to swelling over the last 5 days. The fetus is active.

OBJECTIVE: Current weight today is 145; weight yesterday at home was 142.

B/P = 140/94
Slight edema of the ankles and hands
Urine dip: 2+ protein
Fetus active, left occiput anterior, fetal heart tones (FHTs) in 150 range with positive auscultated acceleration test

ASSESSMENT: r/o preeclampsia

PLAN: The characteristics and implications of preeclampsia were discussed with Mindy. She agreed to have lab work to investigate the possibility of preeclampsia. A CBC, liver function studies, and 24-hour urine were ordered. An NST was done, which was reactive. The consulting physician was brought in to further discuss the diagnosis and to further plan with Mindy and her husband. It was decided that pending laboratory results, Mindy could return home and return to the office tomorrow. She was given instructions on collecting the 24-hour urine sample, on the need for additional rest on her left side for most hours of the day, and on eating a high-quality diet. She was advised to monitor for the onset of headache, dizziness, blurry vision or spots in her eyes, or epigastric pain. Mindy and her husband verbalized understanding of the possible diagnosis and agreed to the immediate plan. She voiced concern about not having a home birth. Her CPM was also consulted and she indicated that Mindy would not qualify for a home birth if she had preeclampsia. Mindy was reassured that her birth wishes would be honored in the hospital setting is she indeed had mild preeclampsia. The CPM was encouraged by the nurse practitioner and physician to remain with her as doula and labor support barring a major change in her condition. Mindy and her husband were reassured and felt their questions were answered fully. They agreed to go home and rest and to return to the office tomorrow with the 24-hour urine collection and to review the laboratory studies done today. The number of the office and emergency contacts were provided and both were encouraged to call with any questions or if Mindy developed headache, dizziness, or vision changes.

References

Abalos, E., Duley, L., Steyn, D., & Henderson-Smart, D. (2007). Antihypertensive drug therapy for mild to moderate hypertension during pregnancy. *Cochrane Database Systematic Review*, (1), CD002252.

ACOG Practice Bulletin No. 125. (2012). Chronic hypertension in pregnancy. *Obstetrics and Gynecology*, 119(2 Pt 1), 396–407.

ACOG Practice Bulletin No. 33. (2002/2008). Diagnosis and management of pre-eclampsia and eclampsia. *Obstetrics and Gynecology*, 99, 159–167.

Aukes, A. M., De Groot, J. C., Wiegman, M. J., Aarnoudse, J. G., Sanwikarja, G. S., & Zeeman, G. G. (2012). Long-term cerebral imaging after pre-eclampsia. *BJOG: An International Journal of Obstetrics & Gynaecology*, 119(9), 1117–1122.

Bellamy, L., Casas, J., Hingorani, A., & Williams, J. (2007). Pre-eclampsia and risk of cardiovascular disease and cancer in later life: Systematic review and meta-analysis. *British Medical Journal*, 335, 974–985.

Centers for Disease Control and Prevention (CDC). (2012). Pregnancy—Related mortality in the United States. Retrieved from http://www.cdc.gov/reproductivehealth/MaternalInfantHealth/Pregnancy-relatedMortality.htm

Cunningham, C., Levano, K., Bloom, S., Hauth, J., Rouse, D., & Spong, C. (2010). *Williams obstetrics* (23rd ed.). New York: McGraw Hill.

Duley, L., Henderson-Smart, J., Meher, S., & King, J. F. (2007). Antiplatelet agents for preventing pre-eclampsia and its complications. *Cochrane Database of Systematic Reviews*, (2), Art. No.: CD004659, doi:10.1002/14651858.CD004659.pub2

Feig, D. S., Shah, B. R., Lipscombe, L. L., Wu, C. F., Ray, J. G., Lowe, J., . . . Booth, G. L. (2013). Preeclampsia as a risk factor for diabetes: A population-based cohort study. *PLoS Medicine*, 10(4), e1001425.

Haram, K., Svendsen, E., & Abildgaard, U. (2009). The HELLP syndrome: Clinical issues and management: A review. *Biomed Central: Pregnancy and Childbirth*, 9, 8. doi:10.1186/1471-2393-9-8

Kelly, M. (1999). Triage and management of the pregnant hypertensive patient. *Journal of Nurse-Midwifery*, 44(6), 558–571.

Leeners, B., Neumaier-Wagner, P., Kuse, S., Mütze, S., Rudnik-Schöneborn, S., Zerres, K., & Rath, W. (2011). Recurrence risks of hypertensive diseases in pregnancy after HELLP syndrome. *Journal of Perinatal Medicine*, 39(6), 673–678.

Meher, S., & Duley, L. (2006). Rest during pregnancy for preventing pre-eclampsia and its complications in women with normal blood pressure. *Cochrane Database of Systematic Reviews*, (2), Art. No.: CD005939, doi:10.1002/14651858.CD005939

National High Blood Pressure Education Program Working Group (NHBPEP). (2000). Report of the national high blood pressure education program working group on high blood pressure in pregnancy. *American Journal of Obstetrics Gynecology*, *183*, S1–S22.

Parretti, E., Lapolla, A., Dalfra, M. G., Pacini, G., Mari, A., Cioni, R., . . . Mello, G. (2006). Preeclampsia in lean normotensive normotolerant pregnant women can be predicted by simple insulin sensitivity indexes. *Hypertension*, *47*, 449–453.

Redman, C. W., & Sargent, I. L. (2010). Review article: Immunology of pre-eclampsia. *American Journal of Reproductive Immunology*, *63*(6), 534–543.

Repke, J. T. (2013). What is new in preeclampsia? Best articles from the past year. *Obstetrics & Gynecology*, *121*(3), 682–683.

Roberts, J. (2008). A randomized controlled trial of antioxidant vitamins to prevent serious complications associated with pregnancy related hypertension in low risk nulliparous women. *American Journal of Obstetrics and Gynecology*, *199*(6), S4.

Saito, S., Sakai, M., Sasaki, Y., Nakashima, A., & Shiozaki, A. (2007). Inadequate tolerance induction may induce pre-eclampsia. *Journal of Reproductive Immunology*, *76*, 30–39.

Seely, E., & Ecker, J. (2011). Chronic hypertension in pregnancy. *New England Journal of Medicine*, *365*, 439–446.

Shamil, C., Edmonds, S., Tong, S., Samarasekera, S., & Whitehead, C. (2011). Characterization and symptoms immediately preceding eclampsia. *Obstetrics & Gynecology*, *118*(5), 995–999. doi:10.1097/AOG.0b013e3182324570

Sibai, B. (1990a). Eclampsia: Maternal-perinatal outcome in 254 consecutive cases. *American Journal of Obstetrics and Gynecology*, *163*(3), 1049–1054.

Sibai, B. (1990b). The HELLP syndrome (hemolysis, elevated liver enzymes, and low platelets): Much ado about nothing? *American Journal of Obstetrics and Gynecology*, *162*(2), 311–316.

Sibai, B. (2002). Chronic hypertension in pregnancy. *Obstetrics and Gynecology*, *100*(2), 369–377.

Sibai, B. (2003). Diagnosis and management of gestational hypertension and preeclampsia. *Obstetrics and Gynecology*, *102*(1), 181–192.

Sibai, B. (2004). Magnesium sulfate prophylaxis in preeclampsia: Lessons learned from recent trials. *American Journal of Obstetrics and Gynecology*, *190*(6), 1520.

Sibai, B., & Cunningham, G. (2009). Prevention of preeclampsia. In M. Lindheimer, J. Robert, & F. Cunningham (Eds.), *Chesleys hypertensive disorders of pregnancy* (3rd ed., p. 215). New York: Elsevier.

Sibai, B., Dekker, G., & Kupferminc, M. (2005). Pre-eclampsia. *Lancet*, *365*, 785–799.

Sibai, B., Mercer, B., & Sarinoglu, C. (1991). Severe preeclampsia in the second trimester: Recurrence risk and long-term prognosis. *American Journal of Obstetrics and Gynecology*, *165*(4 Pt 2), 1408–1412.

Sibai, B., & Stella, C. (2009). Diagnosis and management of atypical preeclampsia-eclampsia. *American Journal of Obstetrics and Gynecology*, *200*(5), 481.e1–481.e7.

Sibai, B. M. (2005). Diagnosis, prevention, and management of eclampsia. *Obstetrics and Gynecology*, *105*(2), 402–410.

Thornton, C. E., Makris, A., Ogle, R. F., Tooher, J. M., & Hennessy, A. (2010). Role of proteinuria in defining pre-eclampsia: Clinical outcomes for women and babies. *Clinical and Experimental Pharmacology and Physiology*, *37*(4), 466–470.

Valdiviezo, C., Garovic, V. D., & Ouyang, P. (2012). Preeclampsia and hypertensive disease in pregnancy: Their contributions to cardiovascular risk. *Clinical Cardiology*, *35*, 160–165. doi:10.1002/clc.2196

van Oostwaard, M., Langenveld, J., Bijloo, R., Wong, K., Scholten, I., Loix, S., . . . Ganzevoort, W. (2012). Prediction of recurrence of hypertensive disorders of pregnancy between 34 and 37 weeks of gestation: A retrospective cohort study. *British Journal of Obstetrics & Gynecology*, *119*(7), 840–847.

Wang, I., Tsai, I. J., Chen, P. C., Liang, C. C., Chou, C. Y., Chang, C. T., . . . Sung, F. C. (2012). Hypertensive disorders in pregnancy and subsequent diabetes mellitus: A retrospective cohort study. *The American Journal of Medicine*, *125*(3), 251–257.

Wiegman, M. J., de Groot, J. C., Jansonius, N. M., Aarnoudse, J. G., Groen, H., Faas, M. M., & Zeeman, G. G. (2012). Long-term visual functioning after eclampsia. *Obstetrics & Gynecology*, *119*(5), 959–966.

Wikström, A. K., Wikström, J., Larsson, A., & Olovsson, M. (2006). Random albumin/creatinine ratio for quantification of proteinuria in manifest pre-eclampsia. *British Journal of Obstetrics & Gynecology*, *113*(8), 930–934.

Workman, J. L., Barha, C. K., & Galea, L. A. (2012). Endocrine substrates of cognitive and affective changes during pregnancy and postpartum. *Behavioral Neuroscience*, *126*(1), 54.

World Health Organization (WHO). (2011). *WHO recommendations for prevention and treatment of pre-eclampsia and eclampsia.* Geneva: WHO. Retrieved from http://www.preeclampsia.org/images/pdf/2011c-who_pe_final.pdf.

Young, B., Levine, R., & Karumanchi, S. (2010). Pathogenesis of preeclampsia. *Annual Review of Pathology*, *5*, 173–192.

Zhang, J., & Patel, G. (2007). Partner change and perinatal outcomes: A systematic review. *Paediatric and Perinatal Epidemiology*, *21*(Suppl. 1), 46–57.

23

Gestational diabetes

Kimberly K. Trout

Relevant terms

Amniotic fluid index (AFI)—measurement of the volume of amniotic fluid (obtained via ultrasound) from adding the largest vertical pockets of fluid from all four maternal quadrants; a normal AFI level is between 5 and 24 cm

Class A1GDM—gestational diabetes in glycemic control with diet and exercise therapy

Class A2GDM—gestational diabetes requiring any medication in addition to diet and exercise therapy to achieve glycemic control

Estimated fetal weight (EFW)—clinical or sonographic estimate of fetal weight

Insulin resistance—a condition in which cells fail to respond to the normal actions of insulin, thereby increasing blood glucose levels

Large for gestational age (LGA)—birth weight greater than the ninetieth percentile for any given gestational age in a defined population

Macrosomia—arbitrarily defined as birth weight >4000 or 4500 g

Overt diabetes—diabetes with onset prior to pregnancy

Introduction

Gestational diabetes mellitus (GDM) is defined as glucose intolerance that is first detected during pregnancy. This simple definition belies the complexity of a condition that spans a spectrum of glycemia, pathophysiology, and clinical effects and for which there is a wide diversity of opinion (Conway, 2007; Kjos & Buchanan, 1999; Metzger et al., 2012). GDM occurs in approximately 7% of all pregnancies and is thought to be increasing due to an increasing prevalence of obesity in the United States and increasing birth rates in ethnic groups at higher risk for GDM (Flegal, Carroll, Kit, & Ogden, 2012; United States Preventive Services Task Force, 2008). The carbohydrate intolerance of GDM may be of varying degrees, with increased perinatal problems with decreasing maternal blood glucose control. This perhaps is the only area of the study of GDM where there is agreement. There are numerous areas of controversy regarding GDM. Much of the debate has focused on the validity of currently used diagnostic criteria and whether identification and treatment of GDM actually improves perinatal outcomes (Crowther et al., 2005; Landon & Gabbe, 2011; Wong, 2013). Association between maternal glucose levels and adverse perinatal outcomes occur on a continuum with no obvious thresholds at which risks increase (HAPO Study Cooperative Research Group, 2008), making the debates particularly complex. Optimal screening methods, result interpretation, antepartum surveillance, and treatment measures are also areas of controversy (O'Neill, & Thorp, 2012).

Pathophysiology and potential problems of gestational diabetes

Pregnancy is characterized by a series of metabolic changes that promote accumulation of adipose tissue in early pregnancy, followed by insulin resistance later in gestation. The hormones of pregnancy affect glucose metabolism by causing increased insulin resistance during the second and third trimesters. Levels of human placental lactogen (HPL), human placental growth hormone, progesterone, cortisol, and prolactin increase

Prenatal and Postnatal Care: A Woman-Centered Approach, First Edition. Edited by Robin G. Jordan, Janet L. Engstrom, Julie A. Marfell, and Cindy L. Farley.
© 2014 John Wiley & Sons, Inc. Published 2014 by John Wiley & Sons, Inc.

and contribute to insulin resistance (Barbour et al., 2007). HPL increases up to 30-fold during pregnancy and promotes insulin release from the pancreas. Tumor necrosis factor alpha (TNFα) and the hormone leptin have also been implicated in insulin resistance of pregnancy (Kirwan et al., 2002; Melczer et al., 2003). The increased insulin resistance during pregnancy poses a challenge to the maternal pancreatic β cells. For most women, this increase in insulin resistance has no adverse effect and actually serves a positive function to provide a steady supply of nutrients to the developing fetus. In those women who eventually develop GDM, there is an inability of the β cells to meet the challenge of secreting the additional amounts of insulin necessary to achieve and maintain euglycemia (Retnakaran et al., 2010).

Glucose passes from maternal to fetal compartments via diffusion facilitated by insulin-dependent glucose transporters (Zoupas, 2007). The delivery of glucose to the fetus beyond normal levels can lead to macrosomia, with the fetus responding to the elevated levels of glucose by becoming hyperinsulinemic. Insulin is an anabolic hormone that promotes cell growth. Most of the potential problems of GDM are related to excessive fetal growth (Table 23.1). Macrosomic infants born to women with gestational diabetes typically have excessive fat on the shoulders and trunk, predisposing them to shoulder dystocia or operative birth (Schafer-Graf et al., 2008). Skeletal growth is largely unaffected. Data from the Australian Carbohydrate Intolerance Study in Pregnant Women (ACHOIS) demonstrated a positive association between elevated fasting glucose levels and relative risk for shoulder dystocia (Athukorala, Crowther, & Willson, 2007). An increased risk for shoulder dystocia is also associated with a maternal body mass index (BMI) >30.

The rates of stillbirth are higher in women with GDM; however, this is related to poor glycemic control during pregnancy (Biggio, Chapman, Neely, Cliver, & Rouse, 2010). The rates of birth defects are increased in women with pregestational diabetes but are not increased in women who develop gestational diabetes after the first trimester (Moore & Catalano, 2009).

Prenatal screening and diagnosis of GDM

All pregnant women should be screened for gestational diabetes by history, clinical risk factors, or lab screening of blood glucose levels. Universal serum screening for GDM has become common practice; however, this type of screening is not recommended by all professional and expert groups (United States Preventive Services Task Force, 2008). Selective serum screening for women based on risk factor evaluation offers individualized care (Table 23.2).

Table 23.1 Potential Problems Related to Gestational Diabetes

Maternal
Operative birth (instrumental and cesarean)
Preeclampsia
Preterm labor
Polyhydramnios (Shoham et al., 2001)
Overt diabetes later in life
Metabolic syndrome later in life

Fetal/neonatal
Macrosomia
Large-for-gestational age (greater than ninetieth percentile)
Shoulder dystocia/birth trauma
Hypoglycemia
Polycythemia
Hyperbilirubinemia
Respiratory distress syndrome
Need for neonatal intensive care unit admission/care

Childhood/adult
Early childhood obesity
Early childhood metabolic syndrome
Type 2 diabetes during adolescence

Table 23.2 Risk Factor Classification for Gestational Diabetes

Low risk	Average risk	High risk
• Age <25 years • Normal prepregnancy BMI • No known diabetes in first-degree relatives • Member of ethnic group with low diabetes prevalence • No history (hx) of poor obstetric outcome • No hx abnormal glucose tolerance test	Any criteria not met for low-risk status	• Overweight or obese; BMI >25 • Prior history of GDM, glycosuria or impaired carbohydrate metabolism • Strong family history of type 2 diabetes (two first-degree relatives) • Prior history of stillbirth, infant with congenital anomalies, or macrosomia • Age ≥40
	Blood screen at 24–28 weeks' gestation	Blood screen at first visit and if normal, repeat screen 24–28 weeks' gestation

Adapted from: International Association of Diabetes in Pregnancy Study Groups (IADPSG) (2010), Metzger (2007).

One-hour oral glucose tolerance testing

The most common screening method used in the United States is a 1-hour oral glucose tolerance test (OGTT) after a 50-g oral glucose load performed between 24 and 28 weeks' gestation. A screening test is considered positive at the level of 130–140 mg/dL. A positive screening result should be followed up by a diagnostic test of a 3-hour glucose challenge test. The screening test threshold at which a diagnostic GTT is recommended is an arbitrary value not determined by scientific study (American College of Obstetricians and Gynecologists, 2001). The higher the threshold glucose level is set, the lower the sensitivity, but the better the specificity and the lower the likelihood of a false positive test result. The lower the threshold glucose level is set, the higher the sensitivity, but the higher the chance of a false positive test result, resulting in the performance of an unnecessary 3-hour diagnostic OGTT. The lower screening level of 130 mg/dL identifies more women with gestational diabetes at the cost of more false positive results. Conversely, a higher cutoff of 140 mg/dL detects fewer women with GDM but reduces the number of false positives, which are common for the 1-hour OGTT. Either value for defining an abnormal initial screening result can be considered correct. Women do not need to be fasting for this test; however, women should be advised that a high-sugar or high-carbohydrate snack or meal just prior to the test can make it more likely to produce false positive results.

The 3-hour, 100-g OGTT is the common diagnostic test used in the United States when a 1-hour screen is positive. A positive diagnosis of GDM requires that two or more threshold glucose levels on the 3-hour test be met or exceeded. The test is administered in the morning after an overnight fast. There are two commonly used criteria to diagnose GDM with the 3-hour GTT (Table 23.3).

Table 23.3 Criteria for Abnormal Result on 100-g, Three-Hour Oral Glucose Tolerance Test in pregnant Women

Blood sample	National Diabetes Data Group criteria	Carpenter and Coustan criteria
Fasting	105 mg/dL (5.8 mmol/L)	95 mg/dL (5.3 mmol/L)
1 hour	190 mg/dL (10.5 mmol/L)	180 mg/dL (10.0 mmol/L)
2 hour	165 mg/dL (9.2 mmol/L)	155 mg/dL (8.6 mmol/L)
3 hour	145 mg/dL (8.0 mmol/L)	140 mg/dL (7.8 mmol/L)

Source: Hillier et al. (2008).

The most recognized diagnostic criteria were established by the National Diabetes Data Group (NDDG) in 1979. This set of values has been challenged in recent years by the Carpenter and Coustan criteria, which designate lower blood glucose values to diagnose GDM. This means more women are diagnosed with GDM. It has been noted that with the NDDG criteria, 3.3% of women are diagnosed with GDM, but with the Carpenter and Coustan criteria, that number rises to 5.1% (Chen, Block-Kurbisch, & Caughy, 2009). The most recent Fifth International Workshop Conference on GDM recommends using the lower Carpenter and Coustan criteria for the 3-hour glucose tolerance test (Zoupas, 2007).

Two-hour oral glucose tolerance testing

The 75-g 2-hour OGGT method is a combined screening and diagnosis method used in many other countries to diagnose GDM. The test basically is the same as the 3-hour test but uses a lower glucose load and draws fasting, 1- and 2-hour postglucose load levels. Only one abnormal value is required for a diagnosis of GDM.

GDM diagnostic criteria 75-g 2-hour OGTT

FBS 92 mg/dL or above
1-hour: 180 mg/dL or above
2-hour: 153 mg/dL or above

Following the recommendations of the International Association of the Diabetes in Pregnancy Study Group (IADPSG), the American Diabetes Association (ADA) endorsed the 75-g 2-hour test to be used as a one-step GDM screening and diagnosis (American Diabetes Association (ADA), 2011). This recommendation was based on results from the Hyperglycemia and Adverse Pregnancy Outcomes (HAPO) study, a prospective observational study of more than 23,000 pregnancies evaluated with a 75-g 2-hour OGTT (HAPO Study Cooperative Research Group et al, 2008). The investigators found a continuum of increasing risk of adverse outcome as each of the three (fasting, 1-hour, and 2-hour) plasma glucose values increased. Because of the lower blood glucose thresholds and the fact that only one abnormal value is required for diagnosis, 75-g 2-hour testing will significantly increase the diagnosed prevalence of GDM. A significant criticism of the IADPSG recommendation for GDM screening and diagnosis is that the decision was made based on expert opinion and consensus rather than on rigorously obtained outcome measures (Langer, Umans, & Miodovnik, 2013). Further debate surrounding these criteria centers on concerns regarding increased costs and resources, and the medicalization of pregnancies previously categorized as normal (ADA, 2011; Langer et al., 2013). A recent analysis found that pregnant women classified as nondiabetic by the Canadian Diabetes Association criteria but considered to have GDM according to the IADPSG criteria have similar pregnancy outcomes as women without GDM (Bodmer-Roy, Morin, Cousinea, & Re, 2012). As of this publication, the American College of Obstetricians and Gynecologists (ACOG) has not endorsed the ADA's recommendation to use the 2-hour one-step test based on the rationale that there is no convincing evidence that outcomes would be improved with this new criteria (ACOG, 2011). Continued support for the ACOG 2-step process was also reaffirmed at a recent National Institutes of Health Consensus Development Conference on the diagnosis of GDM in March, 2013. Screening and testing methods for GDM continue to be the subject of ongoing investigation.

Screening for women at high risk for GDM

Women at high risk for GDM have testing as soon as possible upon entry into prenatal care (Table 23.2). For reasons that are not well established, women who are African-American, Latina, American Indian, or Asian are more likely to develop GDM. Women from these ethnic groups should have blood screening, with the timing dependent on the presence of additional risk factors. Women with polycystic ovarian syndrome (PCOS) also are at higher risk for developing GDM and should have blood screening; however, optimal timing has not been established (Toulis et al., 2009). Women at high risk for GDM should have testing as soon as possible upon entry into prenatal care (Table 23.2). For those women at high risk to develop GDM, the concern is that they may have overt diabetes rather than diabetes with onset in pregnancy. A diagnosis of overt diabetes can be made in women who meet any of the following criteria at their initial prenatal visit (IADPSG, 2010):

- fasting plasma glucose ≥126 mg/dL (7.0 mmol/L) or
- A1C ≥6.5% using a standardized assay, or
- random plasma glucose ≥200 mg/dL (11.1 mmol/) that is subsequently confirmed by elevated fasting plasma glucose or A1C.

The 3-hour glucose tolerance test is not recommended as a diagnostic test in early pregnancy, as this test has not been validated for use in early pregnancy.

Management of gestational diabetes

Basic components of management for gestational diabetes are healthy eating, physical activity, and monitoring blood glucose levels.

Dietary intervention

Dietary modification is the mainstay of treatment for women with GDM. The optimal diet should provide sufficient calories and nutrients for fetal growth and maternal needs while reducing significant postprandial hyperglycemia. Women should be advised to make an appointment with a dietician or a Certified Diabetes Educator (CDE) for diet instruction. However, since this visit may be weeks away, it is important for health-care providers to understand principles of nutrition therapy for the woman diagnosed with GDM since dietary modification should be initiated immediately. Surprisingly, there have been no randomized clinical trials to establish what is the optimal diet for GDM, even though diet therapy is the cornerstone of treatment. A dietary program of 2000–2500 kcal/day, representing approximately 30–35 kcal/kg of present pregnancy weight, is typically initiated (ADA, 2004).

Since carbohydrates are the macronutrients that appear to have the greatest effect on postprandial blood glucose levels, women are advised to monitor carbohydrates more closely than other macronutrients, following a diet of approximately 35–40% complex carbohydrates, eliminating simple sugars, 20–30% protein, and the rest fats. To keep blood sugar even, food is best taken in three meals with two to three snacks with carbohydrates evenly distributed throughout the day, with the exception of breakfast. Moderate use of sweeteners such as aspartame is permitted. Following these dietary guidelines, glucose levels will normalize in around 75–80% of women with gestational diabetes (ADA, 2004). Carbohydrates are generally less well tolerated in the morning due to hormones secreted in the early morning that serve to awaken us such as cortisol and epinephrine. For this reason, fewer carbohydrates are typically consumed at breakfast than with other meals in order to minimize elevation of postbreakfast blood glucose. An important part of nutrition therapy is an evening snack. A bedtime snack consisting of approximately 15–30 g carbohydrate is usually needed to prevent overnight ketosis. For the same reason, the overnight fast should not exceed 10 hours. The dietary reference intake (DRI) for carbohydrates in pregnancy is 175 g/day, the minimal requirement to assure adequate glucose to meet fetal and maternal needs. In order to keep carbohydrate intake in the desired range, it is easy to calculate the actual grams of carbohydrate daily depending on a woman's calorie requirements. There are 4 kcal for each gram of carbohydrate, 4 kcal for each gram of protein, and 9 kcal for each gram of fat. So, for example, if the woman is on a 2000-kcal diet and is attempting to consume 40% carbohydrate: total number of kcal (2000) × 40% = 800 kcals from

Table 23.4   Sample Diet at 2000 Calories with 35–40% Carbohydrate

Breakfast 27 g CHO	1 scrambled egg with 1 slice (1 oz) cheese +1 tsp butter 1 piece toast (15 g CHO) 1 cup skim milk (12 g CHO) Decaf coffee or tea (no sugar)
Snack, mid am 15 g CHO	½ banana–4 oz (15 g CHO) 1 slice turkey bacon
Lunch 46 g CHO	3 oz beef or turkey burger with lettuce and tomato (30 g CHO) Carrots, cucumber, broccoli, celery (10 g CHO) 1 tbs ranch dressing for dip ½ cup skim milk (6 g CHO)
Snack, mid pm 15 g CHO	½ cup fruit salad (15 g CHO) ¼ cup nonfat cottage cheese
Dinner 46 g CHO	3 oz baked chicken breast 1 cup green beans (10 g CHO) 1 cup mashed potato (30 g CHO) 2 tsp butter ½ cup skim milk (6 g CHO)
Snack, bedtime 30 g CHO	2/3 cup fat-free yogurt (12 g CHO) ¾ cup unsweetened cereal (15 g CHO) 1 tbs sugar-free peanut butter (3 g CHO)
Total CHO 179 g CHO	

Table 23.5   Total Daily Carbohydrates for 35–40% of Calories

Kilocalories (kcal)	35% (g)	40% (g)
2000	175	200
2200	193	220
2500	219	250

carbohydrates/4 = 200 g of carbohydrates daily (Table 23.4 and Table 23.5).

Pregnancy weight gain within the Institute of Medicine (IOM) recommendations for BMI should be encouraged (see Chapter 6, "Nutrition before and during Pregnancy"). Severe caloric or carbohydrate restriction should be avoided as this can result in significant ketonuria and ketonemia. Maintaining a food log and recording daily food and fluid intake can help women with GDM monitor their food choices. Some women have reported that this is too time-consuming and cumbersome (K. K. Trout, unpublished data, 2012), but the widespread use of nutritional phone apps has the potential to make this much easier and "doable" for busy women. Interprofessional collaboration with a registered dietician or CDE on nutritional management of GDM can help the woman understand GDM and how to best manage her condition and optimal outcomes.

Exercise therapy

Physical activity is an essential component of treatment for women with GDM, although this is all too often ignored. Regular exercise increases glucose uptake and increases insulin sensitivity, thus decreasing insulin resistance. Research has indicated that 30 minutes of exercise on most days may be comparable to insulin in keeping glycemic control (Brankston, Mitchell, Ryan, & Okun, 2004). The ADA in conjunction with the American College of Sports Medicine recommends at least 150 min/week of moderate-intensity aerobic physical activity (at 50–70% of maximum heart rate) and/or at least 90 min/week of vigorous aerobic exercise (at 70% of maximum heart rate to improve glycemic control) (Colberg et al., 2010). The physical activity should be distributed over at least 3 days/week and with no more than 2 consecutive days without physical activity.

Women should be informed about the benefits of exercise on GDM and instructed in specific exercises. Daily walking, biking, and swimming are excellent exercise options. The use of an exercise bike or a treadmill can be safely recommended for women with no contraindications to exercise. Writing out a "prescription" for the type and amount of exercise may help women recognize the importance of this therapy in managing their GDM. Keeping a daily exercise log can help women track their regimen, correlate activity with blood sugar levels, and emphasize the importance of regular exercise in the treatment of GDM.

Blood glucose monitoring

Surveillance of blood glucose levels is necessary to ascertain that glycemic control has been established. Daily self-monitoring of blood glucose consists of the fasting blood glucose (FBG) and 1- to 2-hours postprandial measures. Some experts advocate the 1-hour postprandial value in lieu of the 2 hour, for that test typically represents peak glucose excursion (Metzger, 2007).

Target capillary blood glucose levels

Fasting : <95 mg/dL
1-hour postprandial: <130 mg/dL
2-hour postprandial: <120 mg/dL
2 am–6 am: >60 mg/dL

A common schedule for self-monitoring of blood glucose is to initially test four times daily. If both fasting and postprandial measures are within normal after several weeks of testing, the testing frequency can be reduced to a schedule tailored to the woman's individual situation. If postprandial blood sugar levels indicate hyperglycemia and poor glycemic control, or if FBG levels are high (diet modification has little effect on fasting glucose levels), then glyburide or insulin therapy is required.

Oral medications for GDM

Oral diabetic medications have several distinct advantages over insulin treatment with regard to ease of use. Oral routes are preferred to self-injection. Establishing the correct insulin dosage is very individualized and depends on several factors, including relative degree of insulin resistance. Knowledge of insulin action based on the type of insulin used, peak and duration of action, and precise matching of insulin to carbohydrate levels can be quite complex. This match can be difficult to initially determine and will quite often need frequent adjustment as increasing pregnancy hormones result in increased insulin resistance. Several studies have found no differences in glycemic control or pregnancy outcomes between insulin and oral hypoglycemic agents (Dhulkotia, Ola, Fraser, & Farrell, 2010; Langer, Conway, Berkus, Xenakis, & Gonzales, 2000).

Glyburide

Glyburide is a second-generation sulfonyurea drug that is now considered an acceptable oral agent for use in pregnancy (Moore, Clokey, Rappaport, & Curet, 2010). It is not thought to cross the placenta in any significant amount. The action of glyburide is to promote increased insulin secretion (insulin secretagogue). Typically, in consultation with a physician, glyburide is started at 2.5 mg prior to breakfast and 2.5 mg prior to the evening meal. If blood glucose values are not within goal range after 1 week of therapy, the evening dose is typically increased to 5 mg, and doses can be increased as needed up to 5 mg in the morning and 5 mg in the evening for a total daily dose that does not usually exceed 10 mg/day (Mazze, Strock, Simonson, & Bergenstal, 2007). Insulin therapy is often the next step if successful blood glucose control is not achieved with doses of 10 mg/day. Hypoglycemia is a possible side effect with glyburide, although not as likely as with insulin. Contraindications to its use include allergy to sulfa drugs and impaired renal function (serum creatinine >2.0 mg/dL).

Metformin

Metformin is another oral agent that has sometimes been used in pregnancy, although it has not been as well studied in pregnancy as glyburide, and it is known to cross the placenta. The primary action of metformin is to decrease output of glucose from the liver. Thus, it is contraindicated with liver or renal dysfunction. The Metformin in Gestational Diabetes (MiG) study comparing pregnancy outcomes in women randomized to metformin or insulin for the treatment of gestational diabetes demonstrated no outcome differences between the two treatments except that women preferred oral therapy (Rowan et al, 2008). As of this publication, both ACOG and the ADA have not recommended using metformin for GDM. The Fifth International Workshop Conference recommends that metformin treatment for GDM be limited to clinical trials, and its use in pregnancy remains controversial (Zoupas, 2007). Metformin has been effectively used for the treatment of polycystic ovarian syndrome (PCOS) to aid with successful conception and reducing rates of spontaneous abortion (Dronavalli & Ehrmann, 2007).

Insulin therapy

Gestational diabetes requiring insulin therapy necessitates medical management by a physician and is therefore beyond the scope of this chapter. Women with a BMI >40 are more likely to need insulin therapy to treat GDM. The woman who requires insulin treatment in order to maintain euglycemia is likely to have increased anxiety about the effects of GDM on her infant's health, along with increased concerns regarding labor and birth. Individual practice configurations will determine to what extent the midwife or NP will be involved with other aspects of the woman's prenatal care.

Fetal surveillance and timing of birth

There is considerable variation in practice with regard to third-trimester fetal surveillance for women with GDM who are well controlled with diet and exercise therapy. When to initiate testing, what type of testing, and the benefits of testing all lack consensus (United States Preventive Services Task Force, 2008). Women with GDM in good glycemic control are at low risk for an intrauterine fetal death and routine nonstress testing is not advocated (Cundy et al., 2000; Landon & Gabbe, 2011). Women who require insulin or an oral antihyperglycemic agent to maintain euglycemia or those with additional risk factors such as hypertension, obesity, or other comorbidities should be managed the same way as women with pregestational diabetes or other conditions placing the pregnancy at an increased risk of an adverse outcome (ACOG, 2001, 2005; Zoupas, 2007). Antenatal testing for these women is initiated in the mid third trimester with biophysical profile testing, nonstress testing, amniotic fluid index (AFI), and/or periodic evaluation of estimated fetal weight (EFW) (Hawkins &

Casey, 2007; Vink, Poggi, Ghidini, & Spong, 2006; Yehuda, Nagtalon-Ramos, & Trout, 2011; Zoupas, 2007).

Macrosomia is a recognized fetal potential problem for women with GDM. Unfortunately, there is no method to evaluate estimated fetal weight that performs well, especially for identifying the large-for-gestational-age (LGA) fetus (Humphries et al., 2002; Idris, Wong, Thomae, Gardener, & McIntyre, 2010; Xiong, Saunders, Wang, & Demianczuk, 2001). Fetal growth monitoring and the investigation of macrosomia is unnecessary for women with GDM controlled by diet and exercise, mainly because high false positive results may lead to unnecessary cesarean sections (Melamed et al., 2011). Fetal weight estimated by ultrasound would have to be ≥4800 g to have at least a 50% chance of predicting an infant being born with a birth weight of 4500 kg or more (McLaren, Puckett, & Chauhan, 1995). If macrosomia is suspected clinically, ultrasound close to term may be done to corroborate the experienced examiners' clinical findings, which have been found to be equivalent to ultrasound findings (Humphries et al., 2002).

Labor and birth

Factors affecting the timing and type of birth for the woman with GDM are both maternal and fetal. Maternal factors include degree of blood glucose control, condition of the cervix, history of any previous births, and presence or absence of any comorbidities. Fetal factors include estimated fetal weight, gestational age, and evidence of fetal well-being. As in women without GDM, spontaneous labor is preferred as the safest option over induction of labor. There are no indications to pursue birth before 40 weeks of gestation in women with good glycemic control unless other maternal or fetal indications are present (ACOG, 2001).

If maternal and fetal factors determine that birth is indicated, induction of labor is a reasonable option if there are no contraindications to vaginal birth or cervical ripening or induction agents. The circumstances under which to offer a scheduled cesarean section to reduce the risk of birth trauma from potential shoulder dystocia are controversial. The anthropomorphic difference in the infant of a diabetic mother increases abdominal and bisacromial diameter and increases risk for shoulder dystocia. These changes distinguish the LGA infant of a mother with diabetes from other LGA infants, thus explaining why induction prior to 40 weeks' gestation or elective cesarean section may be offered as an option at a lower estimated fetal weight than in the woman without diabetes (ACOG, 2000; Horvath et al., 2010). A reasonable approach is to offer elective cesarean section to women with GDM and an estimated fetal weight of 4500 g or more (ACOG, 2001), based on the

woman's history and pelvimetry, and the woman and provider's discussion about the risks and benefits. However, given that ultrasound estimation of fetal weight ≥4800 g is associated with only about a 50% chance that the infant's birth weight will be ≥4500 g, many scheduled cesarean sections will result in birth of infants <4500 g and not at high risk of shoulder dystocia (Chauhan et al., 2005; McLaren et al., 1995). A decision analysis evaluating the cost and efficacy of elective cesarean birth in euglycemic women with a fetus estimated by ultrasound to weigh 4500 g or more found "that 443 cesarean deliveries would need to be performed to prevent one case of brachial plexus injury" (Turok, Ratcliffe, & Baxley, 2003). When counseling women with GDM about suspected fetal macrosomia, the limitations of estimating fetal weight should be included in the discussion. Ultimately, the thoughtful weighing of each woman's individual maternal and fetal risk profile in conjunction with the woman herself is required to determine her best intrapartum path.

Postpartum follow-up

Euglycemia and resolution of disease occurs almost immediately after the delivery of the placenta in most women with GDM (Blackburn, 2013). Women who have been diagnosed with GDM should be advised that the diagnosis itself uncovers a greater risk for development of type 2 diabetes later in life, with many women developing type 2 diabetes within 5 years of diagnosis (Bellamy, Casas, Hingorani, & Williams, 2009). The diagnosis of GDM discloses a relative insufficient amount of insulin secretion when faced with insulin resistance that puts them at risk. Modifiable factors that can decrease the risk of later development of type 2 diabetes such as prolonged breastfeeding, regular exercise, and reaching a normal BMI should be discussed at the postpartum visit.

A 75-g 2-hour GTT at the 6-week postpartum visit is a commonly used test to determine if GDM has resolved. The use of glycosylated hemoglobin (A1C) for diagnosis of persistent diabetes at the postpartum visit is not recommended. Women with prior GDM should be advised to undergo periodic testing for diabetes mellitus.

Postpartum contraception should be discussed to prevent pregnancy before the woman is ready for another baby. Allowing time to achieve a normal BMI for those women with elevated BMI prepregnancy can help to set the stage for a healthier subsequent pregnancy and may prevent GDM in a future pregnancy. The postpartum visit is also an opportunity to discuss healthy lifestyle choices to prevent development of type 2 diabetes.

Women with GDM have a higher rate of postpartum depression than the general population of postpartum women (Kozhimannil, Pereira, & Harlow, 2009) and should be screened for depression at the postpartum visit. See Chapter 28, "Common Complications during the Postnatal Period," for information on screening for postpartum depression.

Scope of practice issues

Prenatal health care providers provide holistic, family-centered care to women with GDM. The care of women with gestational diabetes is commonly managed by midwives, nurse practitioners, and physician assistants. For women with abnormal fasting glucose levels or if <80–90% of postprandial values meet glucose target levels, physician consultation regarding the need for pharmacological therapy should be considered. Collaborative management of women on oral medications, with transfer to physician medical management if insulin therapy is initiated, can be appropriate.

Perspective on GDM risk

The continuous relation between maternal glycemia and macrosomia-related perinatal risks accounts for much of the controversy in the diagnosis and management of GDM. Without a firm biological threshold for risk, it is difficult to establish a superior set of diagnostic criteria or therapeutic guidelines based on maternal glucose alone. The evidence is not clear regarding the best screening and diagnostic testing for GDM, and evidence is lacking on the utility and optimal methods of fetal surveillance in women with GDM (Loomis, Lee, & Tweed, 2006). While GDM is a complication of pregnancy, prenatal care providers need to be mindful of the "most likely" while also being aware of the potential problems. Most women, through healthy eating, physical activity, and self-monitoring, are able to manage their GDM, maintain euglycemia, and are likely to have a normal pregnancy and birth course. However, the prenatal care provider's mindset on GDM may impact perspective and subsequent care. The "knowledge that a woman has GDM may modify the obstetrical practice and increase the risk of cesarean section in this pregnant patient population" (Gorgal et al., 2012, p. 158). GDM is not an indication in itself for cesarean birth; however, the cesarean rate for women diagnosed with GDM is double that of nondiabetic women (Gorgal et al., 2012). To reduce this iatrogenic bias, women who remain in good glycemic control should be cared for during labor in the same way as any other women in labor (Cunningham et al., 2010). Reassurance is especially important for women with GDM who maintain glycemic control with diet and exercise. It is appropriate and important to reassure a woman diagnosed with GDM (especially in women with a normal BMI) that if her blood sugars are within normal limits throughout pregnancy, then her pregnancy course is likely to follow a normal path. A woman confident in her own body's ability certainly has an effect on the birth process. With the current obstetrical medical model emphasis on pathology and potential problems, this may be lost in the discussion, resulting in needless anxiety and intervention.

Case study

Marina Hernandez is a 34-year-old G3, P1011 who presents for a return prenatal visit today at 30 weeks' gestation. Her first baby, Hector, was born in Mexico at home with the assistance of a traditional "partera" (midwife). Marina wants to talk about what to expect in the labor and delivery unit of the hospital where she will be giving birth. Marina states that Hector's birth was scary because "his shoulders got stuck before he came out." Marina stated that Hector weighed 11 lb at birth. Marina had some lab work done 2 weeks ago and the result of her 1-hour glucose screen was 150 mg/dL. The results of her 3-hour GTT were 89-190-175-65. Marina was diagnosed with GDM and met with the midwife and registered dietician for instruction on diet and capillary blood glucose testing. Marina does not have health insurance, so being able to pay for the expensive glucose test strips was a problem. The midwife placed a call to several CDEs in the area and was able to find one from a nearby clinic who had glucose strips available for purchase at a low cost. Marina was doing very well on her 2000-cal diet with 35–40% carbohydrates, once she reduced her portion sizes of rice and increased her beans and nonstarchy vegetables. She was testing four times daily for 3 weeks, and meeting all fasting and postprandial blood glucose targets, so the midwife and Marina jointly decided that it would be fine for Marina to test her BG twice daily, fasting and after dinner. The midwife estimated that Marina's baby was growing appropriately. Marina went on to have a normal, spontaneous vaginal birth of an 8# 10 oz female infant, "Lisbeth," with no delay or difficulty in the birth of Lisbeth's shoulders!

Resources for women and their families

Phone App that maps a walking route, calculates distance: http://www.mapmyrun.com/

Phone App that provides comprehensive nutrition information and tips on healthy eating and exercise: http://www.calorieking.com/

"Share with Women" document with information about Gestational Diabetes from the American College of Nurse-Midwives: http://www.midwife.org/ACNM/files/ccLibraryFiles/Filename/000000000637/Gestational%20Diabetes.pdf

Resources for health-care providers

American Diabetes Association (ADA): http://www.diabetes.org

Centers for Disease Control and Prevention: http://www.cdc.gov/diabetes

National Institute of Diabetes and Digestive and Kidney Diseases, National Institutes of Health: http://www.niddk.nih.gov/

References

American College of Obstetricians and Gynecologists (ACOG). (2000). Fetal macrosomia (Practice Bulletin #22). Washington, DC, Author.

American College of Obstetricians and Gynecologists (ACOG). (2001). Gestational diabetes mellitus (Technical Bulletin #30). Washington, DC, Author.

American College of Obstetricians and Gynecologists (ACOG). (2005). Pregestational diabetes mellitus (Practice Bulletin #60). Washington, DC, Author.

American College of Obstetricians and Gynecologists (ACOG). (2011). Screening and diagnosis of gestational diabetes mellitus (Committee Opinion #504). Washington, DC, Author.

American Diabetes Association. (2004). Gestational diabetes mellitus. *Diabetes Care, 27*(Suppl. 1), S88–S90.

American Diabetes Association (ADA). (2011). Diagnosis and classification of diabetes mellitus. *Diabetes Care, 34*(Suppl. 1), S62–S69.

Athukorala, C., Crowther, C. A., & Willson, K. (2007). Women with gestational diabetes mellitus in the ACHOIS trial: Risk factors for shoulder dystocia. *The Australian and New Zealand Journal of Obstetrics and Gynaecology, 47*(1), 37–41.

Barbour, L. A., McCurdy, C. E., Hernandez, T. L., Kirwan, J. P., Catalano, P. M., & Friedman, J. E. (2007). Cellular mechanisms for insulin resistance in normal pregnancy and gestational diabetes. *Diabetes Care, 30*(Suppl. 2), S112–S119.

Bellamy, L., Casas, J.-P., Hingorani, A. D., & Williams, D. (2009). Type 2 diabetes mellitus after gestational diabetes: A systematic review and meta-analysis. *Lancet, 373*, 1773–1779.

Biggio, J. R., Chapman, V., Neely, C., Cliver, S. P., & Rouse, D. J. (2010). Fetal anomalies in obese women: The contribution of diabetes. *Obstetrics & Gynecology, 115*(2 Pt 1), 290–296. doi:10.1097/AOG.0b013e3181c9b8c3

Blackburn, S. T. (2013). Chapter 16: Carbohydrate, fat, and protein metabolism. In S. T. Blackburn (Ed.), *Maternal, fetal, & neonatal physiology* (4th ed., pp. 560–588). Maryland Heights, MO: Elsevier Saunders.

Bodmer-Roy, S., Morin, L., Cousinea, J., & Re, E. (2012). Pregnancy outcomes in women with and without gestational diabetes mellitus according to the international association of the diabetes and pregnancy study groups criteria. *Obstetrics & Gynecology, 120*(4), 746–752. doi:10.1097/AOG.0b013e31826994ec

Brankston, G. N., Mitchell, B. F., Ryan, E. A., & Okun, N. B. (2004). Resistance exercise decreases the need for insulin in overweight women with gestational diabetes mellitus. *American Journal of Obstetrics and Gynecology, 190*, 188–193.

Chauhan, S. P., Grobman, W. A., Gherman, R. A., Chauhan, V. B., Chang, G., Magann, E. F., & Hendrix, N. W. (2005). Suspicion and treatment of the macrosomic fetus: A review. *American Journal of Obstetrics and Gynecology, 193*, 332–346.

Chen, Y., Block-Kurbisch, I., & Caughy, A. (2009). Carpenter-Coustan criteria compared with the National Diabetes Data Group thresholds for gestational diabetes mellitus. *Obstetrics & Gynecology, 114*(2), 326–334.

Colberg, S. R., Sigal, R. J., Fernhall, B., Regensteiner, J. G., Blissmer, B. J., Rubin, R. R., . . . Braun, B. (2010). Exercise and type 2 diabetes: The American College of Sports Medicine and the American Diabetes Association joint position statement executive summary. *Diabetes Care, 33*(12), 2692–2696.

Conway, D. L. (2007). Obstetric management in gestational diabetes. *Diabetes Care, 30*(Suppl. 2), S175–S179.

Crowther, C. A., Hiller, J. E., Moss, J. R., McPhee, A. J., Jeffries, W. S., & Robinson, J. S.; Australian Carbohydrate Intolerance Study in Pregnant Women (ACHOIS) Trial Group. (2005). Effect of treatment of gestational diabetes mellitus on pregnancy outcomes. *New England Journal of Medicine, 352*(24), 2477–2486.

Cundy, T., Gamble, G., Townend, K., Henley, P. G., MacPherson, P., & Roberts, A. B. (2000). Perinatal mortality in type 2 diabetes mellitus. *Diabetic Medicine, 17*(1), 33–39.

Cunningham, F., Leveno, K., Bloom, S., Hauth, J., Rouse, D., & Spong, C. (2010). *Williams obstetrics* (23rd ed.). New York: McGraw Hill Medical.

Dhulkotia, J. S., Ola, B., Fraser, R., & Farrell, T. (2010). Oral hypoglycemic agents vs insulin in management of gestational diabetes: A systematic review and meta-analysis. *American Journal of Obstetrics and Gynecology, 203*, 457.e1–457.e9.

Dronavalli, S., & Ehrmann, D. A. (2007). Pharmacologic therapy of polycystic ovary syndrome. *Clinical Obstetrics and Gynecology, 50*(1), 244–254.

Flegal, K. M., Carroll, M. D., Kit, B. K., & Ogden, C. L. (2012). Prevalence of obesity and trends in the distribution of body mass index among US adults, 1999–2010. *Journal of the American Medical Association, 307*(5), 491–497.

Gorgal, R., Gonçalves, E., Barros, M., Namora, G., Magalhães, Â., Rodrigues, T., & Montenegro, N. (2012). Gestational diabetes mellitus: A risk factor for non-elective cesarean section. *Journal of Obstetrics and Gynaecology Research, 38*, 154–159. doi:10.1111/j.1447-0756.2011.01659.x

HAPO Study Cooperative Research Group, Metzger, B. E., Lowe, L. P., Dyer, A. R., Trimble, E. R., Chaovarindr, U., . . . Sacks, D. A. (2008). Hyperglycemia and adverse pregnancy outcomes. *The New England Journal of Medicine, 358*(19), 1991–2002.

Hawkins, J. S., & Casey, B. M. (2007). Labor and delivery management for women with diabetes. *Obstetrics and Gynecology Clinics of North America, 34*(2), 323–334.

Hillier, T., Vesco, K., Whitlock, E., Pettitt, D., Pedula, K., & Beil, T. (2008). *Screening for gestational diabetes mellitus. Evidence synthesis No. 60.* AHRQ Publication No. 08-05115-EF-1. Rockville, MD: Agency for Healthcare Research and Quality.

Horvath, K., Koch, K., Jeitler, K., Matyas, E., Bender, R., Bastian, H., . . . Siebenhofer, A. (2010). Effects of treatment in women with gestational diabetes mellitus: Systematic review and meta-analysis. *BMJ (Clinical Research Ed.), 340,* c1395.

Humphries, J., Reynolds, D., Bell-Scarbrough, L., Lynn, N., Scardo, J. A., & Chauhan, S. P. (2002). Sonographic estimate of birth weight: Relative accuracy of sonographers versus maternal-fetal medicine specialists. *The Journal of Maternal-fetal and Neonatal Medicine, 11,* 108–112.

Idris, N., Wong, S., Thomae, M., Gardener, G., & McIntyre, D. (2010). Influence of polyhydramnios on perinatal outcome in pregestational diabetic pregnancies. *Ultrasound in Obstetrics and Gynecology, 36,* 338–343.

International Association of Diabetes in Pregnancy Study Groups (IADPSG). (2010). International association of diabetes and pregnancy study groups recommendations on the diagnosis and classification of hyperglycemia in pregnancy. *Diabetes Care, 33*(3), 676–682.

Kirwan, J. P., Haugel-DeMouzon, S., Lepercq, J., Challier, J.-C.,Huston-Presley, L., Friedman, J. E., . . . Catalano, P. M. (2002). TNF-α is a predictor of insulin resistance in human pregnancy. *Diabetes, 51,* 2207–2213.

Kjos, S. L., & Buchanan, T. A. (1999). Gestational diabetes mellitus. *The New England Journal of Medicine, 341,* 1749–1756. doi:10.1056/NEJM199912023412307

Kozhimannil, K. B., Pereira, M. A., & Harlow, B. L. (2009). Association between diabetes and perinatal depression among low-income mothers. *JAMA: The Journal of the American Medical Association, 301*(8), 842.

Landon, M. B., & Gabbe, S. G. (2011). Gestational diabetes mellitus. *Obstetrics & Gynecology, 118*(6), 1379–1393.

Langer, O., Conway, D. L., Berkus, M. D., Xenakis, E. M.-J., & Gonzales, O. (2000). A comparison of glyburide and insulin in women with gestational diabetes mellitus. *New England Journal of Medicine, 343,* 1134–1138.

Langer, O., Umans, J., & Miodovnik, M. (2013). Perspectives on the proposed gestational diabetes mellitus diagnostic criteria. *Obstetrics and Gynecology, 121*(1), 177–182. doi:10.1097/AOG.0b013e31827711e5

Loomis, L., Lee, J., & Tweed, E. (2006). What is appropriate fetal surveillance of women with diet-controlled gestational diabetes? *The Journal of Family Practice, 55*(3), 238–241.

Mazze, R. S., Strock, E., Simonson, G. D., & Bergenstal, R. M. (2007). *Prevention, detection and treatment of diabetes in adults* (4th ed.). Minneapolis, MN: International Diabetes Center, Park Nicollet Institute.

McLaren, R. A., Puckett, J. L., & Chauhan, S. P. (1995). Estimators of birth weight in pregnant women requiring insulin: A comparison of seven sonographic models. *Obstetrics and Gynecology, 85,* 565–569.

Melamed, N., Yogev, Y., Meizner, I., Mashiach, R., Pardo, J., & Ben-Haroush, A. (2011). Prediction of fetal macrosomia: Effect of sonographic fetal weight-estimation model and threshold used. *Ultrasound in Obstetrics & Gynecology, 38*(1), 74–81.

Melczer, Z., Banhidy, F., Csomor, S., Kovacs, M., Winkler, G., & Cseh, K. (2003). Influence of leptin and the TNF system on insulin resistance in pregnancy and their effect on anthropomorphic parameters of newborns. *Acta Obstetricia et Gynecologica Scandinavica, 82*(5), 432–438.

Metzger, B. E. (2007). Long-term outcomes in mothers diagnosed with gestational diabetes mellitus and their offspring. *Clinical Obstetrics and Gynecology, 50*(4), 972–979.

Metzger, B. E., Gabbe, S. G., Persson, B., Buchanan, T. A., Catalano, P. M., Damm, P., . . . Omori, Y. (2012). International Association of Diabetes & Pregnancy Study Groups (IADPSG) Consensus Panel Writing Group and the Hyperglycemia & Adverse Pregnancy Outcome (HAPO) Study Steering Committee, *Journal of Maternal, Fetal, & Neonatal Medicine, 12,* 2564–2569. doi:10.3109/14767058.2012.718002

Moore, T. R., & Catalano, P. (2009). Diabetes in pregnancy. In R. K. Creasy, R. Resnick, J. D. Iams, C. J. Lockwood, & T. R. Moore (Eds.), *Creasy & Resnick's maternal-fetal medicine: Principles and practice* (pp. 953–994). Philadelphia: Saunders.

Moore, L. E., Clokey, D., Rappaport, V. J., & Curet, L. B. (2010). Metformin compared with glyburide in gestational diabetes: A randomized controlled trial. *Obstetrics & Gynecology, 115*(1), 55–59.

O'Neill, E., & Thorp, J. (2012). Antepartum evaluation of the fetus and fetal well being. *Clinical Obstetrics and Gynecology, 55*(3), 722–730.

Retnakaran, R., Qi, Y., Sermer, M., Connelly, P. W., Hanley, A. J. G., & Zinman, B. (2010). β-Cell function declines within the first year postpartum in women with recent glucose intolerance in pregnancy. *Diabetes Care, 33*(8), 1798–1802.

Rowan, J. A., Hague, W. M., Gao, W., Battin, M. R., & Moore, M. P.; for the MiG Trial Investigators. (2008). Metformin versus insulin for the treatment of gestational diabetes. *The New England Journal of Medicine, 358,* 2003–2015. doi:10.1056/NEJMoa0707193

Schafer-Graf, U. M., Graf, K., Kulbacka, I., Kjos, S. L., Dudenhausen, J., Vetter, K., & Herrara, E. (2008). Maternal lipids as strong determinants of fetal environment and growth in pregnancies with gestational diabetes mellitus. *Diabetes Care, 31*(9), 1858–1863.

Shoham, I., Wiznitzer, A., Silberstein, T., Fraser, D., Holcberg, G., Katz, M., & Mazor, M. (2001). Gestational diabetes complicated by hydramnios was not associated with increased risk of perinatal morbidity and mortality. *European Journal of Obstetrics, Gynecology, and Reproductive Biology, 100*(1), 46.

Toulis, K. A., Goulis, D. G., Kolibianakis, E. M., Venetis, C. A., Tarlatzis, B. C., & Papadimas, I. (2009). Risk of gestational diabetes mellitus in women with polycystic ovary syndrome: A systematic review and a meta-analysis. *Fertility and Sterility, 92*(2), 667–677. doi:10.1016/j.fertnstert.2008.06.045; [Epub 2008 Aug 16].

Turok, D. K., Ratcliffe, S. D., & Baxley, E. G. (2003). Management of gestational diabetes mellitus. *American Family Physician, 68*(9), 1767–1772.

United States Preventive Services Task Force. (2008). Screening for gestational diabetes mellitus: US Preventative Services Task Force recommendation statement. Retrieved from http://www.guideline.gov/summary/summary.aspx?doc_id=12507&nbr=6437&ss=6&xl=999

Vink, J., Poggi, S., Ghidini, A., & Spong, C. (2006). Amniotic fluid index and birth weight: Is there a relationship in diabetics with poor glycemic control? *American Journal of Obstetrics and Gynecology, 195*(3), 848–850.

Wong, V. W. M. (2013). Gestational diabetes mellitus: A review of the diagnosis, clinical implications and management. *Reviews in Health Care, 4*(2), 127–139.

Xiong, X., Saunders, L. D., Wang, F. L., & Demianczuk, N. N. (2001). Gestational diabetes mellitus: Prevalence, risk factors, maternal and infant outcomes. *International Journal of Gynecology & Obstetrics, 75*(3), 221–228.

Yehuda, I., Nagtalon-Ramos, J., & Trout, K. (2011). Fetal growth scans and amniotic fluid assessments in pregestational and gestational diabetes. *JOGNN, 40,* 603–616.

Zoupas, C. (2007). Summary and recommendations of the fifth international workshop-conference on gestational diabetes mellitus. *Diabetes Care, 30*(Suppl. 2), S251–S260.

24

Other complications in pregnancy: Multiple gestation, post-term pregnancy, hyperemesis, and abdominal pain

Tonya B. Nicholson

Relevant terms

Amnion—fetal cells that develop into the amniotic sac

Amniotic fluid index (AFI)—measurement of the amount of amniotic fluid using ultrasonography

Anovulatory cycle—menstrual cycle in which ovulation does not occur

Biophysical profile—fetal evaluation using ultrasound to assess for five factors: fetal movement, fetal tone, fetal breathing movements, fetal heart rate reactivity, and quantity of amniotic fluid

Bishop score—system to evaluate cervical inducibility; scores dilation, effacement, station, cervical consistency, and cervical position

Chorion—fetal cells that develop into the placenta

Dizygotic twins—twins resulting from the fertilization of two separate eggs

Erb's palsy—brachial plexus injury causing weakness or paralysis of the shoulder and upper arm

Glycemic index—measurement of how a given food affects blood glucose levels; a higher glycemic index indicates higher blood glucose levels and may adversely affect glucose control

Kleihauer–Betke test—maternal blood examination that tests for the presence of fetal hemoglobin; the presence of fetal hemoglobin in maternal circulation can alert the practitioner to consider if RhoGAM is indicated and to monitor for fetal complications

Late ovulation—ovulating later than day 14 in the menstrual cycle

Macrosomia—fetal birth weight >4500 g

Meconium aspiration syndrome—complication occurring during the birth process when the fetus aspirates amniotic fluid, which contains meconium; can be associated with fetal acidosis and/or pneumonia

Modified biophysical profile—fetal evaluation composed of nonstress test and amniotic fluid index

Monozygotic twins—twins resulting from the division of a single zygote produced from the fertilization of a single egg

Nonstress test—indirect assessment of fetal well-being in which the fetal heart rate is externally monitored for the presence of accelerations

Oligiohydramnios—decreased amount of amniotic fluid; amniotic fluid index (AFI) <5 cm

Polyzygotic gestation—multiple gestation resulting in three or more fetuses produced by any combination of monozygotic and polyzygotic twinning

Post-term pregnancy—pregnancy lasting more than 42 weeks' gestation

Stripping of the membranes—digital exam of the cervix wherein the examiner sweeps the finger between the cervix and the amniotic sac

Total parenteral nutrition (TPN)—intravenous nutrition including glucose, amino acids, lipids, vitamins, and minerals provided intravenously to prevent malnutrition in patients who are unable to obtain adequate nutrients orally

Twin-to-twin transfusion—syndrome in which the blood of one twin is transfused to the second twin; associated with fetal anemia and discordant growth

Wernicke's encephalopathy—a result of thiamine deficiency due to frequent vomiting

---

Prenatal and Postnatal Care: A Woman-Centered Approach, First Edition. Edited by Robin G. Jordan, Janet L. Engstrom, Julie A. Marfell, and Cindy L. Farley.
© 2014 John Wiley & Sons, Inc. Published 2014 by John Wiley & Sons, Inc.

Abdominal pain in pregnancy

Abdominal pain or discomfort is a common occurrence in pregnancy. A report of abdominal pain in pregnancy should be thoroughly investigated. Abdominal pain or discomfort in pregnancy most often has a normal basis and these conditions should be considered first if appropriate (Table 24.1). Information about comfort measures for these common conditions is found in Chapter 11, "Common Discomforts in Pregnancy." Although normal pregnancy changes explain many cases of abdominal pain, the possibility of pathology should always be considered. A delay in diagnosis of pathological causes of abdominal pain could be life threatening.

Evaluation of abdominal pain includes collection of thorough subjective and objective data. The use of "OLD CAARTS" can be helpful when collecting a history of pain symptoms.

Table 24.1   Normal Causes of Abdominal Pain in Pregnancy

Condition	Physiologic basis
Bloating	Progesterone and enlarged uterus slowing gastrointestinal (GI) motility allowing for increased gas formation
Prelabor (Braxton Hicks) contractions	Normal tightening of the uterine muscle often felt in the late third trimester
Constipation	Progesterone and enlarged uterus slowing GI motility
Heartburn	Progesterone relaxing esophageal sphincter and delayed gastric emptying time
Round ligament pain	Uterine growth causing stretching of ligaments supporting uterus

---

OLD CAARTS mnemonic

O = Onset: when and how the pain started

L = Location: specific location of the pain. Can you put a finger on it?

D = Duration: How long does it last?

C = Characteristics: What is the pain like—cramping, aching, stabbing, burning, tingling, itching, and so on?

A = Alleviating or aggravating factors: What makes the pain better (medication, position change, heat) and what makes it worse (e.g., specific activity, stress)?

A = Associated symptoms: gynecologic (dyspareunia, vaginal discharge, or bleeding), gastrointestinal (constipation, diarrhea), genitourinary (dysuria, urgency, incontinence), and neurological (specific nerve involvement)

R = Radiation: Does the pain move to other body areas?

T = Temporal: What time of day is it worse and better?

S = Severity: on a scale of 1–10.

Other components of the history should include a recent diet history, the presence of any bowel or bladder changes, change or new onset of nausea or vomiting, activity, and history of abdominal trauma such as fall, car accident, and violence.

The abdominal assessment should include fetal heart tones, detection of the presence of epigastric pain, abdominal guarding, overt or rebound tenderness, and the presence of any visible signs and symptoms of trauma. Careful documentation of any signs of trauma is vital.

Objective data that are potentially valuable may include maternal vital signs, complete blood count (CBC), urine analysis, liver enzymes, a Kleihauer–Betke test in cases of abdominal trauma, fetal nonstress testing or biophysical profile depending on gestational age, ultrasound (USN), computed tomography (CT), and other exams as determined with a consulting physician. If a pathological etiology to the woman's report of abdominal pain is suspected, immediate consultation and possible referral of care to a physician is indicated.

Preterm labor or threatened abortion should always be ruled out when presented with a report of abdominal pain in pregnancy depending on gestational age. Signs and symptoms that lead to a concern of preterm labor include the presence of rhythmic abdominal pain after 22 weeks' gestation. Pain related to preterm labor may also be reported as low back pain. Additional possible signs and symptoms of preterm labor include leaking of the amniotic fluid or vaginal bleeding. If a client presents with signs and symptoms that lead to a suspicion of preterm labor, this condition must be ruled out before proceeding to consider other etiologies of the abdominal pain. See Chapter 21 for more information regarding assessment and management of preterm labor.

Two common medical complications that can cause abdominal pain in pregnancy are appendicitis and cholecystitis. These two conditions account for the majority of nonobstetric surgical intervention for abdominal issues during pregnancy. Although both conditions occur rarely during pregnancy, because of the seriousness of potential complications during pregnancy, they should be considered with an unexplained presentation of abdominal pain during pregnancy (Gilo, Amini, & Landy, 2009).

Appendicitis

Appendicitis is the most common indication for non-obstetric surgeries during pregnancies, accounting for 25% of such surgeries (Gilo et al., 2009). Appendicitis occurs at the same rate in the pregnant population as in the nonpregnant population, but the chance of rupture of the appendix is higher during pregnancy. During pregnancy, rupture of the appendix occurs 4–57% of the time while it occurs at a rate of 4–19% in the nonpregnant population (Gilo et al., 2009). Complications of appendicitis in pregnancy include preterm birth and infection. Infectious risks include pneumonia, wound infection, and sepsis. One study reported that 22% of women who had an appendectomy delivered prematurely within 1 week of surgery, with the risk decreasing 1 week postsurgery (Gilo et al., 2009).

The diagnosis of appendicitis during pregnancy is not straightforward. Many of the symptoms of appendicitis can easily be confused with common pregnancy discomforts. General fatigue, mild or nonspecific right lower abdominal pain, and nausea and vomiting are commonly reported in normal pregnancies but are also the presenting symptoms reported with appendicitis. Right lower abdominal pain with rebound and guarding is the most commonly reported symptom of a pregnant woman with appendicitis. Unfortunately, this has led to a high rate of unnecessary surgeries. Among nonpregnant women, negative appendectomies are performed at a rate of 10–26% where within the pregnant population, this occurs at a rate of 40–50% (Gilo et al., 2009). If there is a concern of possible appendicitis, referral to a physician for definitive diagnosis is indicated.

Cholylithiasis

Gallstones are reported in 1–3% of pregnant women (Gilo et al., 2009). However, acute cholescystitis requiring intervention occurs during pregnancy at the same rate as in nonpregnant women. Suspicion of the presence of gallstones should be raised in the pregnant woman who is reporting colicky abdominal pain after consuming a fatty meal. It is important to also consider that up to half of people with gallstones are symptom free. When managing a pregnant woman with gallstones, further concern that there may be a need for intervention should be considered in women who have fever, right upper quadrant pain, elevated white blood cell count, nausea, vomiting, and decreased appetite (Gilo et al., 2009). The addition of these symptoms in the presence of abdominal pain should prompt physical referral for definitive diagnosis and management.

Abdominal trauma

One of the most common and most concerning reasons for abdominal pain in pregnancy is trauma. It is the most common nonobstetric cause of death during the childbearing year, occurring in about 7% of pregnancies (Mirza, Devine, & Gaddipati, 2010). Trauma in pregnancy is most often caused by motor vehicle accidents (MVAs), falls, and physical assault. Pregnant women with a history of substance abuse, younger age, and a history of domestic violence are more likely to experience abdominal trauma during pregnancy (Mirza et al., 2010).

The majority of trauma during pregnancy is caused by MVAs. Many of these MVAs are associated with illicit drug use and/or alcohol use in the pregnant client (Oxford & Ludmir, 2009). This highlights the importance of discussing the use of automobile restraints and the effects of drug and alcohol use with all pregnant women during prenatal care visits.

It is estimated that 7–23% of all pregnant women suffer from domestic violence resulting in trauma during their pregnancy (Oxford & Ludmir, 2009). Many pregnant women who are abused have the abdomen as a target of the violence (Graham-Kevan & Archer, 2011). Midwives and nurse practitioners should routinely screen women for intimate partner violence and provide appropriate counseling and referral (see Chapter 14, "Social Issues in Pregnancy"). Possible complications of trauma during pregnancy include uterine rupture, placental abruption, direct fetal injury, and maternal injury or death.

Women with abdominal trauma should be referred for physician evaluation and management or comanagement if the provider does not have inpatient privileges. Maternal and fetal assessment must be initiated with the ability to intervene for birth if appropriate with regard to findings and gestational age.

Hyperemesis gravidarum (HG)

Nausea and vomiting are common during early pregnancy, experienced by more than 50% of all pregnant women. Although these symptoms are distressing, they are typically benign and self-limited, with most women experiencing relief by 12–14 weeks' gestation. For some women, nausea and vomiting persists and is severe. HG is characterized by persistent and severe nausea and vomiting, dehydration, fluid and electrolyte imbalance, and weight loss. Some women lose 5% or more of their prepregnancy weight (Goodwin, 2008; Ismail & Kenny, 2007; McCormack, 2010). HG negatively affects family, social, and occupational functioning as well as quality of life.

Table 24.2   Possible Etiologies of Hyperemesis Gravidarum (HG)

Factor	Comments
Increase in human chorionic gonadotropin (hCG)	HG is more common in multiple gestation, gestational trophoblastic disease, and in fetuses with Down syndrome, both conditions that increase maternal hCG.
Increase in estrogen	Estrogen decreases intestinal motility, leading to nausea and vomiting. Women carrying female fetuses are more likely to experience HG than those carrying male fetuses.
Increase in thyroid hormone production	High levels of thyroid hormone can cause gestational transient thyrotoxicosis, a condition been observed in up to two-thirds of women with HG.
Helicobacter pylori infection	*H. pylori* infection can exacerbate nausea and vomiting of pregnancy (NVP) and is more common in women with HG

Adapted from: Jueckstock, Kaestner, and Mylonas (2010); Kelly and Savides (2009); Summers (2012).

Etiology and risk factors

The exact cause of HG is unknown, but it likely has a multifactorial etiology (Tan & Omar, 2011) (Table 24.2). Evidence suggests a strong maternal genetic component to HG with many women experiencing recurrence of HD in subsequent pregnancies (Fejzo, MacGibbon, Romero, Goodwin, & Mullin, 2011; Zhang et al., 2011).

An assumption is often made that women with severe nausea and vomiting during pregnancy are transforming psychological distress into physical symptoms. A commonly used explanation for the development of HG was vomiting as a subconscious wish for an abortion or, in a different approach, a conversion disorder underlying the condition (Munch, 2002). Immature personality and pathological attention seeking have also been promoted as psychogenic etiologies of HG. Although these might be the cause in individual cases, the generally accepted perspective is that psychological afflictions are likely a consequence of constant vomiting rather than the source of it (Sheehan, 2007). Focusing entirely on psychogenic factors raises the risk that women are not taken seriously in their suffering and not all existing therapeutic options may be considered with this perspective. Conversely, neglecting the psychosomatic aspects in the development and course of HG in some women has the risk of treating only the symptoms of the condition without further exploration. The psychosomatic aspects of

hyperemesis should be considered, but they are generally not considered a precursor.

Complications of hyperemesis gravidarum

HG affects women of all ethnicities and is the most common cause of hospitalization in the first half of pregnancy, second only to preterm labor for pregnancy hospitalizations overall (Gazmararian et al., 2002). Vomiting-induced esophageal rupture can result in gastrointestinal bleeding. Wernicke's encephalopathy, which normally occurs after several weeks of vomiting, is caused by thiamine deficiency and is a potentially fatal medical emergency. It is reversible but can cause persistent neurological deficits (Chiossi, Neri, Cavazzuti, Basso, & Facchinetti, 2006). Signs and symptoms of Wernicke's encephalopathy are weakness or paralysis of the eye muscles, ataxia, and mental confusion (Ismail & Kenny, 2007). In women with HG, the most common sign of Wernicke's encephalopathy is apathy or confusion (Goodwin, 2008). Persistent vomiting can also cause hyponatremia. Early signs of hyponatremia such as anorexia, headache, nausea and vomiting, and lethargy can be missed since the clinical presentation is similar to HG itself. Fetal complications include fetal growth restriction, preterm birth, and small-for-gestational-age (SGA) infants. The possibility of HG occurring in subsequent pregnancies is approximately 15% (Ismail & Kenny, 2007).

Evaluation

Whenever a pregnant woman has nausea and vomiting, the first priority is a thorough assessment to determine the severity of the problem. See Chapter 11, "Common Discomforts in Pregnancy," for the evaluation of nausea and vomiting severity. The onset of nausea and vomiting related to HG is typically prior to 10 weeks' gestation. Other symptoms of HG include fatigue, exhaustion, ketonuria, and weight loss. Women often report inability to go to work or to perform activities of daily living (ADL). Ptyalism may be present. The urine is examined for the presence of ketones. Other laboratory tests may include a urinalysis, a CBC, electrolytes, liver enzymes, and bilirubin levels. These tests help route the presence of underlying diseases such as gastroenteritis, or pyelonephritis, pancreatitis, cholecystitis, and hepatitis. There is an association between HG and hyperthyroidism; therefore, thyroid levels should be obtained. Multiple pregnancy, trophoblastic disorders, and neoplasias should be excluded by USN.

Care and management

Women presenting with HG have typically attempted dietary and lifestyle measures to reduce nausea and vomiting without success (see Chapter 11). Antiemetics and intravenous (IV) rehydration are important therapies in the management of women with HG. Ondansetron is one of the more commonly used and effective drugs and has relatively few side effects. Diazepam also improves HG due to its sedative properties. A clinical trial demonstrated that a combination of antiemetic therapy and diazepam reduced the need for hospitalization and improved patient satisfaction (Reichmann & Kirkbride, 2008).

The treatment of dehydration is of utmost importance. One or two liters of normal saline often help women feel less nauseated. Volume and electrolyte replacement and parenteral administration of carbohydrate and amino acid solutions are recommended (Jueckstock et al., 2010). Thiamine supplementation should be initiated with IV fluids for women who have had vomiting for longer than 3 weeks duration. Daily oral dosing of 1.5 mg thiamine is started once an adequate diet can be consumed (Wegrzyniak, Repke, & Ural, 2012).

Food is withdrawn until dehydration is corrected and vomiting is reduced. Subsequent food reintroduction is carried out gradually. The diet should consist of low-fat, low-spice foods eaten in small quantities every 2–3 hours. Sleep disturbances often accompany HG, and adequate rest should be promoted with environmental management or brief pharmacological therapy if needed.

Women with HG are often managed on an outpatient basis, even on IV therapy. For those women with severe dehydration, ketonuria, weight loss >5%, and the inability to keep down any food or fluids, inpatient admission may be required.

Advice for women with HG

- Eat dry, bland, low-fat foods if possible every 2–3 hours.
- Eat what will stay down rather than try to follow a diet plan.
- Well-tolerated foods include nongreasy, dry, sweet, and salty foods.
- Separate liquids from solids and alternate every 2–3 hours.
- Cold foods may be better tolerated than warm foods.
- Suck on popsicles throughout the day.
- Avoid nausea triggers such as cooking food odors and cigarette smoke.
- Obtain adequate rest.

For those women with refractory cases of HG, corticosteroids and total parenteral nutrition (TPN) may be useful (Jueckstock et al., 2010). Medical termination of pregnancy is also a consideration for women with severe HG.

HG is a distressing condition and lack of support from care providers and family can increase the distress and affect the psychological disposition of the women. Women are often unable to perform their usual daily activities and have a psychological burden of not feeling well for many weeks or months. Women with HG may feel helpless and incapable and poorly understood by their families, adding to their psychological distress. Secondary depression affects up to 7% of women with HG (Poursharif et al., 2008). Concerns regarding fetal well-being also contribute to maternal emotional distress. Providing care and support, and encouraging family members to do the same, can relieve the psychological burden of the condition. Counseling, psychological support, and evaluation for depression are important components of care to promote positive outcomes for women with HG.

Women with HG may be appropriately managed by nurse practitioners and midwives with physician consultation or comanagement as required by the woman's condition. Women hospitalized with HG may require referral for management if the provider does not have inpatient privileges.

Multifetal pregnancy

Multifetal gestation occurs when the uterus nurtures more than one fetus. Approximately 3% of all pregnancies carry multiple fetuses (Fox et al., 2010). The rate of twin birth has increased by 47% since 1990 primarily due to the increased use of assisted reproductive techniques (Martin et al., 2011). The majority of multiple gestation pregnancies are twin pregnancies with an incidence of approximately 33.2/1000 births (Martin et al., 2011). The triple birth rate has increased approximately 4% to 1.5/1000 births (Martin et al., 2011).

There are three types of multifetal pregnancies. Monozygotic pregnancy occurs when one egg is fertilized and there is subsequent division of this single zygote into two or more zygotes. This pregnancy results in identical twins, with each carrying the same genetic material. Dizygotic twinning occurs when two eggs are released and fertilized by different sperm. Dizygotic twins are commonly referred to as fraternal twins and are the most common kind of multiple birth in humans, occurring in about 1 out of every 80 pregnancies. Polyzygotic twinning is a result from any combination of dizygotic and monozygotic twinning and is most common with assisted reproduction. The timing of the division of the single zygote in monozygotic twinning may result in one or two amnions (amniotic sacs) and one or two chorions (placentas). If the division of the fertilized egg is a little later, conjoined twins can result. Early ultrasonographic evaluation to determine the number of amnions and chorions helps to guide the care of the pregnant woman. Twins that share amnions and/or chorions are at higher risk for complications and should be evaluated by a perinatologist.

Multifetal gestation may be diagnosed at an early prenatal visit via an early dating USN or by USN done as a result of a clinical assessment of uterine size larger than dates. Women with multifetal gestation often report a higher degree of nausea and vomiting than women with a singleton pregnancy. Other common discomforts such as backache, edema, and urinary frequency are greater in correlation with the higher degree of maternal adaptation required in multifetal gestation.

After making an initial diagnosis of a multiple pregnancy, prenatal care must be carefully orchestrated with a specialty physician. Preterm birth is the major reason for higher neonatal morbidity and mortality in multifetal gestation. The risk of low birth weight and very low birth weight increases 10-fold in a multiple pregnancy (Martin et al., 2011). The presence of a multifetal gestation also presents increased maternal risks such as gestational diabetes, gestational hypertension, preeclampsia, acute fatty liver, and pulmonary embolism (American College of Obstetricians and Gynecologists (ACOG), 2004a).

Care of women with multifetal gestation
Decreasing risk of preterm birth

Many of the decisions made in caring for women with multifetal pregnancy are aimed at predicting those at an increased risk for preterm birth and then acting to decrease that risk. In an effort to predict preterm birth, close surveillance of cervical length and/or fetal fibronectin testing is sometimes utilized in collaboration with the consulting physician. Efforts to decrease an individual woman's risk of preterm birth should be aimed at interventions that have potential for change, such as reducing stress, encouraging optimal nutrition, and providing early identification and management of any complications.

A commonly used intervention for multiple pregnancy is the use of modified or complete bed rest. Evidence has not demonstrated this to be of strong benefit in preventing preterm birth (Crowther & Han, 2010) and often induces harm. Side effects of bed rest include muscle atrophy and weakness, depression, decreased maternal weight gain, and fatigue. Many women who were prescribed inpatient bed rest also had the

additional stressor of leaving families at home and this added to maternal anxiety (Maloni, Margevicius, & Damato, 2006).

The administration of progesterone has documented efficacy in decreased preterm birth for women with singleton pregnancies; however, progesterone has no demonstrated benefit in prolonging pregnancy for the woman with a multifetal pregnancy (Dodd, Flenady, Cincotta, & Crowther, 2008). Tocolytics are commonly used in women with multiples in an effort to reduce the risk of preterm birth. Studies have been inconsistent on the effectiveness of this strategy in a woman with multiples and have documented an increased risk of pulmonary embolism (ACOG, 2004a). As with other women experiencing preterm labor, corticosteroids are administered to speed fetal lung maturity. The management of women with multifetal pregnancy in preterm labor should occur under the direction of a physician.

Assessing fetal growth

Serial USNs are indicated in the third trimester to monitor fetal growth. One of the most concerning findings when monitoring a multiple gestation is discordant growth. This has also been referred to as twin-to-twin transfusion. In this situation, the fetuses do not grow at comparable rates. This may occur for many reasons including placental problems, fetal malformation, infection, or umbilical cord differences. If a difference in the estimated fetal weight of 15% or greater is found by USN, this is considered to be discordance in the fetal weights. A multiple pregnancy complicated by this condition should be evaluated and managed by a perinatal specialist.

Fetal surveillance

Women with multifetal pregnancy are at an increased risk of preterm birth, intrauterine growth restriction, and fetal death. Evidence suggests that an increased schedule of fetal surveillance can allow for prolonged pregnancy and yield improved fetal outcomes. Although there is insufficient evidence to recommend a specific schedule for USN assessment of twin gestation, most experts recommend serial USN assessment every 2–3 weeks, starting at 16 weeks of gestation for monochorionic pregnancies and every 3–4 weeks, starting from 18 to 22 weeks for dichorionic pregnancies (Morin & Lim, 2011). A prospective cohort study of 1028 women with twin gestation reported low morbidity and mortality utilizing an intensive monitoring schedule of twice weekly USN examinations starting at 24 weeks for

Table 24.3   Recommended Weight Gain and Caloric Intake in Twin Pregnancy

Prepregnant BMI	Underweight BMI ≤ 18.5	Normal weight BMI = 18.5–24.9	Overweight BMI = 25–29.9	Obese BMI = ≥30
Recommended weight gain for twin pregnancy (lb)	–	37–54	31–50	25–42
Daily caloric needs (calories)	4000	3500	3200	3000

Note that there are no specific weight gain recommendations for underweight women. This information assumes pregnancy duration of 37–42 weeks.
Adapted from: Institute of Medicine (IOM) (2009), Luke (2005).

dichorionic twins and at 16 weeks for monochorionic twins (Breathnach et al., 2012). Evaluation of amniotic fluid volume and biophysical profile scoring are commonly used in multifetal gestation.

Nutritional counseling

Midwives and nurse practitioners may be involved in nutritional counseling of women with a multifetal gestation. Increased maternal weight gain during pregnancy is recommended for the woman carrying more than one fetus. The pattern of weight gain is also important (Table 24.3). For women with a twin pregnancy and a normal body mass index (BMI), a total weight gain of 40–54 lb is recommended with a weight gain pattern of 1–1.5 lb/week from 0 to 20 weeks' gestation, 1.25–1.75 lb/week from 20 to 28 weeks, and 1 lb/week after 28 weeks (Luke, 2005). Nutritional teaching for the mother who is expecting multiple babies is of paramount importance.

Women should be advised that optimal nutrition improves fetal growth and development, reduces risk of perinatal complications, and reduces the risk of preterm labor and birth (Fox et al., 2010). It is appropriate to teach the woman to consider the glycemic index of foods in an effort to combat changes in carbohydrate metabolism during pregnancy (Luke, 2005).

Additional dietary supplementation is often needed to meet increased fetal requirements. Routine supplementation of approximately 30 mg elemental iron daily is advised (Goodnight & Newman, 2009). Supplementation with calcium, magnesium, and zinc has a potential protective effect against the development of hypertensive disorders in pregnancy and preterm birth (Luke, 2005). Supplementation with omega-3 fatty acids is beneficial for fetal neurological development in twin gestation. There are no consensus recommendations for omega-3 fatty acid intake in twin gestation, though amounts of 300–500 mg daily have been advised to accommodate

increased needs in twin gestation (Goodnight & Newman, 2009).

Anticipatory guidance

Women with a multifetal pregnancy should be counseled that they will likely have an increase in the common discomforts of pregnancy due to an even greater increase in hormonal fluctuations, circulating blood volume, fetal mass, and weight gain. The increased size of the uterus may result in increased intra-abdominal pressure and increased difficulty in ambulation. Women with a multifetal gestation will also be seen more frequently for antepartum visits and often give birth prior to term. As the pregnancy progresses and the family is preparing for the birth of the babies, special consideration should be given to identify support and resources for additional help at home. Antepartum lactation consultation can also improve the rate of postpartum breastfeeding in twin pregnancies. She will be facing the demands of more than one newborn and this can lead to increased stress and fatigue. Support for breastfeeding multiples can be sought through local agencies like Healthy Start, LaLeche League, and lactation support counselors.

Post-term pregnancy

Post-term pregnancy is defined as a pregnancy that has progressed beyond 42 completed weeks' gestation. This can also be defined as a pregnancy progressing more than 294 days from the last normal menstrual period (Caughey, Snegovskikh, & Norwitz, 2008). The actual cause of post-term pregnancy is unclear; the etiology and pathophysiology are not completely understood.

Overview

The incidence of post-term pregnancy in the United States is approximately 7% (Cleary-Goldman et al.,

2006). The incidence has decreased in the last decade, most likely due to an increase in the use of early USN for dating pregnancy, resulting in accuracy of pregnancy dating and the obstetrical trends of increased labor induction prior to term. Inaccurate pregnancy dating is the most common reason for post-term pregnancy. Late ovulation or an anovulatory cycle is more common than early ovulation, thus leading to an overestimation of gestational age when using the last menstrual period as the basis for pregnancy dating. An overestimation of gestational age can lead to increased misdiagnosis of post-term pregnancy (Caughey et al., 2011).

Risks factors for experiencing a post-term pregnancy include nulliparity, history of post-term pregnancy, maternal obesity, carrying a male fetus, and having a family history of post-term pregnancies (Mullin & Miller, 2010). Genetic factors may play a role. A woman with a history of one previous post-term pregnancy is more than two times more likely than a woman without a history of a post-term pregnancy to experience a subsequent post-term pregnancy and is almost four times as likely to have a post-term pregnancy if she has had two previous post-term pregnancies (Caughey et al., 2011).

Complications associated with post-term pregnancy

There are maternal and fetal risks associated with pregnancy after 42 weeks' gestation. Maternal risks include dysfunctional labor, operative birth, operative vaginal birth, perineal trauma, and postpartum hemorrhage. These complications are primarily associated with the increased risk of fetal macrosomia in the post-term infant. At 41 weeks' gestation, approximately 4% of infants will be macrosomic (>4500 g) (Mandruzzato et al., 2010). It is also likely that some of these adverse outcomes result from intervening when the uterus and the cervix are not ready for labor.

Fetal macrosomia increases the risk of shoulder dytocia and its associated potential problems. Meconium-stained fluid occurs in 25–30% of post-term pregnancies, increasing the risk of meconium aspiration syndrome. As the placenta begins to age, there are increased areas of infarction and deposition of calcium and fiber within the placental tissue. This creates decreased placental reserve and uteroplacental insufficiency. The volume of amniotic fluid normally begins to decrease after 38 weeks' gestation and may become problematic in post-term pregnancy. The incidence of oligohydramnios is higher after 42 weeks' gestation, which elevates the risk of cord compression and fetal distress during labor.

The incidence of stillbirth in the post-term infant is higher than that of the term infant. The rate of deaths *in utero* and in the early neonatal period in infants carried past 42 weeks' gestation is twice that of infants born before 42 weeks. If the pregnancy progresses to 43 weeks, the rate of perinatal mortality increases to six times higher than the term infant. The incidence of death during the first year of life is also increased for babies born post-term (ACOG, 2004b).

Prevention, intervention, and management options

The most important prevention for preventing post-term pregnancy and its serious risks is accurate pregnancy dating. The use of USN for dating of a pregnancy for women with an uncertain or unknown last menstrual period and in women with irregular cycles is imperative. Evidence suggests that use of first-trimester USN for pregnancy dating reduces the incidence of post-term pregnancy diagnosis (Caughey, Snegovkikh & Norwitz, 2008). Measurements for evaluation of gestational age include crown rump length in the first trimester and a combination of femur length and biparietal diameter in the second trimester. It is necessary, however, to understand the margin of error of USN dating at various times in each trimester. The estimation range using crown rump length is 3–5 days, while the estimation range from 12 to 20 weeks is 7–10 days. The estimation range increases to 14 days between 20 and 30 weeks' gestation. The use of USN for dating a pregnancy after 30 weeks is even less accurate (ACOG, 2004b). The use of first-trimester USN is considered the most accurate with regard to pregnancy dating (see Chapter 7, "Pregnancy Diagnosis and Assessing Gestational Age and Fetal Growth").

It is appropriate to consider management options prior to the postdates or the 42-week gestation mark. There are four options for the management of an impending postdates pregnancy: (1) labor-stimulating activities, (2) initiation of prenatal fetal surveillance, (3) elective induction of labor, and (4) expectant management.

Labor-stimulating activities

Labor-stimulating activities for the pregnancy that has progressed past the estimated date of birth (EDB) include stripping of the membranes. Stripping of the membranes is a mechanical separation of the amniotic membranes away from the wall of the uterus performed manually by the health-care provider. The cervix must be open enough to allow insertion of a finger, and the finger is swept along the wall of the cervix and lower uterus with the intention of gently pulling the membrane slightly away from the tissue. The woman needs to be informed that the process is uncomfortable and may result in some vaginal spotting. Overt bleeding should not occur and would need to be evaluated. Stripping of the membranes may result in the onset of labor but has not been shown to result in a decreased Cesarean section rate or to impact outcomes for mom and baby (Caughey et al., 2011).

Another suggestion to encourage spontaneous onset of labor is for the woman to have unprotected sexual intercourse with her partner. This exposes the uterus to prostaglandins in semen as well as endogenous prostaglandins released in the mother, similar to stripping of the membranes, causing uterine contractions (Caughey et al., 2011). Unprotected intercourse may lead to onset of labor, reduction in post-term pregnancy rates, and reduced rate of induction of labor (Kavanagh, Kelly, & Thomas, 2001; Schaffir, 2006).

Effective labor-stimulating activities

- Stripping of membranes
- Castor oil 60 mg po
- Unprotected intercourse

Castor oil is a potent cathartic derived from the bean of the castor plant. Castor oil is one of the most popular drugs for labor induction, used by many women worldwide outside of the medical setting (Montazeri, Afshary, Souri, & Iravani, 2010), with anecdotal reports dating back to ancient Egypt for use as a labor stimulant. A metabolite of castor oil, ricinoleic acid, activates intestinal and uterine smooth muscle cell activity stimulating the initiation of labor (Tunaru, Althoff, Nusing, Diener, & Offermans, 2012). This traditional method of inducing labor has not been well studied, and its use is very likely underreported. A randomized controlled clinical trial reported a significant increase in the initiation of spontaneous labor in women using one 60 mg oral dose of castor oil at term (Azhari, Pirdaded, Lotfalizadeh, & Shakeri, 2006). Women have added castor oil to other liquids such as juice or ice cream milk shakes to make the taste more palatable. No harmful effects of castor oil to the mother or the fetus have been documented (Boel et al., 2009). Women need to be informed that this method will also cause temporary diarrhea and abdominal cramping. As with other labor induction methods, castor oil is not likely to be effective if the woman's body is not yet physiologically ready for labor.

When discussing effective labor-stimulating strategies, women may bring up other traditional or folk methods, and it behooves midwives and nurse practitioners to be familiar with them. Evening primrose oil (EPO), is obtained by cold expression or solvent extraction from the seeds of the evening primrose plant, *Oenothera biennis*. EPO has been used by women for cervical ripening and labor induction or augmentation. Research to date suggests that EPO does not present post-term pregnancy or shorten labor (National Institutes of Health, 2012).

Fetal surveillance

There is no clear consensus regarding optimal timing to initiate fetal surveillance and which type of fetal surveillance is best. Additionally, there is no consensus in the literature regarding the method, timing, and benefit of routine testing in the postdate and post-term pregnancy (ACOG, 2004b; Divon & Feldman-Leidner, 2008). This makes it challenging for the provider to plan for the post-term pregnancy. It is common practice to initiate twice weekly testing using either biophysical profile or the modified physical profile (Mullin & Miller, 2010).

Prenatal surveillance of fetal well-being is typically initiated before the official post-term period has begun, around 40½–41 weeks' gestation. Physician consultation is indicated at this point to work together toward a plan for the post-term period. Common fetal surveillance options are presented in Table 24.4. Monitoring of amniotic fluid volume via the amniotic fluid index (AFI) or the deepest vertical pocket is an important component of surveillance.

Elective labor induction

Elective induction of labor in a woman with a pregnancy at 41 weeks or beyond and a favorable or inducible cervix are appropriate and have gained popularity. A favorable cervix is defined as achieving a Bishop score of ≥6 (Table 24.5). Most health-care providers agree that most women with known dates at 42 weeks' gestation should be considered candidates for labor induction. However, there is a lack of consensus on optimal management of women with a postdate pregnancy at 41 weeks' gestation. A systemic review of elective induction of labor at 41 weeks of gestation found a decreased risk for cesarean birth and meconium-stained amniotic fluid with elective induction (Caughey et al., 2009). Other studies report an increase in operative birth in low risk pregnancies with elective induction at 41 weeks or later (Oros et al., 2012). It is reasonable to approach each situation of postdate pregnancy within the context of the woman's health, parity, cervical status, estimated fetal weight, and

Table 24.4   Methods of Fetal Surveillance for Women Past Their EDB

Method	Frequency	Comments
Fetal movement count (FMC)	Daily	If pattern of movement decreases, further testing is indicated.
Nonstress test (NST)	Twice weekly	External fetal heart rate (FHR) monitoring. If nonreactive, consultation and further testing is indicated.
Biophysical profile (BPP)	Twice weekly	Performed using external FHR monitoring and ultrasonographic exam. If AFI is low, delivery is indicated even if all other parameters are normal. Consult for nonreassuring results.
Modified biophysical profile	Twice weekly	Performed using ultrasonographic exam; consult for nonreassuring results.
Amniotic fluid index (AFI)	Twice weekly	Combines NST and AFI; consult for nonreassuring results.
Contraction stress test (CST)	Weekly	External monitoring of fetal response to contractions (may be spontaneously occurring or induced by nipple stimulation or pitocin administration). If contractions are induced by the administration of pitocin, FHR must be monitored. This examination must occur in an inpatient setting and requires referral to a midwife or physician who can attend birth.

Table 24.5   Bishop Cervical Scoring

	0	1	2	3
Dilation	Closed	1–2 cm	3–4 cm	≥5 cm
Effacement (%)	0–30	40–50	60–70	≥80
Station	−3	−2	−1	+1, +2
Cervical consistency	Firm	Medium	Soft	–
Cervical position	Posterior	Midline	Anterior	–

preferences for birth. A discussion of risks and benefits can allow her the opportunity to make an informed decision regarding these alternative plans.

In a woman whose cervix is not favorable for induction, cervical ripening with a prostaglandin preparation can be indicated if and when induction of labor is undertaken. The majority of women who reach 42 weeks' gestation have an unfavorable cervix for induction with the Bishop score of less than 7 (Caughey et al., 2011). Several options are available for cervical ripening, each with a different preparation and application. The use of prostaglandins in the form of gel, suppository, or vaginal tablet is a common method of cervical ripening. Mechanical dilation with a Foley balloon catheter or laminaria placed within the cervix is also effective. Consultation or comanagement is common in women who are close to 42 weeks' gestation with an unripe cervix. The management of post-term pregnancy can be complex with multiple decisions to be made by both the health-care provider and the woman.

Resource for health-care providers

The Hypermesis Education and Research (HER) Foundation is the world's largest grassroots network of HG survivors and leading site for HG information on the Internet: http://www.helpher.org/

Resources for women and their families

A consumer Web site on differentiating different types of abdominal pain during pregnancy: http://www.babycenter.com/0_abdominal-pain-during-pregnancy_204.bc

A consumer Web site with information about multiple gestation from the ACOG: http://www.acog.org/~/media/For%20Patients/faq092.pdf?dmc=1&ts=20130324T0816204146

A consumer Web site with information about multiple gestation from the Society for Canadian Obstetrician Gynecologists (SCOG): http://www.sogc.org/health/pregnancy-multiple_e.asp

A "Share with Women" document with information about post-term pregnancy and stripping membranes from the American College of Nurse Midwives: http://www.midwife.org/ACNM/files/ccLibraryFiles/Filename/000000000669/Stripping%20Membranes.pdf

A consumer Web site with information about post-term pregnancy from the ACOG: http://www.acog.org/~/media/For%20Patients/faq069.pdf?dmc=1&ts=20130324T0835212828

Case study: Postdate pregnancy

Alisa is a 16-year-old primigravida who has been coming for prenatal care since her initial visit at 16 weeks' gestation. This is an unplanned pregnancy. Alisa's mother comes to most of her prenatal visits and is supportive.

Due to an unsure last menstrual period and a history of irregular periods, Alisa's pregnancy is dated by a USN at her initial visit. You have discussed with Alisa and her mother the limitations of using a second-trimester USN for establishing a due date. However, as the estimated due date approaches, Alisa and her mother grow insistent that she "can't keep on like this." They are requesting induction of labor and report concerns that the baby will get "too big."

In addressing Alisa's concerns, she's reassured that due dates are estimates, and that it is important to allow her baby to completely and fully develop before being born. Since USN dating of her pregnancy was done in the second trimester, her due date has a range of plus or minus 7–10 days. At 40.3 weeks' gestation, twice weekly nonstress tests (NSTs) and weekly measurements of the amniotic fluid index (AFI) are initiated. Alisa and her mother are reassured that her pregnancy is progressing well and the baby shows no signs of declining health. Alisa's involvement is enlisted by having her do fetal movement counting daily and reporting any change in the baby's fetal movement patterns.

Alisa's mother continues to verbalize concerns that the baby will "get too big." You reassure Alisa and her mother that you are monitoring fetal growth but that USN at this point in pregnancy is highly unreliable for estimation of fetal weight. You further explain that you are watching for extremes of baby's size and that if the baby's size is found to be at an extreme that is concerning, you will be aware and will share that with them.

Alisa's twice weekly visits continue with reactive NSTs and normal AFI findings. At 41.3 weeks' gestation, she is found to be 1–2 cm dilated and 50% effaced. With Alisa's permission, the midwife manually strips her membranes and discusses the probability that she will have increased abdominal cramping and some vaginal spotting following this procedure. Alisa is instructed to call or come in to the birth center with overt vaginal bleeding, leaking of fluid, or decreased fetal movement.

At 41.5 weeks' gestation, Alisa calls into the office to report that she has water running down her legs. She comes into office and rupture of membranes is confirmed, with clear fluid. She is found to be dilated to 3 cm and contracting regularly. She is subsequently admitted to the labor and birth unit and gives birth to a healthy baby girl weighing 7 lb and 9 oz after a 13-hour labor.

References

American College of Obstetricians and Gynecologists (ACOG). (2004a). ACOG practice bulletin number 56: Multiple gestation: Complicated twin, triplet, and high-order multifetal pregnancy. *Obstetrics and Gynecology, 104*(4), 869–883.

American College of Obstetricians and Gynecologists (ACOG). (2004b). ACOG Practice bulletin #55, management of post-term pregnancy. *Obstetrics and Gynecology, 104*(3), 639–646.

Azhari, S., Pirdaded, S., Lotfalizadeh, M., & Shakeri, M.T. (2006). Evaluation of the effect of castor oil on initiation labor in term pregnancy. *Saudi Medical Journal, 27*(7), 1011.

Boel, M. E., Lee, S. J., Rijken, M. J., Paw, M. K., Pimanpanarak, M., Tan, S. O., . . . McGready, R. (2009). Castor oil for induction of labour: Not harmful, not helpful. *Australian and New Zealand Journal of Obstetrics and Gynaecology, 49*(5), 499–503.

Breathnach, F. M., McAuliffe, F. M., Geary, M., Daly, S., Higgins, J. R., Dornan, J., . . . Malone, F. D. (2012). Optimum timing for planned delivery of uncomplicated monochorionic and dichorionic twin pregnancies. *Obstetrics & Gynecology, 119*(1), 50–59.

Caughey, A. B., Chelmow, D., Butler, J., Cowan, B. D., Talavera, F., Legro, R. S., & Gaupp, F. B. (2011). Post dates pregnancy. Medscape Retrieved from http://emedicine.medscape.com/article/261369

Caughey, A. B., Snegovskikh, V. V., & Norwitz, E. R. (2008). Post-term pregnancy: How can we improve outcomes. *Obstetrical and Gynecological Survey, 63*(11), 715–724.

Caughey, A. B., Sundaram, V., Kaimal, A. J., Gienger, A., Cheng, Y. W., McDonald, K. M., . . . Bravata, D. M. (2009). Systematic review: Elective induction of labor versus expectant management of pregnancy. *Annals of Internal Medicine, 151*(4), 252–263.

Chiossi, G., Neri, I., Cavazzuti, M., Basso, G., & Facchinetti, F. (2006). Hyperemesis gravidarum complicated by Wernicke encephalopathy: Background, case report, and review of the literature. *Obstetrical & Gynecological Survey, 61*(4), 255–268.

Cleary-Goldman, J., Bettes, B., Robinson, J. N., Norwitz, E., D'Alton, M. E., & Schulkin, J. (2006). Post-term pregnancy: Practice patterns of contemporary obstetricians and gynecologists. *American Journal of Perinatology, 23*(1), 15–20.

Crowther, C., & Han, S. (2010). Hospitalisation and bed rest for multiple pregnancy. *Cochrane Database of Systematic Reviews, (7),* CD000110.

Divon, M. Y., & Feldman-Leidner, N. (2008). Postdates and antenatal testing. *Seminars in Perinatology, 32*(4), 295.

Dodd, J. M., Flenady, V. J., Cincotta, R., & Crowther, C. A. (2008). Progesterone for the prevention of preterm birth. *Obstetrics and Gyencology, 112*(1), 127–134.

Fejzo, M. S., MacGibbon, K. W., Romero, R., Goodwin, T.M., & Mullin, P.M. (2011). Recurrence risk of hyperemesis gravidarum. *Journal of Midwifery and Women's Health, 56*(2), 132–136.

Fox, N. S., Rebarber, A., Roman, A., Klauser, C. K., Peress, D., & Saltzman, D. H. (2010). Weight gain in twin pregnancies and adverse outcomes. *Obstetrics and Gynecology, 116*(1), 100–106.

Gazmararian, J. A., Petersen, R., Jamieson, D. J., Schild, L., Adams, M. M., Deshpande, A. D., & Franks A. L. (2002). Hospitalizations during pregnancy among managed care enrollees. *Obstetrics and Gynecology, 100*, 94–100.

Gilo, N. B., Amini, D., & Landy, H. (2009). Appendicitis and cholecystitis in pregnancy. *Clinical Obstetrics and Gynecology, 52*(4), 586–596.

Goodnight, W., & Newman, R. (2009). Optimal nutrition for improved twin pregnancy outcome. *Obstetrics and Gynecology, 114*(5), 1121–1134.

Goodwin, T. M. (2008). Hyperemesis gravidarum. *Obstetrics and Gynecology Clinics of North America, 35*(3), 401–417.

Graham-Kevan, N., & Archer, J. (2011). Violence during pregnancy: Investigating infanticidal motives. *Journal of Family Violence, 26*(6), 453–458.

Institute of Medicine (IOM). (2009). *Weight gain during pregnancy: Reexamining the guidelines.* Washington DC: The National Academies Press.

Ismail, S. K., & Kenny, L. (2007). Review on hyperemesis gravidarum. *Best Practice and Research. Clinical Gastroenterology, 21*(5), 755–769.

Jueckstock, J. K., Kaestner, R., & Mylonas, I. (2010). Managing hyperemesis gravidarum: A multimodal challenge. *BMC Medicine, 8*(1), 46.

Kavanagh, J., Kelly, A. J., & Thomas, J. (2001). Sexual intercourse for cervical ripening and induction of labour. *Cochrane Database of Systematic Reviews, 2*, CD003093.

Kelly, T. F. & Savides, T. J. (2009). Gastrointestinal disease in pregnancy. In R. K. Creasy et al. (Eds.), *Creasy and Resnik's maternal fetal medicine: Principles and practice* (6th ed., pp. 1041–1057). Philadelphia: Saunders Elsevier.

Luke, B. (2005). Nutrition and multiple gestation. *Seminars in Perinatology, 29*(5), 349–353.

Maloni, J. A., Margevicius, S. P., & Damato, E. G. (2006). Multiple gestation: Side effects of antepartum bed rest. *Biological Research for Nursing, 8*(2), 115–128.

Mandruzzato, G., Alfirevic, Z., Chervenak, F., Gruenebaum, A., Heimstad, R., Heinonen, S., . . . Thilaganathan, B. (2010). Guidelines for the management of post-term pregnancy. *Journal of Perinatal Medicine, 38*, 111–119.

Martin, J., Hamilton, B., Ventura, S., Osterman, J., Kirmeyer, S., Matthews, T., & Wilson, E. C. (2011). *National vital statistics report; births: Final data for 2009.* Hyattsville, MD: National Center for Health Statistics.

McCormack, D. (2010). Hypnosis for hyperemesis gravidarum. *Journal of Obstetrics and Gynaecology, 30*(7), 647–653.

Mirza, F. G., Devine, P. C., & Gaddipati, S. (2010). Trauma in pregnancy: A systemic approach. *American Journal of Perinatology, 27*(7), 579–586.

Montazeri, S., Afshary, P., Souri, H., & Iravani, M. (2010). Efficacy of castor oil for induction and augmentation of labor. *Iranian Journal of Pharmaceutical Research, 3*(Suppl. 2), 38–39.

Morin, L., & Lim, K. (2011). Ultrasound in twin pregnancies. *Journal of Obstetrics and Gynaecology Canada, 33*(6), 643–656.

Mullin, P. M., & Miller, D. A. (2010). Post-term pregnancy. In T. M. Goodwin, M. Montoro, L. Muderspach, R. Paulson, & S. Roy (Eds.), *Management of common problems in obstetrics and gynecology* (5th ed., Chapter 4, pp. 12–16). Hoboken, NJ: Wiley & Sons.

Munch, S. (2002). Chicken or the egg? The biological–psychological controversy surrounding hyperemesis gravidarum. *Social Science & Medicine, 55*(7), 1267–1278.

National Institutes of Health. 2012. Evening Primrose oil. Retrieved from http://www.nlm.nih.gov/medlineplus/druginfo/natural/1006.html

Oros, D., Bejarano, M. P., Romero Cardiel, M., Oros-Espinosa, D., Gonzalez de Agüero, R., & Fabre, E. (2012). Low-risk pregnancy at 41 weeks: When should we induce labor? *Journal of Maternal-Fetal and Neonatal Medicine, 25*(6), 728–731.

Oxford, C. M., & Ludmir, J. (2009). Trauma in pregnancy. *Clinical Obstetrics and Gynecology, 52*(4), 611–629.

Poursharif, B., Korst, L. M., Fejzo, M. S., MacGibbon, K. W., Romero, R., & Goodwin, T. M. (2008). The psychosocial burden of hyperemesis gravidarum. *Journal of Perinatology, 28*, 176–181.

Reichmann, J. P., & Kirkbride, M. S. (2008). Nausea and vomiting of pregnancy: Cost effective pharmacologic treatments. *Managed Care (Langhorne, Pa.), 17*, 41–45.

Schaffir, J. (2006). Sexual intercourse at term and onset of labor. *Obstetrics and Gynecology, 107*(6), 1310–1314.

Sheehan, P. (2007). Hyperemesis gravidarum: Assessment and management. *Australian Family Physician, 36*(9), 698–701.

Summers, A. (2012). Emergency management of hyeperemesis gravidarum. *Emergency Nurse: The Journal of the RCN Accident and Emergency Nursing Association, 20*(4), 24.

Tan, P. C., & Omar, S. Z. (2011). Contemporary approaches to hyperemesis during pregnancy. *Current Opinion in Obstetrics and Gynecology, 23*(2), 87–93.

Tunaru, S., Althoff, T. F., Nusing, R. M., Diener, M. & Offermans, S. (2012). Castor oil induces laxation and uterus contractions via ricinoleic acid activation prostraglandin EP3 receptors. *Proceedings of the National Academy of Sciences, 109*(23), 9179–9184.

Wegrzyniak, L. J., Repke, J. T., & Ural, S. H. (2012). Treatment of hyperemesis gravidarum. *Reviews in Obstetrics and Gynecology, 5*(2), 78.

Zhang, Y., Cantor, R. M., MacGibbon, K., Romero, R., Goodwin, T. M., Mullin, P. M., & Fejzo, M. S. (2011). Familial aggregation of hyperemesis gravidarum. *American Journal of Obstetrics and Gynecology, 204*, 230.e1–230.e7.

25

Perinatal loss and grief

Robin G. Jordan

Introduction

The term "perinatal loss" encompasses loss of an infant through spontaneous or elective abortion, stillbirth, or early neonatal death (Moore, Parrish, & Perry Black, 2011). There are multiple terms to describe perinatal loss depending primarily on the gestational age at the time of loss. Diagnosis of a perinatal loss may come at a routine prenatal visit when fetal heart tones are not auscultated or may come following a report of decreased fetal movement or trauma. The diagnosis is confirmed by the absence of a heartbeat on ultrasound. After diagnosis is confirmed, the plan is dependent in part upon the gestational age at the time of death. Depression and anxiety are often sequelae in the woman who has had a perinatal loss (Gaudet, 2010). Emotional support and management of physical changes and concerns are integral parts of providing quality care after the diagnosis of a perinatal loss. This chapter focuses primarily on care and management of women experiencing stillbirth and grief reactions. Care and management after early pregnancy loss is covered in Chapter 19, "Bleeding During Pregnancy." Regardless of the timing and even in circumstances when the loss was elective, women and families who have experienced a loss are deeply affected. Women and their partners experience grief reactions after early pregnancy loss and need to receive emotional and supportive care from their nurse practitioner (NP) or midwife as outlined in this chapter.

Stillbirth

Stillbirth is defined as fetal loss after 20 completed weeks gestation and is one of the most common adverse

Prenatal and Postnatal Care: A Woman-Centered Approach, First Edition. Edited by Robin G. Jordan, Janet L. Engstrom, Julie A. Marfell, and Cindy L. Farley.
© 2014 John Wiley & Sons, Inc. Published 2014 by John Wiley & Sons, Inc.

pregnancy outcomes, occurring in approximately 1/160 pregnancies (American College of Obstetricians and Gynecologists (ACOG), 2009). The loss of a child and family member is a devastating experience for families and caregivers who may continue to experience grief for many years after the event. The cause of stillbirth is often difficult to determine with many cases unexplained. Certain risk factors are associated with stillbirth. Some of these include maternal age over 35, maternal obesity, multiple gestation, and African American race.

There are a number of known causes of stillbirth. Sometimes, more than one of these causes may contribute to a stillbirth (Table 25.1).

Other causes of stillbirth include trauma, postdate pregnancy past 42 weeks, Rh incompatibility between the blood of the mother and the baby, and asphyxia during a difficult labor and birth. These causes are uncommon.

Table 25.1   Etiology of Stillbirth

Factor	Comments
Birth defects	About 20% of stillborn babies have one or more birth defects or chromosomal disorders (ACOG, 2009).
Placental problems	Placental problems such as abruption contribute to approximately about 25% of stillbirths (Reddy, 2007). Women who smoke cigarettes or use cocaine during pregnancy are at an increased risk of placental abruption.
Fetal growth restriction	About 40% of stillborn babies have poor growth (Reddy, 2007). Smoking and hypertension are common risk factors for fetal growth restriction.
Infections	Infections involving the mother, the fetus, or the placenta appear to cause about 10–25% of stillbirths and contribute to a significant proportion of early fetal losses (Silver, 2007).
Chronic health conditions	About 10% of stillbirths are related to chronic health conditions such as hypertension, diabetes, kidney disease, and clotting disorders (Silver et al., 2007).
Umbilical cord accidents	Cord accidents such as true knot or abnormal cord insertion in the placenta can cause fetal anoxia and may contribute to about 2–4% of stillbirths (Eller, Branch, & Byrne, 2006).

Breaking the news

If an intrauterine fetal death is suspected, an ultrasound examination is required for diagnosis. If the ultrasound is not done in the office, the midwife or the NP should escort the woman to the ultrasound department for support during the ultrasound examination. Many midwifery and obstetrical care providers hear anecdotes about women being alone with the sonographer who is silent or vague during the examination, while the woman is asking repeatedly, "What's wrong?" Waiting for the arrival of the provider in this situation can cause extreme distress for the woman and is likely to be long remembered as a negative and painful experience. Telling a woman that her unborn infant has died is a difficult task for the prenatal care provider. The news should be given without delay in a private, quiet room. If she is unaccompanied, a call to her support person to come to the office should be offered. Using sympathetic but unambiguous language can prevent misunderstanding. It is appropriate for care providers and staff to express their sorrow for what has happened and can help women feel supported. Unless known, it is best to avoid speculation regarding the cause of death until investigations are complete. When appropriate, reassure the mother that the death was not due to anything she did or did not do. Allow time for the parents to ask questions and to consider their options and make decisions. There is usually no clinical need to expedite birth urgently and hasty intervention may not be in the best long-term interests of the parents. If clinically appropriate, the woman may wish to go home and return for induction at a later date. Some women need some time to adjust and come to believe the diagnosis before the initiation of induction of labor and others feel a sense of urgency to "get it over with."

Care and management of women with stillbirth

After 20 weeks' gestation, fetal loss is typically managed by induction of labor. A systematic review of 14 randomized trials on the use of misoprostol for the management of antepartum fetal death found misoprostol was 100% effective in achieving uterine evacuation within 48 hours in pregnancies between 18 and 28 weeks' gestation (Gómez Ponce de León & Wing, 2009). Induction of labor with pitocin is a common strategy for women with fetal loss after 28 weeks' gestation. Because there is no fetus to consider, pain management can be aggressive during labor induction. The compounding of extreme emotional pain with high levels of physical pain may deplete the woman's coping resources. Providing information to women and their families on how the baby may appear following birth is important in providing anticipatory guidance. Parents' fears are often worse than the reality. Support requests to normalize the birth experience such as cutting the umbilical cord or initiating skin-to-skin contact. Referral and coordination of care with the provider attending the woman during her labor is required. It can be beneficial to provide thorough information about making arrangements for the infant remains after labor induction (Lang et al., 2011).

The proportion of stillbirths that are reported as "explained" increases when there is a systematic comprehensive approach to investigation. Evaluating the cause of stillbirth can facilitate emotional closure for women and couples and can provide a basis for counseling regarding subsequent pregnancies. The evaluation can be facilitated by the midwife, NP, or physician consultant (Table 25.2). Additional evaluation tests may be performed, such as syphilis serology, or thyroid-stimulating hormone, depending on the woman's specific situation.

Table 25.2 Recommended Components of Stillbirth Evaluation

Autopsy
Placental pathology
Fetal karyotype
Klierhauer–Betke test on the mother
Indirect Coombs test for antibodies
Parvovirus B19 IgG and IgM
Toxicology screen
Lupus screen

Adapted from: Silver, 2010.

Grieving and emotional care after perinatal loss

Emotional healing takes longer than physical healing. Caring for a woman during the period following diagnosis of a perinatal loss requires the utilization of a holistic approach. Women who have had a loss at any time in gestation share commonalities in their feelings regarding the loss, though naturally there are variations in grief experience based on gestational age and each woman's individual situation. The depth and intensity of parental grief is variable and can be influenced by the level of prenatal attachment, stress during pregnancy, history of previous losses, and other personal factors (Stolberg, 2011). Emotional attachment to the pregnancy and the

developing fetus typically begins early in the first trimester, and feelings of loss and grief are often more intense than women expected regardless of the gestational age at the time of the loss. Women often feel alone with the sense of loss and unsure of how to grieve. A lack of understanding by others is not an uncommon experience for women who have had an early pregnancy loss. People who have not experienced it themselves may find it difficult to convey empathy, believing that since it was an early loss, the mother would not feel as attached and, thus, would not grieve as deeply. This may lead to unrealistic expectations of the parents' recovery and resolution of grief. The woman may not have even shared the news of her pregnancy and then finds herself needing to explain both events, or not even talk about it at all. The health-care provider may be one of a limited number of individuals with whom the mother can talk to process the experience and express her grief. More than half of women (55%) experiencing first-trimester pregnancy loss presented with significant psychological distress immediately, 25% at 3 months, 18% at 6 months, and 11% at 1 year (Lok, Yip, Lee, Sahota, & Chung, 2010). The pregnancy and the loss cease to be mentioned in conversations often because the subject is too painful or parents sense the discomfort other individuals may have with the topic. This may make the woman feel particularly isolated, contributing to prolonged grief or an interruption in the grieving process. Women who have experienced spontaneous pregnancy loss may find that interaction with pregnant friends and newborns or young children can be painful, leading to avoidance of encounters with certain friends and family, and increasing the sense of isolation.

The manner in which the provider interacts with the family will be remembered and can affect the grieving process (Heazell, 2009). Inappropriate or insensitive responses from the medical professionals can add to the distress and trauma experienced. It is imperative for the health-care provider to recognize and acknowledge the loss to the woman and her family. Appropriate use of language acknowledging that the couple lost a *baby* instead of a *pregnancy*, can be important in setting the stage so that the couple feels that it is acceptable to discuss the loss and the grief that they are experiencing. Statements that contain religious or moral judgments, or that minimize the loss from the parents' perspective (i.e., "Your baby would have suffered anyway") should be avoided (Kavanaugh, 2006). For many parents, the sense of loss related to losing a baby also includes the disappointment of loss of what the child's life might have been. The parents may benefit from the opportunity to discuss the dreams and aspirations that they held for this baby.

Table 25.3 Rights of Parents When a Baby Dies

Rights of parents when a baby dies
• To be given the opportunity to see, hold, touch, and bathe their baby at any time before and/or after death within reason
• To have photographs of their baby taken and made available to the parents or held in a secure place until the parents wish to see them
• To be given as many mementos as possible, for example, crib card, baby beads, ultrasound and/or other photos, lock of hair, baby clothing and blankets, feet and handprints and/or permanent molds, and record of weight and length
• To name their child and bond with him or her
• To observe cultural and religious practices
• To be cared for by an empathetic staff who will respect their feelings, thoughts, beliefs, and individual requests
• To be with each other throughout hospitalization as much as possible
• To be given time alone with their baby, allowing for individual needs
• To be informed of the grieving process
• To be given the option of donating their baby's cartilage, tissue, and/or organs for transplant or donating the baby's body to science
• To request an autopsy; in the case of miscarriage, to request to have or not have an autopsy or pathology exam as determined by applicable law
• To have information presented in terminology understandable to the parents regarding their baby's status and cause of death, including autopsy and pathology reports and medical records
• To plan a farewell ritual, burial, or cremation in compliance with local and state regulations and according to their personal beliefs and religious or cultural tradition
• To be provided with information on support resources that assist in the healing process, for example, local support groups, perinatal loss Internet support, counseling, reading material and perinatal loss newsletters

Source: National Share Pregnancy & Infant Loss Support, Inc.; http://www.nationalshareoffice.com.

Specific care interventions such as encouraging keeping mementos and photos of the baby can help the parents hold on to the short interactions and experiences that they had with the child and can assist in making memories surrounding the birth and death of their child (Table 25.3). This has been found to be significant in the healing process for parents (Stolberg, 2011). Some women may feel a need to perform an act of mothering, such as bathing and dressing the infant, and should be encouraged and supported in these rituals. The NP or midwife can point out physical features that connect them as a family unit. Regardless of the gestational age at the time of loss, the parents appreciate talking about resemblances of the infant to other family members (Kavanaugh & Hershberger, 2005). Guiding parents in participation in the initiation or timing of rituals that are personally meaningful to them can be done by asking such questions as "What's important for you to remember from today?" or "Are there traditions in your family you would have wanted for this baby?" (Kobler, Limbo, & Kavenaugh, 2007).

Parents also need to be made aware of how differently they each may grieve. Although it is important and beneficial for them to grieve together in order to feel less isolated in their grief, their approaches and depth of grief may be vastly different. Women often grieve more deeply and for a longer period of time. Some studies have found that many women are still deeply affected by a perinatal loss after 4 years (Gaudet, 2010). Another area of difference is sexual interest following a loss. Women often find themselves disinterested in sex, while men find sex comforting (Stolberg, 2011). Discussions acknowledging these differences early on in the grieving process can help the partners understand and support one another.

Cultural considerations

It is important for the provider to view each family individually and to determine any cultural or religious customs that could comfort the parents. Cultural or religious beliefs about the destination of the baby's spirit may impact how they grieve. For example, some cultures place great value on male infants and the grief process may be more intense if the baby lost is male. It is appropriate to offer to contact religious or cultural leaders from the family's community to come in to the hospital unit to provide support. Women who have lost infants may still want to carry out any postpartum cultural rituals or guidelines and should be encouraged to do so (Soltesz, 2011).

Physical care after stillbirth

Women need to be informed that they will probably lactate and need to be informed of how to decrease the discomfort of engorged breasts. Appropriate management includes the use of raw cabbage leaves inside the bra to decrease swelling and to help dry the milk. This can be done as often as desired and the cabbage leaves are changed out when they become wilted. Acetaminophen and ibuprofen can also be used to reduce inflammation and discomfort. Pumping or milk expression for discomfort should be used sparingly or not at all as this will encourage the body to make more milk. Some hospitals are linking women who have experienced a stillbirth with donor milk banks; this has been very meaningful for some women in coping with their loss (K. Kavenaugh, personal communication, 2013). Symptoms that would need to be evaluated would include fever, redness in a subscribed area on the breast, or pain in the breasts beyond engorgement.

Lochia following perinatal loss will follow the expected pattern as other postpartum women. The client needs to be informed to call with any signs and symptoms of infection or retained products such as foul-smelling lochia, lochia that is not decreasing in amount over the days after birth, fever, or abdominal pain outside of afterbirth pains.

Follow-up

A postpartum visit or a phone call within the first week after the loss can be beneficial in giving the couple a chance to ask questions and to express their emotions. It is also a good time to evaluate the normalcy of physical changes such as breast and uterine involution. Another visit can be scheduled at 4–6 weeks after birth for routine postpartum care. If genetic testing or an autopsy was performed, results can be reviewed at this time. Although many losses have no clear reason, in cases where there is a clear cause, this can help a woman to feel less guilty and anxious. Autopsies provide a cause of death in only about 10–40% of cases (Moore et al., 2011). At this visit, it is also appropriate to assess a woman's social support system to determine if there is someone with whom the woman can confide her feelings, share her grief, and who will be supportive. Internet support groups are also readily available. These Web-based support groups can provide social support within timing determined by the woman and with a sense of privacy. In-person support groups for women and couples experiencing early or later perinatal loss are often available locally.

Interconception and subsequent pregnancy care

In looking ahead to planning another pregnancy, couples approach this from varying perspectives. Some may need to give themselves time and space to grieve before getting pregnant again. It is not uncommon for many couples to try for another pregnancy immediately, especially after an early pregnancy loss, as this may be part of the healing process for them. Some sources recommend a waiting period after stillbirth before getting pregnant again in order to achieve successful grieving (Moore et al., 2011). Most individuals are able to move through their grief and successfully integrate the experience into their lives, and ultimately decide for themselves ideal timing for a subsequent pregnancy. They can look back on the event with sadness, but are able to move forward.

Interconception care of a woman who has experienced a previous perinatal loss includes acknowledging the loss. Avoiding discussing the loss may actually increase the client's grief and lead to her feeling disconnected from the provider (Moore et al., 2011). Women who have had a stillbirth often worry that this tragedy will happen again. The risk is low for most couples, though the risk is higher than for couples who have not had a stillbirth. Predisposing factors such as chromosomal birth defects, placental problems, and cord accidents are unlikely to occur again in another pregnancy (Eller et al., 2006). The risk for having another stillbirth may be higher if a maternal health condition such as diabetes or a genetic disorder caused the previous stillbirth. A genetic counselor can advise the couple about the risk of stillbirth or other pregnancy complications in another pregnancy. Depending on a woman's individual health status, increased fetal surveillance may be appropriate during a subsequent pregnancy.

In caring for a woman who is pregnant again following a perinatal loss, the provider must be sensitive to meet the individual woman's needs. She may need to discuss the previous loss in a safe and neutral environment. Her anxiety about the current pregnancy may be elevated and her ability to attach to the coming baby may be limited (Gaudet, 2010). The provider should acknowledge these potential feelings, thus giving the woman permission and opportunity to verbalize her needs and emotions. Reassurance of the normalcy of a variety of emotional responses is valid.

Women pregnant again after prior perinatal loss fear another loss and thus protect their emotions and avoid prenatal bonding. This phenomenon is known as "emotional cushioning," and appears to be a complex self-protective mechanism to help women cope with the anxiety, uncertainty, and sense of vulnerability experienced in pregnancies after a prior loss (Cote-Arsenault & Donato, 2011). Minimal prenatal attachment may be present until the woman passes the gestational point at which the previous loss was experienced (Gaudet, 2010). Women should be reassured that this is a normal phenomenon so as not to increase their sense of anxiety. It is also appropriate for the health-care provider to continue to evaluate and promote maternal attachment behaviors as pregnancy progresses.

Summary

Perinatal bereavement is a unique mourning situation. Pregnancy as an exciting time of anticipation turns quickly into one of profound pain and grief. The loss of an infant through stillbirth, miscarriage, or neonatal death is recognized as a traumatic life event and reaction. Men and women grieve differently and intense grief reactions can last weeks, months, and, in some cases, years. The etiology of a pregnancy loss is often never known, adding to parents' sense of guilt, confusion, and sometimes, blame. Health-care providers must be able to therapeutically and skillfully communicate with women and families during the immediate crisis period as well as during the grieving and healing process when support is vital. Encouraging women and their partners to hold their baby as appropriate to each situation and providing support for family rituals to remember their baby can aid family healing. Women experiencing perinatal loss may benefit from follow-up for a period of time after the loss as this event can be a trigger for postpartum depression.

Case study

Sheila presents to you for a routine gynecologic exam. She is a 34-year-old G2P0020 and has recently moved to your community. She was referred to you by a friend. She is trying to get pregnant and wants to discuss this today. You review her history and find that she has been pregnant twice previously within the last 2 years. She miscarried both of these pregnancies at 8 and 10 weeks, respectively. She verbalizes her fear about getting pregnant again and exclaims that her husband "just doesn't get it." She is teary as she discusses her husband's attitude that the pregnancies were early and that she should not feel such grief. She notes warily that her "new friends here don't even know about the pregnancies."

Sheila is immediately reassured that her discussion is confidential and will not be shared with the friend that you have in common. You recognize that Sheila needs to have the opportunity to discuss her feelings and concerns without fear of judgment. You simply ask that she tell you about what happened in her other pregnancies. Sheila proceeds to discuss her joy at becoming pregnant the first time and how she improved her health habits. She reports that she read books about pregnancy; she improved her diet, gave up smoking, and started walking every day. But one evening, she started cramping and bleeding, and then it was "just over. My baby was in the toilet and I was left with nothing."

Sheila goes on to discuss a similar experience with her second pregnancy and discusses her ongoing feelings of emptiness and loss. She cannot understand how her husband just seems to take it all in stride. You share with her that many families find that men and women deal with this kind of loss in very different ways and that what she is describing happens frequently. You acknowledge that it is common for women to experience deep grief reactions after an early pregnancy loss and discuss this in more detail. You encourage Sheila to openly share her feelings with her husband and to consider opening up to a trusted friend. You also provide Sheila with information about grief support groups online and in the community.

Sheila tentatively asks, "So now what? I really want a baby!" You then discuss that at this point, the next step is to prepare to be as healthy as possible going into another pregnancy. You offer a referral to a geneticist as she is 34 years old with a history of two early pregnancy losses. She accepts the referral. You perform a complete health history and gynecological exam and reassure her of your normal findings and prescribe prenatal vitamins with folic acid. You review nutrition and exercise with Sheila and encourage her continued smoking cessation. A depression inventory was administered and was negative. She notes that it "feels good to talk about it."

The week following this initial visit, you place a follow-up call to Sheila and find that she has been talking with a friend that has been supportive and has participated in an online support group that you recommended. She has also discussed her feelings and needs with her husband and is encouraged by his response, and both are attending the meeting with the geneticist next week.

Resources for women and their families

Daily strength—A support site for women who have experienced miscarriage: http://www.dailystrength.org/c/Miscarriage-Stillbirth/support-group

Mommies Enduring Neonatal Death (MEND)—A support organization providing bimonthly newsletters and support groups (1) for those who have recently lost a baby to miscarriage, stillbirth, and infant death; (2) pregnancy group for those who are considering becoming pregnant or are currently pregnant after a loss; (3) father group: http://www.mend.org/

Perinatal Hospice—This group offers perinatal hospice and palliative care and support services to parents who find out during pregnancy that their baby has a life-limiting condition: http://www.perinatalhospice.org/

Share: Pregnancy and Infant Loss Support, Inc.—Supportive resources for those who have experienced pregnancy or infant loss: http://www.nationalshareoffice.com

Resources for health-care providers

Now I Lay Me Down to Sleep (NILMDTS)—This is a nonprofit organization that provides the gift of professional remembrance photography to capture images for bereaved parents in a compassionate and sensitive manner at *no charge* to the families: https://www.nowilaymedowntosleep.org/

Pregnancy Loss and Infant Death Alliance—This group provides resources for health-care providers to provide optimal support to grieving families at http://www.plida.org. Specific practice guidelines include the following:

* Offering the Baby to the Bereaved Parents
* When Bereaved Parents Want to Hold their Baby
* Delaying Postpartum Pathology Studies

References

American College of Obstetricians and Gynecologists (ACOG). (2009). *Evaluation of Stillbirths and Neonatal Deaths.* ACOG Committee Opinion, 383.

Cote Arsenault, D., & Donato, K. (2011). Emotional cushioning in pregnancy after perinatal loss. *Journal of Reproductive and Infant Psychology, 29*(1), 81–92.

Eller, A. G., Branch, D. W., & Byrne, J. L. (2006). Stillbirth at term. *Obstetrics and Gynecology, 108*(2), 442–447.

Gaudet, C. (2010). Pregnancy after perinatal los: Association of grief, anxiety, and attachment. *Journal of Reproductive and Infant Psychology, 28*(3), 240–251.

Gómez Ponce de León, R., & Wing, D. A. (2009). Misoprostol for termination of pregnancy with intrauterine fetal demise in the second and third trimester of pregnancy—A systematic review. *Contraception, 79*, 259.

Heazell, A. (2009). Caring for women after stillbirth—A study of midwives' and obstetricians' knowledge and practice. *MIDIRS Midwifery Digest, 19*(2), 252.

Kavanaugh, K. (2006). Supporting parents after stillbirth or newborn death. *The American Journal of Nursing, 106*(9), 74–79.

Kavanaugh, K., & Hershberger, P. (2005). Perinatal loss in low-income African American parents. *Journal of Obstetric, Gynecologic, and Neonatal Nursing, 34*(5), 595–605.

Kobler, K., Limbo, R., & Kavenaugh, K. (2007). Moments: The use of ritual in perinatal and pediatric death. *Maternal & Child Nutrition, 32*(5), 288–295.

Lang, A., Fleiszer, A. R., Duhamel, F., Sword, W., Gilbert, K., & Corsini-Munt, S. (2011). Perinatal loss and grief: The challenge of ambiguity and disenfranchised grief. *Omega, 63*(2), 183–196.

Lok, I. H., Yip, A. S., Lee, D. T., Sahota, D., & Chung, T. K. (2010). A 1-year longitudinal study of psychological morbidity after miscarriage. *Fertility and Sterility, 93*(6), 1966–1975.

Moore, T., Parrish, H., & Perry Black, B. (2011). Interconception care for couples after perinatal loss: A comprehensive review of the literature. *Journal of Perintatal and Neonatal Nursing, 25*(1), 44–51.

Reddy, U. M. (2007). Prediction and prevention of recurrent stillbirth. *Obstetrics and Gynecology, 110*(5), 1151–1164.

Silver, R. M. (2007). Fetal death. *Obstetrics and Gynecology, 109*(1), 153–167.

Silver, R. M. (2010). Stillbirth workup and delivery management. *Clinical Obstetrics and Gynecology, 53*(3), 681–690.

Silver, R. M., Varner, M. W., Reddy, U., Goldenberg, R., Pinar, H., Conway, D., . . . Stoll, B. (2007). Work-up of stillbirth: A review of the evidence. *American Journal of Obstetrics and Gynecology, 196*(5), 433–444.

Soltesz, P. (2011). Perinatal loss: A doula's perspective. *International Journal of Childbirth Education, 26*(2), 15–17.

Stolberg, J. (2011). "Leaving footprints on our hearts"—How can midwives provide meaningful emotional support after a perinatal death? *MIDIRS Midwifery Digest, 21*(1), 7–13.

Part IV

Postnatal care

26

Physiological alterations during the postnatal period

Kimberly A. Couch and Karen DeCocker-Geist

Relevant terms

Afterpains—uterine contractions that occur after childbirth that produce a range of discomfort perceived as mild to labor-like in intensity

Hyperplasia—enlargement of tissue by an increase in the number of cells

Hypertrophy—enlargement of tissue by the enlargement or growth of cells

Lochia—vaginal discharge resulting from the sloughing of decidual tissue, debris from the products of conception, epithelial cells, red blood cells, white blood cells, and serum

Postpartum—period after birth beginning at the time of complete expulsion of the placenta and membranes, and ending in 6–8 weeks when the reproductive system is returned to nonpregnant status; also known as the puerperium or postnatal period

Uterotonic—substance that induces uterine contractions

Introduction

The postpartum period begins with the expulsion of the placenta after the birth of the infant and continues for 6–8 weeks following birth. This period is characterized by the involution of the reproductive system to its prepregnant state as well as extensive physiological changes throughout the maternal organism. This chapter reviews the normal maternal physiological changes that occur in the maternal body systems during the postpartum period.

Uterus

In a nonpregnant state, the uterus is roughly the size and shape of an inverted pear and weighs only about 100 g or less. During pregnancy, uterine muscle fibers undergo extensive hyperplasia and hypertrophy, increasing uterine weight approximately 10-fold to an average weight of about 1000 g (Katz, 2012).

Immediately after the infant is born, the stretched-to-capacity smooth muscle fibers recoil and contract when the uterus is emptied, resulting in a smaller endometrial surface area. This change in the endometrial surface area leads to placental separation, and the placenta and membranes are usually born shortly thereafter. After the birth of the placenta, the uterus is usually located at about the level or slightly below the maternal umbilicus and remains there for the first two days after birth. The uterus should be firmly contracted and the consistency and size of a softball.

The uterus begins the process of involution at about 2 days after birth and should be completed by 10–14 days postpartum. Involution occurs by a dramatic reduction in the size of the myometrial cells. The process occurs quickly, with the uterus weighing only 500 g at 1 week after birth, 300 g at 2 weeks, and approximately 100 g at 4 weeks (Cunningham et al., 2010). Abdominally, the decrease in the size of the uterus is notable and occurs at a rate of about 1 cm a day. By day 14, the uterus has descended below the rim of the symphysis pubis and is no longer palpable abdominally (Blackburn, 2013).

The uterine contractions that occur after birth are most intense in the first 3 days postpartum and

---

Prenatal and Postnatal Care: A Woman-Centered Approach, First Edition. Edited by Robin G. Jordan, Janet L. Engstrom, Julie A. Marfell, and Cindy L. Farley.

are commonly called afterpains. The contractions are usually more intense in parous women, and most frequently occur during infant suckling due to oxytocin release and when uterotonic agents are administered. These uterine contractions are important in maintaining hemostasis in the postpartum period. Failure of the uterus to involute fully is often related to atony, retained placental fragments, infection, or lacerations (Blackburn, 2013).

After the placenta separates from the endometrium, the uterine muscle fibers contract, effectively ligating the bleeding vessels at the placental site. The compression of these vessels is essential to preventing postpartum hemorrhage. After a normal vaginal birth, maternal blood loss averages about 500 mL and about 1000 mL after a cesarean birth. Without the hemostasis provided by the myometrial contraction, profound hemorrhage can rapidly occur (Blackburn, 2013).

Further blood loss is prevented by the activation of the clotting cascade with placental separation (Osol & Mandala, 2009). This hypercoagulable state remains for the first 2 weeks to aid in healing of the placental site. Involution may be slowed in women who have had a multifetal pregnancy or overdistension from polyhydramnios (Blackburn, 2013).

The endometrium must also be resorted after birth. Excess intracellular proteins as well as intracellular cytoplasm are removed by autolysis with proteolytic enzymes and macrophage degradation (Blackburn, 2013). The placental attachment site takes about 6 weeks to completely exfoliate and regenerate a new endometrial layer.

Lochia

Lochia is a vaginal discharge resulting from the sloughing of decidual tissue and includes debris from the products of conception as well as some bacteria, epithelial cells, and red blood cells. Lochia changes in characteristics as the uterus is emptied of necrotic tissue and new endometrium is regenerated at the basal layer adjacent to the myometrium (Blackburn, 2013). Lochia rubra begins after the expulsion of the placenta and is made up of blood, debris from the placenta, membranes, vernix, lanugo, and decidual tissue. Lochia should not contain large clots; most clots are dime sized and are a result of blood pooling in the vagina. Lochia rubra has a distinctive fleshy odor and lasts about 3 days (Blackburn, 2013).

Lochia serosa is a paler version of lochia rubra and occurs as the uterus begins to regenerate the endometrium and the placental site is exfoliated and remodeled. Lochia serosa lasts about 7–10 days and gradually transitions to a pink, yellow, or white color and is called lochia alba. Lochia alba can last up to 4 weeks (Blackburn, 2013).

Cervix

During labor and birth, each contraction of uterine muscle fibers forces the presenting part of the infant toward and eventually through the cervix and the vagina. Simultaneously, as the muscle fibers shorten with each contraction, the cervix is pulled and stretched over the presenting part, leaving the cervix stretched, edematous, bruised, abraded, and sometimes lacerated (Blackburn, 2013). Within hours of birth, healing of the cervix begins. Although the cervix protrudes into the vagina immediately after birth, shortly thereafter, the contracting uterus begins to pull the cervix back into its usual position. As edema resolves, the cervix shortens, thickens, and the epithelium begins to remodel (Blackburn, 2013). By 1 week postpartum, the cervix is nearly closed and has thickened, and by 6 weeks postpartum, the cervix has almost regained its prepregnant size and shape (Katz, 2012). However, the cervical os of women who have given birth vaginally does not completely regain its nulliparous appearance. The cervix of parous women is usually wider and the cervical os often appears as a transverse slit rather than the more circular os observed in nulliparous women.

Vagina

The vaginal muscles and mucosa are put to the expansion threshold as the infant passes through the vagina and over the perineum. After birth, the vagina is often bruised, swollen, abraded, and lacerated. Immediately postpartum, the vaginal tone is slack and rugae are absent. The vagina begins to heal shortly after birth. By 3 weeks postpartum, the rugae return but are less prominent than before pregnancy. The vaginal epithelium begins to proliferate at about 4 weeks after birth. By 6 weeks postpartum, the vaginal epithelium is usually reconstructed, and vaginal tone is nearly restored. However, like the cervix, the vagina never completely regains its nulliparous tone or shape.

Labia and perineum

The labia and perineum are often bruised and edematous after birth. Abrasions and small lacerations are also common. Lacerations, depending on the severity and the extent of the injury, will vary in healing times from days to weeks. Edema is generally resolved within 3–4 days. The reduction in progesterone aids in the rapid return to vulva tone (Blackburn, 2013).

Additional maternal alterations during the postpartum period

In addition to the dramatic changes observed in the reproductive organs during the postpartum period, alterations occur in other organ systems during the postpartum period (see Table 26.1). Other significant maternal physiological alterations are summarized further. Lactogenesis and the process of breastfeeding are described in detail in Chapter 30.

Endocrine changes

With the delivery of the placenta, immediate changes occur in serum hormone levels. Decreases in estrogen and progesterone are profound. Within 24 hours, estradiol is less than 2% of pregnancy levels; estrogen is almost to prepregnant levels by 7 days; and progesterone

Table 26.1   Maternal Alterations during the Postpartum Period

Physical parameter	Alteration
Venous changes	Increased venous diameter and decreased blood flow velocity take up to 6 weeks to return to prepregnant levels. Women remain at elevated risk for thrombophlebitis and embolism during this time.
Heart rate	Increased in the first hour after birth but returns to prepregnant levels quickly thereafter
Cardiac output	Increased significantly in the first hour after birth and remains elevated for the first 2 days after birth; returns to prepregnant levels in a week but may be longer in some women
Blood pressure	May be slightly elevated during the first 4 days after birth then returns to prepregnant levels
Coagulation	Increased significantly in the first 2 days after birth and remains elevated for approximately 2 weeks
Total blood volume	Remains elevated during the first week after birth but returns to prepregnant level at about 1 week postpartum
Red blood count	Decreased after birth depending on blood loss but returns to prepregnant levels by about 8 weeks postpartum. May appear falsely low immediate postpartum due to fluid overload in labor
Total body water	Remains elevated in the first days after birth; diuresis usually begins on about day 2 and continues through day 5 after birth

Sources: Blackburn (2013), Cunningham et al. (2010), Katz (2012).

is at nonpregnant levels by 24–48 hours (Blackburn, 2013). The return to fertility and the resumption of ovulation and menstruation are described in Chapter 29. The enlarged thyroid gland regresses and the basal metabolic rate is normal by 7 days (Samuels, 2012).

Cardiovascular system

Increased blood volume is needed to ensure an adequate supply to the uterus and placenta during pregnancy. After delivery, the withdrawal of estrogen causes a rapid diuresis for the first 48 hours and a return to normal plasma volume and hematocrit levels. Decreased progesterone leads to removal of excess fluid in the tissues as well as return to normal of the vascular tone. Cardiac output and blood pressure return to prepregnant levels.

Renal system

The pregnancy-related changes in the renal system are reversed in the postpartum period. The kidneys must excrete the excess fluids and the increased breakdown of protein products. With the fall of progesterone levels to prepregnant state, the renal track dilation resolves. The bladder is displaced in labor and the urethra is stretched with delivery, often resulting in temporary loss of bladder tone and transient incontinence (Blackburn, 2013).

Gastrointestinal tract

Smooth muscle tone returns to normal with reduced progesterone circulation, resolving issues with heartburn and reflux quickly. Constipation is relieved by increased bowel tone but may persist due to fear of pain with passing stool if the woman sustained perineal injuries or from immobility from surgical delivery. Fasting plasma insulin levels begin to return to normal at 48 hours and are stable by 6 weeks postpartum (Blackburn, 2013).

Summary

Childbirth may be among the most significant experiences in a woman's life. Typically, it is a joyful time to celebrate the arrival of the baby with family and friends. It is followed by a tender period of adjustment to the new family dynamics, whether it be the first child, second child, or more. The anatomic and physiological changes in pregnancy occur over approximately 40 weeks, while the postpartum recovery takes place in just 40 days. Immediately after childbirth, a woman's body begins the journey of returning to its postpregnant state (Groff, 2011). Health-care providers can make a positive difference by being attentive to the normal progression of postpartum physiological adaptations and by supporting women during these profound changes.

Case study

On postpartum day 1, Catherine, a G2 P2002, who had a third-degree laceration after a 40-minute precipitous birth, is expressing concern about the healing process.

SUBJECTIVE: "I am still stunned by the explosion of this baby from my nether parts. He was crowning during our quick car ride to the hospital. Will I ever be normal down there again?"

OBJECTIVE: Catherine presents her story in a jocular but concerned manner. She is nursing and stroking her baby as she is speaking. Upon inspection and palpation, her fundus is firm and two finger-breadths below the umbilicus. She has a 4-cm diastasis. Her perineal repair is well approximated. Her perineum is bruised, swollen, and tender. All other physical findings are normal.

ASSESSMENT: Catherine is recovering from an unexpected precipitous birth and a third-degree perineal laceration with a healthy baby.

PLAN: Catherine needs reassurance and mental and emotional processing time for the rapid and "explo-

sive" birth that left her with a third-degree laceration. Sit with her and encourage her to share her birth story and her feelings. She will need to tell her story a number of times to incorporate this narrative into her sense of self. Give her positive feedback on her breastfeeding and interaction with her new baby. Share the results of the physical examination of the perineum, which were normal for postpartum day 1, and offer to get a mirror if she would like to see the area. Provide her with systemic and local analgesics as needed. Warmth to the perineal area is indicated on day 1 to enhance circulation and healing and to provide comfort. Some women will prefer herbal baths or compresses to the perineum. Educate her on the natural healing process, including signs of poor healing or infection in the area. Discuss the resumption of regular activities and special concerns regarding bowel movements and sexual intercourse. Follow up with Catherine frequently in the early postpartum period to make sure that her healing is on track.

Resource for women

The new mom: Physical changes: http://www.babies.sutterhealth.org/afterthebirth/newmom/pp_physical.html

Resource for health-care providers

Physiological changes of the postpartum period: http://www.glowm.com/section_view/heading/Postpartum%20Care/item/143#5891

References

Blackburn, S. (2013). *Maternal, fetal, and neonatal physiology: A clinical perspective* (4th ed.). Maryland Heights, MO: Saunders/Elsevier.

Cunningham, F. G., Leveno, K. J., Bloom, S. L., Hauth, J. C., Rouse, D. J., & Spong, C. Y. (2010). Chapter 30. The Puerperium. In F. G. Cunningham, K. J. Leveno, S. L. Bloom, J. C. Hauth, D. J. Rouse, & C. Y. Spong (Eds.), *William's obstetrics* (23rd ed.). New York: McGraw Hill.

Groff, J. (2011). Revisioning postpartum care in the United States: Global perspectives. In C. L. Farley (Ed.), *Final Projects Database*. Philadelphia: Philadelphia University. Retrieved from http://www.instituteofmidwifery.org/MSFinalProj.nsf/a9ee58d7a82396768525684f0056be8d/8f0a029755d12a75852578a1006eaa2c/$FILE/Jade%20Groff%20721-CHAPT1-2FINAL.pdf

Katz, V. (2012). Postpartum care. In S. G. Gabbe, J. R. Niebyl, H. L. Galan, E. R. M. Jauniaux, M. B. Landon, J. L. Simpson, & D. A. Driscoll (Eds.), *Obstetrics: Normal and problem pregnancies* (6th ed., pp. 517–532). Philadelphia: Elsevier.

Osol, G., & Mandala, M. (2009). Maternal uterine vascular remodeling during pregnancy. *Physiology, 24,* 58–71. doi:10.1152/physiol.00033.2008

Samuels, M. (2012). Subacute, silent, and postpartum thyroiditis. *Medical Clinics of North America, 96*(2), 223–233. doi:10.1016/j.mcna.2012.01.003

27

Components of postnatal care

Tia P. Andrighetti and Deborah Brandt Karsnitz

Relevant terms

Boggy—when referring to the uterus, it means soft and not fully contracted

Cystocele—herniation of the bladder into the vagina*

Diastasis—separation of the abdominal rectus muscles

Eschar—area in the uterus where the placenta was attached; at about 10 days postpartum, this "scab" will be released; bright red bleeding for 1–2 hours is normal, then back to previous lochia color and amount

First-degree laceration—tear of the perineum, labia, or vagina involving the superficial layers of tissue**

Fourth-degree laceration—tear that completely lacerates the external and internal anal sphincter**

Fourth trimester—time from birth of the placenta lasting for several months after birth

Fundus—the topmost part of the uterus; felt during abdominal evaluation of the uterus

Homan's sign—maneuver done by placing one hand under the knee and dorsiflexing the foot; elicitation of pain is a positive sign, used to evaluate possible deep vein thrombosis (DVT)**

Involution—normal process the maternal body undergoes after birth; when referred to the uterus, the shrinking back of the uterus to an almost nonpregnant size

Lochia—vaginal blood, tissue, and mucus loss after birth; lasting up to 6 or 8 weeks postpartum

Postpartum blues—feelings experienced by the mother after birth; crying, emotional lability, fatigue, increased or decreased eating; lasts up to 2 weeks postpartum

Postpartum period or puerperium—time from placenta passage until about 6–8 weeks

Rectocele—prolapse of the vaginal wall allowing herniation of the rectum into the vagina*

Second-degree laceration—tear involving the fascia and perineal muscle**

Third-degree laceration—tear involving the perineal muscle as well as the external anal sphincter**

Sources: *Stables and Rankin (2011); **Cunningham et al. (2010).

Introduction

Postnatal care begins with the onset of the postpartum period; it is also referred to as the puerperium. It is generally defined as a 6- to 8-week period beginning with the delivery of the placenta (Blackburn, 2013). Despite this long-standing definition, the postpartum period frequently lasts for several months and is a neglected aspect of modern maternity care. Literature is sparse on the puerperium and when it exists, it deals primarily with abnormal involution and pathology. Respecting and supporting the length of restoration in the postpartum woman has long been the belief and practice in most other developed and developing countries but continues to be frequently overlooked in the United States (Kim-Godwin, 2003).

Postpartum is the culmination of the childbearing year. Many adaptations and adjustments must be made to accommodate the new family member into an already established structure. When health-care providers stress

Prenatal and Postnatal Care: A Woman-Centered Approach, First Edition. Edited by Robin G. Jordan, Janet L. Engstrom, Julie A. Marfell, and Cindy L. Farley.
© 2014 John Wiley & Sons, Inc. Published 2014 by John Wiley & Sons, Inc.

the importance of postpartum care, women and their families will learn to value the significance of a support system, education, surveillance, and interaction. Focus is on assistance for families to maximize their adjustment, surveillance for maladapatation/malinvolution, and education and consultation/collaboration/referral as needed.

Discharge home from the birth facility comes at a time when most women are being bombarded by the sensory overload that accompanies rapid physical and psychological changes after birth. The ability to integrate new information during this time is often diminished and challenges health-care practitioners to find teachable moments. Postpartum teaching ideally begins during the antepartum and continues throughout postpartum. Teaching includes the new mother and family members. Because information is often passed down through family members, inclusion of family during teaching sessions may alleviate confusion or correct inaccurate information.

The degree of postpartum discomfort, adjustment of mother to baby and baby to mother, and degree of support received all affect the recovery and adaptation of the woman to a new role. An important role of healthcare providers includes planning for postpartum recovery and newborn care, identification of social and tangible support, and encouragement of strengths. Anticipatory guidance is approached in a realistic manner. Teaching includes the expected physiological as well as psychological tasks that women face during this time.

Fourth-trimester tasks

- Physical restoration
- Psychological adaptation to a new role
- Development of knowledge and skills to care for a dependent infant
- Establishment of bond with the baby
- Adjustments to lifestyle issues and relationship changes to accommodate a new family member.

The primary concerns of a woman who has recently given birth include learning about infant behavior and care, returning to her prepregnant body, and juggling demands of household, partner, and other children. A mother is able to adapt to her new role faster when the concerns for her own recovery are met. Once a new mother is reassured that the changes she is experiencing are normal, her focus returns to the tasks of infant care.

This chapter will cover normal postpartum care of the mother and family. After initial postpartum care fol-

lowing childbirth, many women are not seen until a 6- to 8-week postpartum visit, thus missing opportunities to assess physical and psychosocial adjustment. Seeing a postpartum mother only at 6–8 weeks can delay interventions for many adjustments/complications. Therefore, a 2-week postpartum visit is recommended. Components of the 2-week as well as the 6-week visit will be discussed. Table 27.1 and Table 27.2 reflect the components covered at each of the 2- and 6-week visits for easy reference. However, it is important to note that postpartum care in the United States is woefully inadequate and a restructuring of current practices is urgently needed.

Table 27.1 Two-Week Postpartum Visit

Two-week postpartum visit	
Subjective assessment	• Maternal physical and emotional adjustment • Birth experience • Family adaptation • Infant feeding • Exercise/activity • Rest/sleep • Diet/fluids • Lochia • Afterbirth pains • Perineal comfort • Diuresis/diaphoresis • Constipation/hemorrhoids • Sexuality/resumption of intercourse • Contraception
Objective assessment	• Vital signs • Weight • Heart/lungs • Breasts • Uterus • CVAT • Perineum/bleeding prn • Extremities/edema • Postpartum depression screening

Plan	• Teaching
	  ○ Family adaptation
	  ○ Maternal role attainment
	  ○ Infant feeding
	  ○ Normal involution
	  ○ Exercise/activity
	  ○ Rest/sleep
	  ○ Diet/fluids
	  ○ Birth control
	  ○ Warning signs
	• Follow-up at 6 weeks and prn
	• Consult, collaborate, refer prn

Table 27.2 Six-Week Postpartum Visit

Six-week postpartum visit	
Subjective assessment	• Maternal physical and emotional adjustment • Birth experience • Family adaptation • Infant feeding • Exercise/activity • Rest/sleep • Diet/fluids • Lochia • Perineal comfort • Constipation/hemorrhoids • Sexuality/resumption of intercourse • Contraception
Objective assessment	• Vital signs • Weight • Heart/lungs • Breasts • Abdomen • Uterus • CVAT • Extremities • Perineum and vagina • Hemorrhoids prn • Postpartum depression screening

Plan	• Teaching
	  ○ Family adaptation
	  ○ Maternal role attainment
	  ○ Normal involution
	  ○ Infant feeding
	  ○ Exercise/activity
	  ○ Rest/sleep
	  ○ Diet/fluids
	  ○ Resumption of menses and ovulation
	  ○ Birth control
	  ○ Warning signs
	• Follow-up at annual exam or prn
	• Consult, collaborate, refer prn

Assessment of maternal physical and emotional adjustment

Postpartum defines a period of many changes and adaptations for a woman and her family. Communication is essential for optimal postpartum adjustment. Healthcare providers should take the opportunity and time to assess feelings and recovery since the birth. This will facilitate noting areas of knowledge deficit as well as areas where support may be needed. Women may not feel comfortable sharing intimate feelings or how their family is adjusting, unless specifically asked.

Communication can be facilitated by asking open-ended questions and giving time to answer, without unduly hurrying onto the physical exam part of the visit. The 2-week visit is about assuring that postpartum involution is proceeding normally, noting psychological adjustment, and determining any maladaptations either physically or emotionally. The 6-week visit is focused on assessing that postpartum involution is complete, that the psychological adjustment of the family is continuing, and that family planning has been addressed.

There are a variety of topics that can facilitate discussion. The health-care provider can start by asking how the woman is feeling both emotionally and physically. Ask the woman to qualify her responses if she gives a short answer. For example, if she answers "good," it can mean very different things to different people. By asking what it means to her specifically, the conversation can continue and a deeper understanding is achieved.

Attaining a realistic balance in life is one of the tasks of the childbearing year. The new mother needs to care for her infant, provide continued attention to siblings, help siblings adjust to a new baby's presence, and maintain her relationships separate from children. Additionally, she may have concerns regarding finances, employment, and the maintenance of daily tasks, such as cleaning, laundry, cooking, and grocery shopping. It is important to the woman's overall health to participate in outside activities and continue to maintain contact with friends; however, this is challenging particularly in the early postpartum weeks. Prioritizing and asking for help are key. Give the woman permission to let things go at home while she prioritizes what is most important to her. For a woman who is really struggling with this concept, write a script noting that her job in the early postpartum period is to care for herself, her baby, and other children. Postpartum doulas are another resource to consider for the early postpartum adjustment; they offer a range of services to help the new mother from breastfeeding support to light housekeeping and meal preparation. Family and friends are often willing to help out and the new mother should be encouraged to graciously accept these offers of help from her extended social network. Paternity or partner leaves for a new baby are an employment benefit for some; these should be explored and arranged in the prenatal period.

Assessing maternal mood at this time is vital since as many as 80% of women will experience postpartum blues (Beck & Indman, 2005). The etiology of postpartum blues is unknown, but many common postpartum aspects such as fatigue, decreased support, hormonal fluctuation, social isolation, and marital or relationship conflict can contribute. It is not unusual for a woman to cry for unexplained reasons, experience anxiety, feel overly fatigued or have trouble sleeping, have an increased appetite or none at all, and have mixed feelings regarding her birth experience (Stables & Rankin, 2011). Symptoms that last 2 weeks or greater should warrant evaluation for postpartum depression. It is important to have a discussion about the woman's emotional state at the 2-week visit, although the onset of postpartum depression can be weeks or months after the birth.

Health-care providers can help women experiencing the postpartum blues in a variety of ways. Sometimes simple active listening can be very therapeutic. Women also need to be reassured that their feelings do not make them a bad parent, but are a normal response to everything going on during this adjustment period. Suggest increased help at home by enlisting family and friends to cook, clean, watch other children, and help care for the baby. Encourage the mother to take some time for herself such as reading a book, taking a bath, visiting with friends, or getting out. Encourage her to sleep when the baby sleeps and take every opportunity to rest, as caring for a newborn is a 24-hour-a-day job. By trying a variety of tactics, the woman can find what coping measures work best for her.

Review of birth experience

A new mother needs to integrate and accept the reality of her own birth and newborn experience while reconciling expectations and fantasies that may have been unmet (Mercer, 1985). Rarely is the birth experience the way the mother imagined it would be. Health-care providers can encourage women to discuss their birth and facilitate the task of integrating their imagined birth with reality. Failure to complete this process can interfere with the mother's ability to become comfortable with her new identity. The psychological task of fitting the pieces of her childbearing experience into her narrative can generate a positive perspective on her experience. A laboring woman is in the midst of a very intense event and her memory of the labor and birth will reflect focused and selected aspects of her experience. She may need help in understanding how her own birth varied from her hopes and expectations. A woman benefits from a birth review in order to make sense of her experience, express her emotions regarding her labor and birth, and incorporate this transformative event into her maternal identity (Affonso, 1977). How a woman feels about her birth can affect her attachment process with her baby.

The "taking-in" phase of postpartum adjustment involves reviewing labor and birth. The time spent with a new mom or her family can help clarify the experience and allow her to progress to the next phase. "Taking hold" follows where the mother assumes tasks of mothering, care of baby and self, along with attention to family and her support network (Ament, 1990; Rubin, 1961). It is important to reflect on the woman's birth experience as well as address current postpartum concerns. Most women enjoy discussing their labor and birth story and will share this over and over again with friends and family.

Family adaptation

The modern family is less likely to consist of the cultural tradition of a married mother and father and their biological offspring than ever before. In the 1960s, 43% of families fell into the nuclear family category, and in 2010, this percent was down to 23%. Family structure affects function; an awareness of the woman's family as she defines it will help the health-care provider give culturally sensitive and realistic information based on her circumstances. Types of families seen today include the nuclear family, single-parent family, unmarried biological or adoptive family, cohabiting family, extended family, and blended family. Do not assume family structure, ask. Regardless of family structure, adjustments will be made to accommodate a new family member and bonding with the new baby will remain an essential feature of this adjustment.

Bonding is the emotional tie that the mother develops with her unborn baby, and later her newborn (see Chapter 16, "Psychosocial Adaptations in Pregnancy"). Bonding can occur between other important members of the family and the newborn, such as father or partner, grandparents, and siblings. This process develops over time and provides a powerful source of motivation for ongoing care-taking activities. The capabilities of parents to recognize their baby's behavioral cues and respond appropriately are influenced by numerous factors and can have lasting ramifications on bonding and attachment (Genesoni & Tallandini, 2009). Strong parent–child bonds can persist throughout a lifetime, despite separation of time and distance.

The stage is set immediately after birth for attachment to the newborn to begin. A cascade of hormones is brought on by the labor and birth process. Endorphins promote an exhilarated sense of achievement about the birth, while prolactin and oxytocin facilitate a peaceful and deepening love for the neonate. However, routine interventions done without medical indication, such as induction of labor, cesarean section, or epidural anesthesia, can mute the hormonal response and can be detrimental to the bonding process.

A healthy newborn should not be separated from the mother after birth. Becoming acquainted with the newly born baby immediately after birth typically proceeds in a progressive journey using gaze, proximity, fingertips, palms, voice, embrace, and movement. The en face position allows optimal eye contact, so mother and child can fixate on the other's features. Women communicate with a high-pitched voice suited to the newborn's hearing range, while babies imitate with mouth and tongue movement (Kennell & Klaus, 1998). This process requires close physical contact and should not be interrupted by hospital procedures that can be done at a later time.

Many factors can affect bonding. Parents' perceptions of their own abilities and skills to care for their newborn can shape their interactions with the baby and each other. Parents are influenced by the way they were parented, both consciously and unconsciously. Parents who are made more aware of their baby's competencies and abilities to communication with them have optimal opportunities for bonding and mutuality. Past experiences with infants influence their expectations and motivation to parent and shape their efforts to nurture, love, and provide for their baby. The personality of the baby and any special needs the baby has can also play a part. Some factors that influence parental behaviors are unalterable, such as the baby's gender, birth order, weight, interfamilial and cultural background, and child-rearing practices they experienced from their own parents. Other events can be influenced positively by the health-care provider, such as providing education, supportive care, and affirming the abilities of both baby and parents.

Fathers and mothers tend to interact differently with their babies; infants shape their caretaker's reaction attachment by their responses. Traditionally, fathers were removed from the daily work of caring for the infant and provided discipline or playtime as the child grew. Mothers assumed primary care of the baby (Schoppe-Sullivan, Brown, Cannon, Mangelsdorf, & Szewczyk-Sokolowski, 2008). A man's relationship with his own mother and father influences his confidence as a parent. Many fathers today want to be more involved with the daily aspects of newborn care and are creating the space in their lives to take on more infant care (Holtslander, 2005; Fagerskiold, 2008; Premberg, Hellstrom, & Berg, 2008).

Sibling adjustment is an important part of family adaptation. Gender, personality, and interests of the older sibling can influence adjustment. Age has traditionally been thought to influence sibling adjustment, but this has not been documented in many studies (Stewart, Mobley, Van Tuyl, & Salvador, 1987). The family's culture, size, setting, and support system may also influence this relationship. Parental factors such as well-being, sense of competence, relationship with each other, and personality also have an effect on sibling adjustment (Sawicki, 1997; Volling, 2012). Parents may be less concerned about their care-taking abilities for an infant, and more concerned with how to manage two or more children adequately.

The addition of a new sibling can be a period of rapid maturation (Anna Freud, 1965, as cited in Stewart et al., 1987). There is a misconception that a great regression occurs with sibling birth. This may be a time of "some disruption, some growth, and no change at all in children's adjustment" (Volling, 2012, p. 26). A child's response involves a whole multitude of factors, many of which are only a small part of having a new sibling. There is also disruption in the mother–firstborn relationship, marital relationship changes, as well as outside influences such as peers and day care. What characteristics a child will display depends on parental characteristics, child characteristics, as well as contextual characteristics (Volling, 2012).

There are a variety of behaviors a sibling may exhibit while adjusting to a newborn. Resorting to newborn behaviors such as mimicry or imitation can occur as the older child attempts to get parental attention. Younger children can evidence behaviors such as increases in pacifier use, toileting accidents, difficulty being left with a sitter, following mom around the house, or aggression to the newborn. Older children can find it hard to play well with other children, have communication difficulties, and may spend more time lying around the house (Sawicki, 1997; Stewart et al., 1987). Many of these behaviors will depend on what developmental milestones are occurring when the new sibling is introduced (Volling, 2012).

In order to help families make this adjustment, education is needed. Sibling prenatal preparation is tailored to their age and development. Some examples of educational strategies are attending sibling classes, allowing participation during antepartum visits by using the tape measure and listening to fetal heart tones, helping with newborn preparations, and talking about "our" baby and what the sibling can expect the baby to do when born in realistic terms, not as a playmate.

Health-care providers can facilitate adjustment by encouraging the belief that this is a time of acclimation versus a time of rivalry. Parents should not scold regressive behavior, but instead offer special time and attention to the older siblings. Visitors should be encouraged to spend time with older siblings when coming to visit the newborn. Parents can keep small gifts on hand for older siblings to decrease jealousy when visitors bring gifts for the newborn. Older siblings should have opportunities to interact with the newborn. Children can help with baby care as desired and age appropriate. It is important to encourage parents to spend time alone with each sibling each day. Finally, it is good to remind parents that open communication and expression of frustration can help prevent aggressive behaviors during this time of sleep and schedule adjustments for the whole family

(Fortier, Carson, Will, & Shubkagel, 1991; Griffin & de la Torre, 1983; Johnsen & Gaspard, 1985; Murphy, 1993; Spero, 1993; Volling, 2005).

Sibling adjustment can have a huge impact on the family as a whole (Feinberg, Solmeyer, & McHale, 2012; Volling, 2012). Relationship conflict and parental frustration can arise due to sibling maladjustment. Future relationships can suffer from early maladjustment as siblings have not learned how to interact with other people. Sibling maladjustment has also been found to increase postpartum depression in the mother and behavioral issues and substance abuse in siblings later in life (Kramer & Bank, 2005; Volling, 2005). Facilitating the adjustment of the whole family to the new baby is a health-promoting practice.

Maternal role attainment is a historical concept used to describe the process a mother goes through as she takes on a new role (Rubin, 1967). The role attainment process may be influenced by culture, personal experiences with being parented, physical condition, socioeconomic status, preparation for this life event, and attitudes about parenting (Meleis, Sawyer, Im, Messias, & Schumacher, 2000). While women begin this journey during pregnancy, continuous changes and honing of the concept of self will occur through transition to the first child and subsequent children. Maternal role attainment is not a static one-time event, but the beginning of a lifelong transformation that is being continually reevaluated and altered.

There are many things that can be done to help women as they evolve their maternal role. The health-care provider can encourage mothers to prepare in advance, trust their instincts about their child, offer suggestions and advice at postpartum and well-child visits, and demonstrate child care practices (Mercer, 2004). Ultimately, this is an important life process for the mother and will influence her self-esteem, satisfaction with her family, as well as set the stage for a nurturing environment for the child where infant development is enhanced.

Infant feeding

Infant feeding method will dictate what topics should be covered and what type of exam is needed. If a woman is bottle-feeding, then a discussion on specifics related to formula should occur. Assessment includes timing, frequency, and amount of feeding. Newborns should formula-feed every 2–3 hours for the first 2 weeks of life and then every 3–4 hours thereafter. Longer periods between feeds at night are fine as long as the infant is gaining weight. After the first 48 hours, the amount of formula taken will increase over the first month to about 12–24 oz/day (Thureen, Deacon, Hernandez, & Hall, 2005). Bottle care and formula storage should be

discussed. Bottles can be washed by hand or in the dishwasher. Sterilization is not necessary. Unused formula should be refrigerated, but a bottle that is half gone should be discarded, not reused for a later feeding.

Breast assessment is important in the woman who is bottle-feeding. Breast engorgement, its resolution, and continuing leakage of milk should be determined. By the 6-week visit, lactation has typically resolved.

If breastfeeding, the health-care provider should assess timing, frequency, and duration. Maternal attitude and acclimation, as well as infant acceptance are important (Blenning & Paladine, 2005). Breastfed babies typically eat at least every 2–3 hours for the first 2 weeks. Feeding on demand is encouraged. Both breasts are used for feeding, but at any given feeding, the baby can get enough supply from one breast (Riordan & Wambach, 2010). Women can check if the baby is getting enough milk by counting the wet diapers, assessing the fontanels (should be firm, not sunken or bulging), and noting sucking and swallowing pattern, as well as demeanor after a feeding.

Women who are breastfeeding should also be taught to assess their nipples after each feeding. This can help determine early signs of nipple breakdown. A crease on the nipple after it is removed from the infant's mouth may signify poor latch. A reddened area may denote malpositioning or a plugged duct. An exam of the breasts by palpation is not essential at the 2-week visit, but should be done based on history as needed. A visual inspection of the nipples can verify the woman's reports of nipple integrity or nipple problems.

Activity/Exercise

Postpartum fatigue is a major concern because of its overall impact on health, as well as the ability to function and care for the newborn. It is difficult in the early postpartum days to recognize differences between what may be normal or what is an early manifestation of an impending problem. Fatigue will impact everything the mother does during this time. The mother needs to prioritize tasks and make time for herself and her other children. Encourage acceptance of help from family and friends. Household chores should be delegated to others. Encourage the mother to nap when the baby naps, as this will bolster her strength for night infant care and feedings.

All women who have given birth should be up and moving relatively soon after birth, even those women who gave birth by cesarean section. Altered clotting factors increase the risk for thrombosis at this time; activity is a preventive practice. Advancement of activity beyond normal walking or house activities will depend on how the woman gave birth. Women who have had a cesarean section should limit activity until their incision is healed. Beginning slowly and building to a normal routine is essential (ACOG Committee on Obstetric Practice, 2002).

Kegel exercises are tightening of the vaginal musculature, specifically the ischiocavernous and transverse perineal muscles, the levator ani and diaphragm muscles, and the pubococcugeal muscles (Varney, Kriebs, & Gegor, 2004). These exercises can begin shortly after birth and should continue throughout life. Kegels can help restore vaginal muscle tone as well as maintain urinary continence. Data suggest a link between pelvic floor muscle training and urinary continence (Hay-Smith, Morkved, Fairbrother, & Herbison, 2008). During the vaginal exam at 6 weeks, have the woman perform a Kegel exercise around the examiner's gloved finger; muscle tone can be assessed and advice given accordingly.

Abdominal musculature has been stretched with the pregnancy and will need work to return to its prepregnant state. Women can begin abdominal strengthening exercises any time after an uncomplicated vaginal birth (Cunningham et al., 2010). These exercises can begin with women lying flat on their backs on the floor with their knees bent pulling their abdomen towards the floor. Once they are able to do this comfortably, women can begin head lifts and progress to curls, as comfort dictates. If a woman had a cesarean birth, then abdominal exercises should be delayed until her incision has healed.

Walking is a wonderful exercise and can begin early in the postpartum period. Going outdoors and getting fresh air benefits the woman, the baby, and possibly other children. Encourage women to start slowly and build back to their normal routine. By monitoring lochial discharge, women can gauge how their body is tolerating the increase in exercise. Heavier or brighter red lochia means they are doing too much and need to slow down.

Progression of the exercise regime should occur once a woman is comfortable doing Kegel exercises, abdominal strengthening, and walking without an increase in bleeding or pain (Varney et al., 2004). The woman may take this time for herself or incorporate her children in this activity. Endorphins released can help improve mood.

Women who regularly exercise vigorously and women athletes require special consideration in advice from health-care providers. Safe limits for vigorous exercise during the early postpartum period have not been determined, so recommendations should be supportive but cautious. Encourage these women to listen to their bodies and remind them of the physiological changes occurring that may need to alter their typical exercise patterns for a brief amount of time.

Warning signs should be reviewed with all women. Women should be cautioned to stop exercising if they experience the following: bright red vaginal bleeding, increased pain, shortness of breath, or light-headedness. If symptoms do not improve with rest, they should seek care.

Diet and nutrition

The woman recovering from childbirth needs excellent, high-quality, well-balanced nutrition. She should follow the ChooseMyPlate guidelines, and not calorie-restrict her diet early in the postpartum period (United States Department of Agriculture, n.d.). Women can visualize what and how much of each food group they should be eating. The dinner plate is divided into quadrants, where vegetables and grains make up the largest quadrants and proteins and fruits make up smaller quadrants. Encouraging food choices with high nutrition value while minimizing empty calorie foods is important for her health. When breastfeeding, the average woman needs approximately 500 calories more than what was needed prepregnancy.

Postpartum discharge instructions from the birth facility usually include continuation of prenatal vitamins and possibly addition of an iron supplement. Nutrients are absorbed better through food, but taking an iron supplement may be necessary to augment a marginal or deficient diet or to replace iron stores. Reviewing how and when the client is taking her supplements is beneficial.

A restriction in caloric intake for weight reduction purposes can occur later in the postpartum period, especially after lactation is well established. According to a Cochrane Review, diet alone can help women shed excess weight after birth (Amorim Adegboye, Linne, & Lourenco, 2007). However, diet in conjunction with exercise facilitates weight loss and has additional health benefits; thus, education on exercise should be undertaken.

Over the first few weeks postpartum, women will naturally lose the excess water retained during pregnancy through increased perspiration and urination. It is important to encourage women to drink when thirsty to maintain hydration. Encouraging water is best for hydration. Soda and fruit juices should be limited, as they contain large amounts of sugar.

Weight loss

Many women are very concerned about returning to their prepregnant weight. Discussion regarding weight management should begin prenatally. Reminding women that they put on pregnancy weight over several months will help them realize that it may take several months for the weight to come off. It is important for women to attain a healthy weight in the first few months postpartum to prevent obesity in subsequent pregnancies and later in life (Amorim-Adegboye et al., 2007). Many women are motivated to remove excess weight but are also adjusting to the demands of a new infant. Taking time to assess diet, lifestyle, risk factors, and current body mass index (BMI) can help facilitate this process. Individual realistic goals are important.

Lochia

Lochia is the vaginal blood, tissue, and mucus loss occurring after birth and often lasting up to 6 or 8 weeks postpartum. Lochia flow progresses through three predictable stages, but timing can vary. Lochia rubra begins after birth and lasts for the first few days postpartum. This bleeding contains erythrocytes, decidua, bacteria, and epithelial cells (Cunningham et al., 2010). Lochia serosa is lighter in color and amount. It usually begins after 4 or so days postpartum. By a week to 10 days, the lochia has become white or yellowish and is termed lochia alba.

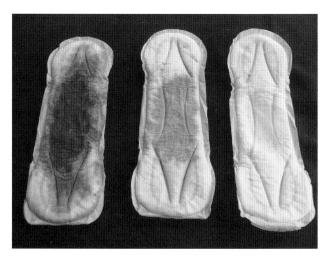

Figure 27.1. Lochia.

Lochial flow	
Average amount of lochia lost during postpartum	8–9 oz, 240–270 mL*
Lochia:	4–8 weeks
Lochia rubra	Lasts 2–4 days postpartum
Lochia serosa	After rubra—up to about 10 days postpartum
Lochia alba	After serosa—up to 4–8 weeks postpartum**

Sources: *Varney et al. (2004); **Cunningham et al. (2010).

Lochia may continue until 4–6 weeks postpartum (Fig. 27.1). Each day, the amount of bleeding should be less and the color lighter. An exception to this rule is eschar bleeding that occurs at about 10 days postpartum. The eschar is the area where the placenta is attached in the uterus. At approximately 10 days, this "scab" will be released. Women can experience heavier, brighter red bleeding which should only last for a few hours. If it persists beyond that time frame, she should be evaluated. It is important to note in the chart when postpartum lochia bleeding stopped. This helps determine whether bleeding at a future date is a return of menses or the continuation of lochial flow.

Afterbirth pain

Afterbirth pains are caused by contractions of the uterus in the process of involution. Afterbirth pains are not usually as strong in most first-time mothers as the uterus stays well contracted after birth. Women who have had more than one birth, or whose uterus had been overdistended due to multifetal gestation, will experience more cramping due to the inability of the uterus to maintain muscle tone and subsequently will often report increased discomfort and pain.

Breastfeeding leads to the release of endogenous oxytocin, which stimulates the uterus to contract (Riordan & Wambach, 2010). This can be very beneficial in decreasing bleeding. It is important to encourage women to empty their bladder prior to breastfeeding. An empty bladder will allow endogenous oxytocin to contract the uterus and keep it contracted during feeding. A full bladder will not allow the uterus to remain contracted and increased cramping with breastfeeding can result.

There are several recommendations to help with cramping. Lying prone is helpful; pressure on the uterus leads to a sustained contraction, keeping the uterus contracted and bringing subsequent relief. Ibuprofen or nonsteroidal anti-inflammatory drugs (NSAIDs) are medications of choice, as they are antiprostaglandins. One recommended dosage schedule is ibuprofen 600 mg po Q 6h prn. Stronger medications, such as narcotics, may be needed to control pain in the first hours or days after birth, but severe afterpains that last longer than that should be evaluated to determine if there is another underlying cause of the pain.

Perineal discomfort

Knowing what type of laceration, or if an episiotomy was performed, will guide the assessment of the perineum. Some lacerations require minimal, if any, suturing, while others may need extensive suturing. By 3 weeks postpartum, most repairs should be well healed and the suture should have resorbed, except for the external knot (Cunningham et al., 2010). The knot will eventually be released when the suture underneath has dissolved.

Early postpartum comfort measures are aimed at reducing perineal swelling and decreasing pain. Ice packs can be used to decrease edema. Topical anesthetics or healing herbs, such as Dermoplast, witch hazel, or comfrey compresses, can also be used. Sitz baths can also offer relief. Sitz baths involve filling a premade tub, which sits in the toilet, with warm or cold water. Cold may be comforting when edema is present. The woman can continue these for as long as is comfortable. Filling a clean tub with a few inches of water can accomplish the same thing, without the necessity of a Sitz bath tub. Kegel exercises help increase circulation to the perineum and can provide comfort with movement after some initial tenderness (Varney et al., 2004).

Each day postpartum, the perineal area should evidence more healing, reflected in increasing comfort in the area. If there is increasing irritation or pain, then an examination is recommended. Diagnoses that are considered include perineal infection, hematoma, and dehiscence of repair. Inquire about activities that could potentially irritate the area, such as intercourse or overexertion. For some women, it can take months for the perineum to feel comfortable again (Blackburn, 2013).

Diureseis/Diaphoresis

Women will begin shedding the excess water, retained during pregnancy, soon after birth. This usually occurs on days 2–5 but may start as early as 12 hours, and last into the second week, especially if large amounts of IV fluid were used in labor. By 21 days postpartum, the diuresis and diaphoresis is complete (Blackburn, 2013).

Diuresis of about 3000 cc/day is common. A single void can be 500 cc or more (Blackburn, 2013). Remind women of the importance of keeping the bladder empty and the uterus contracted, and reassure them that the loss of this extra fluid is a natural part of the postpartum recovery process.

Diaphoresis is another route for shedding excess extracellular fluid. Remind women of its normalcy and discuss comfort measures. Encourage frequent showering or bathing, wearing natural fibers, and dressing in layers. Keep fluids at the bedside and drink to thirst. Explain that weight loss of as much as 5 lb of fluid during this time can be noted (Cunningham et al., 2010)

Constipation/Hemorrhoids

For many women, resumption of normal bowel habits can take up to a week. During birth, many women will push out stool but may be unaware they have done so. Additionally, many women have limited intake during labor and thus have limited stool in the rectum.

Some women will have complaints of constipation and may fear having a bowel movement due to pain or sutures of the perineum. A bowel movement will not disrupt the sutures, so reassurance can be provided. Women should be encouraged to increase fluids, eat high-fiber foods, and get some moderate activity, such as walking. Constipation can be a side effect for women who were instructed to take iron supplementation or are taking pain medications. Over-the-counter mild laxatives or stool softeners can be beneficial.

Hemorrhoids are a common occurrence after birth. Hemorrhoids can develop before or during the pregnancy and are exacerbated or traumatized during birth. Initially, relief measures are aimed at reducing the size and itching of the hemorrhoids. Tucks, or witch hazel compresses, Preparation H ointment, and anesthetic sprays can all offer relief (Blackburn, 2013). Warm sitz baths can also be beneficial. Stool softeners can be used to decrease aggravation. Remind women that preventing constipation will relieve hemorrhoids; so increased fluids, fiber, and exercise, such as walking, are in order.

Sexuality

Resuming intimacy between partners is a very important concern during this time but is often overlooked or not mentioned at all in early postpartum instructions (Johnson, 2011). Resuming intercourse should not be a medical decision but a personal one, stressing the decision is really up to the individual woman and her comfort level. The decision to resume sex is different for every person and every birth experience. Waiting until after the 6-week postpartum visit has no physiological basis and many couples resume intercourse before then; 66% will have resumed intercourse in the first month, and 88% by the second postpartum month (Kennedy & Trussell, 2011). Therefore, having a discussion regarding postpartum resumption of intimate relations in the prenatal and postpartum periods is important (Blenning & Paladine, 2005).

Women should consider many factors when making the decision to resume sex. Readiness to resume intimacy includes factors such as whether the bleeding has decreased, the perineum is comfortable, both partners feel ready, and decisions about family planning and contraception have been made. It is also normal for women to feel less desire for sexual relations due to the close physical and emotional connection with the newborn. The most frequently cited reasons for poor postpartum sexual adjustment include perineal discomfort, vaginal bleeding or discharge, dyspareunia, fatigue on the part of both partners, insufficient lubrication, leaking or tender breasts, fear of waking the infant, fear of injury, fear of pregnancy, and a decreased sense of attractiveness (Blenning & Paladine, 2005; Johnson, 2011).

The partner's reactions to postpartum mothers vary considerably (Williamson, McVeigh, & Baafi, 2008). The partner may have altered attraction to the new mother for physical or emotional reasons. It is helpful to acknowledge this and to foster ways to resolve issues. When sexual interest and desires differ, it is especially important to communicate these feelings (MacAdam, Huuva, & Bertero, 2009). Avoidance behavior and disappointment can be perpetuated when parents avoid talking about emotional and sexual wishes and problems (Von Sydow, 1999). When sexual needs do not coincide, partners can interpret these discrepancies as rejection. Refer couples who struggle with these issues to couples' counseling, and be sure to follow up at subsequent visits.

Vaginal lubrication can be altered postpartally, especially for women who breastfeed (Johnson, 2011; Leeman & Rogers, 2012). Encourage plenty of foreplay, as well as over-the-counter lubricants. Lubricants such as Astroglide and K-Y Jelly are water soluble and therefore safe with latex. Natural oils, such as mineral oil and olive oil, can be used but can weaken the integrity of latex condoms. For a discussion of postpartum contraception, see Chapter 29.

Intimacy can be expressed in various ways, such as holding, touching, caressing, and massaging (Johnson, 2011). The resumption of intimacy does not necessarily signal the resumption of intercourse (MacAdam et al., 2009). Expressing goodwill and humor, creating time and space to be together, feeling nurtured, and getting some sleep can strengthen relationships at this transitional time and can lead to enhanced sexual desire.

Resumption of menses and ovulation

In order to help women anticipate when resumption of menses and ovulation may occur, it is important to take a thorough history. Knowing this woman's lochial flow pattern can help determine if bleeding or spotting is a resumption of lochia or menses. Note whether a woman is breast- or bottlefeeding. Women who breastfeed, even for a short amount of time, may have a delayed

Table 27.3   Resumption of Menses

Nonlactating women	
Resumes	4–6 weeks postpartum
% Anovulatory first month	33%
% Anovulatory months 2–3	15%
Lactating women	
Resumes	Depends on duration and frequency of lactation
% Anovulatory first 3 months	55–67%
% Anovulatory months 4–12	29–36%
% Anovulatory after 12 months	Up to 13%

Source: Kennedy and Trussell (2011).

resumption of menses due to the hormonal shifts that occur to sustain lactation.

There is no certainty as to when menses and ovulation will begin. Women can ovulate prior to their first menses (see Table 27.3) (Blackburn, 2013; Cunningham et al., 2010). Understanding that fertility can return before menses resumes is essential contraceptive teaching. Women who bottle-feed their baby can anticipate a return to menses within 4–6 weeks postpartum (Kennedy & Trussell, 2011). Women who breastfeed their babies can anticipate a delay in the resumption of menses and ovulation, but times vary greatly. Resumption can vary between 2 and 18 months postpartally (Cunningham et al., 2010). Generally, if the woman is exclusively breastfeeding an infant, then the hormonal shift will delay the resumption of ovulation and menses. Teaching emphasis has to be on the unknown nature of the return of ovulation and the ability for ovulation to precede menses, especially for women who want to prevent further or closely spaced pregnancies.

Contraception

Discussion of what contraceptive method will be used after birth should begin in the antenatal period and be affirmed in the very early postpartum period. Postpartum contraceptive education "led to more contraception use and fewer unplanned pregnancies" (Lopez, Hiller, & Grimes, 2010, p. 2). Many women will choose to resume the method they previously used. Method of infant feeding will need to be taken into consideration in this decision. Types of contraception, ease of use, success with prior use, lifestyle, partner responsibilities, and reproductive life plans are important components of discussion.

Women who choose to bottle-feed can use combined hormonal methods. Combined hormonal contraceptives are contraindicated before 21 days postpartum due to the heightened risk of venous thromboembolism (VTE) (Centers for Disease Control, 2011a). Women with risk factors for VTE should be evaluated between days 21 and 42 and included in a risk/benefit analysis regarding contraception decisions. After 42 days postpartum, standard criteria for eligibility for combined hormonal contraceptive are used (Centers for Disease Control, 2011a).

Breastfeeding influences contraception in several ways. First, many exclusively breastfeeding women will experience lactational amenorrhea, which is reliable as a birth control method up until 3 months postpartum (Kennedy & Trussell, 2011). Second, women who are breastfeeding should not use a hormonal method of birth control that contains estrogen. Estrogen can influence the milk supply and lead to earlier cessation of breastfeeding (Riordan & Wambach, 2010). Progestin-only pills are the recommended choice for women who breastfeed and desire oral contraceptives. Finally, some women prefer to limit newborn exposure to exogenous hormones during this time, as progesterone and estrogen can be found in the milk supply (Kennedy & Trussell, 2011). For more information on postnatal contraception, see Chapter 29.

Postpartum physical examination

Breast exam

A breast exam is performed at the 6-week postpartum visit. Historically, it was thought that palpation of the lactating breast would not yield relevant information due to the inherent physical changes. However, since there is an increase in breast cancer found during pregnancy and lactation, the breast exam is now recommended for women while they are breastfeeding. Women who have breast cancer detected in early postpartum often have a worse prognosis than breast cancer detected at another life stage (Johansson, Andersson, Hsieh, Cnattingius, & Lambe, 2011). A delay in evaluation and diagnosis, due to pregnancy and lactation, is thought to be a primary contributor to a poorer prognosis (Bure, Azoulay, Benjamin, & Abenhaim, 2011). Women are instructed to report worrisome changes. Health-care providers need to follow up with any persistent lump.

Women who do not breastfeed will experience breast engorgement on days 2–4 postpartum. Women should be encouraged to refrain from stimulating the breasts in any way. A form-fitting bra should be worn, even to sleep at night. Women can use cold compresses and NSAID pain medications. Lack of breast stimulation will decrease the levels of prolactin and milk production will decline and then cease (Blackburn, 2013; Riordan & Wambach, 2010). This may take several weeks.

For women who choose to breastfeed, the health-care practitioner should visually inspect the breasts and nipples for any areas of breakdown or redness (Riordan & Wambach, 2010). Infant malpositioning and poor latch can lead to nipple breakdown. Observation of a feeding can assist in the assessment for signs of poor latch. Educate women to evaluate their breasts on a regular basis; this can help identify breakdown before it becomes significant. Excessive redness, a break in the skin, or a compressed nipple right after feeding may be signs of a malpositioned infant. While inspecting the breast, assess for warm or reddened areas as well as specific or general breast discomfort. Such areas can indicate mastitis; this is discussed in more detail in Chapter 28.

Palpation of lactating or nonlactating breasts should be done in a standard and thorough manner. Compress the nipple at the end of the exam and observe any discharge. Follow-up and collaboration or referral should be undertaken for any abnormal breast changes or persistent areas of concern.

Abdominal exam

The route of birth will determine expectations and extent of the examination of the woman's abdomen. The abdomen is inspected for sutures or a healing site if she had a cesarean birth. Abdominal inspection postcesarean birth includes assessing for signs of infection (warmth, redness, drainage) and wound dehiscence. Incision staples are usually removed around day 4 postpartum (Cunningham et al., 2010). If there is concern for wound dehiscence, then staples may remain *in situ* for a week or more postpartum.

Involution of the uterus is assessed by location of the fundus compared to the number of days postpartum. Involution of the uterus follows a methodical pattern approximating one fingerbreadth of descent per day from the umbilicus to the pubis symphysis. During the first few days after birth, the uterus should be at or below the umbilicus. If the uterus is above or displaced to the side of the umbilicus, the bladder may be full. Ask the woman to empty her bladder and then reassess. If the uterus remains displaced, then further evaluation of bleeding or clots is warranted (Varney et al., 2004). On day 3 postpartum, the fundus should be about three fingerbreadths below the umbilicus; day 4, four fingerbreadths. By a week, it should be about halfway between the umbilicus and symphysis. The fundus of the uterus should only be palpable abdominally for up to 2 weeks postpartum (Blackburn, 2013). After that time, the involuted uterus sits below the symphysis pubis and is a pelvic organ again (Blackburn, 2013). Palpation of the abdomen is done to ascertain where the fundus is located. If the fundus is not located where anticipated, and her bladder is empty, then further evaluation is needed. It is important to do this exam at 2 as well as 6 weeks postpartum to ascertain normal involution. At the 6-week exam, the uterus will be evaluated on pelvic exam, as it is no longer felt abdominally.

The consistency of the fundus should also be noted. A firm consistency means the myometrial fibers are contracting and there is less blood loss. A soft or boggy uterus means the fibers are relaxed, which can result in heavier bleeding. The fundus is massaged, and any clots expelled which allows the fundus to contract and maintain a firm consistency (Varney et al., 2004).

All women have a certain degree of diastasis of the abdominal recti muscles to accommodate the growing uterus during pregnancy. The degree of diastasis depends on multiple factors including multiple gestation, number of pregnancies, spacing of those pregnancies, and overall abdominal condition of the mother (Varney et al., 2004). To assess the degree of diastasis, have the woman lying supine. Place examining fingers midline on the abdomen. Ask the woman to tighten her abdominal muscles and bring her chin to her chest. A gap is noted in the midline between the two sheaths of abdominal muscles as they contract while the head is lifted. Measure this space in fingerbreadths.

Knowing the degree of diastasis can be a motivating factor to help women resume exercise and regain muscle tone. Encourage chin lifts (like that performed during the exam) with a gradual progression to abdominal curls to help restore abdominal tone. If the woman had a cesarean birth, exercises can begin when all abdominal soreness is gone (Cunningham et al., 2010). Good muscle tone can help alleviate or lessen back pain during subsequent pregnancies. Backache during pregnancy can occur from lax abdominal tone and resultant back muscle compensation.

Costovertebral angle tenderness (CVAT)

Assessing for CVAT is done during the postpartum exam. Women are at an increased risk for urinary tract infection (UTI) postpartally due to events that can occur during labor and birth. Urinary stasis, overdistention of the bladder, and vulvar trauma all increase risk of postpartum UTI (Blackburn, 2013).

Perineal exam

A thorough history noting what happened during her birth will facilitate what to expect when performing a perineal assessment. If the woman had an episiotomy or a laceration, then inspection of the area should be undertaken at the 2- and 6-week visits.

Perineal tissues should be healed by 2–3 weeks postpartum, but it can take up to a few months to be completely healed if extensive tearing occurred or an episiotomy was performed (Blackburn, 2013). Removal of the last knot of suture may be warranted based on complaints and observation. If all remaining repaired tissue is healed, then it is safe to remove the last suture. Granulation tissue may be noted and the use of silver nitrate may offer the woman relief. A faint pinkish line should be noted where the tissues approximated and healed. If there is redness, edema, purulent exudate, or a fever, then a perineal infection should be suspected and appropriate management arranged.

Vaginal and uterine exam

After birth, the vagina can be bruised, lacerated, and edematous. Over the first few days postpartum, increased vaginal tone will be noted as the edema subsides. Rugae return at approximately 3–4 weeks postpartum (Blackburn, 2013). The vagina never fully returns to its prepregnant state, however (Blackburn, 2013; Cunningham et al., 2010). Hymenal remnants can be observed, as well as scars from lacerations and repairs.

A vaginal exam is not essential at the 2-week visit unless the woman is complaining of symptoms indicative of excessive postpartum bleeding or endometritis. If the uterus is larger than anticipated for 2 weeks postpartum, then subinvolution should be diagnosed and the cause is investigated. If she is saturating more than a pad an hour, an exam is performed to determine the cause of postpartum hemorrhage. The management will depend on symptoms and findings.

At 6 weeks postpartum, a speculum exam is done for cultures, or a Pap smear if indicated, and for visual inspection of internal tissues. A vaginal exam is done to assess uterine size, palpate ovaries, and assess vaginal muscle tone. The uterus is approximately the size of a nonpregnant uterus by 6 weeks postpartum (Blackburn, 2013; Stables & Rankin, 2011). Before removing examining fingers from the woman's vagina, ask her to perform a Kegel exercise to assess vaginal tone. Assess for cystocele or rectocele at this time.

Rectal exam

Based on history, some women may need evaluation of their hemorrhoids. Comfort measures are initiated early postpartum, but assessing efficacy and visualizing the hemorrhoids can dictate further treatment. Occasionally, referral to a proctologist will be indicated.

A rectal exam is indicated after a third- or fourth-degree laceration to assess the healing, integrity, and tonus of the internal and external anal sphincters. Any reports of fecal incontinence warrant an assessment of the rectovaginal wall. Occult tears of the anal sphincter during childbirth are emerging as a high-risk litigation area. While rectal exams are used sparingly, it is important to note appropriate healing of all areas traumatized during childbirth. There is debate in the literature on whether a woman with a third- or fourth-degree laceration should have a vaginal birth or cesarean section with a subsequent birth; the general consensus is that cesarean birth should be offered.

Leg exam

Evaluation of the lower extremities occurs at the 2- and 6-week visit. Many women experience varicosities during pregnancy; postpartum assessment can direct further management. An evaluation of any leg pain or tenderness should be done to assess potential deep or superficial venous thrombosis. If a cord-like vessel is noted, or the patient has warmth over an area, edema, or complaints of pain or tenderness, referral is indicated. Homan's sign may or may not be positive (Cunningham et al., 2010). Normal pregnancy edema of the legs has usually dissipated by 2 weeks.

Postpartum depression and domestic violence screening

Postpartum depression occurs in 10–20% of pregnancies (Beck & Indman, 2005; Boyd, Zayas, & McKee, 2006; Gaynes et al., 2005). All women should be screened during every encounter postpartum. This may be at the postpartum visit, a problem visit, or a well-child exam.

Many practices utilize validated screening tools to screen for depression, such as the Edinburgh Postnatal Depression Scale (EPDS) (Committee on Obstetric Practice, 2010). The EPDS screening tool can be given to women as they are placed in an exam room, allowing privacy to complete the tool while waiting to be seen. Health-care practitioners can then score responses and talk to women about their answers. Some women may be ashamed about their feelings, or feel they should be happy since they just had a baby, and may not want to share how they really feel. A self-report screening tool assists women who may be reluctant to self-disclose any negative feelings they may have. The screening tool is used in conjunction with evaluation. A postpartum depression diagnosis is not made based on the screening tool score alone. Further discussion with the woman is done, and her feelings and other symptoms and behaviors are explored. Collaboration with mental health practitioners may be warranted. Postpartum mood and anxiety disorders are discussed in detail in Chapters 28 and 42.

All women should be screened at every encounter to determine if they are safe in their home from intimate partner violence (IPV). Questioning about IPV may occur many times before a woman is comfortable sharing this information. Make IPV questioning a routine part of all encounters, so that women know they can choose to share this information (American College of Obstetricians and Gynecologists (ACOG), 2012).

Postnatal warning signs

The following signs and symptoms that can appear during the postpartum period are linked with a differential diagnosis list to consider in an assessment (see Table 27.4).

Cultural considerations

Cultural traditions and practices are common during childbirth and the postpartum period. Women often

Table 27.4   Postnatal Warning Signs

Symptom	Differential diagnoses
Saturating maxi pad in <1 hour	Postpartum hemorrhage, endometritis, retained products of conception
Passing golf ball-size clots, more than 1	Postpartum hemorrhage, endometritis, retained products of conception
A return of bright red bleeding after that phase of lochia has passed	Eschar bleeding, postpartum hemorrhage, overexertion; endometritis
Temperature >101°F	Endometritis, mastitis, viral infection
Severe headache	Postpartum preeclampsia
Visual disturbances	Postpartum preeclampsia
Seizure	Postpartum preeclampsia
Warm, hard spot on breast	Plugged duct, mastitis
Chest pain	Pulmonary emboli
Warm area, pain, or edema in calf	Deep vein thrombosis, superficial thrombophlebitis
Difficulty or pain with urination	UTI
Pus, redness, foul odor to cesarean section scar	Incision infection, wound dehiscence
Pus, redness, or foul odor of perineum	Endometritis, perineal infection
Hopelessness, despair, or fear of harming self, infant, or other children	Postpartum depression, anxiety, psychosis

look to family members or community for support and guidance. If the woman is removed geographically from her culture or community, an assessment of her resources is needed to help prevent isolation (Johnson Waugh, 2011). Cultural traditions and practices should be honored without interference and encouraged unless safety is a concern. Health-care providers should not make assumptions based on ethnicity. Cultural traditions should be assessed during the prenatal period. Once identified, determine individual needs and facilitate meeting these needs. By gaining a basic understanding of the common cultures in the local community, the practitioner can better care for women during the postpartum period.

Many cultures value postpartum as a time of healing for women and specify a period when she and the baby will remain relatively secluded and cared for by female relatives (Kim-Godwin, 2003). This practice is in contrast to many Western cultures where women are often expected to resume normal activities relatively soon after birth. There may also be specification that sexual intercourse does not resume until all bleeding has stopped or a specified period of time has elapsed. Women are also encouraged to eat particular foods, at certain temperatures or with certain food characteristics that make them hot or cold, in order to help restore their body and help prevent ailments later in life (Holroyd, Katie, Chun, & Ha, 1997; Kim-Godwin, 2003; Lundberg & Thi Ngoc Thu, 2011). By helping facilitate cultural traditions and practices, health-care providers communicate respect for this heritage.

For example, in some Asian cultures, there is the concept of "doing the month" (Holroyd et al., 1997, p. 301; Kim-Godwin, 2003; Matthey, Panasetis, & Barnett, 2002). Women refrain from having visitors, sexual intercourse, reading, crying, bathing/washing their hair, touching cold water, or going out into the sun. They are closely cared for by female relatives. The woman focuses on restoring her body and caring for her baby. Blood is considered hot so when women lose blood through childbirth, they are considered to be in a cold state. Therefore, they need care and foods to restore this balance (Kim-Godwin, 2003; Lundberg & Thi Ngoc Thu, 2011).

Some Hispanic cultures have similar rituals. "La cuarentena" is the time after childbirth for recovery (Johnson Waugh, 2011, p. 732). Heat is very important postpartum and women may be asked to bathe in warm water with herbs, use sitz baths, or have a hot water bottle (Kim-Godwin, 2003). Women in other Hispanic cultures may refrain from bathing during this period of confinement, so it is very important to ascertain what each woman believes. Air currents are considered harmful and women keep scarves and coverings over their body to prevent air currents from causing ailments (Johnson Waugh, 2011). Foods that produce heat, gas, spiciness, heaviness, and acidity should be avoided. Postpartum is seen as a time of the body being susceptible to many things. By following a prescribed regimen, women can close themselves from harmful influences and heal from the ailments of childbirth and prevent illness (Johnson Waugh, 2011).

In most non-Western cultures, the woman is revered as she makes this life-transforming passage into motherhood (Kim-Godwin, 2003). Too much positive attention to the baby is felt to draw the "evil eye" to the child, which may bring harm or bad luck. In contrast, in many Western cultures, the baby is the primary focus and the woman is of little or no focus. Although an accepted practice in the West, lack of support or help may be a source of conflicting emotions for someone who is not raised in this tradition. The woman may feel let down as her rite of passage has not been honored. Health-care practitioners should be aware of this potential conflict and be prepared to assist through active listening and identification of available resources.

Health disparities and vulnerable populations

Health disparities are evident in many populations in the United States. The Pregnancy Risk Assessment Monitoring System (PRAMS) done by the CDC in 11 states and in New York City found that overall, as many as 89% of women attend postnatal visits (Centers for Disease Control, 2007). However, some of the most vulnerable populations are the least likely to get postpartum care: only 71% of women with less than 8 years of education, about 66% with no prenatal care, 71% with late prenatal care, and about 60% of women whose babies also did not have well-child visits. Postpartum teaching, as well as communicating the need for postpartum follow-up visits, is an important aspect of care before discharge following childbirth.

Immigrants, the uninsured or underinsured, homeless women, teen populations, and women who suffer abuse will all need additional considerations during postpartum follow-up. Some women may simultaneously fall into several vulnerable categories, putting them at added risk for problems. The health-care practitioner plays a vital role for many vulnerable women and can offer a safe place to be heard. Helping women learn about care for themselves, their baby, and family can be very challenging when access to information is limited and other living needs take precedence (Sword & Watt, 2005). For some women, attending a postpartum visit may pose many challenges; there may be transportation, childcare, and loss of work issues. Assisting women with available resources or providing incentives for attendance at the postpartum visit may encourage attendance at follow-up visits. Increasing postpartum visit attendance is a Healthy People 2020 objective (U.S. Department of Health and Human Services, 2010).

Immigrant women may not speak the language, understand rites or customs, or be able to negotiate everyday systems such as taking a bus or finding their clinic within a hospital. Food, shelter, and health care can be daunting tasks. Taking time during visits to assess available resources, and supplementing where appropriate, can facilitate optimal health for the whole family. Women struggle to care for themselves and their newborns if they are worried about how to eat or maintain shelter.

The uninsured and underinsured in the United States have many barriers including health-care costs. Health-care practices are often dictated by reimbursement. Lack of reimbursement is the primary reason many practices do not offer a 2-week postpartum visit. Most insurance payers only reimburse for one postpartum visit, which is often part of the global fee. What health insurers have not yet realized is that if women can be screened earlier, and problems averted or determined earlier, then less health-care dollars can be spent to rectify ailments after the fact (Stacy Tsai, Nakashima, Yamamoto, Ngo, & Kaneshiro, 2011). The 2-week appointment is a screening time for the detection of many postpartum problems.

Adolescent mothers face numerous issues during pregnancy as well as postpartum. While teen pregnancy rates are down overall, some groups, such as African Americans, Hispanic teens, and teens living in southern states, continue to have higher rates (Centers for Disease Control, 2011b). Teenage mothers are challenged in the development of the maternal role, as they are going through some of the challenges of adolescent development at the same time. Maternal self-esteem can be an important factor in the developing relationship between teen mother and child. Teenage mothers face social and economic disadvantages. Health-care providers play important roles in education and support. Tailor education and advice to appropriate developmental levels. Praise can go a long way in facilitating positive behaviors. Role modeling of appropriate care and parenting behaviors can also be helpful. Teens are at risk for a repeat teen pregnancy in a short time interval (Wilson, Samandari, Koo, & Tucker, 2011). Postpartum follow-up is essential to help ameliorate this cycle. Facilitation of effective reliable contraception should be done at each postpartum encounter.

Women should be screened for intimate partner violence and asked if they feel safe during the postpartum visit (ACOG, 2012; Garabedian et al., 2011). If women report abuse and are ready to make a change, community resources should be activated. For many women,

pregnancy and childbirth can be a very vulnerable time where abuse escalates. Women can be motivated to seek care due to concerns about the safety of their baby.

There is a fairly high rate of failure to show for postpartum visits. In one large study, as many as 40% of women did not have timely postpartum care (Weir et al., 2011). This is a concern regarding postpartum screening, prevention, and education for these women. Perhaps the message is that many women do not find these postpartum visits meaningful, suggesting a reexamination and restructuring of postpartum care as currently offered. Incorporating home visits and the creative use of social media for monitoring, education, and support holds the promise to enhance and expand postpartum care.

Scope of practice considerations

Health-care providers work within a health-care system where interacting with other providers facilitates optimal care for women and their families. Consultation, collaboration, or referral can occur with physicians, therapists, social workers, lactation consultants, and as well as other providers. Knowing when to bring in the expertise of other professionals with different knowledge and skill sets to serve the woman's needs is an important clinical decision point that all health-care providers need to consider.

There are varying levels of involvement of other providers. Consultation refers to talking with another provider about the care of a patient. This person may have more expertise in a particular area or a consultation may be warranted based on protocols or practicing at the boundaries of scope of practice. An example of a consult situation in postnatal care is when a patient has recurrent plugged ducts in her breasts while breastfeeding. A lactation consultant can be contacted for treatments to ameliorate this problem and prevent mastitis.

Collaboration occurs when each practitioner will be assuming part of the care for the patient. A woman receiving a cesarean section is a good example of when collaborative care may occur. The patient may return to the physician who did the surgery for evaluation of the incision and postsurgical recovery, but may see another practitioner for normal postpartum follow-up and lactation advice.

Referral is necessary when a patient condition dictates that another provider would better serve the patient. Referral is warranted when a patient presents with a high fever, abdominal tenderness, foul smelling lochia, abnormal bleeding, and subinvolution. One practitioner may begin the workup, obtaining cultures or blood work, but the physician will assume care of this woman and treat the severe endometritis requiring hospitalization.

Health-care providers will need to be very cognizant of their own scope of practice, as other practitioners may not be aware of specific guidelines. By reviewing current state practice acts and updating collaborative practice agreements, risk reductions strategies are facilitated ("Understanding Nurse Practitioner Liability," 2010). All members of the health-care team should keep the woman herself at the center of their efforts to provide optimal care for her and her family.

Legal issues

All legal, ethical, and malpractice issues that affect practitioners in other roles also apply to postnatal care. During postpartum, the Family and Medical Leave Act entitles eligible employees of covered employers to take unpaid, job-protected leaves for specified family and medical reasons with continuation of group health insurance coverage under the same terms and conditions as if the employee had not taken leave. Relevant to the postpartum period is the provision of up to 12 work weeks of leave in a 12-month period for the birth of a child and to care for the newborn child within 1 year of birth (United States Department of Labor, 1993). Note that this is an unpaid leave and some eligible parents will not be able to afford this option. Many employers require documentation of a 6-week postpartum exam before women return to work (United States Department of Labor, 1993).

Summary

In the United States, postpartum care is limited in scope and typically completed after the first 6 weeks. This current health-care standard lacks the support required to help a woman and her family adjust to their new roles and responsibilities, and more importantly, to assist the women in their recovery from and adjustment to the anatomic, physiological, and psychological changes after childbirth. The postpartum period follows one of the most significant life-changing experiences in a woman's life. Although during pregnancy it is natural to focus on one's current needs and the preparation for childbirth, little emphasis is placed on educating women about what to expect after giving birth. Many of the physical and emotional problems that women suffer from long term after childbirth arise during the first 2–6 weeks postpartum. An increase in the attention and support women receive during this time can greatly affect their long-term well-being, as well as the health and well-being of their infant and families (Groff, 2011).

Case study

Samantha, a G3P2002, gave birth vaginally 2 weeks ago over a first-degree laceration. She is breastfeeding. She is being seen for her 2-week postpartum visit.

SUBJECTIVE: Samantha is adjusting to sleep disruptions as the baby is nursing frequently, but she is happy that the breastfeeding is going well. She is very pleased with her birth experience—she had wanted to try a water birth and felt that it was everything she had hoped in terms of helping ease her pain and creating a calm and peaceful environment for her baby. Samantha's husband is taking a leave from his job and her mother is helping out with her other children for another week and then her mother-in-law will come for a week to help, so she has lots of tangible and emotional support. Her two children are delighted with the new baby, although they are young enough that she has to keep a close eye on them during their interactions with the baby.

Samantha reports decreased tenderness in the perineal area, small amounts of yellowish to red vaginal discharge, and cramping only with the initiation of breastfeeding. She and her husband have not yet resumed intercourse; she is interested in starting the minipill. She is eating and drinking well. Her activities are primarily self-care, baby care, and family care at this point. She has no difficulty with bowel or bladder elimination.

OBJECTIVE: Samantha's vital signs, BMI, and postpartum depression screening are all normal. She has lost 19 of the 25 lb she gained during pregnancy. A breast exam reveals no masses, expression of mature breast milk, and intact nipples without irritation or trauma. CVAT is not elicited. Upon abdominal exam, the uterine fundus is not palpable and a two-finger-breadth diastasis is elicited. Extremities are negative for edema and Homan's sign. Perineal tissues are pink, healing, and well approximated.

ASSESSMENT: Samantha is a G3P2002 at 2 weeks postpartum with normal findings and successful breastfeeding who desires contraception.

PLAN: Education and support of Samantha's postpartum recovery were given in the following areas: sibling adjustment, exercise, diet/fluids, rest, lubrication with sexual intercourse, and warning signs. Micronor was prescribed to begin at 6 weeks postpartum with condom use encouraged prior to starting Micronor. She is scheduled to return for her 6-week postpartum visit.

Resources for women

Domestic violence: Hotline: 1-800-799-SAFE, Multilingual

Nutrition, exercise, weight loss: https://www.choosemyplate.gov/SuperTracker/#f; http://www.loseit.com/

Perinatal mood and anxiety disorders—Postpartum Support International: http://www.postpartum.net/; 1-800-944-4PPD

Sibling adjustment books: Sears, Sears, Watts, & Kelly. (2001). *Baby on the Way*; Berenstain & Berenstain. (1974). *The Berenstain Bears' New Baby*; Hains. (1992). *My Baby Brother*; Horowitz & Sorensen. (1993). *Mommy's Lap*.

Resources for health-care providers

Edinburgh Postnatal Depression Scale: http://psymed.info/default.aspx?m=Test&id=71&l=3

Nutrition, exercise, weight loss: http://www.choosemyplate.gov/information-healthcare-professionals.html

Patient safety, educational materials, and provider tools: http://fvpfstore.stores.yahoo.net/safetycards1.html; http://www.futureswithoutviolence.org/section/our_work/health/_health_material

Perinatal mood and anxiety disorders—Postpartum Support International: http://www.postpartum.net/Professionals-and-Community/Professional-Tools.aspx; http://www.postpartum.net/Professionals-and-Community.aspx

References

ACOG Committee on Obstetric Practice. (2002, reaffirmed 2009). Exercise during pregnancy and the postpartum period. ACOG Committee Opinion No. 267. *American College of Obstetricians and Gynecologists*, 99, 171–173.

Affonso, D. D. (1977). Missing pieces: A study of postpartum feelings. *Birth and the Family Journal*, 4, 150–164.

Ament, L. (1990). Maternal tasks of the puerperium re-identified. *Journal of Obstetric, Gynecologic, and Neonatal Nursing*, 19(4), 330–335.

American College of Obstetricians and Gynecologists (ACOG). (2012). Intimate partner violence. Committee Opinion No. 518. *Obstetrics & Gynecology*, 119, 412–417.

Amorim Adegboye, A. R., Linne, Y. M., & Lourenco, P. M. C. (2007). Diet or exercise, or both, for weight reduction in women after childbirth. *Cochrane Database of Systematic Reviews*, (3), CD005627, 1–42. doi:10.1002/14651858.CD005627.pub2

Beck, C., & Indman, P. (2005). The many faces of postpartum depression. *JOGN Nursing; Journal of Obstetric, Gynecologic, and Neonatal Nursing*, 34(5), 569–576.

Blackburn, S. (2013). *Maternal, fetal & neonatal physiology* (4th ed.). Maryland Heights, MO: Elsevier Science.

Blenning, C. E., & Paladine, H. (2005). An approach to the postpartum office visit. *American Family Physician*, 72, 2491–2496.

Boyd, R., Zayas, L., & McKee, M. (2006). Mother-infant interaction, life events and prenatal and postpartum depressive symptoms among urban minority women in primary care. *Maternal and Child Health Journal*, 10, 1–10. doi:10.1007/s10995-005-0042-2

Bure, L. A., Azoulay, L., Benjamin, A., & Abenhaim, H. A. (2011). Pregnancy-associated breast cancer: A review for the obstetrical care provider. *Journal of Obstetrics and Gynaecology Canada*, April, 330–337.

Centers for Disease Control. (2007). Postpartum care visits-11 states and New York City, 2004. *MMWR. Morbidity and Mortality Weekly Report*, 56, 1312–1316.

Centers for Disease Control. (2011a). Update to CDC's United States medical eligibility criteria for contraceptive use, 2010: Revised recommendations for the use of contraceptive methods during the postpartum period. *MMWR. Morbidity and Mortality Weekly Report*, 60, 878–883.

Centers for Disease Control. (2011b). Vital signs: Teen pregnancy-United States, 1991–2009. *MMWR. Morbidity and Mortality Weekly Report*, 60, 414–420.

Committee on Obstetric Practice. (2010). Screening for depression during and after pregnancy. ACOG Committee Opinion 453. Retrieved from http://www.acog.org/~/media/Committee%20Opinions/Committee%20on%20Obstetric%20Practice/co453.pdf?dmc=1&ts=20120305T0433158796

Cunningham, F. G., Leveno, K. J., Bloom, S. L., Hauth, J. C., Rouse, D. J., & Young, C. Y. (2010). *Williams obstetrics* (23rd ed.). New York: McGraw Hill.

Fagerskiold, A. (2008). A change in life as experienced by first-time fathers. *Scandinavian Journal of Caring Sciences*, 22, 64–71.

Feinberg, M. E., Solmeyer, A. R., & McHale, S. M. (2012). The third rail of family systems: Sibling relationships, mental and behavioral health, and preventive intervention in childhood and adolescence. *Clinical Child and Family Psychology Review*, 15, 43–57.

Fortier, J. C., Carson, V. B., Will, S., & Shubkagel, B. L. (1991). Adjustment to a newborn. Sibling preparation makes a difference. *JOGN Nursing; Journal of Obstetric, Gynecologic, and Neonatal Nursing*, 20, 73–79.

Garabedian, M. J., Lain, K. Y., Hansen, W. F., Garcia, L. S., Williams, C. M., & Crofford, L. J. (2011). Violence against women and postpartum depression. *Journal of Women's Health*, 20, 447–453.

Gaynes, B. N., Gavin, N., Meltzer-Brody, S., Lohr, K. N., Swinson, T., Gartlehner, G., . . . Miller, W. C. (2005). Perinatal depression: Prevalence, screening accuracy and Screening outcomes. *AHRQ Publication*: US Department of Health and Human Services, 05-E006-2.

Genesoni, L., & Tallandini, M. A. (2009). Men's psychological transition to fatherhood: An analysis of the literature, 1989–2008. *Birth (Berkeley, Calif.)*, 36, 305–317.

Griffin, E. W., & de la Torre, C. (1983). Sibling jealousy: The family with a new baby. *American Family Physician*, 28, 143–146.

Groff, J. (2011). Revisioning postpartum care in the United States: Global perspectives. In C. L. Farley (Ed.), *Final Projects Database*. Philadelphia: Philadelphia University. Retrieved from http://www.instituteofmidwifery.org/MSFinalProj.nsf/a9ee58d7a82396768525684f0056be8d/8f0a029755d12a75852578a1006eaa2c/$FILE/Jade%20Groff%20721-CHAPT1-2FINAL.pdf

Hay-Smith, J., Morkved, S., Fairbrother, K. A., & Herbison, G. P. (2008). Pelvic floor muscle training for prevention and treatment of urinary and faecal incontinence in antenatal and postnatal women. *Cochrane Database of Systematic Reviews*, 4, 1–70.

Holroyd, E., Katie, F. K., Chun, L. S., & Ha, S. W. (1997). Doing the month': An exploration of postpartum practices in Chinese women. *Healthcare for Women International*, 18, 301–313.

Holtslander, L. (2005). Clinical Application of the 15-minute family interview: Addressing the needs of postpartum families. *Journal of Family Nursing, 11,* 5–18.

Johansson, A. L. V., Andersson, T. M.-L., Hsieh, C.-C., Cnattingius, S., & Lambe, M. (2011). Increased mortality in women with breast cancer detected during pregnancy and different periods postpartum. *Cancer Epidemiology, Biomarkers & Prevention, 20,* 1865–1872.

Johnsen, N. M., & Gaspard, M. E. (1985). Theoretical foundations of a prepared sibling class. *JOGN Nursing; Journal of Obstetric, Gynecologic, and Neonatal Nursing, 14,* 237–242.

Johnson, C. E. (2011). Sexual health during pregnancy and the postpartum. *The Journal of Sexual Medicine, 8,* 1267–1284.

Johnson Waugh, L. (2011). Beliefs associated with Mexican immigrant families' practice of la cuarentena during the postpartum recovery. *JOGN Nursing; Journal of Obstetric, Gynecologic, and Neonatal Nursing, 40,* 732–741.

Kennedy, K. I., & Trussell, J. (2011). Postpartum contraception and lactation. In R. A. Hatcher, J. Trussell, A. L. Nelson, W. Cates Jr., D. Kowal, & M. S. Policar (Eds.), *Contraceptive Technology* (20th ed.). New York: Ardent Media.

Kennell, J., & Klaus, M. (1998). Bonding: Recent observations that alter perinatal care. *Pediatrics in Review, 19*(1), 4–12.

Kim-Godwin, Y. S. (2003). Postpartum beliefs & practices among non-Western cultures. *The American Journal of Maternal/Child Nursing, 28,* 75–80.

Kramer, L., & Bank, L. (2005). Sibling relationship contributions to individual and family wellbeing: Introduction to the special issue. *Journal of Family Psychology, 19,* 483–483.

Leeman, L. M., & Rogers, R. G. (2012). Sex after childbirth. *Obstetrics & Gynecology, 119,* 647–655.

Lopez, L. M., Hiller, J. E., & Grimes, D. A. (2010). Education for contraceptive use by women after childbirth. *Cochrane Database of Systematic Reviews,* (1), 1–36. doi:10.1002/14651858.CD001863.pub2

Lundberg, P. C., & Thi Ngoc Thu, T. (2011). Vietnamese women's cultural beliefs and practices related to the postpartum period. *Midwifery, 27,* 731–736.

MacAdam, R., Huuva, E., & Bertero, C. (2009). Fathers' experiences after having a child: Sexuality becomes tailored according to circumstances. *Midwifery, 27,* e149–e155.

Matthey, S., Panasetis, P., & Barnett, B. (2002). Adherence to cultural practices following childbirth in migrant Chinese women and relation to postpartum mood. *Healthcare for Women International, 23,* 567–575.

Meleis, A. I., Sawyer, L. M., Im, E., Messias, D. K. H., & Schumacher, K. (2000). Experiencing transitions: An emerging middle-range theory. *Advances in Nursing Science, 23,* 12–28.

Mercer, R. T. (1985). The process of maternal role attainment over the first year. *Nursing Research, 34*(4), 198–204.

Mercer, R. T. (2004). Becoming a mother versus maternal role attainment. *Journal of Nursing Scholarship, 36,* 226–232.

Murphy, S. O. (1993). Siblings and the new baby: Changing perspectives. *Journal of Pediatric Nursing, 8,* 277–288.

Premberg, A., Hellstrom, A., & Berg, M. (2008). Experiences of the first year as father. *Scandinavian Journal of Caring Sciences, 22,* 56–63.

Riordan, J., & Wambach, K. (2010). *Breastfeeding and human lactation* (4th ed.). Sudbury, MA: Jones and Bartlett.

Rubin, R. (1961). Basic maternal behavior. *Nursing Outlook, 9*(11), 638–687.

Rubin, R. (1967). Attainment of the maternal role. Part 1. Processes. *Nursing Research, 16,* 237–245.

Sawicki, J. A. (1997). Sibling rivalry and the new baby: Anticipatory guidance and management strategies. *Pediatric Nursing, 23,* 298–302.

Schoppe-Sullivan, S. J., Brown, G. L., Cannon, E. A., Mangelsdorf, S. C., & Szewczyk Sokolowski, M. (2008). Maternal gatekeeping, coparenting quality, and fathering behavior in families with infants. *Journal of Family Psychology, 22,* 389–398.

Spero, D. (1993). Sibling preparation classes. *AWHONNS Clinical issues in Perinatal and Womens Health Nursing, 4,* 122–131.

Stables, D., & Rankin, J. (Eds.). (2011). *Physiology in childbearing* (3rd ed.). London: Elsevier.

Stacy Tsai, P.-J., Nakashima, L., Yamamoto, J., Ngo, L., & Kaneshiro, B. (2011). Postpartum follow-up rates before and after the postpartum follow-up initiative at Queen Emma Clinic. *Hawai'i Medical Journal, 70,* 56–59.

Stewart, R. B., Mobley, L. A., Van Tuyl, S. S., & Salvador, M. A. (1987). The firstborn's adjustment to the birth of a sibling: A longitudinal assessment. *Child Development, 58,* 341–355.

Sword, W., & Watt, S. (2005). Learning needs of postpartum women: Does socioeconomic status matter? *Birth (Berkeley, Calif.), 32,* 86–92.

Thureen, P. J., Deacon, J., Hernandez, J. A., & Hall, D. M. (2005). *Assessment and care of the well newborn* (2nd ed.). St Louis, MO: Elsevier.

Understanding Nurse Practitioner Liability. (2010). CNA HealthPro Nurse Practitioner Claims Analysis 1998–2008, Risk management Strategies and Highlights of the 2009 NSO Survey. Retrieved from http://www.nso.com/pdfs/db/Nurse_Practitioner_Claim_Study_02-12-10.pdf?fileName=Nurse_Practitioner_Claim_Study_02-12-10.pdf&folder=pdfs/db&isLiveStr=Y

United States Department of Agriculture. (n.d.). Health and nutrition information for pregnant & breastfeeding women. Retrieved from http://www.choosemyplate.gov/pregnancy-breastfeeding.html

United States Department of Labor. (1993). Health benefits, retirement standards, and workers' compensation: Family and medical leave. Retrieved from http://www.dol.gov/compliance/guide/fmla.htm

U.S. Department of Health and Human Services. (2010). Healthy people 2020. 2020 topics and objectives: Maternal, Infant and Child Health. Retrieved from http://healthypeople.gov/2020/topicsobjectives2020/objectiveslist.aspx?topicId=26

Varney, H., Kriebs, J., & Gegor, C. (2004). *Varney's midwifery* (4th ed.). Sudbury, MA: Jones and Bartlett.

Volling, B. L. (2005). The transition to siblinghood: A developmental ecological systems perspective and direction for future research. *Journal of Family Psychology, 19,* 542–549.

Volling, B. L. (2012). Family transitions following the birth of a sibling: An empirical review of changes in the firstborn's adjustment. *Psychological Bulletin, 138,* 497–528. doi:10.1037/a0026921. Advance online publication.

Von Sydow, K. (1999). Sexuality during pregnancy and after childbirth: A metacontent analysis of 59 studies. *Journal of Psychosomatic Research, 47*(1), 27–49.

Weir, S., Posner, H. E., Zhang, J., Willis, G., Baxter, J. D., & Clark, R. E. (2011). Predictors of prenatal and postpartum care adequacy in a Medicaid managed care population. *Women's Health issues, 21,* 277–285.

Williamson, M., McVeigh, C., & Baafi, M. (2008). An Australian perspective on fatherhood and sexuality. *Midwifery, 24,* 99–107.

Wilson, E. K., Samandari, G., Koo, H. P., & Tucker, C. (2011). Adolescent mothers' postpartum contraceptive use: A qualitative study. *Perspectives on Sexual and Reproductive Health, 43,* 230–237.

28

Common complications during the postnatal period

Deborah Brandt Karsnitz

Relevant terms

Anxiety disorders—generalized anxiety disorder, obsessive-compulsive disorder, panic disorder, and post-traumatic stress disorder

Deep vein thrombosis—inflammation of a vein located deep within a muscle secondary to a blood clot

Delayed postpartum hemorrhage—excessive bleeding occurring after 24 hours until 6 weeks postpartum

Endometritis–metritis—postpartum uterine infection of the functional uterine lining—wall of the uterus

Hematoma postpartum—collection of blood in the tissue, postchildbirth

Maternal morbidity—maternal illness related to childbearing

Maternal mortality—maternal death related to childbearing

Postpartum anxiety disorders—any of the anxiety disorders occurring during the postpartum period

Postpartum blues—sadness, weepiness, mood swings, irritability that occurs in the first few days to 10 days postpartum; lasts less than 2 weeks

Postpartum depression—depression occurring within the first year postchildbirth; lasts longer than 2 weeks

Postpartum infection—infection, usually reproductive structures or abdominal incision postcesarean section postchildbirth

Postpartum preeclampsia/eclampsia—postpartum specific preeclampsia according to standard diagnostic criteria for increasing hypertension or proteinuria/eclampsia—progression to seizure

Postpartum psychosis—psychotic episode (delusions or break with reality) occurring within the first year postchildbirth

Psychotropics—mental health medications—affects mood, behavior, mental activity

Puerperium/postpartum—occurring after the birth—until restoration of body to prepregnancy state

Subinvolution—failure of the uterus to progress to normal size and state postchildbirth

Superficial venous thrombosis—inflammation of a vein located just below the skin's surface secondary to a blood clot

Thyroiditis—inflammation of the thyroid gland

Thyrotoxicosis—overproduction of thyroid hormones to toxic levels

von Willebrand's disease—a type of hemophilia (bleeding disorder)

Introduction

Postpartum represents a time period designed for postchildbirth restoration and recovery, family attachment, and role development. The mother's restoration and recovery are usually uneventful. Despite expected normalcy during this time frame, there may be an occasion when complications arise and recovery becomes complex.

Physiological postpartum complications include late postpartum hemorrhage, infection, late preeclampsia, and various medical complications directly or indirectly influenced by childbearing. Postpartum mood and anxiety disorders are some of the most common complications of childbearing. Postpartum women have increased risk for, or exacerbation of, mood and anxiety

Prenatal and Postnatal Care: A Woman-Centered Approach, First Edition. Edited by Robin G. Jordan, Janet L. Engstrom, Julie A. Marfell, and Cindy L. Farley.

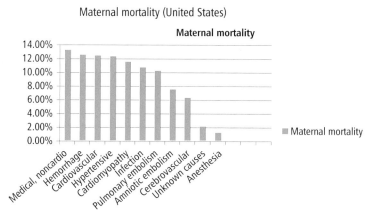

Maternal mortality (United States)

Figure 28.1.   Maternal mortality data, 1998–2005 (Berg et al., 2010).

disorders. Some postpartum complications can be managed by nurse practitioners, nurse midwives, or physician assistants, while others require physician consultation, collaboration, or referral. The significant decrease in postpartum morbidity and mortality is attributed to careful routine practice of hand washing and appropriate and timely management of complications. Unfortunately, the United States still ranks behind many other countries for maternal mortality (Berg, Callaghan, Syverson, & Henderson, 2010; King, 2012). This chapter will describe common postpartum complications, risk factors, assessment, and management.

Postpartum morbidity and mortality

Postpartum recovery often includes relatively common concerns, such as anemia, fatigue, constipation, and hemorrhoids, which are usually mild and easily managed. Health-care practitioners should provide postpartum education and resources to women and families during prenatal care and encourage postpartum follow-up care. Major postpartum complications, with the exception of depression or anxiety disorders, are relatively uncommon. Until the latter half of the twentieth century, the most common causes of maternal deaths were attributed to three complications of childbearing: hemorrhage, postpartum infection, and preeclampsia (Cunningham et al., 2010).

For the past several decades, the Pregnancy Mortality Surveillance System (PMSS) has collected data on pregnancy-related deaths. The most recent report (1998–2005) contains analysis of data collected by reviewing death certificates in relation to birth up to and including within 1 year of pregnancy (Berg et al., 2010). The PMSS analysis found a ratio of 14.5 maternal deaths per 100,000 live births with a low of 12.0 in 1998 and a high of 16.8 in 2003. The mortality ratio increased from 12.9 reported

by the PMSS for 1997 (Berg, Chang, Callaghan, & Whitehead, 2003). The mortality ratio for African American women (37.5) was significantly higher than white women (10.2) and nonwhite and non-African American women (13.4) (Berg et al., 2010). Maternal mortality increased with age and was five times greater for women receiving no prenatal care (Berg et al., 2010). Notably, there has been an increase in maternal mortality from indirect pregnancy-related causes, such as cardiovascular conditions and noncardiovascular medical conditions, and a decrease in historically direct causes related to pregnancy, such as hemorrhage, infection, and hypertensive disorders (Berg et al., 2010). Fig. 28.1 illustrates data from the 1998–2005 analysis.

Recently, the World Health Organization (WHO), United Nations Children's Fund (UNICEF), United Nation's Population Fund (UNFPA), and The World Bank (2012) released their maternal mortality trends report. Despite a significant decrease in global maternal mortality trends, the United States made no progress, has not stabilized, and in fact, continues to see an upward trend. Speculation for the increase in maternal mortality in the United States include emerging trends such as obesity, diabetes, cardiovascular disease, substance use, and possibly, better reporting of direct and indirect causes (Hankins et al., 2012). Additionally, the most recent reports on maternal mortality do not include data on homicide or suicide, making maternal deaths from postpartum depression or intimate partner violence invisible, both of which can exacerbate during pregnancy and/or postpartum (Centre for Maternal and Child Enquiries (CMACE), 2011; Spinelli, 2004).

Postpartum cultural considerations

Most cultures have rich traditions and beliefs surrounding the postpartum period. While some cultures nurture new mothers for 6–7 weeks postpartum, other cultures expect a new mother to resume normal activities in as few as 2 weeks or less (Purnell & Paulanka, 2003). Without adequate time for recovery, complications can occur. Awareness of cultural influences should guide assessment and treatment. Assessment includes identification of the family health-care decision maker. A health-care provider must discover if decision making is shared by family members or has a dominant person making important decisions. Management may be determined by factors such as religious beliefs or traditional folk or herbal medicines. Mental health discussion is important to determine whether or not stigma is a deterrent to treatment. Culture influences diet and exercise during the postpartum period. Some women are encouraged to remain inside their home during a specific time period. Feelings of sadness or despair in the postpartum period can be socially unacceptable in some cultures. The health-care provider needs an understanding of cultural influences and traditions and their impact on postpartum care in order to be sensitive and effective in preventing and treating postpartum disorders.

Postpartum disorders

Puerperal fever (pyrexia)

Puerperal fever is defined as a temperature of 100.4°F (38°C) or greater during the postpartum period. Puerperal fever, often caused by genital tract infection, can also be produced by breast engorgement, dehydration, pyelonephritis, or respiratory illness (Maharaj, 2007). Increased temperature from breast engorgement or dehydration seldom lasts or exceeds 24 hours and will usually not increase greater than 39°C. Occasionally, a slight increase in temperature postpartum can accompany superficial or deep vein thrombosis (DVT). Of note, a woman spiking a fever of 39°C or higher, within 24 hours postcesarean section, can indicate infection with group A Streptococcus (Cunningham et al., 2010). Any fever originating during postpartum warrants investigation for infection.

Puerperal infection (postpartum infection)

Puerperal infection, usually indicated by puerperal fever, generally describes any infection in the female genital tract following birth, miscarriage, or induced abortion. Since the introduction of hand washing, asepsis, and particularly antimicrobial drugs, death from puerperal infection has significantly decreased (Maharaj, 2007; van Dillen, Zwart, Schutte, & van Roosmalen, 2010). The PMSS (1998–2005) reported a maternal mortality infection rate of 10.7%, decreased from 13.2% in the PMSS (1991–1997) report (Berg et al., 2003, 2010).

Historically dreaded for its high rate of mortality, maternal death from puerperal infection has decreased significantly as a result of antimicrobial management (Cunningham et al., 2010). However, puerperal morbidity from infection is still a significant problem. Postpartum women possess an increased risk for infection due to wound or tissue trauma during birth, vulnerability from the placental separation site, and incision from cesarean section (Baxter, Berghella, Mackeen, Ohly, & Weed, 2011). Other potential sites of infection include the urinary tract, breasts, epithelial lining in veins and vulnerability to infection in other sites, such as respiratory or urinary tract infection. Most puerperal infections occur within the first few days or weeks postpartum, a time notoriously devoid of health-care follow-up in both developing and developed countries (Maharaj, 2007).

One of the most common puerperal infections is postpartum uterine infection, often referred to solely as endometritis or simply metritis (Maharaj, 2007). Uterine infection can, however, involve more than the endometrium, including the myometrium (endomyometritis) and the parametrium (endoparametritis). Occurrence for postpartum uterine infection is 1–2% following a vaginal birth and as high as 27% following a cesarean birth (Sweet & Gibbs, 2009). The American College of Obstetricians and Gynecologists (ACOG) recommends antimicrobial prophylaxis for all women undergoing cesarean birth beginning within 60 minutes of initiation of surgery (American College of Obstetricians and Gynecologists (ACOG), 2010b). The addition of antimicrobial prophylaxis has dramatically decreased infection rates overall (Smaill & Gyte, 2010). Nonetheless, it is important to note that infection may occur after cesarean birth despite prophylactic antimicrobials (Sweet & Gibbs, 2009).

There are a number of risk factors for puerperal infection morbidity. Many factors are correlated and exponentially increase the risk for infection. Prolonged labor potentially increases the number of vaginal exams or the need for internal monitoring, both of which are individual risk factors for infection. Amniotomy, if used in conjunction with active labor management, has not been reported to increase the risk of uterine infection. However, amniotomy used in conjunction with prolonged labor and frequent vaginal exams can increase infection rates.

The most common reasons women were readmitted to the hospital in the postpartum period were uterine or wound infection and hypertension, regardless of route of birth (Belfort et al., 2010). Preventing infection in vaginal births may be as simple as decreasing the number of vaginal exams. There are certain standard indications for vaginal exams, such as assessment for presentation

Table 28.1　Common Bacteria in Uterine Infection

Aerobes		
Gram-positive	Gram-negative	Gram-variable
A, B, D streptococci	*Escherichia coli*	*Gardnerella vaginalis*
Enterococcus	*Klebsiella*	
Staphylococcus aureus	*Enterobacter*	
Staphylococcus epidermidis	*Proteus* species	
Anerobes		Others
Peptostreptococcus		*Mycoplasma*
Peptococcus		*Chlamydia*
Bacteroids		*Neisseria gonorrhoeae*
Clostridium		
Fusobacterium		

Adapted from: Cunningham et al. (2010).

and dilatation upon arrival at the birth site during labor. Once this information is obtained, the need for further vaginal exams should be based upon individual indications rather than curiosity or arbitrary time periods.

Once rupture of the amniotic membranes occurs during labor and birth, the uterus becomes more susceptible to colonization and infection. Infection can occur with increased uterine manipulation or exploration during manual removal of the placenta or instrumental birth. Placental site infection most often occurs following a vaginal birth, whereas uterine infection usually comes from an infected cesarean section incision (Cunningham et al., 2010). Any area traumatized during birth is susceptible to infection. Extended infections are the result of localized infections proliferating to additional sites including other pelvic organs (Cunningham et al., 2010). Uterine infections are polymicrobial. Common pathogens implicated in postpartum infections are listed in Table 28.1.

Clinical presentation

Signs and symptoms of uterine infection include elevated temperature (the degree of elevation can be indicative of severity and possible sepsis), general malaise, abdominal pain with uterine tenderness on bimanual exam, lochia with or without a foul smell, and subinvolution. Chills most often accompany severe cases of uterine infection (Cunningham et al., 2010; Sweet & Gibbs, 2009). On occasion, and with certain bacteria

Risk factors for puerperal infection

- Cesarean birth, particularly nonelective
- Prolonged rupture of membranes
- Long labors
- Inadequate hand washing
- Frequent vaginal exams
- Internal fetal or uterine monitoring
- Uterine manipulation or exploration
- Instrumental birth
- Low socioeconomic status
- Obesity
- Medical conditions (diabetes, anemia, immunoinsufficiency, untreated infection prior to birth)

Sources: Belfort et al. (2010), Cunningham et al. (2010).

such as group A or B *Streptococcus*, early signs and symptoms may be more generalized with fever being the only presenting symptom. Differential diagnosis includes pyelonephritis, pneumonia, and appendicitis.

Diagnosis and management

Diagnosis includes physical examination, complete blood count (CBC), blood cultures, aerobic uterine culture, urinalysis and urine culture, and if indicated, chest X-ray. Mild cases of endometritis can be treated

Table 28.2   Uterine Infection

Signs and symptoms (onset, duration, severity)	Diagnostics	Treatment—MD collaboration or referral for IV therapy
Fever (chills)	CBC with differential	Antimicrobial therapy
General malaise	Urinalysis	Clindamycin 900 mg + gentamicin 1.5 mg/kg, q8h IV
Pain/tenderness	Cultures	Clindamycin 900 mg q8h and aztreonam—1–2 g q8h (abnormal renal)
Lochia (odor)	Radiology (if indicated)	Metronidazole 500 mg q12h, PCN, 5 million units q6h
	Ultrasound (if indicated)	Ampicillin 2 g q6h + gentamicin 1.5 mg/kg q8h

Sources: Cunningham et al. (2010), Duff (2007).

with oral antimicrobiotics. Culture of the wound or cervix is rarely necessary to initiate treatment. Moderate to severe cases require hospitalization and treatment with broad-spectrum antimicrobial intravenous therapy (Cunningham et al., 2010).

Physician consultation is recommended for mild cases managed with outpatient oral antimicrobials if secondary to cesarean birth. Physician collaboration or referral is indicated for moderate to severe infections requiring hospitalization (see Table 28.2) (Cunningham et al., 2010; Duff, 2007). Most women will improve markedly within 48–72 hours. Discharge from the hospital can occur after intravenous therapy is discontinued and the woman is afebrile and asymptomatic for 24 hours.

Wound infection

Postpartum wound infections develop most often in the abdominal incision following cesarean section or in a perineal laceration or episiotomy following a vaginal birth. Since the advent of prophylactic antimicrobial management during cesarean section abdominal incision, postsurgical infections are less than 2% (Andrews, Hauth, Cliver, Savage, & Goldenberg, 2003). Risk factors for abdominal and perineal wound infection include similar factors for risk of uterine infection (see Table 28.3).

Abdominal wound infection

Signs and symptoms of abdominal wound infection include localized edema, induration, and erythema, often with exudates and occasionally fever. Management includes wound care, antibiotic treatment, and drainage if necessary. Reclosure of the wound can be indicated if dehiscence is present, although healing by secondary intention is another option, depending on the size, drainage, and other characteristics of the wound. Culture of the wound is rarely necessary for treatment. Common pathogens include *Staphylococcus aureus*, streptococci, and both aerobic and anaerobic bacilli.

Table 28.3   Risk Factors for Venous Thrombosis

Risk factors for venous thrombosis		
Venous stasis	Hypercoagulability	Vascular trauma
Operative vaginal birth	Cesarean birth	Immobilization
Postpartum infection	Coagulopathies	Maternal age >35
Obesity/medical conditions	Smoking	History of thrombosis

Perineal wound infection

Infection of an episiotomy or perineal laceration most often presents with localized edema, erythema, and exudates. Management is similar to other wound infections and includes drainage, removal of sutures, and debridement of the infected area. If cellulitis is apparent, broad-spectrum antimicrobial therapy is indicated. Most infections heal without needing additional sutures. If breakdown of sutures occurs for a third- or fourth-degree episiotomy extension, repair is necessary once infection is eradicated. Studies suggest a reduction occurs in perineal infections post third- and fourth-degree lacerations with the use of prophylactic antimicrobials (Duggal et al., 2008). Women with persistent fever, tachycardia, pain, and tenderness, continuation of symptoms despite several days of treatment should be assessed for complications such as pelvic abscess, septic pelvic thrombophlebitis, and in severe cases, septic shock.

Delayed or late postpartum hemorrhage

Maternal hemorrhage has historically been one of the major causes of maternal mortality. Although dramatically decreased and despite sophisticated understanding and advances in treatment, hemorrhage continues to be one of the leading causes of maternal death (Berg et al., 2010). Hemorrhage occurring after 24 hours and until 12 weeks postpartum is considered a delayed, late, or secondary postpartum hemorrhage (ACOG, 2006). Following childbirth, the uterus is physiologically designed to contract down and stricture the blood vessels. When this natural process is delayed or inhibited, hemorrhage can occur. Approximately 1–2% of postpartum women have secondary postpartum hemorrhage; most of these occur within the first 2 weeks after birth and result from uterine atony and subinvolution (Cunningham et al., 2010). Retained placental fragments do not commonly cause secondary hemorrhage but should be considered during diagnostic workup. Most cases of uterine atony occur without antecedents or risk factors.

Women presenting with secondary postpartum hemorrhage between 2 and 5 days postchildbirth should be screened for von Willebrand's disease (vWD). vWD is the most prevalent of the inherited bleeding disorders (1–2%) in childbearing women (Mannucci, 2004). It is caused by a deficiency of von Willebrand's factor, a protein that causes platelets to adhere. This factor is increased during pregnancy but will drop in the early postpartum period. Subsequently, bleeding is not usually a problem for the initial 48 hours. Risk for bleeding persists for approximately 4 months postpartum.

Management

Treatment for delayed hemorrhage may include uterotonic agents or curettage. Ultrasound can determine if there are significant retained fragments but does not consistently possess a high level of accuracy. If placental fragments or clots are noted on ultrasound, physicians may use suction evacuation to stop bleeding (Katz, 2007). Postpartum curettage is not typically performed because the uterine wall is soft postchildbirth, which increases the likelihood of uterine perforation. Most secondary postpartum hemorrhages will respond to oxytocic agents such as ergonovine, methylergonovine, oxytocin, or a prostaglandin analog (Cunningham et al., 2010).

Postpartum hematoma

Postpartum hematoma is estimated to occur in 1/1000 births. Most often, hematoma formation is associated with episiotomy, instrumental delivery, or nulliparity. Hematoma formation may occur spontaneously, without laceration, and may be delayed in presentation (Cunningham et al., 2010). However, vulvar hematomas are usually related to lacerated vessels. Typically, multiple vessels are involved and surgical repair requires drainage and suturing. If a hematoma is small, expectant management is indicated. Vaginal hematomas appear most often

after instrumental assistance during childbirth and require drainage and packing (Francois & Foley, 2007). Atypical reasons for postpartum hematoma formation include coagulopathies such as vWD. Many hematomas can be prevented with gentle, controlled birth, and appropriate inspection and repair of lacerations or episiotomy.

Clinical presentation and management

Postpartum hematoma should be considered when bleeding persists despite abdominal assessment of a firm uterus. Women characteristically express feeling increased or severe perineal or rectal pain. A hematoma can present in the vulva, vagina, paravaginal, or retroperitoneal areas.

Management varies according to presentation. Small hematomas can reabsorb, while moderate to larger hematomas may need incision and drainage. Subperitoneal hematomas can be more difficult to assess; bleeding and subsequent hypovolemia are of concern. Physician referral is necessary.

Subinvolution

Typical uterine involution is a physiological process of reduction and cellular remodeling of the uterus to a prepregnancy state. When this process is disrupted or incomplete, subinvolution is the result. Uterine subinvolution may be secondary to several factors and differential diagnosis includes retained placental fragments, uterine infection, or excessive maternal activity prohibiting proper recovery. Subjective assessment should include questions pertinent to each possible diagnosis.

Clinical presentation and management

The diagnosis of subinvolution is made clinically. Symptoms include description of irregular bleeding, which can be profuse on occasion. Abdominal and bimanual exam will reveal an enlarged and often boggy uterus.

Once retained placental fragments and infection are ruled out (discussed in other sections), attention to lifestyle issues needed to support healing is indicated. Assessment includes rest, proper nutrition, fluid intake, and a social support system. Along with a short course of methylergonovine (0.2 mg po every 4 hours) for 24–48 hours, women are encouraged to incorporate help at home, get proper rest, nutrition, and hydration with follow-up in 1–2 weeks.

Postpartum preeclampsia–eclampsia

Preeclampsia is a chronic disorder that typically presents during the latter half of pregnancy and resolves within 1–2 days postpartum (Graeber, Vanderwal, Stiller, &

Werdmann, 2005). Postpartum onset of preeclampsia or eclampsia most often occurs within 48 hours postpartum. Late postpartum preeclampsia–eclampsia develops after 48 hours and before 4 weeks postpartum (Sibai & Stella, 2009).

Women diagnosed with gestational hypertension or preeclampsia need close monitoring early postpartum. Evaluation includes observation for signs of worsening disease, monitoring of blood pressure, oxygen saturation, respirations, fluid intake and output, and laboratory indices. Women are at risk for iatrogenic overload of intravenous fluids during labor and birth. Additionally, intravascular fluid volume increases postpartum from physiological extravascular fluid shift. Women with impaired renal function from severe preeclampsia are at risk postpartum for pulmonary edema and worsening hypertension (Sibai, 2007). Development of new-onset seizures can be prevented if prodromal symptoms of preeclampsia are recognized.

Clinical presentation and management

Preeclampsia, eclampsia, or severe hypertension can first present during the postpartum period. Health-care providers should be cognizant of signs and symptoms for early postpartum onset or late postpartum preeclampsia–eclampsia. Women most often present with headaches, visual changes, epigastric pain, or nausea and vomiting. Women with postpartum preeclampsia have an increased risk for pulmonary edema, eclampsia, stroke, or thromboembolism (Hirshfeld-Cytron, Lam, Karumanchi, & Lindheimer, 2006; Sibai & Stella, 2009). Postpartum eclampsia can develop despite treatment with magnesium sulfate during intrapartum and early postpartum (Chames, Livingston, Ivester, Barton, & Sibai, 2002). A previous diagnosis of preeclampsia is not a prerequisite for a postpartum diagnosis (Graeber et al., 2005). Neurological complaints, malaise, and nausea and vomiting are more often reported in women readmitted for postpartum preeclampsia than in mothers with intrapartum preeclampsia. Hypertension and proteinuria do not always present together in late preeclampsia.

Medical management includes hospitalization and administration of magnesium sulfate, as well as antihypertensive therapy. Education regarding signs and symptoms of preeclampsia should be extended after childbirth. Physician referral is indicated.

Postpartum thrombophlebitis

Ambulation soon after childbirth has decreased the incidence of thromboembolic disease during the postpartum period. Currently, the estimated incidence ranges from 1/1000 to 1/2000 women (Pettker & Lockwood, 2007). Risk factors for postpartum thrombosis include

hypercoagulability, venous stasis, and inflammation from venous trauma caused by distension during pregnancy (known as Virchow's triad). Thrombophlebitis is most often diagnosed in women with previous varicosities. However, venous stasis can occur during pregnancy secondary to the effects of progesterone. Thrombosis results from inflammation due to venous distension. Prevention of venous stasis during the intrapartum and postpartum periods can be accomplished by frequent positional changes and ambulation.

Clinical presentation and management

Superficial thrombophlebitis (SVT) presents with increased leg pain, localized edema, erythema, and warmth over the thrombotic site. Physical exam reveals an enlarged and hard, cord-like structure. SVT is managed with support stockings, analgesia (nonsteroidal anti-inflammatory agents), leg rest, and elevation.

DVT may mimic SVT, both characterized by leg pain and inflammation. DVT, however, is usually evidenced by an abrupt onset of symptoms with increased pain elicited with movement or standing. Positive Homan's sign (increase calf pain elicited with dorsiflexion of the foot) may be present but could also be indicative of muscle strain from childbirth. Furthermore, absence of Homan's sign does not rule out DVT. Edema may be more generalized over the leg and thigh; the affected leg may be larger than the other; and at times, a palpable cord may be present over the affected area. Differential diagnosis includes SVT, trauma, ruptured Baker's cyst, muscle strain, vasculitis, or lymphedema.

Venous ultrasonography is the standard diagnostic test, with or without a color Doppler (Pettker & Lockwood, 2007). Laboratory evaluation can include adjunct studies using D-dimer serum concentrations. Management of DVT includes anticoagulant therapy, bed rest with leg elevation, and analgesia. Support stockings should be worn up to when ambulation resumes. Physician management is indicated for DVT (Fig. 28.2).

Postpartum thyroiditis

Transient postpartum thyroiditis does not present in one particular manner, occurring as either hyper- or hypothyroid and sometimes having alternating phases of both disorders. The incidence ranges from 5% to 10% of women. Postpartum thyroiditis can occur anytime during the first year, most commonly between 1 and 4 months postpartum. Because signs and symptoms can be vague and nonspecific, postpartum thyroiditis is sometimes mistaken for other disorders. Postpartum thyroiditis risk increases in women with gestational diabetes and type 2 diabetes. Women with type 1 diabetes can have as much as a 25% increased risk (Neville, 2011).

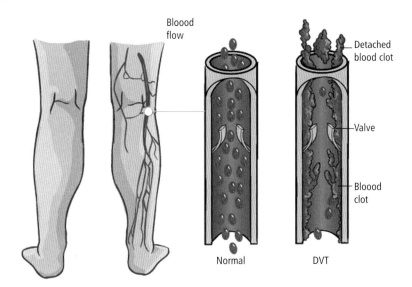

Figure 28.2.   Deep vein thrombosis. Source: National Institute of Health (NIH) Medline Plus.

Clinical presentation and management

Postpartum thyroiditis (inflammation of the thyroid gland) can present with subtle symptoms several months postpartum, which can impede prompt diagnosis. Symptoms of postpartum thyroiditis may resemble some of the stressors experienced by new mothers, such as fatigue, insomnia, anxiety, and weight loss, leading to difficulty in diagnosis. Postpartum women presenting with mild dysphoria can be misdiagnosed with postpartum depression or postpartum psychosis. Thyroid function studies should be performed when suspecting postpartum depression or postpartum psychosis.

Treatment includes beta blockers for hyperthyroid symptoms and thyroid hormone supplementation for hypothyroid symptoms. However, most women have mild symptoms and do not require treatment. If indicated, treatment will not interfere with breast-feeding. Future development of hypothyroidism occurs in 5–30% of women diagnosed with postpartum thyroiditis.

Thyroid storm (thyrotoxicosis) can occur during the first month postpartum and is characterized by abrupt onset, is usually short-lived, but can be life threatening if untreated. Symptoms include fever, nausea, vomiting, diarrhea, tachycardia, and tremor. Without treatment, dehydration can progress to coma. Cardiomyopathy and heart failure can develop secondary to increased T_4 levels (Neville, 2011).

Treatment includes decreasing thyroid hormone production and circulating thyroid hormones, identifying the underlying cause and providing supportive measures. Physician referral is indicated (Neville, 2011).

Postpartum mood and anxiety disorders

Women are more likely than men to suffer from depression, anxiety, somatic illness, and post-traumatic stress syndrome. The childbearing years are a time of increased vulnerability to these disorders (Kessler et al., 2005; Zender & Olshansky, 2009). Mood and anxiety disorders are significant complications during the postpartum period and can result in lifelong effects for the mother and family, at times with dire outcomes (Gaynes et al., 2005; Murray et al., 2011).

Incidence of perinatal depression varies in reports of occurrence from 7% to 20% of pregnancies and 13% during postpartum (Gaynes et al., 2005; Goodman & Tyer-Viola, 2010). A systematic review in 2005 by the Agency for Healthcare Research and Quality (AHRQ) reports a prevalence of 1.0–5.9% for major depression during the first year postpartum (Gaynes et al., 2005). When combining both minor and major depression, prevalence varies between 6.5% and 12.9% during the first year postpartum (Gaynes et al., 2005).

Anxiety disorders, including generalized anxiety disorder (GAD), obsessive-compulsive disorder, panic disorder, and post-traumatic stress disorder (PTSD) have a lifetime prevalence of 28.8% (Kessler et al., 2005). Anxiety disorders have been associated with depression but are more difficult to diagnose due to symptom similarities. Studies have estimated that 58% of women with depression also suffer from comorbid anxiety disorder (Zender & Olshansky, 2009). Most studies utilize validated screening tools to assess depression but omit assessment for comorbid postpartum mood or anxiety disorders (Beck, 2006; Halbreich & Karkun, 2006; Karsnitz & Ward, 2011).

Mood and anxiety disorders can increase with stress, lack of social support, as well as unhealthy lifestyle choices or conditions (Zender & Olshansky, 2009). Coupled with hormonal influences, physiological and social stressors have been indicated as triggers for mood and anxiety disorders (Zender & Olshansky, 2009). In addition to social and economic risk factors, a family or personal history of mood or anxiety disorders increases risk. When accompanied by lack of sleep, demands of a new infant, and routine family activities, risk for mood and anxiety disorders multiplies (Karsnitz & Ward, 2011; Zender & Olshansky, 2009).

The pathophysiology of mood and anxiety disorders is influenced by genetics as well as environment (Alder, Fink, Bitzer, Hosli, & Holzgreve, 2007; Stahl, 2008; Strohle & Holsboer, 2003). Dysfunction between the hypothalamus–pituitary–adrenal (HPA) axis and the noradrenergic and serotonergic systems can result in mood and anxiety disorders. The noradrenergic system has an increased reaction to stress, while the system reacting to serotonin has a decreased response, failing to inhibit serotonin. It is theorized that norepinephrine, dopamine, and serotonin system dysfunctions may individually or in combination initiate or exacerbate underlying mood or anxiety disorders (Stahl, 2008).

A team approach provides the best opportunity for appropriate diagnosis and treatment. Mental health-care providers have expertise in mental health diagnosis and management options and have a list of local psychologists, psychiatrists, and support groups available for clients. Mental health stigma can inhibit symptom disclosure and discussion between health-care providers and women experiencing postpartum mood and anxiety disorders. It has been reported that 57% of women with moderate to severe postpartum depression do not seek health care (Mayberry, Horowitz, & Declercq, 2007).

Women with postpartum depression describe feelings of overwhelming sadness and despair. Isolation may be conditional or self-induced by refusal or inability to admit suffering (Beck, 1993). Failure to disclose the extent of their symptoms leads to inadequate diagnosis and treatment of postpartum mood and anxiety disorders (Beck, 1999). In addition, recognition may be confounded by symptom similarity to normal discomforts and adjustments of postpartum (Gaynes et al., 2005).

Postpartum mood and anxiety disorders affect the entire family. Appropriate interaction between mother and baby, such as timely and sensitive maternal response to infant cues, is often decreased or absent in the depressed mother. Decreased maternal–infant interaction may lead to delayed cognitive skills and long-term emotional effects for the child (Beck & Indman, 2005).

Other children suffer emotional neglect, which may lead to behavior problems.

Postpartum blues

Postpartum mood disorders form a spectrum. At one end, some degree of transient, short-lived mood change, called postpartum blues, occurs in approximately 80% or more of new mothers and most often appears within the first week after birth (Beck & Indman, 2005). Symptoms of postpartum blues comprise several of the following: mood swings, crying, anxiety, insomnia, irritability, and loss of appetite. A new mother may be assisted by family support, periods of uninterrupted rest, exercise, adequate fluids, and nutrition. Herbal remedies and supplements may be helpful but should be discussed with a health-care provider. The health-care provider's role includes active listening, risk assessment, identification, management recommendations, and follow-up. Signs and symptoms are presented in Table 28.4.

Postpartum depression

In the middle of this spectrum is postpartum depression, which is the most prevalent and overlooked postpartum complication. It is estimated that postpartum depression occurs in 10–20% of postpartum women (Centers for Disease Control and Prevention, 2008). Postpartum depression presents in varying degrees with the potential for increased severity without treatment. Postpartum depression can first appear as postpartum blues, subsequently diagnosed as depression when symptoms persist longer than 2 weeks.

Depression can begin during the antepartum period with subtle signs such as fatigue, anxiety, or change in sleep or appetite patterns (all common occurrences during pregnancy), and remains unrecognized until exacerbated during the postpartum period. Although commonly occurring around 4 weeks, postpartum depression may develop anytime within the first year or longer after childbirth. Postpartum depression typically persists for a minimum of 6 months if untreated. Signs and symptoms mimic many symptoms of postpartum blues but include extremes of appetite and sleep disturbances, as well as more severe symptoms including suicide ideations.

Risk factors include a personal or family history of a mental health disorder. Women with a previous or present diagnosis of depression or anxiety disorders before or during pregnancy are at highest risk (Robertson, Grace, Wallington, & Stewart, 2004). Other important risk factors include an array of social and physiological factors. Isolation is often reported and women serving or having a partner serving in the military are at increased risk for postpartum mood disorders (Appolonio & Fingerhut, 2008; Gaynes et al., 2005).

Table 28.4   Postpartum Mood and Anxiety Disorders: Clinical Signs and Symptoms

Postpartum mood disorders

Blues (symptoms <14 days)	Depression	Psychosis
Tearful	Tearful	Hallucinations
Irritability	Irritability or anger	Delusions
Mood swings	Mood swings	Inability to communicate
Fatigue	Fatigue	Rapid mood change
Appetite changes	Lack of interest in the baby	Paranoia
	Sleep disturbances	Inability to sleep
	Appetite disturbances	Hyperactivity
	Guilt or shame	Disorganized thoughts
	Feelings of isolation	
	Hopelessness	
	Loss of pleasure	
	Feelings of harming the baby or self	

Postpartum anxiety disorders

Generalized anxiety	Obsessive-compulsive	Panic	Post-traumatic stress
Excessive worry	Intrusive thoughts	Fear of dying	Flashbacks or nightmares
Sleep disturbances/fatigue	Checking	Dizziness, shortness of breath	Anxiety
Appetite changes	Cleaning	Heart palpitations	Panic attack
Feelings of dread	Hypervigilance of infant	Feeling impending doom	Powerlessness
Physical symptoms		Extreme anxiety	Increased arousal
Restlessness		Irritable bowel	Avoidance of situations
Lack of concentration			Detachment

Depression may be associated with thyroid dysfunction or exacerbated by medical conditions. Substance use is high as women will often try to self-medicate (Hackley, Sharma, Kedzior, & Sreenivasan, 2010). Some women will turn to food for comfort and weight gain can be a feature of depression. Screening for manic episodes is an important part of assessment. Bipolar disorder may present with depressive symptoms.

Differential diagnosis

- Mild to major depression
- Bipolar disorder
- Psychosis
- Anxiety disorders
- Thyroid dysfunction
- Sleep deprivation

Antidepressants (selective serotonin reuptake inhibitors [SSRIs]) are the first-line treatment when choosing psychotropic management. Other psychotherapies such as cognitive-behavioral therapy (CBT) have also been successful. Evidence has not demonstrated one particular mode of treatment as more successful; however, psychotherapy has been shown to decrease relapse particularly in combination with psychotropics (Pampallona, Bollini, Tibaldi, Kupelnick, & Munizza, 2004). Careful consideration is warranted when prescribing antidepressant treatment. Prescribing an antidepressant to women with bipolar disorder can exacerbate a manic episode and potentially trigger a psychosis (King, Johnson & Gamblian, 2011). It is essential to assess for suicidal ideation. If an individual has a suicide plan, immediate referral to a mental health professional is indicated.

Postpartum psychosis

At the opposite end of the spectrum is postpartum psychosis. Postpartum psychosis often occurs within the first few days to 1 week postpartum, with a prevalence of one to two women per thousand (Sit, Rothschild, & Wisner, 2006). Onset can be abrupt and unexpected, although a previous history of mental illness is a common risk factor. Women with bipolar disorder have a significant risk for psychosis (Sit et al., 2006). Other risk factors include sleep deprivation, complications of childbirth, age >35, and other life stressors (Posmontier, 2010). Although diagnosis of psychosis is challenging, the clinical impression is supported by the woman's skewed sense of reality. Family members are the primary source of information and frequently describe unusual behavior and little to no sleep for an extended period of time. Postpartum psychosis is a devastating experience for a family and can have tragic outcomes if not treated. Signs and symptoms are presented in Table 28.4.

Immediate referral to a psychiatric mental health specialist for medication and inpatient treatment at a mental health facility is warranted. The role of the referring health-care provider includes patient and family education and support, assessment, identification, and timely referral.

Generalized anxiety disorder

GAD is defined as an extreme amount of worry that occurs on most days and lasts for at least 6 months (American Psychiatric Association (APA), 2000). For this reason, postpartum generalized anxiety may not be diagnosed if not recognized during the postpartum time frame. Signs and symptoms are presented in Table 28.4. Prevalence of GAD during postpartum is 4.4–8.2% (Ross & McLean, 2006). Risk factors include past or current medical, perinatal, and family history of anxiety, depression, thyroid imbalance, hormonal fluctuations, and life stressors (Vesga-Lopez et al., 2008).

Treatment of choice for GAD includes SSRIs and/or psychotherapy. CBT is often a first-line treatment for anxiety disorder. Once women are able to determine specific triggers that initiate anxious episodes, coping measures, such as relaxation, can be identified (Vythilingum, 2008).

Obsessive-compulsive disorder

Obsessive-compulsive disorder is characterized by an onslaught of intrusive thoughts or rituals. Women are debilitated by the need to perform repetitive physical or mental actions. Cleaning, checking, or counting are the activities most often performed by women to relieve extreme stress (APA, 2000). Postpartum prevalence of obsessive-compulsive disorder is 2.7–3.9% (Ross &

McLean, 2006). Women with postpartum obsessive-compulsive disorder sometimes describe intrusive thoughts of harming their baby. It is important for a health-care provider to note that these thoughts are considered ego-dystonic (not oneself) and should be differentiated from psychosis or homicidal ideation. Determination of ego-dystonic thoughts is established by self-identification and expressions of horror and guilt for having disturbing thoughts (Gangdev, 2002). Many women will not report symptoms of obsessive-compulsive disorder unless asked by a provider.

Treatment includes SSRIs and behavior therapy. Long-term treatment is necessary and often requires higher psychotropic dosages. Referral to a mental health specialist is indicated.

Panic disorder

Panic disorder is exemplified by recurrences of panic attacks, often without provocation. Perinatal prevalence is 1.3–2% (Ross & McLean, 2006). Women with panic disorder are in constant fear of experiencing an attack and will avoid environments if they suspect an attack could occur. Quality of life may be influenced by an inability to hold a job or adequately care for family (Karsnitz & Webster, 2012; Katon, 2006). Risk factors include hormonal fluctuations, which increase the risk for exacerbation postpartum. Panic disorder has been indicated as a risk factor for postpartum depression (Rambelli et al., 2010). Triggers for a panic attack include caffeine, certain substances such as alcohol, and stressful events.

Treatments for most of the mood and anxiety disorders include combining psychotropics and psychotherapy. On occasion, benzodiazepines are effective during an acute phase but should not be used long term as they carry a high risk of abuse (Ham, Waters, & Oliver, 2005).

Post-traumatic stress disorder

PTSD is derived from the experience of a real or perceived threat of death to themselves or another person (APA, 2000). Prevalence of postpartum PTSD is 1.5–5.6% (Beck, 2006). PTSD is characterized by extreme fear and helplessness when exposed to the same or similar environment where the trauma occurred. In addition, women report being plagued by recurring thoughts and dreams (Beck & Watson, 2010; Elmir, Schmied, Wilkes, & Jackson, 2010). Consequences of postpartum PTSD include relationship discord and maternal–child attachment concerns. For example, a mother found herself unable to celebrate her child's first birthday due to memory triggers of her traumatic childbirth experience (Beck, 2006).

While trauma can arise from a variety of past and current life situations, it is important to recognize that some births can be psychologically traumatic to the mother, regardless of the physical outcomes. Health-care providers can encourage birth debriefing and reflection. Debriefing sessions and/or counseling interventions provide opportunities for the mother to describe her experience, discuss her feelings, define occurrences, and obtain validation. There is opportunity for the health-care provider to correct misinformation or misunderstanding about the birth event and to help the woman reframe her narrative to assist in the integration of what she had hoped would happen with what really happened. PTSD has also been linked to postpartum mood and anxiety disorders.

Growing evidence reports the effectiveness of SSRIs for PTSD (Stein, Ipser, & McAnda, 2009). Short-term use of benzodiazepines may also be helpful. Furthermore, psychotherapies have been shown to be an effective treatment and can help women cope with their fears (Feeny, Zoellner, & Kanana, 2009). Although some results are mixed, recent studies report a significant decrease in PTSD symptoms in mothers receiving debriefing, counseling, or CBT after traumatic birth (Elmir et al., 2010; Meades, Pond, Ayers, & Warren, 2011).

Mood and anxiety disorder assessment/screening

Assessment for mental health disorders begins at the initial prenatal visit and should continue throughout postpartum care and beyond. Screening for perinatal mood and anxiety disorders is not standard practice. Although many organizations support assessment for mental health disorders, there are no specific recommendations or guidelines for screening. The American College of Nurse Midwives (ACNM) supports universal screening, treatment, and referral as part of primary care (American College of Nurse-Midwives (ACNM), 2003). The ACOG, in their committee report on depression screening after pregnancy, identifies the need for screening and possible benefits to mother and infant but does not support universal screening at this time (ACOG, 2010a). The American Association of Family Physicians follows the U.S. Preventative Services Task Force (USPSTF), which has no specific recommendations but does support screening if appropriate services are in place (U.S. Preventive Services Task Force (USPSTF), 2009).

Despite a growing network of support for perinatal screening for depression, no specific screening tool has been endorsed as the standard measurement. The screening tool used most often worldwide is the Edinburgh Postnatal Depression Scale (EPDS). The EPDS has been validated in at least 37 studies and has been translated into numerous languages (Gibson, McKenzie-McHarg, Shakespeare, Price, & Gray, 2009). The EPDS is a brief 10-item questionnaire that is easily completed in the office setting and provides a means for continued assessment. The EPDS has a sensitivity of 86% and a specificity of 78%, with a positive predictive value of 73% (Cox, Holden, & Sagovsky, 1987). Other common screening tools include the Postpartum Depression Screening Scale (PDSS), the Center for Epidemiological Studies-Depression Scale (CED-D), the Patient Health Questionnaire (PHQ-9), and the Beck Depression Inventory (BDI) (Gaynes et al., 2005).

Screening for anxiety disorders is not routine practice and few organizations specifically promote screening solely for these disorders. In addition, there are few available screening tools specific for anxiety disorders. The EPDS does not specifically screen for anxiety but does include two questions that may help identify anxiety disorders.

Assessment for mood and anxiety disorders also includes a comprehensive history of pregnancy, labor, birth, and postpartum, including perception and coping measures. Current and past and mental health history for the woman and her family can indicate increased risk. Social assessment should include economic and family stressors, as well as substance use and physical or emotional intimate partner violence and sexual abuse past or present.

Management

Management for postpartum mood and anxiety disorders should incorporate a multifaceted approach. Severity of condition and congruence with the woman's needs and desires guides the health-care provider's plan. Treatment plans may include psychotropics, interpersonal psychotherapy (IPT), as well as various alternative or adjunct therapies.

Consideration of appropriate psychotropic treatment includes past history of psychotropic medication, side effects, and toleration. Cost of medication should be factored into the decision, as well as the woman's personal concerns regarding side effects. Postpartum women usually have increased weight from pregnancy, are often fatigued, and have decreased sexual desire. Choosing a cost-effective medication with the least side effects can increase adherence (Karsnitz & Ward, 2011).

Common psychotropic medications for depression and anxiety are described in Table 28.5.

SSRIs are the most widely prescribed antidepressants as well as treatment of choice for anxiety disorders for postpartum women. In a retrospective study between 1996 and 2005, the use of SSRIs for depression and

Table 28.5 FDA-Approved Common Medications for Depression and Anxiety Disorders

Generic (brand)	FDA approved indications	Dosage	Common side effects	Pregnancy/lactation category	Clinical considerations
Selective serotonin reuptake inhibitors (SSRIs)					
Black box warning (SSRIs)—suicidality in children, adolescents, and young adults up to 25 years (ages of some childbearing women) (King et al., 2011)					
Citalopram (Celexa) Fluoxetine (Prozac)	MDD GAD MDD OCD Panic D/O	Initial dose 20 mg/day; increase by 20 mg/day after 1 week. Maximum is 40 mg/day single dose am or pm. Maximum dose of 20 mg/day for patients >60 years (Stahl, 2008) Initial dose 5 mg/day in am, then increase by 5 mg/week up to 20 mg. Wait a month to assess drug effects before increasing dose, increasing by 20 mg/month; maximum dose generally 80 mg/day (Stahl, 2008)	GI distress, sexual dysfunction, sedation/insomnia (Stahl, 2008) Initial agitation/ sleep disturbance, sedation at high doses, sexual dysfunction (Stahl, 2008)	Pregnancy—C (ACOG, 2008) L3 (Hale, 2008) Pregnancy—C (ACOG, 2008) L2 (infants) (Hale, 2008) L3 (neonates) (Hale, 2008)	Side effects may be dose dependent Not recommended in patients with congenital long QT syndrome (Stahl, 2008) Weight neutral No need to taper for discontinuation (Stahl, 2008)
Paroxetine (Paxil, Paxil CR)	GAD PTSD OCD Panic D/O MDD Social anxiety	Panic disorder: initial 10 mg/day (12.5 mg/day CR); usually wait a few weeks to assess drug effects before increasing dose, but can increase by 10 mg/day (12.5 mg/day CR) once a week; maximum generally 60 mg/day (75 mg/day CR); single dose Other anxiety disorders and MDD: initial 20 mg/day (25 mg/day CR); usually wait a few weeks to assess drug effects before increasing dose, but can increase by 10 mg/day (12.5 mg/day CR) once a week; maximum 60 mg/day (75 mg/day CR); single dose (Stahl, 2008)	Sedation, weight gain, sexual dysfunction (Stahl, 2008)	Pregnancy—D (ACOG, 2008) L2 (Hale, 2008)	Most sedating SSRI and most potential for weight gain Difficult discontinuation A favorite first choice for GAD, PTSD (Stahl, 2008)
Escitalopram (Lexapro)	GAD MDD	Initial 10 mg/day; increase to 20 mg/day if necessary; single dose any time of day; 10 mg of escitalopram may be comparable in efficacy to 40 mg of citalopram with fewer side effects. Give an adequate trial of 10 mg prior to giving 20 mg. (Stahl, 2008)	Sexual dysfunction, G I symptoms, dry mouth, insomnia, sedation, agitation, tremors, headache, dizziness, sweating, bruising, and rare bleeding Rare hyponatremia (mostly in elderly patients—generally reversible when discontinued) (Stahl, 2008)	Pregnancy C (ACOG, 2008) L2 (Hale, 2008)	Relatively expensive Less GI symptoms than citalopram (Stahl, 2008)

(Continued)

Table 28.5 (*Continued*)

Generic (brand)	FDA approved indications	Dosage	Common side effects	Pregnancy/lactation category	Clinical considerations
Sertraline (Zoloft)	MDD OCD Panic D/O PTSD PMDD Social Anxiety	Initial 25 mg/day; increase to 50 mg/day after 1 week thereafter, usually wait a few weeks to assess drug effects before increasing dose; maximum generally 200 mg/day; single dose. (Stahl, 2008) Anxiety associated with PMDD: 25–50 mg in luteal phase of menstrual cycle. Onset is 4.5–8 hours. (King et al., 2011)	GI distress, weight gain, sexual dysfunction (Stahl, 2008)	Pregnancy—C (ACOG, 2008) L2 (Hale, 2008)	Good first choice SSRI. in pregnancy "Zombie" effect common (Stahl, 2008)

Tricyclic antidepressants
Black box warning—suicidality in children, adolescents, and young adults up to 25 years (ages of some childbearing women) (King et al., 2011)

Generic (brand)	FDA approved indications	Dosage	Common side effects	Pregnancy/lactation category	Clinical considerations
Clomipramine (Anafranil)	OCD	Initial 25 mg/day; increase over 2 weeks to 100 mg/day; maximum dose OCD may often require doses at the high end of the range (e.g., 200–250 mg/day) (Stahl, 2008)	GI upset, sedation (Stahl, 2008)	Pregnancy—C (ACOG, 2008) L2 (Hale, 2008)	Take with meals More side effects than SSRIs (Stahl, 2008)
Doxepin (Sinequan)	Anxiety	Initial 25 mg/day at bedtime; increase by 25 mg every 3–7 days 75 mg/day; increase gradually until desired efficacy is achieved; can be dosed once a day at bedtime or in divided doses; maximum dose 300 mg/day (Stahl, 2008)	Sedation (Stahl, 2008)	Pregnancy—C (ACOG, 2008) L5 (Hale, 2008)	Helpful for anxiety with skin/hair/scalp/nail issues (scratchers and pickers) Recent FDA approval as a sleep agent (Stahl, 2008)

Serotonin norepinephrine reuptake inhibitors (SNRIs)
Black box warning (SNRIs)—suicidality in children, adolescents, and young adults up to 25 years (ages of some childbearing women) (King et al., 2011)

Generic (brand)	FDA approved indications	Dosage	Common side effects	Pregnancy/lactation category	Clinical considerations
Venlafaxine XR (Effexor XR)	GAD MDD Panic disorder PPD social anxiety	Initial dose 37.5 mg once daily (extended release) or 25–50 mg divided into two to three doses (immediate release) for a week, if tolerated; increase daily dose generally no faster than 75 mg every 4 days until desired efficacy is reached; maximum dose generally 375 mg/day Usually try doses at 75 mg increments for a few weeks prior to incrementing by an additional 75 mg GAD—150–225 mg/day MDD—75–225 mg/day (Stahl, 2008)	Less sexual dysfunction than SSRIs (Stahl, 2008)	Pregnancy—C (ACOG, 2008) L3 (Hale, 2008)	Difficult discontinuation Monitor for hypertension Helpful for pain syndromes (Stahl, 2008)

Generic (brand)	FDA-approved indications	Dose	Common side effects	Pregnancy/lactation	Clinical considerations
Duloxetine (Cymbalta)	GAD PPD	For generalized anxiety, initial 60 mg once daily; maximum dose generally 120 mg/day (Stahl, 2008)	Nausea (Stahl, 2008)	Pregnancy—C (ACOG, 2008) L3 (Hale, 2008)	Weight neutral Fewer sexual side effects/add to SSRI to decrease sexual dysfunction Hepatotoxicity—watch alcohol intake (Stahl, 2008)

Norepinephrine-dopamine reuptake inhibitors (NDRIs)
Black box warning (NDRIs)—suicidality in children, adolescents, and young adults up to 25 years (ages of some childbearing women) (King et al., 2011)

Generic (brand)	FDA-approved indications	Dose	Common side effects	Pregnancy/lactation	Clinical considerations
Bupropion (Wellbutrin)	MDD	225—450 mg in three divided doses, SR—200–400 mg in two divided doses XL—150–450 mg/day (Stahl, 2008)	Dry mouth, GI symptoms, anorexia, headache, insomnia, sweating, rash, hypertension (Stahl, 2008)	Pregancy—C (ACOG, 2008) L3 (Hale, 2008)	Rise in supine BP (Stahl, 2008)

Other nonbenzodiazepines

Generic (brand)	FDA-approved indications	Dose	Common side effects	Pregnancy/lactation	Clinical considerations
Buspirone (BuSpar)	Anxiety	Initial 15 mg twice a day; increase in 5 mg/ day increments every 2–3 days until desired efficacy is reached; maximum dose generally 60 mg/day (Stahl, 2008)	Nausea, dizziness, restlessness, insomnia (Stahl, 2008)	Pregnancy—B (ACOG, 2008) L3 (Hale, 2008)	Generally not as effective for monotherapy as other agents; may augment SSRIs; recommended as SSRI augment to reduce sexual dysfunction (Stahl, 2008)
Hydroxyzine (Vistaril)	GAD	50–100 mg four times a day (Stahl, 2008)	Sedation, dizziness (Stahl, 2008)	Pregnancy—C (ACOG, 2008) L1 (Hale, 2008)	Can be agitating in some Driving precautions A good augment with SSRIs (Stahl, 2008)

Benzodiazepines
All benzodiazepines have the risk of tolerance and dependency and should be avoided for long-term use (King et al., 2011)

Generic (brand)	FDA-approved indications	Dose	Common side effects	Pregnancy/lactation	Clinical considerations
Lorazepam (Ativan)	Occasional situational anxiety	0.5 mg po (Stahl, 2008)	Sedation, dizziness (Stahl, 2008)	Pregnancy—D (ACOG, 2008) L3 (Hale, 2008)	Short acting, rapid tolerance Acute, short-term use agent; contraindicated for individuals with acute narrow-angle glaucoma, sleep apnea, myasthenia gravis Avoid any use with history of chemical dependency (King et al., 2011)

(Continued)

Table 28.5 (Continued)

Generic (brand)	FDA approved indications	Dosage	Common side effects	Pregnancy/lactation category	Clinical considerations
Clonazepam (Klonopin)	Short-term use while starting SSRI (2–4 weeks) (Stahl, 2008)	0.5 mg po daily, may split dose (Stahl, 2008)	Sedation, dizziness (Stahl, 2008)	Pregnancy—D (ACOG, 2008) L3 (Hale, 2008)	Potential for dependence. Avoided with history of chemical dependency. Contraindicated for individuals with acute narrow-angle glaucoma or hepatic failure. A good choice for the first 2–4 weeks when starting an SSRI for panic symptoms. (King et al., 2011)
Alprazolam (Xanax)	Anxiety	0.25 mg po (Stahl, 2008)	Sedation, dizziness (Stahl, 2008)	Pregnancy—D (ACOG, 2008) L3 (Hale, 2008)	Multiple drug/drug interactions. Risk of tolerance, abuse, dependence is high (King et al., 2011). Avoid use except in extremely limited situations, such as air travel, or needle phobia. Use in collaboration with a mental health specialist (Stahl, 2008)

Adapted with permission from: Karsnitz and Ward (2011).

The current U.S. Food and Drug Administration pregnancy risk categories are as follows: A—Controlled studies show no risk; B— there is no evidence of risk in humans; C—risk cannot be ruled out because animal studies have shown an adverse effect and there are no adequate and well-controlled studies in pregnant women or no animal studies have been conducted, and there are no adequate and well-controlled studies in pregnant women; D—studies, adequate, well controlled, or observational, in pregnant women have demonstrated a risk to the fetus, but the benefits of therapy may outweigh the potential risk; X—adequate, well-controlled trials or observational studies in animals or pregnant women have demonstrated positive evidence that the drug is associated with fetal abnormalities: The use of the drug is contraindicated in women who are or may become pregnant.

Lactation legend:

L1: Safest drug has been taken by a large number of breastfeeding mothers without any observed increase in adverse effects in the infant. Controlled studies in breastfeeding women fail to demonstrate a risk to the infant and the possibility of harm to the breastfeeding infant is remote, or the product is not orally bioavailable in an infant.

L2: Safer drug that has been studied in a limited number of breastfeeding women without an increase in adverse effects in the infant. And/or the evidence of a demonstrated risk which is likely to follow use of this medication in a breastfeeding woman is remote.

L3: Moderately safe. There are no controlled studies in breastfeeding women; however, the risk of untoward effects is possible, or controlled studies show only minimal nonthreatening adverse effects. Drugs should be given only if the potential benefit justifies the potential risk to the infant. New medications that have absolutely no published data are automatically categorized in this category, regardless of how safe they may be.

L4: Possibly hazardous. There is positive evidence of risk to a breastfed infant or to breast milk production, but the benefits from use in breastfeeding mothers may be acceptable despite the risk of the infant (e.g., if the drug is needed in a life-threatening situation or for a serious disease for which safer drugs cannot be used or are ineffective.)

L5: Contraindicated studies in breastfeeding mothers have been demonstrated that there is a significant and documented risk to the infant based on human experience, or it is a medication that has a high risk of causing significant damage to an infant. The risk of using the drug in breastfeeding women clearly outweighs any possible benefit from breastfeeding. The drug is contraindicated in women who are breastfeeding an infant.

FDA, Federal Drug Administration; GAD, generalized anxiety disorder; MDD, major depressive disorder; OCD, obsessive-compulsive disorder; panic D/O, panic disorder; PTSD, post-traumatic stress disorder; PMDD, premenstrual dysphoric disorder; po, by mouth; mg, milligram; GI, gastrointestinal; NDRI, norepinephrine-dopamine reuptake inhibitor.

anxiety disorders in childbearing women ($n = 118,935$) increased from 1.5% to 6.2% (Andrade et al., 2008).

By inhibiting the reuptake of serotonin in the presynaptic cell, the level of serotonin increases in the synapses. There are multiple serotonin receptor cells ($5\text{-}HT_1$–$5\text{-}HT_{15}$). Each SSRI reacts differently on receptor cells causing variable side effects (King, Johnson & Gamblian, 2011). Side effects typically last a few weeks and resolve once the body adapts to the medication. Most practitioners begin treatment with a lower dose, increasing after 1 week or as tolerated (Karsnitz & Ward, 2011; King et al., 2011). Side effects characteristically include gastrointestinal disturbances, headaches, decreased libido, weight gain or loss, sweating, vivid dreams, and agitation. Side effects play an important role in continuation of treatment and should be considered when choosing the appropriate drug therapy. Suicidal ideation has been reported in adolescents and young adults; SSRIs have an Food and Drug Administration (FDA) black box warning for risk of suicidal thoughts for individuals 25 years and younger (King et al., 2011; Stahl, 2008).

Teaching points include dosage, side effects, and importance of provider-guided weaning when discontinuing medication. Serotonin discontinuation syndrome can occur if the drugs are withdrawn abruptly. Symptoms of discontinuation syndrome include dizziness, confusion and tremor, and electric shock-like sensations (King et al., 2011).

Serotonin norepinephrine reuptake inhibitors (SNRIs) have a similar mechanism of action as SSRIs. In addition to inhibiting serotonin, SNRIs also inhibit norepinephrine in the neuronal synapses. Some report SRNIs begin to work more quickly. Side effects are similar to SSRIs but some SRNIs (venlafaxine and duloxetine) can increase blood pressure (Stahl, 2008).

Norepinephrine and dopamine reuptake inhibitors are sometimes a good choice for postpartum women with depression (bupropion) as there are less sedative effects, and they do not cause weight gain or decrease libido. Bupropion can trigger seizures and should not be used in women with a seizure disorder. Although bupropion can be used for depression, it is not helpful for anxiety. Bupropion can be used to treat panic disorder (Stahl, 2008).

Tricyclic antidepressants (TCAs), once the primary medication for treatment of anxiety disorders and depression, are used less frequently today, have increased side effects and many drug to drug interactions. Although helpful for insomnia, women of childbearing age usually respond better to SSRIs. It is important to note that overdose with TCAs can be fatal. Prescriptions should only be written for 7-day increments and are best prescribed by a mental health provider (King et al., 2011).

Psychotherapies are an important treatment modality used alone or in conjunction with pharmacotherapies. CBT utilizes specific behaviors to change a pattern of thinking or redirect negative thoughts. Women identify particular coping mechanisms that effectively interrupt negative or destructive thought processes (Olatunji, Cisler, & Deacon, 2010). IPT focuses on particular conflicts and stress-inducing situations. Postpartum women typically focus on maternal–infant attachment, role transition, or partner conflict and intimacy issues (Mulcahy, Reay, Wilkinson, & Owen, 2009).

Peer support is gaining recognition as evidence shows a decrease in depression scores of individuals receiving support by various means: face-to-face groups, telephone, Internet, and other media (Dennis, 2010; MacArthur et al., 2002; Pfeiffer, Heisler, Piette, Rogers, & Valenstein, 2011). Peer support encourages sharing personal stories, postpartum or daily life stresses, and coping mechanisms. Health-care providers can facilitate peer groups. CenteringPregnancy groups can extend their scheduled sessions into early postpartum and can be an important social support group for new mothers and their families.

Complementary therapies are sometimes used by women who are reluctant to undergo drug therapy. Omega-3 fatty acid supplements, kava root, and St. John's wort have been found to be effective in ameliorating some symptoms of mental health disorders (King et al., 2011). Health-care providers should assess women for use of alternative therapies before starting psychotropic therapy. Most complementary treatments lack an evidence base supporting their effectiveness, benefits, and risks. Teaching includes awareness of label inaccuracy as not all active ingredients or acquisition of substances (leaves, stems, roots) is described. Resources for common herbs and dietary supplements are available through the National Library of Medicine (see "Web Resources for Women and Their and Families").

Summary

Postpartum is a time of restoration and new beginnings. Health-care providers familiar with normal physiological changes during postpartum will be most astute at recognition of complications. Cultural awareness should guide assessment and treatment. Provision of education, regular assessment, and follow-up will increase the likelihood of early identification and treatment. In addition to assessment, health-care providers will diagnose and treat while recognizing when to consult, collaborate, or refer. Development of a local resource and referral list will provide women with options for treatment or assistance and should include supportive social and psychological services in addition to medical services.

Case study

Janine, a 25-year-old Hispanic woman, G1P1, presents to the office today at 5 weeks postpartum. Janine brings her 5-week-old son to the visit. Janine's husband has been deployed to Afghanistan for the past 6 months. She is breastfeeding.

History of present concern

She states that despite having occasional help at home, she feels tired all the time, is rarely hungry, and does not feel like she can accomplish anything throughout the day. Janine states that she cries frequently and, although she loves her baby, does not seem to be able to feel happy. She reports she has been feeling this way since the first week postpartum. She also states that she does not feel comfortable telling her family about how she feels. They dismissed an earlier statement she made about "feeling low," and responded with "you should be happy, you just had a beautiful baby!" She denies suicidal ideation or plans.

Pregnancy history

Her pregnancy was normal without complication. Her labor was 20 hours long with pitocin augmentation to stimulate her labor. She was supported by her mother and sister during labor and birth. She denies depression during this pregnancy.

Family history

Janine's mother has suffered from depression off and on throughout her life.

Current situation history

She takes prenatal vitamins. She denies allergies. Janine does not smoke or use alcohol, prescription drugs, or street drugs. She lives in military housing with her baby, alone while her husband is deployed overseas. Her family lives in another state and came for a 3-week stay around her due date, and left at 2 weeks postpartum.

Evaluation

Janine is alert and oriented to person, place, and time. She appears well nourished. She speaks in monotone but answers appropriately, appearing teary at times. She makes occasional eye contact. A physical exam was done and all parameters, including thyroid, are within normal limits. A depression inventory was administered.

EPDS—*score of 14.*

Assessment: New mother at 5 weeks postpartum with postpartum depression, limited family support available. Consider anemia and postpartum thyroid.

Plan: A discussion with Janine regarding her risk factors for postpartum depression and her EPDS score of 14 was initiated. This score combined with the duration of her symptoms is strongly suggestive of postpartum depression. Treatment options were discussed, including psychotropic medication and referral to a mental health provider for evaluation and behavioral therapy options.

It was explained that she will have two blood tests done to investigate other causes of her symptoms—a CBC and a thyroid stimulating hormone test. Janine was advised to continue her good diet, incorporate daily walks into her routine, and add an omega-3 supplement to her daily prenatal vitamin.

Her need for support from families and friends at this time was discussed. She was encouraged to reach out for support groups available to military families in her area and to stay in frequent contact with her family members.

Janine agreed to start medication and is prescribed Zoloft, 25 mg po every day for 1 week, then increase to 50 mg po every day. A visit with a mental health provider for evaluation and discussion of psychotherapy was scheduled.

Dangers signs were reviewed and she was told to call 911 if suicidal thoughts or plans for self-harm or harm to her baby developed. A return visit to the office was scheduled in 2 weeks for follow-up and a 7-week postpartum exam.

Resource for women and their families

Postpartum Support International: Information regarding Perinatal Mood and Anxiety Disorders: http://postpartum.net/

Resource for health-care providers

Medline Plus [Internet]. Bethesda, MD: National Library of Medicine (US). Herbs and supplements: http:// www.nlm.nih.gov/medlineplus/druginformation.html

References

Alder, J., Fink, N., Bitzer, J., Hosli, I., & Holzgreve, W. (2007). Depression and anxiety during pregnancy: A risk factor for obstetric, fetal and neonatal outcome? A critical review of the literature. *Journal of Maternal-Fetal and Neonatal Medicine, 20*(3), 189–209.

American College of Nurse-Midwives (ACNM). (2003). *Position statement: Depression in women.* Retrieved from http://www.midwife.org

American College of Obstetricians and Gynecologists (ACOG). (2006). Postpartum Hemorrhage. *Practice Bulletin, 76, Obstetrics and Gynecology, 108,* 1039–1047.

American College of Obstetricians and Gynecologists (ACOG). (2008). Practice Bulletin 92. Use of psychiatric medications during pregnancy and lactation: Clinical management guidelines for obstetrician-gynecologists. *Obstetrics and Gynecology, 111,* 1001–1020.

American College of Obstetricians and Gynecologists (ACOG). (2010a). Committee on Obstetric Practice. Committee Opinion No. 453: Screening for depression during and after pregnancy. *Obstetrics and Gynecology, 115*(2 Pt. 1), 394–395.

American College of Obstetricians and Gynecologists (ACOG). (2010b). Antimicrobial prophylaxis for cesarean delivery: Timing of administration. Committee Opinion No. 465. *Obstetrics and Gynecology, 116,* 791–792.

American Psychiatric Association (APA). (2000). *Diagnostic and statistical manual of mental disorders* (4th ed.), Text Revision (DSMV-IV-TR). Washington, DC: American Psychiatric Association.

Andrade, S. E., Raebel, M. A., Brown, J., Lane, K., Livingston, J., Boudreau, D., . . . Platt, R. (2008). Use of antidepressant medications during pregnancy: A multisite study. *American Journal of Obstetrics and Gynecology, 198,* 194.e1–194.e5.

Andrews, W. W., Hauth, J. C., Cliver, S. P., Savage, K., & Goldenberg, R. L. (2003). Randomized clinical trial of extended spectrum antibiotic prophylaxis with coverage for ureaplasma urealyticum to reduce post-cesarean delivery endometritis. *Obstetrics and Gynecology, 101*(6), 1183–1189.

Appolonio, K. K., & Fingerhut, R. (2008). Postpartum depression in a military sample. *Military Medicine, 173*(11), 1085–1091.

Baxter, J. K., Berghella, V., Mackeen, A. D., Ohly, N. T., & Weed, S. (2011). Timing of prophylactic antibiotics for preventing postpartum infectious morbidity in women undergoing cesarean delivery. *Cochrane Database of Systematic Reviews,* (12), CD009516. doi:10.1002/14651858.CD009516

Beck, C. T. (1993). Teetering on the edge: A substantive theory of postpartum depression. *Nursing Research, 42*(1), 42–48.

Beck, C. T. (1999). Postpartum depression: Stopping the thief that steals motherhood. *AWHONN Lifelines, 3,* 41–44.

Beck, C. T. (2006). The anniversary of birth trauma: Failure to rescue. *Nursing Research, 55*(6), 381–390.

Beck, C. T., & Indman, P. (2005). The many faces of postpartum depression. *Journal of Obstetric, Gynecologic & Neonatal Nursing, 34*(5), 569–576.

Beck, C. T., & Watson, S. (2010). Subsequent childbirth after a previous traumatic birth. *Nursing Research, 59*(4), 241–249.

Belfort, M. A., Clark, S. L., Saade, G. R., Kleja, K., Dildy, G. A., Van Veen, T. R., . . . Kofford, S. (2010). Hospital readmission after delivery: Evidence for an increased incidence of nonurogenital infection in the immediate postpartum period. *American Journal of Obstetrics & Gynecology, 202*(1), 35.e1–35.e7.

Berg, C. J., Callaghan, W. M., Syverson, C., & Henderson, Z. (2010). Pregnancy-related mortality in the United States, 1998 to 2005. *Obstetrics and Gynecology, 116*(6), 1302–1309.

Berg, C. J., Chang, J., Callaghan, W. M., & Whitehead, S. J. (2003). Pregnancy-related mortality in the Unites States, 1991–1997. *Obstetrics and Gynecology, 101*(2), 289–296.

Centers for Disease Control and Prevention. (2008). Prevalence of self-reported postpartum depressive symptoms—17 states 2004–2005. *MMWR. Morbidity and Mortality Weekly Report, 57*(14), 361.

Centre for Maternal and Child Enquiries (CMACE). (2011). Saving mothers' lives: Reviewing maternal deaths to make motherhood safer: 2006–08. The Eighth Report on Confidential Enquiries into Maternal Deaths in the United Kingdom. *BJOG: An International Journal of Obstetrics and Gynaecology, 118*(Suppl. 1), 1–203.

Chames, M. C., Livingston, J. C., Ivester, T. S., Barton, J. R., & Sibai, B. M. (2002). Late postpartum eclampsia: A preventable disease? *American Journal of Obstetrics & Gynecology, 186*(6), 1174–1177.

Cox, J. L., Holden, J. M., & Sagovsky, R. (1987). Detection of postnatal depression: Development of the 10-item Edinburgh Postnatal Depression Scale. *British Journal of Psychiatry, 150,* 782–786.

Cunningham, F. G., Leveno, K. J., Bloom, S. L., Hauth, J. C., Rouse, D. J., & Spong, C. Y. (2010). *Williams obstetrics* (23rd ed.). New York: McGraw-Hill Co.

Dennis, C. L. (2010). Postpartum depression peer support: Maternal perceptions from a randomized controlled trial. *International Journal of Nursing Studies, 47,* 560–568.

Duff, P. (2007). Maternal and perinatal infection—bacterial. In S. Gabbe, J. Niebyl, & J. Simpson (Eds.), *Obstetrics: Normal and problem pregnancies* (5th ed., pp. 1140–1155). Philadelphia: Churchill Livingstone.

Duggal, N., Mercado, C., Daniels, K., Bujor, A., Caughey, A. B., & El-Sayed, Y. Y. (2008). Antibiotic prophylaxis for prevention of postpartum perineal wound complications: A randomized controlled trial. *Obstetrics & Gynecology, 111*(6), 1268–1273.

Elmir, R., Schmied, V., Wilkes, L., & Jackson, D. (2010). Women's perceptions and experiences of a traumatic birth: a meta-ethnography. *Journal of Advanced Nursing, 66*(10), 2142–2153.

Feeny, N. C., Zoellner, L. A., & Kanana, S. Y. (2009). Providing a treatment rationale for PTSD: Does what we say matter? *Behaviour Research and Therapy, 47,* 752–760.

Francois, K. E., & Foley, M. R. (2007). Antepartum and postpartum hemorrhage. In S. Gabbe, J. Niebyl, & J. Simpson (Eds.), *Obstetrics: Normal and problem pregnancies* (5th ed., pp. 415–444). Philadelphia: Churchill Livingstone.

Gangdev, P. (2002). The relationship between obsessive-compulsive disorder and psychosis. *Australasian Psychiatry, 10*(4), 405–410.

Gaynes, B. N., Gavin, N., Meltzer-Brody, S., Lohr, K. N., Swinson, T., Gartlehner, G., . . . Miller, W. C. (2005). Perinatal depression: Prevalence, screening accuracy and screening outcomes evidence report/technology assessment (Summary) No. 119. AHRQ Publication No. 05-E006-2.

Gibson, J., McKenzie-McHarg, K., Shakespeare, J., Price, J., & Gray, R. (2009). A systematic review of studies validating the Edinburgh Postnatal Depression Scale in antepartum and postpartum women. *Acta Psychiatrica Scandinavica, 119*(5), 350–364.

Goodman, J. H., & Tyer-Viola, L. (2010). Detection, treatment, and referral of perinatal depression and anxiety by obstetrical providers. *Journal of Women's Health, 19*(3), 477–490.

Graeber, B., Vanderwal, T., Stiller, R. J., & Werdmann, M. J. (2005). Late postpartum eclampsia as an obstetric complication seen in the ED. *The American Journal of Emergency Medicine, 23*(2), 168–170.

Hackley, B., Sharma, C., Kedzior, A., & Sreenivasan, S. (2010). Managing mental health conditions in primary care settings. *Journal of Midwifery & Women's Health, 55,* 9–19.

Halbreich, U., & Karkun, S. (2006). Cross-cultural and social diversity of prevalence of postpartum depression and depressive symptoms. *Journal of Affective Disorders, 91,* 97–111.

Hale, T. (2008). *Medications and mothers' milk* (13th ed.). Amarillo, TX: Hale Publishing.

Ham, P., Waters, D. B., & Oliver, M. N. (2005). Treatment of panic disorder. *American Family Physician, 71*, 733–740.

Hankins, G. D., Clark, S. L., Pacheco, L. D., O'Keeffe, D., D'Alton, M., & Saade, G. R. (2012). Maternal mortality, near misses, and severe morbidity: Lowering rates through designated levels of maternity care. *Obstetrics & Gynecology, 120*(4), 929–934.

Hirshfeld-Cytron, J., Lam, C., Karumanchi, S. A., & Lindheimer, M. (2006). Late postpartum eclampsia: Examples and review. *Obstetrical & Gynecological Survey, 61*(7), 471–480.

Karsnitz, D. B., & Ward, S. (2011). Spectrum of anxiety disorders: Diagnosis and pharmacologic treatment. *Journal of Midwifery and Women's Health, 56*(3), 266–281.

Karsnitz, D. B., & Webster, N. (2012). Mental health during childbearing: The evidence for the midwifery model of care. In B. Anderson & S. Stone (Eds.), *Best practices in midwifery: Using the Evidence for change* (pp. 119–138). New York: Springer Publishing Company.

Katon, W. J. (2006). Panic disorder. *New England Journal of Medicine, 354*(22), 2360–2367.

Katz, V. (2007). Postpartum care. In S. Gabbe, J. Niebyl, & J. Simpson (Eds.), *Obstetrics: Normal and problem pregnancies* (5th ed., pp. 517–532). Philadelphia: Churchill Livingstone.

Kessler, R. C., Berglund, P., Demler, O., Jin, R., Merikangas, K. R., & Walters, E. E. (2005). Lifetime prevalence and age-of-onset distributions of DSM-IV disorders in the National Co-morbidity Survey Replication. *Archives of General Psychiatry, 62*, 593–602.

King, J. C. (2012). Maternal mortality in the United States—Why is it important and what are we doing about it? *Seminars in Perinatology, 36*, 14–18.

King, T., Johnson, R., & Gamblian, V. (2011). Mental health. In T. L. King & M. C. Brucker (Eds.), *Pharmacology for women's health* (pp. 750–786). Sudbury, MA: Jones and Bartlett.

MacArthur, C., Winter, H. R., Bick, D. E., Knowles, H., Lilford, R., Henderson, C., . . . Gee, H. (2002). Effects of redesigned community postnatal care on women's health 4 months after birth: A cluster randomized controlled trial. *The Lancet, 359*(9304), 378–385.

Maharaj, D. (2007). Puerperal pyrexia: A review. Part II. *Obstetrical & Gynecological Survey, 62*, 400.

Mannucci, P. M. (2004). Treatment of von Willebrand's disease. *New England Journal of Medicine, 351*, 683.

Mayberry, L. J., Horowitz, J. A., & Declercq, E. (2007). Depression symptom prevalence and demographic risk factors among U.S. women during the first 2 years postpartum. *Journal of Obstetric, Gynecologic & Neonatal Nursing, 36*, 542–549.

Meades, R., Pond, C., Ayers, S., & Warren, F. (2011). Postnatal debriefing: Have we thrown the baby out with the bath water? *Behaviour Research and Therapy, 49*(5), 367–372.

Mulcahy, R., Reay, R. E., Wilkinson, R. B., & Owen, C. (2009). A randomized control trial for the effectiveness of group interpersonal psychotherapy for postnatal depression. *Archives of Women's Mental Health, 13*, 125–139.

Murray, L., Arteche, A., Fearon, P., Halligan, S., Goodyer, I., & Cooper, P. (2011). Maternal postnatal depression and the development of depression in offspring up to 16 years of age. *Journal of the American Academy of Child & Adolescent Psychiatry, 50*(5), 460–470.

Neville, M. W. (2011). Thyroid disorders. In T. L. King & M. C. Brucker (Eds.), *Pharmacology for women's health*. Sudbury, MA: Jones and Bartlett.

Olatunji, B. O., Cisler, J. M., & Deacon, B. J. (2010). Efficacy of cognitive behavioral therapy for anxiety disorders: A review of meta-analytic findings. *Psychiatric Clinics of North America, 33*, 557–577.

Pampallona, S., Bollini, P., Tibaldi, G., Kupelnick, B., & Munizza, C. (2004). Combined pharmacotherapy and psychological treatment for depression: A systematic review. *Archives of General Psychiatry, 61*, 714–719.

Pettker, C., & Lockwood, C. (2007). Thromboembolic disorders. In S. Gabbe, J. Niebyl, & J. Simpson (Eds.), *Obstetrics: Normal and problem pregnancies* (5th ed., pp. 980–993). Philadelphia: Churchill Livingstone.

Pfeiffer, P. N., Heisler, M., Piette, J. D., Rogers, M. A., & Valenstein, M. (2011). Efficacy of peer support interventions for depression: A meta-analysis. *General Hospital Psychiatry, 33*, 29–36.

Posmontier, B. (2010). The role of midwives in facilitating recovery in postpartum psychosis. *Journal of Midwifery & Women's Health, 55*, 430–437.

Purnell, L. D., & Paulanka, B. J. (2003). The Purnell Model for cultural competence. In L. D. Purnell & B. J. Paulanka (Eds.), *Transcultural health care: A culturally competent approach* (2nd ed., pp. 19–55). Philadelphia: F. A. Davis Co.

Rambelli, C., Montagnani, M. S., Oppo, A., et al. (2010). Panic disorder as a risk factor for post-partum depression: results from the Perinatal Depression-Research & Screening Unit (PND-ReScU) study. *Journal of Affective Disorders, 122*, 139–143.

Robertson, E., Grace, S., Wallington, T., & Stewart, D. E. (2004). Antenatal risk factors for postpartum depression: a synthesis of recent literature. *General Hospital Psychiatry, 26*, 289–295.

Ross, L. E., & McLean, L. M. (2006). Anxiety disorders during pregnancy and the postpartum period: A systematic review. *Journal of Clinical Psychiatry, 67*, 1285–1298.

Sibai, B. M. (2007). Hypertension. In S. G. Gabbe, J. R. Niebyl, & J. L. Simpson (Eds.), *Obstetrics: Normal and Problem Pregnancies* (5th ed.). Philadelphia: Churchill Livinstone.

Sibai, B. M., & Stella, C. L. (2009). Diagnosis and management of atypical preeclampsia-eclampsia. *American Journal of Obstetrics and Gynecology, 200*, 481.e1–e7.

Sit, D., Rothschild, A. J., & Wisner, K. L. (2006). A review of postpartum psychosis. *Journal of Women's Health, 15*, 352–368.

Smaill, F. M., & Gyte, G. M. (2010). Antibiotic prophylaxis versus no prophylaxis for preventing infection after cesarean section. *Cochrane Database of Systematic Reviews*, (1), CD007482, doi:10.1002/14651858,pub2

Spinelli, M. G. (2004). Maternal infanticide associated with mental illness: Prevention and the promise of saved lives. *American Journal of Psychiatry, 161*(9), 1548–1557.

Stahl, S. M. (2008). Essential psychopharmacology online. Retrieved from http://stahlonline.cambridge.org/common_home.jsf

Stein, D. J., Ipser, J., & McAnda, N. (2009). Pharmacotherapy of posttraumatic stress disorder: A review of meta-analyses and treatment guidelines. *CNS Spectrums, 14*(1), suppl 1.

Strohle, A., & Holsboer, F. (2003). Stress responsive neurohormones in depression and anxiety. *Pharmacopsychiatry, 36*, S207–S214.

Sweet, R. L., & Gibbs, R. S. (2009). *Infectious diseases of the female genital tract* (5th ed.). Baltimore, MD: Lippincott Williams & Wilkins.

U.S. Preventive Services Task Force (USPSTF). (2009). Screening for depression in adults: U.S. preventive services task force recommendation statement. *Annals of Internal Medicine, 151*(11), 784–792.

van Dillen, J., Zwart, J., Schutte, J., & van Roosmalen, J. (2010). Maternal sepsis: Epidemiology, etiology and outcome. *Current Opinion in Infectious Diseases, 23*, 249–254.

Vesga-Lopez, O., Schneier, F. R., Wang, S., Heimberg, R. G., Liu, S. M., Hasin, D. S., & Blanco, C. (2008). Gender differences in generalized anxiety disorder: results from the National Epidemiologic Survey on Alcohol and Related Conditions (NESARC). *Journal of Clinical Psychiatry, 69*(10), 1606–1616.

Vythilingum, B. (2008). Anxiety disorders in pregnancy. *Current Psychiatry Reports, 01,* 331–335.

World Health Organization (WHO), United Nations Children's Fund (UNICEF), United Nation's Population Fund (UNFPA), and The World Bank. (2012). *Trends in maternal mortality: 1990 to 2010 WHO, UNICEF, UNFPA and the World Bank estimates.* Geneva, Switzerland: World Health Organization.

Zender, R., & Olshansky, E. (2009). Women's mental health: Depression and anxiety. *Nursing Clinics of North America, 44,* 355–364.

29

Contraception

Patricia Aikins Murphy and Leah N. Torres

Relevant terms

Combined hormonal contraceptives (CHCs)—hormonal contraceptives that contain both estrogen and progestin

Combined oral contraceptives (COCs)—hormonal oral contraceptive pills that contain both estrogen and progestin; also known as "the pill" or "birth control pills"

Emergency contraception (EC)—any contraceptive method used after sexual intercourse to prevent pregnancy; hormonal-based methods are commonly used, but the copper intrauterine device can also be used

Fertility awareness-based methods (FAMs)—a variety of methods that use the woman's natural cycle to determine the fertile period and avoid intercourse during that time; also known as "natural family planning"

Intrauterine contraception (IUC)—small device placed in the uterus to prevent pregnancy

Lactational amenorrhea method (LAM)—temporary contraceptive that can be used during the first months

after birth in women who are exclusively breastfeeding and meet selected other criteria

Long-acting reversible contraceptive methods (LARC)—reversible contraceptive method that provides long-acting protection without requiring the user to do anything on a daily, weekly, or monthly basis; examples include intrauterine devices and contraceptive implants

Medical eligibility criteria (MEC)—evidence-based guidelines about the use of contraceptives in the presence of medical conditions and risk factors for complications, as well as in normal health states such as postpartum and breastfeeding

Progestin-only pills (POPs)—hormonal oral contraceptive pills that contain only progestin; also known as "the minipill"

Sterilization—permanent contraceptive method; intended to *not* be reversible; involves surgical alteration of the fallopian tube in the female or the vas deferens in the male

---

Introduction

Postpartum contraception is important because the successful and appropriate spacing of pregnancies is a critical factor in improving maternal and infant health outcomes in future pregnancies. A meta-analysis of adverse outcomes associated with short interpregnancy intervals showed that intervals shorter than 6 months were associated with a 30–60% increased risk of preterm birth, low birth weight, and small-for-gestational-age infants, and intervals of 18 months or less were associ-

ated with a smaller but still significant increase in the risk of adverse perinatal outcomes (Conde-Agudelo, Rosas-Bermudez, & Kafury-Goeta, 2006).

Thus, it is important to consider contraceptive and family planning methods for women early in the postpartum period. Indeed, counseling and decision making should ideally begin during early pregnancy and continue throughout prenatal care. A recent qualitative study indicated that postpartum women prefer to have frequent sessions of contraceptive counseling throughout the prenatal period, with reinforcement of

Prenatal and Postnatal Care: A Woman-Centered Approach, First Edition. Edited by Robin G. Jordan, Janet L. Engstrom, Julie A. Marfell, and Cindy L. Farley.
© 2014 John Wiley & Sons, Inc. Published 2014 by John Wiley & Sons, Inc.

counseling and family planning decisions after delivery (Yee & Simon, 2011).

Postpartum care and return to fertility after childbirth

The typical postpartum office visit occurs around 6 weeks after delivery. Most women (nearly 90%) have some type of postpartum care visit, although the proportion is much lower in some populations. For example, only about 60% of women in Medicaid managed care programs receive a postpartum care visit (Centers for Disease Control and Prevention [CDC], 2007; Weir et al., 2011). Even if women keep a 6-week postpartum visit appointment, delaying contraceptive counseling until this time does not help the woman prevent an unintended pregnancy. A 2005 Canadian study found that nearly half (47%) of postpartum women had resumed sexual activity by the time of the 6-week visit, with 60% of nonbreastfeeding mothers and about one-third of breastfeeding mothers reporting sexual activity by the time of the visit (Rowland, Foxcroft, Hopman, & Patel, 2005).

Many women think that they are not at risk of ovulation and unintended pregnancy in the first weeks or months after birth, but this assumption is not correct. A 2011 systematic review of the return of ovulation in nonlactating women (Jackson & Glasier, 2011) found that the mean day of first ovulation ranged from 45 to 94 days postpartum, and that 20–71% of first menses were preceded by ovulation, with as many as 60% of these ovulations being potentially fertile. An older study of 22 nonlactating women estimated the mean time from delivery to menses to be about 6 weeks (45 days); none of the women ovulated before 25 days (Gray, Campbell, Zacur, Labbok, & MacRae, 1987). Although a certain proportion of the first bleeding episodes after childbirth are anovulatory and luteal phase abnormalities occur in some early ovulatory cycles, it is not possible to predict which of the first postpartum cycles will be ovulatory and potentially fertile. Thus, clinicians must consider all nonbreastfeeding postpartum women to be at risk of unintended pregnancy as early as 3–4 weeks postpartum.

For breastfeeding women, the return of ovulation is variable (Wang & Fraser, 1994); the pattern of breastfeeding (frequency, timing, and intensity of the infant suckling at the breast) and supplementation of breastfeeding with formula, fluids or foods determines the risk of ovulation, and it is not possible to predict when fertility and the risk of pregnancy will resume. The lactational amenorrhea method (LAM) of family planning is based on the contraceptive effects of full breastfeeding, and a systematic review concluded that

fully breastfeeding women who remain amenorrheic have a very small risk of becoming pregnant in the first 6 months after delivery (Van der Wijden, Kleijnen, & Van den Berk, 2003). In one study of breastfeeding women in China, ultrasonography and basal body temperature were used to determine the return of ovulation after delivery; the mean time to return to ovulation was about 155 days postpartum (about 5 months), but the range was large with ovulation resuming as early as 67 days (about 2 months) (Li & Qiu, 2007).

The fact that the average time of return to ovulation in nonbreastfeeding mothers is about 6 weeks after birth indicates that a proportion of women will ovulate earlier than their 6-week checkup. Research demonstrates that many women will have resumed sexual activity by the time of the 6-week visit, placing them at risk for an unintended pregnancy. Although the return to ovulation is delayed longer in breastfeeding mothers, the variability in breastfeeding practices and an average return to ovulation by 5–6 months (indicating that a proportion of women will ovulate earlier than 5 months) suggest that contraceptive methods should be initiated earlier than typically done to provide adequate protection from an unintended pregnancy.

Family planning experts advise that in fully breastfeeding mothers, a contraceptive method should be initiated by the third postpartum month, and in partial or nonbreastfeeding mothers, a contraceptive method should be initiated by the third postpartum week (Speroff & Darney, 2011). This recommendation is known as the "Rule of Threes."

When to start contraception in the postnatal period: The "Rule of Threes"

In the presence of FULL breastfeeding, a contraceptive method should be used beginning in the *third postpartum month*.

With PARTIAL breastfeeding or NO breastfeeding, a contraceptive method should be used beginning in the *third postpartum week*.

Source: Speroff, L., & Darney, P. (2011). *A clinical guide for Contraception* (5th ed.). Philadelphia: Wolters Kluwer.

Considerations in selecting a postpartum contraceptive method

In addition to recognizing how soon after delivery some women resume ovulation and sexual activity, there are additional considerations in the selection of an appropriate contraceptive method for women who have recently given birth. The stress of new parenthood, whether for a first-time mother or a mother with other children, is well documented (Vernon, Young-Hyman, & Looney, 2010). Lack of time, the responsibilities of caregiving, household tasks and work, lack of child care, and other factors all contribute to challenges in meeting the activities of daily living that may impact a woman's ability to remember to take her birth control pills on time, get to the pharmacy for refills, or even manage an appointment with a clinician for birth control initiation. Loss of interval third party insurance coverage (such as having Medicaid during pregnancy) may also negatively impact a woman's ability to access affordable contraception.

The choice of contraceptive method should not interfere with a woman's ability to breastfeed. Breastfeeding is the optimal feeding method for infants, and there are significant health benefits from breastfeeding for both the mother and the infant (Gartner et al., 2005). Lactogenesis II, the process by which a woman begins to produce copious amounts of breast milk, is initiated in part by the withdrawal of progesterone that occurs when the placenta is delivered, and there are concerns about interfering with this process by the early administration of hormonal, especially progestin, contraceptives (Kennedy, Short, & Tully, 1997). To ensure appropriate initiation of lactogenesis II, it may be prudent to delay the administration of a large progesterone bolus (such as an injection of DMPA or the insertion of the progestin implant) until copious milk production occurs, which usually begins 2–7 days after birth (Hatcher et al., 2011).

In most cases, however, progestin-only contraceptives can be administered in the immediate postpartum period without adverse affects on lactation, and progestin-only contraceptives may even increase milk volume. There is also little evidence that initiating combined hormonal contraceptives (CHCs) after 6 weeks postpartum has an adverse effects on lactation (Kapp, Curtis, & Nanda, 2010). Although some CHCs have been shown to reduce the duration of breastfeeding and diminish the quantity of breast milk, the evidence is limited. No adverse effects on infant growth or development have been described in children breastfed by mothers taking oral contraceptives (Nilsson et al., 1986).

The contraceptive method choice must also be tailored to the normal expected physiological changes of the puerperium. For example, pregnancy is associated with an increased risk of venous thromboembolism, a risk that continues into the postpartum period (4–6 weeks after delivery) before returning to a prepregnancy baseline level of risk (Heit et al., 2005). Estrogen-containing combination hormonal contraceptives are therefore contraindicated for at least 3 weeks after birth or longer, depending on the mother's risk factors for venous thromboembolism (CDC, 2011).

Women who have had perinatal complications need to be carefully evaluated prior to initiating a contraceptive method. For example, the physiological and biochemical changes associated with preeclampsia may persist for several weeks and even months postpartum (Firoz & Melnik, 2011). Women who had gestational diabetes during pregnancy are at a higher risk for developing type II diabetes, a risk that can be increased by the use of progestin-only contraceptives (at least in breastfeeding Latinas) (Kjos et al., 1998). There are also a number of conditions associated with increased risk for adverse health events as a result of unintended pregnancy. These conditions are listed as follows.

Conditions associated with increased risk for adverse health events as a result of unintended pregnancy

Breast cancer
Complicated valvular heart disease
Diabetes: insulin dependent; with nephropathy/retinopathy/ neuropathy or other vascular disease; or of >20 years' duration
Endometrial or ovarian cancer
Epilepsy
Hypertension (systolic >160 mmHg or diastolic >100 mmHg)
History of bariatric surgery within the past 2 years
HIV/AIDS
Ischemic heart disease
Malignant gestational trophoblastic disease
Malignant liver tumors (hepatoma) and hepatocellular carcinoma of the liver
Peripartum cardiomyopathy
Schistosomiasis with fibrosis of the liver
Severe (decompensated) cirrhosis
Sickle cell disease
Solid organ transplantation within the past 2 years
Stroke
Systemic lupus erythematosus
Thrombogenic mutations
Tuberculosis

Source: Medical eligibility criteria for contraceptive use. (2010). Retrieved from: http://www.cdc.gov/reproductivehealth/ unintendedpregnancy/USMEC.htm

---

Medical eligibility criteria (MEC) for contraceptive use have been developed by the World Health Organization (WHO), and are periodically updated by experts at working group meetings held at the WHO (2004). The criteria were established to assist individual countries in the development of guidelines specific to their populations and health systems. The United States developed recommendations for U.S. health-care providers, which were released by the Centers for Disease Control and Prevention (CDC) in 2010 (CDC, 2010). The purpose of these recommendations is to base contraceptive management on the best available evidence and to reduce medical barriers to contraceptive use. All of the contraceptive methods reviewed in the document include recommendations for postpartum and breastfeeding women as well as an extensive array of health conditions. Thus, a health-care professional can use the document to determine the recommendation for whether a particular contraceptive can be used by a woman with a medical condition such as diabetes or a health behavior such as smoking. The recommendations for contraceptive use are summarized into four categories known as the MEC categories. These categories are described as follows.

MEC categories for contraceptive use

Category	Overall recommendation	Recommendation for a specific medical condition or health behavior
1	Use method in any circumstance	No restriction
2	Generally use the method	Advantages generally outweigh the risks
3	Use of method not recommended unless more appropriate methods are not available or acceptable	Theoretical or proven risks usually outweigh advantages
4	Do not use method	Unacceptable health risk

Source: Medical eligibility criteria for contraceptive use. (2010). Retrieved from: http://www.cdc.gov/reproductivehealth/unintendedpregnancy/USMEC.htm.

In summary, contraception is an important consideration and choice for the postpartum woman. Health-care providers need to be aware of all of the modern contraceptive methods and the recommendations for their use in the postpartum period in order to assist women in making appropriate reproductive health choices.

Table 29.1   Contraceptive Methods Grouped by Level of Effectiveness

Level	Effectiveness	Contraceptive methods
Tier one	Most effective methods; failure rates are less than 1 pregnancy per 100 women per year	Male sterilization Female sterilization Intrauterine contraception Implant contraception
Tier two	Very effective methods; failure rates are 6–12 pregnancies per 100 women per year	Injectable contraception Contraceptive patch Contraceptive ring Contraceptive pills
Tier three	Less effective methods; failure rates are 12 or more pregnancies per 100 women per year	Male condom Vaginal diaphragm Female condom Fertility awareness-based methods Withdrawal Spermicides

Source: Hatcher, R. A., Trussel, J., Nelson, A. L., Cates, W., Kowal, D., & Policar, M. S. (2011). *Contraceptive technology* (20th ed.). New York: Ardent Media, Inc.

Contraceptive methods

The effectiveness of contemporary contraceptive methods is usually described by reporting the percentage of women/couples who will experience a pregnancy during the first year of "perfect" or "typical" use. Perfect use refers to correct and consistent contraceptive use at all times; typical use refers to actual use that includes incorrect and inconsistent use of a method (Trussell, 2011). "Typical" effectiveness rates probably have more relevance to the actual likelihood of unintended pregnancy. Methods are then grouped according to their estimated effectiveness in preventing pregnancy, from less effective (about 30 pregnancies per 100 women per year) to most effective (less than 1 pregnancy per 100 women per year). Table 29.1 displays three levels or tiers of contraceptive methods grouped according to their estimated effectiveness. Note that the table only includes methods for which 1-year effectiveness rates can be estimated. Another method pertinent to the postpartum period, the lactational amenorrhea method is not in the table because it is only intended to be used for a maximum of 6 months and, thus, 1-year effectiveness rates cannot be estimated. This method is discussed later in the chapter.

Tier one methods

Tier one contraceptives are the most effective methods of preventing pregnancy. Failure rates are typically much less than 1 pregnancy per 100 women per year. The methods are less susceptible to user error such as forgetting or not using a method at the time of intercourse, forgetting to take a daily pill or to replace a contraceptive patch, or missing an appointment for a repeat contraceptive injection. Once initiated, the methods in this tier provide contraceptive protection for long periods of time without the need for user action.

Permanent methods

Sterilization is the most commonly used contraceptive method in the world. It is intended to be permanent (despite occasional failures) and not reversible. Thus, counseling about the permanency of sterilization is critical to ensuring that the actual sterilization procedure is well understood and that women/couples who choose this method have completed their families.

Female sterilization involves the excision or occlusion of the fallopian tubes. For most procedures, it is effective immediately, and failure rates in the first year after sterilization are less than 1%. Failures do occur, though, and are related to the procedure type, the skill of the operator, and the characteristics of the person being sterilized. For example, the younger a woman is at the time of sterilization, the more likely she is to have a subsequent unintended pregnancy. Over a 10-year period, the cumulative failure rate for female sterilization is about 1.85%, ranging from less than 1% when the procedure is a postpartum tubal excision to over 2% when bipolar coagulation methods are used. Women who experience failure of a tubal sterilization and become pregnant are more likely to have an ectopic pregnancy. Health-care providers must be aware of this risk in any woman presenting with pregnancy who has previously undergone tubal sterilization.

Tubal occlusion can be accomplished abdominally (by laparotomy or laparoscopy) or transcervically. Procedures include electrosurgical methods (which coagulate the tube), use of clips or rings, sclerosing agents to mechanically occlude the tube, or the surgical excision of portions of the tube. Transcervical procedures are not immediately effective; it takes approximately 3 months for tubal occlusion to be complete and a follow-up hysterosalpingogram must be performed to confirm occlusion of both tubes.

Tubal sterilization can be accomplished immediately after birth (before leaving the hospital), or as an interval procedure after the postpartum recovery period (transcervical methods are only done as interval procedures).

There is no evidence of associated major risk or adverse effects on postpartum recovery or lactation from having the procedure performed shortly after birth, other than the usual risks associated with anesthesia and surgery. Similarly, interval procedures carry no additional postpartum specific risks.

The younger a woman is when she undergoes permanent sterilization, the more likely she is to regret the decision later (Curtis, Mohllajee, & Peterson, 2006). Surgical reanastamosis of the tubes to reverse the procedure can be performed, but its success is dependent on the type of procedure and the amount of tube that has been damaged. Counseling should address these issues in addition to those surrounding the risks and benefits of the procedure. The cost of the procedure is also an important consideration since most third party insurers will not cover the cost of this elective procedure.

Minority women are more likely than white women to choose tubal sterilization as a contraceptive method (Borrero et al., 2010). According to the most recent National Survey of Family Growth, which provides nationally representative data of women aged 15–44 years, 22% of black women have been sterilized compared to 15% of white women. On the other hand, regret is experienced more often by minority women (Borrero et al., 2008). Education and counseling about sterilization is important for all women, but the history of the involuntary sterilization of poor and minority women in this country over past decades (Stern, 2005) suggests it may be especially important in this group.

Cost and access are factors to consider with any surgical procedure. Insurance coverage and cost may vary with procedures. For example, interval outpatient procedures may be less expensive than in-hospital procedures; some procedures require additional follow-up testing that is costly (e.g., hysterosalpingogram for transcervical procedures); and there may be varying access to publicly funded or subsidized procedures for women without insurance or financial means. Some types of coverage (particularly federally supported insurance programs) have strict rules about preconsent counseling and timing of consent that must be followed in order for coverage to be secured.

Male sterilization, or *vasectomy*, is also an option for couples to consider. Vasectomy involves the ligation/excision or cautery of the vas deferens and is considered a permanent sterilization method. It is associated with lower risk, lower cost, and a lower failure rate than female sterilization methods (Smith, Taylor, & Smith, 1985). The outpatient procedure commonly uses a "no scalpel" technique that is associated with relatively minor discomfort and bruising. The use of another form of contraception is essential until the man has had at least one negative sperm count, which usually takes at least 3 months and approximately 20 ejaculations to ensure clearance of sperm from the portion of the vas beyond the vasectomy site (Griffin, Tooher, Nowakowski, Lloyd, & Maddern, 2005).

According to the 2002 National Survey of Family, 11.4% of men aged 30–45 years reported having a vasectomy; this represents 14.1% of white men, 3.7% of black men, and 4.5% of Hispanic men, but the reasons for these race/ethnic differences are unknown (Eisenberg, Henderson, Amory, Smith, & Walsh, 2009).

Less than 1% of men who had a vasectomy will request a reversal, but this varies by country. Vasectomy reversals have variable success rates, ranging from 30% to 60%, and the success of reversal attempts diminishes over time. Men sterilized before the age of 30 are more likely to seek a reversal (Michielsen & Beerthuizen, 2010). The issues of cost and access to male sterilization are similar to those of female sterilization.

Long-acting reversible contraceptive (LARC) methods

The permanent nature of sterilization makes that option inappropriate for couples who are not sure whether they have completed their families. Fortunately, these women have the option of using long-acting reversible contraceptive methods that are as effective as sterilization.

Intrauterine contraception (IUC) involves the placement of a small T-shaped device in the uterus to prevent pregnancy. There are two types of intrauterine devices (IUDs) available in the United States at the time this chapter was written: the Copper T 380A (brand name ParaGard®) and the levonorgestrel intrauterine system (LNG IUS, brand name Mirena®). A clinician inserts an IUD during an office visit, providing the additional advantage of avoiding the risks and costs of surgery. Each type of IUD has a string that passes from the uterus through the cervix and into the vagina to facilitate removal as well as provide a visible clue that the device is still in the uterus.

The *copper IUD* is approved for 10 years of contraceptive use, although it may be effective for longer (Sivin, 2007). Once placed, the device produces a sterile inflammatory response within the uterus that creates a hostile environment for sperm, preventing fertilization of the egg. The copper device is effective almost immediately after insertion (indeed, it is used for emergency contraception (EC) up to 5 days after unprotected intercourse) and has a failure rate between 0.5% and 0.8% in the first year. Cumulative pregnancy rates at 7 years and 8–12 years are 1.4–1.6% and 2.2%, respectively (Hatcher et al., 2011). The copper device is associated with an increased amount and duration of bleeding during menses, which

can be up to a 55% increase, as well as increased dysmenorrhea during the first several menstrual cycles (Hatcher et al., 2011). These are the most common reasons for removal of the device in the first year. However, these symptoms are often relieved with the use of nonsteroidal anti-inflammatory drugs (NSAIDs), and the heavier menses rarely leads to anemia. The woman should be counseled regarding these potential side effects.

The *levonorgestrel IUD* is approved for 5 years of contraceptive use, although it may provide protection for up to 7 years (Sivin et al., 1991). Once placed, the device releases a small amount of levonorgestrel into the uterus, producing a thickening of cervical mucus that inhibits sperm motility and function. The steady local hormone effect also produces endometrial atrophy and tubal immobility that prevents transport of the ovum through the tube. Due to the steady systemic absorption of levonorgestrel, ovulation is often inhibited as well. These combined mechanisms effectively prevent fertilization. The levonorgestrel device is presumed to be effective approximately 7 days after placement and, unlike the copper device, cannot be used for EC. The failure rate in the first year of use is between 0.1% and 0.2%, while at 5 years of continuous use, the cumulative pregnancy rate is 0.5–1.1%. The failure rate does not appear to increase at 7 years of use (Hatcher et al., 2011). In contrast to the increased bleeding that can occur with the copper IUD, the levonorgestrel device is associated with a marked decrease in menstrual blood flow.

There are few absolute contraindications to the use of intrauterine contraceptives: active pelvic infection, cervical or endometrial cancer, current breast cancer for the levonorgestrel device, anomalies of the reproductive tract, gestational trophoblastic disease, pelvic tuberculosis, and copper allergy or Wilson's disease for the copper device. However, many clinicians mistakenly think that there are many more contraindications to the use of IUC (Nelson, 2007). Nulliparity, infection with human immunodeficiency virus (HIV), immunocompromise, and adolescent age are *not* contraindications to the use of IUC and are, arguably, populations that should have the most effective methods such as IUC offered to prevent unplanned pregnancy.

There are some preexisting medical conditions that warrant caution with the use of IUC (MEC category 3), but the more common cautions and complications involve the risks of infection, expulsion, and uterine perforation. All of these complications are uncommon but warrant attention particularly for postpartum women. The infection risk associated with IUC is low and primarily associated with insertion, and is likely due to undetected infection at the time. Thus, a woman who has had puerperal sepsis or endometritis after childbirth should not have the device inserted until the infection is completely resolved. Once inserted, the device does not have to be removed should an infection develop, unless the infection is unresponsive to therapy. For women who are at an increased risk of acquiring a sexually transmitted infection, the use of IUC is listed as MEC category 2/3.

Expulsion of the device is uncommon (2–10% within the first year) but can occur and is more common when inserted shortly after childbirth. Devices can be inserted within 10 minutes after the delivery of the placenta ("postplacental" insertion) and within a few days of childbirth, but expulsion rates are higher during these times than if inserted weeks or months after childbirth. In one study of 1933 women receiving postpartum copper IUDs, the expulsion rate in the postplacental insertion group was 9.3%, compared to >30% in the group with insertion at 1, 2, or 3 days postpartum (Chi, Potts, Wilkens, & Champion, 1989). Copper IUD insertion between 4 and 8 weeks postpartum was not associated with increased rate of expulsion, perforation, or other complications (Mishell & Roy, 1982). One study of postplacental insertion of the levonorgestrel device showed a 24% expulsion rate in the postplacental group, compared to 4.4% in the delayed insertion group (Chen et al., 2010). It is important to note that delay in placing the device, though having a reduced risk of expulsion, may impose an additional barrier to the woman having it placed at all. Women are at a higher risk of not receiving the device when asked to return for delayed placement. The social circumstances of a new mother must therefore be considered and the risks and benefits of early and delayed insertion must be discussed. The MEC classification for IUD insertion of both types of devices at 4 or more weeks after birth is category 1.

Perforation of the uterus is uncommon with IUD insertion, 1 per 1000 insertions or less (Hatcher et al., 2011). Concerns that perforations are increased in postpartum breastfeeding mothers are not supported by data, and the MEC categories for insertion of an IUD are the same regardless of whether the mother is breastfeeding (CDC, 2010).

There are no known adverse effects of IUC on maternal postpartum physiology, nor are there known adverse effects on breastfeeding performance in users of either the copper or the levonorgestrel devices. There is no evidence of increased copper concentration in breast milk in users of copper devices, and the transfer of progestin from the mother's milk to the infant is low in women who breastfeed and use a levonorgestrel contraceptive system; there have been no adverse affects reported (Hatcher et al., 2011).

An advantage of intrauterine contraceptive methods is that once placed, the methods require little attention: there are no frequent provider visits or prescription refills to manage, the method is not coitus dependent, and the user does not need to remember daily, weekly, or monthly ingestion, insertion, or reapplication. Fertility returns rapidly once the device is removed. The changes in menstrual bleeding associated with the different devices may vary in their acceptability to women. IUC has been used less by women in the United States than in other countries, but the use of this method in the United States is increasing.

The device itself and the cost of a provider visit for insertion may or may not be covered by third party insurance. Over time, an intrauterine contraceptive device can be one of the least expensive methods because of the potential length of contraceptive protection. However, the entire cost is paid at the initiation of the method and, thus, may be prohibitive.

Implant contraception involves the placement of a subdermal capsule on the inside upper area of the nondominant arm. Once placed, the device can be palpated but is usually not visible. Implants release a small quantity of progestin into the circulation over time. There is one such device available in the United States at the time of this chapter was written (brand name Nexplanon®, formerly known as Implanon®). It is a single flexible rod about 4 cm in length and 2 mm in diameter that releases etonogestrel at a steady rate and provides effective contraception for 3 years. It must be inserted and removed by a trained health-care provider. The method is effective immediately after insertion if inserted early in the menstrual cycle. The failure rate is less than 1 per 1000, and fertility returns rapidly after discontinuation.

The steady release of etonogestrel from the implant suppresses ovulation. In clinical trials, the earliest detected ovulation in women using the implant was after 2.5 years of use. As a consequence, menstrual cycle irregularities are the most commonly reported side effect during use, and irregular bleeding is a primary reason for discontinuing the method. There are no clinically significant metabolic changes noted in users of the device, and the most common reported side effects other than bleeding are mild and hormonally related. The device should not be placed in women experiencing unexplained and unevaluated abnormal uterine bleeding.

There are no studies that assess the effects of immediate postpartum insertion of the implant on maternal physiology. One randomized trial of immediate (within 72 hours) versus delayed (4–8 weeks postpartum) insertion showed little difference in time to lactogenesis II between the groups (Gurtcheff et al., 2011). Because the implant only contains progestin, it is a good choice for women who cannot use estrogen. The only absolute contraindication to implant use is current breast cancer. There are few MEC category 3 cautions for initiation of the method and include women with multiple cardiovascular risk factors and chronic medical conditions such as liver disease. Concomitant use of cytochome P450 enzyme inducing products (such as antiseizure drugs or certain herbal supplements) is a theoretical concern, but there are no research data to address the issue with this product. The MEC classifies concomitant use of certain enzyme inducing drugs as category 2.

As is true of all of the tier one contraceptive methods (Table 29.1), the implant requires little attention, an advantage in the stressful, even chaotic, postpartum adjustment period. The changes in menstrual bleeding may be more or less acceptable to some women. The device and the cost of a provider visit for insertion may or may not be covered by third party insurance. The implant can also be one of the least expensive contraceptive choices because of the potential length of time that contraceptive protection lasts. However, the entire cost is paid at the initiation of the method and thus may be prohibitive for some women. However, when the financial barriers to contraceptive choice are removed, women are more likely to choose a LARC method (Kossler et al., 2011).

Tier two methods

Methods in this category are very effective in preventing pregnancy but are more susceptible to user error in typical use. Typical use accounts for human error such as forgetting to take a daily pill, forgetting to replace a contraceptive patch or ring, or missing an appointment for a repeat injection. Once initiated, the methods in this tier may provide contraceptive protection for shorter periods of time than those in tier one because continued protection is dependent on user action.

Combined hormonal contraceptives (CHCs)

Combined hormonal methods are those that contain both an estrogen-like compound (ethinyl estradiol in most currently available products) and a progestin, of which several types are available in the United States. The dual action of the hormones interferes with the various physiological mechanisms that lead to ovulation and facilitate sperm transport. The contraceptive effect likely operates on several levels given that follicle development and even ovulation have been shown to occur in women taking oral contraceptives. The presence of estrogen in the formulation provides some additional contraceptive effect over that of progestin-only containing methods, and it also stabilizes the endometrium to provide a more regular bleeding pattern than is typically observed with progestin-only methods. In addition to preventing pregnancy, CHCs offer a number of noncontraceptive benefits including a reduced risk or reduced severity of endometrial and ovarian cancers, endometriosis, dysmenorrhea, mood swings, hirsutism, acne, benign breast disease, and iron-deficiency anemia (Hatcher et al., 2011). These additional benefits should be discussed during counseling for women interested in using CHCs.

CHCs are formulated as oral pills, transdermal patches, and vaginal rings. The *oral pills* require remembering to take a pill every day and starting the next month's supply on time. Typically, pill packs contain 21 days of hormonally active pills, followed by 7 days of hormone-free pills; during this 7-day interval, women usually have a light menstrual bleeding episode that is a result of hormone withdrawal. *Transdermal products* deliver hormones via an adhesive patch that is applied to the skin once a week for 3 weeks, followed by a 7-day hormone-free period. The *vaginal ring* releases hormones over a 21-day period; a woman inserts the ring in the vagina and leaves it there for 3 weeks. This is followed by a hormone-free interval of 7 days prior to inserting the next ring.

The longer the hormone-free interval (e.g., if a woman forgets to start the next pill pack, apply a patch, or insert a ring on time), the more likely she will have follicle development in the ovary and ovulate (Zapata, Steenland, Brahmi, Marchbanks, & Curtis, 2013). This observation, coupled with the low doses of hormones in contemporary products, has led to interest over recent years in lengthening the time a woman takes hormonally active pills, and shortening or even eliminating the hormone-free interval. Some newer oral contraceptive products offer different regimens including a 24-day active pill/4-day hormone-free dosing regimen, an 84-day active pill/7-day hormone-free regimen, a continuous dosing for the entire year regimen, and other products that provide a small dose of ethinyl estradiol during the typical hormone-free period or "placebo week." Although there are no such alternative regimens approved for the transdermal or intravaginal delivery systems, some health-care providers instruct women to use these in the same manner to avoid the hormone-free interval. However, such practices are not approved and are considered off-label use of the method.

The failure rate for these methods is estimated at about 9% in a year of typical use. Failure rates for extended regimens have not yet been evaluated in large groups of women.

The vast majority of women can use combined hormonal methods without problems. However, the estrogen content of these products creates more contraindications than is seen with IUD, implants, and progestin-only methods. Women with cardiovascular risk factors, coagulopathies, and certain other medical conditions may not be able to use hormonal methods that include estrogen. The reader is referred to the current CDC MEC for details about specific medical contraindications and reminded that the actual risk of most of these adverse events and contraindicated conditions in women of reproductive age is relatively low. Oral forms of CHCs should be prescribed with caution for women who may not absorb the drug from the gastrointestinal tract, such as in women who have had certain types of bariatric surgery. All combined hormonal forms should be used with caution in women who may metabolize the drugs more rapidly, as with concomitant use of cytochome P450 enzyme inducing products, such as antiseizure drugs or certain herbal supplements. Dual use of such drugs with hormonal contraceptives is classified as category 3 by the MEC.

There are special considerations for all women in the postpartum period. Due to the estrogenic effects of CHCs on the blood coagulation system and the observation that the pregnancy-associated increased risk of thrombosis does not recede completely until about 6 weeks postpartum, estrogen-containing methods are classified as MEC category 4 in the first 21 days after birth for all women (CDC, 2011), and as category 3 through 42 days if they have any elevated risk for thrombosis. After 42 days postpartum, there are no restrictions on CHCs based on postpartum status. CHCs may be started as early as 21 days after delivery if no other medical conditions are present and the mother is not breastfeeding (CDC, 2011). Women who have had gestational hypertension should demonstrate normal blood pressures before beginning CHCs.

Breastfeeding status raises some additional concerns about the use of estrogen-containing hormonal contraceptives. These methods have been associated with lowered quantity and duration of breastfeeding, although there is no evidence of adverse effects on infant growth and development (Kapp & Curtis, 2010). Thus, these methods are classified as category 2 after 42 days postpartum and throughout the duration of breastfeeding.

After assuring that the aforementioned criteria are met, CHCs can be initiated for postpartum women at any time. It is not necessary to wait for menses to begin to initiate any of these methods if there is a reasonable assurance that the woman is not pregnant.

All CHC methods require more user attention than the longer-acting methods in tier one or the contraceptive injection in this tier, which may be a problem for some women with young families during the adjustment period in the months after birth. These methods are less likely to produce irregular bleeding patterns or amenorrhea than progestin-only methods, which may make them more acceptable to some women, although some irregular spotting may occur in the first few cycles of use. The monthly costs of the contraceptive may or may not be covered by third party insurance; however, some federally funded agencies and chain pharmacies offer certain formulations at lower cost.

Progestin-only contraceptives

Progestin-only hormonal contraceptive methods are an alternative for women who cannot or should not use estrogen. Currently, progestin-only methods include the contraceptive implant and the levonorgestrel IUD discussed under tier one methods, and the contraceptive injection and contraceptive pills discussed here in tier two methods. There are some progestin-only contraceptive vaginal rings currently being evaluated, but these are not yet available for use.

The *contraceptive injection* available in the United States at the time this chapter was written is depot medroxyprogesterone acetate (DMPA, trade name Depo-Provera®). It comes in a 150-mg-per-injection formulation for intramuscular injection, or in a 104-mg-per-injection formulation for subcutaneous injection. Both types must be readministered approximately every 12 weeks (with a 10- to 14-week range) for contraceptive protection.

DMPA is a good choice for women who cannot use estrogen. Theoretically, it can be as effective as tier one methods, but in actual practice, the failure rate is estimated at about 6% due to failure to receive repeat injections on time. As is true of other progestin-only methods, there are few absolute contraindications. Breast cancer is always a contraindication for hormonal methods. The MEC category 3 is applied to certain medical conditions such as multiple cardiovascular risk factors and specific chronic medical conditions. Worsening of certain preexisting conditions such as migraine with aura is a reason to discontinue the method. Side effects include weight gain and menstrual cycle irregularities. Nearly all women who use this method experience some irregular and occasionally heavy menstrual bleeding, especially in the first cycles of use. Over time, many women become amenorrheic on this method (46% by 1 year of use according to one systematic review) (Hubacher, Lopez, Steiner, & Dorflinger, 2009).

Immediate injection of DMPA within the first hours or days after childbirth (rather than waiting until several weeks postpartum) has raised theoretical concerns about a negative impact on lactogenesis II. The Food and Drug Administration (FDA)-approved package insert for the drug states that DMPA should be initiated only within the first 5 days postpartum if the woman is not breastfeeding, and if she is exclusively breastfeeding, it should be initiated only at the sixth postpartum week. (http://labeling.pfizer.com/ShowLabeling.aspx?id=522). On the other hand, the U.S. MEC and family planning experts have endorsed the safety of DMPA in the immediate postpartum period as studies have shown no adverse effect on breastfeeding and there are no increased risks of thromboembolism given its lack of estrogen (Hatcher et al., 2011). In a prospective study of 102 women, early administration of DMPA (prior to hospital discharge) showed no differences in breastfeeding rates at 6 weeks compared to women using nonhormonal birth control or progestin-only pills (POPs). Breastfeeding rates were 70% or higher in all groups at 6 weeks postpartum and, of the breastfeeding mothers, two-thirds were supplementing with formula at 6 weeks (Halderman & Nelson, 2002).

Due to concerns about decreased estrogen in DMPA users and its potential adverse effects on bone, in 2004, the FDA placed a "black box" warning on the product to advise health-care providers to be cautious when prescribing this medication. Research and expert opinion, however, suggest that the changes in bone density may not have much lasting clinical impact. Indeed, some research suggests that the effects of this drug on bone mineral density are similar to the effects of breastfeeding; any loss of bone mineral density that occurs during use is rapidly reversed after cessation. Professional recommendations do not call for avoiding the use of the product. This method is classified as MEC category 1 or 2 for women of any age. Concomitant use of cytochome P450 enzyme inducing products (such as antiseizure drugs or certain herbal supplements) is not usually a concern with this contraceptive injection, but there has been no research to evaluate drug levels over time. The MEC classification is category 1.

Some research has suggested an increased risk of developing type II diabetes in Latina women with gestational diabetes who use DMPA (Nelson, Le, Musherraf, & Vanberckelaer, 2008). Others suggest that most of the risk can be explained by preexisting risk factors and increased weight gain during use but warrants observation (Xiang, Kawakubo, Kjos, & Buchanan, 2006). The evidence is unclear as to whether DMPA should be avoided in this population.

Use of DMPA as a contraceptive method requires little attention beyond periodic reinjections, which can be an advantage for women with young families. The changes in menstrual bleeding may be more or less acceptable to some women, and weight gain needs to be monitored in

users. The costs of the drug and provider visits for injection may or may not be covered by third party insurance. In a recent study on choice of methods of birth control, when financial and structural barriers to contraceptive use were eliminated, 35% of women selected a tier two method such as DMPA or hormonal contraceptives (Kossler et al., 2011).

Progestin-only pills, sometimes referred to as the "minipills," are oral pill formulations containing only a small dose of a progestin (about 75% lower than what is in a CHC pill). There is no hormone-free interval with POPs and an active pill must be taken every day at the same time of day. The daily dose of progestin may interfere with hormonal mechanisms that lead to ovulation, but low dosing does not reliably do so and the effect is variable. A recent study showed that 40% or more of women using norethindrone pills (the most commonly available POP in the United States) ovulate normally (Renner & Jensen, 2011). The contraceptive effect is primarily due to the effect of the progestin on cervical mucus thickening and, to a lesser extent, the development of an inactive endometrium and a decrease in tubal motility. The thickening of cervical mucus is the primary contraceptive mechanism for POPs and begins within 2–3 hours of taking the pill. This effect diminishes to baseline within 22–24 hours, allowing sperm to penetrate thereafter (Speroff & Darney, 2011). This underscores the importance of taking the pill as close as possible to the same time of day every day. Taking the pill even a few hours late may compromise its effectiveness, and in such cases, a back-up contraceptive method is recommended.

Irregular, unscheduled bleeding episodes are a common problem with any progestin-only method because of the absence of the estrogen-induced stabilization of the endometrial lining. Although the anovulatory effect is highly variable with POPs, irregular bleeding is a common side effect. The absence of estrogen in the formulation does not inhibit follicle growth, and women using these methods are more prone to develop functional ovarian cysts that usually regress and do not require any intervention.

There are few contraindications to initiating POPs. The primary considerations listed in the WHO's MEC are in women with breast cancer, certain liver tumors or cirrhosis, or malabsorptive bariatric surgery procedures. Women who are taking medications known to increase the metabolism of contraceptive steroids (antiseizure medications, some antiretroviral medications, rifampicin) should use this method with caution. Worsening of migraine with aura or diagnosis of any ischemic cardiovascular event would warrant caution if the method is continued.

In the postpartum period, there is no evidence that bleeding, postpartum involution, or lactogenesis is affected by the use of POPs. In fact, this method is frequently prescribed for breastfeeding mothers. Although small amounts of progestins do pass into breast milk resulting in detectable steroid levels in infant plasma, a recent systematic review found no evidence that maternal use of progestin-only methods of contraception adversely affect breastfeeding performance or infant growth, health, or development (Kapp et al., 2010). Although many health-care providers have women start POPs soon after delivery, data addressing the effects on lactogenesis are sparse. One study found no evidence that early initiation of POPs (within 3 days of delivery) has any adverse effect on lactation (Halderman & Nelson, 2002). Package labeling suggests starting POPs at 6 weeks postpartum for fully breastfeeding women and at 3 weeks postpartum for partially or nonbreastfeeding women; however, this is not considered best practice by family planning experts who stress that progestin-only contraceptive methods, including POPs, may be safely started immediately after birth (Hatcher et al., 2011).

The use of POPs as a contraceptive method requires more attention than tier one methods or contraceptive injections. There is less room for error than with combined hormonal methods due to the rapid disappearance of the cervical mucus effect if pills are not taken at the same time every day. The associated changes in menstrual bleeding may be more or less acceptable to some women. The monthly costs of the contraceptive may or may not be covered by third party payers. However, some federally funded agencies and chain pharmacies offer certain formulations at lower cost, although POPs are often not on the lowest cost formulary.

Lactational amenorrhea method (LAM)

Lactational amenorrhea may be one of the oldest contraceptive methods in existence. Prolonged periods of exclusive breastfeeding after birth have helped to extend the interpregnancy interval in societies across the world and across time. The neuroendocrine effects of frequent and vigorous suckling at the breast maintain prolactin levels above the nonpregnant state and gonadotropin levels remain low. As a result, lactation can suppress ovulation very effectively. The use of lactation as an effective contraception, however, is dependent on certain criteria being met. The woman must be less than 6 months postpartum, she must not have resumed menstruating, and she must be exclusively breastfeeding without or with very little supplementation, and nursing about every 4 hours, including at night. If all of these criteria are met, the LAM is estimated to be 98% effective as a contraceptive method (Kennedy, 2002). Once any of

these requirements are not met, the effectiveness of lactational amenorrhea decreases and the woman is at risk of unintended pregnancy and should begin another method of contraception. The LAM is not listed on tables that categorize and compare contraceptive methods by their 1-year effectiveness rates because the method is only intended to be used for 6 months or less. Nonetheless, LAM has the potential to be a very effective method for this short period of time.

Breastfeeding is more common in the United States now than it was several decades ago. It is important to keep in mind, however, that the requirement for "fully breastfeeding" that predicts the effectiveness of this method may be hard to achieve for many women, especially those who return to work shortly after giving birth. Some experts have posited that expressing or pumping milk is not an acceptable substitute for nursing the infant on the breast due to the lack of suckling stimulation, which is the source of the neuroendocrine effect on prolactin and other hormones that suppress ovulation (Zinaman, Hughes, Queenan, Labbok, & Albertson, 1992). One standard international resource for LAM states that, since manual expression does not elicit the same hormonal response as suckling, the effectiveness of LAM will decrease if expression or supplementation replaces suckling for more than approximately 10% of feedings. (FHI360, 1994).

Women interested in using this method should be counseled about the importance of beginning another contraceptive method as soon as breastfeeding frequency and intensity begin to decline, when supplements to breastfeeding (including formula) are added to the infant's diet, or when she resumes menstruating. As previously noted, while most fully breastfeeding women will not ovulate on average until 5–6 months postpartum, some will ovulate as early as 3 months after delivery. Women for whom a pregnancy would be problematic or medically contraindicated should consider using an additional contraceptive method.

Tier three methods

Methods in this category are effective in preventing pregnancy but are more susceptible to failure and user error than methods in the top two tiers. The methods in this tier are not hormonal and do not alter ovulation patterns, nor are they implanted, injected, ingested, or inserted into the uterus. There is no ongoing protection beyond the individual act of intercourse when they are applied.

Barrier methods

Barrier methods are physical or chemical and function by preventing sperm from entering the reproductive tract (vagina and/or cervix) and/or by inactivating sperm as it enters the vagina.

Male condoms are sheaths made of latex or other synthetic material that fit over the penis and catch the ejaculate after orgasm. They must be used with every act of intercourse and depend on the cooperation of the male partner. They can be purchased without a prescription and offer the added benefit of protection against some sexually transmitted infections. They are subject to breakage or spillage, which raises the risk of sperm entering the reproductive tract. With typical use, the failure rate is estimated at about 18%. EC should be discussed with all women/couples who choose this method. Concomitant use of spermicides (described later) may increase the efficacy of condoms.

Female condoms are polyurethane or nitrile sheaths intended to be placed in the vagina to catch the male ejaculate. They have a closed and sealed ring at one end, which is inserted into the vagina much like a diaphragm or contraceptive ring. An open ring at the other end of the sheath protrudes though the vaginal introitus; penile insertion through this opening ensures that the sheath protects the vaginal mucosa and cervix. Like the male condom, they must be used with every act of intercourse. They can be purchased without a prescription, offer the benefit of protection against some sexually transmitted infections, but are subject to breakage or spillage. With typical use, the failure rate is estimated at about 21%. EC should be discussed with all women/couples who choose this method as an added backup.

Vaginal diaphragms are dome-shaped devices of latex or silicone that are inserted into the vagina to cover the cervix and its surrounding area. The diaphragm is used with a spermicide, creating a chemical as well as physical barrier at the opening of the cervix. Standard diaphragms come in various sizes and must be fit by a clinician. Standard recommendations state that the device should be refit after postpartum involution is complete. A new diaphragm, developed to be a "one size fits all" option that could be purchased in a drugstore without a clinician visit, may soon be available (http://www.path.org/projects/silcs.php). A previous one-size option (Lea's Shield) is no longer on the market, although there may be women who still have the device.

With typical use, the diaphragm failure rate is estimated to be about 12%. Because the diaphragm must be used with a spermicide, it is important to follow standard instructions about how frequently more spermicide must be inserted and how long the device should remain in place after intercourse (recognizing that these instructions have not been derived from data or evidence, but reflect long-standing opinion). There are reports of an increased incidence of urinary tract and vaginal infections with diaphragm use, which may be related to the chemical spermicide.

Cervical caps are smaller dome-shaped devices that are intended to fit over the cervix to create a barrier. Only one cervical cap is currently available in the United States and it is made of silicone. Like the diaphragm, cervical caps are designed to be used with a spermicide. The device holds the spermicide against the cervix to create a chemical as well as physical barrier. Caps come in different sizes and must be fit by a clinician. Failure rates are higher than those of the diaphragm, with multiparous women having more failures than nulliparous women (29% and 14%, respectively) (Mauck, Callahan, Weiner, & Dominik, 1999). As is true of the diaphragm, it is important to follow standard instructions about spermicide use and the length of time the device should remain in place after intercourse. Vaginal infections or irritation may be increased with cap use and may be related to the chemical spermicide.

Contraceptive sponges are small polyurethane foam sponges that carry a spermicide. Only one sponge is currently available in the United States; it contains 1 g of the spermicide nonoxynol-9 (typical dosing in other spermicide products averages about 100 mg per dose). It should be moistened with water before insertion and is designed to protect against pregnancy for 24 hours. The sponge should be left in place for 6 hours after the last act of intercourse. The pregnancy rates associated with the sponge range from 12% to 24%, with the higher rates more common in parous women. Use of the contraceptive sponge is associated with increased vaginal irritation and infection, likely due to the spermicide dose.

Spermicides are chemical agents designed to inactivate or kill sperm by dissolving its cell membrane. All spermicides in the United States have the surfactant nonoxynol-9 as the active ingredient. The nonoxynol-9 is in a carrier such as vaginal film, suppository, foam, gel, or cream. The contraceptive action occurs within a few minutes to half an hour after insertion depending on the carrier. Therefore, the couple must allow the recommended time for tablets, film, or suppositories to melt and disperse before they are effective. The contraceptive effect of spermicides varies with the carrier used, lasting about 1 hour for tablets or suppositories to several hours for gels and foams (Speroff & Darney, 2011). These agents are commonly used with other products such as condoms, the sponge, or with a diaphragm or cervical cap that hold them close to the cervix. When used alone, it is important that the carrier be placed as close to the cervix as possible. Spermicides used alone have a typical use failure rate estimated at 29%.

These products are available without a prescription and are readily accessible to most women. It is important to note that the chemical activity of the spermicide is not specific to sperm, and studies have shown that frequent applications can adversely affect the cervical and vaginal epithelium. Frequent use is associated with increased vaginal irritation and infection in many women, allergy to the chemical or its base, and with increased susceptibility to HIV transmission in high-risk populations. As a result, spermicides are listed as category 3 or 4 in the MEC for any woman with HIV/AIDS or at high risk of acquiring the infection.

Some caveats apply for all of these physical and chemical barrier methods. Their lesser effectiveness makes them a less appropriate choice for women who want to or need to delay pregnancy. People with latex allergies should avoid latex products. Women with a history of toxic shock syndrome should avoid sponges, caps, and diaphragms. Spermicides should be avoided in women with HIV/AIDS or who are at high risk of acquiring the infection. The potential for allergy to or irritation/infection from the use of spermicides and barriers should be noted and women instructed to seek care if symptoms occur. A certain degree of manual dexterity is required for insertion and removal of barrier devices and spermicides, so women who have arthritis or who are severely obese may have difficulty using these products. On the other hand, these contraceptive methods are nonhormonal, inexpensive, and readily available without prescription. Some methods such as male and female condoms have the added benefit of offering protection against sexually transmitted infections. Women using any of these methods should be made aware of the EC option.

Other methods

Withdrawal (coitus interruptus) is a contraceptive method that has been used for centuries if not millennia (it is mentioned in the Bible). It involves withdrawal of the penis from the vagina before ejaculation to avoid depositing the sperm in the reproductive tract. It requires only the ability to recognize imminent ejaculation and act to remove the penis and ejaculate away from the woman's genitalia. Long-held beliefs that withdrawal is ineffective as a contraceptive due to the presence of sperm in pre-ejaculatory fluid may be unfounded; one small study found no evidence to support this (Speroff & Darney, 2011). The typical use failure rate is estimated at 18–22%, roughly equivalent to that of condoms.

Fertility awareness-based methods are based on identifying fertile days in a woman's cycle and avoiding sexual intercourse during that time. There are a number of different approaches, and detailed explanation of each is beyond the scope of this chapter. The Standard Days Method (SDM) counts from day 1 of the cycle, the first day of a menstrual period, and recommends avoidance of intercourse during the presumed fertile period from day 8 to day 19 of the cycle. This calculation is based on extensive data on women's cycles from the WHO. Successful use of the methods is dependent on the woman having a regular and predictable cycle of 26–32 days, which may not be true of postpartum and/or lactating women. There is a product (CycleBeads®) available to help women track their fertile days using the SDM. A calendar days method is similar but requires the woman to track her own cycles for several months to determine her own cycle frequency and probable fertile days. Other methods include monitoring of vaginal secretions to determine likely pre-ovulatory mucus (the TwoDay Method) and monitoring of basal body temperature, which rises around ovulation. The Billings and Creighton methods combine a number of signs and symptoms of fertility into method instructions. Urine testing kits are available that track the rise in hormones such as luteinizing hormone (LH) associated with imminent ovulation.

The typical use failure rates for fertility awareness methods range up to 24%, roughly equivalent to other tier three methods, although lower rates can be achieved by highly motivated couples. Postpartum women may not have regular cycles, especially if they are breastfeeding, which makes these methods difficult to use until ovulation and regular cycling are resumed.

Emergency contraception

EC is any contraceptive method used after sexual intercourse to prevent pregnancy. All women using any of the contraceptive methods that are prone to being forgotten or other user failure (tiers two and three) should be aware of this option, and access to it should be facilitated if needed. The oral form known as the "morning-after pill" is the most commonly used and can be taken at any time during the first 3 days after unprotected sex to prevent pregnancy. It works by inhibiting or delaying ovulation and it will not disrupt an implanted pregnancy; thus, it is not an abortifacient (ACOG, 2010). There are a number of oral products that provide a contraceptive dose of levonorgestrel (a progestin), taken in one or two doses as soon as possible after unprotected sex. These are available without a prescription but are "behind the counter" in pharmacies. A new product, ulipristal acetate (brand name ella®), is available by prescription only and studies have shown this medication to be more effective than levonorgestrel up to 5 days after unprotected intercourse (Glasier et al., 2010). One potential caveat when using these oral products in postpartum women who may still retain some of the weight gained in pregnancy is that the effectiveness of oral EC seems to wane as body mass index increases (Glasier et al., 2011).

There are no restrictions on the use of levonorgestrel in lactating women. One study of 12 women compared levonorgestrel concentrations in milk with those in plasma and found the milk levels were lower with a mean milk-to-plasma ratio of 0.28. The authors estimated the infant's exposure to levonorgestrel as 1.6 μg on the day of dosing and markedly lower (0.2–0.3 μg) on the next 2 days. They concluded that in order to limit infant exposure to maximum excretion in milk, mothers should discontinue nursing for at least 8 hours after taking the medication, but not more than 24 hours (Gainer et al., 2007). However, the U.S. MEC for contraceptive use does not place any restrictions on the use of EC during breastfeeding (CDC, 2010). No studies have examined the excretion of uliprical acetate in human milk, though animal studies have shown that it is detected in milk of lactating rats. Effects, if any, on an infant are unknown. There are no data on ulipristal acetate and lactation and, as a result, the current recommendations are to avoid its use during lactation.

The copper IUD can also be used as an emergency contraceptive up to 5 days after unprotected intercourse and offers the added advantage of continued effective contraception for years after placement. For women who wish to avoid pregnancy for long periods of time and who are using tier two or tier three methods, this should be offered as the first-line EC method.

Summary

Contraception is an important consideration when caring for the postpartum woman. By empowering a woman to plan her next pregnancy, she is also able to maximize her health, the health of her infant, and the health of future pregnancies. Having time to recover physically and emotionally from pregnancy and childbirth, and having the time to devote to a new baby and new family constellation, are critical components of healthy families. All clinicians providing care to postpartum women should be aware of this and ensure that each woman is afforded the opportunity to learn about and choose an effective and appropriate contraceptive method for her.

Clinicians providing contraceptive management should be aware that correct insertion of intrauterine and implant contraception requires training. Such trainings are available and access to an experienced family planning clinician for advice and mentoring will be helpful as a novice provider begins to develop skills in these areas. Initiation of hormonal methods for postpartum women requires prescriptive authority; clinicians

who do not have such regulatory authority will need to collaborate with a provider who has this authority. With each passing year, there is more evidence-based information available about immediate postpartum use of contraceptives, hormonal methods in particular, and some of the guidelines from professional experts may not reflect FDA labeling. Nonetheless, expert guidelines have been developed for contraceptive management that reflect not only the evidence available but also the opinions of experts in the field of family planning.

Finally, this chapter provides an overview of contraception. More comprehensive guidelines for contraceptive initiation and continuation have been adapted from WHO guidelines for U.S. practice and are available from the CDC (2010). Selected practice recommendations for contraceptive management are available from the WHO and are being adapted for U.S. practice by the CDC, and should be available by the time this book is published. A leading and well-known reference for managing contraception is the textbook *Contraceptive Technology* (Hatcher et al., 2011). Another valuable recourse is *A Quick Reference Guide to Contraception*, which is available from the Association of Reproductive Health Professionals (http://www.arhp.org).

Case studies

A 32-year-old woman is at the clinic for her 6 week postpartum visit. She reports no health problems since the birth of her baby and she continues to partially breastfeed the baby. She has two other health children ages 3 and 7. Her health history reveals no health problems. She tells the health-care provider that she is interested in using IUC. She asks if she can have a device inserted today since she has to return to work next week. She tells the nurse practitioner that she has already read the written information about the device and the nurse has already explained the procedures for insertion.

The nurse practitioner completes the physical and gynecologic exam, and determines that the uterus is well involuted and the vagina and cervix are normal with normal secretions. Since the nurse practitioner has received training in the insertion of intrauterine contraceptive devices and has already inserted several devices, she proceeds with the insertion. Had the nurse practitioner not been appropriately trained, arrangements would have been made to refer the woman to someone who was skilled on the placement of intracuterine devices and offered the woman an effective interim "bridge method" of contraception until she can have her device placed.

Resources for women and health-care providers

Association of Reproductive Health Professionals' site known as "Method Match": http://www.arhp.org/MethodMatch/

Centers for Disease Control and Prevention: http://www.cdc.gov/reproductivehealth/UnintendedPregnancy/Contraception.htm

Medical eligibility criteria for contraceptive use. From the Centers for Disease Control and Prevention: http://www.cdc.gov/reproductivehealth/unintendedpregnancy/USMEC.htm

Planned Parenthood offers information about all birth control methods at their site: http://www.plannedparenthood.org/health-topics/birth-control-4211.htm

The National Campaign to Prevent Teen and Unintended Pregnancy Web site known as "Bedsider": http://bedsider.org/

References

ACOG. (2010). ACOG Practice Bulletin No. 112: Emergency contraception. *Obstetrics and Gynecology, 115*(5), 1100–1109. doi:10.1097/AOG.0b013e3181deff2a

Borrero, S., Moore, C. G., Qin, L., Schwarz, E. B., Akers, A., Creinin, M. D., & Ibrahim, S. A. (2010). Unintended pregnancy influences racial disparity in tubal sterilization rates. *Journal of General Internal Medicine, 25*(2), 122–128. doi:10.1007/s11606-009-1197-0

Borrero, S. B., Reeves, M. F., Schwarz, E. B., Bost, J. E., Creinin, M. D., & Ibrahim, S. A. (2008). Race, insurance status, and desire for tubal sterilization reversal. *Fertility and Sterility, 90*(2), 272–277. doi:10.1016/j.fertnstert.2007.06.041

Centers for Disease Control and Prevention (CDC). (2007). Postpartum care visits—11 states and New York City, 2004. *MMWR. Morbidity and Mortality Weekly Report, 56*(50), 1312–1316.

Centers for Disease Control and Prevention (CDC). (2010). U S. medical eligibility criteria for contraceptive use, 2010. *MMWR. Recommendations and Reports: Morbidity and Mortality Weekly Report. Recommendations and Reports, 59*(RR-4), 1–86.

Centers for Disease Control and Prevention (CDC). (2011). Update to CDC's U.S. Medical Eligibility Criteria for Contraceptive Use, 2010: Revised recommendations for the use of contraceptive methods during the postpartum period. *MMWR. Morbidity and Mortality Weekly Report, 60*(26), 878–883.

Chen, B. A., Reeves, M. F., Hayes, J. L., Hohmann, H. L., Perriera, L. K., & Creinin, M. D. (2010). Postplacental or delayed insertion of the levonorgestrel intrauterine device after vaginal delivery: A randomized controlled trial. *Obstetrics and Gynecology, 116*(5), 1079–1087. doi:10.1097/AOG.0b013e3181f73fac

Chi, I. C., Potts, M., Wilkens, L. R., & Champion, C. B. (1989). Performance of the copper T-380A intrauterine device in breastfeeding women. *Contraception, 39*(6), 603–618.

Conde-Agudelo, A., Rosas-Bermudez, A., & Kafury-Goeta, A. C. (2006). Birth spacing and risk of adverse perinatal outcomes: A meta-analysis. *JAMA: The Journal of the American Medical Association, 295*(15), 1809–1823. doi:10.1001/jama.295.15.1809

Curtis, K. M., Mohllajee, A. P., & Peterson, H. B. (2006). Regret following female sterilization at a young age: A systematic review. *Contraception, 73*(2), 205–210. doi:10.1016/j.contraception.2005.08.006

Eisenberg, M. L., Henderson, J. T., Amory, J. K., Smith, J. F., & Walsh, T. J. (2009). Racial differences in vasectomy utilization in the United States: Data from the national survey of family growth. *Urology, 74*(5), 1020–1024. doi:10.1016/j.urology.2009.06.042

FHI360. (1994). Lactational Amenorrhea Methods. Contraceptive Technology and Reprodcutive Health Series. Retrieved from http://www.fhi360.org/sites/default/files/webpages/Modules/LAM/default.htm

Firoz, T., & Melnik, T. (2011). Postpartum evaluation and long term implications. *Best Practice and Research. Clinical Obstetrics and Gynaecology, 25*(4), 549–561. doi:10.1016/j.bpobgyn.2011.03.003

Gainer, E., Massai, R., Lillo, S., Reyes, V., Forcelledo, M. L., Caviedes, R., . . . Bouyer, J. (2007). Levonorgestrel pharmacokinetics in plasma and milk of lactating women who take 1.5 mg for emergency contraception. *Human Reproduction, 22*(6), 1578–1584.

Gartner, L. M., Morton, J., Lawrence, R. A., Naylor, A. J., O'Hare, D., Schanler, R. J., & Eidelman, A. I. (2005). Breastfeeding and the use of human milk. *Pediatrics, 115*(2), 496–506. doi:10.1542/peds.2004-2491

Glasier, A., Cameron, S. T., Blithe, D., Scherrer, B., Mathe, H., Levy, D., . . . Ulmann, A. (2011). Can we identify women at risk of pregnancy despite using emergency contraception? Data from randomized trials of ulipristal acetate and levonorgestrel. *Contraception, 84*(4), 363–367. doi:10.1016/j.contraception.2011.02.009

Glasier, A. F., Cameron, S. T., Fine, P. M., Logan, S. J., Casale, W., Van Horn, J., . . . Gainer, E. (2010). Ulipristal acetate versus levonorgestrel for emergency contraception: A randomised non-inferiority trial and meta-analysis. *Lancet, 375*(9714), 555–562. doi:10.1016/s0140-6736(10)60101-8

Gray, R. H., Campbell, O. M., Zacur, H. A., Labbok, M. H., & MacRae, S. L. (1987). Postpartum return of ovarian activity in nonbreastfeeding women monitored by urinary assays. *The Journal of Clinical Endocrinology and Metabolism, 64*(4), 645–650.

Griffin, T., Tooher, R., Nowakowski, K., Lloyd, M., & Maddern, G. (2005). How little is enough? The evidence for post-vasectomy testing. *The Journal of Urology, 174*(1), 29–36. doi:10.1097/01.ju.0000161595.82642.fc

Gurtcheff, S. E., Turok, D. K., Stoddard, G., Murphy, P. A., Gibson, M., & Jones, K. P. (2011). Lactogenesis after early postpartum use of the contraceptive implant: A randomized controlled trial. *Obstetrics and Gynecology, 117*(5), 1114–1121. doi:10.1097/AOG.0b013e3182165ee8

Halderman, L. D., & Nelson, A. L. (2002). Impact of early postpartum administration of progestin-only hormonal contraceptives compared with nonhormonal contraceptives on short-term breastfeeding patterns. *American Journal of Obstetrics and Gynecology, 186*(6), 1250–1256; discussion 1256–1258.

Hatcher, R. A., Trussel, J., Nelson, A. L., Cates, W., Kowal, D., & Policar, M. S. (2011). *Contraceptive technology* (20th ed.). New York: Ardent Media, Inc.

Heit, J. A., Kobbervig, C. E., James, A. H., Petterson, T. M., Bailey, K. R., & Melton, L. J., 3rd (2005). Trends in the incidence of venous thromboembolism during pregnancy or postpartum: A 30-year population-based study. *Annals of Internal Medicine, 143*(10), 697–706.

Hubacher, D., Lopez, L., Steiner, M. J., & Dorflinger, L. (2009). Menstrual pattern changes from levonorgestrel subdermal implants and DMPA: Systematic review and evidence-based comparisons. *Contraception, 80*(2), 113–118. doi:10.1016/j.contraception.2009.02.008

Jackson, E., & Glasier, A. (2011). Return of ovulation and menses in postpartum nonlactating women: A systematic review. *Obstetrics and Gynecology, 117*(3), 657–662. doi:10.1097/AOG.0b013e3182 0ce18c

Kapp, N., & Curtis, K. M. (2010). Combined oral contraceptive use among breastfeeding women: A systematic review. *Contraception, 82*(1), 10–16. doi:10.1016/j.contraception.2010.02.001

Kapp, N., Curtis, K., & Nanda, K. (2010). Progestogen-only contraceptive use among breastfeeding women: A systematic review. *Contraception, 82*(1), 17–37. doi:10.1016/j.contraception.2010.02 .002

Kennedy, K. I. (2002). Efficacy and effectiveness of LAM. *Advances in Experimental Medicine and Biology, 503*, 207–216.

Kennedy, K. I., Short, R. V., & Tully, M. R. (1997). Premature introduction of progestin-only contraceptive methods during lactation. *Contraception, 55*(6), 347–350.

Kjos, S. L., Peters, R. K., Xiang, A., Thomas, D., Schaefer, U., & Buchanan, T. A. (1998). Contraception and the risk of type 2 diabetes mellitus in Latina women with prior gestational diabetes mellitus. *JAMA: The Journal of the American Medical Association, 280*(6), 533–538.

Kossler, K., Kuroki, L. M., Allsworth, J. E., Secura, G. M., Roehl, K. A., & Peipert, J. F. (2011). Perceived racial, socioeconomic and gender discrimination and its impact on contraceptive choice. *Contraception, 84*(3), 273–279. doi:10.1016/j.contraception.2011.01.004

Li, W., & Qiu, Y. (2007). Relation of supplementary feeding to resumptions of menstruation and ovulation in lactating postpartum women. *Chinese Medical Journal, 120*(10), 868–870.

Mauck, C., Callahan, M., Weiner, D. H., & Dominik, R. (1999). A comparative study of the safety and efficacy of FemCap, a new vaginal barrier contraceptive, and the Ortho All-Flex diaphragm. The FemCap Investigators' Group. *Contraception, 60*(2), 71–80.

Michielsen, D., & Beerthuizen, R. (2010). State-of-the art of non-hormonal methods of contraception: VI. Male sterilisation. *The European Journal of Contraception and Reproductive Health Care, 15*(2), 136–149. doi:10.3109/13625181003682714

Mishell, D. R., Jr., & Roy, S. (1982). Copper intrauterine contraceptive device event rates following insertion 4 to 8 weeks postpartum. *American Journal of Obstetrics and Gynecology, 143*(1), 29–35.

Nelson, A. L. (2007). Contraindications to IUD and IUS use. *Contraception, 75*(6 Suppl.), S76–S81. doi:10.1016/j.contraception.2007 .01.004

Nelson, A. L., Le, M. H., Musherraf, Z., & Vanberckelaer, A. (2008). Intermediate-term glucose tolerance in women with a history of gestational diabetes: Natural history and potential associations with breastfeeding and contraception. *American Journal of Obstetrics and Gynecology, 198*(6), 699 e691–699 e697; discussion 699 e697–698. doi:10.1016/j.ajog.2008.03.029

Nilsson, S., Mellbin, T., Hofvander, Y., Sundelin, C., Valentin, J., & Nygren, K. G. (1986). Long-term follow-up of children breastfed by mothers using oral contraceptives. *Contraception, 34*(5), 443–457.

Renner, R. M., & Jensen, J. T. (2011). Progestin-only oral contraceptive pills. In D. Shoupe (Ed.), *Contraception.* West Sussex: Wiley -Blackwell.

Rowland, M., Foxcroft, L., Hopman, W. M., & Patel, R. (2005). Breastfeeding and sexuality immediately postpartum. *Canadian Family Physician, 51*, 1366–1367.

Sivin, I. (2007). Utility and drawbacks of continuous use of a copper T IUD for 20 years. *Contraception, 75*(6 Suppl.), S70–S75. doi:10.1016/j.contraception.2007.01.016

Sivin, I., Stern, J., Coutinho, E., Mattos, C. E., el Mahgoub, S., Diaz, S., . . . et al. (1991). Prolonged intrauterine contraception: A seven-year randomized study of the levonorgestrel 20 mcg/day (LNg 20) and the Copper T380 Ag IUDS. *Contraception, 44*(5), 473–480.

Smith, G. L., Taylor, G. P., & Smith, K. F. (1985). Comparative risks and costs of male and female sterilization. *American Journal of Public Health, 75*(4), 370–374.

Speroff, L., & Darney, P. (2011). *A clinical guide for contraceptiopn* (5th ed.). Philadelphia: Wolters Kluwer.

Stern, A. M. (2005). Sterilized in the name of public health: Race, immigration, and reproductive control in modern California. *American Journal of Public Health, 95*(7), 1128–1138. doi:10.2105/ ajph.2004.041608

Trussell, J. (2011). Contraceptive failure in the United States. *Contraception, 83*(5), 397–404. doi:10.1016/j.contraception.2011.01.021

Van der Wijden, C., Kleijnen, J., & Van den Berk, T. (2003). Lactational amenorrhea for family planning. *Cochrane Database of Systematic Reviews*, (4), CD001329. doi:10.1002/14651858.cd001329

Vernon, M. M., Young-Hyman, D., & Looney, S. W. (2010). Maternal stress, physical activity, and body mass index during new mothers' first year postpartum. *Women and Health, 50*(6), 544–562. doi :10.1080/03630242.2010.516692

Wang, I. Y., & Fraser, I. S. (1994). Reproductive function and contraception in the postpartum period. *Obstetrical and Gynecological Survey, 49*(1), 56–63.

Weir, S., Posner, H. E., Zhang, J., Willis, G., Baxter, J. D., & Clark, R. E. (2011). Predictors of prenatal and postpartum care adequacy in a Medicaid managed care population. *Women's Health Issues, 21*(4), 277–285. doi:10.1016/j.whi.2011.03.001

WHO. (2004). *Medical eligibility criteria for contraceptive use* (3rd ed.). Geneva: World Health Organization.

Xiang, A. H., Kawakubo, M., Kjos, S. L., & Buchanan, T. A. (2006). Long-acting injectable progestin contraception and risk of type 2 diabetes in Latino women with prior gestational diabetes mellitus. *Diabetes Care, 29*(3), 613–617.

Yee, L., & Simon, M. (2011). Urban minority women's perceptions of and preferences for postpartum contraceptive counseling. *Journal of Midwifery and Women's Health, 56*(1), 54–60. doi:10.1111/j .1542-2011.2010.00012.x

Zapata, L. B., Steenland, M. W., Brahmi, D., Marchbanks, P. A., & Curtis, K. M. (2013). Effect of missed combined hormonal contraceptives on contraceptive effectiveness: A systematic review. *Contraception, 87*, 685–700. doi:10.1016/j.contraception.2012.08.035

Zinaman, M. J., Hughes, V., Queenan, J. T., Labbok, M. H., & Albertson, B. (1992). Acute prolactin and oxytocin responses and milk yield to infant suckling and artificial methods of expression in lactating women. *Pediatrics, 89*(3), 437–440.

30

Lactation and breastfeeding

Marsha Walker

Relevant terms

Alveolus—the milk-secreting unit of the breast; a saclike structure lined by milk-secreting cells; contains a hollow center drained by a small milk duct; surrounded by muscle cells and a rich vascular supply

Colostrum—the milk that is present in the breasts from midpregnancy through the first days after birth

Lactiferous duct or ductule—duct or ductule that transports milk from the alveolus to the nipple; also known as a milk duct

Lactogenesis I—the onset of colostrum production during pregnancy

Lactogenesis II—the onset of copious milk production; usually occurs about 2–4 days after birth

Milk ejection reflex—occurs when the myoepithelial (muscle) cells surrounding the alveolus contract and push the milk into the lactiferous ducts; also known as the "let-down reflex"

Introduction

Lactation is an ancient process, most likely predating placental gestation. Lactation appears to have evolved in incremental steps as part of the innate immune system and acquired its nutritional function later in the evolutionary process. The mammary gland is thought to have first developed as a mucous skin gland that secreted antimicrobial substances to protect the surface of the egg and skin of the newborn. Over time, the mammary epithelium evolved to secrete fat, whey protein, sugar, and water resulting in the unique and complex fluid we call milk (Vorbach, Capecchi, & Penninger, 2006).

Lactation is a robust process that provides both nutrition and immunologic protection to infants and young children. Infants who are not breastfed have increased risk of acute and chronic diseases such as otitis media, lower respiratory tract infections, gastrointestinal infections, necrotizing enterocolitis, sudden infant death syndrome, obesity, types 1 and 2 diabetes, and childhood leukemia (Ip et al., 2007). The lactation process is also important to the mother's health. Women who do not breastfeed have an increased risk of premenopausal breast cancer, ovarian cancer, type II diabetes, hypertension, hyperlipidemia, obesity, and cardiovascular disease (Stuebe & Schwarz, 2010; Wiklund et al., 2011). These diseases are costly. If 90% of U.S. families could comply with the recommendation to breastfeed exclusively for 6 months, the United States would save $13 billion per year and prevent over 900 infant deaths annually (Bartick & Reinhold, 2010).

Central to successful breastfeeding is the support of knowledgeable and skilled health-care providers (U.S. Preventive Services Task Force, 2008). However, many health-care providers receive little training in the provision of evidence-based lactation care in their academic preparation or through continuing education programs. Shortcomings in breastfeeding management skills and knowledge have been identified in nurse practitioners and nurse-midwives (Hellings & Howe, 2000), pediatric nurse practitioners (Hellings & Howe, 2004), clinic and public health nurses (Szucs, Miracle, & Rosenman, 2009), hospital staff nurses (Nelson, 2007), neonatal intensive care nurses (Cricco-Lizza, 2009), pediatricians (Feldman-Winter, Schanler, O'Connor, & Lawrence, 2008), obstetricians (Power, Locke, Chapin, Klein, &

Prenatal and Postnatal Care: A Woman-Centered Approach, First Edition. Edited by Robin G. Jordan, Janet L. Engstrom, Julie A. Marfell, and Cindy L. Farley.

Schulkin, 2003), and family practitioners (Freed, Clark, Curtis, & Sorenson, 1995).

This chapter provides an overview of breastfeeding as a public health issue, the unique properties of human milk, the anatomy and physiology of lactation and breastfeeding, the role of the health-care provider in promoting and supporting breastfeeding, and the basics of breastfeeding support and assessment. The management of common breastfeeding problems is addressed in Chapter 31.

Breastfeeding as a public health issue

Breastfeeding and the provision of human milk provide the foundation of a person's health throughout the life course. Breastmilk programs the infant's immune system and contributes to optimal brain growth and development, while the act of feeding at the breast influences neurodevelopment of the infant. Lactation also provides metabolic and cancer-preventing advantages to the mother. Infant formula and bottle feeding are not equivalent to breastfeeding and lactation, and cannot deliver the same positive health outcomes to mothers and infants.

All major health organizations recommend breastfeeding. The American Academy of Pediatrics (AAP) recommends exclusive breastfeeding for 6 months, followed by the introduction of appropriate complementary foods and continued breastfeeding to 1 year and beyond (Gartner et al., 2005). This recommendation is considered to be the standard of care. It is the goal toward which efforts should be directed to assure the recommended outcome.

There are a few contraindications to breastfeeding and these include classic galactosemia (galactose 1-phosphate uridyltransferase deficiency), mothers who have active untreated tuberculosis disease, mothers who are human T-cell lymphotropic virus (HTLV) type I or II positive, mothers who are receiving diagnostic or therapeutic radioactive isotopes or have had exposure to radioactive materials (until it clears from the milk), mothers who are receiving antimetabolites or chemotherapeutic agents or a small number of other medications until they clear the milk, mothers who are using drugs of abuse, and mothers who have herpes simplex lesions on a breast (infant may feed from other breast if there are no lesions).

In the United States, mothers who are infected with human immunodeficiency virus (HIV) are advised not to breastfeed their infants. However, expressed milk from HIV-positive mothers can be made safe when it is pasteurized (Israel-Ballard et al., 2007). In developing areas of the world with populations at increased risk of other infectious diseases and nutritional deficiencies resulting in increased infant death rates, the mortality risks associated with artificial feeding may outweigh the possible risks of acquiring HIV infection (Gartner et al., 2005).

Increasing the rate of breastfeeding in the United States has been a public health priority for more than a century. The U.S. Department of Health and Human Services (HHS) has promulgated breastfeeding goals for the nation through the Healthy People initiative, which provides science-based, 10-year national objectives for improving the health of all Americans. The breastfeeding objectives for 2020 include improving the breastfeeding initiation and duration rates, raising the exclusive breastfeeding rates, increasing the number of employers who have worksite lactation support programs, reducing the proportion of newborns who receive formula supplementation in the hospital, and increasing the number of infants born in hospitals that provide optimal lactation care.

Breastfeeding initiation rates have increased from a nadir of 26.5% in 1970 to 76.9% in 2012 (Centers for Disease Control and Prevention (CDC), 2012). This increase has taken a concerted effort by federal and state health agencies, breastfeeding and professional health organizations, breastfeeding initiatives, health-care providers, and volunteer breastfeeding counselors.

Contributing to the progress in breastfeeding support over the last 25 years has been the increase in employers who provide time and space to express milk at work, the increase in state legislation mandating worksite support for breastfeeding employees and laws protecting the right to breastfeed in public, expansion in breastfeeding education and training opportunities for health-care providers, the availability of advanced lactation support and services from International Board Certified Lactation Consultants (IBCLCs), and increased research on breastfeeding and human lactation.

While steady progress has been made, there remain many challenges and gaps in care that prevent mothers from meeting their breastfeeding goals. Some public policies have a detrimental effect on breastfeeding. For example, the United States still has no national maternity leave policy resulting in some mothers returning to work within a few weeks of giving birth. A study that examined the impact of work requirements for mothers of young children resulting from the 1996 welfare reform estimated that the national breastfeeding rate 6 months after birth would have been 5.5% higher without the work requirement (Haider, Jacknowitz, & Schoeni, 2003).

The lack of knowledge regarding breastfeeding assessment and the lack of consistent assessment of breastfeeding during the hospital stay increase the risk for poor breastfeeding outcomes and early weaning. Hospital lactation care and services are critical to the successful initiation and continuation of breastfeeding, yet only 6.2% of U.S. infants are born in Baby-Friendly hospitals (CDC, 2012) The Baby-Friendly Hospital Initiative (BFHI) is a program started in 1991 by UNICEF and the World Health Organization (WHO) that recognizes hospitals with best practices in supporting breastfeeding. To be designated as Baby-Friendly, a hospital must implement the WHO/UNICEF Ten Steps to Successful Breastfeeding and comply with the *International Code of Marketing of Breast-milk Substitutes*, which requires hospitals to pay fair market value for infant formula and not promote items detrimental to breastfeeding, including discharge bags that contain formula (UNICEF, 2012).

The 10 steps to successful breastfeeding

1. Have a written breastfeeding policy that is routinely communicated to all health-care staff.
2. Train all health-care staff in skills necessary to implement this policy.
3. Inform all pregnant women about the benefits and management of breastfeeding.
4. Help mothers initiate breastfeeding within 1 hour of birth.
5. Show mothers how to breastfeed and how to maintain lactation, even if they should be separated from their infants.
6. Give newborn infants no food or drink other than breast milk, unless medically indicated.
7. Practice rooming in—allow mothers and infants to remain together 24 hours a day.
8. Encourage breastfeeding on demand.
9. Give no artificial teats or pacifiers to breastfeeding infants.
10. Foster the establishment of breastfeeding support groups and refer mothers to them on discharge from the hospital or clinic.

Source: UNICEF. (2012). The baby-friendly hospital initiative. Retrieved from http://www.unicef.org/nutrition/index_24806.html.

The unique properties of human milk

Human milk has evolved and adapted over the millennia into a living, dynamic fluid that both nurtures and protects the human infant. In contrast, the composition of infant formula does not change and cannot adjust to meet the changing needs of the infant. Formula lacks the enzymes, hormones, disease protective factors, and the myriad of other components that combine to program the immune system and promote the brain growth and development observed in human milk fed infants.

Nutritional properties of human milk

Colostrum is the first milk that is present in the breasts from 12 to 16 weeks of gestation onward. This milk is thicker than mature milk, and its yellowish color is due to the presence of beta-carotene. Colostrum has lower concentrations of fat than mature milk but higher concentrations of protein and minerals. This reverses as the infant matures. Colostrum changes composition and increases in volume over the first several days after birth as it transitions to the composition and volume of mature milk. Since newborns have very small stomachs and digestive systems, colostrum delivers its nutrients in a very concentrated low-volume form. It has a mild laxative effect, which aids in the passing of the infant's first stool, called meconium. Colostrum has a mean energy value of 18.76 kcal/oz, while mature milk is about 21 kcal/oz but can vary widely among women. The volume of colostrum ingested by newborns during the first 3 days of life ranges from 2 to 20 mL per feeding, with about 100 mL of colostrum actually available during the first 24 hours following birth.

Colostrum is higher in protein, sodium, chloride, potassium, carotenoids, and fat-soluble vitamins than mature milk, and lower in sugars, fat, and lactose. Colostrum contains abundant amounts of antioxidants, antibodies, and immunoglobulins, with especially high concentrations of secretory IgA (sIgA). Also present is interferon with its strong antiviral activity, fibronectin that makes certain phagocytes more aggressive, and pancreatic secretory trypsin inhibitor (PSTI) that protects and repairs the delicate intestines of the newborn, preparing this organ to process future foods.

Water makes up the majority of human milk (87.5%) with all of the other components either dissolved, dispersed, or in suspension. Infants consuming adequate amounts of breast milk do not require extra water, even in hot or arid climates (Ashraf, Jalil, Aperia, & Lindblad, 1993). Consuming extra water can depress the infant's appetite and reduces caloric intake, which raises the risk for hyperbilirubinemia, and if given in abundance over a short period of time, can contribute to oral water intoxication. In spite of evidence showing that healthy normal breastfed infants have no need of extra water (Scariati, Grummer-Strawn, & Fein, 1997), this practice persists on hospital maternity units, with 25% of birthing hospitals still engaging in this non-evidence-based practice (CDC, 2009).

Milk lipids or fats provide about 50% of the energy in human milk. The fat content of milk varies throughout a feeding or pumping session. The early milk or foremilk is more dilute, whereas the milk at the end of a feeding or pumping session has a higher fat content. There are several types of fats in breast milk, with triacylglycerols being the most abundant at 98–99% of the total fat. The rest of the fats consist of di- and monoacylglycerols, nonesterified fatty acids, phospholipids, cholesterol, and cholesterol esters. Eighty-five percent of the triacylglycerols are fatty acids of which there are over 200 different types.

Human milk fat contains mostly medium- and long-chain fatty acids, including long-chain polyunsaturated fatty acids (LCPUFAs). The amounts and types of fatty acids are highly dependent on the maternal diet and vary from woman to woman and across cultures. The LCPUFA (particularly docosahexaenoic acid [DHA]) present in human milk is thought to be especially important in the development and maturation of the retina and central nervous system, and is the most abundant omega-3 fatty acid in the brain and retina. DHA has gained much attention in infant feeding since docosahexaenoic acid single-cell oil (DHASCO) and arachidonic acid (AA) were added in 2001 to several brands of premium infant formula sold in North America. However, in spite of the formula industry's marketing claims about these formulas, no consistent beneficial effect on cognitive or visual function has been observed in either term or preterm infants (Schulzke, Patole, & Simmer, 2011; Simmer, Patole, & Rao, 2011). In a study of preterm infants, the beneficial effects of LCPUFAs in breastmilk on cognitive outcomes were blunted when infant formula was used in addition to breastmilk (Isaacs et al., 2011).

Cholesterol is an essential part of all membranes and is required for normal growth and functioning. Breast-fed infants' serum cholesterol levels are higher than those of formula-fed infants. This difference may have a long-term effect on the ability of the adult to metabolize cholesterol. Cholesterol is part of and necessary for the development of the myelin sheath that is involved in nerve conduction in the brain. Formula contains little to no cholesterol.

Human milk proteins have multiple functions that include enhancement of the immune system, defensive duties against pathogens, and stimulation of the growth and development of the gut. The protein content of human milk is approximately 9 g/L. Caseins constitute 10–50% of the total protein and give milk its characteristic white color. Alpha-lactalbumin and lactoferrin are the chief whey fractions. Alpha-lactalbumin has been shown to have antitumor activity (Hakansson, Zhivotovsky, Orrenius, Sabharwal, & Svanborg, 1995) and lactoferrin is thought to alter the properties of the bacterial cell membrane, making it more vulnerable to the killing effects of lysozyme. Immunoglobulins are part of the whey protein fraction, as are enzymes.

The principal carbohydrate in human milk is lactose (galactose + glucose), with others occurring in smaller amounts such as oligosaccharides, monosaccharides, and peptide-bound and protein-bound carbohydrates. Human milk lactose and galactose enhance the colonization of the infant's intestines with microflora that competes with and excludes pathogens, and ensures an adequate supply of galactocerebrosides for optimal brain development. Weaning a breastfed infant to a lactose-free formula removes brain growth nutrients and many layers of disease protection.

The breast cannot synthesize water-soluble vitamins. These are derived from the maternal diet and can vary in concentrations but do not require maternal supplementation in adequately nourished mothers. Vitamin B_{12} is necessary for the infant's developing nervous system and occurs exclusively in animal tissue. A vegan mother who does not consume meat or dairy products will need a supplementary source of vitamin B_{12} to assure adequate amounts of this vitamin in her milk.

Vitamin D comprises a group of fat-soluble compounds with antirachitic (rickets) activity. Vitamin D is not really a vitamin but a precursor of a steroid hormone formed when the skin is directly exposed to ultraviolet B radiation. Less than 10% is derived from food sources, although many people obtain much of their vitamin D from fortified foods and supplements. Human milk has been reported to be deficient in vitamin D, causing the AAP to recommend a supplement of 400 IU/day of vitamin D beginning within the first few days of life and continued throughout childhood (Wagner, Greer, & the Section on Breastfeeding and Committee on Nutrition, 2008). Rickets, poor bone mineralization, and vitamin D deficiency in breastfed infants are rare but do occur. These are associated with dark-skinned children on vegetarian diets, dark-skinned infants exclusively breastfed beyond 3–6 months of age, premature infants, and infants born to mothers who are deficient in vitamin D themselves (Misra, Pacaud, Petryk, Collett-Solberg, & Kappy, 2008).

Exclusive breastfeeding can result in normal infant bone mineral content, but this happens when there is adequate prenatal and postpartum maternal vitamin D status, normal neonatal stores, and regular exposure to small amounts of sunlight. Very high levels of maternal vitamin D supplementation can raise the level of vitamin D in the milk, but this is not a common practice. Currently, vitamin D supplementation of breastfed infants can be viewed as a mechanism to ensure that an adequate substrate for a hormone whose normal production has been adversely affected by the realities of modern living conditions (lack of exposure to sunlight of both mothers and infants, maternal vitamin D insufficiency, and cold climates), not as a treatment for nutritional inadequacy of human milk.

Defense agents in human milk

The defense agents in human milk are composed of an army of components whose interplay is both complex and synergistic. These agents are a compensatory mechanism for the immature immune system of the human newborn with their antimicrobial, anti-inflammatory, and immunoregulatory effects. The antimicrobial proteins in milk include lactoferrin, sIgA, lysozyme, alpha-lactalbumin, lactadherin, defensins, and others. These substances protect the infant from a number of bacteria and also provide some protection from viruses and fungi (Goldman, 2007).

Maternal and infant anatomy and physiology of lactation and breastfeeding

The breast does not become fully developed and functional until pregnancy and lactation. Breast development occurs in stages during fetal development. During puberty, the breast enlarges with about 11 alveolar buds forming clusters at each terminal duct to create a lobule.

The breast completes the majority of its growth and development during pregnancy under the influence the hormones progesterone, prolactin, human placental lactogen, growth hormone, and insulin-like growth factor. Although the breast is capable of secreting colostrum by 12–16 weeks of gestation (lactogenesis I), breast development continues during pregnancy and preterm birth prior to 28 weeks of gestation can interrupt breast development. Lactogenesis II (the onset of copious milk production) may be delayed in mothers of preterm infants and result in diminished amounts of milk during the early weeks following a preterm birth. However, many mothers of preterm infants are able to achieve an adequate milk supply when provided lactation support services and an appropriate breast pump.

The rapid decline in progesterone levels following the expulsion of the placenta, combined with the secretion of prolactin and other permissive hormones such as cortisol and insulin, triggers lactogenesis II. The onset of copious milk production is often described by mothers as the milk "coming in." The size of the breast is not related to its milk-making capacity, although mothers with larger breasts may have a greater milk storage capacity. Breasts that are significantly asymmetrical, tubular, or cone shaped may signal a higher risk for producing reduced amounts of milk, especially when there is more than a 1.5-in. distance between the breasts.

The breast (Fig. 30.1) is composed of glandular tissue surrounded by fatty tissue and supported by fibrous

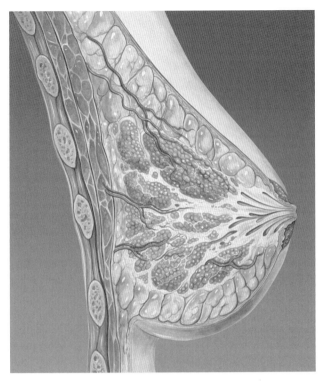

Figure 30.1. Side view of the breast. Illustration by Patrick J. Lynch, medical illustrator; C. Carl Jaffe, MD, cardiologist. Creative Commons. Retrieved from http://commons.wikimedia.org/wiki/File:Breast_anatomy_normal.jpg.

tissue and suspensory ligaments (Cooper's ligaments). Some breast tissue projects into the axilla, called the tail of Spence, and is connected to the breast's ductal system. Between 5 and 10 main ducts branch and extend from the nipple in a complex and intertwined pattern to lobules composed of branching ductules that end in alveolar clusters. The alveolus is the milk-secreting unit and is surrounded by a rich vascular supply and smooth muscle myoepithelial cells. The myoepithelial cells contract under the influence of oxytocin and push the milk down the ductwork to the nipple, an event known as the let down reflex or milk ejection reflex.

Modern ultrasound examinations of the breast have been unable to identify lactiferous sinuses beneath the areola (Ramsay, Kent, Hartmann, & Hartmann, 2005). However, widening of the ducts is commonly observed after the first branching point from the nipple and the ducts appear to widen further under the influence of the milk ejection reflex (Gooding, Finlay, Shipley, Halliwell, & Duck, 2010). Ultrasound imaging also shows localized ductal activity rather than ductal activity in every area of the breast suggesting that not all ductal systems are active during lactation and that the capacity of the breast may exceed the demand for a particular infant (Gooding et al., 2010).

The areola is a circular pigmented area on the center surface of the breast that often enlarges and darkens during pregnancy. It contains Montgomery's tubercles or glands that become prominent during pregnancy and secrete substances such as milk during lactation. The ducts of sebaceous glands often empty near or into the ducts of the Montgomery glands. The nipple sits in the center of the areola and contains 5–10 true lactiferous ducts, which transport milk from the lobules to the nipple tip. Most lactiferous ducts are arranged in a central bundle that narrows to a "waist" approximately 2 mm beneath the skin.

Nipples vary in size and shape. Some nipple variations have the potential for causing a difficult latch such as nipples that are flat, inverted, dimpled, bulbous, bifurcated, or extremely large or mulberry shaped. Prenatal nipple preparation techniques are no longer recommended since they have not been shown to improve nipple protractility or prevent sore nipples.

Sucking at the breast (or sometimes even thinking about the infant) results in the activation of the milk ejection reflex. Oxytocin is released from the posterior pituitary gland and stimulates contraction of the myoepithelial cells and transport of milk to the nipple. Multiple milk ejections typically occur during breastfeeding and milk expression, with the first milk ejection providing the largest amount of milk. Prolactin is secreted in the anterior pituitary gland and facilitates lobuloalveolar growth during pregnancy and promotes lactogenesis II after birth. Prolactin levels double with the sucking stimulus. Once lactation is well established, prolactin is still required for milk synthesis, but its role is permissive rather than regulatory.

Infants bring their own distinctive anatomical structures to the breastfeeding relationship and must coordinate sucking, swallowing, and breathing in order to successfully remove milk from the breast. Evaluation of the infant's oral structures related to breastfeeding is important when providing breastfeeding guidance or managing breastfeeding problems.

Ultrasound studies show that when the posterior part of the infant's tongue is lowered during sucking at the breast, milk ducts in the nipple open and milk flows into the infant's mouth. When the tongue is raised neither milk ducts in the nipple nor milk flow are observed as the milk is captured in the nipple, ready to flow into the infant's mouth when the jaw is lowered (Geddes, Kent, Mitoulas, & Hartmann, 2008). Infants suck in bursts followed by rests. The less mature the infant, the fewer sucks per burst and the longer the rest periods between sucking bursts. Milk intake is related to the number of milk ejections experienced by the mother, rather than by the total time an infant spends at the breast (Ramsay, Kent, Owens, & Hartmann, 2001).

Swallowing involves more than two dozen muscles and is initiated when the milk bolus accumulates between the soft palate and epiglottis. Swallowing should be assessed by both the health-care provider and the mother, especially during the early days of breastfeeding. Even though an infant's jaw may move up and down resembling breastfeeding, jaw movement itself is not a sign of milk transfer. Unless the infant is actually swallowing, he may be receiving little to no milk. Signs of swallowing include deep jaw excursions, audible swallowing sounds, visualization of the throat during a swallow, a small puff of air from the nose, and a "ca" sound from the throat. If a clinician is uncertain whether an infant is swallowing, a small stethoscope can be placed to the side of the larynx to listen for the pharyngeal swallow. In special situations, pre- and postfeed weights can be taken to validate ingestion of milk by the infant.

Promoting and supporting breastfeeding

Health-care providers have an important role in promoting, supporting, and protecting breastfeeding. All health-care providers should have basic core competencies in providing evidence-based breastfeeding care and services as described by the United States Breastfeeding Committee (2010).

There are a number of helpful and unhelpful practices that mothers have identified from their breastfeeding-related interactions with health-care providers. Interventions that mothers have found helpful include prenatal information regarding the realities of breastfeeding, practical help with positioning and latch-on, provision of effective interventions for early problems, and the receipt of evidence-based answers to questions such as how long and how often to breastfeed, when to switch breasts, and whether nipple shields and supplementing with bottles of formula will undermine breastfeeding (Graffy & Taylor, 2005). Remaining with the mother during early feedings, assuring correct latch, and documenting milk transfer offer the mother the type of assistance that is most valuable, making sure that these tasks are demonstrated but allowing the mother to actually perform the task herself (Gill, 2001).

Mothers have described many practices that are not helpful. These include inconsistent advice about breastfeeding techniques, quick intervention with a bottle when feeding difficulties are present, and lack of skilled assistance (McInnes & Chambers, 2008; Mozingo, Davis, Droppleman, & Merideth, 2000; Nelson, 2007). Other unhelpful practices include rough handling of the breast or infant, pushing the breast into the infant's mouth or pushing the baby to the breast), packaged advice that is not tailored to the individual situation, information delivered in a lecture format, and education that consists of literature left at the bedside with no personal explanation (Schmied, Beake, Sheehan, McCourt, & Dykes, 2011). Health-care provider neutrality regarding breastfeeding also negatively affects breastfeeding initiation and duration (DiGirolamo, Grummer-Strawn, & Fein, 2003).

After birth, mothers should have the opportunity to learn and develop the essential breastfeeding knowledge and skills needed to get breastfeeding off to a good start. An essential knowledge and skills checklist is provided in the following textbox.

Checklist of maternal knowledge and skills to be acquired prior to hospital or birth center discharge

- Recognizes infant feeding cues
- Positions the baby correctly at both breasts
- Assists the baby to latch correctly at both breasts
- Does not experience pain during infant sucking
- Can determine when the baby is swallowing milk
- Knows how often to feed the baby
- Knows how long to feed the baby
- Knows when it is time to feed the baby
- Knows how to stimulate feeding when the baby is sleepy
- Knows how many wet and soiled diapers the baby should have each day
- Knows how to determine if the baby is jaundiced
- Knows when to see the infant's health-care provider to check the baby's weight
- Knows when and who to call for help with breastfeeding

Hospital or birth center discharge instructions should be provided so that mothers have a clear plan for breastfeeding when they arrive home. Exemplary discharge instructions for breastfeeding mothers are provided in Figure 30.2.

Once discharged, mothers continue to need help with breastfeeding questions and guidance to prevent premature weaning for problems such as sore nipples, real or perceived insufficient milk, latch issues, and return to employment. Health-care providers can call the mother the day after discharge to check on breastfeeding progress. A sample telephone triage tool is shown in Figure 30.3. Mothers should receive information on how to assess if breastfeeding is going well and a list of community resources to call with questions or problems.

The basics of breastfeeding support and assessment

Proper positioning, latch, suck, and swallow are the foundation for successful breastfeeding. Mothers should be helped into a comfortable position, using pillows if necessary, so they can maintain comfort for the entire feeding. There are a number of effective breastfeeding positions, but mothers do not need to know all of the positions. Prior to hospital discharge, mothers should be able to demonstrate at least one position in which she is comfortable, position the infant by herself, assure proper latch and milk transfer to the infant, and not experience nipple pain.

Position

In the cradle position, the infant is held in the mother's arm, completely facing the mother and slightly angled so that the head is higher than the hips but the head, neck, and trunk are all in a straight alignment (Fig. 30.4). This position should place the infant's nose at the level of the nipple and the lower lip and chin slightly below the nipple. This is the most common breastfeeding position but may be a little awkward when mothers are first learning to breastfeed.

The cross-cradle position (Fig. 30.4) uses the same alignment as the cradle position, but the infant is held with the mother's opposite arm with her hand behind the infant's head. This position is often useful for early breastfeeding sessions and is also appropriate for feeding the late preterm infant, a premature infant, small infants, or any time better head control is needed.

In the football or clutch position, the infant is placed to the side of the mother on a pillow and turned slightly sideways or in a more upright sitting position (Fig. 30.4). Care should be taken not to place a heavy breast directly on top of the infant's chest. This is an easy position to learn and can be useful for small or preterm infants. It provides good control of the infant's head and excellent visualization of the nipple and areola.

The ventral or laid-back position places the infant in a prone position on the mother who is reclining at about a 30° angle. This position is frequently used for positioning sick or preterm infants, late preterm infants, infants with upper airway anomalies, tongue-tied infants, or infants having difficulty handling a fast flow of milk.

A restful way to feed an infant is with the mother lying on her side and the infant on his side completely facing the breast (Fig. 30.4). The infant's body can be supported by the mother's arm or a rolled towel or blanket. Mothers who have experienced a cesarean delivery may find this position helpful.

Building your milk supply:

- Feed early and often, at the earliest signs of hunger.
- 8–12 feedings per 24 hours is expected, although these feedings may not fllow a regular schedule.
- Avoid pacifiers or bottles, at least in the first 4 weeks.
- Frequent feeds, not formula: Only use formula if there's a medical reason.
- Sleep near your baby, even at home, Learn to nurse lying down.

Feed at the earliest signs of hunger:

- Hands to mouth, sucking movements.
- Soft cooing, sighing sounds, or stretching.
- Crying is a late sign of hunger: don't wait until then!

Watch the baby, not the clock.

- Alternate which breast you start with, or start with the breast that feels most full.
- Switch sides when swallowing slows or infant takes himself off.
- It's OK if baby doesn't take the second breast at every feed.
- Help baby open his mouth widely: If you're having trouble with latch, get help promptly.
- If the baby is sleepy: skin-to-skin contact can encourage feeding:
  - ▲ Remove baby's top and place him on your bare chest.

Look for signs of milk transfer:

- You can hear the baby swallowing or gulping.
- There are no clicking or smacking sounds.
- Baby no longer shows signs of hunger after a feed.
- Baby's body and hands are relaxed for a short time.
- You may feel milk let-down:
  - ▲ You may feel relaxed, drowsy,or thirsty, and you may have tingling in your breasts.
  - ▲ You may feel some contractions in your uterus, or your other breast may leak milk.
- You should feel strong tugging, but NOT persistent pain.
- Proper latch prevents pain:
  - ▲ "chin-to-breast, chest-to-chest" "flip lips for a sip:" baby's lips flare outward
  - ▲ wide open mouth: baby's mouth covers most of the areola (dark area of breast)—not just the nipple.
- Baby has adequate weight gain: follow up 2 days after you get home, and again at 2 weeks.

What goes in, must come out, Look for:

- At least 3 poops per day by day 4. Poops change from dark black to green/brown to loose yellow as your milk comes in.
- At least 6 heavy/wet diapers after day 4.
- Urine should be pale yellow as your milk comes in.

Over time:

- All babies have days when they nurse more frequently.
- Breast swelling normally lessens at about 7–10 days and it is NOT a sign of decreased milk supply.
- Your milk may look thin or bluish, but it contains plenty of nutrients.

If you choose to share a bed with your baby:

- Keep the bed away form walls on both sides so the baby won't get stuck.
- Avoid heavy blankets, comforters, or pillows.
- Avoid soft surfaces such as waterbeds, couches, and daybeds.
- Neither parent should be under the influence of alcohol, illegal drugs, or medications that would affect the ability to wake up.
- As with sleeping separately, put the baby to sleep on his back.
- Do not allow the baby to sleep alone on an adult bed.
- Do not allow anyone except the baby's parents to share a bed with the baby.
- Because the risk of Sudden Infant Death Syndrome is higher in children of smokers, parents who smoke should not bedshare, but may sleep with the baby nearby.

Tell your hospital what you think:

- Let your hospital know if you had a good or bad experience with breastfeeding. Suggest they become Baby-Friendly®. You'll be helping other moms!

If you have questions, persistent pain, or can't hear swallowing, ask for help right away!

Massachusetts Breastfeeding Coalition
254 Conant Road, Weston, MA 02493
www. massbreastfeeding.org
©2011 Massachusetts Breastfeeding Coalition
For informational purposes only. This handout does not replace medical advice.

Figure 30.2.   Sample hospital or birth center discharge instructions for breastfeeding mothers. Source: Massachusetts Breastfeeding Coalition. Used with permission. Retrieved from http://massbreastfeeding.org/pdf/Discharge_English_2011.pdf.

Telephone Triage Tool for Neonates

Name of the baby _____

Date of the call: _____ Date/Time of birth: _____ Age of the baby: _____

Nature of the problem _____

Mode of delivery? (c/section, vaginal, vacuum, etc)? _____

Was baby preterm, low birth weight, a multiple, or has other health issues? _____

AAP recommends ALL breastfed babies be seen 48 hours after discharge.

FIRST — Establish if the baby could be in <u>immediate danger</u> and needs to be seen **THAT DAY**, ideally **both** by a Lactation Consultant and the baby's provider.

	Key:	○ Concerning response (be seen today)	❏ OK (can wait 1-2 days)
● Does the baby have fever, vomiting, lethargy, breathing problems, or is refusing to feed?		○ Yes	❏ No
● Press the forehead skin – Is it yellow underneath?		○ Yes	❏ No
● How many times in 24 hours are you nursing?		○ Less than 8	❏ 8 to 12
● How many poopy diapers per 24 hours?		○ Less than 3 by day 3 or 4 by day 4	❏ More than this
● Are poops yellow by day 4?		○ No, poops still dark	❏ Yes, yellow
● How many wet/heavy diapers?		○ Less than 4 by day 4	❏ 4 or more by day 4
● Can you hear the baby swallowing?		○ No, or can't tell	❏ Yes, she hears swallowing
● Is there red staining in the diaper?		○ Yes and it's day 3 or later	❏ Yes before day 3 (normal), or no
● Can you tell if your milk is in?		○ No or can't tell by day 4	❏ Yes

If answers to any of these questions is concerning (left column checked), *she should be seen **that day** and advised to increase number of feedings to 10-12 per 24 hours and massage breast between sucking bursts. Let her know that if she's had a c-section, is obese, or is diabetic, her milk may be delayed coming in.*

Comments: _____

_____

SECOND —If above answers are *adequate*, mom can wait to see a **Lactation Consultant within 1-2 days** .

Learn if there are things mom can do RIGHT NOW until she's seen. *(Further advice in parentheses.)*

If mother complains of not having enough milk:

❐ What makes you concerned that baby isn't getting enough milk?
  ❐ "Baby feeds all the time." *(Ask what she means by this. Review that normal number of feeds is 8-12 per 24 hours)*
  ❐ "Baby is not satisfied after feedings; OR fussy when put down; OR I don't have enough milk." *(Baby may not have effective feeding skills yet. Compress breast to push milk toward nipple during pauses between sucking bursts. Nurse at least 10 times per 24 hours. Feed at the earliest signs of hunger. Encourage skin-to-skin contact- mom's bare chest against baby's bare chest.)*

❐ If you've had your baby's weight checked recently, did his provider say it was OK? *(If no, be seen).*

❐ Is your baby receiving only breast milk? *(Recommend that expressed milk be used before formula. Pump after feedings, tell mom that it's normal if not much milk comes out at this point.)*

❐ Are you on any medications? *(Narcotics, all hormonal contraceptives including mini-pill, sedating antihistamines may cause problems. Ask mom to check with her doctor about the safety of stopping these medications.)*

❐ Do you smoke, drink coffee, or alcohol, including beer? *(Advise stopping. Non-alcoholic beer is OK.)*

❐ Are you sleeping near your baby, in the same room? *(If not, recommend doing so.)*

❐ Are you using a pacifier? *(If so, advise stopping it.)*

If mother complains of painful feedings:

❐ Is breastfeeding very painful even after baby is latched on? Do you have cracked nipples? *(Advise wide open mouth and flip open both lips, position chest to chest, chin to breast. Spread milk on breast and let it dry. It's OK to try lanolin ointment or soothing gel-pads until she's seen.)*

❐ Are you using a pacifier? *(Stop the pacifier.)*

Comments: _____

_____

_____

Massachusetts Breastfeeding Coalition

www.massbfc.org | zipmilk.org

Figure 30.3. Sample telephone triage tool for clinicians. Source: Massachusetts Breastfeeding Coalition. Used with permission. Retrieved from http://massbreastfeeding.org/pdf/TelephoneTriageMBC.pdf.

Breastfeeding positions

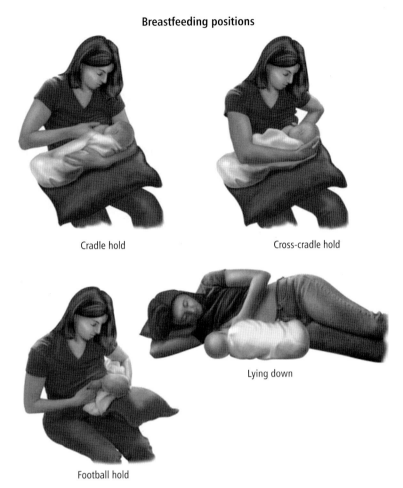

Cradle hold

Cross-cradle hold

Lying down

Football hold

Figure 30.4. Common breastfeeding positions. Retrieved from http://www.ihs.gov/healthed/docs/BF-BreastfeedingPositions%20 Provider.pdf.

Mothers have many options for positioning twins. Many mothers start out feeding one infant at a time so they can learn each infant's manner of feeding and then feed both simultaneously as a time-saving method. The football or clutch is a common position used by mothers of twins.

Many mothers find it helpful to support the breast during the breastfeeding learning period by using the "C" hold. The thumb is placed above the areola and the index finger below the areola, well away from the nipple. This technique allows the weight of the breast to be supported by the mother's hand rather than the infant's jaw.

The "U" hold or "dancer" hand position is the "C" hold rotated 90° such that the infant's chin rests on the space between the thumb and index finger while the palm of the hand supports the breast. This hand position is often used with preterm and late preterm infants, infants with a weak suck, or infants with muscular or neurological challenges that keep them from securely latching to the breast.

Latch

Once positioned correctly, the infant is brought to the breast without the mother leaning down or pushing the breast to the baby. The infant's nose should be at the level of the nipple and the chin contacting the breast as the mouth opens wide and grasps the nipple/areola (Fig. 30.5). Characteristics of a correct latch include the infant's mouth opened wide enough so that the angle at the corner of the mouth is about 160° (Fig. 30.6). The nipple and at least one-fourth to one-half of an inch of the areola should be drawn into the infant's mouth and remain in place during sucking; the infant should not pop on and off the breast during feeding. The nipple should not be flattened or distorted when the baby comes off the breast nor should it be blanched, creased, flattened, or demonstrate blisters, fissures, or cracks.

Swallowing should be either heard or seen and should be documented in the maternal or infant record. Both the upper and lower lips should be flared out, not rolled

Getting your baby to latch:

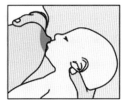

Tickle the baby's lips to encourage him or her to open wide.

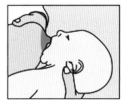

Pull your baby close so that the chin and lower jaw moves into your breast first.

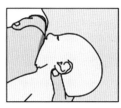

Watch the lower lip and aim it as far from the base of the nipple as possible, so the baby takes a large mouthful of breast.

Figure 30.5.   The correct approach to bringing the infant to the breast to latch. Source: U.S. Department of Health and Human Services. Office on Women's Health.

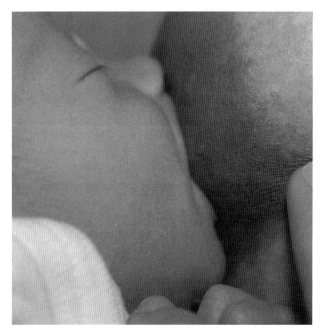

Figure 30.6.   Proper latch. ©B.Wilson-Clay/K.Hoover, from *The Breastfeeding Atlas,* used with permission.

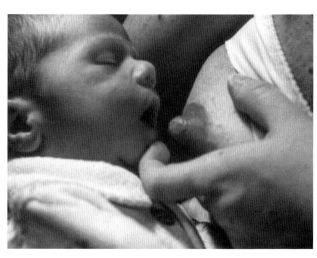

Figure 30.7.   Mother's index finger gently draws the mouth open for a better latch. Photo courtesy of Marsha Walker. Used with permission.

or tucked under. They should form a complete seal with no leakage of milk at the corners of the mouth. The cheeks should not be dimpled or drawn in during sucking, and the cheek line should be a smooth arc. There should be no smacking or clicking sounds during sucking. This indicates that the tongue is losing contact with the nipple/areola. To remedy this, the mother can place her index finger in the soft area under the infant's chin where the tongue attaches and gently push up to provide support.

Correcting the latch may require a position change of the mother and assuring that the infant is in close contact with the mother's body without an arm tucked in between his chest and the breast. The ventral position may be a reasonable choice. If the infant's mouth is not wide open enough or the infant cannot open wide, the mother can use her index finger to gently draw the mouth open as illustrated in Figure 30.7.

Mothers and those assisting her should avoid pushing on the back of the infant's head to achieve latch-on. This does not hasten or improve the latch and can cause the infant to extend the head, bite the nipple, or detach from the breast. A correct latch ensures uniform drainage of all the mammary lobes, avoids nipple discomfort or damage, does not occlude the superficial milk ducts, allows free flow of milk, and ensures maximum milk intake. Proper latch should be checked prior to discharge from the hospital or birth center, especially if the mother complains of sore or damaged nipples, if there is infant weight loss beyond 5–7% of the birth weight, or if the infant appears consistently unsettled following feedings.

Milk production

Lactogenesis II or what mothers describe as the milk coming in, is defined as the onset of copious milk production, which varies widely but is most commonly seen between 32 and 96 hours postpartum (median 66 hours). Delayed onset of lactogenesis refers to the maternal perception of lactogenesis occurring after 72 hours postpartum and the transfer of less than 9.2 g of milk per feeding (Chapman & Perez-Escamilla, 2000). The rapid drop in maternal progesterone levels following the expulsion of the placenta combines with the secretion of prolactin and other permissive hormones such as cortisol and insulin to trigger lactogenesis II.

During the first 3 days postpartum, milk synthesis will occur, even in the absence of a suckling infant or pumping milk. The composition of colostrum is similar in breastfeeding and nonbreastfeeding women over the first 3 days postpartum. However, when milk is not removed from the breast, the women's milk reverts to the composition of colostrum rather than continuing to change to its more mature composition and increase in volume. Thus, efficient milk removal is necessary for continued lactation (Kulski & Hartmann, 1981).

The prevalence of delayed onset of lactation has been reported to range from 33% (Dewey, Nommsen-Rivers, Heinig, & Cohen, 2003) to 44% (Nommsen-Rivers, Chantry, Peerson, Cohen, & Dewey, 2010). There are a number of factors that place mothers at an increased risk for a delayed onset of lactation, including being a first-time mother (the highest risk) (Scott, Binns, & Oddy, 2007), mothers who are overweight or obese (Hilson, Rasmussen, & Kjolhede, 2004), infants who lack effective breastfeeding in the first 24 hours (Nommsen-Rivers et al., 2010), mothers with a retained placenta (Anderson, 2001), preterm delivery (Henderson, Hartmann, Newnham, & Simmer, 2008), unscheduled or emergency cesarean delivery (Nommsen-Rivers et al., 2010), and mothers who are diabetic (Arthur, Smith, & Hartmann, 1989; Neubauer et al., 1993).

During delayed lactogenesis II, infants are at an increased risk for slow or no weight gain, weight loss, dehydration, and jaundice. Some of these factors are amenable to interventions such as assuring effective infant feeding; some are correctable, such as removal of retained placental fragments, but many are conditions that the clinician cannot prevent. These conditions leave the infant and mother in a situation of a prolonged colostral phase where more frequent feedings may be necessary as well as close follow-up after discharge from the hospital. A feeding plan may include 10–12 feedings each 24 hours, use of alternate massage (massaging and compressing the breast during each pause between sucking bursts, on each breast, at each feeding), hand expressing colostrum and spoon feeding it to the infant if breastfeeding is ineffective, and the possible use of donor breast milk, or hydrolyzed infant formula if medically necessary.

Milk production varies widely among mothers, with small volumes of colostrum available during the first 1–3 days (7–123 mL/day) until lactogenesis II occurs and the volume of milk increases rapidly (408 mL on day 3, 625 mL on day 4, 576 mL on day 7). Milk volume continues to increase (750 mL/day at 4 weeks to 800 mL/day at 6 months) until it levels off around 6 months. During the first 1–3 days, the volume of colostrum may seem small relative to the amount of formula an infant can be persuaded to consume from a bottle. This is in keeping with the needs and stores of a newborn infant. The newborn infant's stomach capacity is small and the stomach itself is somewhat noncompliant during the early hours following birth. Over the next 3 days, gastric tone decreases and the stomach becomes more compliant and able to handle larger amounts of milk. The average volume per feeding on day 1 ranges from 5 to 10 mL depending on the size of the infant and increases to approximately 10–20 mL on day 2, 38 mL on day 3, 58 mL on day 4, 65 mL on day 7, and 94 mL at 4 weeks. Clinicians should avoid unnecessary or routine supplementation with infant formula as human milk is rapidly digested and breastfed infants can show hunger signs sooner than 2 or 3 hours after a feeding, especially in the early days after birth.

Milk production is a continuous process and is influenced by a number of control mechanisms. The endocrine system is thought to set an individual woman's maximum potential for milk production, but local control mechanisms actually regulate the short-term synthesis of milk (Hartmann, Sherriff, & Mitoulas, 1998). The endocrine and local mechanisms that control milk production are summarized in Table 30.1.

Breastfeeding patterns

Breastfed infants usually nurse between 8 and 12 times each 24 hours (Gartner et al., 2005). However, this varies depending on the age of the infant, the gestational age of the infant, the condition of the infant, the birth experience, the culture into which the infant is born, and may even show a diurnal pattern. During the first 60 hours of life, breastfed infants may feed approximately seven times each 24 hours with intervals between feeds ranging from 2 to 5 hours. The frequency of feeds may be lower between three and nine in the morning and then gradually increase throughout the day with the highest frequency between nine in the evening and three in the morning (Benson, 2001).

Table 30.1 Factors Regulating Milk Production

Degree of fullness of the breast	Computerized breast measurements have shown that the emptier the breast, the higher the rate of milk synthesis (Daly, Kent, Huynh, Owens, & Hartmann, 1992). Each breast controls its own rate of milk synthesis so one breast may produce more milk than the other.
Infant's demand for milk	The maternal milk supply adjusts to the infant's appetite. Some infants may feed more frequently as their need rises or they may simply consume more milk per feeding.
Storage capacity of the breasts	The size of the breast does not determine the amount of milk that can be produced but larger breasts may be able to store more milk. Mothers whose breasts have a smaller storage capacity make similar amounts of milk in a 24-hour period, but their infant may feed more frequently than infants whose mothers have a larger milk storage capacity (Daly & Hartmann, 1995).
Feedback inhibitor of lactation (FIL)	This is an active milk protein that inhibits milk secretion as milk accumulates in the alveoli. The longer milk remains in the breast, the higher the concentration of FIL, which downregulates milk production.

In a study of feeding characteristics, mothers reported that during the first 2 months, the median frequency of breastmilk feedings was approximately eight feedings per 24 hours. The number of feedings in the early months ranged from 3 to 12 feedings per 24 hours. The rate of decline in frequency of breastmilk feedings per day was gradual throughout the year (Shealy, Scanlon, Labiner-Wolfe, Fein, & Grummer-Strawn, 2008). The average reported length of individual breastfeeding sessions decreased over time. In the first month, approximately half of the respondents estimated that feedings typically lasted less than 20 minutes. The prevalence of feedings of this duration increased throughout the year. Short feedings (<10 minutes) were rare in the first month (Shealy et al., 2008).

Infants may cluster or bunch their feedings toward the end of the day and during the early evening, where intervals between feedings are very short. This is normal and not an indication of insufficient milk or that formula supplementation is necessary. Mothers may ask clinicians questions such as how long should they feed on each side, when should they switch sides, or how do they know when the infant is done on the first side. Rather than using time limits, better indicators of when the infant is done or should switch sides are either when the infant comes off the breast by himself or when the infant will no longer suck and swallow when the breast is massaged and compressed. Infants may feed on one breast per feeding in the early days and do not always take both breasts at each feeding. After lactogenesis II and after the first few days, infants will usually take both sides at most feedings.

Assessing intake

There are a number of tools that have been developed to assess the feeding effectiveness of the breastfed infant (Braun & Palmer, 1986; Jensen, Wallace, & Kelsay, 1994; Matthews, 1988; Mulford, 1992; Nyqvist, Rubertsson, Ewald, & Sjoden, 1996; Shrago & Bocar, 1990; Thoyre, Shaker, & Pridham, 2005; Tsu-Hsin, Keh-Chung, Chung-Pei, Chia-Ting, & Ching-Lin, 2008). These tools vary in their purpose and usefulness, as some are designed to organize the assessment of the actual feeding, while others are more predictive of those infants who are in need of follow-up and referral (Walker, 2011b). Most of the feeding assessment tools are used to identify feeding problems in neonates, and a tool such as the LATCH tool (Jensen et al., 1994) provides a mechanism for clinicians to be consistent when evaluating feedings.

Measuring the actual intake of breast milk in a healthy full-term normal infant is not necessary. Sufficient milk intake is generally verified by diaper output and weight gain. Adequately breastfed infants typically lose about 5–7% of their birth weight during their hospital stay and/or by day 4 after birth (Martens & Romphf, 2007; Mulder, Johnson, & Baker, 2010).

Some adequately breastfed infants will lose more then 5–7% of their birth weight due to the normal diuresis of excess fluid from the maternal fluid load (Mulder et al., 2010) and stooling. The timing and amounts of maternal IV fluids during labor are correlated with neonatal output and newborn weight loss. Neonates appear to experience diuresis and correct their fluid status in the first 24 hours after birth (Noel-Weiss, Woodend, Peterson, Gibb, & Groll, 2011). Intrapartum fluid administration can cause fetal volume expansion and greater fluid loss after birth that is reflected in rapid weight loss after birth (Chantry, Nommsen-Rivers, Peerson, Cohen, & Dewey, 2011). This needs to be accounted for when evaluating feeding parameters and adequacy of intake.

Breastfed infants generally void a median of two times on days 1 and 2, three times on day 3, five times on day 4, six times on day 5, and seven times on days 6 and 7 (Nommsen-Rivers, Heinig, Cohen, & Dewey, 2008). The median number of stools are three on days 1–3, four on days 4 and 5, five on day 5, and six on days 6 and 7 (Nommsen-Rivers et al., 2008).

Breastfed infants who do not have three to five stools per day by 5–7 days of age, or stools not having transitioned to yellow by day 7 following birth should be seen and assessed for adequate weight gain and breastfeeding difficulties (Mulder et al., 2010; Shrago, Reifsnider, & Insel, 2006). Producing less than four stools on day 4 or the delay of lactogenesis II beyond 72 hours postpartum suggests difficulty in establishing breastfeeding. Mothers and infants in this situation should be seen by their health-care provider and an IBCLC. While wet diapers are an indication of hydration, stool output indicates sufficient caloric intake. Assessing that swallowing is taking place at the breast for the majority of the feeding is also an important observation in assessing that adequate breastfeeding is occurring.

After the initial weight loss during the early days following birth, most breastfed infants regain their birth weight by 2 weeks. From 2 to 6 weeks of age, the average breastfed female infant is expected to gain approximately 34 g/day and the male breastfed infant gains about 40 g/day, with a minimum gain of 20 g/day for both male and female infants. A general rule of thumb places weight gain of 4–7 oz (112–200 g) a week during the first month, an average of 1–2 lb (0.5–1 kg)/month for the first 6 months, and an average of 1 lb (0.5 kg)/month from 6 months to 1 year. Infants usually grow in length by about an inch a month (2.5 cm) during the first 6 months, and around 0.5 in./month from 6 months to 1 year.

In 2006, the WHO released new international growth charts for children aged 0–59 months, similar to the 2000 Centers for Disease Control and Prevention (CDC) growth charts. The WHO charts are growth standards describing the growth of healthy children in optimal conditions; the CDC charts are a growth reference describing how certain children grew in a particular place and time. However, in practice, clinicians use growth charts as standards rather than references. The CDC (2010) recommends that clinicians in the United States use the 2006 WHO international growth charts, rather than the CDC growth charts, for children aged <24 months.

The recommendation to use the 2006 WHO international growth charts for children aged <24 months is based on several considerations, including the recognition that breastfeeding is the recommended standard for infant feeding. In the WHO charts, the healthy breastfed infant is intended to be the standard against which all other infants are compared; 100% of the reference population of infants were breastfed for 12 months and were predominantly breastfed for at least 4 months. When using the WHO growth charts to screen for possible abnormal growth, use of the 2.3rd and 97.7th percentiles (or ±2 standard deviations) is recommended, rather than the 5th and 95th percentiles. Clinicians should be aware that fewer U.S. children will be identified as underweight using the WHO charts. Slower growth among breastfed infants during ages 3–18 months is normal, and gaining weight more rapidly than is indicated on the WHO charts may signal early signs of overweight (Grummer-Strawn, Reinold, & Krebs, 2010).

Care of the breastfeeding mother

Breasts and nipples do not need special care unless there are specific problems. There are no particular restrictions or interventions that are required for the lactating breast. Some mothers find that they are more comfortable wearing a well-fitted nursing bra whose cups can contain all of the breast tissue and do not bind or pinch. A well-fitted bra is also snug around the bottom band, which does not ride up and pinch or trap the breast tissue under the breast. The bra should not ride up in back and its straps should keep the breasts elevated without cutting into the shoulders. Some bras have extra wide straps or padded straps for larger sizes.

Nutrition for nursing mothers

Lactation is a normal physiological process for women. While lactation places an extra requirement on the body, women seemed designed to make this adaptation without needing major adjustments in diet or a switch to special diets (Butte, Wong, & Hopkinton, 2001). There are no general food restrictions as long as the mother is not allergic to certain foods and tolerates the food or beverage. There is no need to make breastfeeding seem difficult by providing lists of foods to avoid or strict dietary requirements. Women should not hesitate to breastfeed their babies if their diet is not good or ideal, since most key nutrients will be available in their breast milk.

Weight loss postpartum is more likely for women who breastfeed (Onyango et al., 2011) but depends on activity level, food choices, calories consumed, and individual metabolism. Expected weight loss is about 1 lb/week and mothers can consume as little as 1800 cal/day while still supporting a sufficient milk supply. Once lactation is established, overweight women may restrict their energy intake by 500 kcal/day to promote a weight loss of 0.5 kg/week without affecting the growth of their infants (Lovelady, 2011).

Moderate exercise during lactation does not affect the quantity or composition of breast milk or impact infant growth (Davies et al., 2003). Moderate exercise during lactation improves cardiovascular fitness without affecting the levels of IgA, lactoferrin, or lysozyme in breast milk (Lovelady, Hunter, & Geigerman, 2003). Moderate or even high-intensity exercise during lactation does not impede infant acceptance of breast milk consumed 1 hour postexercise (Wright, Quinn, & Carey, 2002).

Contraception

Breastfeeding mothers have a number of options for contraception (Academy of Breastfeeding Medicine Protocol Committee, 2006) including nonhormonal and hormonal methods. Nonhormonal methods of contraception include some intrauterine devices (IUD), male and female condoms, vaginal diaphragms, cervical caps, contraceptive sponges, spermicides, natural family planning methods, vasectomy, and tubal sterilization. The lactational amenorrhea method (LAM) method of contraception (Labbok, 2000; Labbok et al., 1994) has been shown to be a 98% effective method when the mother can answer "no" to three criteria: (1) Have you had a menstrual bleed? (2) Are you giving any supplemental foods or fluids in addition to breastfeeding? and (3) Is your infant older than 6 months of age? (Labbok, 2000; Labbok et al., 1994). An additional form of contraception should be initiated at any time that the answer to any of these questions becomes affirmative. LAM is not an option for women who are giving their infants regular supplemental feedings. The effectiveness of LAM is slightly less when employed mothers are pumping while away from their infants. IUDs such as the copper IUDs and the progestin IUDs seem to have little effect on breastfeeding.

Hormonal methods of contraception for breastfeeding mothers have raised concern regarding the passage of these drugs into breast milk and the potential effect on the infant. While some of these medications pass into breast milk, there appears to be minimal evidence that the exogenous hormones cause harm (Halderman & Nelson, 2002). The timing of the initiation of hormonal contraception has also been cause for concern (King, 2007), with the recommendation to delay such initiation until 6 weeks postpartum after lactation has been established. There is little data on the effect of hormonal contraceptives on maternal milk supply, although there have been anecdotal reports of decreased milk production in mothers who have been given the long-acting injectable contraceptive depo-medroxyprogesterone acetate (DMPA, Depo-Provera®) prior to 6 weeks after birth. Thus, it may be prudent to wait until the milk supply is fully established before starting any of the progestin-only options such as DMPA injections, progestin-only pills (Micronor® and Nor-QD®), and progestin-only implants (Implanon®). Hormonal contraceptives that contain both estrogen and a progestin such as combined oral contraceptive pills, contraceptive patches (Ortho Evra®), and vaginal rings (NuvaRing®) are best avoided until after the infant has weaned or after 6 months postpartum (Faculty of Family Planning and Reproductive Health Care Guidance, 2004). Hormonal methods of contraception should be avoided for mothers with decreased milk production, a history of milk supply problems, mothers of preterm infants, or in any situation where milk production could be compromised.

Smoking

In spite of messages to the contrary, many women of childbearing age continue to smoke. Nicotine is secreted into breast milk and can have a number of effects on the infant. For example, nicotine in breast milk can decrease heart rate variability in some infants in a dose-dependent manner, altering their autonomic cardiovascular control (Dahlstrom, Ebersjo, & Lundell, 2008). Nicotine can alter the taste of breast milk. Infants spend significantly less time sleeping during the hours immediately after their mothers smoke, with less time spent in active sleep as the nicotine dose increases (Mennella, Yourshaw, & Morgan, 2007). This particular side effect might serve as an incentive to help mothers abstain from smoking. Tobacco smoke exposure or secondhand smoke has been shown to have negative consequences on infant growth, episodes of otitis media, and upper and lower respiratory infections.

While smoking should always be discouraged, if mothers find it impossible to quit, breastfeeding should still be highly promoted to help protect the infant against a number diseases and conditions including sudden infant death syndrome. Nicotine replacement methods to achieve smoking cessation have been used, such as the nicotine patch. It has been shown that the absolute dose of nicotine and its metabolite cotinine decreases by about 70% from when mothers smoke cigarettes or use the 21-mg patch to when they were using the 7-mg patch. The lower-dose patch had no significant impact on milk intake and seems a safer option than continued smoking (Ilett et al., 2003).

Smoking also has the potential to decrease the maternal milk supply as prolactin levels are lower in breastfeeding mothers who smoke (Matheson & Rivrud, 1989). Breastfeeding mothers of preterm infants have also been shown to produce significantly lower amounts of milk at 2 weeks postpartum, 514 mL/day in nonsmokers compared with 406 mL/day in smoking mothers (Hopkinson, Schanler, & Garza, 1992). Smoking mothers should be encouraged to breastfeed more frequently to help offset potential milk supply problems, and infants of smoking mothers should be weighed more frequently to assure that adequate growth is taking place. Smoking is not a contraindication to breastfeeding, but increased vigilance is necessary to assure that infants receive as much breast milk as possible, that breastfeeding occurs frequently, that infants are weighed and checked for adequate growth, and that efforts are made to eliminate smoking from inside the house.

Alcohol and illicit drugs

While alcohol is often considered a recreational beverage, it is a drug that can affect both lactation and the breastfeeding infant (Bowen & Tumback, 2011). Alcohol easily passes into breast milk and its concentration in milk is equal to or greater than the concentration of alcohol in the mother's blood. There is no evidence that alcohol provides any health benefit for mothers or their nursing infants (Koren, 2002). Many cultural beliefs urge mothers to consume various alcoholic drinks as galactogogues or to enhance the milk ejection reflex and help infants relax. However, alcohol blocks the release of oxytocin, which delays the milk ejection reflex and reduces milk yield to the infant. Infants consume an average of 20% less breast milk in the 3–4 hours following their mother's intake of alcohol (Mennella & Garcia-Gomez, 2001).

Women should be encouraged to breastfeed, even if they plan to have an occasional alcoholic drink, as completely forbidding alcohol may serve as a deterrent to breastfeeding. Adverse effects from occasional and moderate drinking can be minimized if mothers are advised to limit the amount of alcohol consumed and to wait 2 hours after ingesting alcohol before breastfeeding the infant.

Illicit drug use and the abuse of legal substances remain a significant problem among women of childbearing age, and there is little research to guide clinicians regarding breastfeeding for these mothers. The Academy of Breastfeeding Medicine has a clinical protocol that outlines recommendations for drug-dependent women, specifying those who should be discouraged from breastfeeding, those who should be supported in their decision to breastfeed, and women whose situations require more careful evaluation (Jansson & The Academy of Breastfeeding Medicine Protocol Committee, 2009).

Medications and breastfeeding

Most medications are compatible with breastfeeding, but there are a few medications that are contraindicated or that should be used with caution. For example, discontinuing breastfeeding for hours or days may be necessary with some medications such as radioactive compounds. Breastfeeding should almost always be recommended, as the risk of not breastfeeding is usually higher than the risk from most medications. Reliance on medication package inserts is an inaccurate source of information regarding the use of drugs in breastfeeding women.

All medications transfer into breast milk to some degree, and for most drugs, the amount transferred is less than 1% of the maternal dose. Medications penetrate into milk more during the colostral phase of milk production and less after the milk matures. Herbal preparations and supplements are also biologically active and should be used with caution. The purity and dosage of many herbal preparations can vary widely. Preterm or unstable infants should be evaluated carefully in terms of their ability to handle even small amounts of medication. For mothers who have been taking medications during pregnancy, the dose of medication in breastfed infants is a fraction of that received by the fetus *in utero*. Both over-the-counter medications and prescribed medications should be evaluated for the absolute dose received by the infant so that abandonment of breastfeeding is not suggested due to anxiety or lack of knowledge on the part of the clinician (Hale, 2012).

Employed nursing mothers

Over half of mothers with infants under 1 year of age return to the workforce, many of them within 4–6 weeks of giving birth. Employment can have a profound effect on breastfeeding, since mothers returning to employment are three times more likely to stop breastfeeding than mothers who are not employed (Duberstein Lindberg, 1996). Many mothers forgo breastfeeding because they feel that breastfeeding and employment are incompatible and cannot imagine how they will be able to combine the two. Mothers identify many challenges to working and nursing that include issues of unpaid maternity leave, stress, cost of a breast pump, finding child care, unsupportive supervisors and coworkers, lack of a place and time to express milk at work, inflexible working hours, lack of sufficient break time, embarrassment, and irregular work hours with long or rotating shifts. Mothers with longer maternity leaves and those who anticipate working part-time are more likely to initiate breastfeeding and breastfeed longer than mothers who plan to return early to work and work full-time.

Until the 2010 Patient Protection and Affordable Care Act (ACA) was passed, breastfeeding employees had little in the way of worksite protection or accommodations for expressing milk. Under this law, employers are required to provide "reasonable break time for an employee to express breast milk for her nursing child for 1 year after the child's birth each time such employee has need to express the milk." Employers are also required to provide "a place, other than a bathroom, that is shielded from view and free from intrusion from coworkers and the public, which may be used by an employee to express breast milk." This law applies only to nonexempt employees (hourly workers who receive payment for overtime work). The requirement for break time for nursing mothers to express breast milk does not preempt state laws that provide greater protections to employees. Twenty-four states currently have laws related to breastfeeding in the workplace (National Conference of State Legislatures, 2011).

Clinicians can provide practical information and resources to help mothers continue breastfeeding after their return to work by assuring that breastfeeding gets off to a good start before the mother returns to work. Planning ahead helps reduce many of the challenges to breastfeeding. Clinicians can help mothers assess the type and extent of breastfeeding support they will need for their particular situation. Mothers should inform their employer that they will be expressing milk when they return to work and should be aware of any worksite protection laws that apply to them. A place to pump milk should be arranged for as well as breaks of sufficient length to accommodate pumping. Childcare arrangements should be made before the infant is born. Some employers allow mothers to bring young infants to work or have onsite childcare. Mothers should obtain a hospital grade electric breast pump with the feature of being able to pump milk from both breasts simultaneously.

Breastfeeding management for mothers with a 2-, 4-, or 6-week maternity leave (or leave from school) may be somewhat different than for mothers with a longer maternity leave. Dwindling milk production and/or insufficient milk supply are often pressing problems if a mother starts back to work soon after giving birth. An approach to avoid insufficient milk is to use the model of initiating and maintaining abundant milk production in the preterm mother. This model promotes a high milk production by 10–14 days postpartum, such that the mother is producing 50% more milk than what the infant actually needs (Hill, Aldag, & Chatterton, 1999). This strategy builds up milk production quickly and serves as a reserve to compensate for any milk volume decrease when the mother starts back to work or school. This excess milk is frozen for use on the first day back to work or school and anytime the mother experiences a fluctuation in the amount of milk she pumps while separated from the infant.

To produce more milk than the baby requires, mothers will need to hand express and/or pump milk several times each day in addition to nursing the baby. Combining hand expression with electric breast pumping during the first days after birth also increases milk production in mothers of preterm infants (Morton et al., 2009).

Additionally, massaging each breast while using an electric breast pump significantly increases the amount of milk pumped at each session (Morton et al., 2007). Time-saving ideas for pumping at work are provided in the textbox below.

Time-saving ideas for pumping at work

- Use of a hands-free bra allows mothers to continue working while pumping if the mother has an office job and a dedicated pumping space.
- Have two or three pump collection kits for use at work; these can be brought home for cleaning instead of having to wash pump collection parts after each use at work.
- Mothers who have access to refrigeration can place the pump collection parts in a sealed, clean plastic bag in a refrigerator between uses and then clean them at home.
- Use sanitizing wipes to quickly clean pump parts if the mother does not have access to running water.
- Pump directly into the bottles that will be used the next day. This eliminates having to transfer milk into other containers.
- Keep nursing pads at work to avoid stains on clothing, especially if the mother is in long meetings or has a long duty assignment that takes her past the regular time she would be pumping. Some mothers keep a change of clothing in their bag, just in case.
- Listen to the baby's sounds while pumping. The sounds can be recorded and played back during pumping. Mothers can also make a slide show with photos and sounds of their baby recorded on an iPhone, iPod, mp3 player, smartphone, or other electronic devices used with earbuds (Roche-Paull, 2010). This provides a relaxed atmosphere and a mechanism to condition the let-down reflex.

Source: Walker (2011a).

Summary

Breastfeeding is widely recognized as the optimal way to nourish the newborn. The health benefits of breast milk are related to its unique nutritional composition, which is ideally suited to the needs of the human infant. Moreover, breast milk contains a number of other components including immunoprotectants, anti-inflammatory agents, and growth factors. Breastfed infants have improved health outcomes and improved cognitive function compared to formula-fed infants. The close physical contact between mother and baby during breastfeeding contributes to maternal–infant attachment and influences infant neurodevelopment. Women also derive long-lasting health benefits from breastfeed-

Case study

LaShanna is a 26-year-old woman who is currently 5 weeks pregnant. At the conclusion of her first prenatal visit, she asks about whether she should consider breastfeeding her baby. She tells the nurse practitioner that she has heard that breastfeeding is healthier for her baby than infant formula, but she has also heard that breastfeeding can be difficult and painful. LaShanna also asks if she should do anything to prepare her breasts for breastfeeding.

The nurse practitioner reviews LaShanna's record and determines that she has no contraindications to breastfeeding and that her breast exam revealed normal, well-developed breasts. The nurse practitioner explains to LaShanna that compared to infant formula, breastfeeding provides superior nutrition and an extensive array of immunoprotectants and anti-inflammatory agents that are associated with improved short- and long-term health outcomes for infants. The improved health outcomes include a reduced incidence of respiratory and gastrointestinal infections, diabetes, allergies, leukemia, and sudden infant death syndrome. The

nurse practitioner also explains that women who breastfeed have improved health outcomes including a reduced risk of ovarian and breast cancers as well as a decreased risk of cardiovascular disease and diabetes.

When addressing LaShanna's concerns about the challenges of breastfeeding, the nurse practitioner explains that breastfeeding should not be painful. She further explains that although breastfeeding is a natural process, women have to learn about breastfeeding and recommends that LaShanna take a breastfeeding class near the end of pregnancy. She also recommends that LaShanna begin reading information about breastfeeding from trusted Web sites such as the Office of Women's Health and the CDC. LaShanna is provided with a list of quality resources about breastfeeding and encouraged to start her reading with "Your Guide to Breastfeeding" from the Office of Women's Health. LaShanna is congratulated on her decision to breastfeed and is reassured that she does not have to do anything special to prepare for breastfeeding.

ing including protection from breast and ovarian cancers as well as a reduced risk of cardiovascular disease and diabetes. Health-care professionals have a responsibility to promote breastfeeding and to develop the knowledge and skills needed to help women initiate and maintain breastfeeding, and cope with common breastfeeding problems.

Resources for women and health-care providers

Academy of Breastfeeding Medicine: http://www.bfmed.org

American Academy of Pediatrics: http://www2.aap.org/breastfeeding/

Baby-Friendly USA: http://www.babyfriendlyusa.org

Centers for Disease Control and Prevention: http://www.cdc.gov/breastfeeding/

Human Milk Banking Association of North America: http://www.hmbana.org/

International Lactation Consultant Association: http://www.ilca.org/i4a/pages/index.cfm?pageid=1

La Leche League International: http://www.llli.org/

United States Breastfeeding Committee: http://www.usbreastfeeding.org

Women, Infants, and Children (WIC) Program U.S. Department of Agriculture, Food and Nutrition Service: http://www.fns.usda.gov/wic/Breastfeeding/mainpage.HTM

Office of Women's Health, U.S. Department of Health and Human Services: http://www.womenshealth.gov/breastfeeding/

United States Lactation Consultant Association: http://www.uslca.org

References

Academy of Breastfeeding Medicine Protocol Committee. (2006). ABM protocol #13: Contraception during breastfeeding. *Breastfeeding Medicine, 1*, 43–51.

Anderson, A. M. (2001). Disruption of lactogenesis by retained placental fragments. *Journal of Human Lactation, 17*, 142–144.

Arthur, P. G., Smith, M., & Hartmann, P. E. (1989). Milk lactose, citrate, and glucose as markers of lactogenesis in normal and diabetic women. *Journal of Pediatric Gastroenterology and Nutrition, 9*, 488–496.

Ashraf, R. N., Jalil, F., Aperia, A., & Lindblad, B. S. (1993). Additional water is not needed for healthy breastfed babies in a hot climate. *Acta Paediatrica Scandinavica, 82*, 1007–1011.

Bartick, M., & Reinhold, A. (2010). The burden of suboptimal breastfeeding in the United States: A pediatric cost analysis. *Pediatrics, 125*, e1048–e1056.

Benson, S. (2001). What is normal? A study of normal breastfeeding dyads during the first sixty hours of life. *Breastfeeding Review, 9*, 27–32.

Bowen, A., & Tumback, L. (2011). Alcohol and breastfeeding: Dispelling the myths and promoting the evidence. *Nursing for Women's Health, 14*, 454–461.

Braun, M. A., & Palmer, M. M. (1986). A pilot study of oral-motor dysfunction in "at-risk" infants. *Physical & Occupational Therapy in Pediatrics, 5*, 13–25.

Butte, N. F., Wong, W. W., & Hopkinton, J. M. (2001). Energy requirements of lactating women derived from doubly labeled water and milk energy output. *The Journal of Nutrition*, *131*, 53–58.

Centers for Disease Control and Prevention (CDC). (2009). CDC National survey of maternity practices in infant nutrition and care (mPINC)—2009. Retrieved from http://www.cdc.gov/breastfeeding/data/mpinc/data/2009/tables2_1a-2_4a.htm

Centers for Disease Control and Prevention (CDC). (2010). Growth charts. Retrieved from http://www.cdc.gov/growthcharts/

Centers for Disease Control and Prevention (CDC). (2012). Breastfeeding report card, 2012: Process indicators. Retrieved from http://www.cdc.gov/breastfeeding/data/reportcard3.htm

Chantry, C. J., Nommsen-Rivers, L. A., Peerson, J. M., Cohen, R. J., & Dewey, K. G. (2011). Excess weight loss in first-born breastfed newborns relates to maternal intrapartum fluid balance. *Pediatrics*, *127*, e171–e179.

Chapman, D. J., & Perez-Escamilla, R. (2000). Lactogenesis stage II: Hormonal regulation, determinants, and public health consequences. *Recent Research in Developmental Nutrition*, *3*, 43–63.

Cricco-Lizza, R. (2009). Formative infant feeding experiences and education of NICU nurses. *MCN. The American Journal of Maternal Child Nursing*, *34*, 236–242.

Dahlstrom, A., Ebersjo, C., & Lundell, B. (2008). Nicotine in breast milk influences heart rate variability in the infant. *Acta Paediatrica*, *97*, 1075–1079.

Daly, S. E. J., & Hartmann, P. E. (1995). Infant demand and milk supply. Part 2: The short-term control of milk synthesis in lactating women. *Journal of Human Lactation*, *11*, 27–37.

Daly, S. E. J., Kent, J. C., Huynh, D. Q., Owens, R. A., & Hartmann, P. E. (1992). The determination of short-term breast volume changes and the rate of synthesis of human milk using computerized breast measurement. *Experimental Physiology*, *77*, 79–87.

Davies, G. A., Wolfe, L. A., Mottola, M. F., MacKinnon, C., Arsenault, M.Y., Bartellas, E., . . . Trudeau, F.; SOGC Clinical Practice Obstetrics Committee, Canadian Society for Exercise Physiology Board of Directors. (2003). Exercise in pregnancy and the postpartum period. *Journal of Obstetrics and Gynaecology Canada*, *25*, 516–529.

Dewey, K. G., Nommsen-Rivers, L. A., Heinig, M. J., & Cohen, R. J. (2003). Risk factors for suboptimal infant breastfeeding behavior, delayed onset of lactation, and excess neonatal weight loss. *Pediatrics*, *112*, 607–619.

DiGirolamo, A. M., Grummer-Strawn, L. M., & Fein, S. B. (2003). Do perceived attitudes of physicians and hospital staff affect breastfeeding decisions? *Birth (Berkeley, Calif.)*, *30*, 94–100.

Duberstein Lindberg, L. (1996). Women's decisions about breastfeeding and maternal employment. *Journal of Marriage and the Family*, *58*, 239–251.

Faculty of Family Planning and Reproductive Health Care Guidance. (2004). Contraceptives choices for breastfeeding women. *The Journal of Family Planning and Reproductive Health Care*, *30*, 181–189.

Feldman-Winter, L. B., Schanler, R. J., O'Connor, K. G., & Lawrence, R. A. (2008). Pediatricians and the promotion and support of breastfeeding. *Archives of Pediatrics and Adolescent Medicine*, *162*, 1142–1149.

Freed, G. L., Clark, S. J., Curtis, P., & Sorenson, J. R. (1995). Breastfeeding education and practice in family medicine. *The Journal of Family Practice*, *40*, 263–269.

Gartner, L. M., Morton, J., Lawrence, R. A., Naylor, A. J., O'Hare, D., Schanler, R. J., . . . American Academy of Pediatrics Section on Breastfeeding. (2005). Breastfeeding and the use of human milk. *Pediatrics*, *115*, 496–506.

Geddes, D. T., Kent, J. C., Mitoulas, L. R., & Hartmann, P. E. (2008). Tongue movement and intra-oral vacuum in breastfeeding infants. *Early Human Development*, *84*, 471–477.

Gill, S. L. (2001). The little things: Perceptions of breastfeeding support. *Journal of Obstetric, Gynecologic, and Neonatal Nursing*, *30*, 401–409.

Goldman, A. S. (2007). The immune system in human milk and the developing infant. *Breastfeeding Medicine*, *2*, 195–204.

Gooding, M. J., Finlay, J., Shipley, J. A., Halliwell, M., & Duck, F. A. (2010). Three-dimensional ultrasound imaging of mammary ducts in lactating women. *Journal of Ultrasound in Medicine*, *29*, 95–103.

Graffy, J., & Taylor, J. (2005). What information, advice, and support do women want with breastfeeding? *Birth (Berkeley, Calif.)*, *32*, 179–186.

Grummer-Strawn, L. M., Reinold, C., & Krebs, NF. (2010). Use of World Health Organization and CDC growth charts for children aged 0–59 months in the United States. Centers for Disease Control and Prevention (CDC). *MMWR. Recommendations and Reports*, *59*(RR-9), 1–15. Erratum in: MMWR Recomm Rep. 2010 Sep 17;59(36):1184.

Haider, S. J., Jacknowitz, A., & Schoeni, R. F. (2003). Welfare work requirements and child well-being: Evidence from the effects on breastfeeding. *Demography*, *40*, 479–497.

Hakansson, A., Zhivotovsky, B., Orrenius, S., Sabharwal, H., & Svanborg, C. (1995). Apoptosis induced by a human milk protein. *Proceedings of the National Academy of Sciences of the United States of America*, *92*, 8064–8068.

Halderman, L. D., & Nelson, A. L. (2002). Impact of early postpartum administration of progestin-only hormonal contraceptives compared with non-hormonal contraceptives on short-term breastfeeding patterns. *American Journal of Obstetrics and Gynecology*, *186*, 1250–1258.

Hale, T. W. (2012). *Medications and mother's milk* (15th ed.). Amarillo, TX: Hale Publishing.

Hartmann, P. E., Sherriff, J. L., & Mitoulas, L. R. (1998). Homeostatic mechanisms that regulate lactation during energetic stress. *The Journal of Nutrition*, *128*, 394S–399S.

Hellings, P., & Howe, C. (2000). Assessment of breastfeeding knowledge of nurse practitioners and nurse-midwives. *Journal of Midwifery and Women's Health*, *45*, 264–270.

Hellings, P., & Howe, C. (2004). Breastfeeding knowledge and practice of pediatric nurse practitioners. *Journal of Pediatric Health Care*, *18*, 8–14.

Henderson, J. J., Hartmann, P. E., Newnham, J. P., & Simmer, K. (2008). Effect of preterm birth and antenatal corticosteroid treatment on lactogenesis II in women. *Pediatrics*, *121*, e92–e100.

Hill, P. D., Aldag, J. C., & Chatterton, R. T. (1999). Effects of pumping style on milk production in mothers of non-nursing preterm infants. *Journal of Human Lactation*, *15*, 209–216.

Hilson, J. A., Rasmussen, K. M., & Kjolhede, C. L. (2004). High pre-pregnant body mass index is associated with poor lactation outcomes among white, rural women independent of psychosocial and demographic correlates. *Journal of Human Lactation*, *20*, 18–29.

Hopkinson, J. M., Schanler, R. J., & Garza, C. (1992). Milk production by mothers of premature infants. Influence of cigarette smoking. *Pediatrics*, *90*, 934–938.

Ilett, K. F., Hale, T. W., Page-Sharp, M., Kristensen, J. H., Kohan, R., & Hackett, L. P. (2003). Use of nicotine patches in breastfeeding mothers: Transfer of nicotine and cotinine into human milk. *Clinical Pharmacology and Therapeutics*, *74*, 516–524.

Ip, S., Chung, M., Raman, G., Chew, P., Magula, N., DeVine, D., . . . Lau, J. (2007). Breastfeeding and maternal and infant health outcomes in developed countries. Evidence Report/Technology Assessment No. 153 (Prepared by Tufts-New England Medical Center Evidence-based Practice Center, under Contract No. 290-02-0022). AHRQ Publication No. 07-E007. Rockville, MD: Agency for Healthcare Research and Quality. April 2007.

Isaacs, E. B., Ross, S., Kennedy, K., Weaver, L. T., Lucas, A., & Fewtrell, M. S. (2011). 10-year cognition in preterms after random assignment to fatty acid supplementation in infancy. *Pediatrics, 128,* e890–e898.

Israel-Ballard, K., Donovan, R., Chantry, C., Coutsoudis, A., Sheppard, H., Sibeko, L., & Abrams, B. (2007). Flash-heat inactivation of HIV-1 in human milk: A potential method to reduce postnatal transmission in developing countries. *Journal of Acquired Immune Deficiency Syndromes, 45,* 318–323.

Jansson, L. M. & The Academy of Breastfeeding Medicine Protocol Committee. (2009). ABM Clinical Protocol #21: Guidelines for breastfeeding and the drug-dependent woman. *Breastfeeding Medicine, 4,* 225–228.

Jensen, D., Wallace, S., & Kelsay, P. (1994). LATCH: A breastfeeding charting system and documentation tool. *Journal of Obstetric, Gynecologic, and Neonatal Nursing, 23,* 27–32.

King, J. (2007). Contraception and lactation. *Journal of Midwifery and Women's Health, 52,* 614–620.

Koren, G. (2002). Drinking alcohol while breastfeeding: Will it harm my baby? *Canadian Family Physician, 48,* 39–41.

Kulski, J., & Hartmann, P. (1981). Changes in human milk composition during initiation of lactation. *The Australian Journal of Experimental Biology and Medical Science, 59,* 101–114.

Labbok, M. (2000). Breastfeeding, fertility and family planning. In J. Sciarra (Ed.), *Gynecology and obstetrics.* Philadelphia: Lippincott.

Labbok, M. H, Perez, A., Valdes, V., Sevilla, F., Wade, K., Laukaran, V. H.,... Queenan, J. T. (1994). The lactational amenorrhea method: A new postpartum introductory family planning method with program and policy implications. *Advances in Contraception, 10,* 93–109.

Lovelady, C. (2011). Balancing exercise and food intake with lactation to promote post-partum weight loss. *The Proceedings of the Nutrition Society, 70,* 181–184.

Lovelady, C. A., Hunter, C. P., & Geigerman, C. (2003). Effect of exercise on immunologic factors in breast milk. *Pediatrics, 111,* e148–e152.

Martens, P. J., & Romphf, L. (2007). Factors associated with newborn in-hospital weight loss: Comparisons by feeding method, demographics, and birthing procedures. *Journal of Human Lactation, 23,* 233–241.

Matheson, I., & Rivrud, G. N. (1989). The effect of smoking on lactation and infantile colic. *JAMA: The Journal of the American Medical Association, 261,* 42–43.

Matthews, M. K. (1988). Developing an instrument to assess infant breastfeeding behaviour in the early neonatal period. *Midwifery, 4,* 154–165.

McInnes, R. J., & Chambers, J. A. (2008). Supporting breastfeeding mothers: Qualitative synthesis. *Journal of Advanced Nursing, 62,* 407–427.

Mennella, J. A., & Garcia-Gomez, P. L. (2001). Sleep disturbances after acute exposure to alcohol in mother's milk. *Alcohol (Fayetteville, N.Y.), 25,* 153–158.

Mennella, J. A., Yourshaw, L. M., & Morgan, L. K. (2007). Breastfeeding and smoking: Short-term effects on infant feeding and sleep. *Pediatrics, 120,* 497–502.

Misra, M., Pacaud, D., Petryk, A., Collett-Solberg, P. F., & Kappy, M. (2008). Vitamin D deficiency in children and its management:

Review of current knowledge and recommendations. *Pediatrics, 122,* 398–417.

Morton, J., Hall, J. Y., Thairu, L., Nomanbhoy, S., Bhutani, R., Carlson, S.,... Stevenson, D. K. (2007). Breast massage maximizes milk volumes of pump-dependent mothers. Abstract. Retrieved from http://www.abstracts2view.com/pasall/view.php?nu=PAS07L1_32

Morton, J., Hall, J. Y., Wong, R. J., Thairu, L., Benitz, W. E., & Rhine, W. D. (2009). Combining hand techniques with electric pumping increases milk production in mothers of preterm infants. *Journal of Perinatology, 29,* 757–764.

Mozingo, J. N., Davis, M. W., Droppleman, P. G., & Merideth, A. (2000). "It wasn't working": Women's experiences with short-term breastfeeding. *MCN. The American Journal of Maternal Child Nursing, 25,* 120–126.

Mulder, P. J., Johnson, T. S., & Baker, L. C. (2010). Excessive weight loss in breastfed infants during the postpartum hospitalization. *Journal of Obstetric, Gynecologic, and Neonatal Nursing, 39,* 15–26.

Mulford, C. (1992). The Mother-Baby Assessment (MBA): An "Apgar score" for breastfeeding. *Journal of Human Lactation, 8,* 79–82.

National Conference of State Legislatures. (2011). Breastfeeding laws. Retrieved from http://www.ncsl.org/issues-research/health/breastfeeding-state-laws.aspx

Nelson, A. M. (2007). Maternal-newborn nurses' experiences of inconsistent professional breastfeeding support. *Journal of Advanced Nursing, 60,* 29–38.

Neubauer, S. H., Ferris, A. M., Chase, C. G., Fanelli, J., Thompson, C. A., Lammi-Keefe, C. J.,... Green, K. W. (1993). Delayed lactogenesis in women with insulin-dependent diabetes mellitus. *The American Journal of Clinical Nutrition, 58,* 54–60.

Noel-Weiss, J., Woodend, A. K., Peterson, W. E., Gibb, W., & Groll, D. L. (2011). An observational study of associations among maternal fluids during parturition, neonatal output, and breastfed newborn weight loss. *International Breastfeeding Journal, 6,* 9.

Nommsen-Rivers, L. A., Chantry, C. J., Peerson, J. M., Cohen, R. J., & Dewey, K. G. (2010). Delayed onset of lactogenesis among first-time mothers is related to maternal obesity and factors associated with ineffective breastfeeding. *The American Journal of Clinical Nutrition, 92,* 574–584.

Nommsen-Rivers, L. A., Heinig, M. J., Cohen, R. J., & Dewey, K. G. (2008). Newborn wet and soiled diaper counts and timing of onset of lactation as indicators of breastfeeding inadequacy. *Journal of Human Lactation, 24,* 27–33.

Nyqvist, K. H., Rubertsson, C., Ewald, U., & Sjoden, P. O. (1996). Development of the preterm infant breastfeeding behavior scale (PIBBS): A study of nurse-mother agreement. *Journal of Human Lactation, 12,* 207–219.

Onyango, A. W., Nommsen-Rivers, L., Siyam, A., Borghi, E., de Onis, M., Garza, C.,... Van den Broeck, J.; WHO Multicentre Growth Reference Study Group. (2011). Post-partum weight change patterns in the WHO Multicentre Growth Reference Study. *Maternal and Child Nutrition, 7,* 228–240.

Power, M. L., Locke, E., Chapin, J., Klein, L., & Schulkin, J. (2003). The effort to increase breastfeeding. Do obstetricians, in the forefront, need help? *The Journal of Reproductive Medicine, 48,* 72–78.

Ramsay, D. T., Kent, J. C., Hartmann, R. A., & Hartmann, P. E. (2005). Anatomy of the lactating breast redefined with ultrasound imaging. *Journal of Anatomy, 206,* 525–534.

Ramsay, D. T., Kent, J. C., Owens, R. A., & Hartmann, P. E. (2001). Ultrasound imaging of milk ejection in the human lactating breast. Society for Reproductive Biology, Proceedings of the Thirty-Second Annual Conference, Gold Coast, Queensland, September 2001, Abstract 30.

Roche-Paull, R. (2010). *Breastfeeding in combat boots: A survival guide to successful breastfeeding while serving in the military*. Amarillo, TX: Hale Publishing.

Scariati, P. D., Grummer-Strawn, L. M., & Fein, S. (1997). Water supplementation of infants in the first month of life. *Archives of Pediatrics and Adolescent Medicine, 151*, 830–832.

Schmied, V., Beake, S., Sheehan, A., McCourt, C., & Dykes, F. (2011). Women's perceptions and experiences of breastfeeding support: A metasynthesis. *Birth (Berkeley, Calif.), 38*, 49–60.

Schulzke, S. M., Patole, S., &Simmer, K. (2011). Long chain polyunsaturated fatty acid supplementation in preterm infants. Retrieved from http://summaries.cochrane.org/CD000375/longchain-poly unsaturated-fatty-acid-supplementation-in-preterm-infants

Scott, J. A., Binns, C. W., & Oddy, W. H. (2007). Predictors of delayed onset of lactation. *Maternal and Child Nutrition, 3*, 186–193.

Shealy, K. R., Scanlon, K. S., Labiner-Wolfe, J., Fein, S. B., & Grummer-Strawn, L. M. (2008). Characteristics of breastfeeding practices among US mothers. *Pediatrics, 122*(Suppl. 2), S50–S55.

Shrago, L., & Bocar, D. (1990). The infant's contribution to breastfeeding. *Journal of Obstetric, Gynecologic, and Neonatal Nursing 19*, 209–215.

Shrago, L. C., Reifsnider, E., & Insel, K. (2006). The neonatal bowel output study: Indicators of adequate breast milk intake in neonates. *Pediatric Nursing, 32*, 195–201.

Simmer, K., Patole, S. K., & Rao, S. C. (2011). Longchain polyunsaturated fatty acid supplementation in infants born at term. Retrieved from http://summaries.cochrane.org/CD000376/longchain-poly unsaturated-fatty-acid-supplementation-in-infants-born-at-term.

Stuebe, A. M., & Schwarz, E. B. (2010). The risks and benefits of infant feeding practices for women and their children. *Journal of Perinatology, 30*, 155–162.

Szucs, K. A., Miracle, D. J., & Rosenman, M. B. (2009). Breastfeeding knowledge, attitudes, and practices among providers in a medical home. *Breastfeeding Medicine, 4*, 31–42.

Thoyre, S. M., Shaker, C. S., & Pridham, K. F. (2005). The early feeding skills assessment for preterm infants. *Neonatal Network, 24*, 7–16.

Tsu-Hsin, H., Keh-Chung, L., Chung-Pei, F., Chia-Ting, S., & Ching-Lin, H. (2008). A review of psychometric properties of feeding assessment tools used in neonates. *Journal of Obstetric, Gynecologic, and Neonatal Nursing, 37*, 338–349.

UNICEF. (2012). The baby-friendly hospital initiative. Retrieved from http://www.unicef.org/nutrition/index_24806.html

United States Breastfeeding Committee. (2010). Core competencies in breastfeeding care and services for all health professionals. Retrieved from http://www.usbreastfeeding.org/LinkClick.aspx?link=Publica tions%2fCore-Competencies-2010-rev.pdf&tabid=70&mid=388

U.S. Preventive Services Task Force. (2008). Primary care interventions to promote breastfeeding: U.S. Preventive Services Task Force Recommendation Statement. *Annals of Internal Medicine, 149*, 560–564.

Vorbach, C., Capecchi, M. R., & Penninger, J. M. (2006). Evolution of the mammary gland from the innate immune system? *Bioessays: News and Reviews in Molecular, Cellular and Developmental Biology, 28*, 606–616.

Wagner, C. L., Greer, F. R., & the Section on Breastfeeding and Committee on Nutrition. (2008). Prevention of rickets and vitamin D deficiency in infants, children, and adolescents. *Pediatrics, 122*, 1142–1152.

Walker, M. (2011a). *Breastfeeding and employment: Making it work*. Amarillo, TX: Hale Publishing.

Walker, M. (2011b). *Breastfeeding management for the clinician: Using the evidence* (2nd ed.). Sudbury, MA: Jones and Bartlett Publishers.

Wiklund, P., Xu, L., Lyytikäinen, A., Saltevo, J., Wang, Q., Völgyi, E., . . . Cheng, S. (2011). Prolonged breastfeeding protects mothers from later-life obesity and related cardio-metabolic disorders. *Public Health Nutrition, 23*, 1–8.

Wright, K. S., Quinn, T. J., & Carey, G. B. (2002). Infant acceptance of breast milk after maternal exercise. *Pediatrics, 109*, 585–589.

31

Common breastfeeding problems

Marsha Walker

Relevant terms

Ankyloglossia—restricted motion of the infant's tongue that interferes with feeding and can cause nipple trauma; also known as "tongue-tie"

Delayed lactogenesis II—delay in the onset of copious milk production beyond the normal interval of 2–4 days after birth

Engorgement—painful swelling of the breasts associated with the sudden increase in milk volume, lymphatic and vascular congestion, and interstitial edema that occurs during the first 2 weeks following childbirth

Flat or inverted nipple—nipple that does not easily protrude from the areola, even with stimulation

Galactagogue—medication or agent that increases the milk supply

Insufficient milk supply—the amount of milk produced is not sufficient to feed an infant

Mastitis—inflammatory condition of the breast that may involve an infection

Oral aversion—infant withdraws from oral stimuli such as feeding; often associated with a history of oral procedures such as suctioning, intubation, gavage feedings

Introduction

Although breastfeeding is the optimal method of feeding an infant and provides improved short- and long-term health outcomes, there are several common problems that pose a challenge to continued and exclusive breastfeeding. The most common breastfeeding problems encountered in the early postnatal period include infant

problems such as fussiness or sleepiness at the breast, low weight gain, and prematurity, and maternal problems such as sore nipples, engorgement, mastitis, and low milk supply. This chapter reviews the management of these common breastfeeding problems.

Common infant-related breastfeeding problems

Fussy baby

Infants who are fussy at the breast, following feedings, or in between feedings can cause a great deal of anxiety for new mothers. Many mothers interpret fussing at the breast as a sign that the infant does not "like" to breastfeed. Infants who are fretful following a feeding may be unnecessarily supplemented with formula because the mother thinks that the infant's fussiness is a sign that the infant is not getting enough milk or that her milk supply is insufficient. Failure to address the cause of a fussy infant can quickly lead to unnecessary supplementation or weaning. Infants who are allowed to cry for prolonged periods of time may not be able to organize themselves to feed well since crying is a late sign of hunger. Factors that may contribute to fussiness include infant pain, oral aversion, medications, and hunger.

Infant pain

Infants can experience pain related to birth injuries such as a fractured clavicle or humerus, a cephalohematoma, or trauma associated with a vacuum extraction or forceps delivery. Positioning an infant with a fractured clavicle can be done with either ventral positioning or in a cradle hold on one breast and then the infant is kept in the same position and moved to the other breast in a cross-cradle

Prenatal and Postnatal Care: A Woman-Centered Approach, First Edition. Edited by Robin G. Jordan, Janet L. Engstrom, Julie A. Marfell, and Cindy L. Farley.
© 2014 John Wiley & Sons, Inc. Published 2014 by John Wiley & Sons, Inc.

hold, keeping the fracture site superior to the unfractured clavicle. Vacuum extraction is a significant contributor to poor feeding mechanics and is a predictor of an increased risk of breastfeeding cessation during the first 10 days after birth (Hall et al., 2002). Mothers may need to try several different positions to find one in which the baby is comfortable feeding.

Oral aversion

Oral aversion to feeding can be caused by the infant's experiences with unpleasant oral experiences such as suctioning, gavage feeding, intubation, or digital assessment of the mouth. Swelling or soreness in the mouth may cause the infant to fuss at the breast. Mothers can encourage the infant to cuddle at the breast and taste expressed drops of colostrum or milk. If the infant refuses the breast, cup feeding of expressed breast milk can be done until the infant can be gently persuaded back to the breast.

Prenatal or perinatal medications or drugs

Infants exposed prenatally to illicit drugs may demonstrate hypertonia, irritability, thrash at the breast, clamp down on the nipple, be difficult to position at breast, or pull away from the breast if experiencing nasal stuffiness (Jansson, Velez, & Harrow, 2004). Tobacco-exposed infants are likely to demonstrate hypertonia, greater excitability, and need more holding (Law, Stroud, LaGrasse, Niaura, & Lester, 2003). Infants whose mothers have been treated prenatally with selective serotonin reuptake inhibitors may demonstrate agitation, tremors, hypertonia, irritability, and sleep disturbances (Jordan et al., 2008). These infants may need to be fed when in a drowsy state and before full crying appears. They may respond to swaddling, soft talking, gentle handling, minimal external stimulation (quiet environment, dim lights), gradual oral stimulation, ventral or side-lying positioning, and skin-to-skin contact.

Hunger

Hunger may be due to poor infant feeding skills or limited milk transfer. Mothers may complain that the infant fusses shortly after a feeding. These infants may be hungry as they may never have really completed a feeding. Some infants, such as late preterm infants and infants of diabetic mothers, have reduced intakes during feedings at breast. Infants who have been exposed to artificial nipples may find it difficult to latch and transfer milk from the breast. It can take time for these infants to develop feeding skills.

Interventions should aim to increase the number of feedings per 24 hours if necessary as well as enhance the amount of colostrum/milk transferred at each feeding. Infants who cannot generate sufficient vacuum such as late preterm infants, newborns affected by maternal prenatal or labor medications, or infants with neurological challenges may be helped to receive more milk per feeding by using alternate breast massage. Alternate massage is also a useful tool for sleepy infants or those who pause for long periods of time between sucking bursts. Alternate massage is done on each breast during each feeding by massaging and compressing the breast each time the infant pauses. This type of breast compression helps elevate the positive pressure within the breast, making a more efficient pressure gradient between the breast and the low pressure within the infant's mouth.

Young infants may cluster their feedings in the late afternoon and early evening, and may feed almost every hour. This is normal and mothers should accommodate these feedings, as some infants "tank up" with milk during this time in order to sleep longer at night.

Some fussy infants exhibit a rapid side-to-side head movement as they approach the breast. This makes it very difficult for the infant to establish a good latch. Clinicians can stop this behavior by placing a small dropper with colostrum or milk in it on the midline of the upper lip and move the infant onto the breast as the infant follows the dropper to the nipple. When the mouth is wide open, a couple of drops of colostrum or milk can be placed on the tongue to elicit sucking and swallowing.

Sleepy baby

Mothers may describe situations such as an infant who does not wake regularly enough to indicate hunger, or the baby may fall asleep at the breast or suck sporadically, or the infant may fall asleep before taking the second breast. The sleepy infant can be a challenge to breastfeed. Mothers and clinicians need to understand that sleeping is not an indicator that an infant has received sufficient amounts of milk. Young infants often do not take both breasts at each feeding, especially during the first few days after birth. If a very young infant does not take the second side, mothers and clinicians may notice feeding readiness signs an hour or so later. Infants should be given the second breast at this time.

Some infants tend to sleep more, such as late preterm infants, jaundiced infants (including those undergoing phototherapy), infants born by cesarean section, and heavier infants of diabetic mothers. Drowsiness at the breast may also be related to the normal release of cholecystokinin (CCK) that occurs when an infant breastfeeds. CCK is a gastrointestinal hormone that is released in response to fat in the diet. CCK enhances gut maturation, promotes glucose-induced insulin release, enhances sedation, and is thought to play a role in regulating food intake by signaling satiety (Marchini & Linden, 1992). Breastfed infants have higher plasma concentrations of CCK during the first 5 days than do formula-fed infants (Marchini, Simoni, Bartolini, & Linden, 1993). During the breastfeeding episode, CCK has the effect of inducing sleepiness in both the mother and the infant (Uvnas-Moberg, Widstrom, Marchini, & Winberg, 1987).

Sleepy infants should be kept skin-to-skin with their mothers as much as possible during the day. Feeding cues of sleepy infants can be quite subtle. These include rapid eye movements under the eyelids, tongue movements, hand-to-mouth movements, body movements, and small sounds. Mothers should put the sleepy baby to breast when they observe these signs. If the infant is skin-to-skin with the mother, she will notice these feeding readiness cues quickly and be able to put the baby to breast when the infant is most likely to feed. Some infants respond well to incentives at the breast that keep them interested in sustaining sucking throughout the feeding. A periodontal syringe or a soft medication dropper can be placed in the side of the baby's mouth to deliver a small amount of colostrum, milk, or water with each suck until the infant demonstrates sustained sucking and swallowing. Butterfly tubing attached to a 10-mL syringe and taped to the breast can also provide such incentives.

Slow weight gain

There are a number of infant and maternal factors that can contribute to slow weight gain in the breastfed infant. These factors are summarized in Table 31.1 and Table 31.2 and should be assessed in an infant with slow weight gain.

Slow weight gain may not in itself be the actual problem, but a manifestation of some other problem or situation that shows up as weight gain issues in the infant. Faulty breastfeeding management should be checked first; use of pacifiers that displace sucking can be eliminated; and then a thorough history and exam should be conducted. Slow weight gain may be a result of a combination of factors.

The health-care provider will also need to determine if supplementation is necessary until the underlying problem is corrected. Powers (2010) suggests that indications for supplementation can be determined by the clinical condition of the infant, the amount of weight loss (greater than 10% in a newborn or young infant), failure to return to birth weight by 2–3 weeks of age, average daily weight gain of less than 20 g, any amount of unexplained weight loss, weight and length curves that are completely flat at any age, and deceleration of head circumference that consecutively crosses percentiles.

Table 31.1   Infant Factors That May Be Associated with Slow Weight Gain

Factor	Effect
Gestational age and size for gestational age	Preterm, late preterm, post-term, small-for-gestational-age, intrauterine growth restricted, and large-for-gestational-age infants may lack mature feeding skills, strength, and stamina to ingest an adequate amount of milk.
Oral anatomy alterations	Ankyloglossia, cleft lip, cleft palate, bubble palate, and craniofacial anomalies may interfere with suckling and result in inadequate milk intake (Forlenza, Paradise Black, McNamara, & Sullivan, 2010).
Neurological alterations	Hypotonia, hypertonia, and neurological abnormalities may interfere with the infant's ability to ingest an adequate amount of milk.
Increased energy requirements	Cardiac disease, respiratory disease, and metabolic disorders may create an increased need for calories.
Infant illness or condition	Infection, cardiac abnormalities, cystic fibrosis, gastrointestinal disorders, and trisomy 21 may be associated with low endurance for feeding and/or high metabolic demands.
Maternal medications	Certain prenatal prescription medications and recreational or illicit drugs may interfere with suckling.
Intrapartum factors	Cesarean birth, fetal hypoxia during labor, maternal medications during labor, epidural analgesia, forceps delivery, and vacuum extraction that may interfere with alertness and ability to feed.
Iatrogenic factors	Separation of mothers and infants, inappropriate supplementation with formula or water, inappropriate pacifier use, and inadequate breastfeeding support can result in reduced milk intake.

Adapted from: Walker, M. (2011) *Breastfeeding management for the clinician: Using the evidence*. Sudbury, MA: Jones and Bartlett Publishing.

Supplemental feedings of the mother's own milk are ideal if the milk supply is sufficient. Infants can start with a minimum of 50–100 mL/kg/day divided into six to eight feedings. Once supplementation has been started, the amount can be increased according to infant appetite and weight gain. Once the mother's milk production has increased and the infant has attained the desired weight,

Table 31.2   Maternal Factors That May Be Associated with Slow Infant Weight Gain

Factor	Effect
Breast alterations	Previous breast surgery including augmentation and reduction, insufficient glandular tissue, and previous breast trauma may result in reduced milk volume
Nipple anomalies	Flat, retracted, inverted, oddly shaped, or dimpled nipples may impair the ability to achieve correct latch and lead to reduce milk intake.
Ineffective or insufficient milk removal	Incorrect breastfeeding position or latch, ineffective sucking, and unresolved engorgement can leave residual milk in the breast and reduce milk supply.
Delayed lactogenesis II	Women who are overweight, obese, diabetic, had a cesarean birth, or retained placental fragments may experience delayed lactogenesis II (Evans, Evans, Royal, Esterman, & James, 2003).
Inappropriate breastfeeding management	Delayed or disrupted early feeding opportunities, separation of mother and infant, too few feedings, failure to pump milk in the absence of an infant suckling at breast, ineffective breast pump, unnecessary formula supplementation, and lack of access to skilled lactation services further contribute to the problem.
Medications	Prescription, over-the-counter, recreational and illicit drugs, labor medications, and intravenous fluids may delay lactogenesis II or may interfere with infant suckling.
Hormonal alterations	Hypothyroidism, polycystic ovarian syndrome, theca lutein cysts (Hoover, Barbalinardo, & Platia, 2002), pituitary disorders, diabetes insipidus, and other endocrine-related problems may interfere with milk production.
Milk ejection problems	Drugs, alcohol, smoking, stress, and pain can inhibit the let-down reflex and reduce the amount of milk available to the infant.
Overlapping pregnancy	Pregnancy can reduce milk production (Marquis, Penny, Diaz, & Marin, 2002).
Other factors	Vitamin B_{12} deficiency in a vegetarian diet, inadequate weight gain during pregnancy, postpartum hemorrhage, and anemia may contribute to an insufficient milk supply.

Adapted from: Walker, M. (2011). *Breastfeeding management for the clinician: Using the evidence.* Sudbury, MA: Jones and Bartlett Publishing.

supplements can gradually be reduced. Clinicians often use a feeding tube device at the breast to both deliver the supplement and increase the mother's milk production.

Preterm and late preterm infants

Infants who are born preterm, those who are ill, or infants with congenital anomalies can and should either breastfeed or be given breast milk. These infants are vulnerable and benefit from human milk's many properties. Preterm infants who are not fed breast milk have higher levels of nosocomial infections (Schanler, 2007), are more likely to develop necrotizing enterocolitis (NEC) (Meinzen-Derr et al., 2009), demonstrate lower scores on tests of visual acuity (Morales & Schanler, 2007) and cognitive performance (Horwood, Darlow, & Mogridge, 2001), have altered immune function (Tarcan, Gurakan, Tiker, & Ozbek, 2004), and increased intestinal permeability and slower intestinal maturation (Taylor, Basile, Ebeling, & Wagner, 2009).

Provision of human milk is important because preterm infants cannot fully digest carbohydrates and proteins. Human milk provides components that aid this process. When preterm infants are fed infant formula, undigested casein can reach the gut, attract neutrophils that provoke inflammation and the opening of the tight junctions between cells, allow intact proteins to engage in systemic invasion, and further damage a fragile gut leading to NEC (Claud & Walker, 2001).

Lack of breastfeeding is a significant predictor of mild and severe cognitive deficiencies in very preterm infants at discharge and at 5 years of age (Beaino et al., 2011). Vohr et al. (2006) found that every 10 mL/kg/day increase in breast milk intake contributed 0.53 points to the Bayley Mental Development Index, conferring a 5.3 IQ point advantage for infants consuming 110 mL/kg/day. This type of effect is a long-term advantage that may optimize cognitive potential and decrease the need for costly early intervention and special education services in childhood. Thus, breast milk feeding for preterm infants is important.

In the absence of an infant who can feed at the breast, mothers need to express or pump their milk, sometimes for weeks or months until their infant is able to feed at the breast or to provide as much breast milk for as long as possible. Mothers need to have an efficient, hospital-grade breast pump that is a fully automated pump that cycles approximately 48–50 times per minute, with vacuum that does not exceed 240 mmHg. A double collection kit that pumps both breasts simultaneously and fits properly should be used. Mothers tend to pump more milk faster when double pumping, especially if breast massage is also used.

Mothers should begin pumping within 6 hours of birth. Morton et al. (2009) demonstrated that in pump-dependent preterm mothers, those that used hand expression greater than five times per day, as well as those using an electric pump five times per day during the first 3 days postpartum produced significantly larger volumes of milk than mothers who only used an electric pump. Furthermore, massaging each breast while using an electric breast pump significantly increased the amount of milk pumped at each session (Morton et al., 2009).

Pumping frequency should be increased to 8 to 12 times per 24 hours until 14 days following birth. Mothers' milk volumes should be carefully monitored using a log that is routinely checked by a health-care provider to assure that the milk supply is adequate. Mothers of preterm infants should receive comprehensive lactation support services from health-care professionals with expertise in breastfeeding and the provision of breast milk for preterm infants.

Late preterm infants (34 0/7 to 36 6/7 weeks of gestation) are also at a disadvantage relative to their feeding skills (Meier, Furman, & Degenhardt, 2007). They are not just smaller versions of full-term infants but present numerous challenges to breastfeeding. Late preterm infants are born with low energy stores, high energy demands, and poor feeding ability; they are sleepy, tire easily when feeding, have a weak suck and low tone, demonstrate an inability to sustain sucking, are easily overstimulated, and take in only small volumes of milk during the early days in the hospital. They are more prone to positional apnea due to airway obstruction and should be breastfed in a clutch, cross-cradle, or ventral position (Walker, 2008). Mothers require specialized lactation support services in the hospital as well as a discharge plan for breastfeeding at home. A sample breastfeeding plan for after hospital discharge is provided in Table 31.3.

Common maternal breastfeeding problems

Breast and nipple problems as well as insufficient milk are some of the most frequently described maternal breastfeeding challenges and are often the cause of decreasing or discontinuing breastfeeding. Even though they are common problems, they need to be addressed immediately to avoid formula supplementation and premature weaning.

Sore nipples

There are a number of factors that contributor to sore nipples. Most notable is improper positioning and latch. Flat or inverted nipples are another common cause.

Ankyloglossia or tongue-tie can also cause substantial nipple damage and pain.

Improper positioning and latch

Improper positioning at the breast has long been thought to be a significant contributor to sore nipples. Clinicians need to check that the infant is latched properly and engaged in correct sucking movements. Positioning of the infant is also important. Proper positioning and latch are reviewed in Chapter 30.

Flat or inverted nipples

Flat or inverted nipples can contribute not only to sore nipples but also to delayed lactogenesis II, poor milk transfer, newborn weight loss, engorgement, and reduced milk production. Flat or inverted nipples fail to protrude sufficiently when an infant latches, so correct attachment to the breast becomes difficult because the nipple/areola cannot be drawn far enough into the mouth (Walker, 2010). Flat nipples can be detected when the areola is compressed and the nipple flattens to the level of the areola or recedes back into the areola.

Most prenatal corrective measures for flat or inverted nipples such as nipple rolling, areolar stretching, and wearing of breast shells do not result in any corrective outcomes (Alexander, Grant, & Campbell, 1992; MAIN Trial Collaborative Group, 1994). Surgery to evert an inverted nipple will correct the problem but may sever too many nerves and milk ducts. Mechanical stretching of the nipple by suction devices such as the Niplette® (McGeorge, 1994) and Supple Cup® (Bouchet-Horwitz, 2011) have a small amount of evidence showing good protrusion after being worn prenatally. The Supple Cups® can be also be used in between or immediately prior to a feeding after the baby is born to increase nipple protractility. Interventions that can be used prior to each feeding are described in Table 31.4.

Ankyloglossia

Ankyloglossia or tongue-tie can restrict or alter tongue movement and contribute to sore and macerated nipples (Ballard, Auer, & Khoury, 2002). When the tongue-tie is released by clipping (frenotomy), most mothers experience immediate relief from pain and see improved sucking (Geddes et al., 2008). Mothers of infants with ankyloglossia need a feeding plan to use until the frenotomy is performed or if a frenotomy will not be done.

Other causes

Other causes of sore nipples that should be explored include eczema, Raynaud's phenomena, nipple bleb, fungal infection (Candida albicans), and if the mother is pumping, a pump flange that is too small.

Table 31.3 Sample Instructions for Breastfeeding a Late Preterm Infant

Feed your baby on cue 8–12 times each 24 hours.

Observe your baby for feeding cues. Feeding cues may not be as obvious in babies born early. Sleeping is *not* a sign that the baby is getting enough milk. Use these signs as a cue to feed if your baby is sleepy:
- sucking movements of the mouth and tongue
- rapid eye movements under the eyelids
- hand-to-mouth movements
- body movements
- small sounds.

Place your baby in a clutch or cross-cradle position. If your baby has difficulty attaching to the breast, flails at the breast, or arches away from the breast, use a semireclining position. Recline to a 30° angle; place your baby on his tummy with his mouth directly over the nipple. This allows gravity to bring his chin and tongue forward and help him latch.

As your baby latches on, make sure his mouth is wide open.

You should hear or feel your baby swallow every one to three sucks during most of the feeding.

Use alternate massage on each breast at each feeding to keep your baby sucking and increase the amount of milk she/he receives at each feeding. Thoroughly massage and compress each part of the breast.

If you are not sure how much milk your baby is getting at each feeding, you can weigh your baby before and after a feeding. This will help you know if you need to offer a supplement.

Record each feeding, whether a supplement is used, the number of wet diapers, and the number of bowel movements on your feeding log until your baby is feeding regularly and gaining weight. Also include the volume of milk pumped.

If your baby does not latch to the breast, try the following:
- Gently roll your nipple between your fingers to make it easier for the baby to grasp.
- As you bring your baby to breast, have a helper place a tube feeding device or dropper in the corner of the baby's mouth and deliver a small amount of milk as the baby attempts to latch. If your baby swallows and attempts to latch again, another small amount of milk can be given. Repeat until your baby no longer attempts to latch. These practice sessions should not last longer than 10 minutes to avoid tiring both you and your baby.
- Finish the feeding by finger or cup feeding.
- If the attempts at latching do not work, you may find that a silicone nipple shield will allow the baby to latch and sustain sucking at the breast. Moisten the shield with warm water, turn it almost inside-out as you apply it to the breast, apply a little breast milk to the outside of the shield, hand express milk into the shield tunnel, and bring the baby to breast. If the baby latches, continue using alternate massage throughout the feeding.

Babies should have at least six wet diapers and three or more bowel movements each day by the fifth day. Bowel movements should start turning yellow by day 4. Meconium diapers on day 5 or the presence of red stains in wet diapers (uric acid crystals) on day 4 may indicate that the baby is not getting enough milk.

Take your baby to see her/his health-care provider 2 days after coming home from the hospital for a weight check and to make sure that she/he is not jaundiced. A weight check every 3 days or so assures that your baby continues to gain about 0.5–1 oz/day.

If your baby cannot feed long enough at each feeding or is not gaining enough weight, supplements of expressed breast milk can be given by tube feeding at the breast, finger feeding, cup feeding, or bottle feeding. If you do not have enough milk to use as a supplement, a hydrolyzed formula can be used until your milk production has increased.

Continue to pump your milk two to three times each day to use as a supplement and to improve your milk supply. Try "power pumping" for an hour once or twice each day. Pump for 5–10 minutes until the milk stops spraying after the first letdown. Wait for 10 minutes or so and pump again until the milk stops spraying. Almost half of the milk that is available in the breast is pumped with the first letdown. Power pumping takes advantage of these "first" letdowns to mimic frequent feedings and helps increase your milk production. Depending on how your baby is feeding at the breast, pumping should continue until she/he is 40–42 weeks corrected gestational age, weaning off the pump over the first month home.

Adapted from: Walker, M. (2009). *Breastfeeding the late preterm infant: Improving care and outcomes.* Amarillo, TX: Hale Publishing.

Table 31.4 Interventions for Flat and Inverted Nipples

Apply cold compresses to the nipple area.

Shape the nipple by rolling it between the fingers.

A breast pump may help extend the nipple. However, a breast pump distributes vacuum over a wide area and may contribute to increasing edema within the nipple and areola, further contributing to latch difficulty.

Breast shells worn between feedings may help displace fluid but can damage underlying tissue if worn for long periods of time in the presence of edema.

A modified 10-mL syringe is a simple and inexpensive tool that can be fashioned by removing the plunger, cutting off the end of the syringe one-fourth of an inch above where a needle would attach, and inserting the plunger through the end that was cut (Kesaree, Banapurmath, Banapurmath, & Shamanur, 1993). The mother then places the smooth end of the syringe directly over her nipple and pulls back gently on the plunger to her comfort for 30 seconds to a minute prior to each feeding. She can repeat this procedure several times each day between feedings to more quickly improve nipple protrusion. An FDA-approved version of this type of device is available—the Evert-It Nipple Enhancer™ (Maternal Concepts).

Flat nipples can also be caused by areolar edema. Reverse pressure softening can be used to expose the nipple in cases or areolar edema (Cotterman, 2004). The mother uses three or four fingertips of each hand to encircle the base of the nipple and push inward for 1–3 minutes with enough pressure to form six to eight pits.

A nipple shield can be applied before or after reverse pressure softening if there appears to be no other way to help the infant latch to the breast.

Management of sore nipples

Dozens of sore nipple treatments have been written about since the seventeenth century with no single agent being clearly superior to others (Morland-Schultz & Hill, 2005). The health-care provider must identify the cause(s) of sore nipples and work to remedy the cause of the problem. Some of the treatments treat bacterial infections, some promote healing, and some relieve pain and increase comfort. Management strategies for uncomplicated sore nipples is outlined in Table 31.5.

The management of sore nipples with evidence of nipple damage is described in Table 31.5. If a break in the skin occurs and the nipple becomes cracked or fissured, there is a high probability for colonization by bacteria and fungal species and additional interventions may be necessary. Cracked nipples also increase the risk for mastitis. *Staphylococcus aureus* is a common pathogen associated with infected nipple cracks. Careful

Table 31.5 Strategies for Preventing and Managing Sore Nipples

Preventive strategies	• Instruct mothers on optimal infant positioning and latch. • Assess latch, suck, swallowing and positioning. • Place infant in ventral position (prone) for gravity assistance to aid latch-on, especially if the infant is tongue-tied. • Check to make sure the infant's mouth is open to 160°, with lips flared outward and neck slightly extended. • If pumping, assure the flange is large enough to prevent nipple strangulation in the flange tunnel. • Provide relief from engorgement. • Assist mothers with flat nipples. • Avoid pacifiers until breastfeeding is well established. • Correct ankyloglossia if present.
Sore nipples without evidence of damage	• Review the preventative strategies described earlier with a special focus on positioning and latch. • Warm water compresses • Warm green tea bag compresses • Coconut oil • Hydrogel dressing • Use a nipple shield if the above measures do not provide relief
Crack in the nipple skin	• Wash the nipples with soap and water once each day. • Apply topical mupirocin. • Avoid pacifier use or wash pacifiers thoroughly with soap and water. • Apply topical low-strength steroids for inflammation.
Exudate, increased erythema, pus, or dry scab is present.	• Systemic antibiotics • If *Candida albicans* is suspected, add 2% miconazole
Persistent or recurrent infection	• Treat the infant with nasal mupirocin. • Culture nipple skin for small colony variants (SCVs) bacteria; send the specimen for culture and sensitivity • If SCVs are present, switch to macrolide therapy. • Use hydrogel dressing for comfort and moist wound healing. • Be watchful for an ascending infection (mastitis).

Adapted from: Walker, M. (2010). *The nipple and areola in breastfeeding and lactation.* Amarillo, TX: Hale Publishing.

washing of the cracked nipples with soap and water followed by a thin application of mupirocin 2% ointment (Bactroban®) may be effective in the early stages of an infection (Livingstone, Willis, & Berkowitz, 1996). Bacteria have a propensity to grow and form colonies that are protected by a biofilm. Biofilms prevent antibiotics from reaching and killing the bacteria and contribute to persistent infections. To disrupt this biofilm, the affected nipple should be washed with soap and water once a day, followed by a coating of mupirocin. This helps penetrate the biofilm and eliminate the infection. The use of lanolin may be considered for sore or abraded nipples, while a hydrogel dressing may be indicated for open sores or cracks with exudate. Coconut oil and Medi-honey® have bactericidal and fungicidal properties and are said anecdotally to produce good results.

Breast engorgement

Engorgement is a physiological process described as the painful swelling of the breasts associated with the sudden increase in milk volume, lymphatic and vascular congestion, and interstitial edema that occurs during the first 2 weeks following childbirth. Engorgement is progressive, as milk production increases rapidly and milk volume can outpace the capacity of the alveoli to store it. If the milk is not removed, engorgement progresses to alveolar overdistension, which can cause the milk-secreting cells to become flattened, drawn out, and even to rupture. The distention can partly or completely occlude the capillary blood circulation surrounding the alveolar cells. Congested blood vessels leak fluid into the surrounding tissue space, contributing to edema. Pressure and congestion obstruct lymphatic drainage of the breasts. Once the system that rids the breasts of toxins, bacteria, and cast-off cell parts becomes stagnated, the breast is predisposed to mastitis (both inflammation and infection).

The areola can also become engorged or edematous with clinical observations of a swollen areola with tight, shiny skin, probably involving overfull lactiferous ducts. A puffy areola is thought to be due to tissue edema. Some degree of breast engorgement is normal.

Severe engorgement is a very painful condition that can be minimized with early frequent feedings, feeding infants on cue, no restriction on sucking times, thorough breast drainage, and correct sucking techniques. Alternate breast massage has been shown to reduce the incidence and severity of engorgement while simultaneously contributing to increased milk intake, increasing the fat content of the milk, and increasing infant weight gain (Bowles, Stutte, & Hensley, 1987–1988; Iffrig, 1968; Stutte, Bowles, & Morman, 1988). Engorgement usually occurs between 3 and 6 days after birth and declines

thereafter. However, some mothers may experience additional episodes of engorgement during the early weeks of breastfeeding. Most mothers find relief from the use of cold compresses (Sandberg, 1998), frequent milk removal by hand expression or pumping, and anti-inflammatory medication for discomfort. The application of chilled cabbage leaves to the breasts may also be beneficial (Roberts, 1995). Lymphatic breast drainage therapy is a gentle massage of the lymphatic drainage channels in the breast that may improve the movement of stagnated fluid and reduce edema (Wilson-Clay & Hoover, 2008). Mothers may need to hand express or pump milk prior to placing the baby at the breast. An edematous areola will benefit from reverse pressure softening for easier latch. However, the application of heat is not recommended and may increase the severity of symptoms (Robson, 1990).

Plugged ducts

Breastfeeding mothers may encounter tender small lumps in their breasts, usually related to the blockage of a milk duct. The lump may also have reddened skin over it, become smaller after a feeding, and be warm to the touch. Poor milk flow may result from the area of the breasts experiencing the blockage, contributing to milk stasis and a firm or hardened area behind the plug. This focal engorgement from a blocked duct may cause a segment of the breast to become swollen, firm, and tender. Milk secretions that are blocked from exiting the breast may become thickened due to absorption of fluid from the milk.

Milk expressed from the breast experiencing plugged ducts may contain material from the plug that is of a fatty composition. Strings that resemble spaghetti or lengths of fatty-looking material have been described. Observation of fatty material in milk has led clinicians to recommend the addition of lecithin to the maternal diet (Lawrence & Lawrence, 2010). Lecithin is a phospholipid used by the food industry as an emulsifier to keep fat dispersed and suspended in water rather than aggregated in a fatty mass. One tablespoon per day of oral granular lecithin has been reported to relieve plugged ducts and prevent their recurrence (Eglash, 1998).

Interventions for plugged ducts include warm compresses and direct massage over the lump while the baby is sucking. Massage over and/or behind the blockage can break up the material obstructing the duct and push the blockage forward. An alternate approach is to massage in front of the lump toward the nipple (Smillie, 2004). The mother begins the massage close to the nipple and repositions the massage farther back until she is massaging directly in front of the blockage (Campbell, 2006). Plugged ducts require prompt attention because they can lead to a series of events that result in breast inflammation and infection (Kinlay, O'Connell, & Kinlay, 2001).

Mastitis

Mastitis is an inflammatory condition of the breast that may involve an infection (Walker, 2004). Mastitis and infection are terms that are often used interchangeably, and mastitis is frequently treated as if it were an infection. Most clinicians rely on a cluster of signs and symptoms to diagnose mastitis due to an infection. The signs and symptoms of mastitis due to an infection are listed as follows.

Signs and symptoms of mastitis due to an infection

Fever of 101°F (38.4°C) or greater
Flu-like aching
Increased heart rate
Nausea
Chills
Pain or swelling at the site
Red, tender, hot area, often wedge shaped
Red streaks on the breast extending toward the axilla
Infant may reject the affected side due to the salty taste of the milk

---

Signs and symptoms of breast problems such as engorgement, plugged ducts, and noninfectious and infectious mastitis sometimes overlap. Each process has some element related to obstructed milk flow, making the differential diagnosis difficult (Betzold, 2007). When breast drainage is blocked, paracellular pathways open, allowing the leakage of cytokines, which contribute to fever, chills, muscle aches, and general malaise. This situation can give the clinical impression of an infection, whether or not that is actually the case. The incidence of mastitis ranges from 2.9% to 24% with the highest occurrence at 2–3 weeks postpartum. However, mastitis can occur at any time during the course of lactation. Risk factors for mastitis are listed in the following textbox.

Risk factors for mastitis

Cracked or damaged nipple
Plugged milk ducts
Milk stasis from unrelieved engorgement or ineffective milk removal
Blocked nipple pore
Infant is a nasal carrier of *S. aureus*
Hyperlactation or a high rate of milk synthesis
Insulin-dependent diabetes mellitus
Nipple piercing

Treatment for mastitis includes recommending that the mother continue to feed or pump on the affected side, rest, a full 10- to 14-day course of antibiotics, and that the cause or precipitating factors of the mastitis be identified and remedied. Frequent feedings and the use of alternate massage will help relieve milk stasis.

Mastitis can recur when the bacteria are resistant or not sensitive to the prescribed antibiotic, when antibiotics are not continued long enough, when an incorrect antibiotic is prescribed, when the mother stopped nursing on the affected side, or when the initial cause of the mastitis was not addressed (such as milk stasis). If mastitis recurs, Lawrence and Lawrence (2010) recommend that milk culture and sensitivity testing be done as well as cultures of the infant's nasopharynx and oropharynx to determine the offending organism as well as what antibiotic it is sensitive to. Milk cultures should be taken if the mastitis is unresponsive to antibiotics after 2 days (Spencer, 2008) because organisms can be resistant to multiple medications (Betzold, 2005). If the infection occurs more than two or three times in the same location, a closer follow-up and evaluation is recommended to rule out an underlying mass (Academy of Breastfeeding Medicine, 2008).

It is important to identify and address the underlying causes of inflammatory signs and symptoms in the breast, which may halt the progression to an infection. If the mother has a low-grade fever, aching, red splotches, and a painful area in the breast, she may find relief from use of a nonsteroidal anti-inflammatory drug such as ibuprofen. If the symptoms do not improve within 8–24 hours, or if the mother continues to run a fever, the fever suddenly increases, she develops flu-like symptoms, feels ill, or has obvious signs of a bacterial infection such as discharge of pus from the nipple, the mother should call her health-care provider. The health-care provider should prescribe a 10- to 14-day course of antibiotics.

Abscess

A breast abscess is a potential complication of mastitis related to untreated, delayed, inadequate, or incorrect treatment of mastitis. Further contributors to this complication are prior episodes of mastitis, avoiding breastfeeding or not pumping on the affected breast, or acute weaning during mastitis. An abscess is a localized collection of pus that becomes walled off and lacks an outlet for the drainage of the collected material. Once this material is encapsulated by the breast, it must be drained surgically. An abscess may appear as a well-defined area of the breast that is hard, red, and tender, or a floculant mass. Breast abscess occurs in about 3% of women with mastitis (Amir, Forster, McLachlan, & Lumley, 2004).

S. aureus is the most common organism isolated in breast abscesses with methicillin-resistant *S. aureus* (MRSA) identified in over 60% of postpartum breast abscesses (Berens, Swaim, & Peterson, 2010; Stafford et al., 2008). Other organisms are less common. Any abscess drainage should be cultured and antibiotic sensitivities determined. It is not always possible to confirm the existence of an abscess by clinical examination or mammography. A diagnostic ultrasound is typically used to confirm the presence of an abscess and to mark the site for either surgical drainage, needle, or catheter aspiration and drainage.

Surgical drainage may be necessary if the abscess is large or there are multiple abscess sites. Breastfeeding should continue during and after the period of treatment as it promotes drainage of the affected segment and helps resolve the infection. Weaning or not breastfeeding or pumping on the affected side may hinder the resolution of the abscess by contributing to the production of increasingly viscid fluid that may promote engorgement. Breastfeeding should continue on the affected side unless the abscess drainage site is so close to the areola that the baby's mouth would cover it during feeding. If the infant will not feed from the affected side, the breast should be pumped. Changes in protein, carbohydrate, and electrolyte concentrations from an affected breast may decrease the level of lactose and cause a rise in sodium and chloride concentrations, making the milk taste salty.

Low milk supply

Insufficient milk supply, either real or perceived, is one of the most frequent reasons for discontinuing breastfeeding (Gatti, 2008). The perception of insufficient milk often has its origin in the hospital during the first 48 hours following delivery. Many clinicians and mothers are unaware that infants need small frequent feedings due to their small stomach capacity, and that the amount of colostrum available to the infant is small. If mothers are pumping their breasts at this time and see small amounts of colostrum, they may incorrectly assume that they have an insufficient milk supply. Mothers may also perceive a lack of milk if the breasts do not feel full, or if the baby feeds frequently, continues to fuss after a feeding, or does not settle between feedings.

Mothers are often worried about infant crying and interpret it as a sign of hunger. Mothers who describe insufficient milk supply most frequently do so because their infant was not satisfied after a feeding and, as a result, offer a bottle of formula to complete the feeding and cause the infant to sleep. While mothers most commonly report infant crying as the cue used to determine

Table 31.6   Common Contributors to Low Milk Supply

Common contributors to low milk supply	
Breastfeeding mismanagement	Limiting the number of feedings, short times at the breast, scheduled feedings that do not coincide with the infant's feeding cues, failure to assess for feeding, unrelieved severe engorgement, inappropriate formula supplementation, use of artificial nipples and pacifiers.
Infant problems	Poor latch, oral anomalies, ankyloglossia, neurological problems, cardiac abnormalities, preterm and late preterm infants, sleepy infants, and infants who are unable to feed at the breast.
Maternal conditions	Hypoplastic breasts, obesity, diabetes, thyroid dysfunction, polycystic ovary syndrome, history of breast surgery, smoking, inverted nipples, postpartum hemorrhage, retained placental fragments, anemia, and selected medications.
Breast pump issues	Use of an inadequate breast pump, poorly fitted flange on a breast pump, or not pumping frequently enough.

insufficient milk, milk production and infant feeding parameters are often not assessed prior to recommending supplementation. When crying is perceived as hunger, mothers and health-care providers often use formula supplementation as a remedy to stop the crying and satisfy the baby (Sacco, Caulfield, Gittelsohn, & Martinez, 2006). However, supplementing with formula can diminish milk production.

There are many contributors to the development of perceived insufficient milk, with the most common contributors related to misinformation and mismanagement of breastfeeding. The common contributors to low milk supply are summarized in Table 31.6.

Insufficient milk supply should be suspected if the infant loses more than 7% of birth weight and fails to regain birth weight by 2 weeks. However, this may also indicate an infant with poor breastfeeding skills who is unable to transfer milk even when there is an abundant milk supply. Weight gain of less than 5 oz/week, concentrated urine in the diapers, passing of dry hard stools, lethargy, and dry mucous membranes signal a potential problem with either milk transfer or milk supply and require immediate assessment and intervention (Amir, 2006). A feeding observation is necessary for infants who sleep excessive amounts, who feed for longer than 45 minutes at a single feeding, or appear to want to nurse continuously. These women should be referred to a

Table 31.7 Interventions for Low Milk Supply

Interventions for low milk supply
Extra feedings, extra pumpings, pumping after a feeding, improving infant positioning, and assisting milk transfer to the infant by using alternate massage.
Mothers can use a tube feeding device at the breast to deliver supplemental milk to the baby while the baby stimulates the breast.
Mothers of preterm infants should be encouraged to engage in skin-to-skin care and pump at their infant's bedside while looking at or touching their infant (Hurst, Valentine, Renfro, Burns, & Ferlic, 1997; Hung & Berg, 2011; Mahmood, Jamal, & Khan, 2011).
If the mother is using a breast pump, assure that it is an effective, electric, hospital-grade breast pump with a double collection kit and properly fitted breast flange. Check the vacuum with a vacuum gauge to assure that the pump is operating efficiently.
Mothers who smoke should be encouraged to quit or reduce the number of cigarettes smoked per day. Smoking should not occur directly prior to a feeding as it may inhibit the let-down reflex.
Evaluate the mother for potential endocrine abnormalities and correct if present.

lactation specialist. Likewise, women who have been pumping regularly should also be referred to a lactation specialist.

Management options for insufficient milk depend on the cause of the milk insufficiency. Clinicians should first assess the infant during a breastfeeding to see if milk transfer is occurring. Pre- and postfeed weights can verify the amount of milk transfer. Faulty sucking skills, oral anomalies, underfeeding, and poor positioning may be recognized and remedied at this time. Interventions for the various causes of insufficient milk supply are summarized in Table 31.7.

Medications known as galactagogues have been used to improve milk production (Gabay, 2002). The efficacy and side effect profile of these products vary (Anderson & Valdes, 2007). Common pharmaceutical galactagogues include metoclopramide and domperidone.

Metoclopramide (Reglan®) is a dopamine antagonist and has been shown to stimulate basal prolactin levels, leading to increased milk production at doses of 30–45 mg/day (Budd, Erdman, Long, Trombley, & Udall, 1993). Metoclopramide is dose dependent and some mothers may not respond if their prolactin levels are normal. Maternal side effects of metoclopramide include gastric cramping, diarrhea, and depression with use

for more than 4 weeks, but few side effects have been reported in infants. Abrupt discontinuation of the medication can result in a precipitous drop in milk production. Thus, tapering the dosage by decreasing it 10 mg/week is recommended.

Domperidone (Motilium®) is a peripheral dopamine antagonist similar to metoclopramide, but it does not cross the blood–brain barrier. This feature reduces the likelihood of central nervous system side effects such as depression. It produces significant increases in prolactin levels and stimulates milk production at doses of 10–20 mg three to four times daily without maternal gastric side effects. Not all mothers respond to the use of domperidone, but for those that do, there is a dose–response relationship with higher doses resulting in more milk production (Wan et al., 2008). There have been no reported effects on the infant and it is considered a better choice as a galactagogue (da Silva, Knoppert, Angelini, & Forret, 2001). Zuppa et al. (2010) consider domperidone the drug of first choice due to its proven efficiency, lack of side effects in infants, and rare side effects in mothers. Domperidone is contraindicated if the mother is taking other medications with anticholinergic properties as these may antagonize the effects on the GI tract. Mothers with cardiac arrhythmias should also avoid taking domperidone. The effects may not be seen for 3–4 days with the maximum effect taking up to 2–3 weeks (Henderson, 2003). Most mothers take the medication for 3–8 weeks. Although not widely available in the United States, compounding pharmacies can formulate domperidone with a prescription. However, the Food and Drug Administration (FDA) has not approved domperidone for use in the United States and has issued a safety warning to consumers and health-care professionals recommending that the drug not be used.

Acupuncture has been successfully used in China since ancient times for insufficient milk (Zhao & Guo, 2006). Clavey (1996) reports over a 90% effectiveness rate when acupuncture is initiated within 20 days of birth but less than an 85% success rate when initiated after 20 days postpartum. The earlier postpartum the treatment is begun, the quicker the results and the more likely that milk production will significantly improve. Electroacupuncture may also be very effective (Wei, Wang, Han, & Li, 2008).

Herbal and botanical preparations have been used since antiquity to stimulate milk production. Varied preparations are widely recommended by clinicians for improving milk output even though there is limited evidence of their effectiveness. Some commonly used herbals include fenugreek, milk thistle, raspberry leaf, nettle, goat's rue, fennel seed, chaste tree seed, fireweed, anise seed, blessed thistle, stinging nettle, and cotton root. Many of these herbs are used in combination in commercial galactagogue preparations.

Fenugreek (*Trigonella foenum-graecum*) is probably the most widely used herbal galactagogue. Fenugreek has been shown to have antianxiety effects, which may contribute to the herb's anecdotally reported effectiveness (Abascal & Yarnell, 2008). The dosage is usually a 1200 mg capsule two to three times daily. Fenugreek is also delivered through tea and has been shown to enhance breastmilk production during the early days following birth (Turkyilmaz et al., 2011).

Goat's rue (*Galega officinalis*) is a common galactagogue (Weiss, 2001) used for insufficient milk. Goat's rue is dosed as 1 tsp of dried herb steeped in 1 cup of water twice daily or 1–2 mL of tincture three times daily.

Other botanical preparations include fennel seed, chaste tree seed, and milk thistle. Fennel seed (*Foeniculum vulgare*) is used to increase milk production at a dose of 5–7 g of seed per day as a tea. Chaste tree seed (*Vitex adnus-castus*) is used at a dosage of 1 tsp of the berries steeped in 1 cup of water three times daily or 2.5 mL of tincture three times daily. Milk thistle (*Silybum marianum*) in a micronized 420 mg dose can significantly increase daily milk production. The micronized form improves its poor bioavailability (Di Pierro, Callegari, Carotenuto, & Tapia, 2008).

Other remedies such as beer (hops), brewer's yeast (vitamin B complex), oatmeal, and various cultural preparations and foods have also been used. Although herbal and botanical preparations are commonly employed, they require some caution. Clinicians can refer to the German Commission E Monographs for safety profiles of botanicals, the American Herbal Products Association (http://www.ahpa.org) for information on manufacturing and labeling standards, and the American Botanical Council (http://www.herbalgram.org) for information on the quality of herbal products. The use of a galactagogue requires close follow-up by the clinician (Academy of Breastfeeding Medicine, 2011).

Summary

Although breastfeeding is the optimal method of infant feeding, there are many challenges to establishing and maintaining breastfeeding. The most common breastfeeding problems encountered during the early postnatal period include infant problems such as fussiness or sleepiness at the breast, low weight gain, and prematurity, and maternal problems such as sore nipples, engorgement, mastitis, and low milk supply. All healthcare professionals who care for women and infants should be familiar with the diagnosis and management of these common breastfeeding problems so that they

Case study

Heather is a 33-year-old new mother who just gave birth to her first child 4 days ago. She and her baby were discharged from the hospital 2 days ago. Heather is calling the office today because she is worried that her baby is "getting enough" to eat. She said that the baby wants to eat often, especially in the afternoon and early evening. Yesterday, the baby nursed 10 times. Heather said that her mother advised giving the baby a little bit of formula after each feeding to help him sleep longer.

Upon questioning, Heather tells the nurse practitioner that the baby had seven wet diapers yesterday and passed a dark sticky stool during three breastfeeding sessions. She reports that the baby is alert during breastfeeding until the very end of the feeding when he falls asleep. She also reports that her breasts feel very full but that the baby appears to latch correctly. When further questioned, she states that she can feel the baby sucking during nursing and can hear the baby swallow. She denies having any nipple pain or redness.

The nurse practitioner reassures Heather that it sounds as if the baby is nursing well and "getting enough" to eat. The nurse practitioner explains that babies eat often during the first days of life and may eat as many as 12 times a day. Other typical feeding behaviors such as nursing more frequently in the early afternoon and evening were also described. The nurse practitioner reassures Heather that the baby is showing signs of being adequately fed by the number of wet diapers and bowel movements as well as by the observation that the baby has periods of alertness coupled with periods of sleep. Hearing the baby's audible swallows during feeding is also a very reassuring sign. Heather is advised to keep assessing the number of wet diapers and bowel movements and is informed that the stool should start to become yellowish in the next day. The nurse practitioner reassures Heather that the baby does not need supplemental formula and explains that feeding formula can interfere with breastfeeding and her milk supply. Heather is reminded to bring the baby in for a weight check tomorrow and is reassured that she should call for any other question or problems.

can provide appropriate care for the breastfeeding mother and infant.

Resources for women and their families

La Leche League International: http://www.llli.org/

Low Milk Supply Web Site: http://www.lowmilksupply .org

Mothers Overcoming Breastfeeding Issues Web Site: http://www.mobimotherhood.org

Stanford School of Medicine—Getting Started with Breastfeeding: http://newborns.stanford.edu/Breast feeding/

Resources for health-care providers

Academy of Breastfeeding Medicine: http://www.bfmed .org

Breastfeeding after Breast Reduction Web Site: http:// www.bfar.org

International Lactation Consultant Association: http:// www.ilca.org/i4a/pages/index.cfm?pageid=1

Late Preterm Infant Toolkit: http://www.cpqcc.org/ quality_improvement/qi_toolkits/care_and_manage ment_of_the_late_preterm_infant_toolkit_rev_febru ary_2013

Office of Women's Health, U.S. Department of Health and Human Services: http://www.womenshealth.gov/ breastfeeding/

Texas Tech University Infant Risk Center: http://www .infantrisk.com/category/breastfeeding

United States Lactation Consultant Association: http:// www.uslca.org

References

Abascal, K., & Yarnell, E. (2008). Botanical galactagogues. *Alternative & Complementary Therapies, 14*, 288–294.

Academy of Breastfeeding Medicine. (2008). ABM clinical protocol #4: Mastitis. *Breastfeeding Medicine, 3*, 177–180.

Academy of Breastfeeding Medicine. (2011). Clinical protocol # 9: Use of galactogogues in initiating or augmenting the rate of maternal milk secretion. *Breastfeeding Medicine, 6*, 41–49.

Alexander, J., Grant, A., & Campbell, M. J. (1992). Randomized controlled trial of breast shells and Hoffman's exercises for inverted and non-protractile nipples. *British Medical Journal, 304*, 1030–1032.

Amir, L. H. (2006). Breastfeeding: Managing supply difficulties. *Australian Family Physician, 35*, 686–689.

Amir, L. H., Forster, D., McLachlan, H., & Lumley, J. (2004). Incidence of breast abscess in lactating women: Report from an Australian cohort. *BJOG: An International Journal of Obstetrics and Gynaecology, 111*, 1378–1381.

Anderson, P. O., & Valdes, V. (2007). A critical review of pharmaceutical galactagogues. *Breastfeeding Medicine, 2*, 229–242.

Ballard, J. L., Auer, C. E., & Khoury, J. C. (2002). Ankyloglossia: Assessment, incidence, and the effect of frenuloplasty on the breastfeeding dyad. *Pediatrics, 110*, e63.

Beaino, G., Khoshnood, B., Kaminski, M., Marret, S., Pierrat, V., Vieux, R., . . . Ancel, P. Y., EPIPAGE Study Group. (2011). Predictors of the risk of cognitive deficiency in very preterm infants: The EPIPAGE prospective cohort. *Acta Paediatrica, 100*, 370–378.

Berens, P., Swaim, L., & Peterson, B. (2010). Incidence of methicillin-resistant *Staphylococcus aureus* in postpartum breast abscesses. *Breastfeeding Medicine, 5*, 113–115.

Betzold, C. M. (2005). Infections of the mammary ducts in the breastfeeding mother. *The Journal for Nurse Practitioners, 1*, 15–21.

Betzold, C. M. (2007). An update on the recognition and management of lactational breast inflammation. *Journal of Midwifery & Women's Health, 5*, 595–605.

Bouchet-Horwitz, J. (2011). The use of Supple Cups for flat, retracting, and inverted nipples. *Clinical Lactation, 2*, 30–33.

Bowles, B. C., Stutte, P. C., & Hensley, J. (1987–1988). Alternate breast massage: New benefits from an old technique. *Genesis (New York, N.Y.: 2000), 9*, 5–9.

Budd, S. C., Erdman, S. H., Long, D. M., Trombley, S. K., & Udall, J. N. (1993). Improved lactation with metoclopramide: A case report. *Clinical Pediatrics, 32*, 53–57.

Campbell, S. H. (2006). Recurrent plugged ducts. *Journal of Human Lactation, 22*, 340–343.

Claud, E. C., & Walker, W. A. (2001). Hypothesis: Inappropriate colonization of the premature intestine can cause neonatal necrotizing enterocolitis. *The FASEB Journal, 15*, 1398–1403.

Clavey, S. (1996). The use of acupuncture for the treatment of insufficient lactation (Que Ru). *American Journal of Acupuncture, 24*, 35–46.

Cotterman, K. J. (2004). Reverse pressure softening: A simple tool to prepare areola for easier latching during engorgement. *Journal of Human Lactation, 20*, 227–237.

da Silva, O. P., Knoppert, D. C., Angelini, M. M., & Forret, P. A. (2001). Effect of domperidone on milk production in mothers of premature newborns: A randomized, double-blind, placebo-controlled trial. *CMAJ, 164*, 17–21.

Di Pierro, F., Callegari, A., Carotenuto, D., & Tapia, M. M. (2008). Clinical efficacy, safety and tolerability of BIO-C (micronized Silymarin) as a galactogogue. *Acta Bio-medica: Atenei Parmensis, 79*, 205–210.

Eglash, A. (1998). Delayed milk ejection reflex and plugged ducts: Lecithin therapy. *ABM News and Views, 4*(1), 4.

Evans, K. C., Evans, R. G., Royal, R., Esterman, A. J., & James, S. L. (2003). Effect of caesarean section on breast milk transfer to the normal term newborn over the first week of life. *Archives of Disease in Childhood. Fetal and Neonatal Edition, 88*, F380–F382.

Forlenza, G. P., Paradise Black, N. M., McNamara, E. G., & Sullivan, S. E. (2010). Ankyloglossia, exclusive breastfeeding, and failure to thrive. *Pediatrics, 125*, e1500–e1504.

Gabay, M. P. (2002). Galactogogues: Medications that induce lactation. *Journal of Human Lactation, 18*, 274–279.

Gatti, L. (2008). Maternal perceptions of insufficient milk supply in breastfeeding. *Journal of Nursing Scholarship, 40*, 355–363.

Geddes, D. T., Langton, D. B., Gollow, I., Jacobs, L. A., Hartmann, P. E., & Simmer, K. (2008). Frenulotomy for breastfeeding infants with ankyloglossia: Effect on milk removal and sucking mechanism as imaged by ultrasound. *Pediatrics, 122*, e188–e194.

Hall, R. T., Mercer, A. M., Teasley, S. L., McPherson, D. M., Simon, S. D., Santos, S. R., . . . Hipsh, N. E. (2002). A breastfeeding assessment score to evaluate the risk for cessation of breastfeeding by 7 to 10 days of age. *The Journal of Pediatrics, 141*, 659–664.

Henderson, A. (2003). Domperidone: Discovering new choices for lactating mothers. *AWHONN Lifelines, 7*, 55–60.

Hoover, K. L., Barbalinardo, L. H., & Platia, M. P. (2002). Delayed lactogenesis II secondary to gestational ovarian theca lutein cysts in two normal singleton pregnancies. *Journal of Human Lactation, 18,* 264–268.

Horwood, L. J., Darlow, B. A., & Mogridge, N. (2001). Breast milk feeding and cognitive ability at 7–8 years. *Archives of Disease in Childhood. Fetal and Neonatal Edition, 84,* F23–F27.

Hung, K. J., & Berg, O. (2011). Early skin-to-skin after cesarean to improve breastfeeding. *MCN. the American Journal of Maternal Child Nursing, 36,* 318–324; quiz 325–326.

Hurst, N. M., Valentine, C. J., Renfro, L., Burns, P., & Ferlic, L. (1997). Skin-to-skin holding in the neonatal intensive care unit influences maternal milk volume. *Journal of Perinatology, 17,* 213.

Iffrig, M. C. (1968). Nursing care and success in breastfeeding. *The Nursing Clinics of North America, 3,* 345–354.

Jansson, L., Velez, M., & Harrow, C. (2004). Methadone maintenance and lactation: A review of the literature and current management guidelines. *Journal of Human Lactation, 20,* 62–71.

Jordan, A. E., Jackson, G. L., Deardorff, D., Shivakumar, G., McIntire, D. D., & Dashe, J. S. (2008). Serotonin reuptake inhibitor use in pregnancy and the neonatal behavioral syndrome. *The Journal of Maternal-Fetal & Neonatal Medicine, 21,* 745–751.

Kesaree, N., Banapurmath, C. R., Banapurmath, S., & Shamanur, K. (1993). Treatment of inverted nipples using a disposable syringe. *Journal of Human Lactation, 9,* 27–29.

Kinlay, J. R., O'Connell, D. L., & Kinlay, S. (2001). Risk factors for mastitis in breastfeeding women: Results of a prospective cohort study. *Australian and New Zealand Journal of Public Health, 25,* 115–120.

Law, K. L., Stroud, L. R., LaGrasse, L. L., Niaura, R., Liu, J., & Lester, B. M. (2003). Smoking during pregnancy and newborn neurobehavior. *Pediatrics, 111,* 1318–1323.

Lawrence, R. A., & Lawrence, R. M. (2010). *Breastfeeding: A guide for the medical profession* (7th ed.). Maryland Heights, MO: Elsevier Mosby.

Livingstone, V. H., Willis, C., & Berkowitz, J. (1996). *Staphylococcus aureus* and sore nipples. *Canadian Family Physician, 42,* 654–659.

Mahmood, I., Jamal, M., & Khan, N. (2011). Effect of mother-infant early skin-to-skin contact on breastfeeding status: A randomized controlled trial. *Journal of the College of Physicians and Surgeons–Pakistan, 21,* 601–605.

Marchini, G., & Linden, A. (1992). Cholecystokinin, a satiety signal in newborn infants? *Journal of Developmental Physiology, 17,* 215–219.

Marchini, G., Simoni, M. R., Bartolini, F., & Linden, A. (1993). The relationship of plasma cholecystokinin levels to different feeding routines in newborn infants. *Early Human Development, 35,* 31–35.

Marquis, G. S., Penny, M. E., Diaz, J. M., & Marin, R. M. (2002). Postpartum consequences of an overlap of breastfeeding and pregnancy: Reduced breast milk intake and growth during early infancy. *Pediatrics, 109,* e56.

MAIN Trial Collaborative Group. (1994). Preparing for breastfeeding: Treatment of inverted and non-protractile nipples in pregnancy. *Midwifery, 10,* 200–214.

McGeorge, D. D. (1994). The "Niplette": An instrument for the nonsurgical correction of inverted nipples. *British Journal of Plastic Surgery, 47,* 46–49.

Meier, P. P., Furman, L. M., & Degenhardt, M. (2007). Increased lactation risk for late preterm infants and mothers: Evidence and management strategies to protect breastfeeding. *Journal of Midwifery and Women's Health, 52,* 579–587.

Meinzen-Derr, J., Poindexter, B., Wrage, L., Morrow, A. L., Stoll, B., & Donovan, E. F. (2009). Role of human milk in extremely low birth weight infants' risk of necrotizing enterocolitis or death. *Journal of Perinatology, 29,* 57–62.

Morales, Y., & Schanler, R. J. (2007). Human milk and clinical outcomes in VLBW infants: How compelling is the evidence of benefit? *Seminars in Perinatology, 31,* 83–88.

Morland-Schultz, K., & Hill, P. D. (2005). Prevention of and therapies for nipple pain: A systematic review. *Journal of Obstetric, Gynecologic, and Neonatal Nursing, 34,* 428–437.

Morton, J., Hall, J. Y., Wong, R. J., Thairu, L., Benitz, W. E., & Rhine, W. D. (2009). Combining hand techniques with electric pumping increases milk production in mothers of preterm infants. *Journal of Perinatology, 29,* 757–764.

Powers, N. G. (2010). Low intake in the breastfed infant: Maternal and infant considerations. In J. Riordan & K. Wambach (Eds.), *Breastfeeding and human lactation* (4th ed.). Sudbury, MA: Jones and Bartlett.

Roberts, K. L. (1995). A comparison of chilled cabbage leaves and chilled gelpaks in reducing breast engorgement. *Journal of Human Lactation, 11,* 17–20.

Robson, B. A. (1990). *Breast engorgement in breastfeeding women* (PhD dissertation). Case Western Reserve University, Cleveland, OH.

Sacco, L. M., Caulfield, L. E., Gittelsohn, J., & Martinez, H. (2006). The conceptualization of perceived insufficient milk among Mexican mothers. *Journal of Human Lactation, 22,* 277–286.

Sandberg, C. A. (1998). *Cold therapy for breast engorgement in new mothers who are breastfeeding* (Master's thesis). College of St. Catherine, St. Paul, MN.

Schanler, R. J. (2007). Mother's own milk, donor human milk, and preterm formulas in the feeding of extremely premature infants. *Journal of Pediatric Gastroenterology and Nutrition, 45*(Suppl. 3), S175–S177.

Smillie, C. M. (2004). The prevention and treatment of plugged ducts. Clinical handout. Stratford, CT: Breastfeeding Resources.

Spencer, J. P. (2008). Management of mastitis in breastfeeding women. *American Family Physician, 7,* 727–731.

Stafford, I., Hernandez, J., Laibl, V., Sheffield, J., Roberts, S., & Wendel, G., Jr. (2008). Community-acquired methicillin-resistant *Staphylococcus aureus* among patients with puerperal mastitis requiring hospitalization. *Obstetrics and Gynecology, 112,* 533–537.

Stutte, P. C., Bowles, B. C., & Morman, G. Y. (1988). The effects of breast massage on volume and fat content of human milk. *Genesis (New York, N.Y.: 2000), 10,* 22–25.

Tarcan, A., Gurakan, B., Tiker, F., & Ozbek, N. (2004). Influence of feeding formula and breast milk fortifier on lymphocyte subsets in very low birth weight premature newborns. *Biology of the Neonate, 86,* 22–28.

Taylor, S. N., Basile, L. A., Ebeling, M., & Wagner, C. L. (2009). Intestinal permeability in preterm infants by feeding type: Mother's milk versus formula. *Breastfeeding Medicine, 4,* 11–15.

Turkyilmaz, C., Onal, E., Hirfanoglu, I. M., Turan, O., Koç, E., Ergenekon, E., & Atalay, Y. (2011). The effect of galactagogue herbal tea on breast milk production and short-term catch-up of birth weight in the first week of life. *Journal of Alternative and Complementary Medicine (New York, N.Y.), 17,* 139–142.

Uvnas-Moberg, K., Widstrom, A. M., Marchini, G., & Winberg, J. (1987). Release of GI hormones in mother and infant by sensory stimulation. *Acta Paediatrica Scandinavica, 76,* 851–860.

Vohr, B. R., Poindexter, B. B., Dusick, A. M., McKinley, L. T., Wright, L. L., Langer, J. C., . . . NICHD Neonatal Research Network. (2006). Beneficial effects of breast milk in the neonatal intensive care unit on the developmental outcome of extremely low birth weight infants at 18 months of age. *Pediatrics, 118*, e115–e123.

Walker, M. (2004). Mastitis in Lactating Women. Unit 2/Lactation Consultant Series Two. Schaumburg, IL: La Leche League International.

Walker, M. (2008). Breastfeeding the late preterm infant. *Journal of Obstetric, Gynecologic, and Neonatal Nursing, 37*, 692–701.

Walker, M. (2010). *The nipple and areola in breastfeeding and lactation.* Amarillo, TX: Hale Publishing.

Wan, E. W., Davey, K., Page-Sharp, M., Hartmann, P. E., Simmer, K., & Ilett, K. F. (2008). Dose-effect study of domperidone as a galactogue in preterm mothers with insufficient milk supply, and its transfer into milk. *British Journal of Clinical Pharmacology, 66*, 283–289.

Wei, L., Wang, H., Han, Y., & Li, C. (2008). Clinical observation on the effects of electroacupuncture at Shaoze (SI 1) in 46 cases of postpartum insufficient lactation. *Journal of Traditional Chinese Medicine, 28*, 168–172.

Weiss, R. F. (2001). *Weiss's herbal medicine* (classic ed.). New York: Thieme.

Wilson-Clay, B., & Hoover, K. (2008). *The breastfeeding Atlas* (4th ed.). Austin, TX: LactNews Press.

Zhao, Y., & Guo, H. (2006). The therapeutic effects of acupuncture in 30 cases of postpartum hypogalactia. *Journal of Traditional Chinese Medicine, 26*, 29–30.

Zuppa, A. A., Sindico, P., Orchi, C., Carducci, C., Cardiello, V., & Romagnoli, C. (2010). Safety and efficacy of galactogogues: Substances that induce, maintain and increase breast milk production. *Journal of Pharmacy and Pharmaceutical Sciences: A Publication of the Canadian Society for Pharmaceutical Sciences, Societe Canadienne Des Sciences Pharmaceutiques, 13*, 162–174.

Part V

Management of common health problems during the prenatal and postnatal periods

32

Respiratory disorders

Janyce Cagan Agruss

Relevant terms

FEV$_1$—volume of air that can forcibly be blown out in 1 second after full inspiration

Inspiratory capacity—the total amount of air that can be drawn into the lungs after normal expiration

Peak expiratory flow rate—the maximum airflow during forced expiration beginning with the lungs fully inflated

Peak-flow meters—portable device that measures air flow or peak expiratory flow rate

Persistent asthma—asthma symptoms at least 2 days a week or 2 nights a month

Residual volume—the volume of air remaining in the lungs after a maximal expiratory effort

Total lung capacity—the maximum volume to which the lungs can be expanded with the greatest possible inspiratory effort

Introduction

When women are pregnant, they are not immune from experiencing some of the more common respiratory disorders such as asthma, pneumonia, and upper respiratory infections (URIs) or colds. This chapter will discuss the management of these common respiratory disorders in pregnancy.

Respiratory physiology and pregnancy

As the uterus enlarges, the level of the diaphragm gradually elevates to about a peak of 4 cm peaking at approximately 37 weeks' gestation. The anterior-posterior and transverse diameter of the thorax and chest circumference increase and the subcostal angle widens. These changes allow lung volume and inspiratory capacity to increase by about 5–10% as the pregnancy progresses. This adaptation assists in preserving total lung capacity throughout the pregnancy as the lungs become displaced by the enlarging uterus.

During pregnancy, the increased level of progesterone resets the hypothalamus to accept a lower level of blood carbon dioxide (PCO$_2$) at closer to 32 mmHg rather than 40 mmHg. This change favors transfer of carbon dioxide from the fetus (higher PCO$_2$) to the mother (lower PCO$_2$). To prevent the fetal transfer from increasing her blood pH levels and causing acidosis, a mild hyperventilation to blow off excess CO$_2$ begins in early pregnancy. The cumulative effect of these changes is often experienced by the pregnant woman as a feeling of being short of breath even without exertion. Women should be informed of these changes and reassured that this sensation is a normal and expected change in pregnancy.

Asthma

Asthma is a chronic inflammatory airway disease characterized by increased reactions of airway inflammation and bronchoconstriction to multiple stimuli such as allergens, irritants, stress, and physical exertion. Symptoms are wheezing, coughing that may worsen at night, chest tightness, and shortness of breath. Asthma is an episodic disease with acute attacks separated by symptom-free periods. Asthma is the most common lung disease in pregnancy with prevalence in pregnant

Prenatal and Postnatal Care: A Woman-Centered Approach, First Edition. Edited by Robin G. Jordan, Janet L. Engstrom, Julie A. Marfell, and Cindy L. Farley.
© 2014 John Wiley & Sons, Inc. Published 2014 by John Wiley & Sons, Inc.

women of approximately 4–8% (Kwon, Triche, Belanger, & Bracken, 2006).

Potential problems

Many women who have asthma find that it actually improves in early pregnancy, and many find that it stays the same. Well-controlled asthma is not associated with significant risk to the mother or the fetus. For about one in three pregnant women, the changes of pregnancy will make their asthma worse (American College of Obstetricians and Gynecologists (ACOG), 2008). Uncontrolled asthma can lead to maternal complications such as hypertension, preeclampsia, preterm labor and birth, and rarely, death. Fetal complications of severe asthma include increased risk of stillbirth, fetal growth restriction (FGR), premature birth, and low birth weight (Dombrowski & Schatz, 2010; Murphy & Gibson, 2011; Murphy et al., 2011). The magnitude of perinatal risk is related to the severity of maternal asthma.

Differential diagnosis

The diagnosis of asthma during pregnancy in a woman without a prior history can be challenging. Other causes of cough and wheezing that can respond to asthma management therapies, such as reactive airway disease, URIs, pneumonia, or gastroesophageal reflux disease can lead to an assumption of asthma as the etiology. Asthma is a disease that can be diagnosed over time after multiple, chronic respiratory events. Pulmonary function testing (PFT) to diagnose asthma is often not done during pregnancy as complications can include hyperventilation or precipitation of an asthmatic episode, unless the provider feels the information gained will guide treatment options.

Common clinical presentation and data gathering

The woman with asthma is typically identified during the initial prenatal visit interview. Some women will report a history of asthma that goes back to childhood and others will report adult onset. The presentation of asthma is the same in the pregnant woman as in the nonpregnant woman. A thorough history includes asthma triggers, symptom characteristics, and medications used currently or in the past for symptom relief.

The physical examination begins with observation to evaluate breathing effort. Auscultation to assess breath sounds should be done in a quiet room and the woman seated comfortably.

For women with moderate to severe asthma, evaluation of respiratory function is recommended at the time of initial prenatal visit and periodically during prenatal visits depending on the course of asthma symptoms

---

> **Common asthma triggers**
>
> - Emotional stress
> - Exercise or physical exertion
> - Animal dander
> - Cigarette smoke, wood smoke, air pollution
> - Pollens
> - Dust mites, cockroach antigen
> - Molds
> - Cold air
> - URI
> - Sulfites in foods
> - Certain medications (aspirin [ASA], nonsteroidal anti-inflammatory drugs [NSAIDs], beta-blockers)

---

during the prenatal period. Measurement of peak expiratory flow (PEF) with a peak flow meter is generally sufficient (National Asthma Education and Prevention Program Working Group (NAEPP), 2005); however, the history of each woman's asthma severity history and possible collaboration with the woman's primary care provider should guide testing recommendations.

Management of asthma during pregnancy

Controlling asthma during pregnancy is a priority to ensure the well-being of both the mother and the developing fetus. The main goal of treatment is to prevent hypoxic episodes in the mother that can cause oxygenation deprivation in the fetus.

Pharmaceutical asthma management

Most pregnant women with asthma can continue using the same medications they used prior to becoming pregnant since the vast majority of asthma medications are safe to use during pregnancy and breastfeeding. Pregnant women have concerns about using medications during pregnancy, and undertreatment of asthma during pregnancy is common (Rey & Boulet, 2007). Women should be informed that it is safer to be treated with asthma medications than to have asthma symptoms and exacerbations (ACOG, 2008). The choice of medication is dependent upon asthma severity. Pregnant women should continue to use their asthma medication in the lowest dose possible to manage symptoms during pregnancy (ACOG, 2008).

Inhaled beta-adrenergic agonists remain the mainstay of treating exacerbations and handling mild forms of asthma in pregnant as well as nonpregnant women. Albuterol is preferred during pregnancy as it has the most well-documented safety record for use in pregnancy

Table 32.1   Medications for Asthma

Step	Step 1	Step 2	Step 3	Step 4
Severity	Mild intermittent asthma	Mild persistent asthma	Moderate intermittent asthma	Severe persistent asthma
Medication	Short-acting inhaled beta$_2$-agonists as needed	Daily low-dose inhaled corticosteroid	1. Daily low-dose inhaled corticosteroid and long-acting inhaled beta$_2$-agonists as needed or 2. Increasing dose of inhaled corticosteroids to medium-dose range	Increase inhaled corticosteroids and addition of oral corticosteroid considered
Preferred medication	Albuterol	Budesonide		

Source: ACOG (2008).

(ACOG, 2008). For moderate-persistent asthma, a beta-adrenergic agonist combined with an inhaled anti-inflammatory agent or inhaled corticosteroid is recommended for treatment (Table 32.1). The inhaled corticosteroids are used to prevent acute asthma attacks. All medication therapy should be tailored to provide pregnant women with the lowest dose necessary to control their asthma.

The stepwise approach to medication use is advocated by the National Heart, Lung and Blood Institute (NHLIB, 2004). The severity of the asthma is classified and corresponding medication plans initiated. The preferred medications listed in Table 32.1 have more pregnancy-use data available than other asthma medications and safety is better established. Other medications may be used safely during pregnancy, especially if women were well controlled by the agents prior to pregnancy (NHLIB, 2004).

This stepwise approach to medication use allows for the dose, administration frequency, and number of medications to increase when needed and to decrease when possible.

Environmental asthma management

Control of environmental asthma triggers is an essential component of asthma management. The health-care provider and the woman should discuss asthma triggers and how to avoid them. Reducing proliferation of indoor allergens can be helpful for women who may not be aware of sources of allergens that may trigger asthma exacerbation.

Smoking cessation

Pregnant women with a history of asthma who also smoke should be counseled on the importance of smoking cessation. In addition to increasing maternal and fetal morbidity (see Chapter 13, "Substance Use during Pregnancy"), smoking predisposes the pregnant

Reducing exposure to indoor allergens

- Keep humidity <50% to reduce dust mites.
- Use covers for mattresses, pillows, comforters, and furniture cushions.
- Reduce sources of animal dander as much as possible.
- Dust and vacuum frequently using vacuum with a high-efficiency air (HEPA) filter.
- Use cockroach traps to reduce infestation and allergen source.
- Identify and remediate household mold.
- Eliminate household smoking.
- Avoid the use of wood stove heaters.

woman to worsening asthma and the potential for increased medication use. The perinatal morbidity of poorly controlled asthma is compounded by smoking during pregnancy, leading to an even higher risk of FGR and preterm birth (Schatz, Zeiger, & Hoffman, 1990).

Educating women about asthma management and how it relates to pregnancy can help women control their symptoms. Asking women to monitor their "personal best" as needed with a peak flow meter can also assist the health-care provider in monitoring asthma status during pregnancy.

Asthma control

1. Minimal or no chronic symptoms day or night
2. Minimal or no exacerbations
3. No limitations on activities
4. Maintenance of (near) normal pulmonary function
5. Minimal use of short-acting inhaled beta$_2$-agonist
6. Minimal or no adverse effects from medications

Source: NHLBI, Managing Asthma during Pregnancy (2004).

Women with asthma should be counseled to start rescue therapy at home if they experience symptoms of asthma flare-up, such as coughing, chest tightness, wheezing, shortness of breath, or labored breathing (ACOG, 2008). The algorithm in Figure 32.1 can be used during pregnancy and the postpartum period and in women who are breastfeeding.

Scope of practice considerations

Women with severe or poorly controlled asthma face higher perinatal risks and should be referred to a physician for surveillance and medication management. A first-trimester ultrasound is often done for women with severe asthma to corroborate pregnancy dating due to

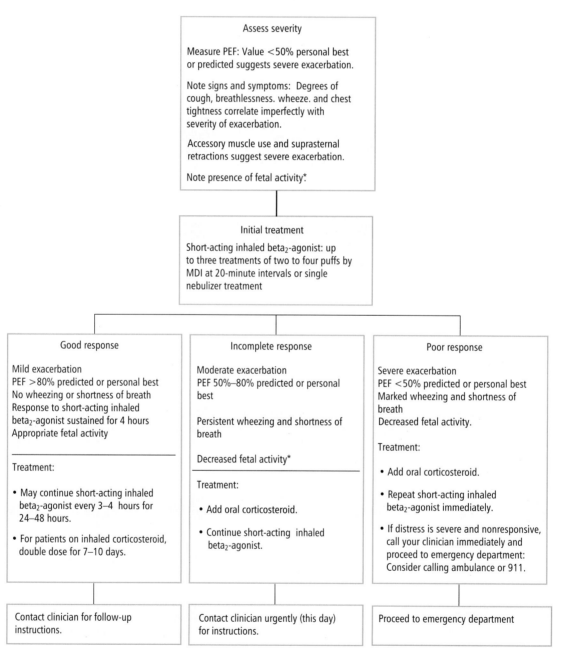

Figure 32.1. Management of asthma exacerbations during pregnancy and lactation: home treatment. MDI, metered-dose inhaler; PEF, peak expiratory flow. *Fetal activity is monitored by observing whether fetal kick counts decrease over time. From NAEPP (2005).

the risk for preterm birth and FGR. Pregnant women with persistent or severe asthma, those with suboptimal asthma control, and those recovering from a severe asthma exacerbation should have periodic ultrasound evaluation for fetal growth in the third trimester (ACOG, 2008; NAEPP, 2005).

Influenza

Influenza is a seasonal contagious respiratory illness that can range from mild to severe. Influenza viruses are spread from person to person primarily through large-particle respiratory droplet transmission. The typical incubation period for influenza is 1–4 days (Centers for Disease Control and Prevention (CDC), 2012). Pregnant women who contract influenza are at an increased risk of developing severe illness, of being hospitalized with acute respiratory disease, and death from influenza than the general population (CDC, 2011). The increased severity of influenza in pregnancy is believed to be related to physiological changes in pregnancy. Pregnancy changes in the cardiovascular and respiratory systems result in increased heart rate and oxygen consumption and decreased lung capacity. Immunologic alterations result in a shift away from cell-mediated immunity, predisposing pregnant women to increased susceptibility to infection and increased illness severity (Jamison, Theiler, & Rasmussen, 2006).

The fetal effects of maternal influenza infection have not been well studied, and some evidence suggests an increase in adverse perinatal outcome such as early pregnancy loss, preterm birth, cesarean birth, and small for gestational age (SGA) (CDC, 2011; Mosby, Rasmussen, & Jamieson, 2011). Adverse fetal effects may be related to maternal fever and hyperthermia. Pregnant women with fever should be promptly treated with acetaminophen.

Clinical signs and symptoms of influenza are the same in pregnant women as in the general population and include fever, chills, cough, rhinorrhea, sore throat, headache, and myalgia. Rapid influenza diagnostic tests either have low sensitivity or take time to provide results (CDC, 2012). Since it is critical to initiate appropriate treatment promptly in pregnant women, the diagnosis of influenza should be made clinically, without waiting for results from diagnostic testing. Treatment consists of symptomatic care and influenza antiviral medications as soon as possible after symptoms are reported. These medications can reduce the severity of illness. Available data suggest no adverse fetal effects from antiviral medications; however, the number of women studied is low (Greer et al., 2010).

Influenza Treatment

Antipyretics	Acetaminophen
Antiviral medication	Oseltamivir—75 mg BID for 5 days Zanamivor—10 mg (two inhalations) for 5 days
Symptomatic relief measures	Increased fluids Increased rest
Infection control	Isolation from other family members Frequent hand washing Household disinfectants used on bedside tables, doorknobs, telephones, and bathrooms while household member is sick

Pregnant women with suspected influenza should be advised to seek emergency care immediately if symptoms such as difficulty breathing, sudden dizziness, confusion, persistent vomiting, or fever not controlled with acetaminophen occur.

During flu season, office settings should have policy measures in place to ensure appropriate triage and care of pregnant women with suspected influenza. Women should be advised of the signs and symptoms of flu and to report them immediately to their health-care provider. Rapid access to telephone consultation should be available. Empiric treatment based on telephone consultation can be considered to facilitate rapid treatment, assuming that hospitalization is not indicated for the woman. In outpatient settings, women should be screened for respiratory symptoms at the front desk and directed to separate waiting areas if they are symptomatic to reduce exposure to others.

Pregnant women should receive the trivalent inactivated influenza vaccine (TIV) as soon as the vaccine is available in the fall. It is safe during any time in gestation. Breastfeeding is not a contraindication for either the live or inactivated influenza immunization (American Academy of Pediatrics, 2012).

Upper respiratory infection

The clinical features, diagnosis, and management of respiratory infections are generally similar in pregnant and nonpregnant populations. Changes in susceptibility to infection, maternal physiology, and the effect of the infection and its treatment on the fetus are considerations in the evaluation and management of pregnant women with URI. URIs are typically caused by viruses

Table 32.2   Common Treatments for the Common Cold

Cough suppressants	Dextromethorphan (Robitussin, Vicks 44 Cough Relief, Delsym)
Decongestants Oral Nasal	Pseudoephedrine after the first trimester (Sudafed) Phenylephrine (Neo-Synephrine) Short-acting phenylephrine (Neo-Synephrine 4-Hour) Long-acting phenylephrine (Afrin spray)
Antihistamines	Diphenhydramine (Benadryl) Chlorpheniramine (Chlor-Trimeton)
Expectorant	Guaifenesin
Nasal corticosteroids	Intranasal cromolyn sodium (NasalCrom)
Symptom relief measures	Increased humidification Increased rest Increased fluids Chicken soup

Source: Manns-James (2011).

and include the common cold, otitis media, sinusitis, and pharyngitis, bronchitis, and pneumonia.

URIs are self-limiting and over-the-counter medications for symptom relief are often all that is required. Antibiotics are not indicated for treatment of the common cold, except in the small subset of patients (less than 2%) with evidence of secondary bacterial sinus infection (Fokkens, Lund, & Mullol, 2007). Analgesics, cough suppressants, decongestants, antihistamines, and expectorants are the most commonly requested over-the-counter medications for relief of cold symptoms. Analgesics such as acetaminophen and ibuprofen are well tolerated and have an excellent safety profile. Non-steroidal anti-inflammatory medication, however, should be avoided in the third trimester as it has been associated with premature ductus arteriosus closure (Erebara, Bozzo, Einarson, & Koren, 2008; Koren, Florescu, Costei, Boskovic, & Moretti, 2006). Cough suppressants, decongestants, antihistamines, and expectorants are all acceptable for short-term use during pregnancy (Erebara et al., 2008) (Table 32.2). Women should be instructed to read the labels of the over-the-counter-medication to avoid products containing alcohol. Single ingredient rather than "multisymptom" medications can be encouraged to avoid unnecessary overmedication. Women with the common cold should be reassured that their symptoms will generally resolve within 3–10 days, although the cough may persist for longer.

Pregnant women with the common cold are at an increased risk of developing sinusitis and otitis media, which has been attributed to congestion from hormonal effects on the nasal mucosa. These women should be evaluated for the need for antibiotics and treated with over-the-counter medications for symptom relief. Pregnant women with any of the following characteristics should generally be given antibiotics: (1) persistent symptoms for 10 days without improvement, (2) severe symptoms or temperature >102.2 for 3–4 days, or (3) worsening symptoms after 5–6 days of improving symptoms (Hickner et al., 2001).

If an antibiotic is required, the medication should be chosen based on coverage of the probable organism, community resistance, and pregnancy category. Acute sinusitis during pregnancy can be treated with amoxicillin-clavulanate (Augmentin) and cefprozil (Cefzil), among others. Additional treatments should include saline nasal spray or saline nasal irrigation. Short-term nasal corticosteroids (beclomethasone) may be initiated in women with rhinitis or sinusitis in need of immediate symptom relief. Intranasal cromolyn sodium improves symptoms of a runny nose and sneezing and has been used safely in pregnancy (Manns-James, 2011). A strep screen is advised for pregnant women who present with symptoms of pharyngitis, and treatment with penicillin, erythromycin, or azithromycin initiated in women with a positive diagnosis.

Bronchitis is a URI of the large airways and manifests as cough that can persist for 10–20 days. As with most URIs, it is caused by a virus and antibiotic therapy is not indicated. Bronchitis can lead to pneumonia; therefore, women whose symptoms worsen or persist should be reevaluated. Pregnant woman are advised to return for follow-up if there is no resolution of symptoms 2–3 days after the start of antibiotic therapy or if symptoms worsen.

Pneumonia

The incidence, clinical manifestations, and diagnosis of pneumonia in pregnancy are the same as in the general population. The classic symptoms of pneumonia are sudden onset of shaking chills, shortness of breath, and cough productive of purulent sputum, though symptom presentation varies. Pneumonia can occur independently or may follow viral URIs such as influenza, bronchitis, or a common cold. *Streptococcus pneumoniae* and *Haemophilus influenzae* are the most common pathogens that cause pneumonia in pregnant women. Chest X-ray is warranted in any woman suspected of having pneumonia during pregnancy. Pregnant women with pneumonia are at risk for preterm birth and pulmonary

Case study

Tiffany is a 29-year-old primigravida and is currently at 21 weeks of gestation. She is vacationing away from her home state over the New Year holiday when she experiences symptoms of fever, chills, body aches, cough, and a runny nose. The day after her symptoms start, she visits an urgent care center to seek help for her symptoms and to check on her baby. Her temperature is 99.8°F, heart rate is 104 per minute, respirations are 18 per minute, and blood pressure is 98/72. Nasal exam indicates red swollen mucosa with copious clear discharge. Examination of the oropharynx reveals reddened mucosa without exudates. Auscultation of the lungs reveals normal breath sounds in all fields. Examination of the abdomen reveals that the uterine fundus can be palpated at the level of the umbilicus and the fundal height measures 21.5 cm. Fetal heart sounds are heard at a rate of 150 per minute. Tiffany reports feeling regular fetal movement.

The nurse practitioner makes a probable diagnosis of influenza. She recommends that Tiffany take two tablets of acetaminophen 325 mg every 4–6 hours until her fever resolves. The importance of resting and consuming adequate fluids such as water, decaffeinated teas, and juices was emphasized. The nurse practitioner also recommends a course of antiviral therapy (oseltamivir 75 mg twice a day for 5 days) to be started immediately because of the increased maternal and perinatal morbidity and mortality associated with influenza. Tiffany is also given detailed instructions about the signs and symptoms of influenza complications. The instructions include a clear warning that Tiffany should proceed promptly to a hospital emergency department if she experiences difficulty breathing; chest pain or pressure, abdominal pain, vomiting, sudden dizziness, or mental confusion.

edema (Bánhidy, Acs, Puhó, & Czeizel, 2008) and consultation or referral for medical management should be initiated.

Summary

Common respiratory disorders include asthma, influenza, URIs, and pneumonia. Pregnant women who contract influenza are at an increased risk of developing severe illness, of being hospitalized with acute respiratory disease, and death from influenza than the general population (CDC, 2011). There is some evidence to suggest influenza during pregnancy may increase adverse perinatal outcome such as early pregnancy loss, preterm birth, cesarean birth, and SGA (CDC, 2011; Mosby et al., 2011). Pregnant women should receive TIV as soon as it becomes available in the fall in an effort to prevent influenza. Women diagnosed with pneumonia during pregnancy are at risk for preterm birth and pulmonary edema (Bánhidy et al., 2008) and consultation or referral for medical management should be initiated. Women with severe or poorly controlled asthma face higher perinatal risks and should be referred for physician management for surveillance and medication management.

Resource for health-care providers

From the National Institutes of Health and Human Services, National Heart Lung and Blood Institute: Managing Asthma during Pregnancy and Lactation:

Recommendations for Pharmacologic Treatment (2005): http://www.nhlbi.nih.gov/health/prof/lung/asthma/astpreg/astpreg_qr.pdf (quick reference); http://www.nhlbi.nih.gov/health/prof/lung/asthma/astpreg/astpreg_full.pdf (full text)

References

American Academy of Pediatrics. (2012). Influenza. In L. K. Pickering, C. J. Baker, D. W. Kimberlin, & S. S. Long (Eds.), *Red book: 2012 report of the committee on infectious diseases* (pp. 439–453). Elk Grove Village, IL: American Academy of Pediatrics.

American College of Obstetricians and Gynecologists (ACOG). (2008). Asthma in pregnancy: ACOG Practice Bulletin. *Obstetrics and Gynecology, 111*, 457–464.

Bánhidy, F., Acs, N., Puhó, E. H., & Czeizel, A. E. (2008). Maternal acute respiratory infectious diseases during pregnancy and birth outcomes. *European Journal of Epidemiology, 23*(1), 29–35. Epub 2007 Nov 20.

Centers for Disease Control and Prevention (CDC). (2011). Maternal and infant outcomes among severely ill pregnant and postpartum women with 2009 pandemic influenza A (H1N1)—United States, April 2009–August 2010. Centers for Disease Control and Prevention (CDC). *MMWR. Morbidity and Mortality Weekly Report, 60*(35), 1193.

Centers for Disease Control and Prevention (CDC). (2012). Evaluation of rapid influenza diagnostic tests for influenza A (H3N2)v virus and updated case count—United States, 2012. *MMWR. Morbidity and Mortality Weekly Report, 61*(32), 619.

Dombrowski, M., & Schatz, M. (2010). Asthma in pregnancy. *Clinical Obstetrics and Gynecology, 53*(2), 301–310.

Erebara, A., Bozzo, P., Einarson, A., & Koren, G. (2008). Treating the common cold during pregnancy. *Canadian Family Physician, 54*, 687–689.

Fokkens, W., Lund, V., & Mullol, J. (2007). European position paper on rhinosinusitis and nasal polyps group. A summary for otorhinolaryngologists. *Rhinology*, *45*(2), 97.

Greer, L. G., Sheffield, J. S., Rogers, V. L., Roberts, S. W., McIntire, D. D., & Wendel, G. D., Jr. (2010). Maternal and neonatal outcomes after antepartum treatment of influenza with antiviral medications. *Obstetrics and Gynecology*, *115*(4), 711.

Hickner, J. M., Bartlett, J. G., Besser, R. E., Gonzales, R., Hoffman, J. R., Sande, M. A., & American Academy of Family Physicians, American College of Physicians-American Society of Internal Medicine, Centers for Disease Control, Infectious Diseases Society of America. (2001). Principles of appropriate antibiotic use for acute rhinosinusitis in adults: Background. *Annals of Internal Medicine*, *134*(6), 498.

Jamison, D. J., Theiler, R. N., & Rasmussen, S. A. (2006). Emerging infections and pregnancy. *Emerging Infectious Diseases*, *12*(11), 1638–1643. Retrieved from http://www.nc.cdc.gov/eid/article/12/11/pdfs/06-0152.pdf

Koren, G., Florescu, A., Costei, A. M., Boskovic, R., & Moretti, M. E. (2006). Nonsteroidal anti-inflammatory drugs during third trimester and the risk of premature closure of the ductus arteriosus: A meta-analysis. *The Annals of Pharmacotherapy*, *40*(5), 824–829.

Kwon, H. L., Triche, E. W., Belanger, K., & Bracken, M. B. (2006). The epidemiology of asthma during pregnancy: Prevalence, diagnosis, and symptoms. *Immunology and Allergy Clinics of North America*, *26*, 29–62.

Manns-James, L. (2011). Pregnancy, Chapter 35. In T. King & M. Brucker (Eds.), *Pharmacology for women's health* (pp. 1066–1067). Boston: Jones and Bartlett.

Mosby, L. G., Rasmussen, S. A., & Jamieson, D. J. (2011). 2009 pandemic influenza A (H1N1) in pregnancy: A systematic review of the literature. *American Journal of Obstetrics and Gynecology*, *205*(1), 10.

Murphy, V., & Gibson, P. (2011). Asthma in pregnancy. *Clinics in Chest Medicine*, *32*(1), 93–110.

Murphy, V., Namazy, J., Powell, H. M., Chambers, C., Attia, J., & Gibson, P. (2011). A meta-analysis of adverse perinatal outcomes in women with asthma. *BJOG: An International Journal of Obstetrics and Gynaecology*, *118*, 1314–1323. doi:10.1111/j.1471-0528.2011.03055.x

National Asthma Education and Prevention Program Working Group (NAEPP). (2005). Managing Asthma During Pregnancy: Recommendations for Pharmacologic Treatment. NAEPP Report: Management of Asthma During Pregnancy. NIH Publication No. 05-5236. Bethesda, MD: U.S. Department of Health and Human Services: National Institutes of Health; National Heart, Lung, and Blood Institute. Retrieved from http://www.nhlbi.nih.gov/health/prof/lung/asthma/astpreg/astpreg_full.pdf

Rey, E., & Boulet, L. P. (2007). Asthma in pregnancy. *BMJ (Clinical Research Ed.)*, *334*(7593), 582–585.

Schatz, M., Zeiger, R. S., & Hoffman, C. P. (1990). Intrauterine growth is related to gestational pulmonary function in pregnant asthmatic women. Kaiser-Permanente Asthma and Pregnancy Study Group. *Chest*, *98*(2), 389.

33

Hematological and thromboembolic disorders

Julie A. Marfell

Relevant terms

Ferritin—storage form of iron; serum ferritin level is the most accurate method of assessing iron status using a simple blood test

Hemoglobin S—an inherited hemoglobinopathy with hemoglobin S rather than the usual hemoglobin A; also known as "sickle cell trait" or "sickle cell disease"

Mean corpuscular hemoglobin (MCH)—average amount of hemoglobin in red blood cells

Mean corpuscular volume (MCV)—average size or volume of red blood cells

Red cell indices—measurements of the red blood cell size and hemoglobin content

Thalassemia—an inherited hemoglobinopathy that causes a reduced synthesis of hemoglobin

Thrombophilia—a group of inherited and acquired disorders that increase the likelihood of thromboembolic disorders

Introduction

Hematological alterations are common in pregnancy. Anemia is the most common hematological disorder, but bleeding disorders and coagulopathies can also complicate pregnancy in otherwise healthy women. This chapter reviews the assessment, differential diagnosis, and management of the common hematological disorders of pregnancy including anemia, bleeding disorders, and coagulopathies.

Anemia

Physiological changes in pregnancy

Pregnancy is characterized by a dramatic increase in blood volume. The increase in blood volume includes a large increase in the plasma volume (about 50%) as well as a substantial but smaller increase in the red cell mass (about 25%) (Samuels, 2012). The disproportionate increase in the plasma volume in contrast to the red cell mass results in decreased hemoglobin, hematocrit, and red cell counts during pregnancy. This decrease is normal and is often described as the physiological or dilutional anemia of pregnancy. These physiological changes necessitate the use of different standards for evaluating common hematological assessments such as the red blood cell count, hemoglobin, and hematocrit during pregnancy (Table 33.1).

Anemia is diagnosed using a complete blood count (CBC) or hemogram. A diagnosis of anemia in pregnancy is made when the hemoglobin is less than 11 g/dL in the first or third trimester, or less than 10.5 g/dL in the second trimester (Curran, 2012).

Diagnosis of anemia during pregnancy

First trimester	Hemoglobin < 11.0 g/dL
Second trimester	Hemoglobin < 10.5 g/dL
Third trimester	Hemoglobin < 11.0 g/dL

Prenatal and Postnatal Care: A Woman-Centered Approach, First Edition. Edited by Robin G. Jordan, Janet L. Engstrom, Julie A. Marfell, and Cindy L. Farley.
© 2014 John Wiley & Sons, Inc. Published 2014 by John Wiley & Sons, Inc.

Once anemia is diagnosed based on the results of a hemogram, the cause of the anemia must be identified. Iron deficiency is the most common cause of anemia during pregnancy, but other causes include vitamin deficiencies such as folate or vitamin B_{12} deficiency, genetic hemoglobinopathies such as hemoglobin S and thalassemia, previous bariatric surgery, gastrointestinal bleeding, alcohol use, side effects from medications, infectious diseases, and unexplained conditions.

The differential diagnosis of anemia begins with a careful examination of the red cell indices to evaluate the size of the red blood cells and hemoglobin content of the cells. Cell size is evaluated using the mean corpuscular volume (MCV). A MCV of less than 80 fL is indicative of microcytic anemia, 80–100 fL normocytic anemia, and greater than 100 fL macrocytic anemia. Cell hemoglobin is evaluated by examining the mean corpuscular hemoglobin (MCH). An MCH of 27–32 pg/cell is normal and is described as normochromic, whereas as MCH less than 27 pg/cell is described as hypochromic.

Evaluation of the red blood cell indices

MCV	Normal 80–100 fL
	Microcytic < 80 fL
	Macrocytic > 100 fL
MCH	Normal 27–32 pg/cell
	Hypochromic < 27 pg/cell

Additional evaluation of hematological parameters may be necessary to determine the cause of the anemia. The measurements most commonly performed include the serum ferritin to assess iron stores, hemoglobin elec-

trophoresis to assess the types of hemoglobin present, and measurement of folate and vitamin B_{12} levels (Table 33.2).

Iron-deficiency anemia

Iron-deficiency anemia (IDA) is the most common cause of anemia in pregnancy, accounting for 75–90% of all cases (Curran, 2012). The high prevalence of IDA during pregnancy is due to the increased iron requirements coupled with inadequate dietary intake. Iron requirements are higher in pregnancy due to increased erythropoiesis and the growth of maternal tissues as well as fetal and placental iron requirements. However, a typical Western diet usually does not contain sufficient iron to meet the needs of pregnancy. Additionally, many women begin pregnancy with low iron stores due to menstrual losses, contraceptive use, recent pregnancy, repeated pregnancies, as well as inadequate dietary intake and absorption.

Women with untreated IDA are more likely to have a shorter gestation and are at greater risk of preterm birth (Banhidy, Nandor, Puho, & Czeizel, 2011). Fetal and neonatal outcomes of maternal IDA include low birth weight and lower mental and psychomotor performance (Ebrahim, Kulkami, Parker, & Atrash, 2010). Decreased iron stores have been noted in infants born to anemic mothers (Cao & O'Brien, 2013). Thus, the identification and treatment of IDA is important during pregnancy.

IDA is a microcytic anemia and is the most likely cause of anemia when the MCV is less than 80 fL. A serum ferritin level should be obtained to evaluate iron stores and to verify the diagnosis of IDA. The range for serum ferritin levels is 10–150 ng/mL in females (Abbassi-Ghanavati, Greer, & Cunningham, 2009). When the ferritin level is lower than 12 ng/mL, the most likely diagnosis is IDA.

Table 33.1   Hematological Findings during Normal Pregnancy

Component	Nonpregnant woman	First trimester	Second trimester	Third trimester
Hemoglobin (g/dL)	12–15.8	11.6–13.9	9.7–14.8	9.5–15.0
Hematocrit (%)	35.4–44.4	31.0–41.0	30.0–39.0	28.0–40.0
MCH (pg/cell)	27–32	30–32	30–33	29–32
MCV (mm)	79–93	81–96	82–97	81–99
Iron (mg/dL)	41–141	72–143	44–178	30–193
Total iron-binding capacity (mg/dL)	251–406	278–403	Not reported	359–609
Ferritin (ng/mL)	10–150	6–130	2–230	0–116
Vitamin B_{12} (pg/mL)	279–966	118–438	130–656	99–526
Folate (ng/mL)	5.4–18.0	2.6–15.0	0.8–24.0	1.4–20.7

Adapted from: Abbassi-Ghanavati et al. (2009) and Cao and O'Brien (2013).

Table 33.2   Hematology Conditions and Differential Laboratory Findings

Condition	MCV	MCH	Ferritin	Hemoglobin	Red blood cells
Iron deficiency	Less than 80 but may be normal	Less than 27 but may be normal	Less than 12	Less than 11 in the first and third trimesters, less than 10.5 in the second trimester	Decreased production
Thalassemia minor	Less than 80	25–27	Normal range		
Thalassemia intermedia	Less than 80	Less than 25	Normal range		
Thalassemia major	Less than 80	Less than 25	Normal range		Increased production
Folate deficiency	Greater than 100		Normal range		Decreased
Vitamin B_{12} deficiency	Greater than 100		Normal range		Decreased

Adapted from: ACOG (2008).

Symptoms noted in IDA may include weakness, fatigue, dizziness, headache, shortness of breath with exertion, restless leg syndrome, palpitations, and irritability. Pica may also be noted. Physical findings are usually not observed except in severe iron deficiency and include angular stomatis, glossitis, and brittle, spoon-shaped fingernails. Skin pallor may also be noted.

Treatment of IDA includes iron replacement and dietary changes. Iron supplementation of 30–60 mg of elemental iron daily is encouraged in all pregnant women (Curran, 2012) and is easily accomplished with a daily prenatal vitamin. For pregnant women with documented IDA, daily supplementation of 60–120 mg of elemental iron is recommended. Iron absorption is affected by the level of iron stores present in the body, the type of iron ingested, and whether the iron is taken with food (Grieger, Katcher, Juturu, & Kris-Etherton, 2011). Absorption is increased if the iron is taken alone on an empty stomach, but this increases the potential for gastrointestinal side effects. Thus, most clinicians recommend taking iron with meals. Common iron formulations are listed below.

Iron supplements

Preparation	Formulation
Ferrous gluconate	34 mg elemental iron per 300 mg tablet
Ferrous sulfate	65 mg elemental iron per 325 mg tablet
Ferrous fumarate	106 mg elemental iron per 325 mg tablet

Source: American College of Obstetricians and Gynecologists (ACOG) (2008).

Iron supplements are associated with significant gastrointestinal side effects and many women stop taking iron due to the side effects. Side effects of iron supplementation include nausea, gastrointestinal distress, constipation, and diarrhea. Supplements that contain lower doses of elemental iron have fewer side effects. Strategies for improving women's tolerance to iron supplements are described in the following text box. All iron supplements should be tightly capped and kept out of children's reach due to the high potential for poisoning and fatality.

Strategies to promote iron supplement tolerance

- Explain the need for increased iron.
- Discuss the side effects of iron.
- Recommend taking the supplement with meals or at bedtime.
- Prescribe supplements with lower concentrations of elemental iron.
- Divide the dose of iron into two doses daily.
- Advise increased dietary fiber intake.
- Recommend increased water intake.
- Encourage increased physical activity.
- Recommend stool softeners as needed.
- Change to a reduced dosing schedule if the side effects of daily dosing are intolerable.

Dietary counseling is a mainstay of treatment for IDA (see Chapter 6, "Nutrition during Pregnancy"). Dietary iron comes in two forms, heme and nonheme. Heme iron is more readily absorbed than nonheme iron. Heme iron is found in animal products such as meat, poultry and fish, with meat having higher iron content than fish. Nonheme iron is found in grains, cereal, eggs, vegetables, fruits, and dairy products. Absorption of nonheme iron is affected by other substances commonly found in nonheme foods such as casein and whey proteins in

Table 33.3 Food Sources of Heme Iron

Food	Milligrams per serving	Percentage of FDA daily value*
Oysters, canned, 3 oz	5.7	32
Beef, chuck, blade roast, lean only, braised, 3 oz	3.1	17
Turkey, dark meat, roasted, 3 oz	2.0	11
Beef, ground, 85% lean, patty, broiled, 3 oz	2.2	12
Beef, top sirloin, steak, lean only, broiled, 3 oz	1.6	9
Tuna, light, canned in water, 3 oz	1.3	7
Turkey, light meat, roasted, 3 oz	1.1	6
Chicken, dark meat, meat only, roasted, 3 oz	1.1	6
Chicken, light meat, meat only, roasted, 3 oz	0.9	5
Tuna, fresh, yellow fin, cooked, dry heat, 3 oz	0.8	4
Crab, Alaskan king, cooked, moist heat, 3 oz	0.7	4
Pork, loin chop, broiled, 3 oz	0.7	4
Shrimp, mixed species, cooked, moist heat, four large	0.3	2
Halibut, cooked, dry heat, 3 oz	0.2	1

*Based on Food and Drug Administration (FDA) recommended daily value of 18 mg.
Source: Office of Dietary Supplements. (2007). Dietary Supplement Fact Sheet: Iron. National Institutes of Health. Retrieved from http://ods.od.nih.gov/factsheets/Iron-HealthProfessional/.

Table 33.4 Food Sources of Nonheme Iron

Food	Milligrams per serving	Percentage of FDA daily value*
Ready-to-eat cereal, 100% iron fortified, ¾ cup	18.0	100
Oatmeal, instant, fortified, prepared with water, one packet	11.0	61
Soybeans, mature, boiled, 1 cup	8.8	48
Lentils, boiled, 1 cup	6.6	37
Beans, kidney, mature, boiled, 1 cup	5.2	29
Beans, lima, large, mature, boiled, 1 cup	4.5	25
Ready-to-eat cereal, 25% iron fortified, ¾ cup	4.5	25
Black-eyed peas, (cowpeas), mature, boiled, 1 cup	4.3	24
Beans, navy, mature, boiled, 1 cup	4.3	24
Beans, black, mature, boiled, 1 cup	3.6	20
Beans, pinto, mature, boiled, 1 cup	3.6	21
Tofu, raw, firm, ½ cup	3.4	19
Spinach, fresh, boiled, drained, ½ cup	3.2	18
Spinach, canned, drained solids, ½ cup	2.5	14
Spinach, frozen, chopped or leaf, boiled ½ cup	1.9	11
Raisins, seedless, packed, ½ cup	1.6	9
Grits, white, enriched, quick, prepared with water, 1 cup	1.5	8
Molasses, 1 tbs	0.9	5
Bread, white, commercially prepared, one slice	0.9	5
Bread, whole-wheat, commercially prepared, one slice	0.7	4

*Percentage based on FDA recommended daily value of 18 mg. Office of Dietary Supplements. (2007). Dietary Supplement Fact Sheet: Iron. National Institutes of Health. Retrieved from http://ods.od.nih.gov/factsheets/Iron-HealthProfessional/.

bovine dairy products, calcium and phosphorus in milk, wheat and maize flour, calcium, zinc and cadmium, and phosphoprotein in eggs. The addition of a serving of heme protein with nonheme protein foods helps with the absorption of iron from the nonheme food due to the presence of meat protein factor, which facilitates iron absorption. Food sources high in heme and nonheme iron are listed in Table 33.3 and Table 33.4.

Dietary counseling includes recommending a serving of meat, poultry, or fish with meals. This will increase the amount of dietary iron as well as help with the absorption of dietary iron obtained from other food sources. Although organ meats such as liver are rich in iron, they are not recommended during pregnancy and should be avoided throughout gestation. Coffee, tea, and carbonated beverages inhibit the absorption of iron and these beverages should not be consumed at mealtime. Including foods rich in vitamin C in meals increases iron absorption. Daily intake of a combination of heme and nonheme foods will help improve the absorption of iron and provide a variety of foods to help balance dietary needs and improve overall nutritional status.

A CBC and serum ferritin level should be repeated in 4 weeks to evaluate the response to therapy. If no improvement is noted, further testing is recommended to rule out blood loss or intestinal parasites. A stool for occult blood should be checked for the possibility of a gastrointestinal bleeding, and a stool for ova and parasites should be obtained to check for parasites. Supplementation at 30 mg of elemental iron daily should continue for 4–6 months after the hemoglobin levels return to normal to rebuild iron stores.

Hemoglobinopathies

Hemoglobinopathies are inherited disorders that affect the structure, function, and production of hemoglobin. These disorders include hemoglobin S and thalassemia.

Hemoglobin S

Hemoglobin S is a genetic hemoglobinopathy and is an autosomal recessive disorder. The structure of hemoglobin S predisposes the cell to become sickle shaped under low oxygen conditions, which leads to sludging in small vessels and potential infarction of the tissues (Samuels, 2012). Individuals who are heterozygous for the gene carry only one copy of the hemoglobin S gene, and these individuals have a mixture of the normal adult form of hemoglobin (hemoglobin A) and hemoglobin S, so their hemoglobin is hemoglobin AS. These individuals are commonly referred to as having sickle cell trait (SCT). Most individuals with SCT do not have any symptoms or health problems. During pregnancy, however, women with SCT may be at higher risk for preeclampsia, having an infant with lower birth weight, and postpartum endometritis (Samuels, 2012). Women with SCT are also at greater risk for urinary tract infection during pregnancy and should be screened as indicated (Samuels, 2012).

Women with SCT should receive genetic counseling regarding their infant's risk of SCT and sickle cell disease (SCD). This requires testing of the fetus's biological father. If both parents have SCT there is a 50% chance that the child will have SCT and a 25% chance of inheriting SCD (Centers for Disease Control and Prevention, 2011). SCT is found in 1 out of 12 African Americans (Curran, 2012) but is also found throughout

the world in individuals of African descent, particularly in persons from the Caribbean, Middle East, India, the Mediterranean, as well as South and Central America (Howard & Oteng-Ntim, 2012). Population migration and better management of the disorder has increased the incidence and changed the geographical distribution.

SCD is the homozygous form of the disorder (hemoglobin SS) and is coinherited from both parents. Anemia and intermittent severe pain in the legs and fingers are symptoms associated with SCD. These symptoms are secondary to decreased hemoglobin oxygen carrying capacity and vascular occlusion caused by irregularly shaped hemoglobin molecules. Symptoms of SCD increase during pregnancy and the condition is associated with serious pregnancy complications including infection, pulmonary complications, preeclampsia, fetal growth restriction, and preterm birth (Howard & Oteng-Ntim, 2012). Thus, women with SCD should be referred for specialized obstetrical and hematological care. Women with SCD comanaged by an interdisplinary team throughout pregnancy, birth, and the postpartum periods have lower maternal and perinatal mortality and morbidity (Howard & Oteng-Ntim, 2012).

During a preconception visit for a woman with SCD, the risk of complications during pregnancy should be discussed. The importance of proper hydration, avoidance of the cold, and decreasing stress in the management of sickle cell crisis should also be emphasized. Medications should be reviewed for possible teratogenic effects. This includes any pain medications such as nonsteroidal anti-inflammatory drugs. These should not be used before 12 weeks of gestation or after 28 weeks of gestation. Women with SCD should take a folic acid supplement of 5 mg daily. If the fetus's biological father has not had genetic screening to determine the presence of hemoglobin S, this should occur as early as possible and, ideally, during the preconception period. Iron supplementation is not recommended for women with SCD unless there is a documented iron deficiency.

Thalassemia

Thalassemia is a genetic hemoglobinopathy caused by an alteration in the synthesis of the globulin chains of the hemoglobin molecule (Samuels, 2012). There are three classifications of thalassemia: minor, which is the carrier or trait status; major; and intermedia. The classification of thalassemia is based on the specific mutations in the globulin chains of the hemoglobin molecule. The condition is prevalent in women from southern Europe, Northern Africa, the Middle East, and southern Asia (Leung & Lao, 2012), but immigration and interethnic marriage have made thalassemia a global issue.

Thalassemia may also appear in persons with another hemoglobinopathy such as hemoglobin S.

Thalassemia should be considered as a differential diagnosis in individuals with hypochromic, microcytic anemia. A MCH is used to differentiate between thalassemia minor, major, and intermedia. In thalassemia minor, the MCH is below 27 but above 25. An individual with an MCH that is below 25 should be screened for thalassemia major and intermedia. A ferritin level as well as a hemoglobin electrophoresis should be completed to rule out IDA and to evaluate the hemoglobin type and structure.

Women diagnosed with thalassemia major or intermedia should be referred for specialized care. These women are at risk for cardiac failure, alloimmunization, viral infections, thrombosis, endocrine, and bone disorders (Leung & Lao, 2012).

Early genetic screening of the biological father of the fetus is advised for a woman with the thalassemia minor. If the couple are both confirmed carriers of the thalassemia genetic mutation, the possibility of the fetus having thalassemia major is one in four (Leung & Lao, 2012). For these couples, further genetic counseling and analysis is performed to determine the specific gene mutation. Fetal diagnostic testing can be performed using chorionic villus sampling or amniocentesis. Supplementation of folic acid 5 mg daily is recommended to prevent neural tube defects and has been shown to increase hemoglobin levels (Leung, Lao, & Chang, 1989).

Folate deficiency

The need for folate is increased in pregnancy due to increased cell turnover and inadequate dietary intake. Folate deficiency has been associated with anemia, placental abruption, pregnancy loss, and neural tube defects. Signs and symptoms of folate deficiency may develop at 12–16 weeks of gestation due to diminished body stores of folate.

Symptoms of anemia, hyperpigmentation of the skin, and a low-grade fever may be present in folate deficiency. Neurological symptoms such as numbness and tingling in the extremities, decreased metal alertness, and memory problems may be seen in folate as well as vitamin B_{12} deficiency. Thus, vitamin B_{12} serum level should be evaluated prior to the beginning of folate supplementation to avoid masking the symptoms of a potential vitamin B_{12} deficiency.

Prevention of folate deficiency consists of supplementation and dietary changes. A dose of folic acid 400 µg (0.4 mg) is recommended for all women during the preconception period and throughout pregnancy. Folate deficiency is treated with folic acid 5 mg daily for 4 months or throughout the pregnancy if the underlying cause is not corrected. A diet rich in green leafy vegetables, lentils, beans, peanuts, and fortified breads and cereals is recommended during pregnancy.

Vitamin B_{12} deficiency

Vitamin B_{12} is needed for the production of red blood cells, neurological function, and DNA synthesis. During pregnancy, there is an increase in cell turnover, cell formation, and red blood cell production. Vitamin B_{12} levels decrease steadily throughout pregnancy with the lowest levels occurring near the term. Women with a history of bariatric surgery or bowel diseases such as Crohn's disease are at increased risk for vitamin B_{12} deficiency as are women who take metformin or proton pump inhibitors (Samuels, 2012). Women with a strict vegetarian diet are also at risk for vitamin B_{12} deficiency (Samuels, 2012). Low maternal levels of vitamin B_{12} increase the risk of birth defects such as neural tube defects. Low maternal vitamin B_{12} levels may lead to vitamin B_{12} deficiency in breastfed infants (Shinwell & Gorodischer, 1982).

Symptoms of vitamin B_{12} deficiency include a change in bowel habits, diarrhea, constipation, fatigue, shortness of breath, and loss of appetite. Clinical signs such as a swollen, red tongue or bleeding gums may be present. Mental slowness, memory deficits, hallucinations, and numbness or tingling of the extremities may also be noted with vitamin B_{12} deficiency (Goonewardene, Shehata, & Hamad, 2012). Laboratory findings include macrocytic anemia, MCV above 100 fL, and a low serum vitamin B_{12} level. Vitamin B_{12} levels should be measured prior to the administration of folate supplements since folate can mask symptoms of vitamin B_{12} deficiency.

Dietary modifications are the best prevention. Vitamin B_{12} is found in foods of animal origin including eggs, milk, and milk products. Pregnant women who follow a vegan diet may benefit from vitamin B_{12} supplementation (Goonewardene et al., 2012). The absorption of vitamin B_{12} requires binding to intrinsic factor in the stomach. In the absence of intrinsic factor, the diagnosis is pernicious anemia. Pernicious anemia should be considered in the differential diagnosis of macrocytic anemia.

Unexplained maternal anemia

Infectious diseases such as HIV, cytomegalovirus, Epstein–Barr virus, parvovirus B19, and hepatitis, though rare, have been associated with anemia during pregnancy. Hidden alcohol use can also be a cause for unexplained anemia during pregnancy. Careful assessment of all possibilities should be considered if there is no clear cause of anemia or if standard therapies do not resolve the anemia (Curran, 2012).

Bleeding disorders

Thrombocytopenia

Thrombocytopenia is defined as a decrease in the serum platelet count below 150,000/mm³. Gestational thrombocytopenia occurs in approximately 6–15% of women in the third trimester and resolves without treatment several weeks after birth and there is no associated neonatal thrombocytopenia (Boehlen, 2006). Gestational thrombocytopenia may be secondary to increased platelet consumption and hemodilution during pregnancy (Curran, 2012).

Other conditions that can cause thrombocytopenia during pregnancy include preeclampsia, HELLP syndrome, and idiopathic thrombocytopenia purpura (ITP). Further investigation is required if the woman has a history of thrombocytopenia prior to pregnancy, if thrombocytopenia occurs in the first or second trimester, if the platelet count is below 75,000/mm³ in the third trimester, or there are complications related to thrombocytopenia (Boehlen, 2006).

Treatment of thrombocytopenia during pregnancy is based on the cause, the severity of the disorder, and the presence of complications. Women with documented thrombocytopenia should be closely monitored for possible complications and referred for specialized obstetric care.

Inherited bleeding disorders

Inherited bleeding disorders include von Willebrand disease, hemophilia A and B, and inherited deficiencies of coagulation factors. The most common inherited bleeding disorder is von Willebrand disease, which occurs in about 1% of women. von Willebrand disease is autosomal recessive. Hemophilia is an X-linked recessive disorder, which means that men inherit the condition and women are carriers. Rare bleeding disorders are typically autosomal recessive disorders.

Inherited bleeding disorders are diagnosed by the evaluation of a CBC, peripheral blood smear, prothrombin (PT), partial prothrombin time (PTT), and platelet function activity (PFA-100). The family history is important especially if there is a history of bleeding in men or a positive family history of any of the disorders. A history of easily provoked bleeding, bruising, petechia, or purpura also requires further evaluation (Ballas & Kraut, 2008). A prolonged PT may be secondary to a deficiency in factor VII. An increased PTT may be

diagnostic for hemophilia A, hemophilia B, and von Willebrand disease. A PFA-100 will provide further evaluation and differentiate von Willebrand disease. The limits of normal for the coagulation profile are presented in Table 33.5.

Preconception counseling and testing will help identify undiagnosed inherited bleeding disorders. This information will help the woman and her partner understand the genetic implications, and provides the opportunity to discuss contraception and pregnancy management. Immunization for hepatitis A and B should be considered in case transfusion is required during the pregnancy.

Prenatal diagnosis is considered primarily in carriers of hemophilia as there is a 50% chance of having a male fetus that is affected and a 50% chance of a female fetus that is a carrier. Diagnosis can be done via chorionic villus sampling or amniocentesis (Chi & Kadir, 2012).

Women with bleeding disorders should be referred for care to an interdisciplinary team with expertise in obstetrics, hematology, and anesthesia. During the antepartum period, clotting factor levels should be closely monitored on a planned schedule. It is recommended that these levels be checked at the first visit and then again at 28 and 34 weeks of gestation (Chi & Kadir, 2012). It is advised that women with inherited bleeding disorders are closely monitored during the third trimester. These women are at an increased risk for bleeding complications during birth and in the postpartum period. A detailed plan for pain management and birth options is needed to decrease the risk of complications for the woman and her infant.

Coagulopathies during pregnancy

Thrombophilia is defined as an increased risk of blood clotting or hypercoagulopathy, and the disorder can be inherited or acquired. Inherited thrombophilias include factor V Leiden mutation, PT *G20210A* mutation, protein C deficiency, protein S deficiency, and antithrombin deficiency (McNamee, Dawood, & Farquharson, 2012). Acquired thrombophilias are due to antiphospholipid antibodies that alone or in groups may cause hypercoagulopathy. Approximately 10% of the world population has thrombophilia. The most common thrombophilias are factor V Leiden and PT mutations (Villa-Fortes Gomes, 2012). The presence of thrombophilia during pregnancy can increase women's risk of deep vein thrombosis (DVT) and pulmonary embolism (PE).

Pregnancy is a hypercoagulatory state. There is an increase in thrombin generation as well as changes to the levels of procoagulant factors. Venous stasis increases secondary to the effects of progesterone on the blood

Table 33.5   Coagulation Profile during Pregnancy

Component	Nonpregnant adult	First trimester	Second trimester	Third trimester
Prothrombin time (PT) (seconds)	12.7–15.4	9.7–13.5	9.5–13.4	9.6–12.9
International normalized ration (INR)	0.9–1.04	0.89–1.05	0.85–0.97	0.80–0.94
Partial prothrombin time (PTT) activated (seconds)	26.3–39.4	24.5–38.9	24.2–38.1	24.7–35.0
Platelet (×10 9th/L)	165–415	174–391	155–409	146–429

vessels and the decrease in venous return due to increasing size of the uterus. Damage to the pelvic vein may also occur due to childbirth. Overall vascular damage can occur secondary to venous distention. All of these factors contribute to an increase in the occurrence of thromboembolic disorders.

Risk factors for thromboembolic disorders include preexisting conditions such as thrombophilia, previous thromboembolism, obesity, parity, smoking, SCD, heart disease, systemic lupus, and varicose veins. Immobility, assisted reproductive therapy, hyperemesis gravidarum, preeclampsia, and multiple pregnancy have also been identified as risk factors. During the postpartum period, the risk for thromboembolic events increases and risk factors include cesarean section, hemorrhage, and infection (Royal College of Obstetricians and Gynaecologists, 2009).

Signs and symptoms of thromboembolic disorders include those that may be associated with pregnancy such as dyspnea and lower leg edema. A DVT may cause a cramping pain in the calf and or a feeling of heaviness in the affected leg. In pregnancy, DVT will occur more frequently in the proximal rather than in the distal veins. The left leg is affected 80% of the time during pregnancy due to compression of the iliac vein by the iliac artery. Isolated swelling as well as a 2-cm difference in leg circumference warrants further investigation. Isolated buttock, groin, flank, or abdominal pain may also be the presenting symptoms of a DVT of the iliac or femoral vein (Gray & Nelson-Piercy, 2012).

A report of chest pain, shortness of breath, a feeling of apprehension, hemoptysis, and/or unexplained tachycardia should be immediately investigated especially in women with noted risk factors for thromboembolic events (Rodger, 2012). A high maternal mortality rate is associated with PE during pregnancy. Thromboembolic events may occur anytime during pregnancy, but the greatest threat is during the postpartum period, during the first 4–6 weeks after birth (Bates, 2007).

Compression ultrasound with Doppler imaging is used to confirm the diagnosis of a DVT. It is noninvasive and does not involve radiation. If there is high clinical suspicion and a negative ultrasound, it is recommended to begin treatment. The ultrasound may be repeated in 1 week or an alternative method of imaging may be utilized to confirm the diagnosis. A D-dimer blood test will reflect the ongoing activation of the hemostatic system. This is frequently used to assist with the diagnosis of DVT but is increased during pregnancy and the postpartum period. Due to the increase, there is no predictive value in this test during pregnancy (Szigeti, 2012).

The diagnosis of a PE is done using a ventilation and perfusion (V/Q) scan. In pregnancy a leg compression ultrasound should be completed prior to the V/Q scan. If positive, therapy will be initiated without the need for radiation exposure. The radiation exposure from a V/Q scan is relatively low, but all radiation exposures should be avoided when possible (Rodger, 2012).

The treatment for thrombophilia during pregnancy is based on an individualized risk assessment. The assessment is based on the type of thrombophilia and the history of a thromboembolic event prior to the current pregnancy. Low-risk thrombophilias include factor V Leiden heterozygous, PT *G20210A*, protein C deficiency, and protein S deficiency. High-risk thrombophilias are antithrombin deficiency, double heterozygous PT *G20210A* and factor V Leiden, factor V Leiden homozygous or thrombin *G20210A* mutation homozygous. Women who are known to have thrombophilia should be advised of the importance of contraception and the risk of thromboembolic events during pregnancy. Women taking warfarin prior to pregnancy should discontinue use and switch to a low-molecular-weight heparin (LMWH) if considering pregnancy or as soon as pregnancy is confirmed if the pregnancy is unexpected.

LMWH and unfractionated heparin (UFH) are safe to use during pregnancy and during breastfeeding. The use of LMWH has been found to be equally effective to UFH and is often preferred due to the dosing schedule of every 12 hours. The side effects of both medications include bleeding, thrombocytopenia, and irritation at the injection site. Heparin is continued for at least 6 weeks postpartum. Table 33.6 outlines thromboprophylaxis for

Table 33.6   Recommended Thromboprophylaxis for Pregnancies Complicated by Inherited Thrombophilias* (ACOG, 2011)

Clinical scenario	Antepartum management	Postpartum management
Low-risk thrombophilia[†] without previous VTE	Surveillance without anticoagulation or prophylactic LMWH or UFH	Surveillance without anticoagulation therapy or postpartum anticoagulation therapy if the patient has additional risks factors[‡]
Low-risk thrombophilia[†] with a single previous episode of VTE—not receiving long-term anticoagulation	Prophylactic or intermediate-dose LMWH/UFH or surveillance without anticoagulation therapy	Postpartum anticoagulation therapy or intermediate-dose LMWH/UFH
High-risk thrombophilia[§] without previous VTE	Prophylactic LMWH or UFH	Postpartum anticoagulation therapy
High-risk thrombophilia[§] with a single previous episode of VTE—not receiving long-term anticoagulation	Prophylactic, intermediate-dose, or adjusted-dose LMWH/UFH regimen	Postpartum anticoagulation therapy or intermediate or adjusted-dose LMWH/UFH for 6 weeks (therapy level should be at least as high as antepartum treatment)
No thrombophilia with previous single episode of VTE associated with transient risk factor that is no longer present—excludes pregnancy- or estrogen-related risk factor	Surveillance without anticoagulation therapy	Postpartum anticoagulation therapy[¶]
No thrombophilia with previous single episode of VTE associated with transient risk factor that was pregnancy or estrogen related	Prophylactic-dose LMWH or UFH[¶]	Postpartum anticoagulation therapy
No thrombophilia with previous single episode of VTE without an associated risk factor (idiopathic)—not receiving long-term anticoagulation therapy	Prophylactic LMWH or UFH[¶]	Postpartum anticoagulation therapy
Thrombophilia or no thrombophilia with two or more episodes of VTE—not receiving long-term anticoagulation therapy	Prophylactic or therapeutic-dose LMWH or prophylactic or therapeutic-dose UFH	Postpartum anticoagulation therapy or therapeutic-dose LMWH/UFH for 6 weeks
Thrombophilia or no thrombophilia with two or more episodes of VTE—receiving long-term anticoagulation therapy	Therapeutic-dose LMWH/UFH	Resumption of long-term anticoagulation therapy

*Postpartum treatment levels should be greater or equal to antepartum treatment. Treatment of acute VTE and management of antiphospholipid syndrome are addressed in other practice bulletins.

[†]Low-risk thrombophilia: factor V Leiden heterozygous; prothrombin *G20210A* heterozygous; protein C or protein S deficiency.

[‡]First-degree relative with a history of a thrombotic episode before age 50 years, or other major thrombotic risk factors (e.g., obesity, prolonged immobility).

[§]High-risk thrombophilia: antithrombin deficiency, double heterozygous for prothrombin *G20210A* mutation and factor V Leiden, factor V Leiden homozygous or prothrombin *G20210A* mutation homozygous.

[¶]Surveillance without anticoagulation is supported as an alternative approach by some experts.

LMWH, low-molecular-weight heparin; UFH, unfractionated heparin; VTE, venous thromboembolism.

Case study

A pregnant woman presents to a clinic for a review of her prenatal laboratory results. Her hemoglobin is 10 g/dL and her MCV is 78 fL. Her serum ferritin is 5 ng/mL. She reports being tired despite adequate rest. Her appetite is good, but she is having some episodes of nausea. She is at 10 weeks of gestation by dates and is currently taking a prenatal vitamin. Her vital signs are as follows: BP 100/60, HR 80, RR 20, and her weight is 132. Her physical exam is within normal. Her history does not contain risk factors for anemia.

Due to a low hemoglobin of 10 g/dL and an MCV less than 80 fL in the first trimester, her diagnosis is IDA. The diagnosis of anemia and implications for pregnancy were discussed with her. She was started on ferrous sulfate 325 mg tablet taken twice daily with orange juice and has an order for a repeat CBC and ferritin level in 4 weeks. Her diet history was reviewed and revealed very limited intake of any vegetables, and only occasional red meat. She has been advised on the benefits of adding leafy green such as spinach, other vegetables high in iron such as sweet potatoes and black eyed peas, and dried fruits to her daily intake. She was strongly encouraged to increase her meat intake at lunch and dinner and to eat iron-fortified cereal for breakfast. She also has 1 cup of coffee every morning. Since caffeine can inhibit iron absorption, she was advised to take her iron supplements and foods high in iron at least 1–3 hours before or after drinking her morning cup of coffee. The side effects of iron supplementation were discussed and she was encouraged to eat several prunes daily and to increase water intake in an effort to avoid constipation. She was encouraged to call the office if she experienced side effects that were difficult to manage.

pregnant women with inherited thrombophilias. The use of intermittent compression devices during periods of immobility has been found to decrease long-term phlebotic syndrome (Rodger, 2012). Women with a history of thrombophilia should be referred for specialized care from an interdisciplinary team.

Summary

In summary, hematological alterations are common in pregnancy and can affect outcomes in pregnancy. Bleeding disorders and coagulopathies can complicate pregnancy in otherwise healthy women, but anemia is the most common hematological disorder. Early identification and management of bleeding disorders are key to good pregnancy outcomes. This chapter has reviewed the assessment, differential diagnosis, and management of the common hematological disorders of pregnancy and coagulopathies.

Resource for women and their families

March of Dimes: Anemia in pregnancy: http://www.marchofdimes.com/pregnancy/complications_anemia.html

Resources for health-care providers

American Society of Hematology: Anemia and pregnancy: http://www.hematology.org/patients/blood-disorders/anemia/5227.aspx

American Society of Hematology: Blood clotting and pregnancy: http://www.hematology.org/patients/blood-disorders/blood-clots/5235.aspx

References

Abbassi-Ghanavati, M., Greer, L., & Cunningham, F. (2009). Pregnancy and laboratory studies: A reference guide for clinicians. *Obstetrics and Gynecology, 114*(6), 1326–1331.

American College of Obstetricians and Gynecologists (ACOG). (2008). Anemia in pregnancy, ACOG practice bulletin clinical management guidelines for obstetrician-gynecologists, number 95. *Obstetrics and Gynecology, 112*(1), 201–207.

American College of Obstetricians and Gynecologists. (2011). Inherited thrombophilias in pregnancy, ACOG practice bulletin clinical management guidelines for obstetrician-gynecologists, number 124. *Obstetrics and Gynecology, 118*(3), 730–740.

Ballas, M., & Kraut, E. (2008). Bleeding and bruising: A diagnostic work-up. *American Family Physician, 77*(6), 1117–1124. Retrieved from http://www.aafp.org/afp

Banhidy, B., Nandor, A., Puho, E., & Czeizel, A. (2011). Iron deficiency anemia: Pregnancy outcomes with or without iron supplementation. *Nutrition (Burbank, Los Angeles County, Calif.), 21*, 65–72.

Bates, S. (2007). Management of pregnant women with thrombophilia or a history of venous thromboembolism. *Hematology/The Education Program of the American Society of Hematology. American Society of Hematology. Education Program*, 143–150.

Boehlen, F. (2006). Thrombocytopenia during pregnancy: Importance of diagnosis and management. *Hamostaseologie, 26*(91), 72–74.

Cao, C., & O'Brien, K. (2013). Pregnancy and iron homeostasis: An update. *Nutrition Reviews, 71*(1), 35–51.

Centers for Disease Control and Prevention. (2011) Sickle cell trait. *Sickle Cell Disease.* Retrieved from http://www.cdc.gov/ncbddd/sicklecell/traits.html

Chi, C., & Kadir, R. (2012). Inherited bleeding disorder in pregnancy. *Best Practice & Research. Clinical Obstetrics & Gynaecology, 26,* 103–117.

Curran, D. (2012) Anemia and Thrombocytopenia in Pregnancy. *Medscape Reference.* Retrieved from http://emedicine.medscape .com/article/261586-overview

Ebrahim, S., Kulkami, R., Parker, C., & Atrash, H. (2010). Blood disorders among women: Implications for preconception care. *American Journal of Preventive Medicine, 38*(4), 459–467.

Goonewardene, M., Shehata, M., & Hamad, A. (2012). Anaemia in pregnancy. *Best Practice & Research. Clinical Obstetrics & Gynaecology, 26,* 2–24.

Gray, G., & Nelson-Piercy, M. (2012). Thromboembolic disorders in obstetrics. *Best Practice & Research. Clinical Obstetrics & Gynaecology, 24,* 53–64.

Grieger, J., Katcher, H., Juturu, V., & Kris-Etherton, P. (2011). Vitamins and minerals. In T. King & M. Brucker (Eds.), *Pharmacology for women's health* (pp. 89–124). Sudbury, MA: Jones & Bartlett.

Howard, J., & Oteng-Ntim, E. (2012). The obstetric management of sickle cell disease. *Best Practice & Research. Clinical Obstetrics & Gynaecology, 26,* 25–36.

Leung, C., Lao, T., & Chang, A. (1989). Effect of folate supplement on pregnant women with beta-thalassemia minor. *European Journal of Obstetrics, Gynecology, and Reproductive Biology, 33,* 209–213.

Leung, T., & Lao, T. (2012). Thalassemia in pregnancy. *Best Practice & Research. Clinical Obstetrics & Gynaecology, 26,* 37–51.

McNamee, K., Dawood, F., & Farquharson, R. (2012). Thrombophilia and early pregnancy loss. *Best Practice and Research. Clinical Obstetrics and Gynaecology, 26,* 91–102.

Office of Dietary Supplements. (2007). *Dietary Supplement Fact Sheet: Iron.* National Institutes of Health. Retrieved from http://ods.od .nih.gov/factsheets/Iron-HealthProfessional/

Rodger, M. (2012). Evidence base for management of venous thrombosis in pregnancy. *Hematology/The Education Program of the American Society of Hematology. American Society of Hematology. Education Program, 1,* 173–180. doi:10.1182/ashedycatuib-2010 .1.173

Royal College of Obstetricians and Gynaecologists. (2009). Reducing the risk of thrombosis and embolism during pregnancy and the puerperium. Retrieved from http://www.rcog.org.uk/files/rcog -corp/GTG37aReducingRiskThrombosis.pdf

Samuels, P. (2012). Hematologic complications of pregnancy. In S. G. Gabbe, J. R. Niebyl, H. L. Galan, E. R. M. Jauniaux, M. B. Landon, J. L. Simpson, & D. A. Driscoll (Eds.), *Obstetrics: Normal and problem pregnancies* (6th ed., pp. 962–979). Philadelphia: Elsevier.

Shinwell, E., & Gorodischer, R. (1982). Totally vegetarian diets and infant nutrition. *Pediatrics, 70*(4), 582–586.

Szigeti, R. (2012) D-dimer. *Medscape Reference.* Retrieved from http:// emedicine.medscape.com/article/2085111-overview#showall

Villa-Fortes Gomes, M. (2012) Thrombophilia. *Vascular Disease Foundation.* Retrieved from http://vasculardisease.org/thrombophilia/

34

Urinary tract disorders

Rhonda Arthur and Nancy Pesta Walsh

Introduction

Upper and lower urinary tract disorders are common in pregnancy. Some of the most commonly encountered urinary tract disorders include urinary tract infection (UTI), pyelonephritis, and nephrolithiasis. UTI during pregnancy may lead to significant morbidity and mortality for both the mother and the fetus (Thomas, Thomas, Campbell, & Palmer, 2010). UTI in pregnancy is an independent risk factor for preterm birth and is also associated with preeclampsia, fetal growth restriction, and

cesarean delivery (Mazor-Dray, Levy, Schlaeffer, & Scheiner, 2009). While the occurrence of nephrolithiasis in pregnancy is no more common than in nonpregnant women, it poses the potential for serious complications to the mother and the fetus, including hypertension, preeclampsia, preterm labor, recurrent abortions, gestational diabetes mellitus, and cesarean delivery (Rosenburg et al., 2011). This chapter will discuss the changes in the urinary tract, physical evaluation, diagnosis, and treatment of common pregnancy-related urinary tract complications.

Urinary tract infection

The definition of UTI depends on the presence or absence of symptoms. In the *asymptomatic* patient, a UTI is defined as the presence of 10^5 colony-forming units (cfu) per milliliter of urine (Johnson, 2012; United States Preventative Services Task Force (USPSTF), 2008). Fewer than 10^5 cfu/mL can be significant in the presence of strong clinical evidence of UTI. These cases are sometimes called low-colony count UTIs (Bryan, 2011).

Prevalence and risk factors

UTIs occur in up to 20% of pregnancies (Sheffield & Cunningham, 2005). The incidence of asymptomatic bacteria in pregnant women ranges from 2% to 7%, and if left untreated, approximately 25–40% of these women will go on to develop acute pyelonephritis (Sheffield & Cunningham, 2005; Smaill, 2007). UTIs during pregnancy are more prevalent among women with lower socioeconomic status (Shrotri, Morrison, & Shrotri, 2007; Whitehead, Callaghan, Johnson, & Williams, 2009),

Prenatal and Postnatal Care: A Woman-Centered Approach, First Edition. Edited by Robin G. Jordan, Janet L. Engstrom, Julie A. Marfell, and Cindy L. Farley.
© 2014 John Wiley & Sons, Inc. Published 2014 by John Wiley & Sons, Inc.

likely due to decreased access to health care and poorer nutritional status. Diabetes, obesity, sickle cell trait, and any condition that requires urinary catheterization place a woman at an even greater risk of UTI. The development of UTI is more common in the second and third trimesters. The prevalence of UTI during pregnancy increases with maternal age.

Pathophysiology

Women have a higher incidence of UTI compared with men due to anatomic differences, such as shorter urethras and the close proximity of the urethra to the perineum. Bacteria ascend from the colonized perineum through the urethra, to the bladder and/or kidneys. For many women, sexual activity increases risk for UTI. Sexual activity causes meatal trauma and can introduce bacteria into the lower urinary tract (Sheffield & Cunningham, 2005).

Anatomic and physiological changes that occur with pregnancy affect the urinary tract system and further increase the risk of UTI. These normal changes include enlargement and displacement of the kidneys, dilation of the renal calyces and ureters, progesterone-related inhibition of ureteral smooth muscle contraction, bladder compression and displacement, hyperemia, and congestion of the uretheral mucosa with decreased contractility of the bladder (Thomas et al., 2010). These changes lead to increased urinary stasis and vesicoureteral reflux. Other pregnancy-related factors contributing to UTI susceptibility include an increase in glomerular filtration rate (GFR), which decreases urine concentration, glycosuria, and the decreased ability to resist invading bacteria due to influence of progestin and estrogen that are present in the urine (Dalzell & Lefevre, 2000). The mechanics of labor and birth, epidural anesthetics, and perineal trauma predispose the postpartum woman to UTIs (Sheffield & Cunningham, 2005).

Common pathogens

Escheria coli is the most commonly identified pathogen in asymptomatic bacteriuria and symptomatic UTI (Millar & Cox, 1997; Schnarr & Smaill, 2008; Sheffield & Cunningham, 2005; Thomas et al., 2010). After *E. coli*, the next most commonly identified pathogens are *Klebsiella*, *Enterobacter*, and *Group B strep* (GBS); *Staphylococcus*, *Enterococci*, and *Gardnerella vaginalis* are additional pathogens found to cause UTI (Dalzell & Lefevre, 2000).

Beta streptococci are important pathogens in pregnancy because early and late complications of neonatal beta-streptococcal infection are well documented. GBS is found in approximately 15–25% of pregnant women (Centers for Disease Control and Prevention (CDC),

2010). GBS is a frequent cause of asymptomatic bacteriuria, UTI, as well as upper genital tract infection and postpartum endometritis. The presence of GBS bacteriuria in any concentration in pregnant women is an indication of heavy vaginal colonization and should be treated appropriately at the time of diagnosis. This finding is an indication for intrapartum antibiotic prophylaxis for prevention of GBS complications in infants and women. There is consensus that symptomatic or asymptomatic women with GBS bacteriuria $\geq 10^5$ cfu/mL during pregnancy should be treated with antibiotics. The utility of treating GBS bacteriuria at colony counts $<10^5$ cfu/mL is uncertain and practice varies. Some health-care providers favor prenatal treatment at lower levels of GBS bacteriuria to prevent UTI, while more recent guidelines advocate antibiotic treatment only during labor for lower levels of GBS bacteriuria (Allen et al., 2012).

Asymptomatic bacteriuria

Asymptomatic bacteriuria is found on urine screening since symptoms are absent. If left untreated, asymptomatic bacteriuria will progress to symptomatic UTI with approximately 25% going on to develop acute pyelonephritis (Millar & Cox, 1997). Routine screening is recommended to detect asymptomatic bacteriuria either by urine culture or urine dip for esterase and leukocytes, followed by a urine culture if results are positive on all pregnant women at the first prenatal visit (Smaill & Vazquez, 2007). However, dipstick tests are not sufficiently sensitive and specific to be used for routine screening of bacteriuria in pregnancy in place of laboratory culture, but may be more cost-effective in low-resource settings (Awonuga, Fawole, Dada-Adegbola, Olola, & Awonuga, 2011). The urine culture is the gold standard for detecting asymptomatic bacteriuria in pregnant women. A urine culture is recommended to be done between 12 and 16 weeks of gestation or at the first prenatal visit if it occurs later during that time frame (USPSTF, 2008). Other guidelines recommend a single urine culture at the first prenatal visit regardless of gestational age. Urine cultures should be done every trimester in women with diabetes and sickle cell trait and can be considered in women at higher risk for preterm labor to improve the detection rate of asymptomatic bacteriuria (McIsaac et al., 2005).

Acute cystitis

Lower UTI, or acute cystitis, is defined as the presence of at least 100,000 cfu/mL of urine with symptoms. The standard definition of a positive urine culture from a clean-catch, midstream, voided specimen is $\geq 100,000$ cfu/mL of a single organism. However, in symptomatic women, the culture sensitivity is increased by lowering the cutoff to 100 cfu/mL of a single organism with a catheter-obtained specimen (Bryan, 2011). Typical symptoms include dysuria, urinary urgency, and frequency. Nocturia, suprapubic pain, and hematuria may also be present. Some women present with vague and mild symptoms. When a woman presents with any combination of these symptoms, a urine dipstick and a urine culture should be obtained. Urinary frequency and urgency are common in normal pregnancy and are not reliable indicators of UTI (Thomas et al., 2010). UTIs are associated with increased risks for pyelonephritis, preterm birth, low birth weight, and perinatal mortality.

Acute pyelonephritis

Acute pyelonephritis is an inflammation of one or both kidneys. Acute pyelonephritis is diagnosed when the woman has significant bacteriuria in the presence of systemic symptoms (Dalzell & Lefevre, 2000). Presenting symptoms may include the symptoms of UTI and also fever, chills, myalgia, anorexia, nausea, vomiting, low back pain, and costovertebral (CVA) tenderness. Women with acute pyelonephritis commonly appear acutely ill. Acute pyelonephritis in pregnancy is serious and can progress to renal failure, acute respiratory failure, and maternal sepsis. Untreated upper UTIs are associated with low birth weight, prematurity, preterm birth, hypertension and preeclampsia, maternal anemia (Hill, Sheffield, McIntire, & Wendel, 2005), fetal growth restriction, and cesarean birth (Mazor-Dray et al., 2009).

Evaluation

The presentation varies according to whether the patient has asymptomatic bacteriuria, a lower UTI (acute cyctitis), or an upper UTI (pyelonephritis).

Health history

A focused health history includes risk factors such as presence of diabetes, sickle cell trait, urinary tract congenital anomaly, frequent or reoccurring UTI, history of previous infant with GBS infection, multiparity, and lower socioeconomic status. A sexual history should be taken. Women should be queried on signs and symptoms of dysuria, urinary urgency, urinary frequency, nocturia, suprapubic pain, and hematuria. Pyelonephritis symptoms can vary and often include fever, shaking chills, loss of appetite, nausea, and vomiting.

Physical examination

Physical examination consists of assessment for suprapubic tenderness and presence of CVA tenderness. In asymptomatic bacteriuria, no physical findings are typically present. Lower UTI may present with tenderness over the bladder. Pyelonephritis signs can vary and often include fever >38°C, shaking chills, and CVA tenderness. Right-side flank pain is more common than left-side or bilateral flank pain due to increased ureteral dilation on the right side with resulting hydronephrosis (Thomas et al., 2010). Assessment of the fetal heart rate is included in the evaluation. If maternal fever is present, the fetal heart rate may be elevated. Depending on presentation, pelvic examination may be considered in symptomatic women to rule out vaginitis or cervicitis.

Laboratory testing

Clinical presentation and the woman's prior history will guide laboratory testing. In the office setting, urinary sediment analysis (UA) and urine dipstick testing offers speed and low cost. Urine dipstick to evaluate for UTI is based on two observations: (1) Normal urine contains nitrates but not nitrites; and (2) about 90% of bacteria causing UTI can convert urinary nitrates to nitrites (Simerville, Maxted, & Pahira, 2005). It is most useful for detecting >10^5 cfu/mL of aerobic gram-negative rods.

Urine culture is more accurate to diagnose UTI; however, it requires 24–48 hours for results and is more costly. Proper collection and handling of urine specimens includes collecting a midstream clean-catch sample and prompt refrigeration if the sample cannot be analyzed within 2 hours of collection (Clinical and Laboratory Standards Institute (CLSI), 2001). Cultures showing mixed gram-positive bacteria, lactobacilli, and *Staphylococcus* species (other than *Staphylococcus saprophyticus*) may be presumed to be contaminants and are not treated (American Congress of Obstetricians and Gynecologists (ACOG), 2011). In women who are extremely obese or unable to void, a catheterized specimen should be collected. Routine catheterization is not recommended because of the risks of introducing bacteria into the urinary tract. Table 34.1 provides guidelines on laboratory testing during pregnancy.

Women with symptoms and with positive urinalysis or dipstick can be treated empirically while awaiting culture results (Table 34.2). Antibiotics should be changed as needed based on urine culture sensitivity profiles. For those women without symptoms and with a positive UA or dipstick, it is appropriate to obtain a urine culture and to treat only if the culture is positive.

Care of women with urinary tract infections

In most pregnant women with aymptomatic bacteriuria and acute cystitis, the prognosis is excellent (Chen, Chen, Li, & Lin, 2011). Long-term sequelae are rare and are due

Table 34.1 Laboratory Testing for Urinary Tract Infection

Test	Timing	Comments	Significant results
Urine culture	All pregnant women at first visit (ACOG) or All pregnant women at 12–16 weeks gestation (USPTF) Any women with UTI symptoms Every trimester in those with history of recurrent UTIs, sickle cell trait	Identify asymptomatic bacteriuria Identifies specific organisms and antibiotic sensitivities	≥100,000 cfu/mL Any amount of GBS in clean catch midstream urine specimen
Urinalysis	Women with symptoms	Faster diagnosis than culture	Positive for nitrites, WBC, RBC, and protein
Urine dipstick	Women with symptoms Often routine at prenatal care visits	Faster screening, inexpensive, unreliable	Positive for nitrites, WBC, RBC

Table 34.2 Urinalysis Results

Findings	Clinical significance	Comments
Nitrites	Gram-negative bacteria like *E. coli* produce nitrites	A negative nitrite does not rule out UTI.
RBCs	>5 RBCs per high-powered field indicate infection	Vaginal secretions can cause contamination.
WBCs	>5 WBCs per high-powered field indicate infection	Vaginal secretions can cause contamination.
WBC casts	Produced in response to cellular injury in distal convoluted tubules	Common in pyelonephritis
Leukocyte esterase	A by-product of WBCs	A negative test means infection is unlikely.
Bacteriuria	Gram-negative strep and staph can be identified	Contamination with multiple dermal bacteria common with midstream clean-catch samples

to complications associated with pyelonephritis such as septic shock, respiratory failure, and hypotensive hypoxia. Adherence to screening for asymptomatic bacteria is key to preventing long-term sequelae.

Antibiotics are very effective at clearing UTIs in pregnancy, and complications are very rare (Morgan, 2004).

There is no consensus on the duration of therapy or choice of antibiotic in pregnancy. Although 1-, 3-, and 5-day antibiotic courses have been evaluated, longer treatment of 7–14 days is usually recommended for use during pregnancy to eradicate the offending bacteria (Johnson, 2012; Widmer, Gülmezoglu, Mignini, & Roganti, 2011). Pregnant women with asymptomatic GBS bacteriuria greater than 100,000 cfu/mL should be treated with a 3- to 7-day course of antibiotic to reduce the incidence of pyelonephritis. Several common medication regimes are noted in Table 34.3. There are no significant differences between pharmacological treatments with regard to efficacy and recurrence of infection (Vazquez & Abalos, 2011). The significant increase in microbial resistance has made appropriate antibiotic selection more challenging. For example, the resistance of *E. coli* to ampicillin and amoxicillin is 20–40%; accordingly, these agents are no longer considered optimal for treatment of UTIs caused by *E. coli* (Johnson, 2012).

For women with symptoms, phenazopyridine should be advised in addition to antibiotics. Phenazopyridine relieves urinary tract pain, burning, urgency, and frequent urination and is available over the counter. However, phenazopyridine is not an antibiotic; it does not cure infections.

An important element of care is educating pregnant women about measures to help reduce symptoms and to prevent UTI recurrence. Women should be advised to call if symptoms worsen and given instructions on recognizing symptoms of preterm labor. Rescreening with a repeat culture should be done to verify cure after completion of antibiotics.

Table 34.3   Medication for Asymptomatic Bacteriuria and Acute Cystitis in Pregnancy

Medication	Dose	Prophylactic dose	Special considerations
Nitrofurantoin macrocrystals (Macrobid, Furadantin)	100 mg BID	100 mg po at bedtime	• FDA pregnancy category B • Concentrates only in urinary tract and causes minimal resistance in gram-negative organisms • Use for suppression. • Avoid use in the first trimester due to inconclusive studies on safety. • Do not use last month of pregnancy
Cephalexin (Keflex)	500 mg QID	250 mg at bedtime	• FDA pregnancy category B • High rates of bacterial resistance
Amoxicillin Ampicillin	500 mg QID	Not advised	• FDA pregnancy category B • High rates of *E. coli* resistance • First choice for GBS in urine
Augmentin	250 mg QID	Not advised	• FDA pregnancy category B • High rates of bacterial resistance
Fosfomycin	3G as a single dose	Not advised	• FDA pregnancy category B • Can be useful for women in uncertain home situations

ACOG (2011); Manns-James (2010). *Pharmacology for women's health.* Jones & Bartlett Learning.

Measures to reduce risk of UTI recurrence

• Drink at least eight glasses of water per day.
• Discourage bubble baths, which can irritate the urethral opening.
• Avoid wearing thongs.
• Wipe front to back after defecation and urination.
• Use good hand washing techniques.
• Void after intercourse.
• Always respond to the initial urge to void.
• Avoid bladder irritants such as coffee and carbonated beverages.
• Complete the entire course of antibiotics as prescribed.
• Cranberry in the form of juice or concentrated tablets daily may decrease the risk of recurrent UTI. Cranberry alters the ability of bacteria to adhere to the walls of the balder and other parts of the urinary tract (Jepson & Craig, 2008).

Recurrent UTI

Approximately one-third of pregnant women diagnosed with UTI will have recurrence (Johnson, 2012). Suppressive therapy is recommended for any pregnant woman with (a) persistent symptomatic or asymptomatic bacteriuria after two antibiotic treatments, (b) all women with a prepregnancy history of recurrent UTIs, (c) a history of acute pyelonephritis during the current pregnancy, and (d) after one lower UTI during pregnancy in women with conditions that potentially increase the risk of complication during episodes of acute cystitis, such as diabetes or sickle cell trait (Epp & Larochelle, 2010). It is also reasonable to use postcoital prophylaxis if UTI is brought on by sexual activity, which is common.

Care of women with suspected acute pyelonephritis

Pyelonephritis is the most common UTI complication in pregnant women, occurring in approximately 2% of all pregnancies (Johnson, 2012). Acute pyelonephritis is characterized by fever, flank pain, and tenderness in addition to significant bacteriuria. Additional symptoms include chills, myalgia, anorexia, nausea, vomiting, and low back pain. Common signs of acute cystitis may or may not be present.

Additional evaluation may include a CBC, chemistry panel, *Chlamydia* cultures, and chest X-ray if dyspnea is present (Johnson, 2012).

Because of increased perinatal risks in women with pyelonephritis, comanagement and/or referral of women presenting with signs and symptoms of pyelonephritis is warranted. The standard course of treatment for pyelonephritis consists of hospital admission and intravenous administration of antibiotics, generally cephalosporins or gentamycin. Outpatient treatment may be an option with carefully selected patients up to 24 weeks' gestation (Schnarr & Smaill, 2008). Women with pyelonephritis can become dehydrated because of nausea and vomiting and often need intravenous hydration. However, they are at high risk for the development of pulmonary edema and acute respiratory distress syndrome (ARDS), and fluids must be administered cautiously. Fever is managed with antipyretics, typically acetaminophen, and antiemetics are given for nausea and vomiting.

Nephrolithiasis

Kidney stones are renal calculi that develop from a combination of naturally occurring chemicals in the body. These chemicals include calcium, oxalate, phosphate, uric acid, and cysteine (National Kidney and Urologic Diseases Information Clearinghouse, 2007). Calcium salts form the majority of the stones identified. Symptomatic nephrolithiasis occurs in 1 in 1500–2000 pregnancies (Rosenburg et al., 2011; Thomas et al., 2010) and is more common in Caucasian women (Lewis, Robichaux, Jaekle, Marcum, & Stedman, 2003). Symptomatic nephrolithiasis is more common in the last two trimesters of pregnancy due to ureteral dilation and compression by the gravid uterus, which allows for more stones to pass through the ureter.

Potential problems associated with nephrolithiasis in pregnancy include hypertension, preeclampsia, preterm birth, and operative birth (Thomas et al., 2010).

Women with nephrolithiasis during pregnancy and postpartum commonly present with acute flank pain, abdominal pain, nausea, vomiting, and hematuria (Thomas et al., 2010). Pyuria may or may not be present. Women with stones in the lower urinary tract may present with frequency, urgency, and dysuria. Approximately 50% of women with kidney stones will have a concomitant UTI (Srirangam, Hickerton, & Cleynenbreugel, 2008). Differential diagnoses can include appendicitis, diverticulitis, placental abruption, pyelonephritis, and round ligament pain.

Evaluation

The problem-focused health history includes prior history of nephrolithiasis, renal disease, hypertension, and assessment of current symptoms. Physical exam includes assessment of CVA tenderness, temperature, abdominal exam, and assessment of fetal heart rate. It should be noted that normal pregnancy-related physical changes may alter the localization of pain and obscure diagnosis (Thomas et al., 2010).

Initial laboratory testing includes UA and dipstick for red blood cells (RBCs), white blood cells (WBCs) to detect concomitant infection. Urine pH should be obtained as a pH greater than 7 or less than 5 may indicate stones of various compositions (Srirangam et al., 2008). Urine culture to identify the presence and sensitivity of a pathogen should be done. Ultrasound is the preferred method to diagnose kidney stones during pregnancy (Srirangam et al., 2008).

Care of women with suspected nephrolithiasis

Management of women with suspected nephrolithiasis requires consultation, collaboration, or referral for medical services, depending on the woman's presentation and the clinician's expertise. The midwife or nurse practitioner should assess and treat a concomitant UTI if the woman is not in acute distress, and promptly initiate services to evaluate for nephrolithiasis. Management is determined by the size, location of stone, and gestational age. Conservative treatment of nephrolithiasis is often first line, which includes oral or IV hydration, pain control, and antibiotics for concomitant infection (Shrotri et al., 2007; Thomas et al., 2010). The majority of women will spontaneously pass kidney stones with conservative treatment (Srirangam et al., 2008), and 50% of the remaining women will pass the stone in the postpartum period (Thomas et al., 2010).

Some pregnant women with stones will need active invasive intervention. Indications for enhanced intervention are the same as nonpregnant women: intractable pain, febrile UTI, obstructive uropathy, nausea, vomiting, acute renal failure, sepsis, or obstruction of a solitary kidney (Shrotri et al., 2007; Thomas et al., 2010).

Summary

UTI, pyelonephritis, and nephrolithiasis are common in pregnancy and, if untreated, may lead to significant morbidity and mortality for both the mother and the fetus (Thomas et al., 2010). In pregnant women, UTIs are an independent risk factor for preterm birth and also are associated with preeclampsia, fetal growth restriction, and cesarean delivery (Mazor-Dray et al., 2009). Nephrolithiasis poses the potential for serious complications to the mother and fetus, including hypertension, preeclampsia, preterm labor, recurrent abortions, gestational diabetes mellitus, and cesarean delivery (Rosenburg et al., 2011). Inter-professional management is appropriate for significant urinary tract complications during pregnancy.

Case study

Asymptomatic bacteriuria

Carolyn L. is a 19-year-old African American G1 P0, at 11 weeks' gestation, presenting for her first prenatal examination.

Her present pregnancy history is positive for amenorrhea, fatigue, mild nausea with rare vomiting, anorexia, and breast tenderness. She states that she has noticed some urinary frequency, but no dysuria or urgency. Her family history, gynecologic history, and review of systems are within normal. She has a history of mild asthma with occasional corticosteroid inhaler use. She has no known allergies.

The physical examination reveals normal vital signs and a body mass index (BMI) of 22.4. A physical exam is performed and is normal. The pelvic exam reveals a uterine size consistent with 11 weeks' gestation; the fetal heart rate is 154 bpm.

Findings on routine urine dipstick

RBCs positive
WBCs positive
Nitrites negative
Bacteria positive
Protein negative
Ketones negative

Results of the dipstick led to the consideration of the diagnosis of asymptomatic bacteriuria. Urine culture is the standard for diagnosis and treatment in pregnancy and was obtained. Since Carolyn was asymptomatic, treatment was deferred until culture and antibiotic sensitivity results were available for most effective treatment. Carolyn was counseled on signs and symptoms of UTI to report until treatment was established.

The culture results came back in 2 days positive for *E. coli*. She called with culture results and was placed on Keflex 500 mg QID for 10 days. Instructions were provided to avoid bubble baths, wearing thong underwear, to wipe from front to back after defecation, to void soon after intercourse, and to complete the entire course of antibiotics. She returned to the office at 14 weeks' gestation and reported taking all of her medication without problems. A repeat clean-catch midstream urine was obtained for a post-treatment test of cure and was negative. Since she has had one episode of asymptomatic bacteriuria, a urine dipstick will be done at each visit to assess for recurrence. A repeat urine culture at 28 weeks' gestation will be done to assess for recurrence.

Resources for women

ACOG: FAQ about group B strep in pregnancy: http://www.acog.org/~/media/For%20Patients/faq105.ashx

ACOG: FAQ about Urinary Tract Infections: http://www.acog.org/~/media/For%20Patients/faq050.ashx?dmc=1&ts=20120119T1613435982

CDC: Group B strep what you need to know patient handout: http://www.cdc.gov/groupbstrep/downloads/GBS_Patient_Info.pdf

CDC: Protect your baby from group B strep handout (in English): http://www.cdc.gov/groupbstrep/resources/downloads/flyer-protect-baby.pdf

Resource for health-care providers

CDC: 2010 Guidelines for the prevention of perinatal group B streptococcal disease: http://www.cdc.gov/mmwr/preview/mmwrhtml/rr5910a1.htm?s_cid=rr5910a1_w

References

Allen, V. M., Yudin, M. H., Bouchard, C., Boucher, M., Caddy, S., Castillo, E., . . . Senikas V., Infectious Diseases Committee, Society of Obstetricians and Gynaecologists of Canada. (2012). Management of group B streptococcal bacteriuria in pregnancy. *Journal of Obstetrics and Gynaecology Canada, 34*(5), 482–486.

American Congress of Obstetricians and Gynecologists (ACOG). (2011). Sulfonamides, nitrofurantoin, and risk of birth defects. Committee Opinion No. 494. American College of Obstetricians and Gynecologists. *Obstetrics and Gynecology, 117,* 1484–1485.

Awonuga, D., Fawole, A., Dada-Adegbola, H., Olola, F., & Awonuga, O. (2011). Asymptomatic bacteriuria in pregnancy: Evaluation of reagent strips in comparison to microbiological culture. *African Journal of Medicine and Medical Sciences* [serial on the Internet], *40*(4), 377–383. [cited July 18, 2012].

Bryan, C. (2011). Urinary Tract Infections, Chapter 7. In Infectious Disease Section of Microbiology and Immunology On-line. Retrieved from http://pathmicro.med.sc.edu/infectious%20disease/Urinary%20Tract%20Infections.htm

Centers for Disease Control and Prevention (CDC). (2010). Prevention of perinatal group B streptococcal disease: Revised guidelines from the CDC. *MMWR. Morbidity and Mortality Weekly Report, 59*(RR10), 1–32.

Chen, Y., Chen, S., Li, H., & Lin, H. (2011). No increased risk of adverse pregnancy outcomes in women with urinary tract infections: A nationwide population based study. *Acta Obstetricia et Gynecologica Scandinavica, 89*(7), 882–888.

Clinical and Laboratory Standards Institute (CLSI). (2001). Urinalysis and collection, transportation, and preservation of urine specimens; approved guideline—Third Edition. Vol. 29. No. 4. Document GP-16A3. Wayne, PA.

Dalzell, J. E., & Lefevre, M. L. (2000). Urinary tract infection of pregnancy. *American Academy of Family Physicians, 61*(3), 713–721.

Epp, A., & Larochelle, A. (2010). Recurrent urinary tract infection, society of obstetricians and gynecologists of Canada (SOGC) clinical practice guideline, NO. 250. *Journal of Obstetrics and Gynaecology Canada, 32*(11), 1082–1090.

Hill, J. B., Sheffield, J. S., McIntire, D. D., & Wendel, G. D., Jr. (2005). Acute pyelonephritis in pregnancy. *Obstetrics and Gynecology, 105*(1), 18–23.

Jepson, J. P., & Craig, J. C. (2008). Cranberries for preventing urinary tract infections. *Cochrane Database of Systematic Reviews*, (1), CD 001321.

Johnson, E. K. (2012). Overview of UTIs in Pregnancy. Retrieved from http://emedicine.medscape.com/article/452604-overview

Lewis, D. F., Robichaux, A. G., Jaekle, R. K., Marcum, N. G., & Stedman, C. M. (2003). Uriolithiasis in pregnancy. *The Journal of Reproductive Medicine, 48*(2), 28–32.

Manns-James, L. (2011). Pregnancy, Chapter 35. In T. King & M. Brucker (Eds.), *Pharmacology for women's health* (pp. 1066–1067). Boston: Jones and Bartlett.

Mazor-Dray, E., Levy, A., Schlaeffer, F., & Scheiner, E. (2009). Maternal urinary tract infection: Is it independently associated with adverse pregnancy outcomes? *The Journal of Maternal-Fetal and Neonatal Medicine, 22*(2), 124–128.

McIsaac, W., Carroll, J. C., Biringer, A., Bernstein, P., Lyons, E., Low, D. E., & Permaul, J. A. (2005). Screening for asymptomatic bacteriuria in pregnancy. *Journal of Obstetrics and Gynaecology Canada, 27*, 20–24.

Millar, L. K., & Cox, S. M. (1997). Urinary tract infections complicating pregnancy. *Infectious Disease Clinics of North America, 11*(1), 13–26.

Morgan, K. L. (2004). Management of UTIs. *MCN. The American Journal of Maternal Child Nursing, 29*(4), 254–258.

National Kidney and Urologic Diseases Information Clearinghouse. (2007). Kidney stones in adults. Retrieved from http://kidney.niddk.nih.gov/Kudiseases/pubs/stonesadults/#what

Rosenburg, E., Sergienko, R., Abu-Ghanem, S., Wiznitzer, A., Romanowsky, I., Neulander, E. Z., & Sheiner, E. (2011). Nephroli-

thiasis during pregnancy: Characteristics, complications and pregnancy outcomes. *World Journal of Urology, 29*(6), 743–747.

Schnarr, J., & Smaill, F. (2008). Asymptomatic bacteriuria and symptomatic urinary tract infection in pregnancy. *European Journal of Clinical Investigation, 38*(S2), 50–57.

Sheffield, J. S., & Cunningham, G. (2005). Urinary tract infection in women. *Obstetrics and Gynecology, 106*(5), 1085–1092.

Shrotri, K. N., Morrison, I. D., & Shrotri, N. C. (2007). Urological conditions in pregnancy: A diagnostic and therapeutic challenge. *Journal of Obstetrics and Gynaecology, 27*(7), 648–654.

Simerville, J. A., Maxted, W. C., & Pahira, J. J. (2005). Urinalysis: A comprehensive review. *American Family Physician, 71*(6), 1153–1162.

Smaill, F. (2007). Asymptomatic bacteriuria in pregnancy. *Best Practice and Research. Clinical Obstetrics and Gynaecology, 21*(3), 439–450.

Smaill, F., & Vazquez, J. C. (2007). Antibiotics for asymptomatic bacteriuria in pregnancy. *Cochrane Database of Systematic Reviews, 2*(2).

Srirangam, S. J., Hickerton, B., & Cleynenbreugel, B. V. (2008). Management of urinary calculi in pregnancy: A review. *Journal of Endourology/Endourological Society, 22*(5), 867–875.

Thomas, A. A., Thomas, A. Z., Campbell, S. C., & Palmer, J. S. (2010). Urologic emergencies in pregnancy. *Urology, 76*(2), 453–460.

United States Preventative Services Task Force (USPSTF). (2008). Guide to preventive services. Retrieved from http://www.uspreventiveservicestaskforce.org/uspstf08/asymptbact/asbactrs.htm

Vazquez, J. C., & Abalos, E. (2011). Treatments for symptomatic urinary tract infections during pregnancy. *Cochrane Database of Systematic Reviews*, (1), CD002256. doi:10.1002/14651858.CD002256.pub2

Whitehead, N. S., Callaghan, W., Johnson, C., & Williams, L. (2009). Racial, ethnic and economic disparities in the prevalence of pregnancy complications. *Maternal and Child Health Journal, 13*, 198–205.

Widmer, M., Gülmezoglu, A. M., Mignini, L., & Roganti, A. (2011). Duration of treatment for asymptomatic bacteriuria during pregnancy. *Cochrane Database of Systematic Reviews*, (12), CD000491. doi:10.1002/14651858.CD000491.pub2

35

Gastrointestinal disorders

Audra C. Malone and Karen DeCocker-Geist

Relevant terms

Appendicitis—acute inflammation of the appendix; may be associated with complications such as gangrene, perforation, or abscess formation

Cholestasis—a pregnancy-related liver condition in which bile flow is blocked from the liver

Cholelithiasis—formation of a stone within the gallbladder caused by accumulation of bile components

Gastroenteritis—an acute, self-limiting gastrointestinal illness characterized by diarrhea that may or may not be accompanied by fever, nausea, and vomiting; gastroenteritis is commonly referred to as the stomach flu or food poisoning

Jaundice—a yellow color of the skin, mucous membranes, or eyes caused by excessive bilirubin

McBurney's point—the point on the right lower quadrant of the abdomen over the appendix, midway between the anterosuperior iliac spine and umbilicus; used as a landmark to evaluate tenderness in suspected appendicitis

Murphy's sign—a sign of gallbladder disease in which the woman is asked to inhale while the examiner's fingers are hooked under the liver border at the bottom of the rib cage; the inspiration causes the gallbladder to descend onto the fingers, producing pain if the gallbladder is inflamed

Introduction

Approximately 80% of pregnant women will experience gastrointestinal distress during their pregnancy (Kametas & Nelson-Piercy, 2007). Many of the gastrointestinal symptoms reported during prenatal care are associated with normal physiological changes of pregnancy such as nausea, vomiting, constipation, and heartburn. The assessment and management of these conditions are described in Chapter 11. Pregnancy may also be associated with a more serious form of nausea and vomiting known as hyperemesis gravidarum, which is addressed in Chapter 24. This chapter reviews the signs and symptoms, and evaluation of women presenting with abnormal gastrointestinal conditions during pregnancy including gastroenteritis, intraheptic cholestasis of pregnancy (ICP), cholecystitis, and appendicitis.

Gastroenteritis

Gastroenteritis, commonly referred to as stomach flu or food poisoning, is an acute, self-limiting disorder characterized by diarrhea. It causes irritation and inflammation of the gastrointestinal tract. Gastroenteritis can be caused by infectious agents including viruses (e.g., noroviruses), bacteria (e.g., *Escherichia coli*), and protozoa (e.g., *Giardia lamblia*). Parasitic infections and food-borne toxins may also cause gastroenteritis. Most cases of acute gastroenteritis are self-limiting and benign. However, more harmful causes of gastroenteritis are *Listeria*, *Salmonella*, *E. coli*, *Shigella*, and *Clostridium difficile*.

Evaluation and management

Diagnosis of gastroenteritis is generally based on history and clinical symptoms. Gastroenteritis commonly presents as acute diarrhea, nausea, and vomiting, with or without fever. Women with gastroenteritis may experience cramping abdominal pain, bloating, mucus or blood in the stool, and decreased urination.

Prenatal and Postnatal Care: A Woman-Centered Approach, First Edition. Edited by Robin G. Jordan, Janet L. Engstrom, Julie A. Marfell, and Cindy L. Farley.
© 2014 John Wiley & Sons, Inc. Published 2014 by John Wiley & Sons, Inc.

Subjective data gathering for women presenting with gastroenteritis

- Gestational age of the pregnancy
- Fetal movement patterns
- Presence of any uterine contractions
- Current symptoms
- Recent travel
- Exposure to animals
- Recent meals
- Anyone else in the home with same symptoms
- Contact with potentially contaminated food or water

Objective data gathering for women presenting with gastroenteritis

- General status and level of distress
- Vital signs
- Mucous membranes, skin turgor, orthostatic changes
- Abdominal palpation for tenderness and signs of acute abdomen
- Fetal heart tones
- Signs of uterine irritability
- Urine ketones, leukocytes, and nitrites

Differential diagnoses for gastroenteritis depend on the severity of the signs and symptoms as well as the gestational age of the pregnancy. The differential diagnosis should include ectopic pregnancy, hyperemesis gravidarum, appendicitis, and urinary tract infection. Extensive diagnostic testing is not usually indicated in healthy pregnant women with diarrhea and gastrointestinal distress. Urine dipstick or urinalysis for ketones to detect signs of dehydration and bacteruria can be performed. Microbiological stool samples are considered if the woman has signs of more severe illness such as bloody stool, prolonged fever, and neurological involvement such as paresthesia, severe dehydration, or suspicion of exposure to food toxins (Operario & Houpt, 2011).

Oral rehydration therapy is the recommended mode of administration, but this depends on the hydration status and clinical presentation of the pregnant woman. If the woman can tolerate oral fluids, rehydration with an over-the-counter (OTC) oral rehydration solution is recommended to maintain baseline need for hydration as well as to replace fluids that have been lost in diarrhea. The woman should be instructed to drink a rehydration solution slowly, consuming small amounts hourly as opposed to trying to quickly replace fluids. Intravenous fluid replacement may be indicated if the symptoms are severe and dehydration is present. A gradual return to a normal diet, starting with bland foods, should be encouraged as symptoms subside.

Antibiotics may be required based on the results of the stool culture and sensitivity. Azithromycin is recommended to use empirically for travelers' diarrhea and is safe to use in pregnancy. It is important to note that loperamide is not recommended in pregnancy for the treatment of acute diarrhea because it may cause complications in diarrheal illnesses associated with bacterial infections such as ileus or toxic megacolon. In addition, loperamide is contraindicated for bloody diarrhea and immunocompromised patients. *Listeriosis* is treated with penicillins or with sulfamethoxazole/trimethoprim (Bactrim) if the patient has an allergy to penicillin. OTC probiotics may be recommended since they can help prevent diarrhea and restore positive flora that are often destroyed during antibiotic use (Dugoua et al., 2009).

Scope of practice issues

Most pregnant women with gastroenteritis recover without intervention or complications. Obstetrical consultation is warranted for women presenting with severe and persistent nausea and vomiting with diarrhea, signs of preterm labor, or fetal distress.

Intraheptic cholestasis of pregnancy

Prenatal cholestasis, also known as ICP, affects approximately 1 in 700 pregnant women (Cuckson & Germain, 2011). It is characterized by symptoms of severe pruritis and impaired liver function. ICP has no clear etiology, and it is thought to be a multifactorial disorder caused by hormonal, genetic, immune, and environmental factors. The condition has a strong familial component and is more common in relatives and offspring of women who experience ICP during pregnancy (Kingham, 2006). The normal physiological changes of pregnancy may predispose some women to ICP. The elevated levels of progesterone during pregnancy slow gallbladder emptying during pregnancy, resulting in bile stasis. The stasis may be so severe in some women that the excess bile acids may enter the circulation. The elevated levels of estrogen during pregnancy also influence gallbladder function, redisposing women to ICP (Geenes & Williamson, 2009).

Typically, ICP presents in the third trimester but can begin at any time during the pregnancy. Severe itching, especially of the hands and feet, and reports of very dark urine are common with ICP. Bowel movements may be light colored. Jaundice may develop but is usually seen after several weeks of ICP or in severe cases. The pruritis of ICP generally worsens at night. It may be of such intensity that it becomes intolerable and interferes with the woman's ability to function. In these cases, labor induction is considered as early as 35–37 weeks of gestation (Pathak, Sheibani, & Lee, 2010). Questions about pruritus should be a routine component of the prenatal assessment during the last trimester of pregnancy and, when women report symptoms, the condition should be evaluated promptly. ICP is associated with high rates of preterm birth (30–60%) and fetal distress (33%), and is also associated with an increased risk of intrauterine fetal death (2–5%) (Geenes & Williamson, 2009; Milkiewicz et al., 2002). Thus, prompt diagnosis and referral are imperative.

The diagnosis of ICP is based on physical examination, clinical presentation, and laboratory findings. ICP is usually a diagnosis of exclusion. Other differential diagnoses include dermatitis, hepatitis, pancreatitis, or pre-eclampsia. Laboratory testing should include a liver panel that includes asparate aminotransferase (AST), alanie aminotransferase (ALT), gamma-glutamyl transpeptidase (GGT), alkaline phosphatase (ALP), and total bilirubin. Coagulation studies such a prothrombin time (PT), partial thromboplastin time(PTT), and international normalized ratio (INR) should also be performed. Serum bile acid levels are an essential component of the evaluation of a woman with suspected ICP.

Once a diagnosis of ICP has been made, close fetal surveillance by nonstress testing and biophysical profile is indicated to monitor fetal health. Total serum bile acid levels are followed every 2–3 weeks to guide therapy and the timing of birth. Ursodeoxycholic acid (UDCA), more commonly known as Urso, improves clinical symptoms and liver parameters in ICP. Symptomatic relief can be offered through the use of antihistamines such as diphenhydramine (Benadryl). Oatmeal-based lotions and baths may temporarily soothe the skin and relieve itching.

Scope of practice issues

Laboratory screening should be performed immediately for pregnant women with suspected ICP. Consultation and referral to obstetrical services is essential if laboratory testing reveals ICP due to a significant risk of preterm birth, fetal distress, and fetal death. All women with ICP should have a plan for the continued assessment of fetal well-being and ongoing monitoring of maternal status and liver function.

Cholecystitis

Cholecystitis is the acute inflammation of the gallbladder usually resulting from bile accumulation when the cystic duct becomes occluded by gallstones or biliary sludge. As the obstruction persists, the gallbladder becomes thickened and inflamed, which can lead to a secondary infection caused by organisms commonly found in the bowel,

and results in necrosis or gangrene. Approximately 1 in 1000 pregnant women are affected by acute cholecystitis (Gilo, Amini, & Landy, 2009). Acute cholecystitis is the second most common nonobstetrical surgical emergency in pregnant women after acute appendicitis (Mendez-Sanchez, Chavez-Tapia, & Uribe, 2006).

The normal hormonal changes that occur during pregnancy predispose the women to the formation of gallstones and the development of biliary sludge. Estrogen contributes to increased cholesterol formation and progesterone causes decreased soluble bile acid secretion, which favors the formation of gallstones (Gilo et al., 2009). Progesterone causes decreased smooth muscle contractility of the gallbladder, which delays bladder emptying and exacerbates bile stasis. After the woman gives birth, the more soluble forms of bile acids are secreted; however, this return to the prepregnancy state may take months (Gilo et al., 2009). The risk of gallstones increases with the number of pregnancies and with age.

Evaluation and management

Pregnant women with acute cholecystitis usually present with epigastric pain that can vary from minimal to severe. The woman may report colicky pain located in the upper right quadrant, nausea, vomiting, and heartburn, especially after eating a high fat content meal (Gilo et al., 2009). The woman's general appearance and level of distress should be noted and the skin and sclera observed for jaundice. A fever may be present in women with acute cholecystitis. The differential diagnosis of cholecystitis includes appendicitis, pancreatitis, peptic ulcer disease, pyelonephritis, HELLP syndrome, hepatitis, and acute fatty liver (Gilo et al., 2009).

Palpation of the abdomen should be done to assess right upper quadrant tenderness and to determine Murphy's sign. To elicit Murphy's sign, the examiner asks the woman to take in a deep inspiration as the examiner's fingers are hooked under the liver border at the bottom of the rib cage. The inspiration causes the gallbladder to descend onto the fingers, producing pain if the gallbladder is inflamed. Guarding and tenderness are positive responses.

Laboratory testing for women with suspected cholecystitis

Complete blood count (CBC)—assess for infection
ALT/AST—assess liver function
Total bilirubin—may be elevated in cholecystitis
Alkaline phosphatase—may be elevated in cholecystitis
Amylase/lipase—rule out pancreatitis

Ultrasound is effective in diagnosing gallstones and is safe during pregnancy. Once a diagnosis of cholecystitis is made, clinical management is dependent upon the gestational age of the pregnancy and the severity of symptoms. Conservative treatment includes intravenous hydration, bowel rest, broad-spectrum antibiotics, and analgesia (Cuckson & Germain, 2011). Fetal assessment and uterine monitoring are indicated, depending on the gestational age of the pregnancy. Surgical intervention may be delayed into the second trimester to avoid the risk of spontaneous pregnancy loss in the first trimester; however, surgical laparoscopic techniques have improved and are more commonly used to treat women with gallstones in all trimesters of pregnancy (Corneille et al., 2010).

Scope of practice issues

A targeted evaluation by history, physical examination, and laboratory screening should be initiated immediately for pregnant women with suspected cholecystitis. Consultation and referral to obstetrical services is essential since the differential diagnosis of cholecystitis includes potentially life-threatening complications such as HELLP syndrome. Additionally, the treatment plan will be determined by obstetric consultation and surgical intervention may be required.

Appendicitis

Appendicitis is an inflammation of the appendix, a 3.5-in.-long tube of tissue that extends from the large intestine. Acute appendicitis affects approximately 1 out of 1000 pregnant women and is the primary cause of nontraumatic acute abdomen in pregnancy (Brown, Wilson, Coleman, & Joypaul, 2009). Acute appendicitis can occur any time during pregnancy and is considered a surgical emergency due to the increased risk for poor outcomes for both the mother and the fetus. A major risk for acute appendicitis in pregnancy is perforation, abscess formation, and peritonitis (Brown et al., 2009). Perinatal complications from appendicitis include preterm labor and birth, increased maternal morbidity, and fetal loss. A perforated appendix often leads to uterine contractions and premature labor. Maternal mortality rate is as high as 4%, while fetal death is estimated at 43% of pregnancies complicated by a perforated appendicitis (Murariu, Tatsuno, Hirai, & Takamori, 2011).

Evaluation and management

Evaluation of a pregnant woman presenting with acute abdominal pain warrants a careful workup due to the possible risks for the fetus and the mother. The diagnosis of appendicitis is made on the basis of clinical signs and symptoms, laboratory tests, and noninvasive imaging (Brown et al., 2009). The classic presentation of abdominal pain in appendicitis is a sharp midabdominal pain that increases over time, becoming more localized to the right lower quadrant. The woman may present with a report of abdominal pain, nausea, vomiting, and decreased appetite.

Pregnant women are less likely to have a classic presentation of appendicitis than nonpregnant women (Gilo et al., 2009). The normal physiological changes that accompany pregnancy make the diagnosis of appendicitis challenging. For example, typical symptoms of appendicitis such as nausea and vomiting are common occurrences for most pregnant women during the early months of pregnancy. Additionally, the enlarging uterus moves the appendix upward, displacing the location of pain and tenderness on palpation. The presentation may mimic that observed in women with preterm labor, lower or upper urinary tract infection, placental abruption, or cholecystitis.

The woman's general status and level of distress should be evaluated. Hydration status should be evaluated by assessing mucous membranes, skin turgor, and orthostatic changes, and fetal heart tones are documented. Abnormal vital signs such as tachycardia and fever can indicate pain and infection. Abdominal palpation may reveal tenderness and signs of an acute abdomen. Pain and tenderness are generally localized to the right side and may be in either the upper or lower quadrant. Uterine tone and the presence of any contractions should be noted.

There is no laboratory testing that is diagnostic for acute appendicitis in pregnancy. Laboratory testing generally includes a CBC, cryoreactive proteins (CRP), and urinalysis, along with liver function studies to rule out other etiologies. In the nonpregnant population, leukocytosis in the presence of right upper or lower quadrate pain should raise suspicion of acute appendicitis. In pregnant women, the normal leukocytosis of pregnancy (white blood cell [WBC] count as high as 16,000/μL) might mask signs of infection, making the WBC a less effective parameter than in nonpregnant women (Brown et al., 2009).

Scope of practice issues

As soon as acute appendicitis is suspected in a pregnant woman, prompt obstetrical and surgical evaluation should be initiated. Treatment of appendicitis is by surgical exploratory laparotomy or laparoscopic appendectomy.

Case study

Louise is a 34-year-old G3P2 at 32 weeks' gestation. She presents at the office for an urgent appointment with a report of right lower quadrant abdominal pain. The pain started last night and has been constant and increasing in intensity. Currently, her pain is rated 7/10. She has felt "warm" but did not take her temperature. Louise reports that she has felt nauseated but has not vomited. She reports no appetite. She appears to be in mild distress and anxious. She reports no precipitating event and denies substance use and trauma. Her chart is reviewed and reveals no risk factors, allergies, or contributory medical or family history. Her prepregnancy body mass index (BMI) is 26.6 and her total weight gain to date is 26 lb. Her vital signs are as follows: temperature 101.6°F oral, pulse 92, respirations 18 and nonlabored, and BP 128/70.

Findings on routine UA: negative for RBC's, WBC's, nitrites, bacteria, protein; Positive ketones; Specific gravity 1.036

An abdominal exam was done. Her fundal height is 33 cm and fetal heart tone 144 bpm. Positive bowel sounds are present in all quadrants; she is tender to palpation in the right mid quadrant, and rebound tenderness is present. There is no significant guarding; the uterus is soft, and no contractions are noted.

Her elevated temperature and abdominal findings are consistent with possible appendicitis. You discuss this possible diagnosis with her and advise her that you will bring in a consulting obstetrician to further evaluate. Louise is first sent to the lab for a CBC, CRP, and liver studies. When she returns to the office, the consulting obstetrician talks with Louise and reviews her exam findings, and initiates a general surgery consult for possible appendicitis while awaiting the lab results.

Summary

Many of the gastrointestinal symptoms reported during prenatal care are associated with normal physiological changes of pregnancy such as nausea, vomiting, constipation, and heartburn. The health care-provider must conduct a targeted history and physical examination in each woman to rule out gastrointestinal pathology. Laboratory evaluation may be required with abnormal findings. Prompt diagnosis and referral can reduce maternal and fetal complications associated with abnormal gastrointestinal conditions.

Resource for women and their families

A Center for Disease Control and Prevention (CDC) Web site on viral gastroenteritis: http://www.cdc.gov/ncidod/dvrd/revb/gastro/faq.htm

References

Brown, J. J. S., Wilson, C., Coleman, S., & Joypaul, B. V. (2009). Appendicitis in pregnancy: An ongoing diagnostic dilemma. *Colorectal Disease, 11*, 116–122. doi:10.1111/j.1463-1318.2008.01594.x

Corneille, M. G., Gallup, T. M., Bening, T., Wolf, S. E., Brougher, C., Myers, J. G., . . . Stewart, R. M. (2010). The use of laparoscopic surgery in pregnancy: Evaluation of safety and efficacy. *American Journal of Surgery, 200*(3), 363.

Cuckson, C., & Germain, S. (2011). Hyperemesis, gastrointestinal and liver disorders in pregnancy. *Obstetrics, Gynaecology and Reproductive Medicine, 21*(3), 80–85.

Dugoua, J., Machado, M., Zhu, X., Chen, X., Koren, G., & Einarson, T. (2009). Probiotic safety in pregnancy: A systematic review and meta-analysis of randomized controlled trials of *Lactobacillus, Bifidobacterium*, and *Saccharomyces* spp. *Journal of Obstetrics and Gynaecology Canada, 31*(6), 542–552.

Geenes, V., & Williamson, C. (2009). Intrahepatic cholestasis of pregnancy. *World Journal of Gastroenterology, 15*, 2049–2066.

Gilo, N., Amini, D., & Landy, H. (2009). Appendicitis and cholecystitis in pregnancy. *Clinical Obstetrics and Gynecology, 52*(4), 586–596.

Kametas, N., & Nelson-Piercy, C. (2007). Hyperemesis gravidarum, gastrointestinal and liver disease in pregnancy. *Obstetrics, Gynaecology and Reproductive Medicine, 18*(3), 69–75.

Kingham, J. G. C. (2006). Liver disease in pregnancy. *Clinical Medicine (London, England), 6*(1), 34–39.

Mendez-Sanchez, N., Chavez-Tapia, N. C., & Uribe, M. (2006). Pregnancy and gallbladder disease. *Annals of Hepatology, 5*(3), 227.

Milkiewicz, P., Gallagher, R., Chambers, J., Eggington, E., Weaver, J., & Elias, E. (2002). Obstetric cholestasis. *BMJ (Clinical Research Ed.), 324*(7330), 123–124.

Murariu, D., Tatsuno, B., Hirai, C. A., & Takamori, R. (2011). Case report and management of suspected acute appendicitis in pregnancy. *Hawaii Medical Journal, 70*(2), 30.

Operario, D. J., & Houpt, E. (2011). Defining the causes of diarrhea: Novel approaches. *Current Opinion in Infectious Diseases, 24*(5), 464–471. doi:10.1097/QCO.0b013e32834aa13a

Pathak, B., Sheibani, L., & Lee, R. H. (2010). Cholestasis of pregnancy. *Obstetrics and Gynecology Clinics of North America, 37*(2), 269–282.

36

Obesity

Cecelia M. Jevitt

Introduction

In the United States, one-third of women over age 15 and older are obese (Centers for Disease Control and Prevention (CDC), 2012a). The incidence of obesity is increasing and obesity during pregnancy is becoming a common condition. Maternal pregravid obesity is a significant risk factor for adverse perinatal outcomes. This chapter covers the special prenatal care issues relevant to the pregnant woman with a body mass index (BMI) $\geq$ 30.

Overview

A common folk lore saying is "Pregnant women eat for two." This perspective may actually contribute to overeating in pregnancy. A more accurate saying would be "Pregnant women eat for 1.1" because fetal growth and the increased metabolic demands of pregnancy only require an extra 300 cal/day.

Obese individuals are at high risk for a variety of poor health outcomes and risk increases linearly as excess weight increases. Obesity can also be defined by a waist circumference greater than 35 in. (88 cm) in nonpregnant women. Abdominal adipose tissue is the most metabolically active adipose tissue producing a variety of inflammatory cytokines and hormones. Therefore, the greater the waist circumference, the higher the risk for obesity-related diseases. Waist circumference loses its usefulness in pregnancy; therefore, BMI has become the international measurement used to describe the relationship of weight to height during pregnancy. The Institute of Medicine (IOM) recommends a gain of 11- to 20-lb total for women in the obese category, with women

Prenatal and Postnatal Care: A Woman-Centered Approach, First Edition. Edited by Robin G. Jordan, Janet L. Engstrom, Julie A. Marfell, and Cindy L. Farley.
© 2014 John Wiley & Sons, Inc. Published 2014 by John Wiley & Sons, Inc.

Table 36.1   IOM Recommendations for Total Pregnancy Weight Gain for Women with BMI > 30

Prepregnancy obesity class		Optimal weight gain
Obese: BMI ≥ 30		11–20 lb
Class 1	BMI 30.0–34.9	
Class 2	BMI 35.0–39.9	
Class 3	BMI 40+	

in higher obesity classes gaining at the lower end of the range (Table 36.1).

Prevalence

Obesity during pregnancy is now a common condition affecting approximately one of five pregnant women (CDC, 2012a). Prior to 1970, obesity was uncommon in the United States and other industrialized nations. Between 1980 and 2000, mean maternal weight at the first prenatal visit increased by 20% and the incidence of women who were obese at the first prenatal visit tripled (Lu et al., 2001). Currently, 30% of reproductive age women in the United States are overweight, while another 30% are obese (Ogden, Caroll, Bit, & Flegal, 2012). Older adults have a higher incidence of obesity than youth (17%), suggesting that nutritional interventions for the young may be effective in reducing age-related weight gain. Additionally, following the national focus on reducing obesity, obesity rates did not increase from 2007–2008 to 2009–2010 for adults or children (Ogden et al., 2012). While obesity is associated with increased perinatal potential problems, it should be remembered that many pregnant women with obesity have a normal pregnancy and birth course.

Health disparities and cultural considerations

Large disparities exist in obesity and associated health impacts across racial and ethnic groups in the United States. Racial and ethnic differences in obesity did not change significantly from 1988 through 2008, with black and Mexican American women having a higher prevalence of obesity than white women. The higher the income in white women, the lower the prevalence of obesity (CDC, 2011). This relationship is weaker among other groups. Racial and ethnic differences in the prevalence of obesity persist after controlling for income, suggesting differing cultural norms in perceived health and genetic differences in metabolism. The elevated rate of extreme obesity in black women may account for a

portion of the black–white disparity in neonatal mortality (Salihu et al., 2008).

Low socioeconomic status is an independent risk factor for obesity. In the United States, women with higher incomes and higher levels of education have lower BMIs. High rates of obesity are linked to lower incomes and education. Women who are uninsured prior to their pregnancy or who are on Medicaid are at a higher risk of being overweight or obese (Wang & Chen, 2012).

Many cultural and environmental factors affect the risk for obesity. Weight acceptance is based upon cultural norms. Children raised in families where the parents are obese learn to view this body type as beautiful and the cultural norm (Everette, 2008), contributing to generational obesity patterns.

In some immigrant groups coming from countries where starvation is widespread, being overweight is a sign of health and prosperity. Mothers from these areas may purposefully overfeed themselves and their children, attempting to look prosperous. In other communities where HIV/AIDS caused weight loss and wasting, having excess adipose tissue is a sign of being HIV free.

Food preferences are also culturally based. Meal times are social opportunities. All cultures use food in celebratory ceremonies. Individuals learn to associate food with happiness and prosperity. Conversely, limiting intake or dieting is viewed as punitive or restrictive. Food habits are among the hardest habits to change.

Personal and family considerations

Some women, particularly young women and women with low incomes, have little control over their food choices. They may eat at the home of their mothers or sisters when they have no money to buy their own food and have little choice in what is served. Women who qualify for Women, Infants, and Children's (WIC) supplemental foods or the Supplemental Nutrition Assistance Program (SNAP), formerly known as food stamps, may share their foods with other family members who do not qualify for assistance. The clinician can suggest that the mother mark these foods "for the baby."

Full service groceries are not common in low-income neighborhoods where convenience food stores are more often found. Convenience stores stock processed foods with long shelf lives that are calorie dense but nutrient poor. High-fat, high-sugar processed foods are less expensive than fresh fruits and vegetables, prompting families with tight budgets to purchase less nutritious food. Transportation barriers to full service groceries are common for low-income families. Risk factors for pregestational obesity are noted below.

Risk factors for obesity

Maternal factors
Having an obese mother
Maternal diabetes during pregnancy
Excessive maternal weight gain during pregnancy
Birth weight > 4000 g

Environmental factors
Low family income
Low education
Food insecurity
Unsafe/urban neighborhoods

Health factors
Hypothyroidism
Polycystic ovary syndrome
Psychiatric medication use

Psychiatric medications shown to cause weight gain

Clozapine
Olanzapine
Quetiapine
Risperidone
Iloperidone
Ziprasidone
Asenapine tricyclic antidepressants
Monoamine oxidase inhibitors
Some selective serotonin reuptake inhibitors (especially paroxetine)

Source: Nihalani et al. (2011).

Obesity physiology

Food intake greater than that used by basal metabolic needs and calories burned during daily activity is initially stored as muscle glycogen. When not used for immediate energy needs, it is converted into stored fat. Stored fat is deposited around the body. Adipose tissue is metabolically active, particularly retroperitoneal fat, which produces inflammatory cytokines such as tumor necrosis factor alpha (TNFα). The production of inflammatory cytokines may account for the rise in diseases, such as hypertension with increasing BMI. Excess adipose tissue increases cardiac workload. Coupled with the increased circulatory demands of pregnancy, the increased cardiac demands of obesity increase risk for hypertensive disorders of pregnancy (Helmreich, Hundley, & Varvel, 2008).

Insulin is a growth hormone in pregnancy. Women with BMIs ≥30 are insulin resistant. Many pregnancy hormones such as estrogen and human placental lactogen promote insulin resistance. As gestation progresses, the metabolic demands of pregnancy outstrip pancreatic ability to produce insulin. Insulin resistance from obesity and pregnancy hormones contribute to the increased risk for gestational diabetes (GDM). Excess cytokine production, increased cardiac demand and increasing insulin resistance contribute to a variety of conditions that often accompany obesity in pregnancy.

Many psychotropic drugs are known to increase weight gain even obesity (Nihalani, Schwartz, Siddiqui, & Megna, 2011). The association of mental health problems, low income, and food insecurity makes weight management especially challenging.

Potential problems associated with obesity in childbearing women

The risks of adverse pregnancy outcomes increase as maternal BMI increases beyond the normal range (Table 36.2). Conception can be more difficult for obese women because they are less likely to ovulate regularly, have decreased fertility, and have increased risk of miscarriage. GDM affects as many as 20% of pregnancies in women who are obese, a fourfold increase compared to normal-weight women (Kim et al., 2010). Hypertension in pregnancy is more frequent in obese women. The risk of preterm birth in obese women is also elevated, likely in part because of their increased risk of preeclampsia. Recent investigations indicate that obesity prior to pregnancy is the strongest predictor of whether a mother will give birth to a large infant, even if the woman did not develop GDM (Black, Sacks, Xiang, & Lawrence, 2012; Retnakaran et al., 2012). This research suggests that reducing obesity prior to pregnancy may be

---

Common comorbidities of obesity in pregnancy

Pregestational type 2 diabetes
Pregestational type 1 diabetes
GDM, class A1 (diet controlled)
GDM, class A2 (hypoglycemic agent necessary)
Polycystic ovary syndrome
Chronic hypertension
Gestational hypertension
Preeclampsia
Hypothyroidism
Candidal vaginitis
Intertrigo
Dysthymia
Depression
Bulimia

Table 36.2   Potential Problems Associated with Obesity in Pregnancy

Prenatal potential problems	Intrapartum potential problems	Postpartum potential problems
• Spontaneous abortion • Neural tube defects • Anencephaly • Anemia • Gestational diabetes • Pregestational diabetes • Urinary tract infection • Genital tract infection • Prolonged pregnancy • Stillbirth • Preeclampsia • Pregnancy hypertension • Placental abruption • Intrauterine growth restriction	• Dysfunctional labor • Induction of labor • Pitocin labor augmentation • Forceps- or vacuum-assisted birth • Macrosomia • Shoulder dystocia • Cesarean section • Lower Apgar scores • Epidural failure • Increase use of general anesthesia • Immediate postpartum hemorrhage	• Wound dehiscence • Wound infection • Postpartum hemorrhage • Endometritis • Deep vein thrombosis • Urinary tract infection • Breastfeeding problems • Anemia • Excessive weight retention

Sources: ACOG (2013), Beyerlein et al. (2011).

more effective in reducing the incidence of large for gestational age (LGA) than treatment for GDM. Obese women are also at an increased risk for other perinatal problems such as birth defects and failure to initiate breastfeeding.

Management of pregestational obesity

Nondiscriminatory language

Many health-care providers dislike acknowledging women's weight issues, often fearing that they will alienate women from their practices. Weight and body image are sensitive issues; however, their effect on health can be so deleterious that clinicians who fail to address unhealthy weights are ignoring their patients' most pressing health-care needs. Using pejoratives such as "fatness" or "morbid obesity" is demeaning, while using euphemisms such as "big boned" or "plus sized" avoids the issue. The Obesity Society recommends using BMI descriptors or terms such as excess weight in place of pejorative language. The term "obesity" may be used in scientific writing but may be offensive in writing for the general public.

Assessment of the obese pregnant woman

Problem-focused health history

Obesity is diagnosed at the first prenatal visit using prepregnancy height and weight. Maternal recall may overestimate height and underestimate weight; therefore, accurate BMI calculations depend on a measured height and weight at the first prenatal visit. If the first prenatal visit is within the first 12 weeks of pregnancy, the health-care provider may decide to use the first clinic weight

measurement as the prepregnancy weight as some women may not remember a prepregnancy weight. Waist measurements for women exceeding 35 in. also indicate obesity. Waist measurement can be useful in the first trimester in diagnosing obesity in women with BMIs between 28 and 31. Muscle is more dense than fat. Well-muscled women, such as marathon runners, may have BMIs between 25 and 30 but have little adipose tissue. A waist measurement less than 35 in. paired with a BMI of 25–30 indicates increased muscle mass. Waist measurement may also be useful in the assessment of postpartum weight loss.

In addition to the elements of a routine prenatal history the clinician will want to take a detailed diet history (see Chapter 6). Physical activity during the work day, frequency of fast-food meals, and eating patterns should be explored. The woman's affect should be assessed carefully for signs of dysthymia or depression, such as avoidance of eye contact, flat affect, disparaging or self-deprecating comments, exhaustion, and inability to sleep. If the woman describes wide weight fluctuations, binging and purging eating practices should be explored.

Physical examination

Excess adipose tissue, particularly that deposited around the waist, confounds physical examination. In the first and early second trimester, the health-care provider may be unable to palpate the size of the uterus during the bimanual exam. Special long speculums may be needed to visualize the cervix.

Prenatal breast growth is a common cause of shoulder and back pain in obese women. Those with pendulous breasts should be encouraged to purchase well-fitting, supportive brassieres when breast growth is complete at about 20 weeks' gestation.

Ultrasound imaging is limited by obesity (Dashe, McIntire, & Twickler, 2009). Visualization during early screening, such as a 12- to 13-week nuchal translucency screening, may be incomplete and may require repeat exams outside of the best screening time frame. Fetal anatomy scans in the second trimester may need to be repeated depending on the depth of suprauterine adipose tissue.

Doppler assessment of early fetal heart tones may be delayed depending on adipose depth. Where heart tones can be auscultated by Doppler at 10–12 weeks on lean women, they might not be audible until 14–16 weeks in some obese women. If the mother has a large pannus (adipose apron) the fetal heart tones might be found by having the mother lift up the pannus and searching for the heart tones above the pubic bone. A referral for transvaginal ultrasound to rule out fetal death *in utero* may be needed if the fetal heart tones are inaudible.

Fundal height measurements are inaccurate in women with BMIs ≥30, and often exceed 40 cm in the last trimester. Palpation of fetal lie and position becomes more difficult as BMI exceeds 30, and the health-care provider may be unable to reach the presenting part to verify position. An ultrasound exam in late gestation may be necessary to verify position and can be useful to estimate fetal weight in obese women as needed.

Laboratory testing

Women with BMIs ≥30 at the first prenatal visit should have an early 1-hour GDM screen, either between or at the next prenatal visit. If that first screen is normal (blood glucose ≤ 130–140 mg/dL depending on practice guidelines), the gestational glucose screen should be repeated at 26–28 weeks' gestation. Lipid screening is not done during pregnancy or lactation as lipids are physiologically elevated during these periods. Thyroid function screening tests are not part of routine prenatal testing for pregnant women; however, serum thyroid-stimulating hormone (TSH) values should be obtained early in pregnancy in women with BMIs of 40 or greater as they have a higher risk for overt hypothyroidism (Stagnaro-Green et al., 2011).

Management principles

Women who are obese are encouraged to reduce weight before starting a pregnancy through behavior modification, reducing intake, and increasing activity level (ACOG, 2013). In the absence of a successful preconception program for weight loss, helping women achieve optimal prenatal weight gain begins at the first prenatal

---

Management of obesity in pregnancy

- Measure height with a stadiometer.
- Measure weight. Ask the woman to recall her prepregnancy weight. If the first prenatal visit is in the first trimester, consider using the weight at the first prenatal visit for the BMI calculation.
- Calculate the BMI.
- Assess psychological risk factors, depression, and potential eating disorders. Refer for counseling if necessary.
- Advise a pregnancy weight gain consistent with the 2009 IOM recommendations (Table 36.1) (Institute of Medicine, 2009). Document the target weight and counseling in the medical record.
- Assess comorbidities of obesity and patterns of previous weight gain and loss.
- Perform a nutritional assessment.
- Have woman identify one to two nonnutritious foods that could be dropped or changed immediately for more nutritious foods.
- Provide nutritional counseling.
- Refer for nutrition counseling if available.
- Obtain 1-hour oral glucose tolerance test (OGTT) at the first prenatal visit in women without pre-GDM. If normal, rescreen at 26–28 weeks.
- If the mother has pre-GDM or a history of GDM, assess HgA1C at the first prenatal visit. The percent of glycosolated hemoglobin should be less than 6%.
- Offer early screening for neural tube defects (NTDs) including early serum screening and ultrasound at 11–13 weeks to assess nuchal translucency. Obesity often limits ultrasound visualization and women may need to be rescheduled 1–2 weeks later, past the ideal nuchal translucency evaluation time.
- Schedule frequent visits every 2 weeks for regular weight gain assessment and nutrition counseling. Visits in addition to routine prenatal visits can be coded as other visits.

Source: ACOG (2013), Jevitt (2009).

---

visit. The desired outcomes include the woman having a prenatal weight gain within the IOM guidelines, to breastfeed for 1 year, and to have a gradual loss of all pregnancy weight gained by 9 months postpartum. Nutritional assessments and patient-centered counseling are time-consuming. Some practices have obese women return after the first visit for a separate nutrition counseling session. Nutrition and activity advice sessions are done most efficiently in group settings whether the groups are scheduled specifically for weight gain management in addition to prenatal care or integrated into group prenatal care.

Nutrition

Women with BMIs ≥30 have the same nutritional needs as pregnant women with lower BMIs. Generally, pregnant women do not need more than about an extra 300 cal/day after 16 weeks' gestation for proper fetal growth. Researchers have divided calorie recommendations by trimester with women needing an extra 20 kcal/day in the first trimester, 85 kcal/day in the second trimester, and 310 kcal in the third trimester (Thomas & Bishop, 2007). Some women with BMIs exceeding 35 may have been eating more than 4000 cal on many days and will not need to increase food intake to gain weight.

Obese women have the same elevated risk of congenital malformations as women with type 2 diabetes, particularly neural tube and cardiac defects (Blomberg & Kallen, 2010; Kennedy & Koren, 2012). Therefore, obese women ideally should start folic acid 4 mg orally daily before conceiving. If not started prenatally, extra folic acid should begin at the first prenatal visit and continue through the first trimester. Increased folic acid ingestion reduces the incidence of NTD in obese pregnant women; however, their risk remains elevated above normal-weight women (Ray, Wyatt, Vermeulen, Meier, & Cole, 2005).

Weight loss concerns

Weight loss is not recommended during pregnancy, even for women in the obese weight category. Some pregnant women who begin eating low-fat foods and increase fruit and vegetable consumption during pregnancy, reduce their daily calorie intake and lose weight. In the third trimester, obese women may feel as if they do not have enough room to eat their usual prepregnancy meals. Research regarding pregnancy weight reduction and outcomes has been inconclusive. Some experts have advocated for weight loss in obese women during pregnancy, citing improved immediate outcomes such as reduced operative birth, reduced incidence of GDM, and fetal macrosomia (Blomberg, 2011). Other studies indicate that women who lose weight during pregnancy have a decreased risk of pregnancy hypertension but an increased risk of preterm birth and SGA (Beyerlein, Schiessl, Lack, & Von Kries, 2011). Weight loss leads to a state of chronic ketosis from the breakdown of body fat. Ketones circulate in the woman's bloodstream and pass to the fetus. Studies suggest that fetal ketone exposure is associated with negative neurological effects and should be avoided. Animal studies have documented lower brain weight and reduced neurological development in offspring exposed to maternal ketones (Bhasin & Shambaugh, 1982). The

IOM recommends a pregnancy weight gain between 11 and 20 lb during pregnancy for obese women. Until long-term effects of maternal weight loss on the fetus are established, it may be prudent to discourage weight loss or weight maintenance during pregnancy.

Physical activity

Pregnant obese women should be encouraged to increase physical activity. Most pregnant women can walk 30 minutes a day regardless of weight. Walking provides non-insulin-mediated glucose use by muscle, helping to stabilize blood glucose (Swartz et al., 2003), and improves fitness for labor. Women with BMIs ≥40 or those with long-standing obesity should be evaluated for knee or back problems before starting a walking regimen. All women should start additional activity gradually and increase activity as tolerated.

Walking can be done in three 10-minute periods, two 15-minute periods, or continuously for 30 minutes (CDC, 2012a). This walking is done in addition to any waking done during the woman's regular work. Contemporary work has become sedentary, which can significantly reduce the physical activity of pregnant women.

Getting more sleep instead of using sleep time for increased physical activity is counterintuitive; however, sleep deprivation causes insulin resistance, lowering blood glucose levels and increasing appetite. Sleeping at least 7 hours a night is essential for weight maintenance (Gunderson et al., 2008). Overall, 30.0% of non-military-employed U.S. adults (approximately 40.6 million workers) report average sleep durations of ≤6 hours/day (CDC, 2012b). The real first step in activity advice for weight optimization is to have women rearrange their daily schedules to assure 7 hours of sleep or more as needed.

Comfort measures

Comfort measures for women with BMIs ≥30 are both psychological and physical. Obese women may be reluctant to come for timely care because of the social stigma associated with excessive weight. Weight measurement should be done in a private area. Large exam gowns should be used that give appropriate coverage. Office settings and birthing areas should have several rooms with bariatric-sized chairs, exam tables, and beds. Health providers should be aware that excess weight can amplify pregnancy common discomforts. Pregnancy stresses joints, particularly the low back, pelvis, knees, and ankles. These joints are already stressed by excess weight. Occasional acetaminophen, hot or cold packs, or soaking in a warm tub may provide some relief.

Common pregnancy discomforts exacerbated by obesity

Backache
Knee pain
Dependent edema
Dyspnea
Gastroesophageal reflux
Sleep disturbances

Bariatric surgery

The obesity rate among women of childbearing age is expected to rise from about 24% in 2005 to about 28% in 2015 (Sassi, Devaux, Cecchini, & Rusticelli, 2009), and the number of women having weight loss surgery is increasing. Pregnancy in women who have had bariatric surgery is safer than pregnancy in morbidly obese women (Hezelgrave & Oteng-Ntim, 2011). A recent review examined previous studies to assess the safety, limitations, and advantages of bariatric surgery prior to pregnancy and during and after surgery (Khan, Dawlatly & Chappatte, 2013). Bariatric surgery reduces pregnancy risk in extremely obese women, and most women experienced no complications during their pregnancy. However, early pregnancy loss is higher in women who become pregnant soon after surgery, and it is recommended that women should wait at least 1 year after bariatric surgery to attempt pregnancy. This waiting time allows for the weight loss phase to be completed and nutritional deficiencies to be corrected.

There are two types of bariatric surgery procedures commonly performed in the United States: (1) restrictive (laparoscopic gastric banding or LAP-BAND) and (2) restrictive/malabsorptive (Roux-en-Y gastric bypass [RYGB]).

In caring for pregnant women who have had bariatric surgery, it is important to know the type of procedure done. LAP-BAND slippage and movement can occur during pregnancy and result in severe vomiting (Vrebosch, Bel, Vansant, Guelinckx, & Devlieger, 2012). Some advocate for deflating the band prior to pregnancy to allow for adequate nutrition, though there are no guidelines of consensus (ACOG, 2009).

Prenatal nutrition in women who have had bariatric surgery is extremely important. As with all women, pregnancy weight gain recommendations are based on pre-pregnancy BMI. The RYGB procedure can drastically alter the absorption of food and medications and can lead to nutritional deficiencies in iron, vitamin B_{12}, folate, vitamin D, calcium, and protein. Anemia is common and can be severe in women who have undergone RYGB. A broad evaluation for deficiencies in micronutrients should be considered at the beginning of pregnancy in women who have had bariatric surgery, and supplements should be initiated if any deficits are present. If no deficits are noted, a complete blood count and measurement of iron, ferritin, calcium, and vitamin D levels every trimester should be considered (Armstrong, 2010).

Women who have had the RYGB procedure should avoid oral glucose challenge testing due to dumping syndrome. Assessment for GDM can be done by either following fasting and postprandial blood glucose levels after breakfast for 1 week (ACOG, 2009) or obtaining a Hgb A1C and assuming diabetes if >6.5 for women with prior RYGB surgery (Vrebosch et al., 2012). Fetal growth assessment by ultrasound may be appropriate in the third trimester if weight gain has been limited.

Optimal care of pregnant women after bariatric surgery includes multiple health-care providers such as dieticians and perinatal or obstetrical consultants.

Scope of practice considerations

Pregestational obesity and excessive gestational weight gain without comorbidities are within the scope of practice for midwives and for nurse practitioners with additional training.

Collaboration, consultation, and/or referral to obstetrical services depend more on comorbid conditions such as hypertension or GDM than on pregestational obesity or excessive prenatal weight gain. Many women with uncomplicated obesity and a weight gain within IOM ranges may have an otherwise normal pregnancy and birth. Obese women are at high risk for induction or augmentation of labor or cesarean birth, conditions requiring obstetrical consultation, comanagement, or referral. Difficulty in placing intravenous and epidural catheters and intubation increase with increasing BMI; therefore, many anesthesiologists request a prenatal consult.

Legal and liability issues

Pregestational obesity and excessive prenatal weight gain are both linked with diabetes and fetal macrosomia, which are, in turn, linked with shoulder dystocia. Improper management of shoulder dystocia with permanent brachial plexus injury is one of the most common claims against midwives. Tort claims have included improper management of prenatal weight gain and diabetes during pregnancy that has a potential contributory factor in poor birth outcomes.

Obesity should be identified at the first prenatal visit, and informed consent regarding the potential pregnancy problems related to obesity and pregnancy should be documented. A weight gain management plan also needs to be established and documented along with associated counseling. Women who receive appropriate weight gain counseling and continue to gain excessive amounts of weight may be held responsible for contributory negligence in the event of a poor birth outcome.

Intrapartum and postpartum issues

Obesity is linked with labor complications that increase the risk for a surgical birth or increase the difficulty of a vaginal birth (Table 36.2). No evidence-based management recommendations have been developed to counteract the effect of obesity on labor and birth. Complications related to obesity continue in the postpartum period. The most common obesity-related complications in the postpartum period are postcesarean wound infection and dehiscence. Incision openings must heal from the bottom up, which requires daily cleaning and packing. This is a painful, difficult process for women, particularly those who are trying to establish breastfeeding. The skin incision may be below the pannus, making it impossible for the woman to visually examine the wound and to pack it herself.

Postpartum deep vein thrombosis (DVT) is the most lethal of obesity-related postpartum complications and is a leading cause of postpartum mortality. DVT prevention includes early postpartum ambulation, use of alternating pressure cuffs on lower extremities, and prenatal anticoagulation with Lovenox or heparin for those with prior thrombus formation.

Obesity is associated with delayed onset of milk production (lactogenesis II), maternal perceptions of insufficient milk production, and early cessation of breastfeeding (Anstey & Jevitt, 2011). Mothers with BMIs ≥30 need extra support in the early postpartum period. Extra stimulation with double pumping and frequent feeding may increase the supply of colostrum and later milk. Extra large shields may be needed for breast pumps as shields that are too small can strangulate and bruise the nipple. Obese mothers need chairs and beds that are large enough to comfortably position the feeding newborn with supportive pillows (Jevitt, 2010; Jevitt, Hernandez, & Groer, 2007).

Because lactation uses about 500 cal of energy daily, if mothers restrict intake, they will have a gradual reduction in weight without affecting milk quality of infant growth (Lovelady, 2011).

Summary

Obesity during pregnancy is now a common condition that affects approximately one of five pregnant women in the United States. Prepregnancy obesity increases risk for birth defects, stillbirth, and prenatal maternal complications such as hypertensive disorders and GDM. Intrapartum and postpartum risks are increased as well for women who are obese. Specific dietary and exercise plans are primary components of care for pregnant women with BMIs over 30. Cultural and family dietary practices need to be considered when counseling women about changing eating and activity patterns. Providing guidance and assistance to achieve appropriate weight gain is especially important for obese pregnant women and requires a multidisciplinary approach, time during prenatal visits, focused effort, and adequate support to help achieve optimal perinatal outcomes.

Resources for women and their families

Patient resources related to obesity are available at: http://www.cdc.gov/obesity/resources/factsheets.html
The CDC also offers physical activity guidelines and tracking devices for individuals at: http://www.cdc.gov/physicalactivity/everyone/guidelines/pregnancy.html
The U.S. Department of Agriculture Web site contains resources for individuals, families and health-care providers. Included on the Choose My Plate site is a customizable program where women can receive individualized meal plans and recipes. Data can be saved for continuous use. The program can be adjusted for pregnancy and breastfeeding. There is also a Super-Tracker than can track intake and physical activity. The health-care provider sections contain clinical information to assist in weight management, printable nutrition handouts and graphics. The Choose my Plate program is available at: http://www.choosemyplate.gov/

Resources for health-care providers

Nutrition and physical activity advice can be augmented by printable, color pamphlet pdf files on numerous topics. These can be obtained at: http://www.cdc.gov/obesity/resources/factsheets.html
The CDC also offer BMI calculators as downloadable widgets that can be placed on web sites or smart phones at: http://www.cdc.gov/healthyweight/assessing/bmi/index.html
The latest U.S. obesity data are available from the Centers for Disease Control (CDC) in reports, maps

Case study: Mary, the primigravida

Mary, a 23 year-old medical assistant, was 61 in. tall and weighed 165 lb at her first prenatal visit at 10 weeks' gestation. Her BMI was 31.2. This was her first pregnancy and she had no chronic health problems. During the physical examination, a clinical assessment of Mary's nutritional status was done and a 24-hour diet recall was taken. On the 24-hour recall, Mary described eating a Mambo sandwich with a bottle of water and a can of chocolate drink for breakfast. Mary listed the sandwich ingredients as a 12-in. piece of Cuban bread filled with eggs scrambled with onions, peppers, and sausage. Half laughing but a little defensively, she said, "Well eggs, onions and peppers are good for you, right?" Lunch consisted of a ½ lb cheeseburger with two strips of bacon, a small order of potato wedges and 12 oz of cola. Dinner was a large plate of spaghetti with tomato sauce and meatballs, garlic bread, a slice of chocolate cake, and iced tea. She noted snacking at her desk during work on candy, chips, or baked goods.

Based on the initial evaluation of her diet recall, the midwife determined that Mary's diet was inadequate in the areas of calcium, omega-3 fatty acids, fruits, and vegetables, and excessive in fats, calories, sugar, and processed foods. The midwife reviewed Mary's diet with her and explained the amounts of each food group needed daily during pregnancy. She showed Mary the MyPlate food plate diagram, recommending that half a plate be fruits and vegetables. The midwife estimated that Mary took in twice as many calories as needed in a day and asked Mary what she thought she could drop to reduce intake. Mary decided to drop colas and chocolate drinks and do without bacon on her cheeseburgers. The midwife recommended that instead of eating a 12-in. sandwich, Mary share half with a coworker or save half for breakfast the next morning. She also suggested reducing the size of the hamburger. Instead of totally denying herself sweets, Mary was encouraged to have dessert twice a week.

Pregnancy weight gain was discussed. Mary was advised to gain 11–20 lb but to try and stay closer to 11 lb. Mary was encouraged to add 20–30 minutes of walking a day to her routine. She said, "I'm so tired when I get home from work. I just want to put my feet up." Her partner did most of the cooking. The midwife helped Mary plan a new evening routine where she would put her feet up for 30 minutes while her partner cooked dinner. They would eat a leisurely dinner, clean the kitchen, and then walk for 20–30 minutes. Mary was also encouraged to increase her sleep from 6 to at least 7 hours a night. After initial nutrition counseling, the midwife set up a series of visits with the nutritionist to help with diet counseling and motivation. The midwife reviewed pregnancy potential problems associated with obesity and the importance of adequate

weight gain. A 1-hour OGTT was explained and scheduled. A daily prenatal vitamin was prescribed.

At her second prenatal visit at 14 weeks' gestation, Mary had gained 6 lb over the last 4 weeks. At that rate, Mary could gain 45 lb by her due date. Mary was surprised at her own weight gain but said her family and coworkers were pushing her to eat for the baby. She indicated she was not walking after work every day but was encouraged to do so by her unexpectedly high weight gain. Diet and weight gain counseling were reinforced, and Mary expressed motivation and continued interest in gaining the appropriate amount of weight. First visit labs were reviewed and were normal.

At 18 weeks' gestation, Mary had a total weight gain of 10 lb. She had checked her own 1-hour postprandial blood glucose at work and was shocked to find it was 172 mg/dL. The midwife ordered a 3-hour glucose tolerance test, which was normal. The HgA1C was 5.9%. Mary was motivated to place herself on an American Diabetic Association diet using the ChooseMyPlate method and targeting 2200 cal/day.

Mary was seen every 2 weeks between 18 and 28 weeks specifically for weight management. She slowed her weight gain and had a total gain of 16 lb at 28 weeks. Her glucose levels at that point were normal. Between 35 and 36 weeks' gestation, Mary became too tired to walk after work and admitted eating coke and fries occasionally at lunch.

Mary started labor at 40 weeks and 6 days' gestation with a fundal height of 44 cm and an estimated fetal weight of 8 lb by ultrasound. Her total gestational weight gain was 21 lb. She was normotensive and nonedematous. Mary had a prolonged prelabor labor period and, after 2 days of irregular contractions at 2 cm of dilatation, received a pitocin augmentation of labor. After a 2.25-hour second stage of labor, she gave birth to an 8 lb 11 oz boy.

Mary desired to breastfeed and a consultation with the hospital lactation counselor was initiated right after birth by the midwife. The nurses and the lactation counselor worked together to help position the baby at Mary's breast at most feedings while she was in the hospital to provide her with information, support, and encouragement. At 4 weeks postpartum, she indicated she was bottle-feeding as her breasts never felt full and her family was worried the baby "wasn't getting enough." At her 6-week postpartum checkup, contraceptive counseling was done and Mary chose to use oral contraceptives. She was given positive feedback for continuing to walk for 15–30 minutes most days of the week and for maintaining some of the healthy diet habits initiated during pregnancy. A long-term weight loss plan was made with referral to a nutritional specialist and a bariatric physician.

and PowerPoint slides that can be downloaded free of charge at: http://www.cdc.gov/obesity/data/trends.html

The U.S. Department of Agriculture provides a wealth of resources in printable, pdf format available from http://www.choosemyplate.gov/ including MyPlate posters, brochures encouraging patients to make half their plate fruits and vegetables, sample meal plans for 2000 cal a day, and sample recipes.

References

American College of Obstetricians and Gynecologists (ACOG). (2009). ACOG practice bulletin no. 105: Bariatric surgery and pregnancy. *Obstetrics and Gynecology*, 113(6), 1405–1413. doi:10.1097/AOG.0b013e3181ac0544

American College of Obstetricians and Gynecologists (ACOG). (2013). Obesity in pregnancy. ACOG Committee Opinion #549. Washington, DC: ACOG.

Anstey, E., & Jevitt, C. (2011). Maternal obesity and breastfeeding: A review of the evidence and implications for practice. *Clinical Lactation*, 2–3, 11–16.

Armstrong, C. (2010). Practice Guidelines ACOG Guidelines on Pregnancy after Bariatric Surgery. *American Family Physician*, 81(7), 905–906.

Beyerlein, A., Schiessl, B., Lack, N., & Von Kries, R. (2011). Associations of gestational weight loss with birth-related outcome: A retrospective cohort study. *BJOG : An International Journal of Obstetrics and Gynaecology*, 118, 55–61. doi:10.1111/j.1471-0528.2010.02761

Bhasin, S., & Shambaugh, G. E. (1982). Fetal fuels V. ketone bodies inhibit pyrimidine synthesis in the fetal rat brain. *The American Journal of Physiology*, 243(3), F234–F239.

Black, M. H., Sacks, D. A., Xiang, A. H., & Lawrence, J. M. (2012). The relative contribution of prepregnancy overweight and obesity, gestational weight gain, and IADPSG-defined gestational diabetes mellitus to fetal overgrowth. *Diabetes Care*, 36(1), 56–62. Published ahead of print August 13, 2012, doi:10.2337/dc12-0741

Blomberg, M. (2011). Maternal and neonatal outcomes among obese women with weight gain and the new Institute of Medicine recommendations. *Obstetrics and Gynecology*, 117(5), 1065–1070.

Blomberg, M. I., & Kallen, B. (2010). Maternal obesity and morbid obesity: The risk for birth defects in the offspring. *Birth Defects Research. Part A, Clinical and Molecular Teratology*, 88(1), 35–40.

Centers for Disease Control and Prevention (CDC). (2011). CDC health disparities and inequalities report-United States, 2011. *MMWR. Morbidity and Mortality Weekly Report*, 60(6). Retrieved from http://www.cdc.gov/mmwr/pdf/ss/ss6006.pdf

Centers for Disease Control and Prevention (CDC). (2012a). Physical activity for everyone: Healthy pregnant and postpartum women. Retrieved from http://www.cdc.gov/physicalactivity/everyone/guidelines/pregnancy.html

Centers for Disease Control and Prevention (CDC). (2012b). Short sleep duration among workers-United States, 2010. *MMWR. Morbidity and Mortality Weekly Report*, 61(16), 281–285. Retrieved from http://www.cdc.gov/mmwr/pdf/wk/mm6116.pdf

Dashe, J., McIntire, D., & Twickler, D. (2009). Maternal obesity limits the ultrasound evaluation of fetal anatomy. *Journal of Ultrasound in Medicine*, 28, 1025–1030.

Everette, M. (2008). Gestational weight and dietary intake during pregnancy: Perspectives of African-American women. *Maternal and Child Health Journal*, 12, 718–724.

Gunderson, E., Rifas-Shiman, S., Oken, E., Rich-Edwards, J., Kleinman, K., Taveras, E., & Gillman, M. (2008). Association of fewer hours of sleep at 6 months postpartum with substantial weight retention at 1 year postpartum. *American Journal of Epidemiology*, 167, 178–187.

Helmreich, R., Hundley, V., & Varvel, P. (2008). The effect of obesity on heart rate (heart period) and physiologic parameters during pregnancy. *Biological Research for Nursing*, 10, 63–78.

Hezelgrave, N. I., & Oteng-Ntim, E. (2011). Pregnancy after bariatric surgery: A review. *Journal of Obesity*. doi:10.1155/2011/501939

Institute of Medicine. (2009). *Weight gain during pregnancy: Reexamining the guidelines*. Washington, DC: The National Academies Press.

Jevitt, C. (2009). Pregnancy complicated by obesity: Midwifery management. *Journal of Midwifery and Women's Health*, 54, 445–451.

Jevitt, C. (2010). Lactation support for women with raised BMIs. In Y. Richens & T. Lavender (Eds.), *Prenatal and postpartum obesity management*. London: Quay Books.

Jevitt, C., Hernandez, I., & Groer, M. (2007). Lactation complicated by overweight & obesity: Supporting the mother & newborn. *Journal of Midwifery & Women's Health*, 56(6), 606–613.

Kennedy, D., & Koren, G. (2012). Identifying women who might benefit from higher doses of folic acid in pregnancy. *Canadian Family Physician Medecin de Famille Canadien*, 58(4), 394–397.

Khan, R., Dawlatly, B., & Chappatte, O. (2013). Pregnancy outcome following bariatric surgery. *The Obstetrician & Gynaecologist*, 15(1), 37–43.

Kim, S. Y., England, L., Wilson, H. G., Bish, C., Satten, G. A., & Dietz, P. (2010). Percentage of gestational diabetes mellitus attributable to overweight and obesity. *American Journal of Public Health*, 100, 1047–1052.

Lovelady, C. (2011). Session 1: Balancing intake and output: Food v. exercise. Balancing exercise and food intake with lactation to promote postpartum weight loss. *Proceedings of the Nutrition Society*, 70(2), 181–184.

Lu, G. C., Rouse, D. J., DuBard, M., Cliver, S., Kimberlin, D., & Hauth, J. C. (2001). The effect of the increasing prevalence of maternal obesity on perinatal morbidity. *American Journal of Obstetrics and Gynecology*, 185(4), 845–849.

Nihalani, N., Schwartz, T., Siddiqui, U., & Megna, J. (2011). Weight gain, obesity, and psychotropic prescribing. *Journal of Obesity*. doi:10.1155/2011/893629

Ogden, C. L., Caroll, M. D., Bit, B. K., & Flegal, K. M. (2012). Prevalence of Obesity in the United States 2009–2010. NCHS data brief no. 82. Hyattsville, MD: National Center for Health Statistics.

Ray, J., Wyatt, P. R., Vermeulen, M. J., Meier, C., & Cole, D. E. (2005). greater maternal weight and the ongoing risk of neural tube defects after folic acid flour fortification. *Obstetrics and Gynecology*, 105(2), 261–26.

Retnakaran, R., Ye, C., Hanley, A. J., Connelly, P. W., Sermer, M., Zinman, B., & Hamilton, J. (2012). Effect of maternal weight, adipokines, glucose intolerance and lipids on infant weight among women without gestational diabetes mellitus. *CMAJ: Canadian Medical Association Journal = Journal de l'Association Medicale Canadienne*, 184(12), 1353–1360. doi:10.1503/cmaj.111154

Salihu, H., Alio, A., Wilson, R., Sharma, P., Kirby, R., & Alexander, G. (2008). Obesity and extreme obesity: New insights into the black-white disparity in neonatal mortality. *Obstetrics and Gynecology*, 111, 1410–1416.

Sassi, F., Devaux, M., Cecchini, M., & Rusticelli, E. (2009), The Obesity Epidemic: Analysis of Past and Projected Future Trends in Selected OECD Countries. *OECD Health Working Papers*, No. 45, OECD Publishing. doi:10.1787/225215402672

Stagnaro-Green, A., Abalovich, M., Alexander, E., Fereidoun, A., Mestman, J., Negro, R., . . . Wiersinga, W. (2011). Guidelines of the American Thyroid Association for the diagnosis and management of thyroid disease during pregnancy and postpartum. *Thyroid*, *21*(10), 1081–1125.

Swartz, A., Strath, S., Bassett, D., Moore, J. B., Redwine, B., Groer, M., & Thompson, D. (2003). Increasing daily walking improves glucose tolerance in overweight women. *Preventive Medicine*, *37*, 356–362.

Thomas, B., & Bishop, J. (2007). Pregnancy. In B. Thomas & J. Bishop (Eds.), *Manual of dietetic practice* (4th ed., pp. 256–266). Oxford: Blackwell Publishing Ltd.

Vrebosch, L., Bel, S., Vansant, G., Guelinckx, I., & Devlieger, R. (2012). Maternal and neonatal outcome after laparoscopic adjustable gastric banding: A systematic review. *Obesity Surgery*, *22*(10), 1568–1579.

Wang, Y., & Chen, X. (2012). How much of racial/ethnic disparities in dietary intakes, exercise, and weight status can be explained by nutrition- and health-related psychosocial factors and socioeconomic status among US adults? *Journal of the American Dietetic Association*, *111*(12), 1904–1911.

37

Endocrine disorders

Elizabeth Gabzdyl

Introduction

The endocrine system is a network of glands that are vitally important for the regulation of many body functions including metabolism, growth, brain function, and cell and tissue activity (Coad & Dunstall, 2011). The most commonly encountered disorders in pregnant women are hypothyroidism, hyperthyroidism, and diabetes both overt (pregestational) diabetes and gestational diabetes (GDM). There are numerous differential diagnoses for hypothyroidism and hyperthyroidism, underscoring the necessity of referral in the case of a new diagnosis for further development of a diagnosis and treatment plan (Avery & Baum, 2007). This chapter will review the most common thyroid disorders as well as present an overview of pregestational diabetes and pregnancy.

Thyroid disorders in pregnancy

Thyroid disorders are the second most common endocrinologic disorders found in pregnancy (Shah, Mehta & Viradia, 2013). Uncorrected thyroid dysfunction in pregnancy has adverse effects on fetal and maternal well-being. The negative effects of thyroid dysfunction can also extend to affect neurointellectual development in the early life of the child. Demand for thyroid hormones increase during pregnancy, which may cause a previously unnoticed thyroid disorder to worsen and become symptomatic for the first time. The common causes of thyroid dysfunction are noted in Table 37.1. A brief review of thyroid physiology during pregnancy is presented as a foundation for understanding the specific thyroid disease in pregnancy.

Thyroid physiology in pregnancy

To meet the challenge of increased metabolic needs during pregnancy, the thyroid adapts through changes in thyroid hormone economy and in the regulation of the hypothalamic–pituitary–thyroid axis. The hypothalamic–pituitary–thyroid network produces and regulates thyroid hormones via a negative feedback control system. The hypothalamus responds to the level of circulating T_4 and T_3. If the levels are rising, it signals the pituitary to decrease production of thyroid-stimulating hormone (TSH), which will decrease the production of T_4 and T_3. If decreasing levels of T_4 and T_3 are perceived, the hypothalamus will produce thyroid-releasing hormone (TRH), which will stimulate the pituitary to increase TSH production to produce more

Prenatal and Postnatal Care: A Woman-Centered Approach, First Edition. Edited by Robin G. Jordan, Janet L. Engstrom, Julie A. Marfell, and Cindy L. Farley.
© 2014 John Wiley & Sons, Inc. Published 2014 by John Wiley & Sons, Inc.

Table 37.1   Causes of Thyroid Dysfunction and Expected Laboratory Findings

Diagnosis	TSH	Free T$_4$	Free T$_3$	Antibodies
Hypothyroidism				
Hashimoto's thyroiditis (autoimmune hypothyroidism)	↑	↓	Varied	Present
Post-thyroid ablation therapy	↑	↓	↓	Absent
Subclinical hypothyroidism	↑ (slightly)	Normal	Normal	Absent
Hyperthyroidism				
Graves' disease (autoimmune hyperthyroidism)	↓	↑	↑	Present
Subclinical hyperthyroidism	↓	Normal	Normal	Absent
Thyroid storm	↓↓	↑↑	↑↑	Variable
Postpartum thyroiditis	↓ then ↑	↑ then ↓	↑ then ↓	Present

Sources: Avery & Baum (2007), Society for Maternal-Fetal Medicine (SMFM) (2012), Stagnaro-Green (2011).

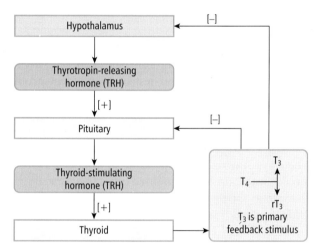

Figure 37.1.   Hypothalamic–pituitary–thyroid interactions. [+], stimulation; [–], inhibition. Source: Laposata, M., Aleryani, S., & Woodworth, A. (2010). In M. Weitz & R. Pancotti (Eds.), *Laboratory medicine: The diagnosis of disease in the clinical laboratory* (p. 395). New York: McGraw Hill.

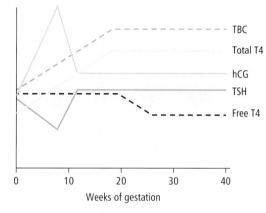

Figure 37.2.   Thyroid hormone and human chorionic gonadotropin fluctuations throughout pregnancy. Source: Casey, B., & Leveno, K. (2006). Thyroid diseases in pregnancy. *Obstetrics and Gynecology, 108*(5), 1284.

Diagnosing thyroid disorders

The serum TSH is a simple, accurate, and economical screening test for thyroid disorders (Table 37.1). Because of the changes in thyroid physiology during pregnancy, the Guidelines of the American Thyroid Association (ATA) recommend using trimester-specific reference ranges for TSH, and method and trimester-specific reference ranges for serum free T$_4$ (FT$_4$).

thyroid hormones, T$_4$ and T$_3$ (Coad & Dunstall, 2011). Figure 37.1 diagrams this system.

The thyroid gland is often slightly enlarged in the early weeks of pregnancy, reflecting the increased pregnancy-related metabolic demands. Pregnancy-associated goiters are much more common in iodine-deficient areas of the world and are relatively uncommon in the United States. The thyroid hormones exhibit normal fluctuations during pregnancy, especially in the first trimester. This may make it especially difficult to know when it is appropriate to screen for thyroid disease and how to interpret the values. Figure 37.2 shows the normal thyroid hormone fluctuations throughout pregnancy in the mother.

> **Reference ranges for TSH (mU/L) by trimester**
>
> - First trimester: 0.1–2.5
> - Second trimester: 0.2–3.0
> - Third trimester: 0.3–3.0
>
> Source: Fitzpatrick and Russell (2010).

The physical symptoms that many women experience in early pregnancy, such as fatigue and weight gain, are very similar to those noticed when experiencing symptoms of thyroid disease, making it very challenging at times to make a clear diagnosis (Avery & Baum, 2007).

Common signs and symptoms of pregnancy and thyroid disease		
Hypothyroidism	**Hyperthyroidism**	**Common pregnancy symptoms**
Weight gain	Weight loss	Appetite increase and weight gain
Cold intolerance	Heat intolerance	Increased sense of warmth
Fatigue	Nervousness/anxiety	Fatigue
Depression	Insomnia	Insomnia
Constipation	Diarrhea	Constipation
Dry skin, thin hair	Bulging of the eyes	

Source: American Thyroid Association (2012).

Overt hypothyroidism

Hashimoto's thyroiditis, also called chronic lymphocytic thyroiditis, is an autoimmune thyroid disorder, first described by Hakaru Hashimoto in 1912. Hashimoto's thyroiditis is the most common cause of overt hypothyroidism in pregnancy, accounting for approximately 80–90% of all cases of hypothyroidism (Laposata, Aleryani, & Woodworth, 2010; Stagnaro-Green et al., 2011). Overt hypothyroidism is defined as the presence of an elevated TSH concentration during gestation in conjunction with a decreased FT$_4$ concentration. Historically, the reference range for serum TSH was established from the serum of healthy, nonpregnant individuals and was set at values less than 4.0 mIU/L. More recently, data from healthy pregnant women suggest the upper reference range may approximate 2.5–3.0 mIU/L (Stagnaro-Green et al., 2011). Overt hypothyroidism is estimated to occur in 0.3–0.5% of pregnant women. Subclinical hypothyroidism (SCH) appears to occur in 2–3%, and hyperthyroidism is present in 0.1–0.4% of pregnant women (Abalovich et al., 2007).

Maternal and fetal risks

When thyroid hormone levels are well managed, maternal and neonatal outcomes will be the same as in pregnancies without thyroid disease. Adverse outcomes are related to the degree of thyroid hormone abnormalities, highlighting the importance of preventing deficiency whenever possible to minimize perinatal risks. The most common maternal complication of poorly controlled hypothyroidism is hypertensive disorders such as preeclampsia and gestational hypertension.

Perinatal complications of hypothyroidism	
Maternal	**Neonatal**
Preeclampsia	Low birth weight
Gestational hypertension	Preterm birth
Preterm birth	Cognitive impairment
Increased rate of cesarean section	Increased morbidity and mortality
Postpartum hemorrhage	

There is no indication for antenatal surveillance with serial ultrasound, nonstress test of biophysical profile testing when hypothyroidism is being treated and is well controlled (Stagnaro-Green et al., 2011).

Clinical presentation

When hypothyroidism is present, an enlarged thyroid may be noted, up to two to three times the normal size. Changes in the thyroid gland may also be nonpalpable. Other findings may include dry skin and hair, and a patient report of fatigue, constipation, weight gain, and intolerance to cold. The initial presentation can consist of nonspecific symptoms, and subsequently, hypothyroidism may be misdiagnosed as depression premenstrual syndrome, chronic fatigue syndrome, or fibromyalgia.

Laboratory testing, diagnosis, and management

The TSH will be elevated, usually between 2.5 and 10 mIU/L, and the T$_4$ will be decreased (De Groot et al., 2012; Stagnaro-Green et al., 2011). Women with TSH levels of 10.0 mIU/L or above, irrespective of their FT$_4$ levels, are also considered to have overt hypothyroidism. Antithyroid antibodies (ATAs) will be present in all women with Hashimoto's thyroiditis. For women under treatment for hypothyroidism, early prenatal care is advised to enable early thyroid function screening and medication adjustment as necessary.

Hypothyroidism should be treated with thyroid hormone when the TSH concentration is between 2.5 and 10.0 mIU/L (Stagnaro-Green et al., 2011). Levothyroxine is generally started at 25–50 mcg or even up to

100 mcg/day. The TSH should be assessed every 4–6 weeks and the levothyroxine dose should be adjusted until the TSH value is normal, between 0.5 and 2.5 mIU/L. A pregnant woman newly diagnosed with hypothyroidism should see a physician for the development of a plan of care and a treatment regimen (Avery & Baum, 2007). The goal of treatment is to maintain the pregnant woman's serum TSH in the trimester-specific reference range.

For a woman entering prenatal care with a history of ongoing treatment for stable hypothyroidism, TSH testing should be done at the first visit. The majority of these women will need higher dosing of thyroxin replacement to maintain a normal TSH secretion. During pregnancy, a woman's total T_4 concentrations should increase by 20–50% in order to meet the demands of pregnancy. In a woman with hypothyroidism, the thyroid is unable to respond to the hormonal cues to increase T_4 production in pregnancy, resulting in a need for an increased dosage of thyroid hormone replacement medication. Dose requirements may increase by as much as 50% during pregnancy, and the increase occurs as early as the fifth week of gestation (Alexander et al., 2004). One recommended strategy is to increase a levothyroxine by two tablets weekly to nine tablets weekly as soon as conception occurs (De Groot et al., 2012; Stagnaro-Green et al., 2011). The TSH should then be rechecked every 4–6 weeks during the first 20 weeks of pregnancy, then again between 26 and 32 weeks (Stagnaro-Green et al., 2011). Medication should be adjusted to maintain trimester-specific levels. Postpartum, the woman should immediately resume taking the prepregnancy dose of levothyroxine and her TSH level rechecked at 6 weeks postpartum. Medication dose is then adjusted if indicated (De Groot et al., 2012; Stagnaro-Green et al., 2011). Again, the goal is to maintain serum TSH within the trimester-specific reference range.

Subclinical hypothyroidism

Although it is well accepted that untreated overt hypothyroidism is linked to adverse perinatal outcomes, researchers are now focusing on the potential impact of SCH on maternal and fetal health. SCH is clinically defined as an elevated TSH with normal FT_4. SCH occurs in approximately 5% of childbearing aged women (ACOG, 2007). Compared to overt hypothyroidism, data on perinatal outcomes are variable. There is some high-quality evidence suggesting that SCH is associated with increased risk of adverse pregnancy outcomes such as early pregnancy loss or fetal death (Ashoor, Maiz, Rotas, Jawdat, & Nicolaides, 2010), maternal hypertensive disorders (Wilson, Casey, McIntire, Halvorson, & Cunningham, 2012) and the development of gestational diabetes

(Tudela, Casey, McIntire, & Cunningham, 2012). It is unclear if treatment is warranted in pregnant women with SCH. For women who are diagnosed with SCH in pregnancy and are not initially treated, they should be monitored for progression to overt hypothyroidism with a serum TSH and FT_4 approximately every 4 weeks until 16–20 weeks' gestation and at least once between 26 and 32 weeks' gestation (Stagnaro-Green et al., 2011).

Screening for hypothyroidism in pregnancy

At the initial prenatal appointment, the health-care provider should determine through history taking and physical exam if the woman is at risk for thyroid dysfunction and would benefit from thyroid screening. All pregnant women already on levothyroxine for hypothyroidism should have serum TSH, T_3, and T_4 screening.

Risk factors for thyroid dysfunction: TSH screening should be done in early pregnancy

1. History of thyroid dysfunction or prior thyroid surgery
2. Age >30 years
3. Symptoms of thyroid dysfunction or the presence of goiter
4. Thyroid antibody positive
5. Type 1 diabetes or other autoimmune disorders
6. History of miscarriage or preterm birth
7. History of head or neck radiation
8. Family history of thyroid dysfunction
9. Morbid obesity (body mass index [BMI] > 40 kg/m²)
10. Use of amiodarone or lithium or recent administration of iodinated radiologic contrast
11. Infertility
12. Residing in an area of known moderate to severe iodine insufficiency

Source: Stagnaro-Green (2011).

The universal screening of asymptomatic pregnant women for hypothyroidism during the first trimester of pregnancy is controversial and is the subject of much expert debate. Current consensus is that there is insufficient evidence to support universal screening of pregnant women without risk factors or symptoms (ACOG, 2007; SMFM, 2012; Stagnaro-Green et al., 2011). However, this view is being challenged by recent research. Routine screening results in approximately 200–300 women per 100,000 pregnant women screened diagnosed with hypothyroidism (Laurberg, Andersen, Pedersen, Andersen, & Carlé, 2013). Additionally, most pregnant women diagnosed with thyroid disease by routine screening have no symptoms (Shah et al., 2013) and routine screening is cost effective compared to selective screening (Dosiou et al., 2012).

Preconception care of a woman with hypothyroidism

Ideally, a woman with hypothyroidism planning a pregnancy receives preconceptional counseling to discuss her thyroid disorder, her medical history, and the management plan for her thyroid disorder prior to conception. The current state of her thyroid function is established and consultation or referral done as needed. The target preconception serum TSH level is <2.5 mU/L (Stagnaro-Green, 2011). It may be necessary to advise her to postpone pregnancy during treatment and stabilization, often up to 3–6 months, if she is taking medications or requires surgery to manage hyperthyroidism.

Hyperthyroidism

Graves' disease, or overt hyperthyroidism, is an autoimmune cause of hyperthyroidism, named for Sir Robert Graves who first described the condition in the early nineteenth century. It is relatively uncommon during pregnancy, affecting 0.1–0.4% of all pregnant women (Krarras, Poppe, & Glinoer, 2010). Hyperthyroidism (supression of TSH, elevation of FT_4 and/or T_3) is not frequently diagnosed during pregnancy because conception is much more difficult and pregnancy loss is more frequent with undetected Graves' disease (Galofre & Davies, 2009). Ideally, women with Graves' hyperthyroidism will be diagnosed and treated prior to conceiving. If the diagnosis of Graves' disease occurs at the time of confirmation of pregnancy, accurate and prompt diagnosis, development of a management plan, and stabilization of thyroid hormones are crucial since adverse outcomes for the mother and the fetus may be significant when the hyperthyroidism is untreated or poorly controlled.

Maternal and fetal risks

Extremely high levels of thyroid-stimulating immunogloblulins (TSIs) are produced in Graves' disease to stimulate the thyroid gland. These antibodies cross the placenta and can interact with the baby's thyroid, resulting in neonatal thyroid dysfunction.

When excessive thyroid hormones are present during pregnancy, neonatal complications may include a significantly higher rate of spontaneous abortion, decreased birth weight, stillbirth, preterm birth, and neonatal mortality. Maternal adverse outcomes may include GDM,

preeclampsia, thyroid storm, and congestive heart failure (Stagnaro-Green, 2011).

Clinical presentation

Upon physical exam, when hyperthyroidism is present, tachycardia, palpitations, anxiety, and a fine tremor may be noted. A failure to gain weight is frequently seen, in spite of sufficient calorie intake. An enlarged thyroid (goiter) is almost always present, between two and six times the normal size. Exophthalmos may be seen in 20–40% of individuals with Graves' disease, showing upper lid retraction, edema, and the eyes may have the appearance of protruding (Avery & Baum, 2007; Stagnaro-Green et al., 2011).

Laboratory testing, diagnosis, and management

A definitive diagnosis is based on laboratory results. The TSH will be very low, perhaps even undetectable, and the T_4 will be very elevated. ATAs will be present (Stagnaro-Green et al., 2011).

The goal of treatment is to maintain T_4 levels as close to normal as possible. Propylthiouracil (PTU) and Methimazole (MMI) are the preferred medications used to treat Graves' disease. Both act to block production of T_3 and T_4 (Avery & Baum, 2007). PTU is often preferred, especially in the first trimester, since use of MMI in the first trimester is associated with possible fetal abnormalities (De Groot et al., 2012; Stagnaro-Green et al., 2011). Due to the small but serious risk of liver toxicity, the U.S. Food and Drug Administration (FDA) has recommended changing to MMI once a woman is in her second trimester of pregnancy (De Groot et al., 2012; Stagnaro-Green et al., 2011). While on PTU, liver function studies should be monitored every 3–4 weeks and warning signs should be reviewed with the woman so she is aware of what adverse symptoms to report (De Groot et al., 2012). Women with moderate to severe disease may also be treated with beta blockers to reduce symptoms (Bahn-Chair et al., 2011).

A reduction in symptoms and improvement of thyroid laboratory values are usually seen within several weeks of beginning therapy. Thyroid values are closely monitored during the prenatal period. Many women are able to decrease and even discontinue their antithyroid medication in the final weeks prior to labor and birth (De Groot et al., 2012). This helps to decrease the incidence of neonatal hypothyroidism from exposure to the higher doses of maternal medications prior to birth due to the normal fluctuations of thyroid hormones in pregnancy. Thyroidectomy (subtotal or total) may be indicated if there is a medication allergy, low medication compliance, or a very large goiter. Radioactive iodine treatment to ablate the thyroid is contraindicated in pregnancy (De Groot et al., 2012).

The fetus should be monitored for thyroid dysfunction by periodic ultrasound to determine if there is evidence of thyroid enlargement, growth restriction, hydrops, tachycardia, or heart failure. If fetal hyperthyroidism is suspected, the mother's physician could prescribe PTU or MM to treat the condition in the fetus (De Groot et al., 2012). After birth, depending on the stability of the woman's hyperthyroidism, the baby may have transient hypothyroidism, which should resolve spontaneously.

Scope of practice considerations

Collaboration and referral to obstetrical or maternal–fetal medicine services are recommended for women with hyperthyroidism for the development of a long-term plan of care (Stagnaro-Green, 2011). Newly diagnosed pregnant women are best managed by physician specialists as their plan of care is often complex, and medication regimens must be determined and monitored closely. These women will require follow-up throughout pregnancy and continued close follow-up until the thyroid laboratory studies once again stabilize.

Subclinical hyperthyroidism

This condition is noted when the TSH is decreased and the T_4 is normal and the woman is asymptomatic. Since there are no adverse maternal or fetal outcomes associated, there is no treatment required (SMFM, 2012). However, if TSH values fall below 0.1 mIU/L, it may be prudent to treat (Avery & Baum, 2007). In pregnant women with diagnosed subclinical hyperthyroidism, monitoring TSH and FT_4 every 4–6 weeks during pregnancy can assess for change in stability. Mild hyperthyroidism during pregnancy often only requires period monitoring and no intervention.

Thyroid storm

Thyroid storm is a rare but life-threatening form of hyperthyroidism in which the body is in a hypermetabolic state. This condition is associated with a 20–30% mortality rate and must be treated quickly and aggressively. Symptoms include high fever (over 103°F), tachycardia, nausea and vomiting, and symptoms of congestive heart failure. The T_4 will be very elevated and the TSH very low. Treatment is based on constellation of symptoms rather than laboratory values and should be initiated under physician care in an intensive care unit, where the woman will be given supportive therapy.

> The prevention and/or treatment of overt hypothyroidism and overt hyperthyroidism during pregnancy, especially in the first trimester, are important to childhood health since the intellectual ability of the fetus may be compromised if these conditions were present during fetal development (Laposata et al., 2010; Stagnaro-Green, 2011).

Postpartum thyroiditis

Postpartum thyroiditis (PPT) is a transient autoimmune thyroid disorder associated with the presence of thyroid antibodies. This occurs in postpartum women within 6 months to 1 year after giving birth. These women typically do not demonstrate any signs or symptoms of thyroid disease prior to pregnancy. They usually present with symptoms of hyperthyroidism for 1–2 months before their symptoms develop into hypothyroidism symptoms for 4–6 months until they resolve completely (De Groot et al., 2012; Stagnaro-Green et al., 2011).

There is an increased incidence of PPT in women who have other autoimmune disorders, type 1 diabetes, stable Graves' disease, or chronic viral hepatitis and almost always occurs in women who are thyroid antibody positive (De Groot et al., 2012; Stagnaro-Green et al., 2011). Twenty to fifty percent of women found to have PPT will go on to develop a permanent hypothyroidism condition in the future (Stagnaro-Green et al., 2011). The most common symptoms tend to be mild and vague and may include fatigue, irritability, tachycardia, dry skin, or palpitations. A mildly enlarged thyroid may be noted.

Laboratory evaluation, diagnosis, and management

PPT is typically diagnosed infrequently since it is a condition that occurs several months postpartum. Abnormalities usually resolve spontaneously. PPT may present with either hyperthyroidism or hypothyroidism, although the usual presentation is hyperthyroidism. The T_4 may be elevated or decreased (Laposata et al., 2010). Most women will present with hyperthyroidism between 2 and 6 months, although some will present with hypothyroidism first then develop hyperthyroidism. In virtually all cases, the hyperthyroidism resolves spontaneously by the end of the first postpartum year (Stagnaro-Green et al., 2011). Women who have risk factors for PPT should have a screening TSH at 3 and 6 months postpartum (De Groot et al., 2012).

If the TSH is elevated between 4 and 10 mIU/L and a woman is symptomatic, a physician may prescribe

Table 37.2 Diabetes Mellitus Classifications, Etiology, Onset, and Usual Treatment

Classification	Etiology	Onset	Treatment options
Type 1	Autoimmune destruction of β cells in pancreas	Childhood, adolescence, young adult	Insulin
Type 2	Insulin deficiency or insulin resistance	Adult	Diet Medication Insulin
Gestational diabetes	Uncertain etiology	Pregnancy	Diet Medication Insulin
Others	• Genetic defects of β cells, insulin action • Diseases of pancreas, endocrinopathies • Drug, infection, or chemical induced	Variable	Diet Medication Insulin

Source: ADA (2012).

levothyroxine for her if she is hypothyroid or a beta blocker if she is hyperthyroid for symptom management. Abnormal thyroid levels and symptoms will resolve spontaneously, usually within 2–12 months, and drug tapering to discontinue may be done once the woman is asymptomatic and thyroid levels are stable (De Groot et al., 2012).

Pregestational diabetes

Diabetes mellitus is a group of metabolic disorders that cause hyperglycemia and is the most common of all endocrine disorders. It is estimated that 18.8 million people in the U.S. had been diagnosed with diabetes and 7.0 million remained undiagnosed (Centers for Disease Control and Prevention (CDC), 2011). The prevalence of pregestational diabetes is increasing due to the increase in type 2 diabetes in women of childbearing age.

Classifications

There are four classifications of diabetes mellitus with three of them considered "pregestational diabetes." Type 1 diabetes (formerly known as insulin dependent diabetes or juvenile diabetes) typically occurs in childhood or adolescence. Type 1 is caused by is autoimmune destruction of pancreatic β cells and accounts for 5–10% of all diabetes in the United States. Insulin is always necessary for the management of type 1 diabetes and should be initiated by a physician (American Diabetes Association (ADA), 2012; Handelsman et al., 2011). Although the only treatment option is insulin, it is possible to choose various types of injection regimens to reduce hypoglycemic episodes. Insulin pumps are an option for continuous infusion, now used by 20–30% of patients with type 1 diabetes in the United States (Handelsman et al., 2011) (Table 37.2).

Type 2 diabetes, (formerly known as non-insulin dependent diabetes) is the most common type of diabetes, accounting for 90–95% of all cases, occurring more frequently in women with a prior history of GDM. Although the precise etiology is not known, it is thought that the cause is likely to be either an insulin deficiency or an insulin resistance. Individuals with type 2 diabetes tend to be obese with increased abdominal body fat distribution. Type 2 diabetes tends to develop gradually over an extended period of time. Often, classic symptoms are not clearly seen, making these individuals at greater risk of developing complications such as microvascular and macrovascular disease (ADA, 2012). It is possible to have type 2 diabetes for many years before diagnosis because of the lack of symptoms, or the symptoms are so subtle they are not easily or quickly noticed and the onset is gradual (Avery & Baum, 2007).

Gestational diabetes (GDM) affects approximately 7% of all pregnant women. In this type of diabetes, glucose intolerance is first recognized during pregnancy (ADA, 2012). Certain ethnic groups including Native American, Hispanic, Asian, Pacific Island, and African women are at greater risk of developing GDM. It is estimated that 20% of women with GDM will develop diabetes mellitus within 10 years (Göbl et al., 2011). GDM is addressed in detail in Chapter 23.

A small number of diabetes cases are caused by other varied conditions which create a hyperglycemic state, thereby causing diabetes mellitus and associated risks. Some examples of these include genetic defects of β cells or insulin action, diseases of the pancreas, and endocrinopathies; drugs or chemicals such as toxins, glucocorticoids, α-interferon; infections such as certain viruses, congenital rubella, cytomegalovirus, mumps, and genetic syndromes such as Turner, Down, and Klinefelter (ADA, 2012).

Perinatal risks of pregestational diabetes

Women with pregestational diabetes are at higher risk for maternal and fetal/neonatal complications. The risk of major congenital malformations is doubled in women with pre gestational diabetes and is thought to be related to the degree of maternal hyperglycemia during the embryonic period (Metzger et al., 2007).

Adverse pregnancy outcome in women with pregestational diabetes

- Spontaneous early pregnancy loss
- Macrosomia
- LGA
- Shoulder dystocia
- Polyhydramnios
- Preeclampsia
- Preterm birth
- Unexplained stillbirth
- Respiratory distress
- Hyperbilirubinemia
- Neonatal death
- Congenital anomalies
  - Congenital heart defects
  - Neural tube defects
  - Renal agenesis/caudal dysgenesis syndrome

Women with pregestational diabetes are at risk for other comorbidities such as thyroid disease, hypertension, and cardiac disease. These women benefit from specialty medical care by those with expertise in diabetes during pregnancy. Members of the optimal interprofessional team include nurses, dieticians, and endocrinologists with referrals initiated early in pregnancy as needed. Woman with pregestational diabetes may seek care for pregnancy-related issues unrelated to her diabetes. Midwives and nurse practitioners (NPs) may attend to those needs as part of her health-care team within the provider's level of expertise and scope of practice.

Preconception counseling and care of women with pregestational diabetes

Efforts should be made to achieve the best maternal glycemic control prior to conception to lower the risk of fetal malformation. This is challenging since more than 50% of pregnancies in the United States are unintended. Glycemic control plays an important role in reducing the frequency of fetal and neonatal complications. Glycated hemoglobin (A1C) values, which reflect the average blood glucose concentration over the previous 8–12 weeks, are useful in evaluating glycemic control before conception and throughout pregnancy.

Preconception counseling considerations for women with pregestational diabetes

- Regular medical visits for diabetes management
- Medication and insulin regimens carefully followed
- Target prepregnancy A1C values of <6.1%
- Self-blood glucose monitoring
- Diet therapy for glucose regulation
- Addition of folic acid 400 μg daily preconceptionally and through the first trimester
- Exercise and weight management
- Comprehensive ophthalmic exam to evaluate vascular changes.

Glycemic control needs to be achieved preconceptionally to maximize prevention of adverse outcomes. Therefore, the major goals of preconception care of women with pregestational diabetes are to evaluate glycemic control and to recommend adjustments in diet, medications, and lifestyle to achieve euglycemia.

Summary

This chapter has reviewed the most common thyroid disorders in pregnancy as well as an overview of pregestational diabetes- pregnancy. The most commonly encountered disorders in pregnant women are hypothyroidism, hyperthyroidism, and diabetes, and both overt diabetes and GDM. Due to the complexity of the diagnosis of hypothyroidism and hyperthyroidism, it is recommended that a referral be obtained for all pregnant women with a new endocrine diagnosis for the development of a treatment plan

Resources for women and health-care providers

Agency for Healthcare Research and Quality: http://www.ahrq.gov/

American Diabetes Association: http://www.diabetes.org/

American Thyroid Association: http://www.thyroid.org

Centers for Disease Control and Prevention: http://www.cdc.gov/diabetes/

Centers for Disease Control and Prevention. *National diabetes fact sheet, 2011:* http://www.cdc.gov/diabetes/pubs/pdf/ndfs_2011.pdf

National Diabetes Education Program: http://www.ndep.nih.gov/

National Diabetes Information Clearinghouse (NDIC): http://diabetes.niddk.nih.gov/

National Endocrine and Metabolic Diseases Information Service (NEMDIS): http://www.endocrine.niddk.nih.gov/

The Endocrine Society: http://www.endo-society.org

Case study

A 28-year-old primigravida, at 10 weeks' gestation is here for her first prenatal visit. She reports that she is very fatigued, having problems sleeping, and is also constipated. These symptoms started relatively recently, but she is not sure exactly when because she has a busy and stressful job and works long hours. She is wondering if these are normal symptoms for early pregnancy.

What are your consider and data gathering? Her symptoms are all normal physiologic symptoms during early gestation, however consideration must be given to hypothyroid disorder. Has she noticed any of the following symptoms: weight gain or loss, intolerance to heat or cold, depression, dry skin, or hair thinning prior to pregnancy? Is there any family history of thyroid disorders of any type? Does she have any history of thyroid dysfunction or thyroid surgery? What is her BMI (over 40 is a risk factor)? Does she have a history of any autoimmune disorders? (Refer to text box, "Risk Factors for Thyroid Dysfunction" for the full list of risk factors for thyroid dysfunction). If she responds positively to any of the questions, TSH screening should be done to rule out thyroid dysfunction. Diagnosis and treatment decisions should be made on the basis of laboratory results, physical exam, and the woman's symptoms.

References

Abalovich, M., Amino, N., Barbour, L. A., Cobin, R. H., De Groot, L. J., & Glinoer, D. (2007). Management of thyroid dysfunction during pregnancy and postpartum: An Endocrine Society Clinical Practice Guideline. *The Journal of Clinical Endocrinology and Metabolism*, *92*(8 Suppl.), S1–S47.

Alexander, E. K., Marquesee, E., Lawrence, J., Jarolim, P., Fischer, G. A., & Larsen, P. R. (2004). Timing and magnitude of increases in levothyroxine requirements during pregnancy in women with hypo fibroidism. *The New England Journal of Medicine*, *351*, 241.

American College of Obstetricians and Gynecologists (ACOG). (2007). Committee Opinion, Number 381: Subclinical hypothyroidism in pregnancy. *Obstetrics and Gynecology*, *110*(4), 959–960.

American Diabetes Association (ADA). (2012). Diagnosis and classification of diabetes mellitus. *Diabetes Care*, *35*(1), S64–S71. doi:10.2337/dc12-s064

American Thyroid Association. (2012). Hyperthyroidism FAQ. Retrieved from http://www.thyroid.org/faq-hyperthyroidism/

Ashoor, G., Maiz, N., Rotas, M., Jawdat, F., & Nicolaides, K. H. (2010). Maternal thyroid function at 11 to 13 weeks of gestation and subsequent fetal death. *Thyroid*, *20*, 989–993.

Avery, M. D., & Baum, K. D. (2007). Endocrine. In B. Hackley, J. M. Kriebs, & M. E. Rousseau (Eds.), *Primary care of women: A guide for midwives and women's health providers* (pp. 559–596). Sudbury, MA: Jones & Bartlett.

Bahn-Chair, R. S., Burch, H. B., Cooper, D. S., Garber, J. R., Greenlee, M. C., Klein, I., . . . Stan, M. N.; American Thyroid Association, American Association of Clinical Endocrinologists. (2011). Hyperthyroidism and other causes of thyrotoxicosis: Management guidelines of the American Thyroid Association and American Association of Clinical Endocrinologists. *Thyroid*, *21*(6), 593.

Centers for Disease Control and Prevention. (2011). *National diabetes fact sheet: National estimates and general information on diabetes and prediabetes in the United States*. Atlanta, GA: U.S. Department of Health and Human Services, Centers for Disease Control and Prevention. Retrieved from http://www.cdc.gov/diabetes/pubs/estimates11.htm#8

Coad, J., & Dunstall, M. (2011). *Anatomy and physiology for midwives* (3rd ed.). St. Louis, MO: Churchill Livingston.

De Groot, L., Abalovich, M., Alexander, E. K., Amino, N., Barbour, L., Cobin, R. H., . . . Sullivan, S. (2012). Management of thyroid dysfunction during pregnancy and postpartum: An Endocrine Society clinical practice guideline. *The Journal of Clinical Endocrinology and Metabolism*, *97*(8), 2543–2565. doi:10.1210/jc.2111-2803

Dosiou, C., Barnes, J., Schwartz, A., Negro, R., Crapo, L., & Stagnaro-Green, A. (2012). Cost-effectiveness of universal and risk-based screening for autoimmune thyroid disease in pregnant women. *Journal of Clinical Endocrinology & Metabolism*, *97*(5), 1536–1546.

Fitzpatrick, D. L., & Russell, M. A. (2010). Diagnosis and management of thyroid disease in pregnancy. *Obstetrics and Gynecology Clinics of North America*, *37*, 173.

Galofre, J., & Davies, T. (2009). Autoimmune thyroid disease in pregnancy: A review. *Journal of Women's Health*, *18*(11), 1847–1856. doi:10.1089/jwh.2008.1234

Göbl, C. S., Bozkurt, L., Prikoszovich, T., Winzer, C., Pacini, G., & Kautzky-Willer, A. (2011). Early possible risk factors for overt diabetes after gestational diabetes mellitus. *Obstetrics & Gynecology*, *118*(1), 71–78.

Handelsman, Y., Mechanick, J., Blonde, L., Grunberger, G., Bloomgarden, Z., Bray, G., . . . Wyne, K. (2011). American Association of Endocrinologists medical guidelines for clinical practice for developing a diabetes mellitus comprehensive plan. *Endocrine Practice*, *17*(Suppl. 2), 1–53.

Krarras, G. E., Poppe, K., & Glinoer, D. (2010). Thyroid function and reproductive health. *Endocrine Reviews*, *31*, 702.

Laposata, M., Aleryani, S., & Woodworth, A. (2010). *Laboratory medicine: The diagnosis of disease in the clinical laboratory*, M. Weitz & R. Pancotti (Eds.). New York: McGraw Hill.

Laurberg, P., Andersen, S. L., Pedersen, I. B., Andersen, S., & Carlé, A. (2013). Screening for overt thyroid disease in early pregnancy may be preferable to searching for small aberrations in thyroid function tests. *Clinical Endocrinology*.

Metzger, B. E., Buchanan, T. A., Coustan, D. R., De Leiva, A., Dunger, D. R., Hadden, D. R., . . . Zoupas, C. (2007). Summary and recommendations of the fifth International Workshop-Conference on Gestational Diabetes Mellitus. *Diabetes Care*, *30*(Suppl. 2), S251–S260. doi:10.2337/dc07-s225

Shah, J. M., Mehta, M. N., & Viradia, H. B. (2013). Screening for thyroid dysfunction during pregnancy. *Thyroid Research and Practice*, *10*(2), 65.

Society for Maternal-Fetal Medicine (SMFM). (2012). Screening for thyroid disease during pregnancy. *Contemporary OB/GYN*, *57*(8), 45–47.

Stagnaro-Green, A. (2011). Overt hyperthyroidism and hypothyroidism during pregnancy. *Clinical Obstetrics and Gynecology*, *54*(3), 478–487.

Stagnaro-Green, A., Abalovich, M., Alexander, E., Azizi, F., Mestman, J., Negro, R., . . . Wiersinga, W., for The American Thyroid Association Taskforce on Thyroid Disease During Pregnancy and Postpartum. (2011). Guidelines of the American Thyroid Association for the diagnosis and management of thyroid disease during pregnancy and postpartum. *Thyroid*, *21*(10), 1081–1125. doi:10.1089/thy.2011.0087

Tudela, C. M., Casey, B. M., McIntire, D. D., & Cunningham, F. G. (2012). Relationship of subclinical thyroid disease to the incidence of gestational diabetes. *Obstetrics & Gynecology*, *119*(5), 983–988.

Wilson, K. L., Casey, B. M., McIntire, D. D., Halvorson, L. M., & Cunningham, F. G. (2012). Subclinical thyroid disease and the incidence of hypertension in pregnancy. *Obstetrics & Gynecology*, *119*(2, Pt 1), 315–320.

38

Neurological disorders

Tonya B. Nicholson

Relevant terms

Absence seizure—brief seizure that includes loss of consciousness and occasional clonic movements; also known as petit mal seizures

Acquired seizure disorder—seizure disorder occurring due to a known and identifiable cause such as a head injury

Active seizure disorder—seizure activity present within the last 5 years

Aura—sensory, motor, or visual changes that occur immediately preceding or at the onset of a migraine headache

Chronic migraine—ongoing pattern of frequent migraine headaches (daily or almost every day) over several months or years

Chronic tension headache—ongoing pattern of daily or near daily tension-type headache

Clonic movements—involuntary muscle movement

Cluster headache—severe, unilateral headache with pattern of short duration and "cluster" periods of frequent headaches

Idiopathic seizure disorder—seizure disorder occurring with no known or identifiable cause

Migraine headache—moderate to severe headache often with associated gastrointestinal or neurological symptoms, and may be accompanied by aura

Partial seizure—seizure involving no loss of consciousness but including the presence of motor, sensory, or psychiatric symptoms; also known as focal seizures

Photophobia—sensitivity to light

Preeclampsia—complication of pregnancy or early postpartum period characterized by hypertension and proteinuria

Tension headache—usually described as achy, viselike, nonpulsatile headache or mild to moderate intensity; minimal or no associated gastrointestinal or neurological symptoms

Tonic–clonic seizure—seizure that involves loss of consciousness and involuntary muscle contractions

---

Introduction

The most commonly encountered neurological disorders in the pregnant woman are seizure disorders, multiple sclerosis, and headache. In most circumstances, a pregnant woman with a seizure disorder or multiple sclerosis can be cared for by the nurse practitioner or midwife with physician collaboration. Headaches in pregnancy can usually be managed independently by the advanced practice nurse or midwife.

Care of the pregnant woman with seizure disorders

Seizure disorders, also known as epilepsy, can be divided into two categories: acquired or idiopathic. Acquired seizure disorders occur as a result of some insult to the neurological system due to trauma or illness. More commonly, the seizure disorder has no identifiable cause and is classified as idiopathic.

Seizures are categorized as partial (also known as focal) or generalized. Women with partial or focal

---

Prenatal and Postnatal Care: A Woman-Centered Approach, First Edition. Edited by Robin G. Jordan, Janet L. Engstrom, Julie A. Marfell, and Cindy L. Farley.
© 2014 John Wiley & Sons, Inc. Published 2014 by John Wiley & Sons, Inc.

seizures have symptoms that may be motor, sensory, or psychiatric in nature, but, regardless of the type of symptoms, the woman remains conscious throughout the seizure. Generalized seizures include loss of consciousness and are further described as tonic–clonic (grand mal) or absence (petit mal). Tonic–clonic seizures have the distinguishing characteristic of loss of physical control with the classic musculoskeletal rigidity and jerking motions. Petit mal seizures are short in duration and do not include loss of physical control. Pharmacological treatment is determined by the seizure type and patient response to the medication.

Most seizures that happen during pregnancy occur in women with a preexisting seizure disorder. Other reasons for seizures during pregnancy are eclampsia, acute fatty liver of pregnancy, and amniotic fluid embolism. Signs and symptoms of preeclampsia and acute fatty liver of pregnancy are discussed in detail in Chapter 22, "Hypertensive Disorders in Pregnancy." New onset of seizure activity in the pregnant woman should be managed by the obstetrician in coordination with a neurologist. New onset of seizure activity in early pregnancy is suggestive of a seizure disorder and necessitates transfer of care to a physician. If the onset of seizure activity occurs during the third trimester of pregnancy, eclampsia is the most likely etiology, which necessitates emergent care and immediate comanagement with a physician.

Less than 1% of all pregnancies occur in women with a history of seizure disorder; approximately one-fourth of those women experience a decrease in seizures and one-third experience an increase in seizures during pregnancy (Karnad & Guntupalli, 2005). The higher blood volume and increased hepatic metabolism of antiepileptic drugs (AEDs) during pregnancy, and decreased medication compliance due to fetal concerns are thought to play a significant role in the increased seizure activity in some pregnant women. Therefore, it is important to be vigilant in the management of seizure disorders in pregnant women. However, it is also important to recognize that the vast majority of pregnant women with a seizure disorder have a normal pregnancy course and the obstetrical care can be comanaged when appropriate. The vast majority of women with epilepsy will have good perinatal outcomes. An interprofessional team approach including maternity care providers, neurologists, and pediatricians allows for optimal prenatal and postnatal care of women with seizure disorders.

A pregnant woman who has an active seizure disorder or with an uncontrolled seizure disorder is at higher risk for seizures during pregnancy (American College of Obstetricians Gynecologists (ACOG), 1997). These women should be referred to a physician for care during pregnancy. Many times, a woman will present for

prenatal care having taken AEDs for several years and been declared seizure free, but has not been reevaluated by a neurologist. A pregnant woman in this situation would benefit from a reevaluation by a neurologist to determine whether continuation of medication therapy is indicated or whether it would be reasonable to discontinue pharmacological treatment.

Ideally, women with a seizure disorder should be evaluated by a neurologist before pregnancy. In addition to evaluating a woman's seizure activity and need for continued medication, the preconception period is an ideal time to change medications and to monitor the woman's response to the medications. Some of the AEDs commonly used to manage seizure disorders in nonpregnant women are known to be increase the risk for birth defects (Table 38.1). Because of the known risks of some AEDs, women with seizure disorders should be advised to consult with their neurologist and pregnancy care provider for medication management before becoming pregnant.

Women with seizure disorders may also have a slightly increased risk of developing other complications during pregnancy, labor, and postpartum. A recent study concluded that pregnant women with a seizure disorder have a slightly increased risk of hypertensive disorders, labor induction, cesarean section, and postpartum hemorrhage (Borthen & Gilhus, 2012). However, most pregnancies are not adversely affected by the presence of a seizure disorder (Crawford, 2009). The most compelling question is whether the slightly increased risk of perinatal complications is due to the seizure disorder or the use of AEDs (Borthen, Eide, Daltveit, & Gilhus, 2011).

Pertinent issues to address with pregnant women who have seizure disorders include the use of AEDs and potential fetal risks, the need for genetic screening, and measures for seizure prevention (Crawford, 2009). The woman should be advised to maintain a regular sleep pattern, take AEDs as prescribed, and take folate supplementation. It is well documented that sleep deprivation increases seizure activity. Medication adjustments should be considered in women with pregnancy-related nausea and vomiting to the degree that might adversely affect medication delivery. In cases where nausea and vomiting may interfere with absorption of AEDs, the woman should be advised to cease operation of motor vehicles. Women should also be advised that the use of antacids can interfere with absorption of AEDs. Additionally, the effects of pregnancy on serum concentrations seem to vary considerably individually and are thus difficult to predict, thus making periodic AED monitoring important (Tomson, Landmark, & Battino, 2013).

A pregnant woman with a seizure disorder has a 4–6% risk of having a baby with the birth defect, which is

Table 38.1 Maternal and Fetal Effects of Commonly Prescribed Antiepileptic Medications

Medication	FDA pregnancy category	Lactation risk category	Potential fetal and neonatal effects	Potential maternal effects
Carbamazepine (Tegratol®)	D	L4	Facial malformations, neural tube defects, hypoplasia of distal phalanges, hypospadias, developmental delays	Drowsiness, leucopenia, ataxia, liver toxicity, anemia
Ethosuximide (Zarontin®)	C	L4	No known fetal effects	Agranulocytosis, leukopenia, depression, drowsiness, ataxia, anorexia
Gabapentin (Neurontin®)	C	L2	No known neonatal effects, animal studies show fetal effects	Leukopenia, ataxia, drowsiness, nystagmus, thrombocytopenia
Lamotrigine (Lamictal®)	C	L3	Facial clefting when used in first trimester, no effects in animal studies	Leucopenia, anemia, serious rashes, drowsiness, ataxia thrombocytopenia
Levetiracetam (Neurontin or Gralise®)	C	L3	No known fetal effects, animal studies show developmental effects	Depression, leukopenia, neutropenia, aggressive behavior, drowsiness, ataxia, infection, anorexia
Oxcarbazepine (Trileptal®)	C	L3	No known fetal effects, animal studies show fetal effects	Hyponatremia, leucopenia, aplastic anemia, drowsiness, ataxia, nystagmus
Phenobarbitol	D	L3	Decreased vitamin K-dependent clotting factors, neonatal withdrawal, possible fetal abnormalities	Anemia, drowsiness, ataxia
Phenytoin (Dilantin®)	D	L2	Decreased vitamin K-dependent clotting factors, facial clefting, hypoplasia of distal phalanges	Nystagmus, ataxia, hirsutism, megoplastic anemia
Primidone (Mysoline®)	D	L3	Decreased vitamin K-dependent clotting factors, neonatal withdrawal, possible birth defects	Drowsiness, ataxia, nausea, anemia, anorexia, thrombocytopenia
Tiagabine (Gabitril®)	C	L3	No known fetal effects	Weakness, serious rash, drowsiness, ataxia
Topiramate (Topamax®)	D	L3	Oral clefting, hypospadias	Metabolic acidosis, osteomalacia, leucopenia, anemia, anorexia, drowsiness, ataxia
Valproic acid (Depacon®, Depakene®, Stavzor®)	D	L2	Facial malformations, neural tube defects, impaired cognitive development; malformation rates with valproate have consistently been found to be two to three times higher compared with carbamazepine or lamotrigine (Tomson & Battino, 2009)	Drowsiness, ataxia, hair loss, liver involvement, thrombocytopenia, pancreatitis, anemia
Zonisamide (Zonegran®)	C	L5	No known fetal effects, animal studies show fetal effects	Aplastic anemia, agranulocytosis, depression, drowsiness, ataxia, anorexia

Adapted from: Gedzelman and Meador (2012), Williams and Kehr (2012).

slightly higher than the 2–3% risk for a woman without a seizure disorder (Yerby, 2001). This risk may be related to the seizure disorder or the medication used to treat the disorder. AEDs negatively impact folic acid absorption making increased folic acid supplementation imperative for pregnant women with seizure disorder. Due to this impaired folic acid absorption, evaluation for macrocytic anemia should be done preconceptually, at the first visit, and at approximately 28 weeks' gestation. Folic acid deficiency has a well-documented association with an increase in risk for fetal neural tube defects. Although the research on whether folate supplementation actually decreases the incidence of fetal malformations due to epilepsy in not conclusive, there is consensus that it is reasonable to increase folic acid supplementation in women taking AEDs. The recommended dose for at risk women is 4 mg daily. This addition of folic acid may alter metabolism of AEDs, so it is imperative to monitor serum medication levels. Additionally, vitamin D and vitamin K supplementation should be considered (ACOG, 1997).

When possible, a single medication regime for seizure prevention should be chosen. The risk of birth defects is dose dependent, increases with multimedication regimes, and is influenced by the type of AED used. The most commonly encountered fetal malformations are cleft lip/palate and defects of the cardiovascular system. It is widely accepted that the use of medications for seizure disorder results in higher incidence of fetal malformations. However, the risk of an uncontrolled seizure disorder is even higher and has even more deleterious risks for the fetus and the mother (Table 38.1). Serial AED levels before pregnancy, during each trimester, and during the postpartum state may help guide appropriate dose augmentation or reduction (St Louis, 2009). Presently, there is no consensus as to the frequency that drug levels should be drawn during pregnancy however a monthly schedule has been proposed (Williams & Kehr, 2012).

Women with seizure disorders should be offered early and comprehensive genetic counseling and screening for neural tube defects. Screening tests offered will be dependent on the gestational age at which a woman presents to prenatal care. If presentation to care occurs before 20 weeks, serum screening that includes maternal serum alpha-fetoprotein (MSAFP) should be offered along with ultrasonography. A comprehensive fetal ultrasound (USN) for malformations should be offered at 18–22 weeks. Due to the risk of fetal growth abnormalities, fetal growth should be monitored carefully. If there are concerns about fundal height measurements or difficulty in obtaining accurate growth assessment due to maternal obesity, serial USNs are indicated to accurately monitor fetal growth.

The following principles should be adhered to when caring for the pregnant patient with a seizure disorder: Use the lowest effective dose of the AED; use single drug therapy when possible; and monitor medication levels at regular intervals in each trimester. Anticipatory guidance for the woman with a seizure disorder should also include teaching that vaginal birth is considered safest unless there are other complications. Breastfeeding should not be discouraged because the mother is taking AEDs. Although AEDs do transfer into breast milk, this has not been found to be harmful to infants unless there is excessive neonatal sedation (ACOG, 1997). Additionally, breastfeeding may also serve as a method of gradually withdrawing the infant from an AED (Rousseau, 2008). Medication levels must be carefully monitored in the postpartum period and often need to be decreased. Women should also be counseled that many AEDs can decrease the effectiveness of hormonal contraception. Women with active seizure disorders need information on safety precautions related to newborn care before they are discharged home (Rousseau, 2008).

Safety precautions for mothers with seizure disorders

- Potentially hazardous activities (e.g., ironing or cooking) should be avoided until another adult is present.
- Do not carry the baby when alone in case of a fall during a seizure. A small "umbrella" stroller maneuvers easily through the home.
- To limit stair climbing, keep baby supplies on each floor.
- Bathe the baby in a tub only if another person is present and watching.
- When alone and baby needs washing, give sponge bath on the floor with a separate container of water.
- Perform other infant care activities (e.g., dressing and diaper changes) on the floor to decrease the risk of a fall during a seizure.

Adapted from: Rousseau (2008).

A commonly asked question is whether the infant will be at an increased risk for epilepsy. Teaching should include the fact that the baby will be four times more likely to have a seizure disorder. However, a paternal seizure disorder has not been shown to increase incidence in offspring (ACOG, 1997).

Care of pregnant women with headache

A commonly reported concern during pregnancy is the onset of a headache. Headaches are more common during the first and third trimesters. The etiology of headaches during pregnancy includes hormonal changes and an increase in blood volume during the first trimester, tension headaches, postural changes and related muscle strain, and the development of preeclampsia during the third trimester.

Headaches are divided into two major classifications: primary and secondary. Primary headaches are then further divided into subcategories of tension type: migraine, cluster, and other. Secondary headaches occur in response to another condition such as trauma, bleeding in the brain, tumor, or encephalitis. Determination of headache type is the initial step in the evaluation and treatment of headaches.

The assessment and diagnosis of headache symptoms are largely based on a thorough history pertinent to headache in pregnancy. It is essential to assess for other signs and symptoms of preeclampsia in any woman reporting a headache in the third trimester (refer to Chapter 22, "Hypertensive Disorders in Pregnancy"). For women whose headache does not have a clear etiology, completion of a headache diary can provide information on headache triggers, severity, and the impact on the woman's life. A sample headache diary is displayed in Table 38.2.

Tension-type headaches

Tension-type headaches are the most commonly reported type of headache in both pregnant and nonpregnant

Table 38.2 Headache Diary

Date
Time of onset
Location of pain
Pain rating (1–10)
How long did pain last?
Any aura or warning? Describe if present
Describe pain (stabbing, aching, dull, sharp, pressure etc.)
Other symptoms (nausea, sensitivity to light, etc.)
Foods and drinks before onset
Activity before and at onset
Amount of sleep last night
Stress/mood before onset
Treatments (medication, massage, bath, etc.)
Effectiveness of treatment(s) above
Notes

women. Tension-type headaches are generally mild to moderate in intensity, are usually perceived bilaterally, and have minimal or no associated symptoms such as nausea, visual disturbances, or photophobia. Tension-type headaches can further be categorized based upon the frequency (Table 38.3).

The frequency, duration, and the presence or severity associated signs and symptoms influence the treatment plan for tension headaches. In most instances, tension-type headaches are relieved by conservative interventions such as massage, heat, and oral acetaminophen. In cases where these measures do not provide adequate relief, the episodic use of opioids or acetaminophen with opioids can be considered if symptoms are severe and unresponsive to more conservative treatment. Chronic tension-type headaches may be managed prophylactically in collaboration with a consulting physician.

Migraine headaches

Migraine headaches can be divided into the subcategories of migraine without aura, migraine with aura, and chronic migraine. Migraines are more commonly experienced by women than men. The higher prevalence of migraine in women is thought to be due to hormonal fluctuations. Most women find that they have a decrease in frequency and intensity of migraine headaches during pregnancy, with the most significant reduction during the second and third trimesters (Kvisvik, Stovner, Heide, Bovim, & Linde, 2011). Women with migraines have an increased risk of developing preeclampsia (Cripe, Frederick, Qui, & Williams, 2011).

A minority of pregnant women will have their first migraine during pregnancy and this is most likely to occur during the first trimester. Postpartum headaches are very common and occur in 30–40% of all women. The first week following birth is the most common time for postpartum migraine headaches to occur (Kvisvik et al., 2011).

Nonpharmacological headache management

For all headache types, nonpharmacological measures should be the first choice for pregnant woman (Table 38.4) Magnesium supplementation has been shown as beneficial for the prevention of headaches and is safe for use during pregnancy. Although supplements such as riboflavin and alphalipoic acid have recently been shown to have possible prophylactic properties against migraines, controlled studies of the use of these substances in pregnant women have not been conducted. The herbal supplement feverfew has possible benefits for migraine relief; however, it has known potentially harmful side effects for pregnant women and should be avoided (Sun-Edelstein & Mauskop, 2011).

Table 38.3 International Headache Society Criteria for Tension Headaches

Classification	Frequency	Duration	Characteristics
Infrequent episodic tension type	• 10–12 episodes per year • <1 episode each month	30 minutes to 7 days	At least two of the following: • Bilateral location • Pressing/tightening (nonpulsating) quality • Mild/moderate intensity • Not aggravated by routine physical activity Both of the following: • No nausea or vomiting • Not attributed to another disorder Only one of the following: • Photophobia • Phonophobia
Frequent episodic tension type	• ≥10 episodes per month occurring on 1–14 days/month • Occurs for at least 3 months	30 minutes to 7 days	Same as above
Chronic tension type	• ≥15 days/month • Occurs for at least 3 months	• 30 minutes to 7 days or • Lasting hours or continuous	Same as above with the following changes: • Neither moderate or severe nausea or vomiting Only one of the following: • Photophobia • Phonophobia • Mild nausea

Source: The International Headache Society (IHS), http://ihs-classification.org/en/02_klassifikation/02_teil1/.

Common headache triggers

Inadequate or excessive sleep
Smoke
Change in caffeine intake
Stress
Hormonal fluctuations
Eyestrain
Sensory overload (odors or noise)
Very cold foods/drinks
Foods containing monosodium glutamate (MSG)
Chocolate
Foods containing tyramine (examples):
 Aged cheeses
 Canned or processed meats
 Olives
 Pickles
 Canned soups
Alcohol
 Red wine
 Champagne
 Whiskey
 Beer

Source: Martin and MacLeod (2009).

Lifestyle changes that encourage better overall health should be encouraged by the health-care provider. Maintaining regular and adequate sleep patterns will help many headache sufferers. Lifestyle changes such as smoking cessation and regular exercise can also contribute to better headache control. A consistent daily routine for eating, activity, and sleeping may also be beneficial in headache prevention. Dietary modifications such as not skipping meals and avoidance or minimal use of foods and beverages that can trigger headaches is often all that is needed to reduce headache incidents in pregnancy. Avoiding common headache triggers can also be beneficial. Massage therapy is effective for headache relief. Migraine sufferers receiving massage therapy once a week for 5 weeks had greater improvements in sleep quality and reduction in migraine frequency compared to control participants (Lawler & Cameron, 2006).

Pharmacological treatment of migraine headaches

Women with a history of migraine headaches should be encouraged to treat the headache at the first onset of symptoms. Treatment early in the progression of the headache is more likely to be effective. Appropriate pharmacological treatment at this juncture would be analgesics such as acetaminophen. Aspirin and

Table 38.4   Nonpharmacological Treatment of Headaches

- Relaxation
  - Breathing exercises
  - Meditation
  - Visual or guided imagery
  - Progressive relaxation (tense and relax muscle groups)
    - Rationale: stress and muscle tension can result in increased headache activity which can be ameliorated with client relaxation
    - Evidence: especially useful when combined with biofeedback, no supporting evidence of relaxation alone being effective
- Acupuncture
  - Performed by skilled practitioners with the goal to restore and maintain equilibrium in the body
    - Rationale: control pain receptors
    - Evidence: 2009 Cochrane Review supports acupuncture as an effective treatment for migraines
- Cognitive-behavioral therapy
    - Rationale: target thinking patterns that contribute to stress and headaches and train client to control these thinking patterns
    - Evidence: supported by the U.S. Headache Consortium as effective
- Physical therapy
  - Massage
  - Transcutaneous nerve stimulation (TENS)
  - Chiropractic manipulation
  - Hot and cold packs
    - Rationale: decreasing muscle tension that may decrease headache pain
    - Evidence: weak evidence to support benefits
- Biofeedback
  - Physical indicators of stress such as changes in skin temperature, heart rate, and muscle activity are signaled to the client, who then responds.
    - Rationale: voluntary recognition of tension and reactionary ability of client to decrease the tension and thereby decrease headache
    - Evidence: supports this therapy as effective
- Oxygen therapy
  - Inhalation of normobaric oxygen through face mask
    - Rationale: increasing oxygen to constricted vessels will decrease pain
    - Evidence: conflicting

Sources: Bendtsen et al. (2010), Sun-Edelstein and Mauskop (2011).

other nonsteroidal anti-inflammatory drugs (NSAIDs) should be avoided during pregnancy due to its association with fetal bleeding and cardiac problems. There is also recent research to indicate that NSAIDs should be avoided during the first trimester due to an increased risk of miscarriage. The risk of spontaneous abortion in women using NSAIDs has been found to be twice that of unexposed pregnant women (Nakhai-Pour, Broy, Sheehy, & Brard, 2011). If the use of acetaminophen is ineffective or if the headache is severe, antiemetics along with opioid pain relief may be effective. Ongoing use of opioid-containing agents should be avoided particularly during the third trimester due to the possibility of fetal dependency. Ergot alkaloids should not be used during pregnancy because of their association with fetal birth defects (Jamil, 2004). Other management options for acute and severe headaches include intravenous hydration and intramuscular or intravenous magnesium.

Triptans are widely accepted as treatment for migraine headache. Although there are no data indicating triptans are problematic during pregnancy, there is limited evidence about the safety of this group of medications (ACOG, 2009). In limited cases, prophylactic treatment for women with frequent migraines is appropriate and should be undertaken in collaboration with a consulting physician. Pregnant women who do not respond adequately to commonly used medications and lifestyle changes should be referred for further evaluation and treatment.

Postpartum headaches

Headaches in the early postpartum period must first be evaluated to eliminate the possibility that the headache is associated with preeclampsia. If there is no indication of preeclampsia, the health-care provider should consider the possibility of anesthesia complications if the woman had epidural pain management in the intrapartum period. If this is not the likely cause of the headache, primary headache management principles should be undertaken. Nonpharmacological measures should be the primary intervention with the addition of medications as needed using acetaminophen as an initial mediation choice. Safety to the infant should be taken into consideration if the mother is breastfeeding.

Cluster headaches

Cluster headaches are rare and occur more commonly in men than in women. Cluster headaches are very severe and most often unilateral in nature. Patterns of cluster headaches range from short duration headaches that occur frequently over several weeks or months followed by long headache-free periods to a more chronic pattern of daily or almost daily headaches. Cluster headaches are often associated with symptoms such as excessive tearing on the affected side and nasal stuffiness. The pregnant woman with cluster headaches should be referred to a neurologist or other health-care providers who specialize in the treatment of cluster headaches.

Care of pregnant women with multiple sclerosis

Multiple sclerosis (MS) is a chronic neurological disease that affects more women than men. It is the most commonly found neurological disorder not caused by injury among young adults. MS causes demyelinization of central nervous system myelin sheaths, which leads to neurological symptoms such as muscle weakness, parasthesias, and visual changes. MS is diagnosed when magnetic resonance imaging shows areas of demyelinization of the central nervous system.

Approximately 20–33% of women diagnosed with MS will subsequently bear a child (van der Kop et al., 2011). MS has not been consistently shown to have an adverse effect on pregnancy and birth. Most women with MS have healthy, uneventful pregnancies with no significantly increased risk of miscarriage, prematurity, or cesarean birth (Karnad & Guntupalli, 2005). Women with MS may have an increased risk of spontaneous abortion, a small-for-gestational-age infant, antepartum hospital admissions, and cesarean birth (Signore, Spong, Krotoski, Shinowara, & Blackwell, 2011).

Many women with MS may be treated with interferon outside of pregnancy. Most brands of interferon treatment are labeled as pregnancy risk category C however, due to increased risk of spontaneous abortion. Evidence supports the discontinuation of interferon treatment for women attempting pregnancy. This can be discussed at the time of preconceptual counseling. For the woman who presents for confirmation of pregnancy and has continued her interferon treatment, the medication should be discontinued at that time. A recent study found that the only long-term effect in women with unintentional interferon exposure in pregnant women was an increase incidence of assisted vaginal birth (Lu et al., 2012).

Prenatal care for the woman with MS should follow the usual pattern of care with the added component of treatment aimed at providing symptomatic relief as needed. This is usually possible with the use of analgesics. If the woman has bladder involvement, it is wise to monitor her carefully for urinary tract infections and to teach her signs and symptoms of infection.

Women with MS are more often overweight compared with women without MS and should be counseled appropriately regarding increased risk of pregnancy complications associated with a high body mass index (van der Kop et al., 2011). These risks include gestational diabetes, fetal macrosomia, assisted vaginal birth, cesarean section, and shoulder dystocia. Women with MS during pregnancy who are overweight should be monitored for appropriate weight gain and nutrition and advised accordingly. If gestational diabetes is diagnosed, vigilant monitoring and strict control of blood sugars are a priority.

Women with MS have a decreased risk of disease relapse during pregnancy. However, there is an increased rate of relapse in the first 3 months postpartum. The pattern of relapse usually returns to the prepregnancy level at about 4 months after birth (Finkelsztejn, Brooks, Paschoal, & Fragoso, 2011).

A unique focus of prenatal care for the woman with MS is directed at teaching and preparing the woman to function as a mother while coping with treatment and management of her MS symptoms. Discussions regarding the challenges that she faces as a woman with MS can lead to discussions about functioning as a new mother with MS. Identification of resources and support systems should be encouraged. Utilization of a multidisciplinary approach to pregnancy and postpartum care should optimize care during the childbearing year.

Summary

The most commonly encountered neurological disorders in the pregnant woman are seizure disorders, headache, and MS. This chapter has covered the assessment, diagnosis, and management of these disorders. The pregnant woman with a seizure disorder or MS can in some instances be managed in collaboration with a physician or may require referral depending on the stability of the disorder and/or the time of the initial diagnosis. Headaches that occur during pregnancy are usually managed independently by the nurse practitioner or midwife.

Case study

Candace is a G1P0 who presents for an initial prenatal visit at 6 weeks' gestation. Candace did not plan this pregnancy and the pregnancy was discovered incidentally when she had a USN for vaginal bleeding. Candace is adjusting to the idea of being pregnant but is extremely concerned about her antiseizure medications and how these might "hurt my baby." Candace is accompanied by her mother, who echoes these concerns.

Candace was diagnosed with a tonic–clonic seizure disorder when she was 14 years old. She is now 25 and has not had a seizure since she was 19. She was placed on Neurontin at that time. Her Neurontin is renewed each year by her primary care physician. Further investigation reveals that she has not seen a neurologist since her last seizure activity at 19 years of age.

It was discussed with Candace and her mother that there are risks with any medication and that overall, women with seizure disorder are at an increased risk of having a baby with malformations. However, the current medication that Candace is taking has been shown to be one of the safest to take during pregnancy and has not been associated with the problems most commonly found with the use of antiseizure medications. The risks of seizure activity during pregnancy were discussed and reassurance was given that keeping Candace seizure free is an important goal during pregnancy. A plan was developed to compare the risks associated with taking Neurontin compared to the risks of possible reoccurrence of seizure activity. A referral to the neurology department was instituted for thorough evaluation of Candace's current medication regime and seizure history. Candace and her mother seem relieved by this plan.

Candace was seen again at 8 weeks' gestation after her visit with the neurologist. The neurologist determined that Candace should remain on Neurontin with a dose adjustment. Early genetic screening and testing options and the role of MSAFP screening in the

identification of malformations associated with the use of antiseizure medications were discussed. Candace chooses to have a quad screen at 16 weeks and an anatomical screening USN at 20 weeks' gestation. Candace was encouraged to choose a health-care provider for her baby and to make a visit before birth to discuss breastfeeding and the use of her medications.

Candace's quad screen is negative and her USN at 20 weeks reveals no signs of fetal malformations. Fetal growth is found to progress as expected using fundal height measurements until Candace's 33-week appointment. Her fundal height at this visit is found to be 29 cm. At her last visit 2 weeks ago, it was 28 cm. Candace's weight gain has been steady but on the low end of normal. A USN was ordered for growth; the baby's size is in the ninth percentile. A consultation with the obstetrician was done and the plan is to monitor Candace more often.

Candace is scheduled for twice weekly visits with nonstress tests (NST) and biweekly USN for growth and measurement of the amniotic fluid index. Adequate nutrition and increased caloric intake was encouraged and Candace was given a medical leave from her job at a local convenience store. The goal of conserving calories for the baby's growth by taking rest breaks during the day and eating well was discussed.

Candace's care is comanaged for the remainder of her pregnancy. Each visit, the USN and NST results are reviewed with the consulting physician. At 37 weeks, it was agreed that an induction of labor is indicated due to deterioration of the placenta as evidenced by a nonreactive NST and a biophysical profile score of 4.

Candace's labor was induced with Cytotec and pitocin and she gives birth to a healthy baby boy weighing 5 lb, 2 oz. She successfully initiated breastfeeding and was discharged home with a postpartum visit appointment in 6 weeks to review contraception options.

Resources for women and their families

ACOG—A question-and-answer informative webpage about seizure disorders and pregnancy: http://www.acog.org/~/media/For%20Patients/faq129.pdf?dmc=1&ts=20130110T1811472673

March of Dimes—A consumer-oriented overview of headaches in pregnancy and relief measures: http://www.marchofdimes.com/pregnancy/yourbody_headaches.html

References

American College of Obstetricians and Gynecologists (ACOG). (1997). ACOG educational bulletin Number 231: Seizure disorders in pregnancy. *International Journal of Gynaecology and Obstetrics*, 56, 279–286.

American College of Obstetricians and Gynecologists (ACOG). (2009, reaffirmed in 2012). Migraines and other headache disorders. *Clinical Updates in Women's Health Care*, 1(3).

Bendtsen, L., Evers, S., Linde, M., Mitsikostas, G., Sandrini, G., & Schoenen, J. (2010). EFNS guidelines on the treatment of tension-type headache—Report of an EFNS task force. *European Journal of Neurology*, *17*, 1318–1325.

Borthen, I., Eide, M., Daltveit, A., & Gilhus, N. (2011). Obstetric outcome in women with epilepsy: A hospital-based, retrospective study. *BJOG: An International Journal of Obstetrics and Gynaecology*, *118*(8), 956–965.

Borthen, I., & Gilhus, N. E. (2012). Pregnancy complications in patients with epilepsy. *Current Opinion in Obstetrics and Gynecology*, *24*(2), 78–83.

Crawford, P. M. (2009). Managing epilepsy in women of childbearing age. *Drug safety*, *32*(4), 293–307.

Cripe, S. M., Frederick, I. O., Qui, C., & Williams, M. A. (2011). Risk of preterm delivery and hypertensive disorders of pregnancy in relation to maternal co-morbid mood and migraine disorders during pregnancy. *Paediatric and Perinatal Epidemiology*, *25*(2), 116–123.

Finkelsztejn, A., Brooks, J., Paschoal, F., & Fragoso, Y. (2011). What can we really tell women with multiple sclerosis regarding pregnancy? A systematic review and meta-analysis of the literature. *BJOG: An International Journal of Obstetrics and Gynaecology*, *118*(7), 790–797.

Gedzelman, E., & Meador K.J. (2012). Antiepileptic drugs in women with epilepsy during pregnancy. *Therapeutic Advances in Drug Safety*, *3*(2), 71–87.

Jamil, T. (2004). Migraines in pregnancy. *Pulse*, *64*(34), 30.

Karnad, D. R., & Guntupalli, K. K. (2005). Neurologic disorders in pregnancy. *Critical Care Medicine*, *33*(10), S362–S371.

Kvisvik, E. V., Stovner, L. J., Heide, G., Bovim, G., & Linde, M. (2011). Headache and migraine during pregnancy and puerperium: The MIGRA- study. *Journal of Headache and Pain*, *12*, 443–451.

Lawler, S. P., & Cameron, L. D. (2006). A randomized controlled trial of massage therapy as a treatment for migraine headache. *Annals of Behavioral Medicine*, *32*(1), 50–59.

Lu, E., Dahlgren, L., Sadovnick, A. D., Sayao, A., Synnes, A., & Tremlett, H. (2012). Perinatal outcomes in women with multiple sclerosis exposed to disease-modifying drugs. *Multiple Sclerosis Journal*, *18*(4), 460–467.

Martin, P. R., & MacLeod, C. (2009). Behavioral management of headache triggers: Avoidance of triggers is an inadequate strategy. *Clinical Psychology Review*, *29*(6), 483–495.

Nakhai-Pour, H. R., Broy, P., Sheehy, O., & Brard, A. (2011). Use of nonaspirin nonsteroidal anti-inflammatory drugs during pregnancy and the risk of spontaneous abortion. *Canadian Medical Association Journal*, *183*(15), 1713–1720.

Rousseau, J. (2008). Meeting the needs to postpartum women with epilepsy. *MCN. The American Journal of Maternal Child Nursing*, *32*(2), 84–89.

Signore, C., Spong, C. Y., Krotoski, D., Shinowara, N., & Blackwell, S. (2011). Pregnancy in women with physical disabilities. *Obstetrics and Gynecology*, *117*(4), 935–937.

St Louis, E. K. (2009). Monitoring antiepileptic drugs: A level-headed approach. *Current Neuropharmacology*, *7*, 115–119.

Sun-Edelstein, C., & Mauskop, A. (2011). Alternative headache treatments: Nutraceuticals, behavioral and physical treatments. *Headache*, *51*(3), 469–483.

Tomson, T., & Battino, D. (2009). Teratogenic effects of antieplileptic medications. *Neurologic Clinics*, *27*(4), 993–1002.

Tomson, T., Landmark, C. J., & Battino, D. (2013). Antiepileptic drug treatment in pregnancy: Changes in drug disposition and their clinical implications. *Epilepsia*, *53*(3), 405–414.

van der Kop, M. L., Pearce, M. S., Dahlgren, L., Synnes, A., Sadovnick, D., Sayao, A. L. & Tremlett, H. (2011). Neonatal and delivery outcomes in women with multiple sclerosis. *Annals of Neurology*, *70*(1), 41–50.

Williams, S. H., & Kehr, H. A. (2012). An update in the treatment of neurologic disorders during pregnancy—Focus on migraines and seizures. *Journal of Pharmacy Practice*, *25*(3), 341–351.

Yerby, M.S. (2001).Teratogenicity of anticonvulsant medication. In J. M. Pellock, W. E. Dodson, & B. F. D. Bourgeois (Eds.), *Pediatric Epilepsy: Diagnosis and Treatment*. New York: Demos.

39

Dermatological disorders

Gwendolyn Short and Elizabeth Powell Holcomb

Relevant terms

Herpetiform—resembling herpes: raised, red blisters or macules that crust to form a papule

Iris or target lesions—a series of concentric rings with a dark or blistered center

Papule or Papula—circumscribed, solid elevation of skin that does not contain pus

Plaque—broad papule or confluence of papules

Urticaria—red, raised skin rash, also known as hives

Introduction

Numerous physiological changes occur within a woman's body throughout pregnancy, most of which are the normal changes in response to the pregnant condition. The skin is not spared in this adaptation response. The common benign conditions occur primarily as a result of the dramatic hormonal changes that take place during pregnancy and the immediate postpartal period (see Chapter 11, "Common Discomforts in Pregnancy"). Preexisting skin conditions can also be impacted by the pregnant state. Atopic dermatitis (AD), acne, psoriasis, and eczema are the most notable of these.

Even though the majority of these skin changes are benign in nature, there are several pathological skin conditions occurring in pregnancy that are associated with significant maternal discomfort and may be associated with poor fetal outcomes. Prurigo of pregnancy (PP), pruritic urticarial papules and plaques of pregnancy (PUPP), also known as polymorphic eruption of pregnancy (PEP), and pruritic folliculitis of pregnancy (PFP) are all conditions that can cause significant discomfort to the pregnant woman. All of these conditions are self-limiting with symptoms resolving following birth. There are no associations between these conditions and the health of the fetus or newborn. In contrast, pemphigoid gestationis (PG), impetigo herpetiformis (IH), and intrahepatic cholestasis of pregnancy (ICP) are all conditions that may negatively impact the mother and the fetus, and so increased antepartum surveillance is recommended (Tunzi & Gray, 2007). It is important for the health-care provider to be able to differentiate among these various skin conditions when arriving at an accurate diagnosis and treatment plan. This chapter covers AD, PP, and the pathological skin conditions occurring during pregnancy. Table 39.1 displays common abbreviations for the skin disorders covered in this chapter.

Atopic dermatitis

Acne, psoriasis, and eczema are all conditions of AD and can be altered by the pregnant state. In some cases, these conditions improve, but most often, symptoms worsen during the pregnant condition (Thurston & Grau, 2008). AD is the most common pregnancy dermatosis but is not specific to pregnancy. Differentiating AD from the specific dermatoses of pregnancy is a challenge because of lack of clarity in diagnostic criteria for many of the pregnancy-related dermatoses (Koutroulis, Papoutsis, & Kroumpouzos, 2011). There is significant overlap in presenting symptoms between AD, PP, and PFP that has prompted some researchers to recategorize

---

Prenatal and Postnatal Care: A Woman-Centered Approach, First Edition. Edited by Robin G. Jordan, Janet L. Engstrom, Julie A. Marfell, and Cindy L. Farley.
© 2014 John Wiley & Sons, Inc. Published 2014 by John Wiley & Sons, Inc.

Table 39.1Table 39.1   Abbreviations for Skin Disorders in Pregnancy

AD	Atopic dermatitis
AEP	Atopic eczema (or eruption) of pregnancy
EP	Eczema of pregnancy
GP	Gestational pemphigoid
ICP	Intrahepatic cholestasis of pregnancy
IH	Impetigo herpetiformis
PEP (PUPP)	Polymorphic eruption of pregnancy
PF	Pruritic folliculitis
PG	Pemphigoid gestationis
PP	Prurigo of pregnancy
PUPP (PEP)	Pruritic urticarial papules and plaques of pregnancy

certain of the dermatoses (Ambros-Rudolph, Müllegger, Vaughan-Jones, Kerl, & Black, 2006) under the umbrella term of atopic eruption of pregnancy.

Current research in the area of AD explores the prevalence of "new AD," or AD that develops during the pregnancy, compared to AD that was present prior to pregnancy. Several researchers noted that 20–40% of patients with AD in pregnancy have a preexisting history of eczema with the remainder experiencing new symptoms while pregnant (Ambros-Rudolph et al., 2006). Approximately 24% of women experience improvement of AD symptoms during pregnancy, and 52% experience worsening of the disorder (Kemmett & Tidman, 1991).

Assessment

AD in pregnancy typically presents with lesions on the flexor surfaces of the upper and lower extremities, less so on the trunk, and even less so on the hands, feet, and nipples. The lesions of AD are often more widespread than that seen in PP (Ingber, 2010).

Differential diagnoses

Differentiating AD from other dermatoses seen in pregnancy can be challenging as there is much overlap in symptoms presentation. Differentiation from the specific dermatoses of pregnancy can often be made by assessing the history of atopic symptoms, and timing of symptom onset, as AD will typically present early in the pregnancy (Koutroulis et al., 2011).

Treatment and management

Use of emollients to avoid skin dryness is a safe and effective management of AD, as is the use of oral antihistamines. First-generation antihistamines (diphenhydr-

amine and chlorpheniramine) and second-generation formulations (loratadine and cetirizine) are all pregnancy category B and so are not found to be harmful during pregnancy. This should be the first-line approach. The use of ultraviolet light has also been found to be effective and safe.

Topical steroids that are mild to moderate in strength (pregnancy category B) can be used safely in pregnancy, as long as they are used judiciously, in small areas, and used sparingly during the first trimester (Koutroulis et al., 2011). Some studies show an association between high potent topical steroid use and small-for-gestational-age (SGA) infants (Katz, Thorp, & Bowes, 1990). Oral steroids are an option for symptoms that are resistant to treatment, but should be used in the lowest possible dose. Referral to dermatology services is always an option for those women whose symptoms fail to improve with use of mild-to-moderate-strength topical corticosteroid preparations and antihistamines. A stronger topical steroid or oral steroids may be indicated for those women with severe cases of AD. Women should be advised that preexisting AD may improve or worsen during pregnancy and reassured that it is a self-limiting condition.

Prurigo of pregnancy

PP, also known as eczema of pregnancy (EP), is a skin disorder not clearly categorized. It has commonly been associated with pregnancy; however, it may be a condition that is already present and with worsening symptoms during pregnancy (Table 39.2). PP is estimated to affect one in every 300–450 pregnancies (Ambros-Rudolph et al., 2006).

Assessment

The classic presentation of PP appears in grouped, crusted, erythematous papules, patches, and plaques, often with excoriations, and typically located on the extensor surfaces of arms and legs, and on the abdomen (Bremmer et al., 2010). Onset of symptoms is usually earlier than other pregnancy-related dermatoses, occurring midpregnancy between 25 and 30 weeks' gestation, but onset has been seen in all trimesters. The lesions disappear within weeks after birth but can remain for up to 3 months postpartum (Roth, 2011).

Differential diagnoses

PP can be easily mistaken for the PUPP and can manifest overlapping symptoms. Differentiation can be made from preexisting atopic symptoms or from conditions totally unrelated to pregnancy, such as scabies, eczema, drug rashes, or insect bites.

Table 39.2   Skin Disorders of Pregnancy: Defining Characteristics

Disorder	Defining characteristics	Diagnostic aides	Pregnancy risk
PP	Excoriated papules/nodules on Extensor surfaces of arms, legs, abdomen Weeks 25–30	Diagnosis based on history and physical	None known
PUPP/ PEP	Excoriated papules Abdominal striae, thighs, buttocks, arms, legs Last trimester or immediately postpartum	Diagnosis based on history and physical	None known
PFP	Follicular papules or pustular eruptions Chest Second or third trimester	Diagnosis based on history and physical	None known
PG	Severe pruritis with erythematous papules Periumbilical area and extremities Second or third trimester	Biopsy is needed for definitive diagnosis, with direct immunofluorescence (DIF)	Increased risk of low birth weight, prematurity, neonatal skin lesions
IH	Erythematous plaques with greenish yellow pustules, no pruritis Inner thighs, flexor surfaces, groin Second half of pregnancy	Diagnosis based on history and physical Lab measurements: ESR and WBC may be elevated; vitamin D and calcium may be low.	Increased fetal morbidity
ICP	Intense pruritis without lesions Palms of hands, soles of feet Third trimester	Laboratory measurements: Elevated serum bile acids is diagnostic; AST and ALT may be elevated; vitamin K may be low.	Preterm birth, fetal distress, meconium-stained amniotic fluid, intrauterine fetal demise

Adapted from: Tunzi and Gray (2007).

Treatment and management

Effective treatment often consists of a moderate-strength topical corticosteroid cream and an oral antihistamine. Emollients containing 3–10% urea is another suggested treatment (Roth, 2011). Narrow band ultraviolet B (NBUVB) phototherapy has also been suggested as an effective treatment (Jang et al., 2011).

Pruritic urticarial papules and plaques of pregnancy

PUPP is also known as PEP. Clinical manifestations include wheals, papules, erythematous plaques, vesicle, and target or iris lesions (Fig. 39.1) (Table 39.2). This disorder is the most common skin disorder that occurs in pregnancy, with an incidence rate of 1 in every 160 pregnancies worldwide (Paunescu, Feier, & Paunescu, 2008; Roth, 2011). A relationship between asthma, eczema, and seasonal allergies and the development of PUPP may be present (Roth, 2011). Multiple gestation pregnancies and excessive maternal weight are significantly associated with PUPP (Rudolph, Al-Fares, & Vaughan-Jones, 2006). No definitive cause for this disorder has yet been clearly identified, and no diagnostic test

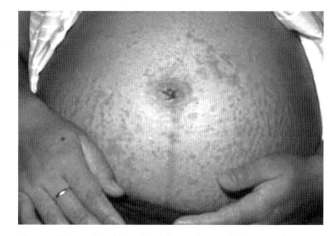

Figure 39.1.   Pruritic urticarial papules and plaques of pregnancy (PUPP). The papules often first localize in the abdominal striae.

exists. Subsequent pregnancies do not seem to be affected at a higher rate.

Assessment

PUPP typically appears during the third trimester or immediately postpartum. The clinical manifestation is most often pruritic urticarial papules along the abdominal striae, spreading to the thighs, buttocks, arms, and legs; the face, palms, soles, umbilicus, and mucous membranes are typically not affected. In up to 50% of the cases, as the disorder progresses, papular lesions are joined by wheals, plaques, vesicles, and target lesions (Roth, 2011).

Differential diagnoses

There are no diagnostic tests for PUPP, making timing of symptom onset and location a primary clue to an accurate clinical diagnosis. Lesions are often located in the periumbilical area in PG, while this area is spared in PUPP (Bremmer et al., 2010). PUPP can easily be mistaken for other dermatoses of pregnancy, such as PP or PFP. To exclude a diagnosis of pemphigus gestationis (PG), histopathologic and immunopathologic (both direct immunoflouresence or direct immunofluorescene [DIF], and indirect immunofluorescene [IIF]) tests can be performed (Roth, 2011). To exclude the diagnosis of IHCP, total serum bile acid levels must be normal.

Treatment and management

Symptomatic treatment is all that is typically needed when managing this skin disorder. Topical corticosteroids, oral antihistamines (loratadine and ceftirizine are safe in pregnancy), emollient creams, and antipruritic medication (menthol) are all possible treatments that have been shown to be safe and effective.

Women should be reassured that the pruritic lesions of PUPP are benign and self-limiting and typically resolve between 1–6 weeks postpartum. There may be occasional flaking of the skin, though there is generally no scarring.

Pruritic folliculitis of pregnancy

PFP is a benign dermatological condition of pregnancy that presents with papules and pustules surrounding the hair follicles. Initially, the lesions appear on the abdomen and then spread to the extremities (Roth, 2011). PFP most commonly occurs in the second or third trimester of pregnancy (Tunzi & Gray, 2007).

The incidence of PFP is about 1 in every 3000 pregnancies (Bremmer et al., 2010), though as a result of misdiagnosis as acne and bacterial folliculitis, the incidence is probably higher (Roth, 2011). The pathophysiology of PRP is largely unknown.

Assessment

Typically, the lesions initially appear as small (3–5 mm) erythematous papules on the upper trunk spreading to the lower extremities. Interestingly, pruritus may be absent or mild or it can be severe (Roth, 2011). This is a self-limiting disorder that usually clears in the last weeks of gestation. Complete resolution should occur by at least 2 weeks postpartum. There is no reported recurrence in subsequent pregnancies (Bremmer et al., 2010).

Differential diagnosis

Other dermatoses of pregnancy warrant consideration with this type of presentation. The absence of bullous lesions, striae, and urticarial lesions helps differentiate this from PG and PEP. PFP, unlike PP, has follicular lesions and first appears on the chest and abdomen (Table 39.2). An absence of comedones and lesions on the face helps differentiate this condition from acne. Bacterial folliculitis can be differentiated from PFP by culture. Drug reaction is also a consideration and warrants a thorough medication history (Roth, 2011).

Treatment and management

In the absence of pruritis, no specific treatment is indicated. For symptomatic presentation, the use of low-to-moderate-potency topical corticosteroids, such as triamcinolone or desonide, is indicated. Benzol peroxide wash has also been shown to be effective (Bremmer et al., 2010; Roth, 2011). Ultraviolet B (UVB) is another recommended therapy (Roth, 2011).

Pemphigoid gestationis

PG is a rare autoimmune blistering skin disorder occurring in 1 in 40,000–50,000 pregnancies (Lipozencic, Ljugojevic, & Bukvic-Mokos, 2012; Roth, 2011; Ruiz-Villaverde, Sánchez-Cano, & Ramirez-Tortosa, 2011; Tunzi & Gray, 2007). This disorder was originally referred to as herpes gestationis because of the herpetiform appearance of the lesions (Tunzi & Gray, 2007). Since there is no association with herpes virus infection, the name was later changed to PG. PG is an immune response that directs immunoglobin (IgG) to attack a hemidismosome transmembrane glycoprotein. This targeted protein accounts for several blistering skin disorders, including PG (Bremmer et al., 2010) (Fig. 39.2).Women with a history of PG have a higher incidence of autoimmune diseases including Graves disease, Hashimoto thyroiditis, pernicious anemia, and autoimmune thrombocytopenia (Lipozencic et al., 2012; Roth, 2011).

The disease generally appears in a first pregnancy and in the second (34%) or third (34%) trimester of pregnancy. However, a smaller percentage (14%) initially appears in the immediate postpartum period (Roth, 2011). Since exacerbation can occur with contraceptive use (Roth, 2011), it is believed that hormonal factors play a role in this condition. There is a high recurrence rate in subsequent pregnancies with an earlier onset of symptoms (Roth, 2011).

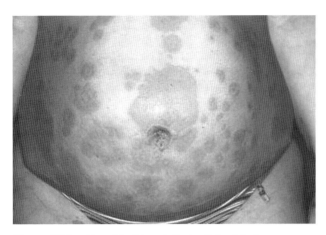

Figure 39.2. Pemphigoid gestationis: Urticarial plaques progress to generalized tense bullae on erythematous base.

Unlike other skin disorders, in PG the first immunological response occurs in the placenta and not the skin. As a result of IgG1 antibodies crossing over the placenta, up to 10% of newborns develop a mild form of the disease with urticarial or vesicular skin lesions (Bremmer et al., 2010). These lesions tend to disappear in several days to weeks after the birth while antibodies slowly decline during the first 3 months of life. The newborn can also have subclinical disease where antibody tests are positive but there are no skin lesions. In addition, there is an increased risk of having a baby that is premature or SGA, both of which are suggestive of placental insufficiency (Roth, 2011). No lasting morbidity or mortality has been noted in these infants (Bremmer et al., 2010).

Assessment

The woman with PG initially presents with severe pruritus and urticarial erythematous papules most often located in the periumbilical area or extremities (Bremmer et al., 2010; Roth, 2011). Even though the entire skin area can be involved, the face, palms, soles, and mucous membranes are usually spared (Roth, 2011). As the condition progresses over days and weeks, the papules become plaques and tense blisters develop. Once the blisters rupture, eroded areas covered by yellowish or hemorrhagic crusts are left behind. In the majority of cases, PG worsens close to the time of birth and improves after birth (Bremmer et al., 2010). The bullous eruptions generally disappear at 4 weeks postpartum, while the urticaria can persist for up to 14 weeks following birth. Rarely, the condition can be severe and can last for years after birth (Roth, 2011).

A definitive diagnosis of PG is reached through biopsy of skin tissue surrounding the lesions. DIF shows complement component protein C3 deposits along the basal membrane zone in patients with PG. This is

detected in 100% of all cases. In addition, IgG can be seen in 25–30% of women with PG. Serum enzyme-linked immunosorbent assay (ELISA) for PG antibody, with its high sensitivity and specificity, can also be useful in arriving at a diagnosis (Lipozencic et al., 2012; Roth, 2011).

Differential diagnosis

Other diagnoses with similar presentations that need to be considered include PEP, PUPP, and ICP (Table 39.2). Prior to blister formation, it may be difficult to differentiate PC from PEP. An absence of striae gravidarum and the presence of skin lesions in the umbilical area can be suggestive of PG and assist in ruling out PEP. It is also necessary to rule out other bullous conditions that can occur without pregnancy such as bullous pemphigoid, erythema multiforme, drug eruptions, and contact dermatitis. DIF can play a role in excluding these disorders (Roth, 2011).

Treatment and management

High-potency corticosteroids, along with emollients in the mild preblistering stage, can be used to treat PG (Roth, 2011). Treatment with oral corticosteroids during the preblistering stage can also be effective (Bremmer et al., 2010). Prednisone 20–60 mg/day is the recommended drug and dose. Prednisone at these doses given over a short period of time has not been associated with any congenital problems (Roth, 2011).

Oral prednisone is advised once blisters begin to appear. The recommended dosage is 0.5–1 mg/kg/day. This dosage should reduce pruritus and prevent the formation of new blisters. If improvement is not satisfactory, the dosage can be increased to 2 mg/kg/day. Women on this regimen should experience symptom relief in approximately 2 weeks. At that time, the dosage can be tapered until the lowest effective dose is achieved. The woman is then maintained on this lowest dose until just prior to the EDB. Since there is a characteristic flare-up of symptoms at this time and early postpartum, a higher dose is administered (Roth, 2011).

Oral antihistamines are also recommended as pruritus can be debilitating and can interrupt sleep (Bremmer et al., 2010). The type of antihistamine is dependent on the stage of pregnancy. Older sedating antihistamines (e.g., chlorphenamine) are recommended in the first trimester with newer nonsedating antihistamines (e.g., loratadine) being recommended for the later trimesters.

Newborn treatment consists only of skin care since the condition is usually mild and self-limiting. Even though adrenal insufficiency can occur in infants whose mothers have been treated with high doses of systemic corticosteroids over an extended period of time, fetal adrenal suppression is thought to be a rare occurrence (Roth, 2011).

Reevaluation within 2 weeks of therapy initiation should be done or sooner if symptoms fail to improve or worsen. Oral contraceptives can result in flare-ups and are not recommended for women with a history of PG (Roth, 2011).

Collaboration, consultation, and referral

Due to the potential for adverse fetal consequences (Bremmer et al., 2010; Roth, 2011), the management of women with PG should be done by or in collaboration with an obstetrical or perinatal specialist. Failure to respond to conventional treatment warrants referral to a dermatologist for possible intravenous IgG (Bremmer et al., 2010; Ruiz-Villaverde et al., 2011).

Impetigo herpetiformis

IH, also known as acute pustular psoriasis of pregnancy, is a rare pustular dermatosis with usual onset in the second half of pregnancy (Rebora, 2011; Roth, 2011). There is debate about IH's status as a pregnancy-induced dermatosis. Rather, it is widely considered as a manifestation of ordinary psoriasis, which happens to be related to pregnancy. Unlike ordinary psoriasis, IH occurs in women with no personal or family history of the disease. The incidence and pathophysiology of this disorder is largely unknown (Bremmer et al., 2010; Roth, 2011).

Assessment

The lesions of IH appear as erythematous plaques with superficial greenish yellow pustules arranged in a herpetiform pattern. As the pustules in the center rupture, they are replaced by crusting. Pruritus is usually not present (Roth, 2011). The lesions commonly first appear on the inner thighs, flexor areas, and groin but then spread to the trunk and extremities. The face, hands, and feet are usually spared (Bremmer et al., 2010; Roth, 2011). Onycholysis of the nails may also occur. Associated signs and symptoms consist of mild pruritus, pain, flu-like symptoms, and lymphadenopathy (Bremmer et al., 2010; Roth, 2011) (Table 39.2). After the lesions disappear, hyperpigmentation of the previously inflamed areas may occur. IH usually resolves following birth but has been reported to continue several weeks postpartum and to recur with subsequent pregnancies.

Diagnosis is based primarily on clinical presentation. Blood cultures of the pustules are negative. Laboratory findings may show leukocytosis, elevated erythrocyte sedimentation (ESR), low-serum calcium, and low levels of vitamin D (Bremmer et al., 2010; Roth, 2011).

Differential diagnosis

IH must be distinguished from pityriasis, drug reactions, eczema, lupus, and lichens simplex chronicus (Bremmer et al., 2010).

Treatment and management

The first line of treatment with IH is systemic corticosteroids. Initial treatment with prednisone at a 15–30 mg/day is recommended. The dosage may be increased to 50–60 mg/day until relief of symptoms is achieved (Bremmer et al., 2010). If limited relief is seen with the higher dosages, cyclosporine 100 mg twice daily is an acceptable alternative (Bremmer et al., 2010; Roth, 2011). Even though cyclosporine is a category C drug, there is little data to support fetal malformations and risk of this drug appears minimal (Bremmer et al., 2010; Roth, 2011).

IH has been associated with fetal growth restriction, hypocalcemia, stillbirth, and neonatal death (Bremmer et al., 2010; Roth, 2011). Since the condition is so rare, lack of data impedes good evidence to support the actual incidence of sequelae (Bremmer et al., 2010).

Collaboration, consultation, and referral

Because of potential complications, management should be done by or occur in close collaboration with an obstetrical or perinatal specialist.

Intrahepatic cholestasis of pregnancy

ICP is also known as cholestasis of pregnancy, recurrent or idiopathic jaundice of pregnancy, obstetric cholestasis, and pruritus gravidarum (Bremmer et al., 2010). ICP is a reversible condition occurring during pregnancy in which the substances normally excreted into bile, such as conjugated bilirubin and bile salts, are retained within the liver. The increased serum bile acids are deposited within the skin, causing intense pruritus.

ICP is a rare disorder affecting approximately 0.5–1% of pregnant women in the United States (Roth, 2011). Onset of this condition is most often in the third trimester (Tunzi & Gray, 2007), with 75–80% of diagnoses made after the thirtieth week of gestation (Bremmer et al., 2010). A family history of ICP is often present and may recur in up to 70% of subsequent pregnancies. ICP has no clear etiology, and it is believed to be a multifactorial disorder with environmental, hormonal, and genetic contributions. Women with twin pregnancies are five times more likely to develop ICP than women with a singleton pregnancy (Roth, 2011), lending support to the increased levels of estrogen and progesterone and their metabolites as contributing factors to the condition.

Maternal outcomes are typically good, with no long-term sequelae; however, fetal outcomes can be devastating. ICP is associated with premature birth, fetal distress, fetal demise and stillbirth, and may be caused by decreased fetal elimination of toxic bile salts (Ambros-Rudolph et al., 2006). Sudden fetal death, sometimes within hours of normal fetal heart rate tracings, is a particular concern with ICP. The risk of intrauterine fetal demise rises as the total bile acid level is elevated and/or jaundice is present, but it rarely occurs prior to 36 weeks' gestation.

Assessment

The classic symptom presentation of ICP is intense, generalized pruritus without skin lesions or rash with sudden onset in the third trimester. The pruritus is first noticed on the palms of the hands and soles of the feet, and tends to be more severe at night, resulting in significant insomnia. The itching spreads to other areas of the body, most commonly to the shins, lower arms, and abdomen. Secondary skin infections can develop as a result of itching. Jaundice may develop in 17–75% of women with ICP and typically develops 1–4 weeks after the onset of pruritus (Roth, 2011).

In the presence of classic symptoms, the diagnosis is supported by physical examination and laboratory findings, and is often a diagnosis of exclusion. If ICP is suspected, a liver panel and a total bile acid level should be obtained. The most specific and sensitive marker of ICP is total serum bile acid levels greater than 10 mcmol/L. There is no uniform agreement on the bile acid level criteria for diagnosing ICP. The average value for bile acids in a woman with ICP is 47 mcmol/L compared to pregnancy normal values of 6.6–11 mcmol/L (Bremmer et al., 2010). A correlation is noted between increases in adverse outcomes in women with bile acid levels of 40 mcmol/L or greater (Glantz, Marschall, & Mattsson, 2004). Most laboratories have a turnover time of 3–4 days for bile acid level results, making immediate management decisions based solely on bile acid levels difficult. Liver function tests often show mild abnormalities, with alanine aminotransferase (ALT) the most likely to show an increase and aid in diagnosis (Bremmer et al., 2010; Roth, 2011). In severe cases of ICP, prolonged cholestasis and jaundice may cause vitamin K deficiency and coagulopathy (Kroumpouzos & Cohen, 2003).

Differential diagnoses

Other dermatological disorders such as PP, PG, PFP, and PUPP need to be excluded (Table 39.2). Skin disorders that are not related to pregnancy must also be considered, including allergic dermatitis and bacterial and viral rashes. Scabies infestation can also occur in pregnancy and mimic scratching-induced excoriations of ICP. Exclusion of these other disorders can be reliably done by determining the absence of primary lesions and elevated serum levels of bile acid (Roth, 2011). Women presenting with jaundice should be evaluated for other conditions such as hepatitis, metabolic and hemolytic diseases, or conditions causing hyperbilirubinemia.

Treatment and management

Once the diagnosis of ICP is made, treatment should be initiated immediately. Serum bile acid levels correlate with the severity of and the duration of pruritus. The goals of treatment of IHCP are to lower the bile acid levels to decrease maternal symptoms and to reduce adverse fetal outcome.

Ursodeoxycholic acid (Ursodiol) has been shown to be effective in accomplishing both treatment goals and is considered a primary component of therapy. Despite its efficacy and safety to treat ICP, ursodeoxycholic acid has not been approved by the Federal Drug Administration to treat this condition, so special approval must be obtained to use it off-label (Roth, 2011). It has a pregnancy category B, and common dosing is 13–15 mg/kg/day (or 1 g/day, independent of weight) as a single dose or divided into two to three doses daily. This dosing is continued until postpartum. Mild cases may respond to supportive treatment such as soothing baths, topical antipruretics, emollients, and evening primrose oil. Antihistamine use at bedtime may help to promote sleep but is rarely effective in reducing pruritis of ICP.

Fetal surveillance is indicated with a diagnosis of ICP. Umbilical artery Doppler studies, nonstress tests, and biophysical profile testing starting at 34–35 weeks' gestation have been suggested to reduce the incidence of fetal demise. The risk of fetal demise is greatest between weeks 37 and 39 (Bremmer et al., 2010; Geenes & Williamson, 2009), and can range from 2% to 11% even with treatment. Additionally, maternal pruritus can be so intense and intolerable that quality of life is severely compromised. For these reasons, many experts advocate labor induction at 37 weeks' gestation (Mays, 2010). Maternal symptoms typically resolve after birth.

Collaboration, consultation, and referral

Collaboration and referral to an obstetrician or perinatal specialist are recommended once ICP is suspected or diagnosed. Once referred, the woman may also benefit from the clinical expertise of a gastroenterologist to assist with her clinical care (Bremmer et al., 2010).

Summary

Pregnancy causes significant changes in the skin that are often a temporary cosmetic nuisance. Common skin conditions during pregnancy generally can be separated into three categories: hormone related, preexisting, and pregnancy specific. Most of the skin changes seen in pregnancy are due to the effects of hormones and resolve postpartum and only require symptomatic treatment. Rapid evaluation and diagnosis can be challenging due to many overlapping features of the various skin conditions; however, it can be especially important for women demonstrating symptoms of PG, IH, and ICP as those conditions can affect maternal and fetal health. Antepartum surveillance and collaboration as indicated by each situation can also be important care components for these skin disorders.

Resources for health-care providers

DermAtlas.org: a searchable database of over 12,000 dermatology images.

Dermatology Online Journal: an open-access, refereed publication intended to meet reference and education needs of the international dermatology community.

Case study

A 32-year-old woman presents to her primary health-care provider, a family nurse practitioner, with a recent onset of abdominal itching and rash. She is 35 weeks pregnant with her first child and is due to visit her midwife next week for ongoing prenatal care. Thus far, her pregnancy has been uneventful. Her weight gain has been within the recommended guidelines, and her vital signs have been normal at all of her visits. She reports today that her only concern is this itchy rash. Her past medical history is significant for childhood asthma and rare episodes of eczema that recur on the flexor surfaces of her elbows, primarily in the winter.

On physical examination:

Vital signs—weight: 140 lb; height: 5 ft 5 in.; BP 120/66; P 82; R 14
General—pleasant, comfortable, no distress
HEENT—normocephalic, eyes anicteric with +light reflex bilaterally; ear canals clear with pearly gray tympanic membranes, nares patent, posterior pharynx pink with +clear postnasal drainage, no adenopathy or thyromegaly
Lungs clear to auscultation bilaterally
CV—RRR w/o murmur or extra sounds
Abdomen—pregnant abdomen, +scattered papular lesions grouped along the abdominal striae, with fewer lesions scattered between the striae; a few excoriations noted due to scratching
Skin—few papular lesions noted on upper, inner thighs bilaterally

Differential diagnoses for this presentation include

1. PP
2. PFP
3. PG
4. AD exacerbation
5. PUPP.

Discussion

Of those differentials listed earlier, the timing of onset does not fit with PP, as PP typically appears between 25 and 30 weeks' gestation. PFP can be ruled out because of the absence of the follicular lesions in PFP that first appear on the chest and abdomen. PG is not a likely diagnosis because in this condition, the erythematous papules are located in the periumbilical area, which is not evident in this woman. This rash is either an exacerbation of known AD, or the PUPP. Because of the timing of symptom onset, a sensible working diagnosis would be PUPP. However, treatment of both AD and PUPP is similar, and neither condition warrants concern about fetal outcome.

Treatment

A low-to-moderate-strength topical cortisone cream or ointment (hydrocortisone, triamcinolone, betamethasone) and a pregnancy category B antihistamine (diphenhydramine, loratadine, cetirizine) are indicated to control the symptoms. The patient was advised that this is a benign problem that does not harm the fetus and that her symptoms can be managed with medication that is safe to take during pregnancy. She was prescribed hydrocortisone valerate 0.2% for BID application and Dermaveen shower wash: a soap free cleanser with colloidal oatmeal. Comfort measures to relieve itching included the use of cool, soothing baths; urea-containing emollients; wet soaks; and light cotton clothing. She was advised to take over-the-counter (OTC) Benadryl if she experienced insomnia due to itching. A medical note describing the details of the visit was transcribed and sent to the patient's midwife.

Dermnet.com: a searchable reference for skin diseases.
Dermnetnz.org: the Web site for the New Zealand Dermatological Society, containing facts and images for numerous skin disorders.

References

Ambros-Rudolph, C. M., Müllegger, R. R., Vaughan-Jones, S. A., Kerl, H., & Black, M. M. (2006). The specific dermatoses of pregnancy revisited and reclassified: Results of a retrospective two-center study on 505 pregnant patients. *Journal of the American Academy of Dermatology, 54*(3), 395–404.

Bremmer, M., Driscoll, M., & Colgan, R. (2010). The skin disorders of pregnancy: A family physician's guide. *The Journal of Family Practice, 59*(2), 89–96.

Geenes, V., & Williamson, C. (2009). Intrahepatic cholestasis of pregnancy. *World Journal of Gastroenterology, 15*, 2049–2066.

Glantz, A., Marschall, H., & Mattsson, L. A. (2004). Intrahepatic cholestasis of pregnancy: Relationships between bile acid levels and fetal complication rates. *Hepatology (Baltimore, Md.), 40*, 467–474.

Ingber, A. (2010). Atopic eruption of pregnancy. *Journal of the European Academy of Dermatology and Venereology, 24*, 974.

Jang, M. S., Baek, J. W., Kang, D. Y., Kang, J. S., Kim, N. T., & Suh, K. S. (2011). Successful treatment with narrowband UVB phototherapy in prurigo pigmentosa associated with pregnancy. *European Journal of Dermatology, 21*(4), 634–635.

Katz, V. L., Thorp, J. M., Jr., & Bowes, W. A., Jr. (1990). Severe symmetric intrauterine growth retardation associated with the topical use of triamcinolone. *American Journal of Obstetrics and Gynecology, 162*(2), 396–397.

Kemmett, D., & Tidman, M. J. (1991). The influence of menstrual cycle and pregnancy on atopic dermatitis. *British Journal of Dermatology, 125*, 59–61.

Koutroulis, I., Papoutsis, J., & Kroumpouzos, G. (2011). Atopic dermatitis in pregnancy: Current status and challenges. *Obstetrical and Gynecological Survey, 66*(10), 654–663.

Kroumpouzos, G., & Cohen, L. M. (2003). Specific dermatoses of pregnancy: An evidence-based systematic review. *American Journal of Obstetrics and Gynecology, 188*(4), 1083–1092.

Lipozencic, J., Ljugojevic, S., & Bukvic-Mokos, Z. (2012). Pemphigoid gestationis. *Clinics in Dermatology, 30*, 51–55. doi:10.1016/j.clindermatol.2011.03.009

Mays, J. K. (2010). The active management of intrahepatic cholestasis of pregnancy. *Current Opinion in Obstetrics and Gynecology, 22*(2), 100–103.

Paunescu, M. M., Feier, V., & Paunescu, M. (2008). Dermatoses of pregnancy. *Acta Dermatovenerologica Alpina, Panonica, et Adriatica, 17*(1), 4–11.

Rebora, A. (2011). Shape and configuration of skin lesions: Grouped herpetiform. *Clinics in Dermatology, 29*, 509–510. doi:10.1016/j.clincermatol.2010.09.018

Roth, M. (2011). Pregnancy dermatosis: Diagnosis, management, and controversies. *American Journal of Clinical Dermatology, 12*(1), 25–41.

Rudolph, C., Al-Fares, S., & Vaughan-Jones, S. (2006). Polymorphic eruption of pregnancy: Clinicopathology and potential trigger factors in 181 patients. *British Journal of Dermatology, 154*, 54–60.

Ruiz-Villaverde, R., Sánchez-Cano, D., & Ramirez-Tortosa, C. L. (2011). Pemphigoid gestationis: Therapeutic response to pre- and postpartum immunoglobulin therapy. *Actas Dermo-Sifiliograficas, 102*, 735–747.

Thurston, A., & Grau, R. (2008). An update on the dermatoses of pregnancy. *Journal of the Oklahoma State Medical Association, 101*(1), 7–11.

Tunzi, M., & Gray, G. (2007). Common skin conditions during pregnancy. *American Family Physician, 75*(2), 211–218.

40

Infectious diseases

Jacquelyne Brooks and Elizabeth A. Parr

Relevant terms

Arthropathy—joint pain or joint disease

Avidity testing—measures antibody maturity to detect recent primary infection

Congenital—present at birth; may or may not be hereditary

Congenital anomaly—structural or functional health problem present at birth that varies from the standard presentation (also known as congenital abnormality, congenital malformation, or birth defect)

Enzyme-linked immunosorbent assay (ELISA)—common serological test for the presence of particular antigens (direct) or antibodies (indirect)

Herd immunity—immunity for the whole population when a certain threshold number of the population is protected via vaccination from an infectious disease

Hyperechogenic—increased amplitude of sound waves

Immunoglobulins—proteins produced by the immune system in response to antigens like bacteria and viruses (also known as antibodies)

IgM antibodies are expressed on the surface of B cells and excreted to eliminate pathogens in the early stages of humoral immunity before there is sufficient IgG

IgG antibodies provide the majority of antibody-based immunity against pathogens in a long-term response and is the only antibody capable of crossing the placenta to give passive immunity to the fetus

Polymerase chain reaction (PCR)—diagnostic tool that facilitates the detection of DNA or RNA of pathological organisms

Protozoan—single-celled, microscopic organisms that can perform all necessary functions of metabolism and reproduction

Reference laboratory—laboratory facilities that provide standard and well-defined measures for testing and for interpretation of testing

Reservoir—a reservoir of infection is the environment in which an infectious agent lives and multiplies and from which it can spread to cause disease

Seroconversion—the new development of detectable specific antibodies to microorganisms in the blood serum as a result of infection or immunization from a previously negative state

Seroprevalence—the proportion of the population that has developed antibodies in response to exposure to an infectious agent

Teratogen—any agent or factor that induces or increases the incidence of abnormal prenatal development

Vertical transmission—transmission of a disease, condition, or trait either genetically or congenitally; vertical transmission of an infection, also known as perinatal transmission, occurs *in utero*, during the birth process, or with breastfeeding

---

Introduction

Infections in pregnancy can have more serious sequelae than in the nonpregnant state because of the potential for congenital or perinatal infection in the fetus or newborn. Congenital and perinatal infections can result in devastating consequences, including fetal anomalies and fetal or neonatal death. Long-term disabilities that result from congenital anomalies have a significant impact on individuals, families, health-care systems, and

Prenatal and Postnatal Care: A Woman-Centered Approach, First Edition. Edited by Robin G. Jordan, Janet L. Engstrom, Julie A. Marfell, and Cindy L. Farley.
© 2014 John Wiley & Sons, Inc. Published 2014 by John Wiley & Sons, Inc.

societies. The woman who acquires an infection during pregnancy can be asymptomatic; therefore, the knowledge of risk factors and appropriate screening is imperative for prenatal care providers. The timing of infection and whether it is a primary or secondary infection must be considered to determine the potential risk to the fetus. This chapter discusses the perinatal infections caused by cytomegalovirus (CMV), group B *Streptococcus* (GBS), hepatitis, parvovirus B19, rubella, toxoplasmosis, and varicella.

Cytomegalovirus

CMV, a ubiquitous member of the herpesvirus family, is the most common cause of congenital infections in developed countries (McCarthy, Giles, Rowlands, Purcell, & Jones, 2011; Pass, 2002). Humans are the only known hosts of CMV, which is transmitted via bodily fluids such as semen, cervicovaginal secretions, saliva, urine, and breast milk. Sexual transmission of the virus is common. Infected children shed CMV in their urine for months following infection, which is why transmission is common in daycare settings and between young children and parents or siblings (Cannon, 2009; Cannon et al., 2012). Secondary infections are caused by reactivation of dormant infections or infection by different strains of CMV (Society of Obstetricians and Gynaecologists of Canada (SOGC), 2010).

An estimated 50–80% of women in the United States are infected with CMV by the time they are 40 (Centers for Disease Control and Prevention (CDC), 2010a; Reddy, Fry, Pass, & Ghidini, 2004). Women with low-to-middle incomes and black and Hispanic women are more likely to have both higher seroprevalence of CMV and birth prevalence of congenital CMV (Adler, 2011; Cannon, 2009). Approximately 1–4% of uninfected women will have a primary CMV infection during their pregnancies (CDC, 2010a). The probability of intrauterine transmission is 20–50% when there is a primary infection during the pregnancy and 10–15% when there is a secondary infection. Most congenital CMV infections and related disabilities result from primary infections during pregnancy (Cannon, 2009; Duff, 2010).

Each year in the United States, approximately 30,000 children are born with congenital CMV and 5000 children experience some type of disability (CDC, 2010a). The most severe fetal injuries occur as a result of intrauterine transmission in the first 8 weeks of pregnancy. The risk of congenital infection is much lower during the first trimester, however, because viral excretion increases as the pregnancy progresses (Lazzarotto, Guerra, Gabrielli, Lanari, & Landini, 2011).

Potential problems

Infection with CMV is not a health concern for the general population as it usually does not result in clinical illness. Although congenital CMV rarely results in health problems, more children suffer serious disabilities caused by congenital CMV than by other, better-known maladies such as Down syndrome or fetal alcohol syndrome (Cannon, 2009). Sensorineural hearing loss is the most common CMV-related disability, but infected children can also have vision loss or neurodevelopmental disabilities (Cannon, 2009; Colugnati, Staras, Dollard, & Cannon, 2007). Five to fifteen percent of infants with congenital CMV are symptomatic at birth and may exhibit intrauterine growth restriction (IUGR), hepatosplenomegaly, jaundice, thrombocytopenia with resultant petichiae, microcephaly, chorioretinitis, sensorineural hearing loss, and/or cerebral calcifications. Eighty-five to ninety-five percent of infants with congenital CMV have no signs or symptoms at birth, but 10–15% will develop associated disabilities that become apparent when the child is of school age (Duff, 2010).

Clinical presentation and assessment

The woman with primary or secondary CMV infection will most likely be asymptomatic. Occasionally, the client will exhibit signs and symptoms that mimic mononucleosis or the flu, including malaise, persistent fever, myalgia, and cervical lymphadenopathy. A diagnosis of maternal CMV infection should be considered in the presence of these findings.

Congenital CMV should also be considered when there are abnormal ultrasound results that include IUGR, placental enlargement, oligohydramnios or polyhydramnios, echodensities of the bowel or liver, hydrocephalus, microcephaly, ascites or hydrops, or calcified lesions in the brain (Adler, 2011; Duff, 2010; SOGC, 2010).

A focused health history includes household and employment, particularly when it involves care of young children or infants, recent CMV infection in the home, workplace, or day care in which the client has children; and sexual risk factors, including age at first intercourse, number of partners, condom usage, and history of sexually transmitted infections, and patient report of symptoms. A targeted physical examination consists of vital signs, including temperature, evaluation for hepatosplenomegaly, lymphadenopathy, arthralgia, and routine prenatal surveillance, including fundal height.

Laboratory testing is recommended only if the woman presents with a mononucleosis-type illness, when a fetal anomaly is detected, or upon maternal request (CDC, 2008). Depending on presentation, the practitioner should consider testing for both the Epstein–Barr virus and influenza. Active infection with CMV can be diagnosed by polymerase chain reaction (PCR) or viral culture taken from urine, saliva, oropharynx, or other body tissues, but these tests are expensive and are not widely available (CDC, 2010a). Seroconversion of IgG antibodies is diagnostic of primary maternal infection, but, in the absence of universal screening, initial seronegative data are rarely available (Adler, 2011).

Serological assays for IgM and IgG antibodies are obtained when primary maternal infection is suspected. Because IgG avidity has been shown to reliably detect recent primary CMV infection, this test should also be performed, if available (Adler, 2011; CDC, 2008). Serological assays can be confusing because the IgM antibody can remain positive for 9–12 months following acute infection and can be detected in 10% of recurrent infections. The presence of the IgM antibody is not diagnostic of primary CMV infection but is useful in determining the timing of infection (Adler, 2011; Duff, 2010).

Tests for the diagnosis of maternal CMV

Type of infection	Serum PCR	Urine PCR	IgG
Acute	Positive	Positive	Absent on low-avidity antibody
Recurrent or reactivated	Usually negative	May be positive	Positive for high-avidity antibody

Adapted from: Duff (2010).

When maternal testing detects primary maternal CMV infection or when a fetal anomaly is detected, congenital infection is identified by both viral culture and PCR to detect CMV in the amniotic fluid (Adler, 2011). Amniocentesis should be performed at least 7 weeks after presumed timing of maternal infection and after 21 weeks of gestation because a detectable quantity of the virus is not present in amniotic fluid until 5–7 weeks following transmission (Duff, 2010; SOGC, 2010). It should be noted that detection of fetal CMV infection does not predict newborn disease (Adler, 2011).

Management

Treatments for CMV are either not approved for pregnant women or have not been shown to prevent or treat congenital CMV infections. However, there are promising studies that show the efficacy of both CMV hyperimmune globulin and antiviral agents (Adler, 2011; Adler, Nigro, & Pereira, 2007; Duff, 2010). Depending on the

gestational age, pregnancy termination may be an option in the presence of congenital CMV or fetal anomalies.

Consultation or collaboration should be considered in the presence of primary maternal infection or fetal anomalies for amniocentesis, serial ultrasounds, or available treatments. Counseling and support should be provided, when appropriate, and based on the following:

- For women who have young children in their homes or care, hygienic measures have been shown to reduce CMV transmission.
- Congenital CMV usually does not result in health problems, but potential problems and resources for the woman and child can be discussed.
- With a secondary infection, congenital infection rate is very low.
- There are no recommendations against vaginal birth or breastfeeding when maternal CMV is detected.

Prevention

Most women have not heard of CMV and are unaware of how it is transmitted, the appropriate preventative measures, or the risks of congenital infection (Jeon et al., 2006; Ross, Victor, Sumartojo, & Cannon, 2008). Currently, two CMV vaccines are under investigation (Adler et al., 2007; Duff, 2010; Steininger, 2012). Because there is evidence that education may prevent maternal CMV infection, both the American College of Obstetricians and Gynecologists (ACOG) and the Centers for Disease Control and Prevention (CDC) recommend educating women about reducing their risk of infection. The health-care provider should take advantage of annual exams, preconceptual counseling, or new OB visits to educate women about measures to prevent infection (Adler, 2011; Cannon, 2009). Prevention is aimed at common sources of infection, including urine or saliva of young children and sexual activity.

Prevention of CMV infection

- Wear gloves and wash hands after changing diapers.
- Wash hands after feeding a young child, wiping a young child's nose or drool, or handling a child's toys.
- Avoid sharing cups or utensils with a young child, contact with tears or saliva when kissing a child, putting a pacifier in her own mouth, or sharing a toothbrush with a young child.
- Clean toys, countertops, and other surfaces that come in contact with a child's urine or saliva.
- Practice safe sex, including limiting the number of partners and correct use of condoms.

Group B *Streptococcus*

GBS, or *Streptococcus agalactiae*, remains the leading cause of neonatal and meningitis in the first week of life (CDC, 2010c). *S. agalactiae* is a gram-positive, beta hemolytic bacterium that causes invasive disease primarily in infants, and in pregnant or postpartum women (CDC, 2009a). In 1996, the CDC announced prevention strategies for GBS disease of the newborn. The guidelines were updated in 2002 and again in 2010, and are used to prevent early-onset disease. The use of increased prevention strategies in the 1990s and universal prenatal screening in 2002 led to a decrease in the incidence of newborn disease from 1.7 cases per 1000 live births in the 1990s to 0.34–0.37 cases per 1000 live births in recent years. Racial disparities persist with the incidence among blacks approximately twice that of non-blacks (CDC, 2010c).

Group B *Streptococci* colonize the vaginal and gastrointestinal tracts in 15–45% of healthy women (Nandyal, 2008). Colonization can be transient, intermittent, or persistent (Hansen, Uldbjerg, Kilian, & Sorensen, 2004). Neonates can acquire the organism by vertical transmission *in utero* or during the birth process. Although the transmission rate is 50% when the colonized woman delivers vaginally, only 1–2% of the infected neonates develop GBS disease (Nandyal, 2008). Risk factors for early-onset GBS disease are maternal intrapartum GBS colonization, gestational age <37 completed weeks, prolonged duration of membrane rupture, intra-amniotic infection, young maternal age, and black race. Available data do not confirm association between obstetric procedures and GBS disease (CDC, 2010c).

Potential problems

Maternal GBS colonization is not a clinical illness. Maternal infection with GBS is rare but can result in sepsis, amnionitis, and urinary tract infection (CDC, 2012b).

Early GBS disease in infants often presents within 24 hours of the birth but may not be apparent for up to 7 days postpartum. Late GBS disease becomes apparent between 1 week and 3 months postpartum and can be the result of perinatal transmission or infection from another source (CDC, 2012b). Early-onset GBS disease of the newborn typically presents as sepsis or pneumonia. Meningitis can occur with early-onset disease but is more common in late-onset GBS, which is also characterized by sepsis.

Regardless of timing, GBS disease can result in deafness and developmental disabilities (CDC, 2012b). The mortality rate from GBS disease of the newborn is approximately 20% (Sendi, Johansson, & Norrby-Teglund, 2008). Because of the continued burden of disease, the health-care practitioner must be knowledge-

able about current recommendations for GBS screening, prevention, and treatment.

Assessment

Maternal GBS colonization is usually asymptomatic but adherence to CDC (2010c) guidelines for screening is essential to prevent GBS infection in the newborn. Focused health history includes assessment of a prior history of early-onset GBS disease in another infant, history of GBS bacteriuria during any trimester of the current pregnancy, current GBS culture results, and amniotic fluid status, including client-reported leaking of amniotic fluid.

Laboratory testing consists of universal screening for maternal GBS colonization at 35–37 weeks' gestation with the use of a single swab (Martinez de Tejada et al., 2010). To collect the GBS specimen, the practitioner should swab the lower vagina (vaginal introitus), then the rectum, inserting the swab through the anal sphincter. The woman can obtain the culture herself, following appropriate instruction. Cervical, perianal, perirectal, or perineal specimens are not acceptable and a speculum should not be used for culture collection (CDC, 2010c).

Management

Universal screening and the prophylactic use of antibiotics have been effective at reducing the incidence of perinatal GBS disease. When a woman colonized with GBS receives antibiotics in labor, there is a 1 in 4000 risk of perinatal transmission; if she does not receive antibiotics, the risk increases to 1 in 200 (CDC, 2010c).

Prophylactic antibiotics are administered when the woman is in labor when there is a positive GBS culture in the current pregnancy (except in the case of a cesarean birth with intact membranes), history of GBS bacteriuria in the current pregnancy, or history of previous infant with GBS invasive disease. The current CDC (2010c) recommendations for intrapartum prophylaxis are to administer penicillin, with ampicillin being an acceptable alternative. When GBS colonization is identified in a woman with a high-risk penicillin allergy, antimicrobial susceptibility should be performed since resistance to clindamycin, the most common agent used in this population, is increasing (CDC, 2010c; Schrag et al., 2000).

Consultation or collaboration is typically not warranted when GBS colonization is identified but should be initiated according to the practitioner's scope of practice when a woman presents with preterm labor or premature rupture of membranes. Women who are GBS-positive during pregnancy should receive counseling and information based on the following (CDC, 2010c):

- GBS is part of the normal vaginal flora.
- GBS is not sexually transmitted.
- Most cases of maternal GBS colonization do not result in infant disease.
- Treatment before labor and treatment with oral antibiotics are not effective at eradicating GBS colonization.
- GBS colonization in a previous pregnancy is not diagnostic of colonization in the current pregnancy and screening is advised, in the absence of risk factors identified in the current pregnancy.
- GBS bacteriuria in a previous pregnancy is not an indication for treatment in the current pregnancy.
- When intrapartum antimicrobial therapy is indicated, intravenous access will be required.
- In the absence of known GBS status and the presence of intrapartum risk factors, for example, prolonged rupture of membranes or maternal fever, antibiotic prophylaxis should be administered.
- Intrapartum GBS prophylaxis is not indicated when a cesarean birth is performed before the onset of labor and in the presence of intact amniotic membranes, regardless of GBS colonization status.
- Strategies to decrease the incidence of early-onset disease are not effective at decreasing late-onset disease.

Hepatitis infections

Hepatitis A

Hepatitis A virus (HAV) is a small RNA virus transmitted by the fecal–oral route, either by person-to-person contact or by consumption of contaminated food or water. It is typically self-limited and does not result in chronic infection. The incubation period for hepatitis A is approximately 28 days after exposure, with a range of 15–50 days (CDC, 2010d). The virus replicates in the liver and is shed in feces from 2 weeks before to 1 week after the onset of clinical symptoms. While 80% of adults infected with HAV are symptomatic, the symptoms are usually mild and nonspecific, and rarely include jaundice.

HAV was responsible for about one-third of acute hepatitis cases in the United States until vaccination programs were introduced in the 1990s; the incidence has steadily declined since then. The incidence of acute HAV infection in pregnancy is approximately 1 : 1000 (Contag, 2012).

Risk factors for HAV include exposure to contaminated food or water, substandard hygiene or sanitation, illegal drug use, and having children in day care. Those who have emigrated from or have recently traveled to high-risk countries are also at an increased risk for HAV.

An updated list of areas of concern for HAV infection is maintained by the CDC at http://www.cdc.gov/travel/contentdiseases.aspx.

Potential problems

Hepatitis A does not cause chronic liver disease, and acute liver failure is extremely rare. However, 10–15% of patients can experience a relapse of symptoms during the 6-month period after they have been acutely infected (American College of Obstetricians and Gynecologists (ACOG), 2007; CDC, 2010d).

There is a minimal risk associated with HAV in pregnancy. Transmission to the fetus is negligible because maternal anti-HAV IgG antibodies cross the placenta and protect the infant after the birth (Contag, 2012).

Assessment

HAV is diagnosed by serological testing. IgM anti-HAV antibodies appear early in the disease process and persist for several months. IgG antibodies, which predominate during the convalescent period, persist and provide immunity for life against reinfection. IgG antibodies will also be present after vaccination.

Management

Hepatitis A vaccines have been available since 1995 and are the most effective means of preventing transmission. The ACOG (2007) recommends vaccination for high-risk adults. Both the HAV vaccine, made of inactivated HAV, and the HAV immune globulin are safe in pregnancy. Vaccines are available as a single antigen (HAV) or as a combination with hepatitis B antigen.

Pregnant women who have close personal (household or sexual) contact with infected individuals should receive postexposure prophylaxis by a single intramuscular dose of HAV immune globulin (0.02 mL/kg) and the HAV vaccine. When the immune globulin is given within 2 weeks of exposure, it confers protection for up to 3 months with 80–90% efficacy. The vaccine may be as effective when given alone as when combined with immune globulin, and some experts recommend the vaccine alone for postexposure prophylaxis in women under age 40 (ACOG, 2007).

Management of pregnant women with hepatitis A infection is primarily supportive. Physical activity should be limited in order to avoid trauma to the liver, and a healthy diet should be encouraged. Particular care should be taken to avoid alcohol and medications that are potentially hepatotoxic.

There is no known transmission from the mother to the fetus. Even so, an infant born to an infected mother should be given HAV immune globulin within 48 hours of the birth to prevent infection. Infected mothers can safely breastfeed their infants with appropriate hygienic precautions.

Prevention

Vaccines are the most effective means of prevention of HAV infection. Additional preventive measures include good hygiene, ensuring clean water, and counseling travelers to high-risk countries regarding sanitary precautions. Heating food to about 185°F for 1 minute and disinfecting surfaces with dilute bleach can decrease the risk of food contamination (ACOG, 2007).

Hepatitis B

Hepatitis B virus (HBV) is a highly contagious infection caused by a small DNA virus transmitted by blood and sexual contact. Its incubation period is 6 weeks to 6 months from the time of initial exposure. HBV is transient in 90% of HBV infected adults, and they experience complete resolution of the disease with protective antibody levels. Approximately 5–10% of infected adults will develop chronic infection (Contag, 2012). Most individuals with chronic hepatitis are asymptomatic, although some will complain of fatigue, anorexia, and malaise. Of those individuals with chronic HBV, 15–25% will die prematurely from cirrhosis or hepatocellular carcinoma (CDC, 2010e). The risk of developing chronic infection is inversely related to age; 90% of infants who acquire HBV perinatally will develop chronic disease if they do not receive prophylaxis.

The incidence of HBV in the United States has declined significantly since 1991, when prevention programs for maternal screening and universal vaccination at birth were implemented (CDC, 2005b, 2009b). It is estimated that approximately 5% of individuals in the United States have ever been infected with HBV and 1–2% of the population has chronic HBV infection (CDC, 2010d).

The highest concentration of HBV is found in blood, but it is also found in semen, vaginal secretions, saliva, and wound exudate. The primary risk factors for HBV are injectable drug use and sexual contact with at-risk and/or multiple partners. Sexual transmission of the virus is quite efficient, and 25% of individuals with infected sexual partners will become infected themselves. In the United States, Asian women have the highest rate of infection (Degli-Esposti, 2010). Others at risk include health-care workers, hemodialysis patients, and travelers to high-risk areas.

Potential problems

Chronic hepatitis infection carries a much higher mortality rate (15–25%) than acute hepatitis (1%) (ACOG, 2007). Most chronic carriers of HBV are asymptomatic and can transmit the virus unknowingly for many years. Chronic disease can persist for decades, slowly progressing to cirrhosis or hepatocellular carcinoma. More than 80% of hepatocellular carcinomas are associated with HBV.

Acute HBV is the most common cause of jaundice in pregnancy. It is usually mild and well tolerated, with only 1% of acutely infected pregnant women developing severe liver disease (Reddick, Jhaveri, Gandhi, James, & Swamy, 2011). There does not appear to be any increased risk of mortality or teratogenicity with acute HBV in pregnancy, although there are some reports of an increased incidence of low birth weight and prematurity (Lee & Lok, 2013).

Most pregnant women with chronic HBV tolerate pregnancy well, but hepatitis flares may occur. Chronic HBV in pregnancy may be associated with an increased risk of gestational diabetes, preterm birth, and antepartum hemorrhage, but the data are not clear, and the risk of obstetric complications is low (Lee & Lok, 2013).

HBV cannot cross the placenta; transmission *in utero* is infrequent and occurs only with a break in the maternal–fetal barrier. Most perinatal transmission occurs at the time of birth, with exposure of the infant's mucosal membranes to maternal blood or secretions. Infants who are uninfected at birth and do not receive prophylaxis are at risk for infection during the postpartum period through close contact with an infected mother (Degli-Esposti, 2010).

The risk of perinatal transmission is higher in women who are HBeAg positive (90% risk, compared to 10–20% in HBeAg negative women), have a high viral load, have a history of threatened preterm labor, and who acquired the infection in pregnancy. The risk of transmission is highest when HBV is acquired in the third trimester (80–90%); in the first trimester, only up to 10% of neonates are infected (ACOG, 2007).

Those infants who acquire HBV perinatally from HBeAg-positive mothers have a 90% chance of chronic disease if they do not receive immunoprophylaxis, and 15–20% of them will go on to die in adulthood of cirrhosis or hepatocellular carcinoma. Those whose mothers were HBeAg negative are less likely to be infected and have a lower risk (40–70%) of chronic disease.

Assessment

HBV is evaluated by testing for the presence of specific antigens and antibodies, as follows:

- *Hepatitis B surface antigen (HBsAg)*—HBsAg is present in both acute and chronic infections and indicates that the individual is infectious. It is the only serological marker that can be detected during the first 3–5 weeks in newly infected persons, before the onset of symptoms. HBsAg clears after acute infection in 3–4 months but persists in chronic carriers.

- *Antihepatitis B surface antibody (anti-HBs)*—Anti-HBs appears during convalescence from acute infection after HBsAg has cleared and continues to increase for up to 10–12 months. It can remain positive for the lifetime of those who have recovered from acute infection; it indicates immunity. It is also present in the serum of those who have been successfully vaccinated. In chronic carriers, anti-HBs is negative, but HBsAg is positive.
- *Antihepatitis B core antibody (anti-HBc)*—Anti-HBc is only present in a previous or ongoing natural infection; it is not present after vaccination. IgM anti-HBc appears with the onset of symptoms during an acute infection and persists for up to 6 months if the disease resolves. IgG anti-HBc appears during convalescence and usually persists for life.
- *HBe antigen (HBeAg)*—HBeAg is present in acute or chronic infection and indicates active viral replication and high infectivity.
- *Antihepatitis Be antibody (Anti HBe)*—This antibody appears during recovery of the acute phase and indicates decreased infectivity.

Management

All pregnant women should be tested for HBV at the first prenatal visit, even if they were previously vaccinated or tested. High-risk women (those with a sexually transmitted infection, who have had more than one sex partner in the last 6 months, have a history of injection drug use, or a have an HBV-positive sex partner) should be screened on admission for delivery, as should those whose HBV status is unknown.

Pregnant women who are HBsAg negative but are at risk for HBV should be vaccinated with three doses of the HBV vaccine at 0-, 1-, and 6-month intervals. If a pregnant woman is exposed to HBV, she should have immediate screening for HBsAg and anti-HBs; if she is not immune, she should receive both Hepatitis B immune globulin (HBIG) and HBV vaccine (CDC, 2005b; Wood & Isaacs, 2012).

Pregnant women with a positive HBsAg screen should be reported to state and local hepatitis prevention programs, and referred to a specialist in liver disease. Management of women who have acute HBV infection in pregnancy is primarily supportive. They should be counseled to maintain good nutrition and to limit their activity to prevent upper abdominal trauma (ACOG, 2007). Periodic monitoring of liver biochemical tests is recommended (Lee & Lok, 2013). Hospitalization may be required for those who become seriously ill.

Pregnant women with chronic HBV may experience hepatitis flares, even if they were previously asymptomatic, and should be monitored for viral load and liver biochemical tests periodically (Lee & Lok, 2013). They

should be hospitalized if they show any signs of liver decompensation.

Antiviral medications are not teratogenic, but there is limited data on their safety in pregnancy. They are rarely recommended in acute HBV infection unless the woman is severely affected; they are typically reserved for those with chronic HBV, or with high viral load (greater than 6–10,000 copies/mL, depending on the protocol). Initiating antiviral medications such as telbivudine and tenofovir (both pregnancy category B) 6–8 weeks prior to birth allows time for the viral load to decline and reduces the risk of perinatal transmission (Lee & Lok, 2013).

Immediate immunoprophylaxis of infants of infected mothers reduces the risk of vertical transmission by 85–95%. These infants should receive HBIG and the first dose of the hepatitis B vaccine intramuscularly in two different sites within the first 12 hours of birth. The remaining two injections in the series should be administered within the first 6 months of life. If the maternal status is unknown, the woman should undergo screening, and the infant should receive vaccine within 12 hours of birth.

The risk of perinatal transmission of HBV with amniocentesis appears low, but should be avoided if at all possible (Lee & Lok, 2013). There is no advantage to birth by cesarean section in women with hepatitis B. Breastfeeding in HBV-positive mothers is safe as long as they are not taking antiviral medication, and the infant has received prophylaxis with HBIG and vaccine. Women with bleeding nipples should abstain from breastfeeding until they are healed.

Prevention

All health-care providers caring for pregnant women should follow the national guidelines for screening and immunization. The incidence of HBV infection has improved dramatically with the implementation of national prevention strategies (see CDC, 2010e). Routine screening of all pregnant woman is recommended because screening based on risk factors will detect only 60% at most of HBV carriers. When the recommended immunoprophylaxis is followed, the risk of perinatal transmission decreases from 90% to as low as 5–10%.

Both HBIG and the hepatitis B vaccine are safe in pregnancy. There are two single antigen vaccines available that contain HBsAg, and a combination vaccine for both hepatatis A and B. Over 95% of those vaccinated become immune (ACOG, 2007). HBIG contains anti-HBS and is recommended for those who experience a specific exposure to HBV, and those who have not responded to the HBV vaccine. When given within 24 hours of exposure, it provides protection for 3–6 months. Measures to prevent transmission of HBV to others should be discussed with women who are infected.

Transmission preventive measures for HBV-positive women

- Avoid alcohol and potentially hepatotoxic medications.
- Avoid sharing household articles that could be contaminated with blood.
- Use condoms with sex partners.
- Identify household, sexual, and needle-sharing contacts so they can be tested and vaccinated.
- Inform all health-care providers of their HBV status.

Hepatitis C

Hepatitis C virus (HCV), a single-stranded RNA virus, is the most common blood-borne infection in the United States and the leading cause of chronic liver disease (CDC, 2009b). The incidence of HCV has decreased significantly due to screening of blood donors, which has been mandated since 1992. Over 3 million people have chronic HCV infection in the United States, (CDC, 2011) and it is found in approximately 1% of pregnant women (Contag, 2012). The majority of those infected with HCV are asymptomatic. Clinical symptoms occur in approximately 25% of exposed individuals. The onset is 2–24 weeks after exposure and may include fatigue, joint pain, jaundice, myalgia, and generalized pruritis. The illness is generally mild and may often be ignored or mistaken for transient viral illness. Chronic HCV infection develops in the majority of individuals who are positive for HCV. Most individuals with chronic HCV have no symptoms and are unaware they are infected, and thus may unknowingly transmit HCV to others. At least 20% of chronic HCV carriers progress to cirrhosis within 10–20 years, and of those, 20% will develop hepatocellular cancer, decades after the initial infection (Contag, 2012).

Transmission of HCV is primarily parenteral, with risk factors being either intravenous drug use or having received a blood transfusion before 1992. Although it is not effectively transmitted sexually, 15–20% of those infected report sexual contact as their only exposure to HCV (CDC, 2011, 2012a). The risk of sexual transmission is higher in those who are HIV positive and have multiple sexual partners.

Risk factors for HCV infection

- History of intravenous drug use
- History of blood transfusion received before 1992
- History of body tattoos or body piercings
- Health-care workers, especially those experiencing needlestick injury
- Multiple sexual partners
- History of prior sexually transmitted disease
- HIV infection

Potential problems

Pregnant women with HCV are at higher risk for cholestasis, premature rupture of membranes, preterm birth, congenital malformations, placental abruption, gestational diabetes, and overall perinatal mortality (Le Campion, Larouche, Fauteux-Daniel, & Soudeyn, 2012; Reddick et al., 2011). Their infants are more likely to be of low birth weight or to be admitted to a neonatal intensive care nursery (Arshad, El-Kamary, & Jhaveri, 2011).

The risk of perinatal transmission varies; the best predictor is a maternal HCV viral load. HCV positive women who do not have detectable HCV RNA in their blood are unlikely to transmit HCV to their infants, but those who do carry a 4–7% risk of transmission. The risk of transmission is increased in women with higher viral titers (>100,000 copies/mL), women with HIV infection (two to three times higher), and those whose alanine aminotransferase (ALT) levels were elevated in the year preceding the pregnancy (Arshad et al., 2011). Some studies suggest that perinatal transmission may be increased with invasive fetal monitoring, amniocentesis, and rupture of membranes for over 6 hours (Arshad et al., 2011).

Assessment

Routine screening for HCV during pregnancy is not recommended, though it is recommended for all adults born between 1945 and 1965 (U.S. Preventive Services Task Force (USPSTF), 2013). At-risk women such as those using IV drugs should be screened for antibody to HCV. Women who test positive should have hepatitis C viral RNA testing to check for current infection and to evaluate their viral load.

HCV is diagnosed by an enzyme-linked immunosorbent assay (ELISA) screening test for HCV-specific antibodies. HCV antibodies appear 6–10 weeks after the onset of illness and are present in more than 97% of infected persons within 6 months after exposure (CDC, 2013). Women with a positive ELISA screen should undergo specific testing of hepatitis C viral RNA, which is positive within 1–3 weeks after exposure.

Management

There is no treatment for HCV in pregnancy other than expectant management, as the medications that are typically used, pegylated interferon and ribafarin, are contraindicated in pregnant women. Infected women should be referred to a specialist who treats chronic liver disease, and counseled to abstain from alcohol and potentially hepatotoxic medications.

Vaginal birth and breastfeeding are not contraindicated. HCV has been detected in breast milk at very low levels; however, the virus is inactivated in the infant's gastrointestinal tract (Arshad et al., 2011). If the woman has cracked or bleeding nipples, she should abstain from breastfeeding until she is healed to prevent neonatal ingestion of maternal blood.

Pregnant women infected with HCV should be counseled regarding possible transmission to sexual partners. They should not share personal items that could be contaminated with blood and should cover any open cuts. For secondary prevention of chronic liver disease, infected women should be counseled to avoid alcohol and hepatotoxic drugs, and should receive vaccinations for hepatitis A and B. Unlike hepatitis A and B, there is no effective vaccine against HCV.

Parvovirus B19

Parvovirus B19, often referred to as fifth disease, or erythema infectiosum, is a single-stranded DNA virus of the Parvoviridae family (Corcoran & Doyle, 2004). Infections are more common in the winter and spring with respiratory spread as the most common route of transmission. Outbreaks often occur where there is high opportunity for exposure such as in schools and daycare centers. Transmission by hand-to-mouth contact and blood products is also possible. Most infected individuals are asymptomatic. If symptoms are present, they are likely to be mild and nonspecific, and can include fever, arthralgia, coryza, headache, and nausea, occurring approximately 1–2 weeks after exposure (Servey, Reamy, & Hodge, 2007). In the third week after exposure, a bright facial exanthema, or rash, appears over the cheeks, giving the characteristic "slapped cheek" appearance. A lacy red rash may also appear on the trunk and extremities.

An ultrasound done for another reason during the second or third trimester may demonstrate a hyperechogenic focus in the fetal liver (ACOG, 2000). While this can occur with other fetal complications, it can also indicate possible fetal infection with parvovirus B19.

Potential problems

Approximately 50–65% of women of reproductive age have developed immunity to parvovirus B19 (CDC, 2012c). Pregnant women who are not immune are at risk for contracting parvovirus B19. Infection with parvovirus B19 affects 1 in 400 pregnant women (Goff, 2005). The majority of pregnant women who become infected with parvovirus B19 have no adverse pregnancy outcome, while approximately 3% of infected women experience miscarriage, severe fetal anemia, or nonimmune hydrops fetalis (Rodis et al., 1998; Staroselsky, Klieger-Grossmann, Garcia-Bournissen, & Koren, 2009). Parvovirus B19 replicates rapidly in red blood cells and is a potent inhibitor of erythropoiesis, and is the etiology of anemia and hydrops (Young & Brown, 2004). Since most pregnant

women who become infected with parvovirus B19 are asymptomatic, an accurate determination of the risk of fetal infection and miscarriage is difficult. The highest risk of fetal infection occurs between the ninth and twentieth week of gestation and within 2–4 weeks of maternal infection (Staroselsky et al., 2009).

Assessment

Laboratory testing should be performed when the pregnant women is exposed to or develops symptoms of parvovirus B19, or when abnormal ultrasound findings suggest congenital infection. Serology consists of ELISA testing for IgG and IgM antibodies. If the IgG is present but the IgM is negative, immunity is demonstrated. If both are negative, and the test was performed after the incubation period, the woman is not immune and has not been infected. If both antibodies are positive, the woman has been infected in the previous 7–120 days (SOGC, 2002). Pregnant women who have been exposed to parvovirus B19 during a known outbreak are understandably concerned. Initial counseling should be accurate, informative, and reassuring.

> **Counseling pregnant women about parvovirus**
>
> - Most women of reproductive age have already been exposed and are immune.
> - A lab test can determine the presence or absence of immunity.
> - If no immunity is present, individuals with viral symptoms should be avoided.
> - There is very low risk to the fetus for long-term sequelae from congenital parvovirus B19 infection (Vogel et al., 1997).
> - Animal strains of parvovirus do not infect humans.
> - The woman with a congenitally infected fetus should be reassured that most infants do not exhibit long-term sequelae.

Management

There is no treatment for the pregnant woman with parvovirus B19 infection. Serial ultrasounds are done to evaluate for the presence of hydrops. If hydrops is found, further care is managed by an obstetrician or perinatologist, and can include cordocentesis to determine fetal hemoglobin and reticulocyte count, possible intrauterine transfusion, and early delivery.

Rubella

Rubella is an acute, mild viral disease that typically affects susceptible children and young adults. Rubella infection, also known as German measles or three-day measles, is transmitted by direct person-to-person contact or by airborne droplets from the respiratory secretions of an infected individual. Replication of the virus occurs in the nasopharynx and regional lymph nodes (CDC, 2001; Mayo Clinic Staff, 2012). The incubation period is usually about 2 weeks but can be as long as 3 weeks (WHO, 2008). Individuals are most contagious in the first days after the rash appears. However, individuals can transmit the virus during the incubation period. About 50% of rubella cases are asymptomatic and these individuals are also contagious (CDC, 2013).

Rubella is usually a mild illness but complications can occur and are more common in adults than in children. Complications of rubella infection include arthralgia, hemorrhagic arthritis, and encephalitis (CDC, 2013; WHO, 2008). Rubella encephalitis has an associated mortality as high as 50% (WHO, 2008).

In addition to the potentially serious complications associated with rubella infection, the virus can be transmitted to the fetus during pregnancy and can cause congenital rubella syndrome (CRS). CRS can result in spontaneous abortion, fetal death, low birth weight, and preterm birth. Hearing impairment is the most common manifestation of CRS, but other congenital anomalies including cataracts and other eye defects, cardiac anomalies, hepatosplenomegaly, and neurological abnormalities can occur. Congenital infection is most severe when it occurs early in gestation. Manifestations of CRS may not be apparent until early childhood when complications such as autism, progressive encephalopathy, and diabetes may be identified (CDC, 2005a; WHO, 2011).

Fortunately, the rubella vaccination program has been very successful and fetal infection is relatively rare in the United States (ACOG, 2002; CDC, 2013). However, cases have occurred sporadically in the United States in areas with lower vaccination rates and in women from countries with less effective vaccination programs (CDC, 2013).

Presentation and assessment

Rubella infection is associated with lymphadenopathy in the postauricular, deep cervical, and suboccipital lymph nodes, which persists for 3 weeks. Lymphadenopathy is followed by the appearance of a fine, maculopapular pink rash that begins on the face and spreads to the trunk and then the extremities. The rash resolves in the same sequence. Other presenting signs and symptoms include headache, conjunctivitis, nasal congestion, mild pyrexia, and arthralgia. An estimated 50% of infections are subclinical (SOGC, 2008).

CRS is not usually identified until after birth. However, CRS may be considered in the differential diagnosis of abnormal ultrasound findings such as cardiac anomalies, microcephaly, and IUGR (Merz, 2005).

The focused health history should include the following: symptom review, rubella vaccination history, and recent occurrence of rubella infection in the home or place of employment. The physical examination consists of vital signs, including temperature, and evaluation for rash, lymphadenopathy, conjunctivitis, congested nose, and arthralgia. Routine prenatal assessment such as listening for heart sounds and evaluating uterine and fetal size are also performed.

Routine prenatal laboratory testing should include serological rubella IgG to determine whether the woman has immunity to rubella. When there is suspicion of either maternal or fetal infection in the absence of documented maternal immunity, further laboratory testing should be performed. Enzyme immunoassays are typically used for serological testing and are convenient, sensitive, and accurate. Serological testing to detect IgG and IgM antibodies should be performed 7–10 days after the onset of the rash and repeated 2–3 weeks later (McLean, Redd, Abernathy, Icenogle, & Wallace, 2012; SOGC, 2008).

IgM antibodies can usually be detected 4–30 days after the onset of illness, and often for longer. The presence of IgM antibodies is indicative of rubella infection. However, because the incidence of rubella is low, the presence of IgM can be a false positive result (McLean et al., 2012). False positive results are more likely to occur in cases of parvovirus or mononucleosis (White, Boldt, Holditch, Poland, & Jacobson, 2012). A fourfold rise in the IgG antibodies supports the diagnosis of acute rubella infection (White et al., 2012).

The rubella virus can be cultured or identified by PCR analysis of specimens from the nose, throat, urine, blood, and cerebrospinal fluid, with the best results obtained from throat swabs (McLean et al., 2012). A positive culture or PCR analysis is considered positive evidence of rubella infection. If acute maternal rubella infection is identified early in the pregnancy, PCR on chorionic villi sampling can identify fetal infection. Amniotic fluid or fetal blood sampling can be used later in the pregnancy (SOGC, 2008).

Management

There is no treatment for acute rubella except supportive care and symptomatic relief. The woman with acute infection has an excellent prognosis. There is no evidence to support the use of immune globulin to decrease transmission to the fetus, although it can be offered to women with known rubella exposure who decline pregnancy termination (CDC, 1999; White et al., 2012).

Consultation or collaboration should be obtained when caring for a woman with suspected rubella infection or fetal anomalies that may be associated with CRS. When immunity is demonstrated by serological testing, there is virtually no risk of acquiring rubella for the woman or her fetus. CRS is very unlikely when infection occurs after the 20 weeks of gestation.

Prevention of rubella and CRS

Adherence to the recommended childhood immunization schedule is the first step in preventing rubella and CRS. Women of reproductive age should be tested to document their rubella immunity or lack thereof before becoming pregnant. The ideal times to screen women are during routine well-women health-care visits, family planning visits, and preconception visits. Women who are not immune to rubella should be offered vaccination unless they are planning on becoming pregnant in the next 4 weeks. Vaccination should also be offered to nonimmune postpartum women regardless of whether they are breastfeeding or have received Rh immune globulin.

In recent years, more parents are choosing to refuse or delay vaccinations of all kinds for their children. A primary reason for this relates to concerns regarding the adverse effects of vaccines. The success of vaccines in eradicating various infectious diseases has also played a role; thus, the current generation of parents has no reference point for the devastating consequences of these infections. The concept of herd immunity, defined as immunity for the whole population when a certain threshold number of the population is protected via vaccination from an infectious disease, is thought to be at work here. However, isolated outbreaks of these diseases are occurring; if current trends in declining vaccinations continue, there is a public health concern for reemergence of these infections on a broader scale. While women have a right to decline vaccination for themselves and their children, make sure that this is an informed refusal with the latest evidence available for their consideration.

Toxoplasmosis

Toxoplasmosis is a common infection caused by the protozoan parasite *Toxoplasma gondii*, which can be carried by many warm-blooded animals. Cats are the definitive hosts of the parasite and shed *T. gondii* oocytes in their feces (Montoya & Remington, 2008). Human infection results from ingestion of raw or undercooked infected meats, ingestion of oocytes inadvertently transferred from cat litter and soil, and congenital transmission, as illustrated in Figure 40.1 (CDC, 2000).

Toxoplasmosis is one of the most common infections in humans. In certain geographic areas, an estimated 95% of people have been infected. Approximately 22.4% of those aged 12 and older in the United States have been infected with *T. gondii* (CDC, 2010b). Cases of congenital toxoplasmosis are estimated to occur at a rate of 400–4000 each year in the United States (CDC, 2000).

Congenital toxoplasmosis can occur when a previously uninfected woman acquires the infection during or just prior to pregnancy. Congenital infection occurs in 30% of fetuses of newly infected women (Jones, Lopez, Wilson, Schulkin, & Gibbs, 2001; Mayo Foundation for Medical Education and Research, 2013). The frequency of vertical transmission increases with gestational age; however, the greatest damage to the fetus results if infection occurs in the first trimester (Montoya & Remington, 2008). Approximately 750 deaths are attributable to toxoplasmosis infection yearly, and 50% of those are the result of eating contaminated meats (CDC, 2000).

Potential problems

Maternal infection usually does not result in clinical illness (Remington, McLeod, Thuilliez, & Desmonts, 2006). Congenital toxoplasmosis is the primary concern. Severe sequelae can result from infection of the developing brain and include mental retardation, hydrocephalus or microcephaly, chorioretinitis, hepatosplenomegaly, jaundice, and seizures. Many infants are asymptomatic at birth, but most will develop learning and visual disabilities later in life if left untreated. Congenital toxoplasmosis is one of the most important causes of ocular infection that can result in retinochoroiditis later in life. Congenital infection in the first trimester can result in miscarriage or stillbirth (CDC, 2000; Mayo Foundation for Medical Education and Research, 2013).

Clinical presentation and assessment

The pregnant woman with toxoplasmosis will most likely be asymptomatic but may present with self-limiting symptoms that mimic mononucleosis, including headache, fever, myalgia, and cervical lymphadenopathy. Rarely, the woman may present with visual changes that result from chorioretinitis (Garweg, Scherrer, Wallon, Kodjikian, & Peyron, 2005). A diagnosis of maternal toxoplasmosis should be considered in the presence of these findings. Prenatal detection of fetal toxoplasmosis infection should be considered when abnormal ultrasound findings indicate fetal anomalies or hydrops (Remington et al., 2006).

Prompt and accurate diagnosis of toxoplasmosis is important in order to reduce the risk to the fetus with maternal treatment. A focused health history includes recent history or habit of eating undercooked meat (especially pork, lamb, and venison), produce handling

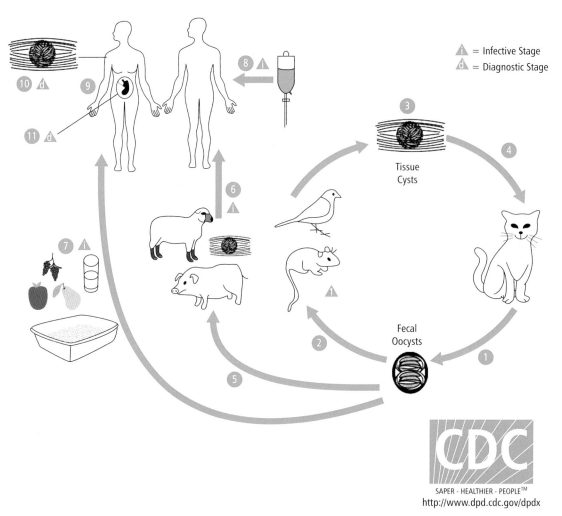

Figure 40.1. Life cycle of *T. gondii*. The only known definitive hosts for *T. gondii* are members of the family Felidae (domestic cats and their relatives). Unsporulated oocysts are shed in the cat's feces ①. Although oocysts are usually only shed for 1–2 weeks, large numbers may be shed. Oocysts take 1–5 days to sporulate in the environment and become infective. Intermediate hosts in nature (including birds and rodents) become infected after ingesting soil, water, or plant material contaminated with oocysts ②. Oocysts transform into tachyzoites shortly after ingestion. These tachyzoites localize in neural and muscle tissue and develop into tissue cyst bradyzoites ③. Cats become infected after consuming intermediate hosts harboring tissue cysts ④. Cats may also become infected directly by ingestion of sporulated oocysts. Animals bred for human consumption and wild game may also become infected with tissue cysts after ingestion of sporulated oocysts in the environment ⑤. Humans can become infected by any of several routes:

- eating undercooked meat of animals harboring tissue cysts ⑥
- consuming food or water contaminated with cat feces or by contaminated environmental samples (such as fecal-contaminated soil or changing the cat litter box) ⑦.
- blood transfusion or organ transplantation ⑧.
- transplacentally from the mother to the fetus ⑨.

In the human host, the parasites form tissue cysts, most commonly in skeletal muscle, myocardium, brain, and eyes; these cysts may remain throughout the life of the host. Diagnosis is usually achieved by serology, although tissue cysts may be observed in stained biopsy specimens ⑩. Diagnosis of congenital infections can be achieved by detecting *T. gondii* DNA in amniotic fluid using molecular methods such as PCR ⑪. Source: Image and information courtesy of DPDx of the CDC's Division of Parasitic Diseases and Malaria (2010). http://dpd.cdc.gov/dpdx/HTML/Image_Library.htm

Table 40.1 Interpretation of Results of Serological Tests for Toxoplasmosis

IgG test result	IgM test result	Interpretation
Negative	Negative	No infection; serial testing during pregnancy is advised.
Positive	Negative	Most often reflects prior infection
Negative	Positive or equivocal	Can indicate acute or prior infection; positive or equivocal IgM test results should be followed by confirmatory testing at a *Toxoplasma* reference laboratory.
Positive	Positive or equivocal	Same as above

Adapted from: Montoya and Remington (2008).

practices in the home, gardening, presence of cats in the home, and a review of pertinent symptoms. The focused physical examination consists of vital signs, including temperature; neurologic exam, including neurologic deficits, visual field deficits, gait disturbances, and abnormalities in speech, cognitive, or affective functions; and assessment for cervical lymphadenopathy.

Routine toxoplasmosis screening is performed in countries with high rates of *T. gondii*. In the United States, where prevalence is low, laboratory testing for toxoplasmosis should be performed if abnormal fetal findings are detected on ultrasound, including hydrocephaly, central nervous system abnormalities, symmetric fetal growth restriction, or nonimmune hydrops, and should be considered in a woman who is immunocompromised or demonstrates lymphadenopathy in the absence of a positive mononucleosis testing (Montoya & Remington, 2008). The primary diagnostic method is detection of *Toxoplasma*-specific antibodies, but serological testing lacks specificity. Initially, an IgG titer should be drawn. If the IgG is positive, an IgM is drawn and the titers of both are analyzed and interpreted as follows (Table 40.1).

IgM antibodies appear at the initial infection and may persist for years (Montoya & Remington, 2008). The serological testing lacks specificity, creating false positive results. The true value of IgM testing is in ruling out the presence of acute infection. Because of the significant potential of misinterpreting a positive IgM test result, confirmatory testing should be performed. Confirmatory tests include toxoplasma serological profile (TSP), the Sabin–Feldman dye test (DT) and avidity testing. Avidity testing can differentiate between antibodies from a recent infection and remote infection. If there is a high avidity in the first 12–16 weeks of pregnancy, antenatal acquisition is ruled out and the fetus is essentially not at risk for congenital infection. A low IgG avidity can persist for months and is not diagnostic of recent infection (CDC, Division of Parasitic Diseases and Malaria, 2009; Montoya & Remington, 2008). The Food and Drug Administration (FDA) has recommended that sera with positive IgM test results obtained at nonreference laboratories should be sent to a toxoplasma reference laboratory.

When maternal toxoplasmosis is suspected or diagnosed, amniocentesis and PCR after 18 weeks' gestation are used for the diagnosis of congenital toxoplasmosis. Ultrasound is recommended to evaluate the presence of fetal anomalies. In addition to ultrasound, computed tomography (CT) or magnetic resonance imaging (MRI) may be used to identify fetal brain calcifications and other anomalies (Montoya & Remington, 2008).

Management

Prenatal treatment of women with *toxoplamsa* can reduce the incidence of severe sequelae in the newborn, with the most benefit from treating promptly upon diagnosis. For women found to be infected prior to 18 weeks' gestation, vertical transmission to the fetus can be decreased with the use of spiramycin, though clinical trials are lacking. Spiramycin is considered an experimental drug in the United States and must be obtained through the FDA. Other treatments include the use of sulfadiazine, pyrimethamine, and folinic acid (Montoya & Remington, 2008). Depending on fetal status, consultation or collaboration may be considered in the presence of maternal infection for maternal and fetal surveillance and maternal treatment plans. If fetal infection is found, referral to specialty care should be initiated.

Information for women about toxoplasmosis

- Wash vegetables and fruit thoroughly before consuming.
- Wash hands, utensils, and cooking surfaces after touching uncooked meat and unwashed produce.
- Cook all meat to a safe temperature using a food thermometer.
- Wear gloves when gardening.
- Wash hands with soap and warm water if there is contact with soil or sand.
- Keep outdoor sandboxes covered.
- Avoid changing cat litter when possible and use gloves and hand washing when it cannot be avoided
- Indoor cats that do not hunt and are not fed raw meat pose little risk for toxoplasmosis infection.
- There is no risk of toxoplasmosis infection through intact skin.

Prevention

Information about modes of transmission and prevention of *toxoplasma* infection should be provided during preconception visits and during routine prenatal care.

Varicella

Varicella zoster virus (VZV) is one of eight herpes viruses known to infect humans. Primary VZV infection leads to varicella (chickenpox) and establishes latency in dorsal root ganglia. Reactivation of VZV causes herpes zoster (HZ), commonly called shingles (CDC, 2007). VZV is transmitted by direct contact with vesicular fluid or respiratory droplets (CDC, 2011; SOGC, 2012). The incubation period is 10–21 days and the disease is infectious 48 hours before the rash appears until the vesicles have crusted over (Tyring, 1992). Owing to varicella vaccination programs in the United States, the mortality rate from VZV infection is as low as 0.4 per 1 million population. Mortality rates increase with age (Nguyen, Jumaan, & Seward, 2005; SOGC, 2012). The annual incidence of HZ in the United States is approximately 1 case per 4000 (CDC, 2012d).

It is estimated that over 90% of pregnant women are seropositive for VZV IgG antibody and are therefore immune to infection. Approximately 2 to 3 of every 1000 pregnancies are complicated by VZV each year (CDC, 2007). Congenital varicella syndrome (CVS) is a rare complication of maternal varicella infection. The rate of CVS is 0.4–2% of fetuses of women who become infected with VZV in the first or second trimesters (CDC, 2007; Ramachandra, Metta, Haneef, & Kodali, 2010).

Neonatal varicella is caused by maternal varicella acquired during the last 3 weeks of pregnancy, occurring primarily when symptoms of maternal infection occur between 5 days before birth and 2 days after birth. This period correlates with the development of maternal IgG antibodies and is too brief to provide transplacental passive immunization to the fetus or neonate (SOGC, 2012). Neonatal varicella that occurs in the first 10–12 days of life is usually the result of transplacental transmission of the virus. When neonatal varicella occurs after this time, it is most likely due to postnatal infection (Sauerbrei & Wutzler, 2001). In the absence of treatment, newborns with neonatal varicella can develop severe neonatal varicella infection (CDC, 2007).

Potential problems

Pregnant women are at an increased risk for complications from VZV infection compared to nonpregnant adults. Complications include secondary bacterial infec-

tion of the skin, central nervous system manifestations, such as meningoencephalitis or cerebellar ataxia, and pneumonia or pneumonitis, either viral or bacterial. Less common complications include hepatitis, hemorrhagic complications, thrombocytopenia, and nephritis (CDC, 2007). Approximately 5–10% of pregnant women with VZV infection develop pneumonitis, particularly women who smoke or who have a profuse numbers of lesions (Harger et al., 2002; Paryani & Arvin, 1986). Mortality in pregnant women is higher than in nonpregnant adults, and death usually results from respiratory disease (CDC, 2007; SOGC, 2012).

Maternal VZ can result in HZ ophthalmicus when the ophthalmic division of the trigeminal nerve is involved, and can lead to chronic ocular complications, reduced vision, and blindness. Varicella zoster (VZ) can also lead to neurological and dermatologic complications for the pregnant woman. Maternal VZ has not been shown to cause fetal sequelae (SOGC, 2012).

The newborn with CVS may present with low birth weight, cutaneous scars, lesions, localized absence of skin on a limb, hypoplasia of one or more limbs, malformed digits, or various ocular and central nervous system abnormalities (Puder, Treadwell, & Gonik, 1997). Neonatal varicella is fatal in 20–23% of cases (Sauerbrei & Wutzler, 2001).

Clinical presentation and assessment

The pregnant woman with primary varicella can develop a prodrome of fever, malaise, headache, and abdominal pain 1–2 days before a rash appears. The rash typically consists of three or more successive crops of lesions that develop over several days. Each crop progresses from macules to papules, vesicles, and pustules, then crusts over, so that any part of the body may have lesions in different stages (CDC, 2007; SOGC, 2012). The rash usually starts on the face and trunk then spreads to the extremities. It takes 4–7 days for all lesions to become crusted (CDC, 2007).

VZ has a prodromal period marked by headache, photophobia, malaise, fever, abnormal skin sensations, and excruciating pain. The VZ rash is typically unilateral, involving one to three adjacent dermatomes, and possibly ophthalmic involvement. The rash is initially erythematous and maculopapular and then forms vesicles over several days that crust over. Full resolution of VZ takes 2–4 weeks, but the postherpetic pain may persist for months or even years. Occasionally, a rash does not develop (zoster sine herpete) (CDC, 2012d).

Ultrasound findings for the fetus with CVS appear after the maternal VZV infection has subsided and can represent virus-specific deformation or nonimmune hydrops. The deformation sequence consists of some combination of limb hypoplasia, skin lesions, microph-thalmos, and abnormal positioning of limbs. Nonim-mune hydrops findings include hepatosplenomegaly, ascites, pleural effusion, pericardial effusion, and liver calcification (Puder et al., 1997).

The incidence of varicella disease is declining as a result of vaccination programs, making clinical diagno-sis more uncommon and more challenging. The focused health history should include history of varicella infec-tion in the home or workplace; documentation of vari-cella immunity by documentation of age-appropriate vaccination, laboratory evidence of immunity, or history of varicella disease or HZ; and a review of reported symptoms or prodrome. The focused physical examina-tion consists of vital signs, including temperature, and examination of lesions, including type and crusting.

Laboratory testing is used to determine susceptibility to varicella or confirm varicella infection. PCR testing of skin lesions is accurate and convenient. If the lesions have resolved, PCR of oral specimens can sometimes aid in the diagnosis of varicella disease (Leung et al., 2010). The use of single IgM or IgG results cannot be used to confirm infection. In the presence of a rash and positive IgM, the clinician can interpret the findings as confirmation of varicella. A positive IgM ELISA result is suggestive of primary infection but does not exclude reinfection or reactivation of latent VZV. Serology for IgM is considerably less sensitive then PCR testing of skin lesions; commercial IgM assay may not be reliable; and false negative IgM results are common (CDC, 2007).

Management

Varicella zoster immunoglobulin (VZIG) has been shown to lower varicella infection rates and to reduce maternal complications in nonimmune women. VZIG should be administered as soon as possible after expo-sure but may be effective if administered as late as 96 hours after exposure (CDC, 2007; Enders, Miller, Cradock-Watson, Bolley, & Ridehalgh, 1994; Royal College of Obstetricians and Gynecologists, 2007). The intramuscular dose for VZIG is 125 units per 10 kg, with a maximum of 625 units. Serology should, if possible, precede the use of VZIG (SOGC, 2012).

The pregnant woman with varicella pneumonitis should be referred for treatment with antiviral agents, which may be administered orally or intravenously if the illness warrants. Acyclovir is a synthetic nucleoside analog that inhibits replication of human herpes viruses, including VZV, and crosses the placenta to transplacental passage of the virus to the fetus (CDC, 2007; SOGC, 2012). When administered within 24 hours of onset of the rash, acyclovir has been demonstrated to be effective

in reducing varicella-associated morbidity and mortality in the pregnant population (CDC, 2007).

Consultation or collaboration should be considered for women who develop varicella in pregnancy for detailed ultrasound and follow-up to screen for fetal consequences of infection. If pneumonitis develops, referral to specialty care and hospital admission is war-ranted. The neonatal care team should be informed of peripartum varicella exposure in order to optimize early neonatal care with VZIG.

Counseling and support are based on the following:

Key counseling points on varicella infection

- A positive IgG ELISA result indicates antibodies to VZV either from past varicella or vaccination and may be obtained as part of preconception or prenatal care.
- Varicella vaccination is recommended for all nonimmune women as part of prepregnancy and postpartum care. Nonpregnant women who get vaccinated should wait 1 month to attempt pregnancy.
- A woman who acquires a varicella infection during pregnancy should be made aware of the potential adverse maternal and fetal sequelae, the risk of transmission to the fetus, and the options for testing.
- Breastfeeding of infants infected with or exposed to VZV is encouraged.
- If siblings at home have varicella, a newborn baby should be given VZIG if the mother is seronegative.

Summary

While vaccines and antibiotics have made remarkable strides in preventing or treating the progression and serious sequelae of many infections, it is important to remember that infectious disease remains a leading cause of death worldwide and is the third leading cause of death in the United States. The hope of new drugs and vaccines to further reduce disease burden from infection is balanced by the rapid mutation of certain microbes and the reemergence of infectious agents resistant to standard treatments.

Due to the normal physiological changes in pregnancy that allow the woman's body to accept the semiallograft of the fetus, pregnant women are more vulnerable to infection. And infection in the pregnant woman renders her fetus vulnerable as well. Health-care providers need to remain vigilant to signs and symptoms of their clients so that they can intervene in a timely manner to infec-tious processes. Basic hygiene is of vital importance and should be practiced by health-care providers and women alike.

Case study

Rebecca is a 34-year-old white female and is 28 weeks pregnant. She is a G2P1001. Her first child, a boy, is 22 months old. She comes in for a routine visit. She says that she thinks she has poison ivy on her breast area as she has blisters that itch and are somewhat painful. She attributes the pain to the sensitive location of the blisters.

SUBJECTIVE: Upon further questioning, Rebecca has recently been hiking in the woods and is quite sensitive to oils from the poison ivy plant, and she thinks this oil was transferred from her clothing to her breast. She has noticed these lesions for about a week. She reports good fetal movement and no concerns other than her blisters. She has a history of receiving the measles–mumps–rubella (MMR) vaccination series and had chicken pox as a child.

OBJECTIVE: Upon examination, the blisters are unilateral and wrap around from her left breast along her left rib area to her spine in a classic dermatome pattern. Multiple lesions are present, mostly located on the right upper quadrant of the left breast. They are in various stages—some blistered, some open and weeping, others crusted over.

Her fundal height is 27 cm; her fetus is in vertex position with activity palpated and fetal heart tones are 140.

ASSESSMENT: This is a woman with a 28-week intrauterine pregnancy who has varicella zoster or shingles.

PLAN: Because Rebecca is in the middle of her pregnancy with prior immunity, she can be given reassurance that her fetus will most likely be fine. Rebecca should keep the blistered areas clean and dry and covered and should practice careful hand washing so that her 22-month-old son is not exposed. Discuss pain management options with her, recommending acetaminophen with the thought that the use of stronger medications may be warranted.

An ultrasound is ordered to assess fetal well-being; consultation with a physician colleague is done and testing options to verify the diagnosis can be initiated, with PCR testing of skin lesions as the preferred test in this case. Rebecca is likely to have concerns now and later as she processes this information at a factual and emotional level. She is provided with resources, emotional support, and a number to call for concerns between now and her next visit.

Resources for women

March of Dimes pregnancy complications: http://www.marchofdimes.com/pregnancy/complications.html
MedlinePlus infections and pregnancy: http://www.nlm.nih.gov/medlineplus/infectionsandpregnancy.html

Resources for health-care providers

CDC interpretation of Hepatitis B serological results: http://www.cdc.gov/hepatitis/HBV/PDFs/SerologicChartv8.pdf
CDC 2010 STD Treatment Guidelines: http://www.cdc.gov/std/treatment/2010/
National Institute of Allergy and Infectious Diseases: http://www.niaid.nih.gov/Pages/default.aspx

References

Adler, S. P. (2011). Screening for cytomegalovirus during pregnancy. *Infectious Diseases in Obstetrics and Gynecology, 2011,* Article ID 942937, 9 pages. doi:10.1155/2011/942937. Retrieved from http://www.hindawi.com/journals/idog/2011/942937/#B33

Adler, S. P., Nigro, G., & Pereira, L. (2007). Recent advances in the prevention and treatment of congenital cytomegalovirus infections. *Seminars in Perinatology, 31,* 10–18. Retrieved from http://congenitalcmv.org/recent.pdf

American College of Obstetricians and Gynecologists (ACOG). (2000). Clinical management guidelines for obstetrician-gynecologists. ACOG guidelines No. 20. Retrieved from http://www.fifthdisease.org/cmsFiles/acog_guidelines.pdf

American College of Obstetricians and Gynecologists (ACOG). (2002). Rubella vaccination. ACOG Committee Opinion No. 281. *Obstetrics and Gynecology, 100*(6), 1417. Retrieved from http://journals.lww.com/greenjournal/Fulltext/2002/12000/ACOG_Committee_Opinion_No__281__Rubella.46.aspx#

American College of Obstetricians and Gynecologists (ACOG). (2007, reaffirmed 2012). Viral hepatitis in pregnancy. ACOG Committee Opinion No. 86. *Obstetrics and Gynecology, 110,* 941–955.

Arshad, M., El-Kamary, S. S., & Jhaveri, R. (2011). Hepatitis C virus infection during pregnancy and the newborn period are they opportunities for treatment? *Journal of Viral Hepatitis, 18*(4), 229–236.

Cannon, M. J. (2009). Congenital cytomegalovirus (CMV) epidemiology and awareness. *Journal of Clinical Virology, 46S,* S6–S10.

Cannon, M. J., Westbrook, K., Levis, D., Schleiss, M. R., Thackeray, R., & Pass, R. F. (2012). Awareness of and behaviors related to child-to-mother transmission of cytomegalovirus. *Preventive Medicine, 54*(5), 351–357. Retrieved from http://www.sciencedirect.com.ezproxy.midwives.org/science/article/pii/S0091743512000916

Centers for Disease Control and Prevention (CDC). (1999). Rubella prevention. Recommendations of the immunization practices advisory committee (ACIP). *MMWR. Recommendations and Reports, 39*(RR-15), 1–18.

Centers for Disease Control and Prevention (CDC). (2000). Preventing congenital toxoplasmosis. *MMWR. Recommendations and Reports, 49*(RR02), 57–75. Retrieved from http://www.cdc.gov/mmwr/preview/mmwrhtml/rr4902a5.htm

Centers for Disease Control and Prevention (CDC). (2001). Control and prevention of rubella: Evaluation and management of suspected outbreaks, rubella in pregnancy women, and surveillance for congenital rubella syndrome. *MMWR. Recommendations and Reports, 50*(RR12), 1–23. Retrieved from http://www.cdc.gov/MMWR/PREVIEW/mmwrhtml/rr5012a1.htm

Centers for Disease Control and Prevention (CDC). (2005a). Achievements in public health: Elimination of rubella and congenital rubella syndrome-United States, 1969–2004. *MMWR. Recommendations and Reports, 54*(11), 279–282. Retrieved from http://www.cdc.gov/mmwr/preview/mmwrhtml/mm5411a5.htm

Centers for Disease Control and Prevention (CDC). (2005b). A comprehensive immunization strategy to eliminate transmission of hepatitis B virus infection in the United States. *MMWR. Recommendations and Reports, 54*(RR-16), 1–39. Retrieved from http://www.cdc.gov/mmwr/pdf/rr/rr5416.pdf

Centers for Disease Control and Prevention (CDC). (2007). Prevention of varicella. *MMWR. Recommendations and Reports, 56*(RR-4), 1–40.

Centers for Disease Control and Prevention (CDC). (2008). Knowledge and practices of obstetricians and gynecologists regarding cytomegalovirus infection during pregnancy—United States, 2007. *MMWR. Morbidity and Mortality Weekly Report, 57*(03), 65–68. Retrieved from http://www.congenitalcmv.org/knowledge.pdf

Centers for Disease Control and Prevention (CDC). (2009a). Trends in prenatal group B Streptococcal disease-United States, 2000–2006. *MMWR. Morbidity and Mortality Weekly Report, 58,* 109–112.

Centers for Disease Control and Prevention (CDC). (2009b). Viral hepatitis statistics and surveillance. Retrieved from http://www.cdc.gov/hepatitis/Statistics/SurveillanceGuidelines.htm

Centers for Disease Control and Prevention (CDC). (2010a). Cytomegalovirus (CMV) and congenital CMV infection. Pregnant women. Retrieved from http://www.cdc.gov/cmv/risk/preg-women.html

Centers for Disease Control and Prevention (CDC). (2010b). Parasites-Toxoplasmosis (*Toxoplasma* infection). Epidemiology & risk factors. Retrieved from http://www.cdc.gov/parasites/toxoplasmosis/epi.html

Centers for Disease Control and Prevention (CDC). (2010c). Prevention of perinatal group B Streptococcal disease. Revised guidelines from CDC, 2010. *MMWR. Recommendations and Reports, 59*(RR10), 1–32. Retrieved from http://www.cdc.gov/mmwr/pdf/rr/rr5910.pdf

Centers for Disease Control and Prevention (CDC). (2010d). Hepatitis A information for health professionals. Retrieved from http://www.cdc.gov/hepatitis/hav/index.htm

Centers for Disease Control and Prevention (CDC). (2010e). Hepatitis B information for health professionals. Retrieved from http://www.cdc.gov/hepatitis/HBV/StatisticsHBV.htm

Centers for Disease Control and Prevention (CDC). (2011). Chickenpox and pregnancy. Retrieved from http://www.cdc.gov/pregnancy/infections-chickenpox.html

Centers for Disease Control and Prevention (CDC). (2012a). 2011 sexually transmitted diseases surveillance. Retrieved from http://www.cdc.gov/std/stats11/tables/1.htm

Centers for Disease Control and Prevention (CDC). (2012b). Group B Strep infections in newborns. Retrieved from http://www.cdc.gov/groupbstrep/about/newborns-pregnant.html

Centers for Disease Control and Prevention (CDC). (2012c). Parvovirus B19 and fifth disease: Pregnancy and fifth disease. Retrieved from http://www.cdc.gov/parvovirusb19/pregnancy.html

Centers for Disease Control and Prevention (CDC). (2012d). Shingles (herpes zoster). Retrieved from http://www.cdc.gov/shingles/hcp/clinical-overview.html

Centers for Disease Control and Prevention (CDC). (2013). Hepatitis C information for health care professionals. Retrieved from http://www.cdc.gov/hepatitis/hcv/

Centers for Disease Control and Prevention, Division of Parasitic Diseases and Malaria. (2009). Toxoplasmosis: Antibody detection. Retrieved from http://dpd.cdc.gov/dpdx/HTML/Toxoplasmosis.htm

Colugnati, F., Staras, S., Dollard, S. C., & Cannon, M. J. (2007). Incidence of cytomegalovirus infection among the general population and pregnant women in the United States. *BMC Infectious Diseases, 7*(71), 1–10. Retrieved from http://www.biomedcentral.com/content/pdf/1471-2334-7-71.pdf.

Contag, S. (2012) Hepatitis in pregnancy. Retrieved from http://emedicine.medscape.com/article/1562368-overview#a1

Corcoran, A., & Doyle, S. (2004). Advances in the biology, diagnosis & host-pathogen interactions of paravovirus B19. *Journal of Medical Microbiology, 53,* 459–475.

Degli-Esposti, S. (2010). Hepatitis B transmission re-evaluated in pregnancy. *Gastroenterology & Endoscopy News, 61,* 10.

DPDx of the CDC's Division of Parasitic Diseases and Malaria. (2010). Retrieved from http://dpd.cdc.gov/dpdx/HTML/Image_Library.htm

Duff, P. (2010). Diagnosis and management of CMV in pregnancy. *Perinatology, 1,* 1–6. Retrieved from http://www.perinatology.com/exposures/Infection/CMV/Cytomegalovirus.htm#PREVENTION

Enders, G., Miller, E., Cradock-Watson, J., Bolley, I., & Ridehalgh, M. (1994). Consequences of varicella and herpes zoster in pregnancy: Prospective study of 1739 cases. *Lancet, 343*(8912), 1548–1551.

Garweg, J. G., Scherrer, J., Wallon, M., Kodjikian, L., & Peyron, F. (2005). Reactivation of ocular toxoplasmosis during pregnancy. *BJOG, 112,* 241–242.

Goff, M. (2005). Parvovirus B19 in pregnancy. *Journal of Midwifery and Women's Health, 50,* 536–538.

Hansen, S. M., Uldbjerg, N., Kilian, M., & Sorensen, U. B. (2004). Dynamics of *Streptococcus agalactiae* colonization in women during and after pregnancy and in their infants. *Journal of Clinical Microbiology, 42,* 83–89.

Harger, J. H., Ernest, J. M., Thurnau, G. R., Moawad, A., Momirova, V., Landon, M. B., . . . Von Dorsten, P. (2002). Risk factors and outcome of varicella-zoster virus pneumonia in pregnant women. *Journal of Infectious Diseases, 185*(4), 422–427.

Jeon, J., Victor, M., Adler, S. P., Arwady, A., Demmler, G., Fowler, K., . . . Cannon, M. J. (2006). Knowledge and awareness of congenital cytomegalovirus among women. *Infectious Diseases in Obstetrics and Gynecology, 2006,* 1–7. doi:10.1155/IDOG/2006/80383

Jones, J. L., Lopez, A. L., Wilson, M., Schulkin, J., & Gibbs, R. (2001). Congenital toxoplasmosis: A review. *Obstetrical and Gynecological Survey, 56*(5), 296–305. Retrieved from http://www.cimerman.com.br/artigos/Pediatria/toxo%20congentia%20revis%C3%A0o.pdf

Lazzarotto, T. T., Guerra, B. B., Gabrielli, L. L., Lanari, M. M., & Landini, M. P. (2011). Update on the prevention, diagnosis and management of cytomegalovirus infection in pregnancy. *Clinical Microbiology and Infection, 17*(9), 1285–1293. doi:10.1111/j1469-0691.2011.03564.x

Le Campion, A., Larouche, A., Fauteux-Daniel, S., & Soudeyns, H. (2012). Pathogenesis of hepatitis C during pregnancy and childhood. *Viruses, 4*(12), 3531–3550.

Lee, H., & Lok, A. S. F. (2013). Hepatitis B and pregnancy. Wolters Kluwer Health: Up to Date. Retrieved from http://www.uptodate.com/contents/hepatitis-b-and-pregnancy

Leung, J., Harpaz, R., Baughman, A. L., Heath, K., Loparev, V., Vazquez, M., . . . Schmid, D. S. (2010). Evaluation of laboratory methods for diagnosis of varicella. *Clinical Infectious Diseases, 51*(1), 23–32. Retrieved from http://cid.oxfordjournals.org/content/51/1/23.long

Martinez de Tejada, B., Pfister, R. E., Renzi, G., Francois, P., Irion, O., Boulvain, M., & Schrenzel, J. (2010). Intrapartum group B Streptococcus detection by rapid polymerase chain reaction assay for the prevention of neonatal sepsis. *Clinical Microbiology and Infection, 17*, 1786–1791. doi:10.1111/j.1469-0691.2010.03378.x

Mayo Clinic Staff. (2012). Rubella. Retrieved from http://www.mayoclinic.com/health/rubella/DS00332/DSECTION=symptoms

Mayo Foundation for Medical Education and Research. (2013). Toxoplasmosis. Retrieved from http://www.mayoclinic.com/health/toxoplasmosis/DS00510/DSECTION=symptoms

McCarthy, F. P., Giles, M. L., Rowlands, S., Purcell, K. J., & Jones, C. A. (2011). Antenatal interventions for preventing the transmission of cytomegalovirus (CMV) from the mother to fetus during pregnancy and adverse outcomes in the congenitally infected infant. *Cochrane Database of Systematic Reviews,* (3), CD008371. doi:10.1002/14651858.CD008371.pub2

McLean, H., Redd, S., Abernathy, E., Icenogle, J., & Wallace, G. (2012). Rubella. In S. W. Roush, L. McIntyre, & L. M. Baldy (Eds.), *Manual for the surveillance of vaccine-preventable diseases* (pp. 1–7). Atlanta, GA: Centers for Disease Control and Prevention. Retrieved from http://www.cdc.gov/vaccines/pubs/surv-manual/chpt14-rubella.html

Merz, E. (2005). *Ultrasound in obstetrics and gynecology,* Vol. 1. New York: Georg Thieme Verlag.

Montoya, J. G., & Remington, J. S. (2008). Management of *Toxoplasma gondii* during pregnancy. *Clinical Infectious Diseases, 47*(4), 554–566. Retrieved from http://cid.oxfordjournals.org/content/47/4/554.full

Nandyal, R. R. (2008). Update on group B Streptococcal infections: Perinatal and neonatal periods. *Journal of Perinatal and Neonatal Nursing, 22*(3), 230–237.

Nguyen, H. Q., Jumaan, A. O., & Seward, J. F. (2005). Decline in mortality due to varicella after implantation of varicella vaccination in the United States. *New England Journal of Medicine, 352,* 450–458.

Paryani, S. G., & Arvin, A. M. (1986). Intrauterine infection with varicella-zoster virus after maternal varicella. *New England Journal of Medicine, 314*(24), 1542–1546.

Pass, R. F. (2002). Cytomegalovirus infection. *Pediatrics in Review, 23,* 163–170.

Puder, K. S., Treadwell, M. C., & Gonik, B. (1997). Ultrasound characteristics of in utero infection. *Infectious Diseases in Obstetrics and Gynecology, 5,* 262–270. Retrieved from http://www.ncbi.nlm.nih.gov/pmc/articles/PMC2364537/pdf/IDOG-05-262.pdf

Ramachandra, S., Metta, A. K., Haneef, N. S., & Kodali, S. (2010). Fetal varicella syndrome. *Indian Journal of Dermatology, Venereology and Leprology, 76*(6), 724. doi:10.4103/0378-6323.72475

Reddick, K. L., Jhaveri, R., Gandhi, M., James, A. H., & Swamy, G. K. (2011). Pregnancy outcomes associated with viral hepatitis. *Journal of Viral Hepatitis, 18*(7), e394–e398. doi:10.1111/j.1365-2893.2011.01436.x

Reddy, U., Fry, A., Pass, R., & Ghidini, A. (2004). Infectious diseases and perinatal outcomes. *Emerging Infectious Diseases* [serial on the Internet]. Retrieved from http://dx.doi.org/10.3201/eid1011.040623_10

Remington, J. S., McLeod, R., Thuilliez, P., & Desmonts, G. (2006). Toxoplasmosis. In J. S. Remington, J. O. Klein, C. B. Wilson, & C. Baker (Eds.) *Infectious diseases of the fetus and newborn infant* (6th ed., pp. 947–1091). Philadelphia: Elsevier Saunders.

Rodis, J. F., Borgida, A. F., Wilson, M., Egan, J. F. X., Leo, M. V., Odibo, A. O., & Campbell, W. A. (1998). Management of parvovirus infection in pregnancy and outcomes of hydrops: A survey of the Society of Perinatal Obstetricians. *American Journal of Obstetrics and Gynecology, 179*(4), 985–988. Retrieved from http://www.ajog.org/article/S0002-9378(98)70203-0/abstract

Ross, D. S., Victor, M., Sumartojo, E., & Cannon, M. J. (2008). Women's knowledge of congenital cytomegalovirus: Results from the 2005 HealthStyles survey. *Journal of Women's Health, 17*(5), 849–858.

Royal College of Obstetricians and Gynecologists. (2007). Chickenpox in pregnancy (Green-top 13). Retrieved from http://www.rcog.org.uk/womens-health/clinical-guidance/chickenpox-pregnancy-green-top-13

Sauerbrei, A., & Wutzler, P. (2001). Neonatal varicella. *Journal of Perinatology, 21*(8), 545–549.

Schrag, S. J., Zywicki, S., Farley, M. M., Reingold, A. L., Harrison, L. H., Lefkowitz, L. B., . . . Schuchat, A. (2000). Group B streptococcal disease in the era of intrapartum antibiotic prophylaxis. *New England Journal of Medicine, 342,* 15–20. Retrieved from http://www.nejm.org/doi/full/10.1056/NEJM200001063420103

Sendi, P., Johansson, L., & Norrby-Teglund, A. (2008). Invasive group B Streptococcal disease in non-pregnant adults: A review with emphasis on skin and soft-tissue infections. *Infection, 36*(2), 100–111.

Servey, J. T., Reamy, B. V., & Hodge, J. (2007). Clinical presentations of parvovirus B19 infection. *American Family Physician, 75*(3), 373–376. Retrieved from http://www.aafp.org/afp/2007/0201/p373.html

Society of Obstetricians and Gynaecologists of Canada (SOGC). (2002). Parvovirus B19 infection in pregnancy. SOGC Clinical Practice Guidelines, No. 119. *Journal of Obstetrics and Gynaecology Canada, 24*(9), 1–8. Retrieved from http://www.sogc.org/guidelines/public/119e-cpg-september2002.pdf

Society of Obstetricians and Gynaecologists of Canada (SOGC). (2008). Rubella in pregnancy. SOGC Clinical Practice Guidelines, No. 203. *Journal of Obstetrics and Gynaecology Canada, 30*(2), 152–158. Retrieved from http://www.sogc.org/guidelines/documents/guiJOGC203CPG0802.pdf

Society of Obstetricians and Gynaecologists of Canada (SOGC). (2010). Cytomegalovirus infection in pregnancy. SOGC Clinical Practice Guidelines, No. 240. *Journal of Obstetrics and Gynaecology Canada, 32*(4), 348–354. Retrieved from http://www.sogc.org/guidelines/documents/gui240CPG1004E.pdf

Society of Obstetricians and Gynaecologists of Canada (SOGC). (2012). Management of varicella infection (chickenpox) in pregnancy. SOGC Clinical Practice Guidelines, No. 274. *Journal of Obstetrics and Gynaecology, 34*(3), 287–292. Retrieved from http://www.sogc.org/guidelines/documents/gui274CPG1203E.pdf

Staroselsky, A., Klieger-Grossmann, C., Garcia-Bournissen, F., & Koren, G. (2009). Exposure to fifth disease in pregnancy. *Canadian Family Physician, 55*(12), 1195–1198.

Steininger, C. (2012). Cytomegalovirus vaccine: Light on the horizon. *The Lancet Infectious Diseases, 12*(4), 257–259.

Tyring, S. K. (1992). Natural history of varicella zoster virus. *Seminars in Dermatology, 11,* 211–217.

U.S. Preventive Services Task Force (USPSTF). (2013). Screening for Hepatitis C Virus Infection in Adults. AHRQ Publication No. 12-05174-EF-2. Retrieved from http://www.uspreventiveservicestaskforce.org/uspstf/uspshepc.htm

Vogel, H., Kornman, M., Ledet, S. C., Rajogopalan, I.., Taber, L., & McClain, K. (1997). Congenital parvovirus infection. *Pediatric Pathology and Laboratory Medicine, 17*(6), 903–912.

White, S. J., Boldt, K. L., Holditch, S. J., Poland, G. A., & Jacobson, R. M. (2012). Measles, mumps, and rubella. *Clinical Obstetrics and Gynecology, 55*(2), 550.

Wood, N., & Isaacs, D. (2012). Hepatitis B vaccination in pregnancy. *Expert Review of Vaccines, 11*(2), 125–127. doi:10.1586/erv.11.185

World Health Organization. (2008). Progress towards eliminating rubella and congenital rubella syndrome in the western hemisphere, 2003–2008. *Weekly Epidemiological Record, 83*(44), 395–400.

World Health Organization. (2011). Rubella vaccines: WHO position paper, No. 29. *Weekly Epidemiological Record, 86*, 301–316.

Young, N. S., & Brown, K. E. (2004). Mechanisms of disease: Parvovirus B19. *New England Journal of Medicine, 350*, 586–597. doi:10 .1056/NEJMra030840

41

Sexually transmitted infections and common vaginitis

Meghan Garland and Barbara P. Brennan

Relevant terms

Antibodies—proteins in the blood produced in reaction to foreign substances, such as bacteria and viruses that cause infection

Chancre—a sore caused by syphilis and appearing at the place of infection

Chlamydia—sexually transmitted infection (STI) caused by infection with *Chlamydia trachomatis* and is the most frequently reported bacterial sexually transmitted infection in the United States

Chorioamnionitis—an acute inflammation of the membranes and chorion of the placenta

Gonorrhea—STI caused by infection with the *Neisseria gonorrhoeae* bacterium; *N. gonorrhoeae* infects the mucous membranes of the reproductive tract and the mucous membranes of the mouth, throat, eyes, and anus

Herpes simplex virus—STI caused by the herpes simplex viruses type 1 (HSV-1) or herpes simplex virus type 2 (HSV-2)

Human papillomavirus (HPV)—genital HPV is the most common STI; there are more than 40 HPV types that can infect male and female genitalia

Pelvic inflammatory disease (PID)—an infection of the uterus, fallopian tubes, and nearby pelvic structures

Sexually transmitted infections (STIs)—also known as sexually transmitted diseases (STDs); these are infections that are spread by sexual contact

Syphilis—STI caused by the bacterium *Treponema pallidum*

Trichomonas—STI with a protozoan parasite called *Trichomonas vaginalis*

Introduction

Five out of the top 10 reportable diseases in the United States are sexually transmitted infections (STIs) (Rompalo, 2011). The nature of human reproduction provides opportunities for the spread of infectious pathogens. Intercourse, birth, and breastfeeding all break down usual physical barriers that protect against infection. Normal changes in maternal immunity during pregnancy increase susceptibility to STIs. There are four major classes of infectious agents: bacterial, viral, fungal, and parasitic. Reproductive health can be adversely affected by any of these. Infectious disease has been implicated in many pregnancy complications including spontaneous abortion, birth defects, fetal infection, premature rupture of membranes, preterm birth, growth

restriction, perinatal mortality, intrapartum infection, cesarean birth, and postpartum infection.

Infection and inflammation are strongly associated with preterm birth. Up to 75% of placentas from preterm births demonstrate evidence of chorioamnionitis and up to 90% of preterm births prior to 24 weeks show histological evidence of chorioamnionitis (Baecher-Lind, Miller, & Wilcox, 2009). The mechanisms that lead from infection to preterm birth are not fully understood; however, inflammation is believed to play a significant role. Bacterial infection of the amniotic membranes, amniotic fluid, or placenta causes increased prostaglandin production. Prostaglandins are associated with increased uterine activity, cervical softening, and dilation that may ultimately result in preterm labor and birth. A positive feedback loop perpetuates prostaglandin

Prenatal and Postnatal Care: A Woman-Centered Approach, First Edition. Edited by Robin G. Jordan, Janet L. Engstrom, Julie A. Marfell, and Cindy L. Farley.

formation through a diffuse inflammatory response; a cascade of cytokines and interleukins encourages more prostaglandin release. However, clinical trials of antibiotic treatment in women at high risk for preterm birth have not consistently demonstrated efficacy and some clinical trials have suggested harm.

Pregnancy is a frequent point of entry into the healthcare system and screening for STI is a routine part of prenatal care. This chapter will review STIs including chlamydia, gonorrhea, syphilis, herpes simplex virus (HSV), human papillomavirus (HPV), and trichomonas. Human immunodeficiency virus (HIV/AIDS) is covered in Chapter 40, "Infectious Diseases." Bacterial vaginosis (BV) and candida vaginitis are common vaginal conditions in pregnancy and are covered in this chapter.

Sexually transmitted bacterial infections

Chlamydia trachomatis

Chlamydia is a largely asymptomatic sexually transmitted infection. Women presenting with symptoms report vaginal discharge, postcoital bleeding, dysuria, and vague lower abdominal pain. Mucopurulent cervical discharge and tenderness on bimanual exam are common. Numerous white blood cells may be noted on wet mount, though this is not diagnostic.

The greatest disease burden is among adolescents and young adults. The rate of chlamydia infection among African American women is eight times greater than Caucasian women (Wiehe, Roseman, Wang, Katz, & Fortenberry, 2011). *C. trachomatis* has been associated with an increased risk of preterm birth and premature rupture of membranes. Past infection may destroy tubal cilia and may lead to fibrosis of the fallopian tubes, resulting in ectopic pregnancy. Chlamydial infection is thought to account for half of all tubal pregnancies worldwide (Baecher-Lind et al., 2009). It can also lead to neonatal conjunctivitis and pneumonia. Generally, neonatal infection is associated with vaginal birth but may also occur following cesarean birth especially after prolonged rupture of membranes. Women with active chlamydial infection at the time of vaginal birth have a 50–75% chance of passing the infection to the neonate (Baecher-Lind et al., 2009).

Pregnancy testing and treatment

Pregnant women should be screened for chlamydia at the first prenatal visit. Nucleic acid hybridization testing (NATTs) with an endocervical swab is sensitive and specific. Urine testing can also be done. Women who are at high risk for chlamydia, including those whose age is less than 25 years, and those with new sexual partners or multiple partners, should be retested in the third

trimester. Women who test positive at the first prenatal visit should be retested 3–6 months later, preferably in the third trimester (CDC, 2010).

Preferred treatment in pregnancy is 1 g azithromycin as a one-dose treatment or amoxicillin 500 mg three times daily for 7 days. Alternative regimens include erythromycin base 500 mg four times daily for 4 days or erythromycin ethylsuccinate 800 mg four times daily for 7 days. Partners should receive testing for chlamydia, gonorrhea, and HIV, as well as treatment if positive. Partners should abstain from sexual contact until 7 days after completion of antibiotic therapy.

Neisseria gonorrhoeae

Like chlamydia, gonorrhea may be asymptomatic. Women presenting with symptoms report vaginal discharge, dysuria, urinary frequency, and tenderness in the area of Bartholin's or Skene's glands and lower abdominal tenderness. Mucopurulent discharge and tenderness on abdominal exam may be noted.

Gonorrhea is associated with preterm birth in a limited number of studies. It has also been linked to fetal growth restriction in populations with high rates of infection (Baecher-Lind et al., 2009). Past infection is also associated with ectopic pregnancy. Gonorrhea is transmitted from mother to baby during vaginal birth at rates of 30–50% (Baecher-Lind et al., 2009). The neonatal conjunctiva is the most common site of infection. Other neonatal manifestations include polyarticular arthritis, gonococcemia, and genital infection. In the United States, routine screening for chlamydia and gonorrhea and routine newborn erythromycin eye prophylaxis have dramatically decreased neonatal ophthalmic infection.

Pregnancy testing and treatment

All women should be tested for gonorrhea at the first prenatal visit by endocervical swab. Concurrent chlamydia is typically tested by the same sample with the NATT test as these infections have similar presentations and persons affected by one pathogen may be infected with the other. For women testing positive, a repeat test should be performed 3–6 months later, preferably in the third trimester (CDC, 2010). Unaffected women should be retested in the third trimester if risk factors such as age less than 25 years, infection with another sexually transmitted disease (STD), previous gonorrhea infection, new sexual partner, multiple partners, drug use, inconsistent condom use, or employment as a commercial sex worker are present. Because these infections have similar presentations and persons affected by one pathogen may be infected with the other chlamydia and gonorrhea, testing should be obtained concurrently.

Pregnant women should be treated with 250 mg ceftriaxone intramuscularly *and* 1 g azithromycin orally. If allergy prevents cephalosporin administration, 2 g of azithromycin orally is the alternative. Partners should be tested for chlamydia and HIV and receive treatment as outlined previously, and both partners should abstain until 7 days after treatment.

Syphilis

Syphilis is caused by the gram-negative spirochete bacterium *Treponema palladium*. After decades of decline due to the discovery of penicillin, syphilis has reemerged as a worldwide health threat. The incidence of syphilis has nearly doubled in the United States since 2000 (Aadland, Finnoff, & Huang, 2012), with the highest increases seen in black men.

Primary syphilis presents as a painless ulcer with that has a raised, indurated border found at the site of infection, usually the genitals. It resolves spontaneously in 3–6 weeks. Infected women may be unaware of lesions especially inside the vagina or on the cervix. Secondary syphilis presents within weeks or months of the primary phase. It is a systemic disease characterized by a maculopapular rash especially on the palms, soles, and mucous membranes. Andenopathy, fever, anorexia, weight loss, and flesh-colored genital lesions called condylomata lata that are highly infectious may also be present. Symptoms resolve spontaneously in 2–6 weeks. Tertiary syphilis is a rare complication characterized by gummatous lesions, aortic aneurysm, seizures, and dementia. Recognizing how syphilis presents clinically and understanding how it moves from latent to active infection can be challenging even for experienced clinicians. It does not always move through consecutive clinical stages, and a person with secondary or tertiary syphilis may present with no recollection of prior symptoms. Women testing positive for syphilis should be tested for other STIs including HIV, hepatitis B, and hepatitis C.

Syphilis easily crosses the placenta and is devastating to the developing fetus. Congenital syphilis can affect any organ system but is often associated with infections of the bone, brain, heart, lungs, and abdominal organs. It is the leading cause of stillbirth and neonatal death in the developing world (Rompalo, 2011). Neonatal acquisition is most likely within the first 4 years after acquisition when the spread of spirochetes through the blood is most likely if the infection is not sufficiently treated. Approximately 1 million pregnancies are affected worldwide by syphilis annually with nearly half ending in miscarriage or neonatal death, one-quarter ending in preterm birth, and one-quarter of neonates acquiring congenital syphilis (Baecher-Lind et al., 2009).

Pregnancy testing and treatment

A serological test for syphilis should be performed at the first prenatal visit. Some states and areas where syphilis is more common require repeat testing after 28 weeks of gestation and/or upon admission for labor (CDC, 2010). Syphilis is unique among STIs as it cannot be cultured or genetically manipulated (Rompalo, 2011). Commercially available diagnostic serological tests for syphilis measure IgG and IgM antibodies. Current tests are unable to distinguish between recent or remote infections or among the various stages of infection. Women who present with symptoms of syphilis can be tested using dark field microscopy. Samples should contain exudates or tissue for most accurate results.

Because of the inability to culture *T. palladium*, antibiotic sensitivities have never been done. Treatment recommendation for parenteral penicillin is based on past treatment success as defined by clinical resolution of symptoms and prevention of sexual transmission (Rompalo, 2011) (Table 41.1). Pregnant women who are penicillin allergic should have skin testing to confirm allergy. If true allergy exists, the woman should undergo desensitization therapy prior to treatment. No alternative to penicillin treatment is considered adequate in pregnancy.

Sexually transmitted viral infections

Herpes simplex

HSV is one of the most prevalent STDs, affecting more than one in six people aged 14–49 years (CDC, 2012). The HSV viruses are similar to the viruses that cause varicella zoster shingles. After an initial infection, the virus moves to nerve cells where they remain until a recurrence is triggered. Infected persons may transmit the infection during periods of asymptomatic viral shedding. Most infected persons are not aware of their infection. HSV may present as genital or rectal sores accompanied by one or more of the following: pruritis, pain, burning, edema, dysuria, myalgia, headache, and fever. Subsequent outbreaks tend to be mild and have

Table 41.1   Syphilis Treatments in Pregnancy

Primary and secondary syphilis	Benzathine penicillin G 2.4 million unit single dose
Early latent syphilis	Benzathine penicillin G 2.4 million unit single dose
Late latent syphilis or syphilis of unknown duration	Benzathine penicillin G 2.4 million units once weekly for 3 weeks

Table 41.2 Classification of Genital HSV Infections

Clinical designation	Description
Primary genital HSV infection	Newly acquired antibodies to HSV-1 or 2 in the absence of preexisting antibodies
Nonprimary first-episode genital HSV infection	Newly acquired antibodies to HSV-1 or 2 in the presence of preexisting antibodies to the other type
Recurrent genital HSV infection	Reactivation of genital HSV with HSV type recovered from the lesion the same as serum HSV type

Adapted from: Westhoff, G. L., Little, S. E., & Caughey, A. B. (2011). Herpes simplex virus and pregnancy: A review of the management of antenatal and peripartum herpes infections. *Obstetrical & Gynecological Survey, 66*(10), 629–638.

fewer systemic symptoms. Lesions or vesicles may be noted on inspection and tender inguinal lymph nodes may be present.

Classification of genital HSV infection can be divided into three categories: primary, nonprimary first episode, or recurrent (Table 41.2). The incidence of primary HSV infection during pregnancy is thought to be between 0.5% and 2% (Baecher-Lind et al., 2009). There are multiple strains of herpes simplex viruses type 2 (HSV-2) and infection with one does not confer immunity to other strains of HSV-2.

Fetal infection is associated with recent maternal primary HSV infection, prolonged rupture of membranes, or disruption of fetal skin or mucous membranes during labor or birth. Fetal infection can occur *in utero* by transmission of the virus through the placenta. Fetal infection from transplacental HSV is called congenital herpes, and neonatal infection acquired during birth is called neonatal herpes. Intrauterine infection is associated with spontaneous abortion and stillbirth as well as neurological damage, congenital cataracts, and skin vesicles. About 30% of neonates with disseminated disease will die (Baecher-Lind et al., 2009).

Approximately 75% of pregnant women infected with HSV experience a recurrence during pregnancy (Baecher-Lind et al., 2009). It is helpful to correctly classify the type of HSV infection to effectively counsel women about the risk of vertical transmission. However, this is not necessarily easy especially in populations with limited health-care resources.

Primary HSV infection may be asymptomatic, minor, or severe. Generally, symptomatic primary HSV infections have an incubation period of about 4 days and lesions may occur 2–12 days after exposure. Primary

lesions tend to be larger, more numerous, pustular, ulcerating, and bilateral as compared to nonrecurrent primary or recurrent infections. Lesions generally disappear after 3 weeks. Most women with symptomatic primary infection also present with systemic symptoms including fever, headache, malaise, and myalgia. Severe cases of primary HSV infection may include aseptic meningitis, distant skin lesions, urinary retention secondary to autonomic sacral nerve dysfunction, and rarely, systemic infection may lead to encephalitis or hepatitis. Occasionally disseminated disease may be confused with HELLP syndrome due to hepatic dysfunction and abdominal tenderness.

Non-primary, first-episode infection occurs most frequently when a person has a newly acquired HSV-2 infection in the presence of a pre-existing herpes simplex viruses type 1 (HSV-1) infection. HSV-1 antibodies can be partially protective against HSV-2. Conversely, HSV-2 antibodies are highly protective against new HSV-1 infection (Westhoff, Little, & Caughey, 2011) making nonprimary first epidode infection with HSV-1 very unlikely. Non-primary first-episode infections tend to have fewer systemic symptoms, less pain, a shorter period of viral shedding, and a more rapid resolution of symptoms.

Recurrent genital infections are more common with HSV-2 than with HSV-1. Women with HSV-2 have an average of four recurrences in the first year after infection compared to one recurrence for women infected with HSV-1 (Hollier & Wendel, 2008). Recurrent infections are typically less severe. Prodromal symptoms of tingling, shooting pain, burning, or itching at the site of infection are common. Recurrent infections also tend to be unilateral and have fewer lesions. These lesions may not have the classic vesicular appearance and instead appear as fissures or simply vulvar irritation.

Pregnancy testing and treatment

Pregnant women presenting with symptoms of HSV infection should have serological testing for HSV-1 and HSV-2 IgG and IgM in addition to viral culture, polymerase chain reaction (PCR), or direct antibody fluorescence to identify the subtype of HSV infection (Westhoff et al., 2011). The latter two tests have limited availability. IgG and IgM can help determine whether the episode is primary or recurrent as well as identify the infection subtype to better characterize the risk of vertical transmission. Antibodies to HSV infection develop relatively late, about 2–12 weeks after infection, and cannot be used alone to diagnose acute infection.

The mainstays of antenatal treatment for HSV are famicyclovir, acyclovir, and valacyclovir (Table 41.3). All are category B medications and are not associated with

Table 41.3   Recommended Treatments for HSV Outbreaks in Pregnancy

Indication	Drug	Dosage	Duration	Alternative
Primary infection	Acyclovir	400 mg TID	7–10 days	200 mg five times daily
	Valacyclovir	1000 mg BID	7–14 days	
	Famciclovir	400 mg TID	7–14 days or until lesions disappear	
Recurrent disease	Acyclovir	400 mg TID	5 days	200 mg five times daily or
	Valacyclovir	500 mg BID	3 days	800 mg BID for 5 days or
	Famciclovir	250 mg BID	5 days	1000 mg daily for 5 days
Severe disease	Acyclovir	5–10 mg/kg IV Q 8h	2–7 days or until clinical improvement followed by oral acyclovir for a total of 10 treatment days	

Adapted from: Westhoff, G. L., Little, S. E., & Caughey, A. B. (2011). Herpes simplex virus and pregnancy: A review of the management of antenatal and peripartum herpes infections. *Obstetrical & Gynecological Survey, 66*(10), 629–638.

adverse neonatal or fetal effects. All three are considered safe in the first trimester. Suppressive therapy using the same medications for women with primary or recurrent HSV starting at 36 weeks of pregnancy has proven effective in reducing the risk of HSV recurrence at the time of labor (ACOG, 2007). Women with one or more genital HSV outbreaks during pregnancy should begin suppressive therapy starting at 36 weeks. Clinical data are lacking for those women with a history of nonrecurrent genital HSV and no outbreaks in the current pregnancy. Suppressive therapy regimen can be used for these women and is believed to be cost-effective.

The primary goal of prenatal and intrapartum care for women with a history of genital HSV infection is to prevent transmission to the neonate. About 14% of women with HSV will present in labor with either clinical signs of HSV or report prodromal symptoms (Hollier & Wendel, 2008). Maternal transmission is thought to be almost exclusively through contact with virus containing vaginal secretions during birth, although *in utero* and postnatal infection may occur rarely (Westhoff et al., 2011). Although much of the effort toward preventing vertical transmission is aimed at women with recurrent HSV-2, this is not the primary etiology of the estimated 1500 cases of neonatal HSV infection that occur annually in the United States (Westhoff et al., 2011). It is thought that <1% of neonatal infection is due to recurrent HSV-2 and this suggests a very protective role for maternal antibodies.

The greatest risk of vertical transmission is for seronegative women who contract either HSV-1 or HSV-2 near term. In this population, the risk of transmission is estimated between 20% and 50%. Infection with HSV-1 (either primary or recurrent) appears to be more easily transmitted to the neonate than HSV-2 (Westhoff et al., 2011). Other risks for HSV transmission during birth

include internal fetal monitoring, birth prior to 38 weeks' gestation, HSV isolated from the cervix, and maternal age less than 21.

When women with a history of HSV infection present in labor, a careful examination of the vulva, vagina, and cervix should be performed and a detailed history of the presence of prodromal symptoms should be obtained. Women presenting with lesions near but not on the genital area (such as the buttocks) should birth vaginally, and an occlusive dressing over the site is recommended. Asymptomatic viral shedding at the time of birth has been a concern; however, studies of PCR testing in labor to screen for this have failed to demonstrate a health or cost benefit (Westhoff et al., 2011).

Pregnant women at term or in labor with active lesions or prodromal symptoms such as vulvar pain or burning should have a cesarean section to reduce the risk of neonatal transmission. No studies have demonstrated a benefit of cesarean birth for women with recurrent HSV, but the benefit is inferred from broader studies (Westhoff et al., 2011). More research is needed to determine the actual risk to the neonate from recurrent HSV-2. It may be that the risks associated with cesarean birth outweigh the risks of vaginal birth if the risk of transmission is very low.

Human papillomavirus

HPV is prevalent among sexually active adults. The prevalence of HPV is 35% in women age 14–19, 29% in women 20–30, and between 6% and 11% in women 30–65 years old (Lacour & Trimble, 2012). HPV is often subclinical and asymptomatic, although some women may experience pruritis or pain associated with genital warts.

Tiny abrasions in surface epithelium allow HPV to infect the basal layer of squamous epithelial cells. The squamocolumnar junction of the cervix and the oropharynx are also targets. There are five phases of the HPV life cycle: infection and uncoating, proliferation, genomic phase, viral synthesis, and shedding. Another possible phase is latency. After initial infection, the host immune system may induce a regression in the life cycle and the virus remains latent in the basal epithelium. Although nonsexual transmission is possible, the primary mechanism of infection is through sexual contact. Oral lesions in young children are primarily caused by HPV 6 and 11 contracted at the time of birth (Lacour & Trimble, 2012).

Approximately 30–40% of pregnant women harbor HPV DNA (Baecher-Lind et al., 2009). Coinfection with multiple HPV strains is common (Koskimaa et al., 2012). Genital warts may appear and become larger and more numerous during pregnancy. This may be due to altered maternal immunity associated with pregnancy as well as high levels of estrogen and progesterone. Neonatal acquisition of HPV types associated with genital warts may result from aspiration of genital tract secretions during birth and may result in laryngeal papillomatosis. However, cesarean birth is not recommended because a high proportion of babies birthed by cesarean also demonstrate HPV infection.

There are contradictory data about the rate of vertical transmission, ranging from 1% to 80%. This is largely due to differences in study methodology. Most studies place the rate of transmission between 16% and 69% (Koskimaa et al., 2012). Several mechanisms of vertical transmission have been proposed but are not well understood (Lacour & Trimble, 2012). HPV DNA has been isolated from the vas deferens, seminal fluid, and sperm. In studies of mother–baby pairs, HPV DNA concordance is nearly perfect. However, this concordance starts to diverge just 3 days after birth (Koskimaa et al., 2012). Prenatal transmission is suspected because infants have been born with condyloma and HPV DNA has been isolated from amniotic fluid prior to rupture of membranes. This suggests ascending infection rather than transplacental infection. HPV can also be transmitted after birth during bathing and diapering.

Pregnancy testing and treatment

Generally, diagnosis is made after clinical observation of genital warts. They are typically flesh colored and may be flat or raised, or have a cauliflower-like appearance. Treatment is not medically necessary during pregnancy and complete resolution may not be possible until after pregnancy due to changes in maternal immunity and the presence of increased estrogen. If treatment is desired, once weekly application of 80–90% tricholoacetic acid (TCA) or bichloroacetic acid (BCA) may clear lesions especially in the second half of pregnancy. The acid is applied directly to the lesion until a frosted white appearance is obtained. Petroleum or lidocaine jelly can be applied to the surrounding healthy tissue to prevent injury to healthy tissue. Excessive acid application can be neutralized with soap or bicarbonate. Weekly treatments can be repeated until the lesions resolve. The presence of HPV at birth is not an indication for cesarean birth unless the lesions are obstructive.

Fungal infection

Vaginal candidiasis

Candidiasis is a common concern during pregnancy. Women may present with a thick, white discharge, dysuria, vaginal soreness, and pruritis. On exam, the vulva may appear edematous and red. Excoriation and fissures may also be present. Discharge may be scant or copious and adherent or may have a curdled appearance. Foul or fishy odor is not a defining characteristic of this disorder. Diagnosis is made by observation of candidiasis hyphae and buds, which appear as long, translucent strands on wet mount with 10% potassium hydroxide solution. Vaginal ph should be normal (less than 4.5). Candidiasis can also be cultured. Recommended treatment during pregnancy is a 5 g, seven-night course of vaginal Clotrimazole 1% or miconazole 1% cream. Other acceptable methods include prescription terconazole 0.4% 5 g intravaginally each night for seven nights.

Candidiasis colonization rates during pregnancy are approximately 40%, roughly twice that of nonpregnant women. This may be due to increased levels of estrogen and progesterone. There is some evidence that treating cadidiasis in pregnancy may be associated with decreased rates of preterm birth and late miscarriage (Hay & Czeizel, 2007). *Candida* itself is unlikely to be directly responsible for poor pregnancy outcomes. The effect of *Candida* on vaginal flora may provide an indirect contribution to these adverse effects through its role in creating an environment conducive to BV development.

Sexually transmitted parasitic infection

Trichomonas vaginalis

T. vaginalis is a very common parasitic infection of the lower genital tract. Women may be asymptomatic or conversely present with intensely symptomatic vaginitis with profuse purulent discharge that is white, yellow, green, or frothy. Puritis, burning, postcoital bleeding, urinary frequency, or dysuria may be present. The external genitalia and vagina may appear red, inflamed, and excoriated from scratching. The cervix may be friable and petichiae may be observed. The pelvis and abdomen may be tender, and tender inguinal lymph nodes may also be noted.

Trichomonas can reliably be detected on a saline slide 40–80% of the time compared to culture, generally through observation of motile organisms. Cervical cytology also detects trichomonas 60–70% of the time compared to culture. Most strains of *T. vaginalis* are susceptible to metronidazole. More than 90% of women will be cured by a single 2 g dose or 400 mg twice daily for 5 days. Tindazole 2 g can also be used. The sexual partners of infected women should be screened for STI and treated for trichomonas with the same regimen of antibiotics.

T. vaginalis is associated with adverse pregnancy outcomes including premature rupture of membranes, preterm birth, and low birth weight. Vertical transmission is thought to occur in about 5% of pregnancies. Most cases of neonatal infection resolve within 1 month after birth without treatment. Paradoxically, treatment for *T. vaginalis* during pregnancy may be associated with an increase in the rate of preterm birth (Hay & Czeizel, 2007). Current consensus is that symptomatic women and their partners should be treated to relieve suffering, though it remains unclear if this course of action prevents or promotes preterm birth.

Practice points

- Symptomatic trichomoniasis or candidiasis in pregnancy should be treated adequately.
- Although trichomoniasis is associated with preterm birth, the role of treatment in reducing this risk is not yet established and may even be harmful.
- Routine screening for and treatment of vaginal colonization by trichomoniasis or candidal species is not recommended.

Sexually transmitted bacterial infection

Bacterial vaginosis

BV is the most common lower genital tract disorder among both pregnant and nonpregnant women of reproductive age, affecting 15–30% of nonpregnant women and an estimated 20–50% of pregnant women (Laxmi, Agrwal, Raghunandan, Randhawa, & Saili, 2012). In-office diagnosis can be made using Amstel's criteria. BV is clinically described as a homogenous grayish-white discharge, bacterial overgrowth, pH > 4.5, and an amine "fish" odor released when vaginal dis-

charge is treated with 10% potassium hydroxide solution (KOH). A defining criteria is the presence of "clue cells," with greater than 20% of vaginal epithelial cells with such a heavy coating of bacteria that the peripheral borders are obscured. A minimum of three of the four criteria must be met to make a diagnosis of BV. Women symptomatic for BV may report an increase in white discharge with a strong "fishy" odor. These symptoms are often only noticeable or worsen after intercourse.

Amstel criteria

- An adherent and homogenous vaginal discharge
- Vaginal ph greater than 4.5
- Detection of clue cells (vaginal epithelial cells with such a heavy coating of bacteria that the edges are obscured) on wet mount
- An amine odor after the addition of potassium hydroxide (positive whiff test)

BV is associated with increased risk for acquiring STIs including HIV and developing pelvic inflammatory disease (PID). It has also been implicated as a causal factor for preterm birth premature rupture of membranes and spontaneous abortion. Multiple behaviors and demographic factors have been associated with BV including douching, frequent intercourse, female receptive oral sex, use of vaginal products, as well as low socioeconomic status. The African American race is associated with a threefold risk of developing BV compared to the Caucasian race (Denney & Culhane, 2009).

The alteration in the composition in vaginal flora from an acidic one predominated by lactobacilli to a basic one predominated by other bacterial species is thought to produce irritating symptoms and to trigger the mucosal immune system. The immune reaction to altered vaginal microflora is considered the triggering mechanism for adverse pregnancy outcomes. It is theorized that a genetic predisposition to mount a pathological inflammatory response in the presence of BV may contribute to adverse pregnancy outcomes (Denney & Culhane, 2009). Lactobacilli may play a protective role in preventing the inflammatory response that leads to intrauterine infection and related perinatal sequel (Denney & Culhane, 2009).

Pregnancy testing and treatment

The laboratory method of diagnosing BV is called Nugent score. The Nugent score (Table 41.4) looks at Gram-stained samples of vaginal secretions and rates

Table 41.4   Nugent Scoring System for Gram-Stained Vaginal Smears

Score	Lactobacillus morphotypes	Gardnerella and Bacteroides spp. morphotypes	Curved gram-variable rods
0	4+	0	0
1	3+	1+	1+
2	2+	2+	2+
3	1+	3+	3+
4	0	4+	4+

several characteristics including presence or relative absence of lactobacilli associated with vaginal health, plus the number of curved gram-variable rods and *Bacteriodes* species morphotypes such as *Mobiluncus* spp., *Gardnerella vaginalis*, *Mycoplasma hominis*, and *Peptostreptococcus* spp. Each item is scored on a scale of 0–4 depending on the frequency of observation. A final Nugent score of 0–12 is assigned. A score of 0–3 is considered negative, 4–6 is considered intermediate or partial BV, and 7–12 is considered positive for BV (Anderson et al., 2011).

BV is treated with oral metronidazole 500 mg twice daily for a week. Clindamycin 300 mg orally twice daily is also acceptable. Vaginal medication is equally effective in relieving symptoms but has not demonstrated efficacy in reducing preterm birth. Systemic treatment may be needed to eradicate vaginosis-associated bacteria from both the upper and lower genital tract to prevent adverse pregnancy outcomes (Yudin & Money, 2008). Metronidazole is not teratogenic or mutagenic and is considered safe for use in pregnancy.

Evidence is conflicting on benefits of BV screening in pregnant women before 20 weeks gestation. Meta-analysis and reviews have not demonstrated that treatment of low-risk pregnancies decreases risk of preterm birth and is not recommended (Iams, Romero, Culhane, & Goldenberg, 2008; Sangkomkamhang, Lumbiganon, Prasertcharoensook, & Laopaiboon, 2009). Some reports suggested that harm may be associated with treating asymptomatic women, especially those of low risk (Laxmi et al., 2012; Nygren et al., 2008; Simcox, Wing-To, Seed, Briley, & Shennan, 2007). Harm may also be associated with antibiotic resistance and disruption of vaginal flora (Simcox et al., 2007). It is theorized that antibiotics that are not selective microbicides produce alteration of vaginal flora, specifically loss of lactobacilli, which may encourage the growth of more pathological bacteria.

BV as an ecological disorder

Donders et al. (2009) describes BV an "ecological disorder" where lactobacilli are replaced by large numbers of bacteriodes. Abnormal vaginal flora is described as any condition that is characterized by a lack of lactobacilli in the absence of other diagnostic criteria for BV or other infections such as chlamydia or gonorrhea. Aerobic vaginitis is described as the replacement of lactobacilli and infection of the parabasal cells by intestinal microflora such as *Escherichia coli*, enterococci, and group B *Streptococcus*. Aerobic vaginitis presents clinically as inflamed vaginal mucosa, sticky yellowish discharge, pH > 6, and a foul (not fishy) odor. Severe symptoms are rarely seen in pregnancy, but less severe forms may be encountered. Both abnormal vaginal flora and aerobic vaginitis would have intermediate Nugent scores of 4–6 and meet some but not all Amstel criteria for diagnosis of BV.

Women with normal vaginal flora have a 75% decrease in the risk of preterm birth before 35 weeks compared to women with abnormal vaginal floras (Donders et al. 2009). The risk of preterm birth is elevated in women with ecological disorders marked by the absence of lactobacilli and the presence of mixed flora with relatively few clue cells (partial BV).

BV is often a chronic condition characterized by short-term relief of symptoms after appropriate antibiotic treatment, only to have bothersome symptoms return in weeks or months. Metronidazole efficiently kills anaerobic bacteria but not aerobic bacteria. Intermediate BV may be primarily composed of aerobic bacteria. This observation may explain why some studies have failed to demonstrate that metronidazole treatment of BV in pregnancy reduces preterm birth and premature rupture of membranes.

The vagina is a unique microenvironment that is poorly understood. It is complex and dynamic. The vast majority of women are colonized by gram-negative rods and cocci as well as several species of anaerobic and as yet unnamed bacteria (Rompalo, 2011). It is believed that a healthy vaginal floral composition is more than 95% lactobacilli. The vaginal microbiome is affected by hormonal changes throughout the reproductive years and during pregnancy. Hydrogen peroxide producing *Lactobacillus* species are believed to be very important in maintaining an acidic environment that controls bacterial counts. BV is associated with a loss of lactic acid producing bacteria and an overgrowth of anaerobic bacteria. There is limited knowledge of the fluctuations and composition of the vaginal microbiome. It is not yet understood how protective vaginal microbes are maintained or how shifts in composition increase susceptibility to adverse health outcomes (Rompalo, 2011).

BV practice points

- BV, especially when found early in pregnancy, is associated with late miscarriage, preterm premature rupture of membrane (PPROM), preterm labor (PTL), preterm birth (PTB), chorioamnionitis, and postpartum endometriosis.
- Administering antibiotics to women with asymptomatic BV does not improve obstetric outcomes but may reduce late miscarriage rates.
- BV spontaneously resolves in approximately 50% of pregnant women.
- Mainstay treatment for symptomatic BV is metronidazole or clindamycin.
- Women with symptomatic BV should be considered at an increased risk of poor obstetric outcomes.
- Treatment of women with symptomatic BV may result in reducing the risk of adverse pregnancy outcomes.
- Condom use may be protective.
- Women with BV should be counseled about the increased risk of contracting STIs.
- BV is not considered an STI but is most common in sexually active women.

Partner treatment of an STI

Data are limited whether partner notification decreases the STI exposure or if it reduces the community burden of these infections (CDC, 2010). However, partner treatment reduces the risk of reinfection. The importance of partner notification should be discussed and specific community resources for partner testing and treatment provided. Encouraging women to bring their partners to the office to discuss diagnosis and treatment may provide an opportunity for counseling about the diagnosis, treatment, and preventing reinfection.

For women who indicate that their partner is unlikely to seek treatment, the Centers for Disease Control and Prevention (CDC) recommends patient-delivered partner therapy (PDPT) by providing multiple prescriptions to the woman, one for herself and for her partner(s). This is a form of expedited partner therapy (EPT), when treatment is given without diagnosis or counseling. EPT is legal in most states and prohibited in others, making it important for midwives and nurse practitioners to be aware of state EPT regulations.

Legal requirements for reporting STI diagnosis

Accurate and timely reporting of STI infections helps public health departments to assess trends, notify partners, and allocate precious resources wisely. Reportable diseases vary somewhat from state to state. Syphilis, gonorrhea, chlamydia, HIV/AIDS, and chancroid are reportable in every state. Nurse practitioners and midwives should be aware of reporting requirements where they practice. Local and state health departments are able to provide information on reporting requirements. STI reporting can be initiated by either the laboratory where the STI was identified or by the clinician receiving the STI diagnostic report.

Psychosocial impacts of STI diagnosis

Effects on the individual

Diagnosis of sexually transmitted infections has profound impacts on an individual's concept of self and how she relates to others in her social support network, family, and relationships. It is not unusual for a woman to be diagnosed for the first time with an STI during pregnancy, causing significant maternal concern and guilt regarding fetal health.

Regardless of the nature of the infection, either bacterial, which can be "cured" with antibiotics, or viral infection, which may linger in the body for years or perhaps a lifetime, the impact of diagnosis alters a person's self-image from that point forward. Newer testing modalities such as serological testing for HSV-1 and HSV-2 and HPV DNA testing mean more women are being diagnosed with sexually transmitted infections in the absence of symptoms. Additionally, the absence of symptoms and variable latency periods, sometimes lasting years, means that very little information can be given to women about when or how they contracted an infection.

Surprise and denial are common short-term reactions to STI diagnosis after serological testing in the absence of clinical symptoms Confusion about the meaning of STI diagnosis is also frequently expressed because of the lack of symptoms.

The stigma associated with contracting an STI is significant for many women (Duncan, Hart, Scoular, & Bigrigg, 2001). Long-term reactions include feeling like "damaged goods." Women report negative impacts on their sexual relationships. Pregnant women and women with children also express fear of transmitting the infection to their fetus or other children (Melville et al., 2003). For women currently pregnant, their primary concern is preventing transmission to their baby and this remains true throughout pregnancy. Feelings of shock, denial, self-disgust, anxiety and fear of rejection by her partner, and concerns about future reproductive health are also common. Anger toward the individual believed to have infected them and feelings of guilt for possibly transmitting the infection to others are often present (Melville et al., 2003).

STI diagnosis can strongly impact an individual's feeling of sexuality and desirability. This can range from feelings of being unworthy of attention from intimate partners to complete cessation of sexual activity (Newton & McCabe, 2008). Disclosure of STI status is fraught with anxiety and fear. The initial reaction of intimate partners may have long-term consequences on individual coping and the likelihood of individual disclosure of STI status to future intimate partners (Newton & McCabe, 2005).

These emotional aspects of STI care should be addressed. Nurse practitioners and midwives counseling women newly diagnosed can address the common nature of the STIs to help reduce feelings of stigma and isolation. Clarifying misinformation about STIs and providing resources for women to learn how to cope with infection are essential elements of care.

Discussing STI diagnosis

- Avoid using medical jargon.
- Tailor counseling to the woman's literacy level.
- Take time to listen to her questions and concerns.
- Provide consumer-friendly handouts in addition to basic facts.
- Limit the amount of information given at the time of diagnosis.
- Ask her to describe in her own words her understanding of the diagnosis to evaluate comprehension.
- Use a respectful, caring, and sensitive approach.
- Provide telephone access for follow-up questions.

Adapted from: Bertram, C., & Magnussen, L. (2008). Informational needs and the experiences of women with abnormal Papanicolaou smears.

STI prevention within relationships

Studies of adult heterosexual couples demonstrate discordance between perception of monogamy and the practice of monogamy. There is a clear association between lack of awareness regarding a partner's nonmonogamy and acquisition of sexually transmitted infection. This is particularly true for women who believe they are in a monogamous relationship, but in reality, their partner is involved in other sexual relationships. Studies of concordance in heterosexual couples suggest that between 3% and 48% of women are unaware that their sexual partner has concurrent sexual partners (Eyre, Flythe, Hoffman, & Fraser, 2012; Witte, El-Bassel, Gilbert, Wu, & Chang, 2010), and 10% of women in monogamous relationships are unaware that their partner had been diagnosed with an STI in the previous 90 days (Witte et al., 2010). This lack of awareness can create a false estimate of STI acquisition risk. In the office setting, creating a safe place for couples to discuss STI diagnosis may help with disclosure and allow appropriate treatment and prevention strategies to be discussed.

These issues and others are felt even more keenly by women in abusive relationships. Estimates of intimate partner violence (IPV) during pregnancy range from 0.9% to 20%. Pregnancy may also be viewed by the abuser as a means of increasing dependence, and episodes of IPV may increase or decrease (Humphreys, 2011). Women experiencing IPV are at greater risk of contracting an STI through a combination of lack of control over sexual encounters and a lack of knowledge about STI transmission. It is incumbent on health-care providers to not assume that women with formal educations also have adequate knowledge about STIs, contraception, or IPV (Humphreys, 2011). Women in abusive relationships may place themselves in jeopardy of further violence if they suggest condom use or avoid sex as a method of STI prevention.

Adolescents, especially those involved with the father of their children, use condoms inconsistently or not at all to protect themselves from sexually transmitted infection (Kershaw et al., 2010). Using no contraception or withdrawal is common (Hensel & Fortenberry, 2011). Adolescents are less likely to use condoms with partners who are older or who they consider a trusted intimate partner (Foulkes, Petttigrew, Liningston, & Niccolai, 2009). This is despite the fact that studies of adolescent women who reported they were in monogamous relationships were unaware that their male partner had other concurrent sexual relationships 37% of the time (Witte et al., 2010). Diagnosis of an STI appears to have no effect on this behavior. Hensel and Fortenberry (2011) suggest that counseling for adolescent mothers diagnosed with STIs needs to be tailored to include information to dispel myths about future susceptibility to reinfection or new infections. Young women need information about how to integrate condoms into sexual practices as well as strengthening condom negotiation skills with her sexual partners.

Eyre et al.'s (2012) qualitative study of African American couples age 19–22 suggest a framework for counseling couples after STI diagnosis to reduce risk of reinfection or new STI acquisition. Erye suggests that young adult relationships can be categorized as main relationships and side relationships. Main relationships are characterized by a sense of trust and commitment, foster interpersonal growth and bonding, and frequently involve unprotected sex. Concurrently with the main relationship, side relationships might also exist that may not involve consistent condom use and involve types of sex acts that increase risk for STI acquisition. Often oral and anal sex are part of a side relationship. Because the risk of pregnancy is perceived to be nonexistent, condoms may not be used. Additionally, side partners who wish to supplant the main partner may discourage condom use in order to become pregnant.

Entreaties to use condoms in all sexual encounters do not acknowledge that, although main relationships may not be mutually monogamous, insistence on condoms undermines the characterization of trust implied in the main relationship. Maintenance of an illusion of commitment is important to both partners. Instead, tailoring counseling to acknowledge the relationship dynamics, especially the male partner, may foster consistent condom use in side relationships, thus reducing the risk of STI acquisition by the main partner. Partners work to keep knowledge of side relationships from main partners. STI prevention counseling might be more efficacious if tailored to suggest that consistent condom use for all sex acts with side partners will reduce the risk of the main partner becoming aware of side relationships through prevention of STI acquisition and unintended pregnancy.

CDC (2010) recommends the consistent use of latex male condoms during all types of sex acts as the best method of preventing STI infection. Sex research has focused very little on how male condom use affects sexual experiences. Pleasure is the main reason why people seek out sexual experiences, and reduction in pleasure is one of the main reasons people give for not using male condoms (Graham, 2012). Reduction of pleasure appears to be more important to men than women, but both sexes cite it as a barrier to condom use. Loss of erection for men and difficulty reaching orgasm in men and women can occur with condom use, increasing the likelihood that the male condom will be removed before sex is over (Graham, 2012).

Condom slippage and breakage can also occur (Crosby & Bounse, 2012; Crosby, Milhausen, Yarber, Sanders, & Graham, 2008). These issues may be amenable to teaching the proper application of condoms. Data suggest that incorrect condom use can be as high at 40–50% among users (Shih et al., 2011). Health-care providers routinely teach women to apply other methods of contraception including diaphragms and contraceptive rings, yet often correct use of condoms is not discussed or demonstrated. Health-care providers should be comfortable teaching men and women how to correctly and efficiently apply male condoms. Adding a liberal amount of water-based lubricant both before and during intercourse may relieve condom-associated discomfort.

An often overlooked and forgotten barrier method of contraception and STI protection is the female condom. *In vitro* data on effectiveness suggest lower leak rates than male condoms and the female condom is impermeable to cytomegalovirus (CMV) and HIV. Since the female condom covers the external genitalia as well as the vagina, it may prove useful in preventing transmission of HSV and HPV, though this has not been verified (Gallo, Kilbourne-Brook, & Coffey, 2012). Like male condoms, studies of female condom failures demonstrate a wide range from 2.5% to 25% of acts (Gallo et al., 2012). Lack of provider awareness and inclusion of the female condom among contraceptive barrier methods that also protect against STI also inhibits acceptability.

Female condoms have advantages over male condoms. Female condoms can be used with oil-based lubricants. Male partners do not report decreased sensation as often; some men and women report that the external and internal rings enhance sexual pleasure. Because erection is not required to apply the female condom, it can be placed at any point during sexual activity. Having women practice with pelvic models in the office can dramatically reduce rates of insertion difficulty and device failure (Mantell et al., 2011). Proper training about use of the female condom is the first step toward increasing client awareness and acceptance.

STI prevention strategies

- Screen for domestic violence. Positive screen increases risk of STI acquisition.
- Adolescents and young adults are more likely to have partners outside of the main relationship. Counseling must be tailored to prevent reinfection and new STI acquisition.
- Advising condom use for all sexual encounters may not be an effective strategy for all women.
- Both male and female condoms reduce the risk of STI acquisition when used correctly.
- Clinicians should be comfortable with instructing men and women about the proper use of male and female condoms.
- Penis models and pelvic models for demonstration of condom application should be available in the clinic setting.

Summary

Many STIs pose the risk of a number of adverse pregnancy outcomes including miscarriage, stillbirth, preterm birth, low birth weight, and ophthalmia neonatorum. Effective management is imperative as STIs can be detrimental to both the mother and baby and can result in very costly complications. Risk assessment for STIs should be initiated at the first prenatal visit, and screening protocols during prenatal care should follow current evidence. Drugs selected for treatment should not be contraindicated in pregnant women, should have a high efficacy, and should be well tolerated. National guidelines for the management of STIs during pregnancy are produced and regularly updated by the CDC.

Case study

Cara is a 22-year-old G1P0 who came to the office 5 days ago for her first prenatal visit at 9 weeks' gestation. Her cervical cultures returned positive for chlamydia. Cara was called at home and was informed of the culture results and the need for treatment. Cara expressed concern for her baby, anger at her boyfriend "for infecting her," and wanted to be treated immediately. Cara was further queried about her sexual partners and practices. She states that she is monogamous with her boyfriend, but she knows he has not been, even though he denies other sexual partners. Cara states she can talk with her boyfriend about this even though she is angry with him, and will give him the information about the infection and need for treatment. She was strongly advised to use condoms at each sexual encounter with her boyfriend to prevent reinfection. Cara stated that she would definitely do this. After determining she had no allergies, 1 g azithromycin as a one-dose treatment was called into her pharmacy. The same treatment was called in for her boyfriend as well. Cara was advised that she would be retested at her next visit in 3 weeks to determine if her infection has cleared, and then again 3 months later during her pregnancy and in the last trimester. Cara had no additional questions and stated she would pick up the medication right away. She had her next appointment in 3 weeks.

Resources for health-care providers

CDC information on the legal status of EPT in various states: http://www.cdc.gov/std/ept/legal/default.htm
CDC treatment guidelines for STDs, including treatment during pregnancy: http://www.cdc.gov/std/treatment/2010/

Resource for women and partners

CDC Fact Sheets for consumers on pregnancy and specific STIs: http://www.cdc.gov/std/healthcomm/fact_sheets.htm

References

Aadland, D., Finnoff, D., & Huang, K. X. (2013). *The equilibrium dynamics of economic epidemiology* (No. 13-00003). Vanderbilt University Department of Economics.

ACOG. (2007). Management of herpes in pregnancy. ACOG Practice Bulletin. *Obstetrics & Gynecology, 109*(6), 1489–1498.

Anderson, B., Zhao, Y., Andrews, W., Dudley, D., Sibai, B., Iams, J., . . . O'Sullivan, M. (2011). Effect of antibiotic exposure on Nugent score among pregnant women with and without bacterial vaginosis. *Obstetrics and Gynecology, 117*(4), 844–849.

Baecher-Lind, L., Miller, W., & Wilcox, A. (2009). Infectious disease and reproductive health: A review. *Obstetrical and Gynecological Survey, 65*(1), 53–65.

Bertram, C., & Magnussen, L. (2008). Informational needs and the experiences of women with abnormal Papanicolaou smears. *Journal of the American Academy of Nurse Practitioners, 20*, 455–462. doi:10.1111/j.1745-7599.2008.00341.x

CDC. (2010). Sexually transmitted disease treatment guidelines, 2010. *Morbidity and Mortality Weekly Report, 59*, 1–112.

CDC. (2012). Legal Status of Expedited Partner Therapy. Retrieved from http://www.cdc.gov/std/ept/legal/default.htm

Crosby, R., & Bounse, S. (2012). Condon effectiveness: Where are we now? *Sexual Health, 9*, 10–17.

Crosby, R., Milhausen, R., Yarber, W., Sanders, S., & Graham, C. (2008). Condon turn offs among adults: An exploratory study. *International Journal of STD and AIDS, 19*(9), 590–594.

Denney, J., & Culhane, J. (2009). Bacterial vaginosis: A problematic infection from both a perinatal and neonatal perspective. *Seminars in Fetal and Neonatal Medicine, 14*, 200–203. doi:10.1016/j.siny.2009.01.008

Donders, G. G., Van Calsteren, K., Bellen, G., Reybrouck, R., Van den Bosch, T., Riphagen, I., & Van Lierde, S. (2009). Predictive value for preterm birth of abnormal vaginal flora, bacterial vaginosis and aerobic vaginitis during the first trimester of pregnancy. *BJOG: An International Journal of Obstetrics & Gynaecology, 116*(10), 1315–1324.

Duncan, B., Hart, G., Scoular, A., & Bigrigg, A. (2001). Qualitative analysis of psychosocial impact of diagnosis of chlamydia trichomonas: Implications for screening. *British Medical Journal, 322*, 195–199.

Eyre, S., Flythe, M., Hoffman, V., & Fraser, A. (2012). Concepts of infidelity among African American emerging adults: Implications for HIV/STI prevention. *Journal of Adolescent Research, 27*(2), 231–255. doi:10.1177/0743558411417865

Foulkes, H., Petttigrew, M., Liningston, K., & Niccolai, L. (2009). Comparison of sexual partnership characteristics and associations with inconsistent condom use among a sample of adolescents and adult women diagnosed with *Chlamydia trachomatis*. *Journal of Women's Health (2002), 18*(3), 393–399. doi:10.1089/jwh.2008.0840

Gallo, M., Kilbourne-Brook, M., & Coffey, P. (2012). A review of the effectiveness and acceptability of the female condom for dual protection. *Sexual Health, 9*, 18–26.

Graham, C. (2012). Condom use in the context of sex research: A commentary. *Sexual Health, 9*, 103–108.

Hay, P., & Czeizel, A. (2007). Asymptomatic *Trichomonas* and *Candida* colonization and pregnancy outcomes. *Best Practice and Research. Clinical Obstetrics and Gynaecology, 21*(3), 403–409. doi:10.1016/j.bpobgyn.2007.02.002

Hensel, D., & Fortenberry, D. (2011). Adolescent mothers' sexual, contraceptive, and emotional relationship content with the fathers of their children following a first diagnosis of sexually transmitted infection. *Journal of Adolescent Health, 49,* 327–329. doi:10.1016/j .jadohealth.2010.12.020

Hollier, L., & Wendel, G. (2008). Third trimester antiviral prophylaxis for preventing maternal genital herpes simplex virus recurrences and neonatal infection. *Cochrane Database of Systematic Reviews,* (1), CD004946. doi:10.1002/14651858.cd004946.pub2

Humphreys, J. (2011). Sexually transmitted infections, pregnancy, and intimate partner violence. *Health Care for Women International, 32,* 23–38. doi:10.1080/07399332.2010.529211

Iams, J., Romero, R., Culhane, J., & Goldenberg, R. (2008). Primary, secondary and tertiary interventions to reduce morbidity and mortality of preterm birth. *Lancet, 371,* 164–175.

Kershaw, T., Ethier, K., Niccolai, L., Lewis, J., Milan, S., Meade, C., & Ickovics, J. (2010). Let's stay together: Relationship dissolution and sexually transmitted diseases among parenting and non-parenting adolescents. *Journal of Behavioral Medicine, 33,* 454–465. doi:10 .1007/s10865-010-9276-6

Koskimaa, H., Waterboer, T., Pawlita, M., Grenman, S., Syrjanen, K., & Syrjanen, S. (2012). Human papillomavirus genotypes present in the oral mucosa of newborns and their concordance with maternal cervical human papillomavirus genotypes. *Journal of Perdiatrics, 160*(5), 837–843.

Lacour, D., & Trimble, C. (2012). Human papillomavirus in infants: Transmission, prevalence, and persistence. *Journal of Pediatric and Adolescent Gynecology, 24,* 93–97. doi:10.1016/j.jpag.2011.03.001

Laxmi, U., Agrwal, S., Raghunandan, C., Randhawa, V., & Saili, A. (2012). Association of bacterial vaginosis with adverse fetomaternal outcome in women with spontaneous preterm labor: A prospective cohort study. *Journal of Maternal-Fetal and Neonatal Medicine, 25*(1), 64–67. doi:10.3109/1467058.2011.565390

Mantell, J., West, B., Sue, K., Hoffman, S., Exner, T., Kelvin, E., & Stein, Z. (2011). Health care providers: A missing link in understanding acceptability of the female condom. *AIDS Education and Prevention, 23*(1), 65–77.

Melville, J., Sniffen, S., Crosby, R., Salazar, L., Whittington, W., Dithmer-Schreck, D., . . . Wald, A. (2003). Psychosocial impact of serological diagnosis of herpes simplex virus type 2: A qualitative assessment. *Sexually Transmitted Infections, 79,* 280–285.

Newton, D., & McCabe, M. (2005). The impact of stigma on couples managing a sexually transmitted infection. *Sexual and Relationship Therapy, 20*(1), 51–63.

Newton, D., & McCabe, M. (2008). Sexually transmitted infections impact on individuals and their relationships. *Journal of Health Psychology, 13*(7), 864–869. doi:10.1177/1359105308095058

Nygren, P., Rongvei, F., Bongalsos, C., Klebanoff, M., Freeman, M., & Guise, J. (2008). Evidence of benefits and harms of screening and testing pregnant women who are asymptomatic for bacterial vaginosis: An update review for the U.S. Preventative Services Task Force. *Annals of Internal Medicine, 148*(3), 220–233.

Rompalo, A. (2011). Preventing sexually transmitted infection: Back to basics. *Journal of Clinical Investigation, 121*(12), 4580–4583. doi:10.1172/jci61592

Sangkomkamhang, U., Lumbiganon, P., Prasertcharoensook, W., & Laopaiboon, M. (2009). Antenatal lower genital tract infection screening and treatment programs for preventing preterm delivery. *Cochrane Database of Systematic Reviews,* (2), CD006178. doi:10 .1002/14651858.cd006718.pub2

Shih, S., Kebodeaux, C., Secura, G., Allsworth, J., Maddn, T., & Peipert, J. (2011). Baseline correlates of inconsistent and incorrect condom use among sexually active women in the contraceptive choice project. *Sexually Transmitted Diseases, 38*(11), 1012–1019. doi:10 .1097/olq.0b013e318225f8c3

Simcox, R., Wing-To, A., Seed, P., Briley, A., & Shennan, A. (2007). Prophylactic antibiotics for the prevention of preterm birth to women at risk: A meta-analysis. *Australian and New Zealand Journal of Obstetrics and Gynaecology, 47,* 368–377. doi:10.1111/j .1479-828x.2007.00759.x

Westhoff, G., Little, S., & Caughey, A. (2011). Herpes simplex virus and pregnancy: A review of the management of antenatal and peripartum herpes infections. *Obstetrical and Gynecological Survey, 66*(10), 629–638.

Wiehe, S., Roseman, M., Wang, J., Katz, B., & Fortenberry, J. (2011). Chlamydia screening among young women: Individual and provider level differences in testing. *Pediatrics, 127,* e336. doi:10.1542/ peds.2010-0967

Witte, S., El-Bassel, N., Gilbert, L., Wu, E., & Chang, M. (2010). Lack of awareness of partner std risk among heterosexual couples. *Perspectives on Sexual and Reproductive Health, 42*(1), 49–55. doi:10 .1363/4204910

Yudin, M., & Money, D. (2008). Screening and management of bacterial vaginosis in pregnancy. *Journal of Obstetrics and Gynaecology Canada, 211,* 702–708.

42

Psychological disorders

Heather Shlosser

Relevant terms

Anhedonia—inability to derive pleasure from normally enjoyable activities

Catatonia—an awake state of apparent unresponsiveness to external stimuli, seen in severe mania

Epstein anomaly—rare heart defect of tricuspid valves, associated with prenatal use of carbamazepine

Hypomania—set of distinct behaviors that are part of bipolar disorder. Hypomania is a milder form of mania. The person remains able to function well in day-to-day activities. Psychosis does not happen in hypomania.

Mania—seen in severe bipolar disorder, may include psychotic features such as hallucinations, delusion of grandeur, suspiciousness, catatonic behavior, aggression, and a preoccupation with thoughts and schemes that may lead to self-neglect

Melancholy—seen in depression, a gloomy or sad state of mind

Overview

It is estimated that psychiatric illness affects 500,000 pregnant women per year with approximately one-third of women being exposed to some type of psychotropic medication at some point during her pregnancy. When maternal psychiatric illness goes unrecognized or inadequate treatment occurs, this results in fewer prenatal care visits, inadequate nutrition, and potential exposure to additional medications, herbal remedies, alcohol and tobacco use, and substance use. Subsequently, the lack

of psychiatric illness identification and intervention can result in poor mother–infant bonding, adverse neonatal outcomes, and other disruptions and dysfunction within the family unit (American College of Obstetricians and Gynecologists (ACOG), 2008; Marcus, 2009). This chapter will discuss the assessment and treatment of depression, bipolar disorder, and anxiety disorder during pregnancy (Table 42.1).

Depression during pregnancy

Women are at an appreciably greater risk than men to develop major depressive disorders (MDDs) at some point in their lives with studies indicating that depression occurs twice as frequently in women as in men (American Psychiatric Association (APA), 2000). The prevalence of MDD in women is highest during the childbearing years, with the average age of onset in the mid-20s (APA, 2000). Approximately 14–23% of women will experience depressive symptoms during pregnancy (ACOG, 2008). In the primary care setting, depression is not recognized by health-care providers in 50% of cases (Yonkers et al., 2009). Although there is more awareness about postpartum depression today than in the past, depression during pregnancy has received less focus despite the potential for depression to affect perinatal outcomes.

Multiple factors have been found to contribute to a woman's risk of prenatal depression. A prior history of depression or anxiety, extensive life or work stressors, lack of social support, unintended pregnancy, intimate partner violence, low socioeconomic status, limited education, smoking, lack of a partner, interpersonal

---

Prenatal and Postnatal Care: A Woman-Centered Approach, First Edition. Edited by Robin G. Jordan, Janet L. Engstrom, Julie A. Marfell, and Cindy L. Farley.

Table 42.1 Definitions and Classifications of Select Mood Disorders

Definition and classification of mood disorders	
Major depressive disorder (MDD)	Five or more of the following symptoms present during the same 2-week period and represent change from previous function and are not related to a medical condition: 1. Depressed mood most of the day, nearly every day 2. Anhedonia 3. Weight change (increase or decrease), not related to pregnancy or other medical conditions; loss of food enjoyment 4. Fatigue 5. Feelings of worthlessness or inappropriate guilt 6. Psychomotor agitation or retardation nearly every day 7. Inability to think clearly or to make decisions 8. Recurrent thoughts of death, suicidal ideation with or without plan or suicide attempt
Dysthymic disorder	Depressed mood for most of the day, for more days than not for at least 2 years Person has never been without the symptoms for more than 2 months at a time No MDD present during the first 2 years of the disturbance Presence of depression plus two or more of follow symptoms for at least 2 years: 1. Poor appetite or overeating 2. Insomnia or hypersomnia 3. Fatigue 4. Feelings of hopelessness 5. Difficulty making decisions or poor concentration 6. Low self-esteem
Manic episode	Abnormal, persistently elevated, expansive, or irritable mood lasting at least 1 week plus at least three symptoms (not due to substances, medical condition, antidepressant treatment): 1. Grandiosity or inflated self-esteem 2. Decreased need for sleep 3. Distractibility, attention easily drawn to irrelevant outside stimuli 4. Flight of ideas 5. Increased goal-directed activity 6. Increased talkativeness or pressure to keep talking 7. Excessive involvement in pleasurable activities with potential for painful consequences Causes marked impairment in occupational function, relationships, necessitates hospitalization, or has psychotic features
Hypomanic	Abnormal, persistently elevated, expansive, or irritable mood lasting at least 4 days plus at least three symptoms: 1. Grandiosity or inflated self-esteem 2. Decreased need for sleep 3. Distractibility, attention easily drawn to irrelevant outside stimuli 4. Flight of ideas 5. Increased goal-directed activity 6. Increased talkativeness or pressure to keep talking 7. Excessive involvement in pleasurable activities with potential for painful consequences Symptoms are not due to substances, medical condition, or antidepressant treatment. Episode is not severe enough to cause marked impairment in social or occupational functioning, no hospitalization, and no psychotic features.
Bipolar disorder I	One or more manic episodes or mixed episodes, often one or more MDD episodes
Bipolar disorder II	One or more MDD episodes accompanied by at least one or more hypomanic episodes

Adapted from: American Psychiatric Association (2000). *Diagnostic and statistical manual of mental disorders, fourth edition*, Text Revision. Washington, DC: American Psychiatric Association.

violence, and poor interpersonal relationships have all been found to increase the possibility of the development or exacerbation of depression during pregnancy (Lancaster et al., 2010; Price & Proctor, 2009). Pregnancy itself can also be a risk factor for depression and may trigger recurrence of depressive symptoms in vulnerable women.

Potential problems of prenatal depression

Untreated prenatal depression has been linked with adverse perinatal outcomes in both the mother and the offspring (Table 42.2). Antenatal stress may interfere with the development of the hypothalamic–pituitary–adrenal axis, the limbic system, and the prefrontal cortex in the developing fetus. Cortisol, which crosses the placenta, may be a prime mediator of these effects. Increased cortisol levels that accompany depression have been implicated with higher rates of preterm birth and preeclampsia as well as higher rates of childhood cognitive and behavioral impairments (Field, 2011; Field, Diego, & Hernandez-Reif, 2006). It is difficult to determine precise influences of maternal depression on neonatal outcomes because of the comorbidities that often occur with maternal depression such as substance use and confounders such as limited prenatal care and low income.

Screening for prenatal depression

Early detection of depression during pregnancy is critical since depression can adversely affect birth outcomes and neonatal health and, if left untreated, can persist after the birth. Pregnant women should be screened for depression at the first prenatal visit (ACOG, 2010; Akkerman et al., 2012; American College of Nurse Midwives (ACNM), 2013). Women can be screened by routine data gathering about signs and symptoms of depression and/or by formalized depression inventories. All pregnant women should have a direct assessment of mental health history and current mental health status. Social support system and coping methods should be evaluated. If women report a positive history for depression, treatment modalities and efficacy should be assessed and formal screening performed.

Some experts advocate that all women be screened in early pregnancy with a recommended screening tool (Breedlove & Fryzelka, 2011). Findings from the Agency for Healthcare Research and Quality (AHRQ) evidence report on perinatal depression suggest that the Edinburgh Postnatal Depression Scale (EPDS) and the Center for Epidemiologic Studies Depression Scale (CES-D) provide the highest level of specificity and sensitivity for depression screening during pregnancy (Gaynes et al., 2005).

Signs and symptoms of depression

- Feelings of isolation, despair, worthlessness
- Fatigue prior to pregnancy
- Insomnia
- Multiple somatic complaints/symptoms
- Weight changes (often loss) unrelated to pregnancy
- Limited eye contact
- Flat general affect
- Suicide ideation

Management of prenatal depression

An integrative approach to treatment will offer optimal symptom relief for pregnant women with depression. A variety of effective nonpharmacological approaches exist, which can be used alone or in combination with pharmacological intervention. Use of cognitive-behavioral therapy (CBT), interpersonal therapy, supportive therapy, and mind–body modalities have been utilized as part of an integrative plan for the patient with prenatal depression. For women with mild-moderate depression, CBT, exercise, and light therapy can improve depression symptoms. Massage therapy improved mood, reduced anxiety, and improved perinatal outcomes in a cohort of pregnant women with depression compared with a control group (Field, Diego, Hernandez-Reif, Schanberg, & Kuhn, 2004). Yoga has been reported to improve depression symptoms in nonpregnant populations and can be safely used as an adjunctive therapy in pregnancy.

Effective measures to treat depression

Exercise—Exercise reduces the depression hormone cortisol, provides a feeling of accomplishment, enhances self-esteem, and increases serotonin levels in the brain.
CBT—CBT is a form of psychotherapy and is an essential part of a successful depression treatment regime.
Light therapy—sitting in front of a special light box for about 30 minutes every day can alleviate symptoms of depression in pregnant women (Oren et al., 2002; Wirz-Justice et al., 2011).

CBT has demonstrated efficacy in the nonpregnant and pregnant population for mild to moderate depression (Yonkers et al., 2009). Current guidelines suggest psychotherapy should be considered as a primary treatment option for depression during pregnancy (ACOG, 2008). CBT may be short or long term and done by a clinical psychologist, psychiatrist, social worker, psychiatric and mental health nurse practitioner (PMHNP), and psychotherapist.

Table 42.2 Untreated Depression and Maternal/Child Outcomes

Untreated depression and maternal/child outcomes	
Maternal	Neonatal/child
Poor nutrition	Preterm birth
Inadequate weight gain	Low birth weight
Substance use: alcohol, tobacco, drugs	Fetal growth restriction
Anxiety	Increased mental health problems
Insomnia	Behavioral problems
Impaired maternal–infant bonding	
Worsening of depression	
Suicide ideation and suicide	
Postpartum depression	
Preterm birth	
Preeclampsia	

Sources: Bonari et al. (2004), Grote et al. (2010), Wisner et al. (2009).

Women with moderate to severe depression are likely to require additional treatment with antidepressants to relive symptoms. The most commonly used antidepressants are selective serotonin reuptake inhibitors (SSRIs) and the serotonin and norepinephrine reuptake inhibitor, venlafaxine (Table 42.3). Paroxetine (Paxil) should be avoided by pregnant women and women who plan to become pregnant because of an increased risk for cardiac malformations (ACOG, 2008). Fetal echocardiography should be considered for women exposed to paroxetine during early pregnancy.

Starting medications

The largest amount of safety data on antidepressants in pregnancy is found for tricyclic antidepressants (TCAs) and SSRIs; however, TCAs are rarely used due to the greater risk of adverse reactions. SSRIs are more commonly used with sertraline, which is the preferred first-line agent. It has been demonstrated that sertraline has lower maternal serum levels and almost undetectable levels in breast milk (Hackley, 2010). Starting an antidepressant at a low dose and titrating slowly upward until remission is achieved is the approach recommended by the American College of Obstetricians and Gynecologists and the American Psychiatric Association (Hackley, 2010).

Pregnant women currently taking antidepressants

The decision about whether to stop or change medications is complex. Pregnant women often feel quite uncertain and conflicted in making a decision to continue or

Table 42.3 Pharmacological Considerations in Treating Psychological Disorders during Pregnancy

Pharmacological considerations in treating psychological disorders during pregnancy

Antidepressants
- Selective serotonin reuptake inhibitors (SSRIs)
  - Most SSRIs are pregnancy category C.
  - Fluoxetine is the best studied SSRI in terms of safety and efficacy.
  - Sertraline and citalopram may be associated with an increased risk of septal heart defects; however, further studies are needed in this area.
  - Sertraline is found in very low doses in breast milk, while fluoxetine is found in high amounts (very long half-life).
  - SSRI use in late pregnancy may cause self-limited neonatal behavioral syndrome.
  - Conflicting studies regarding the development of persistent pulmonary hypertension in the neonate exposed to SSRIs after 20 weeks' gestation
  - Paroxetine—category D: thought to cause fetal heart defects when taken during the first trimester
- Serotonin norepinephrine reuptake inhibitor (SNRI)
  - Venlafaxine can cause elevated blood pressure at higher doses and difficulty with withdrawal
  - Pregnancy category C
- Norepinephrine and dopamine reuptake inhibitor (NDRI)
  - Buproprion
  - Pregnancy category C
  - Not indicated for use in anxiety or panic disorder
  - Higher doses can lower seizure threshold
    - Do not use in women with anorexia, bulimia, or seizure disorder
- Tricyclic antidepressants (TCAs)
  - Lowest known risks during pregnancy (amitriptyline, imipramine, notriptyline)
  - Overdose attempts with TCA can be fatal
  - Amitriptyline pregnancy category C

Sources: ACOG (2008), National Institute for Health and Clinical Excellence (NICE) (2007) Guidelines.

discontinue medication for depression during pregnancy. Women should be cautioned that the risk of relapse of depression is high. One study found that women who maintained antidepressant medication use throughout the pregnancy had a 26% relapse of major depression, compared to 68% of those who discontinued antidepressant medication (Cohen et al., 2006). Sixty percent of women who discontinued antidepressant treatment at the beginning of pregnancy restarted it during pregnancy. A reduced dose does not appear to reduce fetal risk, and the risk of relapse is substantial for women on medications if the dose is subtherapeutic (Cohen et al., 2006). Women should be advised to take the prescribed amount to achieve remission of symptoms.

Some women want to stop taking an antidepressant as soon as pregnancy is discovered. Women who discontinue or reduce their doses of antidepressants are at a particularly high risk for prenatal depression. However, if the initial depression was mild and the woman is motivated to implement lifestyle changes to reduce depression symptoms, this strategy can be appropriate. Withdrawal from an SSRI should be done slowly in a tapered fashion (by 25% every 1–2 weeks) to avoid SSRI withdrawal symptoms. She should be encouraged to use exercise, light therapy, and/or other modalities, and be monitored for signs and symptoms of recurring depression. A strategy of tapering off antidepressants in the third trimester to reduce neonatal withdrawal symptoms in women with moderate to severe depression has been reported; however, there is no evidence that tapering or discontinuing antidepressant medication near term is effective in terms of preventing transient neonatal complications. Indeed, in some women with depression, doses need to be increased in the second half of pregnancy because of the metabolic changes during pregnancy (Sit, Perel, Helsel, & Wisner, 2008).

In an effort to reduce prenatal exposure to pharmaceuticals, women may turn to herbal therapies to treat depression. St John's wort (*Hypericum perforatum*) has been featured in lay literature as a natural alterative for depression treatment. Studies on this herb have been short term and not well controlled. Herbal supplements are not regulated by the Food and Drug Administration (FDA), and no standard for uniformity of dose or amounts and types of ingredients exists. St John's wort has a long half-life (Organization of Teratology Information Specialists (OTIS), 2010) and can make other medications less effective, including some antidepressant and anticonvulsant medications (Henney, 2000). There is lack of safety data to recommend use during pregnancy or breastfeeding.

Initial and ongoing evaluation of women diagnosed with depression will include (1) establishing patient safety, (2) establishing the most appropriate treatment setting, (3) assessment of patients' level of functioning and support network, and (4) care coordination and planning (APA, 2010). Collaboration with the woman, close follow-up and consultation, and referrals with mental health providers as needed are crucial to safely caring for women with prenatal depression. The risk of treatment with an antidepressant needs to be compared with risk of not treating her depressive illness in each individual woman.

Bipolar disorder in pregnancy

Bipolar disorder, formerly known as manic depression, is a chronic condition characterized by periods of mania,

depression, or a combination of both states. Bipolar disorder is a spectrum disorder with several different diagnostic categories. *Bipolar I* is defined as having one or more manic or mixed episodes, and is usually accompanied by major depressive episodes. *Bipolar II* is characterized by one or more major depressive episodes accompanied by at least one hypomanic episode. *Cyclothymia* is defined as the presence of at least 2 years of numerous periods of hypomanic and depressive symptoms. Bipolar disorder has an average age of onset from the late teens to early 20s (APA, 2000; Viguera et al., 2007). The risk of relapse is not reduced during pregnancy and increases substantially after childbirth (Swann et al., 2005).

The cause of bipolar disorder is unknown, although it is clear that it is highly heritable (APA, 2000; McGuffin et al., 2003). There has been little research devoted to methods of screening and treatment of this disorder in the pregnant woman. Bipolar disorder in the pregnant woman has been associated with increased risks of antepartum hemorrhage, prematurity, low birth weight, and intrauterine growth restriction (Galbally, Snellen, Walker, & Permezel, 2010). Women with bipolar disorder are at high risk for experiencing a mood episode during pregnancy as well as exacerbation during the postpartum period (Viguera et al., 2007, 2011). Abrupt discontinuation of medications, younger age, unplanned pregnancy, and primaparity are risk factors associated with bipolar mood disorder episode or psychosis events (Cohen et al., 2006; Doyle et al., 2012; Viguera et al., 2007, 2011).

Signs and symptoms of bipolar disorder

Symptoms of bipolar disorder vary depending on the phase of the illness cycle. The depressive phases tend to outnumber the manic phases and typically last 2–3 months (Benazzi, 2007). Women with bipolar disorder depression often describe being unable to get out of bed (Ward & Wisner, 2007). Manic episodes are characterized by periods of high activity, excitability, and impulsive behavior in varying degrees. The manic phase may last from days to months. These symptoms of mania occur with bipolar disorder I. In people with bipolar disorder II, the symptoms of mania are similar but less intense. Table 42.4 outlines the symptoms of bipolar disorder.

Mixed episodes are those in which both manic and depressive symptoms occur together. A woman may feel energized and irritable while at the same time feel sad, hopeless, and suicidal. Mixed episodes are often severe and impair daily functioning and relationships. They can last from 1 week to several months and are generally followed by a depressive episode (APA, 2000).

Table 42.4 Bipolar Disorder Symptoms

Symptoms of mania or a manic episode	Symptoms of depression or a depressive episode
Mood changes • A long period of feeling "high," or an overly happy or outgoing mood • Extremely irritable mood, agitation, feeling jumpy or wired • Increased energy • Racing thoughts • Talking a lot	**Mood changes** • A long period of feeling worried or empty • Daily low mood or sadness • Feeling worthless, hopeless, or guilty • Loss of self-esteem

Behavioral changes
• Talking very fast, jumping from one idea to another, having racing thoughts
• Being easily distracted
• Increasing goal-directed activities, such as taking on new projects
• Being restless
• Sleeping little
• Poor judgment
• Poor temper control
• Having an unrealistic belief in one's abilities
• Reckless impulsive behavior
  ○ Binge eating or drinking, and/or drug use
  ○ Sex with many partners
  ○ Spending sprees
	Behavioral changes
	• Feeling tired or "slowed down"
	• Having problems concentrating, remembering, and making decisions
	• Being restless or irritable
	• Loss of interest in activities once enjoyed, including sex
	• Changing eating habits
	• Trouble getting to sleep or sleeping too much
	• Pulling away from friends or activities that were once enjoyed
	• Thinking of death or suicide, or attempting suicide

Sources: U.S. National Library of Medicine, Bipolar Disorder (2012), National Institute of Mental Health, Bipolar Disorder (2013).

Because of the variable presentation of bipolar disorder and recurrent depression as part of the disorder, women with bipolar disorder are often inadequately screened, diagnosed, and/or appropriately treated for many years. The mood criterion symptoms for hypomania can be used as a simple screen in the prenatal office setting. Asking questions such as "Have you ever had 4 continuous days in which you felt so good, high, excited, or 'hyper' that other people thought you were not your usual self or you got into trouble? Have you ever had 4 continuous days when you were so irritable you found yourself shouting at people, or starting fights or arguments?" (Swann et al., 2005). Asking about suicide ide-

ation is very important in women who exhibit symptoms of bipolar mood disorder. Women who screen positive should be referred to a psychiatric professional for expert screening, evaluation, and treatment.

Management of pregnant women with bipolar disorder

The goal of therapy for bipolar disorder is to reduce the frequency and severity of episodes, promote optimal functioning, and reduce the risk for self-harm. Both pharmacological and psychosocial interventions assist in reducing bipolar disorder episode relapses and suicidal risk (Viguera et al., 2007). Decisions to continue or initiate pharmacological intervention during pregnancy should be made in collaboration with a mental health professional and should balance the risks versus benefits. The risk–benefit decision-making model directs the treatment structure of bipolar disorder during pregnancy based on the risk of no treatment versus reproductive toxicity in five domains: intrauterine fetal death, physical malformations, growth impairment, behavioral teratogenicity, and neonatal toxicity (Ward & Wisner, 2007). Mood stabilizing drugs are typically first-line medications used to treat bipolar disorder, and in general, treatment with these medications is continued for years. Except for lithium, many of these medications are anticonvulsants, such as valproic acid and neurontin. Some women maintained on lithium may be advised to taper off the medication before conception, and then gradually restarted after organogenesis is complete (ACOG, 2008). This is balanced with the understanding that stopping medications, either suddenly or gradually, greatly increases the risk that bipolar symptoms will recur during pregnancy (Viguera et al., 2007).

Antidepressant medications, particularly SSRIs, are sometimes used to treat symptoms of depression in bipolar disorder. Currently, there is no expert consensus on best medication, best timing, or optimal dose of SSRIs to treat bipolar depression during pregnancy.

When caring for women with psychological disorders during pregnancy, it is important to be aware that antidepressant medications can induce episodes of hypomania and even psychotic episodes in those women who have bipolar disorder. This is a particular problem for those women with undiagnosed bipolar disorder and depression symptoms.

Generalized anxiety disorder (GAD)

GAD is a disorder characterized by excessive worries and anxieties about a number of different areas that are difficult to control and cause significant distress and impairment. Twice as many women are affected by GAD compared to men (Grant et al., 2005). The majority of individuals with GAD are found to have concomitant psychiatric disorders such as panic disorder, social phobia, specific phobia, substance disorders, and most notably, MDD (APA, 2000).

Definition and characteristics of GAD

GAD is defined as excessive anxiety and worry occurring most days for at least 6 months. The individual finds it difficult to control the worry. Anxiety and worry are associated with three or more of the following:

1. restlessness or feeling on edge
2. fatigue
3. difficulty concentrating
4. irritability
5. muscle tension
6. sleep disturbance.

Anxiety, worry, or physical symptoms are causing a significant disturbance in social, occupational, and other areas of functioning.

Adapted from: American Psychiatric Association. (2000). *Diagnostic and statistical manual of mental disorders, fourth edition*, Text Revision. Washington, DC: American Psychiatric Association.

Risk factors for GAD include low socioeconomic status, medical illness, substance abuse, adverse life events and stressors, history of physical or emotional trauma, and family history of GAD (Fricchion, 2004; Weisberg, 2009). There are few data regarding the risk to the fetus of untreated anxiety disorders during pregnancy. High levels of perinatal anxiety have been associated with preterm birth, postpartum depression, and behavioral inhibition in infants (Coleman, Carter, Morgan, & Schulkin, 2008). Prenatal anxiety has been implicated as an independent risk for behavioral and emotional impairments in children (O'Connor, Heron, Glover, & ALSPAC Study Team, 2002).

Screening for GAD

There are significant cultural variations in the expression of anxiety that should be taken into account with all screenings and diagnostics around anxiety. There is limited research regarding specific anxiety screening tools to utilize, assess, and monitor for perinatal GAD. Three brief screening tools that have been validated in the primary care population and have been commonly utilized in the perinatal population include the GAD-7, Hamilton Anxiety Rating Scale (HAM-A), and Zung

Self-Rating Anxiety Scale. An excessive number of physical symptoms are expressed more often by women with anxiety disorders (Kelly, Russo, & Katon, 2001); therefore, pregnant women with multiple somatic symptoms should be screened for anxiety disorders.

Management of GAD

Psychotherapy and medications are commonly used to treat GAD. Research has established that CBT is highly effective for anxiety disorders, although little study has been done on examining the efficacy of CBT in pregnant women. First-line medications for GAD are SSRIs and serotonin norepinephrine reuptake inhibitors (SNRIs). As in women with depression, sertraline is the preferred drug to use during pregnancy.

Benzodiazapines are used to treat GAD. The U.S. FDA has categorized benzodiazepines into either category D or X, meaning potential for harm in the unborn has been demonstrated. Maternal use of benzodiazepines shortly before birth is associated with floppy infant syndrome (i.e., hypothermia, lethargy, poor respiratory effort, and feeding difficulties), and withdrawal syndromes may persist for several months after birth in infants whose mothers took alprazolam (Xanax), chlordiazepoxide (Librium), or diazepam (ACOG, 2008). Expert groups note that benzodiazapines do not pose a significant increase in long-term risk and can be safely used (ACOG, 2008; OTIS, 2010).

Given the fact that psychotropic drugs readily cross the placenta and could have important implications for the developing fetus, it is necessary to balance the possible effects of medication against the potential effects on both the mother and fetus if GAD is left untreated. When working with women with GAD, an engaging and nonjudgmental therapeutic relationship should be used to explore the woman's worries and to investigate treatment options using a patient-centered shared decision-making philosophy of care (National Guideline Clearinghouse (NGC), 2011).

Scope of practice considerations

Initial interventions and reassessments should always start with the patient safety evaluation, assessment of the most appropriate treatment environment, and functional assessment and evaluation of supports. Frequent reevaluation is necessary throughout pregnancy and during the postpartum period. A clear risk versus benefits analysis of intervention versus no-intervention is essential and should be provided both verbally and in writing with the information being presented at the woman's education level, preferred language, and with cultural consideration (ACOG, 2008; NGC, 2011).

Women with prenatal depression, bipolar disorders, or GAD are at a higher risk for postpartum depression and benefit from postpartum assessment of mental health status (Sutter-Dallay, Giaconne-Marcesche, Glatigny-Dallay, & Verdoux, 2004). Chapter 28 covers postpartum depression is detail.

Interprofessional collaboration, referral, and/or comanagement with a mental health-care professional is imperative for women who have a high-risk score on one of the screening tools, indications of suicidal ideation, self-disclosure of concern, previous treatment in a pregnancy, or ineffective response to current regimens. Certain medication regimes and medication changes in pregnancy are decisions that are best made within interprofessional collaboration. For all psychological conditions occurring during pregnancy, CBT should be encouraged and facilitated.

Summary

Although pregnancy is often a time of emotional well-being, recent studies suggest that approximately 20% of women suffer from mood or anxiety disorders during pregnancy. Particularly vulnerable are those women with histories of psychiatric illness who discontinue psychotropic medications during pregnancy. All women should be screened for depression during pregnancy and again postpartum. Although data accumulated over the last 30 years suggest that some medications may be used safely during pregnancy, knowledge regarding the risks of prenatal exposure to psychotropic medications is incomplete. A growing body of literature suggests that the risk of adverse effects of untreated depression in pregnancy is high. When advising women about treatment options, the severity of illness, history of symptoms off medications, current medications, and plans for breastfeeding are important considerations. The presence of a stable support system and the availability of child care assistance during the postpartum period are also important. Counseling is often an important component of a well-considered treatment plan. All treatment decisions should be carefully documented and discussed with the woman as well as with other collaborating or treating health-care providers.

Case study

Adele is a 32-year-old G2P1 who is here for her first prenatal visit at 9 weeks' gestation. She has a 5-year history of depression that began 2 years before the birth of her first child. She reports that she has been treated successfully with ecitalopram (Lexapro) and has participated in counseling at various periods over the 5 years. Adele and her husband are satisfied with their relationship; her history reveals no specific additional stressful lifestyle issues other than parenting a toddler and working full time. She has a healthy lifestyle and is not taking any medication other than Lexapro at this time. On further questions on the symptoms that prompted her to start the medication, Adele reveals that she had symptoms of anxiety, insomnia, and dark moods. At her "lowest point," she found herself missing work for a few days each week because she was "just unable to get out of bed." It was at this point that with the support of her husband, she sought help from a psychotherapist.

Adele is very concerned about continuing her ecitalopram during this pregnancy and expressed a strong desire to discontinue the medication. Depression and pregnancy was discussed with Adele. She was advised that more than half of the women who discontinue SSRIs during pregnancy may experience relapse, and that untreated prenatal depression is linked with adverse effects such as low birth weight and postpartum depres-sion. She was further advised that there are limited data on the safety of ecitalopram taken during pregnancy; however, there is no data to suggest that it causes fetal malformations. Adele was informed that some data suggest an increase in low birth weight and an increased risk for persistent pulmonary hypertension in newborns exposed to SSRIs during pregnancy. Information about additional treatment modalities for depression such as light therapy and exercise was also provided. She was informed that if she chose to stop taking her medication, the medication should be tapered slowly to prevent serotonin syndrome and off slowly, and she would be closely monitored for depression relapse. An appointment for Adele was then made in the office with the prescribing psychotherapist to discuss her depression history and medication with a request made to have the report sent to the midwives office. Written information was provided to Adele about depression and SSRIs in pregnancy. Adele planned to continue with her SSRIs for now and was leaning toward discontinuing her medication in a planned manner after discussion with her psychotherapist. Adele expressed renewed interested in trying alternative treatment modalities that she had not implemented before, in an effort to reduce dependence on medication during pregnancy. Her efforts were supported, and a 4-week revisit appointment was made.

Resources for women and their families

Health Resources Service Administration. (2006). *Depression during and after pregnancy: A resource for women, their families, and friends.* Rockville, MD: U.S. Department of Health and Human Services. Available at: http://www.mchb.hrsa.gov/pregnancyandbeyond/depression

Self-help book for childbearing age women about depression: Nonacs, R. (2006). *A deeper shade of blue: A woman's guide to recognizing and treating depression in her childbearing years.* New York: Simon & Schuster.

Resources for health-care providers

Center for Epidemiologic Studies Depression Scale (CES-D), English Version available at: http://media.mycme.com/documents/13/mdd-centerforepidemiologicscal_3060.pdf

Center for Epidemiologic Studies Depression Scale (CES-D), Spanish Version available at: http://patienteducation.stanford.edu/research/cesdesp.pdf

Edinburgh Postnatal Depression Scale (EPDS), English Version available at: http://www.fresno.ucsf.edu/pediatrics/downloads/edinburghscale.pdf (Source: Cox, J. L., Holden, J. M., & Sagovsky, R. (1987). Detection of postnatal depression: Development of the 10-item Edinburgh Postnatal Depression Scale. *British Journal of Psychiatry, 150,* 782–786.

Personal Health Questionnaire—Depression (PHQ-9) English Version available at http://patienteducation.stanford.edu/research/phq.html

Personal Health Questionnaire—Depression (PHQ-9) Spanish Version available at http://patienteducation.stanford.edu/research/phqesp.html

References

Akkerman, D., Cleland, L., Croft, G., Eskuchen, K., Heim, C., Levine, A., . . . Westby, E. (2012 Jul). Routine prenatal care. Bloomington (MN): Institute for Clinical Systems Improvement (ICSI). 115 p. [314 references].

American College of Nurse Midwives (ACNM). (2013). Position Statement. Depression in women. Division of Women's Health Policy and Leadership.

American College of Obstetricians and Gynecologists (ACOG). (2008). Use of psychiatric medications during pregnancy and lactation. *ACOG Practice Bulletin, no. 92. Obstetetrics Gynecology, 111,* 1001–1020. doi:10.1097/AOG.0b013e31816fd910

American College of Obstetricians and Gynecologists (ACOG). (2010). Committee Opinion No. 453: Screening for depression during and after pregnancy. *Obstetrics Gynecology, 115,* 394–395.

American Psychiatric Association (APA). (2000). *Diagnostic and statistical manual of mental disorders, fourth edition,* Text Revision. Washington, DC: American Psychiatric Association.

American Psychiatric Association (APA). (2010). Treating major depressive disorder: A quick guide. *Psychiatry Online.* Retrieved from http://psychiatryonline.org/content.aspx?bookid=28&sectionid=1663263

Benazzi, F. (2007). Bipolar disorder—Focus on bipolar II disorder and mixed depression. *Lancet, 369*(9565), 935–945.

Bonari, L., Bennett, H., Einarson, A., & Koren, G. (2004). Risks of untreated depression during pregnancy. Motherisk. Retrieved from http://www.motherisk.org/women/updatesDetail.jsp?content_id=683

Breedlove, G., & Fryzelka, D. (2011). Depression screening during pregnancy. *Journal of Midwifery and Women's Health, 56,* 18–25. doi:10.1111/j.1542-2011.2010.00002.x

Cohen, L. S., Altshuler, L. L., Harlow, B. L., Nonacs, R., Newport, D. J., Viguera, A. C., . . . Stowe, Z. N. (2006). Relapse of major depression during pregnancy in women who maintain or discontinue antidepressant treatment. *JAMA, 295*(5), 499.

Coleman, V. H., Carter, M. M., Morgan, M. A., & Schulkin, J. (2008). United States obstetrician-gynecologists' screening patterns for anxiety during pregnancy. *Depression and Anxiety, 25,* 114–123.

Doyle, K., Heron, J., Berrisford, G., Whitmore, J., Jones, L., Wainscott, G., & Oeybode, F. (2012). The management of bipolar disorder in the perinatal period and risk factors for postpartum relapse. *European Psychiatry, 27,* 563–569.

Field, T. (2011). Prenatal depression effects on early development: A review. *Infant Behavior and Development, 34*(1), 1–14.

Field, T., Diego, M. A., & Hernandez-Reif, M. (2006). Prenatal depression effects on the fetus and newborn: A review. *Infant Behavior and Development, 29*(3), 445–455. ISSN 0163-6383. doi:10.1016/j.infbeh.2006.03.003

Field, T., Diego, M. A., Hernandez-Reif, M., Schanberg, S., & Kuhn, C. (2004). Massage therapy effects on depressed pregnant women. *Journal of Psychosomatic Obstetrics and Gynaecology, 25*(2), 115–122.

Fricchion, G. (2004). Clinical practice. Generalized anxiety disorder. *New England Journal of Medicine, 351,* 675–682.

Galbally, M., Snellen, M., Walker, S., & Permezel, M. (2010). Management of antipsychotic and mood stabilizer medication in pregnancy: Recommendations for antenatal care. *Australian and New Zealand Journal of Psychiatry, 44*(2), 99–108.

Gaynes, B. N., Gavin, N., Meltzer-Brody, S., Lohr, K. N., Swinson, T., Gartlehner, G., . . . Miller, W.C. (February 2005). Perinatal depression: Prevalence, screening accuracy, and screening outcomes. Evidence Report/Technology Assessment No. 119. AHRQ Publication No. 05-E006-2. Rockville, MD: Agency for Healthcare Research and Quality.

Grant, B. F., Hasin, D. S., Stinson, F. S., Dawson, D. A., Ruan, W., Golstein, R. B., . . . Huang, B. (2005). Prevalence, correlates, co-morbidity, and comparative disability of DSM-IV generalized anxiety disorder in the USA: Results from the national epidemiologic survey on alcohol and related conditions. *Psychological Medicine, 35,* 1747–1759.

Grote, N. K., Bridge, J. A., Gavin, A. R., Melville, J. L., Iyengar, A., & Katon, W. J. (2010). A meta-analysis of depression during pregnancy and the risk of preterm birth, low birth weight, and intrauterine growth restriction. *Archives of General Psychiatry, 67,* 1012–1024.

Hackley, B. (2010). Antidepressant medication use in pregnancy. *Journal of Midwifery and Women's Health, 55*(2), 90–100.

Henney, J. E. (2000). From the Food and Drug Administration: Risk of drug interactions with St John's wort. *JAMA, 283*(13), 1679.

Kelly, R. H., Russo, J., & Katon, W. (2001). Somatic complaints among pregnant women cared for in obstetrics: Normal pregnancy or depressive and anxiety symptom amplification revisited? *General Hospital Psychiatry, 23*(3), 107–113.

Lancaster, C. A., Gold, K. J., Flynn, H. A., Yoo, H., Marcus, S. M., & Davis, M. M. (2010). Risk factors for depressive symptoms during pregnancy: A systematic review. *American Journal of Obstetrics and Gynecology, 202*, 5–14.

Marcus, S. M. (2009). Depression during pregnancy: Rates, risks and consequences. *Canadian Journal of Clinical Pharmacology, 16*, 15–22.

McGuffin, P., Rijsdijk, F., Andrew, M., Sham, P., Katz, R., & Cardno, A. (2003). The heritability of bipolar affective disorder and the genetic relationship to unipolar depression. *Archives of General Psychiatry, 60*, 497–502.

National Guideline Clearinghouse (NGC). (2011). Generalised anxiety disorder and panic disorder (with or without agoraphobia) in adults. Management in primary, secondary and community care. London: National Institute for Health and Clinical Excellence (NICE); 56 p. (Clinical guideline; no. 113). Retrieved from http://www.guideline.gov/content.aspx?id=34280

National Institute for Health and Clinical Excellence (NICE). (2007). Quick reference guide: Antenatal and postnatal mental health. Clinical management and service guidance. London: National Collaborating Centre for Mental Health.

O'Connor, T. G., Heron, J., Glover, V., & ALSPAC Study Team. (2002). Antenatal anxiety predicts child behavioral/emotional problems independently of postnatal depression. *Journal of the American Academy of Child and Adolescent Psychiatry, 41*(12), 1470–1477.

Oren, D. A., Wisner, K. L., Spinelli, M., Epperson, C. N., Peindl, K. S., Terman, J. S., & Terman, M. (2002). An open trial of morning light therapy for treatment of antepartum depression. *American Journal of Psychiatry, 159*, 666–669.

Organization of Teratology Information Specialists (OTIS). (2010). St John's wort (*Hypericum perforatum*) and pregnancy. Retrieved from http://www.otispregnancy.org/files/stjohnswort.pdf

Organization of Teratology Information Specialists (OTIS). (2010). Benzodiazapines and pregnancy. Retrieved from http://www.otispregnancy.org/files/benzodiazepines.pdf

Price, S. K., & Proctor, E. K. (2009). A rural perspective on perinatal depression: Prevalence, correlates, and implications for help-seeking among low-income women. *Journal of Rural Health, 25*, 158–166.

Sit, D. K., Perel, J. M., Helsel, J. C., & Wisner, K. L. (2008). Changes in antidepressant metabolism and dosing across pregnancy and early postpartum. *Journal of Clinical Psychiatry, 69*(4), 652.

Sutter-Dallay, A. L., Giaconne-Marcesche, V., Glatigny-Dallay, E., & Verdoux, H. (2004). Women with anxiety disorders during pregnancy are at increased risk of postnatal depressive symptoms: A prospective survey of the MATQUID cohort. *European Psychiatry, 19*, 459–463.

Swann, A. C., Geller, B., Post, R. M., Altshuler, L., Chang, K. D., DelBello, M. P., . . . Juster, I. A. (2005). Practical clues to early recognition of bipolar disorder: A primary care approach. *Primary Care Companion to the Journal of Clinical Psychiatry, 7*(1), 15.

Viguera, A. C., Tondo, L., Koukopoulos, A. E., Reginaldi, D., Lepri, B., & Baldessarini, R. J. (2011). Episodes of mood disorders in 2,252 pregnancies and postpartum periods. *American Journal of Psychiatry, 168*, 1179.

Viguera, A. C., Whitfield, T., Baldessarini, R. J., Newport, D. J., Stowe, Z., Reminick, A., . . . Cohen, L. S. (2007). Risk of recurrence in women with bipolar disorder during pregnancy: Prospective study of mood stabilizer discontinuation. *American Journal of Psychiatry, 164*, 1817–1824.

Ward, S., & Wisner, K. (2007). Collaborative management of women with bipolar disorder during pregnancy and postpartum: Pharmacologic considerations. *Journal of Midwifery and Women's Health, 52*(1), 3–13.

Weisberg, R. B. (2009). Overview of generalized anxiety disorder: Epidemiology, presentation, and course. *Journal of Clinical Psychiatry, 70*, 4–9.

Wirz-Justice, A., Bader, A., Frisch, U., Stieglitz, R. D., Alder, J., Bitzer, J., . . . Riecher-Rössler, A. (2011). A randomized, double-blind, placebo-controlled study of light therapy for antepartum depression. *Journal of Clinical Psychiatry, 72*(7), 986.

Wisner, K. L., Sit, D. K., Hanusa, B. H., Moses-Kolko, E. L., Bogen, D. L., Hunker, D. F., . . . Singer, L. T. (2009). Major depression and antidepressant treatment: Impact on pregnancy and neonatal outcomes. *American Journal of Psychiatry, 166*(5), 557–566.

Yonkers, K. A., Wisner, K. L., Stewart, D. E., Oberlander, T. F., Dell, D. L., Stotland, N., . . . Lockwood, C. (2009). The management of depression during pregnancy: A report from the American Psychiatric Association and the American College of Obstetrics and Gynecologists. *Obstetrics and Gynecology, 114*, 703–713.

Index

Page references followed by *f* denote figures. Page references followed by *t* denote tables.

AAP (American Academy of Pediatrics), 77–78
AAT (auscultated acceleration test), 182
Abdomen enlargement, as probable sign of pregnancy, 128–129
Abdominal exam, postpartum, 433–434
Abdominal pain in pregnancy, 398–399
  abdominal trauma, 399
  appendicitis, 399
  cholylithiasis, 399
  normal causes, 398*t*
  OLD CAARTS mnemonic, 398
Abdominal strengthening exercises, 429
Abdominal trauma, 399
Abdominal wound infection, 445
ABM (Academy of Breastfeeding Medicine), 253
ABO incompatibility, 45
Abortion
  aspiration, 144
  defined, 409
  dilation and evacuation (D & E) procedure, 144
  habitual, 341
  medical, 144
  spontaneous (*see* Spontaneous pregnancy loss)
Abscess, breast, 507–508
Absolute risk, 149, 153
Abuse Prevention and Treatment Act, 252
Academy of Breastfeeding Medicine (ABM), 253, 493
Acceptance of pregnancy, 297–301
ACEI (angiotensin converting enzyme inhibitors), 232*t*
Acetaminophen
  after stillbirth, 413
  asthma association, 196
  for back or pelvic girdle pain, 196
  for carpal tunnel syndrome, 198
  for headaches, 575, 576
  incidence of use by pregnant women, 224
Acetylcholinesterase (AChE), 168

ACFP (American College of Family Physicians), 77
ACHOIS (Australian Carbohydrate Intolerance Study in Pregnant Women), 388
Acidemia
  defined, 176
  fetal, 361
  prediction of, 182, 184, 187
Acidosis, 176
Acne, 580
ACNM. *See* American College of Nurse-Midwives
ACOG. *See* American College of Obstetricians and Gynecologists
Acquired seizure disorder, 570
Acrosome reaction, 19–20
ACTH. *See* Adrenocorticotropic hormone
Active labor
  ambulation in early labor, 330
  case study, 331
  coping strategies and comfort measures for early labor, 330
  data collection, 327–328
  defined, 325
  determining, 327
  timing of admission to birth setting, 326
Active seizure disorder, 570–571, 573
Active transport, 19, 23, 24*t*
Acupressure
  for nausea and vomiting of pregnancy, 218
  for nausea relief, 209*f*
Acupuncture
  for headaches, 576*t*
  for stimulation of milk production, 509
Acute cystitis, 536–538
Acute pustular psoriasis of pregnancy. *See* Impetigo herpetiformis (IH)
Acyclovir, for herpes simplex virus (HSV), 611–612, 612*t*
Adaptation
  defined, 291
  psychosocial in pregnancy, 291–309

Addiction
  ASAM definition, 240
  counseling for, 241
  terminology, 239–240
Adequacy of Prenatal Care Utilization (APNCU) Index, 79
Adequate intake, 99
ADH (antidiuretic hormone), 46
Adipose tissue, 551–552
Admission to birth setting, timing of, 326
Adolescents
  cognitive development of, 314–315
  intimate partner violence, 265
  nutrition, 116–117
    assessment, 116
    counseling, 116–117
    recommended intakes of nutrients, 116
    strategies for dietary change, 116–117
  postnatal care, 436–437
  prenatal health education, 314–315
  preventing STIs, 617
Adoption
  counseling, 143–144
  positive language for discussing, 144
Adrenal gland, function changes during pregnancy, 47
Adrenarche, 5, 13
Adrenocorticotropic hormone (ACTH), 46–47
  chorionic, 25, 26*t*
Adult education principles, 315
Adverse drug reaction, 223
AFAFP (amniotic fluid alpha-fetoprotein), 168
Affective state, 291
AFI. *See* Amniotic fluid index
AFP (alpha-fetoprotein), 160, 162, 168
Afterbirth pain, 430
Afterpains, 419–420
AFV. *See* Amniotic fluid volume
AGA (appropriate for gestational age), 358

Prenatal and Postnatal Care: A Woman-Centered Approach, First Edition. Edited by Robin G. Jordan, Janet L. Engstrom, Julie A. Marfell, and Cindy L. Farley.
© 2014 John Wiley & Sons, Inc. Published 2014 by John Wiley & Sons, Inc.

Agency for Healthcare Research and
    Quality (AHRQ), 77
  on depression prevalence, 448
  on screening for depression during
    pregnancy, 623
Age of viability, 365
Ainsworth, Mary, 293
Albuterol, for asthma, 518–519, 519*t*
Alcohol
  breastfeeding and, 254*t*, 493
  in early gestation, 110–111
  pregnancy implications of, 241–242
  prenatal health promotion and
    education, 92
  prevalence of use, 239
  screening for use, 242, 245, 245*t*
  T-ACE questionnaire, 92
  teratogenicity of, 233*t*
Alcohol-related birth defects (ARBDs),
    92, 242
Alcohol-related neurodevelopmental
    disorders (ARNDs), 92, 242
Aldosterone, 47
Allantois, 19, 28, 29*f*
Allograft, fetus as, 43–44
Alpha-fetoprotein (AFP), 160, 162, 168
Alpha-linolenic acid (ALA), 104, 106*t*,
    118
Alphalipoic acid supplements, for
    headache, 574
Alpha-thalassemia, genetic screening for,
    166*t*, 167
Alprazolam
  FDA approved indications, 456*t*
  side effects, 456*t*
Alveolus, 482
Amenorrhea
  defined, 125
  presumptive sign of pregnancy, 128
American Academy of Pediatrics (AAP),
    77–78, 479
American Botanical Council, 510
American College of Family Physicians
    (ACFP), 77
American College of Nurse-Midwives
    (ACNM), 77
  on mood and anxiety disorder
    screening, 452
  position statements on prenatal
    substance use, 240
American College of Obstetricians and
    Gynecologists (ACOG), 77–79
  on alcohol use, 242
  Committee on Genetics, 168
  on cytomegalovirus education, 591
  on Doppler velocimetry, 188
  exercise recommendations, 274, 276
  on gestational diabetes, 390
  on hepatitis A virus (HAV)
    vaccination, 593

  on mood and anxiety disorder
    screening, 452
  position statements on prenatal
    substance use, 240
  on shackling incarcerated women in
    labor, 264
American College of Sports Medicine,
    391
American Dietetic Association, 117
American Herbal Products Association,
    510
American Society of Addiction Medicine
    (ASAM), 240
American Thyroid Association (ATA),
    561
Ammonia, fetal, 105
Amniocentesis, 168
Amnion
  defined, 397
  in multifetal pregnancy, 401–402
  stripping of the membranes, 397,
    404–405
Amniotic fluid
  dynamics, 353–354
  fetal swallowing of, 354
  meconium-stained amniotic fluid
    (MSAF), 356
  turnover rate, 354
Amniotic fluid alpha-fetoprotein
    (AFAFP), 168
Amniotic fluid disorders, 354–358
  oligohydramnios, 354–357
  polyhydramnios, 357–358
  resources for health-care providers,
    363
  resources for women and their
    families, 363
  terminology, 352–353
Amniotic fluid index (AFI), 354–355, 356*f*
  defined, 352, 387, 397
  in gestational diabetes (GDM), 392
  in post-term pregnancy, 405, 406*t*, 407
Amniotic fluid volume (AFV)
  assessment, 183, 184*t*
  defined, 352
  dynamics, 353–354
  fetal contributions to, 353
  as function of gestational age,
    353–354, 353*f*
  in post-term pregnancy, 404
Amoxicillin
  resistance to, 539
  for urinary tract infection, 540*t*
Amphetamines
  breastfeeding and, 254*t*
  pregnancy implications of use, 244
Ampicillin
  for group B *Streptococcus* (GBS), 592
  resistance to, 539
  for urinary tract infection, 540*t*

Ampulla, 5
Amstel criteria for bacterial vaginosis,
    614
Anabolic, 34, 41
Anagen, 34, 42
Anal sphincter, occult tears of, 434–435
Anal triangle, 8*f*
Anatomy
  breast, 482–483, 482*f*
  external genitalia, 6–8, 7*f*
  female reproductive, 6–11
  internal genitalia, 8–11, 9*f*
  superficial muscles of the perineum,
    8, 8*f*
Androgens, adrenal, 47
Anemia, 525–529
  diagnosis, 525–526
  folate deficiency, 527*t*, 530
  hemoglobinopathies, 527*t*, 529–530
  iron deficiency, 106, 526–529,
    527*t*–528*t*
  physiological changes in pregnancy,
    525–526
  restless leg syndrome and, 210
  Roux-en-Y gastric bypass and,
    555
  unexplained, 530–531
  vitamin B$_{12}$ deficiency, 527*t*, 530
Anencephaly, 161
Aneuploidy. *See also* Trisomy 18; Trisomy
    21
  defined, 160
  screening options for, 162–165
Angiogenesis, 19, 25, 26*t*
Angiotensin converting enzyme
    inhibitors (ACEI), 232*t*
Angiotensin II antagonists, teratogenicity
    of, 232*t*
Anhedonia, 621, 622*t*
Ankyloglossia, 499, 503
Anorexia nervosa, 118–119
Anovulatory cycle, 397, 404
Antacids, 203
Antenatal fetal testing
  amniotic fluid volume (AFV)
    assessment, 183, 184*t*
  biophysical profile (BPP), 183–187
  contraction stress test, 183
  Doppler velocimetry, 187–188
  education and counseling, 188
  fetal heart rate (FHR) monitoring,
    180–183, 181*f*
  fetal movement counts (FMCs),
    178–180, 180*f*
  methods, 178–188
  nonstress test, 180–183
  oxytocin challenge test (OCT), 183
  physiological principles and
    indications for, 177
  terminology, 176

Antibiotics
    for gastroenteritis, 545
    for group B *Streptococcus* (GBS), 592
    for mastitis, 507
    for pyelonephritis, 541
    for upper respiratory infection, 522
    for urinary tract infection, 539–540,
        540*t*
    for uterine infection, 445
    for wound infections, 445
Antibodies
    defined, 608
    in sexually transmitted infections,
        610–612
Anticipatory guidance, 317
    defined, 193
    for discomforts of pregnancy, 194
    for onset of labor, 327
    for pregnant women who are
        substance dependent, 249
    for women who will give birth while
        incarcerated, 264
    in multifetal pregnancy, 403
Antidepressants, 624–625, 624*t*
    for postpartum depression, 450
    teratogenicity of, 232*t*
Anti-D immunoglobulin (RhoGAM),
    340
Antidiuretic hormone (ADH), 46
Antiepileptic medications, 571, 572*t*, 573
Antihistamines
    for atopic dermatitis, 581
    for intrahepatic cholestasis of
        pregnancy (ICP), 586
    for pemphigoid gestationis (PG), 584
    for prurigo of pregnancy, 582
    for pruritic urticarial papules and
        plaques of pregnancy (PUPP),
        583
    for upper respiratory infection, 522,
        522*t*
Antimicrobial compounds, in human
    milk, 482
Antineoplastic agents, teratogenicity of,
    232*t*
Antioxidants, for preeclampsia
    prevention, 383
Antithyroid antibodies, 562
Antithyroid drugs, teratogenicity of, 232*t*
Anxiety, defined, 291
Anxiety disorders
    defined, 441
    postpartum, 448–457
        assessment and screening, 452
        generalized anxiety disorder (GAD),
            450*t*, 451, 626–627
        management, 452–457, 453*t*–456*t*
        obsessive-compulsive disorder, 450*t*,
            451
        panic disorder, 450*t*, 451

        post-traumatic stress disorder
            (PTSD), 450*t*, 451–452
        signs and symptoms, 450*t*
    prevalence of, 448
APNCU (Adequacy of Prenatal Care
    Utilization) Index, 79
Apocrine sweat glands, 41
Apoptosis, 19–20
Appendicitis, 40, 399
    case study, 548
    definition, 544
    evaluation and management, 547
    scope of practice issues, 547
Appropriate for gestational age (AGA),
    358
ARBDs (alcohol-related birth defects),
    92
Areola, 483, 506
ARNDs (alcohol-related
    neurodevelopmental disorders),
    92, 242
Arsenic exposure, 282
Arterial Doppler flow velocity
    waveforms, 352
Arteriovenous (AV) nicking, 375
Arthropathy, 589
Artificial sweeteners, 111
ASAM (American Society of Addiction
    Medicine), 240
"Ask me 3" program, 316
Aspartame, 229
Asphyxia, 176–177
Aspiration abortion, 144
Aspirin
    for headaches, 575
    for preeclampsia prevention, 383
Association of Women's Health,
    Obstetric and Neonatal Nurses
    (AWHONN), 264
Asthma, 517–521, 519*t*, 520*f*
    acetaminophen association, 196
    clinical presentation, 518
    data gathering, 518
    differential diagnosis, 518
    management during pregnancy,
        518–520
        environmental, 519
        exacerbations of, 520, 520*f*
        pharmaceutical, 518–519, 519*t*
        smoking cessation, 519
    persistent, 517
    potential problems, 518
    scope of practice considerations,
        520–521
    triggers, 518
Astroglide, 432
Asymptomatic bacteriuria, 537, 542
ATA (American Thyroid Association),
    561
Atopic dermatitis, 580–581

Atresia, 5, 11
Attachment
    defined, 291
    maternal, 292–301
    partner, 302–305, 302*t*
    sibling, 301–302
Attitude, defined, 291
Attributable risk, 149, 153
AUDIT C screening tool, 245
Augmentin (amoxicillin-clavulanate)
    for upper respiratory infection, 522
    for urinary tract infection, 540*t*
Aura, 570, 574
Auscultated acceleration test (AAT),
    182
Auscultation of the fetal heart, 85, 132,
    132*f*
Australian Carbohydrate Intolerance
    Study in Pregnant Women
    (ACHOIS), 388
Autosomal recessive conditions, 167
Avidity testing, 589, 591, 601
AWHONN (Association of Women's
    Health, Obstetric and Neonatal
    Nurses), 264
Azithromycin
    for chlamydia, 609
    for gastroenteritis, 545
    for gonorrhea, 610

Baby-Friendly Hospital Initiative (BFHI),
    480
Baby shower, 299
Background risk, 223, 228
Back pain, 194–196
    assessment, 195
    causes and symptoms, 194–195
    incidence of, 194
    relief and preventative measures,
        195–196, 195*t*
Baclofen, 243
Bacterial infection
    gastroenteritis, 544–545
    group B *Streptococcus* (GBS), 592–593
    sexually transmitted infections (STIs),
        609–610
    urinary tract infection (UTI),
        536–541, 539*t*–540*t*
Bacterial vaginosis (BV), 614–616
    Amstel criteria, 614
    as ecological disorder, 615
    Nugent scoring system, 614–615, 615*t*
    practice points for, 616
    preterm birth and, 370
    prevalence of, 614
    testing and treatment, 614–615
Bacteriuria. *See also* Urinary tract
    infection (UTI)
    asymptomatic, 370, 537, 542
    defined, 536

Ballantyne, John, 73, 74

Bariatric surgery, 555

Barker, David, 102

Barker hypothesis, 102

Barrier methods of contraception, 472–474

Bartholin gland, 8, 8*f*

Basal body temperature (BBT)
  change for gestational age estimation, 138
  defined, 125
  for pregnancy diagnosis, 131

Basal metabolic rate (BMR), 41, 103

"Bath salts," 244

Bayley Mental Development Index, 502

BBT. *See* Basal body temperature

BDI (Beck Depression Inventory), 88

Beck Depression Inventory (BDI), 88, 452

Beclomethasone, for upper respiratory infection, 522

Behind-the-counter (BTC) drug, 223

Benzodiazepines
  breastfeeding and, 254*t*
  drug-drug interactions and, 248
  FDA approved indications, 455*t*–456*t*
  floppy infant syndrome, 627
  for generalized anxiety disorder (GAD), 627
  for post-traumatic stress disorder, 452
  side effects, 455*t*–456*t*
  teratogenicity of, 232*t*

Benzoyl peroxide, for pruritic folliculitis of pregnancy, 583

Beta-human chorionic gonadotropin (β-hCG)
  discriminatory levels for, 337*t*
  for ectopic pregnancy diagnosis, 342
  in gestational trophoblastic disease, 344
  for pregnancy diagnosis, 131–132
  serial, 337, 342, 344

Beta-thalassemia, genetic screening for, 165, 166*t*, 167

Bichloroacetic acid, for human papillomavirus (HPV), 613

Biliary sludge, 546

Billings method, of fertility awareness, 474

Bimanual pelvic examination
  pregnancy diagnosis, 129–130
  uterine size and shape, 130

Binge drinking
  defined, 238
  prevalence of, 239

Binge eating, 119

Bioequivalent, 223

Biofeedback, for headaches, 576*t*

Biofilms, 506

Biophysical profile (BPP), 183–187
  algorithm for use, 187*f*
  defined, 352, 397
  interpretation and management of score, 186*t*
  intrauterine growth restriction and, 361
  key points of, 187
  Manning scoring criteria, 185*t*
  modified, 187, 187*f*, 352, 361, 397, 406*t*
  in post-term pregnancy, 406*t*
  in preeclampsia management, 380
  Vintzileos scoring criteria, 185*t*

Biparietal diameter, gestational age estimation by, 140

Bipolar disorder, 622*t*, 625–626, 626*t*
  classification, 622*t*, 625
  management of, 626
  risks associated with, 625
  signs and symptoms, 625–626, 626*t*

Birth defects. *See also* Teratology
  baseline risk of, 160
  etiology of, 228, 228*f*

Birth experience, review of, 426

Birth fear, 153

Birth order, 302

Birth plan, defined, 312

Birth weight
  average, 30
  classifications, 358
  macrosomia, 361–362

Bishop score, 397, 406, 406*t*

Bisphenol A (BPA)
  exposure to, 283
  preconception counseling about, 60–61

Black box warning, 223

Bladder infection. *See also* Urinary tract infection (UTI)
  increased susceptibility during pregnancy, 39

Blastocyst, 19, 20–21, 21*f*

Bleeding, 335–351
  benign causes of, 336, 336*t*
  case studies, 349–350
  delayed postpartum, 441, 445–446
  differential diagnosis, 345
  ectopic pregnancy, 341–343
    diagnosis, 342
    incidence, 342
    management of, 342–343, 343*t*
    maternal death and, 342
    recurrence risk, 343
    risk factors for, 342, 342*t*
    signs and symptoms, 342, 342*t*
  evaluation, 336–337
    diagnostic testing, 337
    laboratory evaluation, 337, 337*t*

physical exam, 336–337
    problem-focused history, 336
  during first half of pregnancy, 335–336
  gestational trophoblastic disease (GTD), 343–344
    diagnosis and management, 344
    incidence of, 344
    potential problems, 344
    presentation, 344
    recurrence risk, 344
    risk factors for, 344*t*
    types, 343*t*
  gums, 196
  implantation, 19, 22
  inherited disorders, 531
  leiomyomas, 337
  placental abruption, 346–348
    defined, 335, 346
    incidence of, 346
    potential problems, 347
    presentation, 347–348
    risk factors for, 347*t*
    types, 347, 347*f*
  placenta previa, 345–346, 346*f*, 346*t*
    differential diagnosis, 346
    potential problems, 345–346
    presentation, 346
    risk factors for, 346*t*
    types, 345, 346*f*
  postpartum, 420
  potential problems of unexplained early, 341
  prevalence of, 336
  resources for women and their families, 348
  scope of practice considerations, 344–345, 345*t*, 348
  during second half of pregnancy, 345
    causes, 345–348
    diagnosis and management, 348
    family considerations, 348
    scope of practice considerations, 348
  spontaneous pregnancy loss, 337–341
    classification of first-trimester loss, 338*t*
    defined, 335, 338
    diagnosis, 339
    differential diagnosis, 338–339, 339*t*
    family considerations, 340–341
    follow-up care, 340
    incidence of, 338
    management, 339–340
      expectant management, 339–340
      medical, 340
      surgical, 340
    recurrent, 341

risk factors for, 338, 339*t*
signs and symptoms, 339*t*
subchorionic hemorrhage or
hematoma, 337
terminology, 335
thrombocytopenia, 531
Bloating, 398*t*
Blood glucose monitoring, in gestational
diabetes (GDM) management,
391–392
Blood pressure. *See also* Hypertensive
disorders
maternal alterations during pregnancy,
37–38
supine hypotensive syndrome, 37–38
Blood supply
to cervix, 9
uterine, 11
Bloom syndrome, genetic screening for,
167
Blues, postpartum, 423, 425–426, 441,
449
BMI. *See* Body mass index
BMR (basal metabolic rate), 41, 103
Body hair changes during pregnancy,
213
Body image
clothing as extension of, 306
defined, 291
postpartum, 306
in pregnancy, 305–306
social comparison, 305
Body mass index (BMI), 99
defined, 549
insulin resistance and, 551
obesity and, 549–556, 550*t*
Bonding, 47, 426–427. *See also*
Attachment
Borg rating of perceived exertion (RPE),
277, 277*f*
Botanicals, 224–225, 234
defined, 223
for stimulation of milk production,
509–510
Bottle-feeding, 428
Bowlby, John, 293
BPA. *See* Bisphenol A
BPP. *See* Biophysical profile
Bradley method, 75, 313
Braxton Hicks contractions, 130, 325,
331, 398*t*
Brazelton, T. Berry, 294
Breast
abscess, 507–508
anatomy, 482–483, 482*f*
changes as presumptive signs of
pregnancy, 128
development, 482
engorgement, 499, 506–507
exam, postpartum, 433

physiology of lactation and
breastfeeding, 482–483
skin changes, 212
Breast cancer genes (BRCA1 and
BRCA2), 61
Breastfeeding, 478–495
anatomy and physiology of, 482–483,
482*f*
asthma exacerbations, management of,
520, 520*f*
basics
latch, 487–488, 488*f*
position, 484, 487, 487*f*
care of breastfeeding mother,
491–494
alcohol use, 493
contraception, 433, 492
employed nursing mothers,
493–494
illicit drug use, 493
medications, 493
nutrition, 429, 491–492
smoking, 492–493
case study, 495
checklist of maternal knowledge and
skills acquired before discharge,
484
contraception and, 433, 492
contraindications to, 479
defense agents in human milk, 482
discharge instructions for, 484, 485*f*
estrogen-containing contraceptives
and, 470
flavor learning, 102
intake, assessing, 490–491
lactational amenorrhea method
(LAM) of contraception,
462–463, 472
maternal nutrition/diet and, 429,
491–492
milk production, 489, 490*t*
neonatal abstinence syndrome and,
252
nutritional properties of human milk,
480–482
patterns, 489–490
postnatal assessment, 428
preconception counseling, 60
problems (*see* Breastfeeding problems)
promoting and supporting, 483–484
as public health issue, 479–480
return to ovulation, 463
steps to successful, 480
substance use and, 253–254, 254*t*, 493
swallowing by infant, 483
telephone triage for clinicians, 484,
486*f*
terminology, 478
voiding by infants, 490–491
weight gain by infants, 491

Breastfeeding problems, 499–511
case study, 510
infant related, 499–503
fussy baby, 499–500
hunger, 500
infant pain, 499–500
late preterm infants, 503, 504*t*
oral aversion, 499–500
prenatal or perinatal medications,
500
preterm infants, 502–503
sleepy baby, 500–501
slow weight gain, 501–502,
501*t*–502*t*
maternal, 503–510
abscess, breast, 507–508
breast engorgement, 499,
506–507
low milk supply, 499, 508–510,
508*t*–509*t*
mastitis, 499, 507
plugged ducts, 506–507
sore nipples, 503–506, 505*t*
resources for health-care providers,
511
resources for women and their
families, 511
terminology, 499
Breast tenderness, 196–197
assessment, 197
causes and symptoms, 196–197
relief and preventative measures,
197
Breath, shortness of, 211–212
Breckinridge, Mary, 73
Broad ligament, 9*f*
Bronchitis, 522
BTC (behind-the-counter) drug, 223
Budesonide, for asthma, 519*t*
Bulbocavernosus muscle, 8
Bulb of the vestibule, 8*f*
Bulbospongiosus muscle, 8*f*
Bulimia nervosa, 118–119
Buprenorphine
breastfeeding and, 254*t*
drug-drug interactions and, 248
for opioid dependence, 250–251
Buprenorphine/naloxone combination
therapy, 250
Bupropion, 246, 253
black box warning, 455*t*
for depression, 457
FDA approved indications, 455*t*
side effects, 455*t*
Buspirone
FDA approved indications, 455*t*
side effects, 455*t*
BV. *See* Bacterial vaginosis
B vitamin deficiency, in vegetarian/vegan
diet, 118

Caffeine
    content of select coffee brands, 111
    intake during pregnancy, 111
Calcium
    demands of pregnancy, 45
    dietary intake during pregnancy, 106t,
        107
    levels in pregnancy, 39, 45–46
    in vegetarian/vegan diet, 118
Calcium supplements, for preeclampsia
    prevention, 383
Calf muscles, stretching to prevent leg
    cramps, 205–206, 205f
Caloric intake, during pregnancy, 103
Calorie density, 99
Campylobacteriosis, 110
Canavan's disease, genetic screening for,
    87t, 166t, 167
Cancer survivors, preconception care for,
    61
Candidiasis, vaginal, 613–614
Capacitation, 19, 20
Carbamate, exposure to, 283
Carbamazepine
    maternal and fetal effects of, 572t
    teratogenicity of, 232t
Carbohydrates
    in gestational diabetes (GDM)
        management, 390–391, 391t
    in human milk, 481
    metabolism changes during pregnancy,
        41
Carbonic anhydrase, 38
Cardiac output, increase during
    pregnancy, 37
Cardiff "count to ten" method of fetal
    movement counts (FMCs), 179
Cardinal ligament, 9–10
Cardiovascular system
    maternal alterations during pregnancy,
        37–38, 37t
        blood pressure, 37–38
        heart changes, 37, 37t
        supine hypotensive syndrome,
            37–38
        vascular adaptations, 37
    physiological alterations during
        postnatal period, 421, 421t
"Caring for Our Future: The Content of
    Prenatal Care," 75–77
Carpal tunnel syndrome (CTS), 197–198
    assessment, 197–198
    causes and symptoms, 197
    relief and preventative measures, 198
Carrier screening, 167
Case study
    appendicitis, 548
    asymptomatic bacteriuria, 542
    breastfeeding, 495
    breastfeeding problems, 510

contraception, 475
depression, 458
dermatological disorders, 580
endocrine disorders, 568
fetal growth disorders, 363
fetal well-being, assessment of, 190
gastrointestinal disorders, 548
genetic screening, 172
gestational diabetes (GDM), 394
health education, 322
heartburn and sleep deprivation, 219
hematological disorder, 534
hypertensive disorders, 385
infectious diseases, 604
influenza, 523
labor onset, 331
nausea and vomiting during
    pregnancy, 218
neurological disorders, 578
nutrition, 120–121
obesity, 557
perinatal loss and grief, 414
perineal laceration, 422
physiological alterations during
    postnatal period, 422
physiological changes of pregnancy,
    47
postnatal care, 438
postnatal complications, 458
preeclampsia, 385
pregnancy diagnosis and gestational
    age assessment, 145
prenatal care, 96
preterm birth (PTB), 372
psychological disorders, 628
psychosocial adaptations in pregnancy,
    309
reproductive tract structure and
    function, 18
respiratory disorders, 523
risk assessment and management,
    157
social issues in pregnancy, 269
substance use, 255
vaginal bleeding, 349–350
Castor oil, 405
Catabolism, 34, 41
Catatonia, 621
CBT. See Cognitive-behavioral therapy
CDC. See Centers for Disease Control
    and Prevention
CDE (Certified Diabetes Educator), 390
CDER (Center for Drug Evaluation and
    Research), 225
Cefprozil, for upper respiratory infection,
    522
Ceftirizine, for pruritic urticarial papules
    and plaques of pregnancy
    (PUPP), 583
Ceftriaxone, for gonorrhea, 610

Cell-mediated immunity, 44
Center for Drug Evaluation and Research
    (CDER), 225
Center for Epidemiologic Studies
    Depression Scale (CES-D), 88,
    452, 623
Centering Healthcare Institute (CHI),
    81
CenteringPregnancy, 80–81, 81t, 314
Centers for Disease Control and
    Prevention (CDC)
    contraception recommendations, 465,
        475
    on cytomegalovirus education, 591
    growth charts, 491
    on physical abuse, 265
    reproductive life plan and, 141
    on smoking and low birth weight
        births, 242
Central tendon of the perineum, 8
Cephalexin, for urinary tract infection,
    540t
Cephalosporins, for pyelonephritis, 541
Cerclage, cervical, 365, 371
Certified Diabetes Educator (CDE), 390
Cervical canal, 9f
Cervical caps, 473
Cervical cerclage, 365, 371
Cervical changes, as probable signs of
    pregnancy, 129
Cervical insufficiency, 365
Cervical length measurement, for
    predicting preterm birth, 368
Cervical motion tenderness (CMT), 335
Cervical mucus, 8, 10
Cervical pain, 198
Cervical ripening agents, 340, 406
Cervix, 5
    anatomy, 9–10, 9f
    Bishop score, 397, 406, 406t
    cancer of, 10
    effacement, 325, 327–328
    elective labor induction and, 405–406,
        406t
    mechanical dilation, 406
    physiological alterations during
        postnatal period, 420
Cesarean birth
    incidence of, 152
    overuse of, 152
    placental abruption and, 346
    rate among late preterm birth, 366f
Cetirizine, for atopic dermatitis, 581
Chadwick's sign, 10, 125, 129
Chancre, 608, 616
Chaste tree seed, for stimulation of milk
    production, 510
CHCs (combined hormonal
    contraceptives), 462, 464,
    469–470

CHI (Centering Healthcare Institute), 81
Chicken pox. *See* Varicella zoster virus (VZV)
Childbirth classes, 299
Childbirth confidence, 306–308
  influence of witnessing a birth on, 300
  self-efficacy and, 306–308
  strategies to enhance, 308
Childbirth education
  Bradley Method, 313
  defined, 312
  hospital-based classes, 313
  hypnobirthing, 313
  Lamaze, 313
  prenatal visit approach to, 314
  reading material, 314
  reality television shows, 314
  sources and quality of, 312–314
Childbirth Education movement, 75
Childbirth fear (tocophobia), 214
Childbirth without Fear, 75
Childhood sexual abuse (CSA)
  assessment, 266
  incidence, 266
  providing care, 268
  signs and symptoms of, 267t
Children's Bureau, 73–74
Child Support Enforcement Office, state, 263
Chills, uterine infection and, 444, 445t
Chlamydia, 608, 609
  case study, 619
  pregnancy testing and treatment, 609
  screening recommendations, 58t
Chlorpheneriamine
  for atopic dermatitis, 581
  for pemphigoid gestationis (PG), 584
Choice, illusion of, 154
Cholasma, 212, 212f
  as presumptive sign of pregnancy, 128
Cholecystitis, 399, 546–547
Cholecystokinin (CCK), 500–501
Cholelithiasis, 399, 544
Cholestasis
  defined, 544
  intrahepatic cholestasis of pregnancy (ICP), 545–546
Cholesterol
  in human milk, 481
  levels in third trimester, 41
ChooseMyPlate guidelines, 114, 429
Chorioamnionitis, 608
Chorion, 19, 22, 28
  defined, 397
  in multifetal pregnancy, 401–402
Chorion frondosum, 19, 22
Chorionic villi, 19, 21

Chorionic villus sampling (CVS), 168
Chorion leave, 19
Chromosomal microarray analysis (CMA), 169
Chronic diseases
  defined, 51
  preconception care for women with, 61–65, 63t
    cancer survivors, 61
    chronic hypertension, 61, 64
    diabetes, 64
    epilepsy, 64
    HIV infection, 64
    mental illness, 64
    thyroid disorders, 64
Chronic hypertension, 375–376, 376t
  preconception care for, 61, 64
  preecalmpsia superimposed on, 376t, 377
Chronic migraine, 570, 574
Chronic tension headache, 570, 574, 574t
Cigarettes. *See* Smoking
Citalopram
  FDA approved indications, 453t
  side effects, 453t
Class A1GDM, 387
Class A2GDM, 387
Cleavage, 19, 20–21, 21f
Clindamycin
  for bacterial vaginosis (BV), 615
  for group B *Streptococcus* (GBS), 592
  resistance to, 592
Clinical pelvimetry, 85
Clinical trials, 223
Clitoris, 5, 6, 6f–8f
Cloacal membrane, 19, 27, 29f, 31f
Clomipramine
  FDA approved indications, 454t
  side effects, 454t
Clonazepam
  FDA approved indications, 456t
  side effects, 456t
Clonic movements, defined, 570
Clonidine, 243
Closed neural tube defects, 160
Clostridium sordellii infection, 144
Clothing, as extension of body image, 306
Clotrimazole, for candidiasis, 61
Clotting factors, changes during pregnancy, 36, 36t
Cluster headache, 570, 574, 576–577
CMA (chromosomal microarray analysis), 169
CMT (cervical motion tenderness), 335
CMV. *See* Cytomegalovirus
Coagulation factors
  changes during pregnancy, 36, 36t
  deficiencies, 531

Coagulopathies, 531–534, 533t
Cocaine
  breastfeeding and, 254t
  pregnancy implications of use, 243
  teratogenicity of, 232t
COCs (combined oral contraceptives), 462
Cod liver oil, 104
Coelom, 19, 22, 28, 31f
Coffee, caffeine content of, 111
Cognition, defined, 291
Cognitive-behavioral therapy (CBT)
  for cocaine addiction, 243
  for depression, 623
  for generalized anxiety disorder, 451, 627
  for headaches, 576t
  for mood and anxiety disorders, 457
  for obsessive-compulsive disorder, 451
  for postpartum depression, 450
  for post-traumatic stress disorder, 452
Coitus, 5
Colorado clinical guidelines for preconception and interconception care, 54f–55f
Colostrum, 197, 480, 489
Combined hormonal contraceptives (CHCs), 462, 464, 469–470
Combined oral contraceptives (COCs), 462
Comfrey, for perineal discomfort, 431
Common cold, 522, 522t
Complement factors, increase in pregnancy, 44
Complications
  common postnatal, 441–458 (*see also* Postpartum complications)
  in pregnancy, 397–407 (*see also* *specific conditions*)
Conception, 20
Conception process, preconception counseling on, 60
Conceptus, transport, 20–21, 21f
Condoms
  female, 473, 618
  male, 473
    incorrect use of, 618
    STI prevention and, 617–618
Confined placental mosaicism, 160
Congenital, defined, 589
Congenital anomaly
  defined, 589
  nutrition in pregnancy and, 100
Congenital rubella syndrome (CRS), 227, 598–599
Congenital varicella syndrome (CVS), 602
Conization, history of prior, 368
Connective tissue changes during pregnancy, 42

Consent, 169. *See also* Informed consent
Constipation, 40, 198–199, 199*t*, 398*t*
    assessment, 198
    causes and symptoms, 198
    incidence of, 198
    postnatal care, 431
    relief and preventative measures,
        198–198, 199*t*
Continuous labor support, 325, 330
Contraception, 462–476
    adverse health events with unintended
        pregnancy, 464
    barrier methods, 472–474
    for breastfeeding women, 433, 492
    case study, 475
    emergency, 462, 474–475
    medical eligibility criteria (MEC),
        462, 464–465
    methods, 465–474
        barrier methods, 472–474
        cervical caps, 473
        combined hormonal contraceptives
            (CHCs), 462, 464, 469–470
        contraceptive sponges, 473
        effectiveness, grouping by, 465, 465*t*
        female condoms, 473, 618
        female sterilization, 466
        fertility awareness-based methods
            (FAMs), 462, 474
        implant contraception, 468–469
        intrauterine contraception, 462,
            467–468
        lactational amenorrhea method
            (LAM), 462–463, 472
        long-acting reversible contraceptive
            methods (LARC), 462, 467–469
        male condoms, 473, 617–618
        male sterilization (vasectomy),
            466–467
        permanent, 466–467
        progestin-only contraceptives, 462,
            470–472
        spermicides, 473–474
        sterilization, 462, 466–467
        tier one methods, 465*t*, 466–469
        tier three methods, 465*t*, 472–474
        tier two methods, 465*t*, 469–472
        vaginal diaphragms, 473
        withdrawal, 474
    postpartum, 432–433, 462–476
        considerations in method selection,
            463–465
        interpregnancy intervals, 462
        lactational amenorrhea method
            (LAM), 462–463
        return to fertility after childbirth,
            463
        "Rule of Threes," 463
        when to start, 463
    resources for women and health-care
        providers, 476
    STI prevention and, 617–618
    terminology, 462
Contraceptive sponges, 473
Contraceptive Technology (Hatcher),
        475
Contractions, 325–331
    assessment of, 328
    Braxton Hicks, 130, 325, 331, 398*t*
    defined, 325
    determining onset of labor, 325–326
    false labor and, 326–327
    postpartum, 419–420
Contraction stress test (CST), 183, 406*t*
Control, fear of loss in labor, 300
Controlled substance, 223, 225, 226*t*
Coping, defined, 291
Copper IUD, 467, 468, 475
Cordocentisis, 168
Corneal edema, 45
Cornua, 5, 11
Corona radiata, 15, 19, 20
Coronary heart disease, low birth weight
        linked to, 102–103
Corpus albicans, 15
Corpus luteum
    formation of, 15
    involution of, 15, 16
    life span of, 14
    progesterone secretion by, 16–17
Corticosteroids
    for asthma, 519, 519*t*, 520*f*
    for atopic dermatitis, 581
    for hyperemesis gravidarum, 401
    for impetigo herpetiformis (IH),
        585
    nasal for upper respiratory infection,
        522, 522*t*
    for pemphigoid gestationis (PG),
        584
    for preeclampsia management, 380
    for prurigo of pregnancy, 582
    for pruritic folliculitis of pregnancy,
        583
    for pruritic urticarial papules and
        plaques of pregnancy (PUPP),
        583
    teratogenicity of, 232*t*
Corticotropin-releasing hormone (CRH),
        25, 47
Cortisol, 47
    in prenatal depression, 623
    striae gravidarum color and, 42
Costovertebral angle tenderness (CVAT),
        434
Costs, risk assessment and, 152–153
Cough suppressants, for upper
        respiratory infection, 522, 522*t*
Coumarin, teratogenicity of, 232*t*
Counseling
    adoption, 143–144
    antenatal fetal testing, 188
    genetic
        perspective on, 171–172
        pretest counseling, 170
        referrals to genetic counselor, 169
    on parvovirus B19, 597
    preconception, 57–61
        conception process, 60
        diet, 57, 59
        environmental exposure to toxins,
            60–61
        exercise, 59
        infections, 60
        in pregestational diabetes, 567
        preparation for pregnancy and
            childbirth, 60
        substance use and abuse, 59–60
        supplementation, 59
        vaccinations, 61, 62*t*
        weight, 59
    pregnancy diagnosis, 140–145
        adoption counseling, 143–144
        after negative pregnancy test, 141
        after positive pregnancy test, 141
        delivery of test results, 140–141
        ethics and standards for
            reproductive options counseling,
            142
        evidence-based information about
            pregnancy options, 143
        pregnancy termination, 144–145
        steps in pregnancy options
            counseling, 143
        for unintended pregnancy, 141–143
    prenatal nutrition, 57, 59, 114, 116
        in adolescent pregnancy, 116–117
        in multifetal pregnancy, 403, 403*f*
    on sexuality in pregnancy, 285–286
    substance abuse, 248
    on varicella infection, 603
    on working during pregnancy, 287–288
Court order of protection, 266
Couvade, 303
Couvade syndrome, 303
Couvelaire uterus, 335, 347
CRAFFT screening tool, 245
C-reactive protein, increase in pregnancy,
        44
Creighton method, of fertility awareness,
        474
CRH (corticotropin-releasing hormone),
        25, 47
Crisis, pregnancy as, 292–293
Crisis pregnancy centers, 143
Critical periods in human development,
        228–229, 230*f*
Cromolyn sodium, for upper respiratory
        infection, 522, 522*t*
Crown-rump length, gestational age
        estimation by, 140
CRS (congenital rubella syndrome), 227,
        598–599

CSA. *See* Childhood sexual abuse
CST (contraction stress test), 183, 406*t*
CTS. *See* Carpal tunnel syndrome
Cultural considerations
    in obesity, 550
    in postnatal care, 435–436
    in postnatal complications, 442–443
Culture
    defined, 291
    health education and, 321
    nutrition and, 111–112
    substance use and, 254
Curettage, for delayed postpartum
        hemorrhage, 446
CVAT (costovertebral angle tenderness),
        434
CVS (chorionic villus sampling), 168
CVS (congenital varicella syndrome),
        602
Cyclosporine, for impetigo herpetiformis,
        585
Cyclothymia, 625
Cystic fibrosis (CF) screening, 87*t*, 165,
        166*t*
Cystitis, acute, 536–538
Cystocele, 423
Cytochrome P450 enzymes, 235*t*
    defined, 223
    progesterone stimulation of, 40
Cytokines, 34, 43–44
    inflammatory, 551
    produced by adipose tissue, 551
Cytomegalovirus (CMV), 590–591
    clinical presentation and assessment,
        590–591
    congenital, 590–591
    management, 591
    potential problems, 590
    prevalence of infection, 590
    prevention, 591
    testing for, 590–591
Cytotrophoblast, 19, 21–22, 27*f*, 354

DEA (Drug Enforcement
        Administration), 225, 250
Decidual hemorrhage, preterm birth and,
        367
Decidual reaction, 19, 22, 25
Decongestants, 206, 522, 522*t*
Dedifferentiation, 296
Deep vein thrombosis (DVT), 37, 448*f*,
        531–532
    defined, 441
    in obese women, 556
    postpartum, 447, 556
    risk factors for venous thrombosis,
        445*t*
    as sequelae to IV drug use, 241
    symptoms, 447
Defensive care practices, by obstetrician
        gynecologists, 152

Dehydration
    in hyperemesis gravidarum, 401
    in nausea and vomiting of pregnancy,
        207
Dehydroepiandrosterone sulfate
        (DHEA-S), 25, 26*t*, 47
Delayed lactogenesis II, 499
Delayed postpartum hemorrhage, 441,
        445–446
Dendritic cells, 43–44
Dependence, opioid, 250
Depot medroxyprogesterone acetate
        (DMPA), 470–471, 492
Depression. *See also* Bipolar disorder
    case study, 458
    comorbid with substance use, 241
    postpartum, 435, 449–450
        assessment and screening, 452
        differential diagnosis, 450
        Edinburgh Postnatal Depression
            Scale (EPDS), 435, 452
        management, 450, 452–457,
            453*t*–456*t*
        prevalence of, 448–449
        risk factors for, 449
        signs and symptoms, 449, 450*t*
        thyroid function studies and, 448
    during pregnancy, 621–625, 622*t*,
        624*t*
        case study, 628
        contributing factors, 621, 623
        incidence of, 621
        management of, 623–625
        outcomes of untreated, 623, 624*t*
        pharmaceutical considerations in
            treating, 624*t*
        problems of, 623, 624*t*
        screening for, 623
    with pregnancy loss, 341
    screening tools, 435, 452
    signs and symptoms of, 622*t*, 623
    sleeplessness and, 287
Dermatological disorders, 580–588
    abbreviations for skin disorders,
        581*t*
    atopic dermatitis, 580–581
    case study, 580
    defining characteristics of, 582*t*
    impetigo herpetiformis (IH), 582*t*,
        585
    intrahepatic cholestasis of pregnancy
        (ICP), 582*t*, 585–586
    pemphigoid gestationis (PG), 582*t*,
        583–585, 584*f*
    prurigo of pregnancy (PP), 581–582,
        582*t*
    pruritic folliculitis of pregnancy (PFP),
        582*t*, 583
    pruritic urticarial papules and plaques
        of pregnancy (PUPP), 582–583,
        582*f*, 582*t*

resources for health-care providers,
        587–588
    terminology, 580
Dermoplast, for perineal discomfort,
        431
DES (diethylstilbestrol), 74, 232*t*
Designer drugs, 244
Desonide, for pruritic folliculitis of
        pregnancy, 583
Detection rate, defined, 160
Development
    breast, 482
    chorionic and amniotic membranes,
        22–23
    cleavage, 20, 21*f*
    embryo, 27–29
        folding, 28, 31*f*
        gastrulation, 27, 27*f*
        neurulation, 28
        notochord formation, 28, 29*f*
        organogenesis, 28–29
        primitive streak, 27–28, 27*f*
    fetus, 29–30
    implantation, 21
    placenta
        functions, 23–25, 24*t*, 26*t*
        structure, 21–22
    umbilical cord, 23
Developmental phase, pregnancy as,
        292–293
DHA (docosahexaenoic acid), 104, 106*t*,
        118
DHEA-S (dehydroepiandrosterone
        sulfate), 25, 26*t*, 47
DIA (dimeric inhibin A), in genetic
        screening, 163
Diabetes mellitus
    classifications, 566, 566*t*
    etiology, 566, 566*t*
    gestational diabetes (GDM)
        decrease risk with exercise, 275
        incidence of, 566
        preconception care for, 64
        pregestational, 566–567
            adverse pregnancy outcomes and,
                567
            classifications, 566
            glycemic control, 567
            perinatal risks of, 567
            preconception counseling, 567
Diagnostic testing, prenatal care,
        87–88
Diaphoresis, 431
Diaphragms, vaginal, 473
Diarrhea, in gastroenteritis, 544–545
Diary, headache, 574
Diastasis, 423, 434
DIC. *See* Disseminated intravascular
        coagulation
Dickinson's sign, 125, 130
Dick-Read, Grantly, 73, 75, 313

Diet. *See also* Nutrition
  for gestational diabetes (GDM)
      management, 390–391, 391*t*
  for headache control, 575
  postpartum, 429
  preconception counseling, 57, 59
Dietary counseling, in iron-deficiency
     anemia, 527–529, 528*t*
Dietary reference intake (DRI), 99, 100
  for carbohydrates in pregnancy,
     390–391
Diethylstilbestrol (DES), 74, 232*t*
Dilation, 325–328
Dilation and evacuation (D & E)
     procedure, 144
Dimeric inhibin A (DIA), in genetic
     screening, 163
Diphenhydramine, 329, 581
Diploid, 19–20
Disabilities, preconception care for
     women with, 65
Discharge instructions for breastfeeding,
     484, 485*f*
Discomforts of pregnancy, 193–220
  back pain and pelvic girdle pain,
     194–196
    assessment, 195
    causes and symptoms, 194–195
    relief and preventative measures,
     195–196, 195*t*
  bleeding gums, 196
    assessment, 196
    causes and symptoms, 196
    relief and preventative measures, 196
  breast tenderness, 196–197
    assessment, 197
    causes and symptoms, 196–197
    relief and preventative measures,
     197
  carpal tunnel syndrome (CTS),
     197–198
    assessment, 197–198
    causes and symptoms, 197
    relief and preventative measures, 198
  cervical pain, 198
  constipation, 198–199, 199*t*
    assessment, 198
    causes and symptoms, 198
    relief and preventative measures,
     198–198, 199*t*
  dizziness/syncope, 199–200
    assessment, 199
    causes and symptoms, 199
    relief and preventative measures,
     199–200
  edema, 200
    assessment, 200
    causes and symptoms, 200
    relief and preventative measures,
     200

emotional changes, 200–201
  assessment, 201
  causes and symptoms, 200
  relief and preventative measures,
    201
epistaxis, 206–207
fatigue, 201
  assessment, 201
  causes and symptoms, 201
  relief and preventative measures, 201
flatulence, 201–202
  assessment, 201–202
  causes and symptoms, 201
  relief and preventative measures,
    202
headache, 202–203
  assessment, 202
  causes and symptoms, 202
  relief and preventative measures,
    202–203
heartburn, 203–204
  assessment, 203
  case study, 219
  causes and symptoms, 203
  relief and preventative measures,
    203–204
heart palpitations, 204
  assessment, 204
  causes and symptoms, 204
  relief and preventative measures, 204
hemorrhoids, 204
  assessment, 204
  causes and symptoms, 204
  relief and preventative measures,
    204
increased warmth and perspiration,
    204–205
leg cramps, 205–206
  assessment, 205
  causes and symptoms, 205
  relief and preventative measures,
    205–206, 205*f*
leukorrhea, 205
  assessment, 205
  causes and symptoms, 205
  relief and preventative measures, 205
nasal congestion, 206
  assessment, 206
  causes and symptoms, 206
  relief and preventative measures,
    206
nausea and vomiting of pregnancy
    (NVP), 207–209, 208*t*–209*t*, 209*f*
  assessment, 207, 208*t*
  case study, 218
  causes and symptoms, 207
  relief and preventative measures,
    207–208, 208*t*–209*t*, 209*f*
in obese women, 555
overview signs and symptoms, 193–194

ptyalism, 209–210
  assessment, 210
  causes and symptoms, 209
  relief and preventative measures,
    210
  resources for health-care providers
    and women and their families,
    220
restless leg syndrome (RLS), 210–211
  assessment, 210
  causes and symptoms, 210
  relief and preventative measures,
    210–211
round ligament pain, 211, 211*f*
  assessment, 211
  causes and symptoms, 211
  relief and preventative measures, 211
shortness of breath, 211–212
  assessment, 211–212
  causes and symptoms, 211
  relief and preventative measures,
    212
skin changes, 212–214
  assessment, 213
  hair and nail changes, 213
  hyperpigmentation, 212–213, 212*f*
  relief and preventative measures,
    213–214
  striae gravidarum, 212–213, 213*f*
  vascular changes, 213
sleep disturbances, 214–215
  assessment, 214
  case study, 219
  causes and symptoms, 214
  relief and preventative measures,
    214–215
supine hypotension syndrome (SHS),
    215
  assessment, 215
  causes and symptoms, 215
  relief and preventative measures, 215
terminology, 193
urinary frequency, 215
  assessment, 215
  causes and symptoms, 215
  relief and preventative measures, 215
urinary incontinence, 216
  assessment, 216
  causes and symptoms, 216
  relief and preventative measures, 216
varicosities, 216–218
  leg, 216–217
  vulvar, 217–218, 217*f*
visual changes, 219–220
  assessment, 219
  causes and symptoms, 219
  relief and preventative measures, 220
Discrimination in the workplace, 287
Discriminatory drug screening policies,
    240

Disseminated intravascular coagulation
(DIC)
defined, 375
in preeclampsia, 377
Diuresis, 431
Dizygotic twins, 397, 401
Dizziness/syncope, 199–200
assessment, 199
causes and symptoms, 199
incidence of, 199
relief and preventative measures,
199–200
DMPA (depot medroxyprogesterone
acetate), 470–471, 492
Docosahexaenoic acid (DHA), 104, 106*t*,
118
Domestic violence. *See also* Intimate
partner violence
screening, postpartum, 435
substance abuse and, 248–249
Domperidone, for stimulation of milk
production, 509
Doppler flow studies, intrauterine
growth restriction and, 361
Doppler ultrasound, for auscultation of
fetal heart, 85, 132, 553
Doppler velocimetry
antenatal fetal testing, 187–188
defined, 352
Doulas, postpartum, 425
Down syndrome. *See* Trisomy 21
Doxepin
FDA approved indications, 454*t*
side effects, 454*t*
DRI. *See* Dietary reference intake
Drug Addiction Treatment Act of 2000,
250
Drug-drug interaction, for substance
exposed pregnancies, 248
Drug Enforcement Administration
(DEA), 225, 250
Drug resistance, defined, 223
Duloxetine
FDA approved indications, 455*t*
side effects, 455*t*
Dumping syndrome, 549
DVT. *See* Deep vein thrombosis
Dysthymic disorder, 622*t*
Dystocia, 325, 327
Dysuria, 536, 538

Early labor. *See also* Labor onset
ambulation in, 330
coping strategies and comfort
measures for, 330
defined, 325
determining active labor, 327
plan of care, 328–329
self-care, 329
sleep and rest in, 329–330

timing of admission to birth setting,
326
Early pregnancy loss, defined, 409
Eating disorders, 118–119
Eating disorders not otherwise specified
(EDNOS), 118–119
Eccrine sweat glands, 41
Eclampsia, 376–377
laboratory manifestations of, 381*f*
postpartum, 441, 446–447
Ectoderm, 19, 21–22, 27–28, 27*f*, 29*f*
Ectopic pregnancy, 341–343
defined, 335
diagnosis, 342
incidence, 342
management of, 342–343, 343*t*
maternal death and, 342
recurrence risk, 343
risk factors for, 342, 342*t*
signs and symptoms, 342, 342*t*
Ectropion, 5
Eczema, 580–581
Eczema of pregnancy. *See* Prurigo of
pregnancy (PP)
EDB (estimated date of birth), 82,
125–126, 137–138
EDC (estimated date of confinement),
125–126
EDCs (endocrine-disrupting chemicals),
274, 283
EDD (estimated date of delivery or
estimated due date), 125–126
Edema, 200
assessment, 200
causes and symptoms, 200
in preeclampsia, 379
relief and preventative measures,
200
Edinburgh Postnatal Depression Scale
(EPDS), 88, 452, 623
Education. *See* Health education
Edwards syndrome. *See* Trisomy 18
Effacement, 325, 327–328
EFM (electronic fetal monitor), 181
EFW. *See* Estimated fetal weight
Eicosapentaenoic acid (EPA), 104, 106*t*,
118
fish consumption guidelines, 104–105,
105*t*
Elastic stocking, 217
Electroacupuncture, for milk production
stimulation, 509
Electronic fetal monitor (EFM), 181
ELISA. *See* Enzyme-linked
immunosorbent assay
Embryo development, 27–29
folding, 28, 31*f*
gastrulation, 27, 27*f*
neurulation, 28
notochord formation, 28, 29*f*

organogenesis, 28–29
primitive streak, 27–28, 27*f*
Emergency contraception, 462, 474–475
Emollients
for atopic dermatitis, 581
for pemphigoid gestationis (PG), 584
for prurigo of pregnancy, 582
for pruritic urticarial papules and
plaques of pregnancy (PUPP), 583
Emotion
defined, 291, 301
effects of events/influences, 301
Emotional changes, 200–201
assessment, 201
causes and symptoms, 200
relief and preventative measures, 201
Emotional cushioning, 409, 413–414
Employment, of nursing mothers,
493–494
Endocervical canal, 5, 9–10
Endocrine disorders, 560–568
case study, 568
pregestational diabetes, 566–567
adverse pregnancy outcomes and,
567
classifications, 566
glycemic control, 567
perinatal risks of, 567
preconception counseling, 567
resources for women and health-care
providers, 567
terminology, 560
thyroid disorders, 560–566
causes and expected laboratory
findings, 561*t*
diagnosing, 561–562
hyperthyroidism, 561*t*, 564–565
hypothyroidism, 561*t*, 562–564
postpartum thyroiditis (PPT), 561*t*,
565–566
signs and symptoms, 562
thyroid physiology in pregnancy,
560–561, 561*f*
Endocrine-disrupting chemicals (EDCs),
274, 283
Endocrine pregnancy test, 125, 131–132
Endocrine system
maternal alterations during pregnancy,
46–47
adrenal function changes, 47
anatomical changes, 46
pituitary function changes, 46–47,
46*t*
thyroid function changes, 47
physiological alterations during
postnatal period, 421
Endoderm, 19, 21–22, 27–28, 27*f*
Endometrial cycle, 15–17, 17*f*
Endometritis, 441, 443. *See also* Uterine
infection

Endometrium, 5, 9*f*
  anatomy, 10
  decidual reaction, 22
  postpartum changes, 420
Endorphins, exercise and, 429
Engorgement, breast, 499, 506–507
Environmental and Occupational Health
    History Profile, 280, 281*t*
Environmental exposures, 279–284
  assessment of, 280, 281*t*
  to endocrine-disrupting chemicals
    (EDCs), 283
  Environmental and Occupational
    Health History Profile, 280,
    281*t*
  to metals and metalloids, 280, 282
  to organic solvents, 282
  to pesticides, 283
  preconception counseling on, 60–61
  preconception risk assessment and
    screening, 56, 57*f*
  reducing, 283–284
  Resources on pregnancy and
    environmental exposure for
    women, 288
  Resources on pregnancy and
    environmental exposure for
    health-care providers, 288
  Resource on work during pregnancy
    for women, 288
Enzyme-linked immunosorbent assay
    (ELISA)
  defined, 589
  for hepatitis C, 596
  for parvovirus B19, 597
  for varicella zoster, 603
EP (eczema of pregnancy). *See* Prurigo
    of pregnancy (PP)
EPA. *See* Eicosapentaenoic acid
EPDS (Edinburgh Postnatal Depression
    Scale), 88
Epigastric pain, 546
Epilepsy. *See* Seizure disorders
Epistaxis, 206–207
Epstein anomaly, 621
Epulis, 34, 40
Erb's palsy, 397
Ergonovine, for delayed postpartum
    hemorrhage, 446
Erythema infectiosum, 597
Erythrocyte sedimentation rate, increase
    in pregnancy, 44
Erythromycin, for chlamydia, 609
Erythropoiesis, 35
Eschar, 423
Escherichia coli
  antibiotic resistance, 539
  in urinary tract infections, 537, 539
Escitalopram
  FDA approved indications, 453*t*
  side effects, 453*t*

Escutcheon, 5–6
Estimated date of birth (EDB), 30, 82,
    125–126, 137–138
Estimated date of confinement (EDC),
    125–126
Estimated date of delivery or estimated
    due date (EDD), 125–126
Estimated fetal weight (EFW), 362
  defined, 387
  in gestational diabetes (GDM),
    392–393
  labor-stimulating activities, 404–405
  in multifetal pregnancy, 402
Estriol, 25
Estrogen(s)
  adrenal, 47
  in combined hormonal contraceptives
    (CHCs), 462, 464, 469–470
  corpus luteum secretion of, 15
  follicle production of, 15
  functions of, 25, 26*t*
  influence on milk supply, 433
  postpartum levels, 421
  puberty onset and, 13
  rising at end of menses, 17
Ethanol. *See* Alcohol
Ethinyl estradiol, 469
Ethnic disparities, in risk of prenatal
    death, 189
Ethnicity-based genetic screening,
    165–167, 166*t*
Ethosuximide, maternal and fetal effects
    of, 572*t*
Etonogestrel, 468
Evening primrose oil, 405
Exercise(s)
  abdominal strengthening, 429
  in gestational diabetes (GDM)
    management, 391
  Kegel exercises
    for hemorrhoids, 204
    for pelvic girdle pain, 195*t*
    for perineal discomfort, 431
    postpartum, 429
    for urinary incontinence, 216
  during lactation, 491–492
  pelvic floor and pelvic tilt, 195,
    195*t*
  postnatal, 428–429
  preconception counseling on, 59
  in pregnancy, 274–279
    benefits of, 275–276
    contraindications to, 275–276
    for depression, 623
    exercise activities, 277
    general advice for, 278–279
    guidelines for, 277–278, 277*f*
      exercise intensity, 277, 277*f*
      interval-type exercise, 277–278
      strength exercises, 278
    for headache control, 575

  motivating women, 276–277, 276*t*
  in obese women, 554
  physiological changes of pregnancy
    and, 274–275
  "talk test," 278
  terminology, 274
  transtheoretical stages of change
    and, 276–277, 276*t*
  warning signs to stop, 279
  prenatal health promotion and
    education, 93–94
  reasons to discontinue or decrease,
    93–94
Exercise intensity, 277, 277*f*
Exophthalmos, 560, 564
Expectation, 291
Expected date of birth (EDB). *See*
    Estimated date of birth
Expectorants, for upper respiratory
    infection, 522, 522*t*
Expert Panel on the Content of Prenatal
    Care, 75–79, 81, 84–85, 92
Expressing breast milk, 493–494
External anal sphincter, 8, 8*f*
External genitalia, anatomy of, 6–8, 7*f*
External os, 9*f*
External urethral orifice, 6*f*–8*f*
Extraembryonic somatic mesoderm, 19,
    22
Eye changes during pregnancy, 45

Facilitated transport/facilitated diffusion,
    19, 23, 24*t*
Fallopian tubes, 10–11
False labor, 326–327
False negative rate, 160
False positive rate, 160
Famciclovir, for herpes simplex virus
    (HSV), 611–612, 612*t*
Familial dysautonomia, genetic screening
    for, 87*t*, 166*t*, 167
Family
  defined, 291
  genetic risk evaluation, 161
  in poverty, 263
Family adaptation, postnatal care
    assessment of, 426–428
Family history, 84
Family Medical Leave Act (FMLA), 94
FAMs (fertility awareness-based
    methods), 462, 474
Fanconi's anemia, genetic screening for,
    167
Fantasy, in maternal role taking, 296
FAS (fetal alcohol syndrome), 242
FASD (fetal alcohol spectrum disorder),
    59, 92, 242
Fas/FasL, 34, 43
Fasting blood glucose (FBG), in
    gestational diabetes (GDM)
    management, 391–392

Fathers
    postnatal adjustment, 427
    psychosocial adaptation and
        attachment, 303–304
    signs and symptoms of pregnancy,
        303
Fatigue, 201
    assessment, 201
    causes and symptoms, 201
    from lack of sleep, 214
    postpartum, 428
    reduction for preterm birth
        prevention, 371
    relief and preventative measures,
        201
    work-associated, 286–287
Fats, 99
    in human milk, 480–481
    metabolism changes during pregnancy,
        41, 41t
    omega-3 fatty acids, 104–105
    recommendations in pregnancy,
        103–105
Fatty acids, in human milk, 481
FBG (fasting blood glucose), in
        gestational diabetes (GDM)
        management, 391–392
FDA. See Food and Drug Administration
Fear
    of childbirth (tocophobia), 153
    defined, 291
    of loss of control in labor, 300
    of loss of self-esteem in labor, 301
    predisposing variables to extreme,
        301
    of sexual activity in pregnancy,
        284–285
Federal Trade Commission (FTC), 225
Female condom, 473, 618
Female sterilization, 466
Feminist movements, 73
Femur length, gestational age estimation
        by, 140
Fennel seed, for stimulation of milk
        production, 510
Fenugreek, for stimulation of milk
        production, 510
Fern test, 352, 357
Ferritin
    defined, 525
    hematological findings during normal
        pregnancy, 526t
    in hematology conditions, 527t
    in iron-deficiency anemia, 526, 527t,
        529
Fertility, return after childbirth, 463
Fertility awareness-based methods
        (FAMs), 462, 474
Fetal alcohol spectrum disorder (FASDs),
        59, 92, 242
Fetal alcohol syndrome (FAS), 242

Fetal assessment for substance exposed
        pregnancies, 249
Fetal death, 409. See also Pregnancy loss;
        Stillbirth
    conditions related to increased risk of,
        177, 178t
Fetal fibronectin (fFN) testing, 368
Fetal growth and development, prenatal
        teaching regarding, 294
Fetal growth disorders, 358–362. See also
        specific disorders
    case study, 363
    determination of growth disorders,
        358–359
    fetal weight percentiles throughout
        gestation, 359f
    intrauterine growth restriction,
        359–361
    macrosomia, 361–362
    resources for health-care providers,
        363
    resources for women and their
        families, 363
    terminology, 352–353
Fetal growth restriction (FGR), 100
Fetal heart activity
    defined, 125
    identification of, 132, 132f
Fetal heart rate (FHR), 132
    accelerations, 180–183
    baseline, 176
    monitoring, 180–183, 181f
    variability, 176
Fetal heart sounds
    defined, 125
    maternal obesity and assessment of,
        553
    timing of hearing, 132
Fetal movement, detection of, 132–133,
        134f
Fetal movement count (FMC), 178–180,
        180f
    education on, 179
    factors influencing maternal perception
        of fetal movement, 179
    key points on fetal movement, 180
    in post-term pregnancy, 406t
    techniques for, 179
Fetal/neonatal withdrawal, opioid,
        249–252
Fetal origins of disease hypothesis,
        102–103
Fetal well-being, assessment of, 176–190
    antenatal fetal testing
        amniotic fluid volume (AFV)
            assessment, 183, 184t
        biophysical profile (BPP), 183–187
        contraction stress test, 183
        Doppler velocimetry, 187–188
        fetal heart rate (FHR) monitoring,
            180–183, 181f

    fetal movement counts (FMCs),
        178–180, 180f
    methods, 178–188
    nonstress test, 180–183
    oxytocin challenge test (OCT), 183
    physiological principles and
        indications for, 177
    case study, 190
    conditions related to increased risk of
        fetal death, 177, 178t
    cultural, personal, and family
        considerations, 188–189
    education and counseling, 188
    health disparities and vulnerable
        populations, 189
    legal and liability issues, 189–190
    overview, 176–177
    scope of practice considerations,
        177–178
    terminology, 176
Fetoscope, 125, 132, 132f
Fetotoxicity, 227
Fetus development, 29–30
FEV₁, 517
Fever, puerperal, 443
Feverfew, for headache, 574
fFN (fetal fibronectin) testing, 368
FGR (fetal growth restriction), 100
Fiber, 99
    for constipation, 199, 199t
    for hemorrhoids, 204
Fibrinogen, 36
Fibrinolysis, 34, 36
Fibroadenomas, 193
Fibroids. See Uterine fibroids
Fifth disease, 597
Fimbriae, 5, 9f, 11
Financial security, 263
First-degree laceration, 423
First polar body, 5, 12, 12f
Fish, mercury in, 282
Fish consumption guidelines, 104–105,
        105t
Fish oil supplements, 104
5A's and 5 R's model of smoking
        cessation, 91, 92t, 246, 247t
Flat nipples, 499, 503, 504t
Flatulence, 201–202
    assessment, 201–202
    causes and symptoms, 201
    relief and preventative measures, 202
Flavor learning, prenatal, 102–103
Floppy infant syndrome, benzodiazepine
        use associated with, 627
Fluid requirements during pregnancy,
        103
Fluid retention in pregnancy, 39
Fluoxetine
    drug-drug interactions and, 248
    FDA approved indications, 453t
    side effects, 453t

FMC. *See* Fetal movement count
FMLA (Family Medical Leave Act), 94
Folate, 106–107, 106*t*
 hematological findings during normal
  pregnancy, 526*t*
 requirement changes during
  pregnancy, 36
 supplementation, 530
Folate-deficiency anemia, 527*t*, 530
Folic acid antagonists, teratogenicity of,
 233*t*
Folic acid supplementation, 141, 162,
 224
 preconception counseling on, 59
 for women taking gabapentin, 211
Folinic acid, for toxoplasmosis, 601
Follicles, 11, 12*f*, 14–15, 14*f*
Follicle-stimulating hormone (FSH), 13,
 14*f*
 newborn's, 12
 ovarian cycle and, 14
 puberty onset, 13
Follicular phase, of ovarian cycle, 13–15
Food and Drug Administration (FDA)
 categories for drugs in pregnancy,
  229, 231, 231*t*
 Center for Drug Evaluation and
  Research (CDER), 225
 defined, 223
 DES and, 74
 DHA supplementation of infant
  formula, 104
 fish consumption advice, 105*t*
 folic acid supplementation of grain
  products, 106
 oversight of pharmaceutical agents,
  225
 preapproval drug trials, 229
 thalidomide and, 227–228
Food-borne illness, 99, 110
Food cravings, 40
Food groups and subgroups, 100, 101*t*
Food insecurity, 99, 261, 262
Food safety, 109–111
 alcohol, 110–111
 food-borne infections, 110
 foods and beverages to avoid,
  109*t*
 safe food handling, 109
Food stamps, 550
Food Tracker, 114
Food units, 100
Formula-feeding, 428
Fornix (fornices), 5, 8
Fortification, 99
 with folic acid, 106, 162
 with vitamin B₁₂, 118
Fosfomycin, for urinary tract infection,
 540*t*
Fourchette, 5

4Ps Plus screening tool, 245
Fourth-degree laceration, 423
Fourth trimester, 423
Fragile X syndrome, carrier screening
 for, 167
Frenulum of the clitoris, 6
FSH. *See* Follicle-stimulating hormone
FSH-releasing factor, 13, 14
FTC (Federal Trade Commission),
 225
Fundal height measurements, 138–139,
 139*f*
 defined, 125
 maternal obesity and, 553
Fundus
 defined, 423
 postpartum assessment of, 434
Fungal infections
 vaginal candidiasis, 613–614
Fussy baby, breastfeeding problems
 and, 499–500

Gabapentin
 maternal and fetal effects of, 572*t*
 for restless leg syndrome, 211
GAD. *See* Generalized anxiety disorder
GAD-7 screening tool, 627
Galactoceles, 193
Galactagogue, 499, 509–510
Gallstones, 40, 399, 546–547
Gametes, 19, 20
Gaskin, Ina May, 73, 75
Gastroenteritis, 544–545
Gastroesophageal reflux disease, 193.
 See also Heartburn
Gastrointestinal disorders
 appendicitis, 544, 547–548
 case study, 548
 cholecystitis, 546–547
 gastroenteritis, 544–545
 incidence of, 544
 intrahepatic cholestasis of pregnancy
  (ICP), 545–546
 resources for women and their
  families, 548
 terminology, 544
Gastrointestinal system
 adaptations during pregnancy, 39–40
  anatomical, 39–40
  functional changes, 40
  liver and biliary adaptations, 40,
   40*t*
 physiological alterations during
  postnatal period, 421
Gastrulation, 19, 27, 27*f*
Gaucher's disease, genetic screening for,
 167
GBS. *See* Group B *Streptococcus*
GDM. *See* Gestational diabetes mellitus
Gender, embryo, 11

Generalized anxiety disorder (GAD),
 626–627
 management of, 627
 postpartum, 450*t*, 451
 risk factors for, 627
 screening for, 627
Genetics, preconception risk assessment
 and, 56
Genetic screening, 56, 160–173
 carrier screening, 167
 case study, 172
 chromosomal microarray analysis
  (CMA), 169
 for cystic fibrosis, 165
 development in testing options,
  168–169
 diagnostic procedures, 167–168
  amniocentesis, 168
  chorionic villus sampling (CVS),
   168
  percutaneous umbilical blood
   sampling (PUBS), 168
 ethical considerations, 169
 ethnicity-based, 165–167, 166*t*
 family history and risk evaluation,
  161, 161*t*
 for fragile X syndrome, 167
 genetic counseling
  perspective on, 171–172
  pretest, 169
 for neural tube defects, 161–162
 noninvasive prenatal testing (NIPT),
  168–169
 offered to all pregnant women,
  161–165, 163*t*
 prenatal, 86, 87*t*
 psychosocial effects in, 170–171
 purposes, 160
 referrals to genetic counselor, 169
 resources for health-care providers,
  173
 resources for women and their
  families, 173
 scope of practice considerations, 169
 for spinal muscular atrophy (SMA),
  167
 "tentative pregnancy" and, 171
 terminology, 160
 for trisomy 21 and trisomy 18, 162–165
  first-trimester screening, 163–164,
   163*t*
  integrated screening, 163*t*, 164
  penta screen, 163*t*, 164
  quad screen, 163*t*, 164
  second-trimester screening, 164
  ultrasound, 164–165
Gentamycin, for pyelonephritis, 541
German measles. *See* Rubella
Germ layers, 28. *See also* Ectoderm;
 Endoderm; Mesoderm

Gestational age
    defined, 125
    genetic screening and, 161
Gestational age assessment, 133–140
    devices used to calculate, 136–137
    early, 126
    methods of estimating, 137–140
        basal body temperature change, 138
        fundal height measurements,
            138–139, 139f
        known date of conception, 138
        last menstrual period (LMP),
            137–138
        ultrasound, 139–140
    resources for health-care providers, 145
    resources for women and their
        families, 145
    terminology, 125, 133, 136
    timing of events in gestation, 135t–136t
Gestational age wheels, 82
Gestational diabetes mellitus (GDM),
        387–395
    assessment after Roux-en-Y gastric
        bypass, 555
    case study, 394
    decrease risk with exercise, 275
    defined, 387
    fetal surveillance and timing of birth,
        392–393
    incidence of, 566
    management of, 390–392
        blood glucose monitoring, 391–392
        dietary intervention, 390–391, 391t
        exercise, 391
        glyburide, 392
        insulin therapy, 392
        metformin, 392
        oral medications, 392
    nutrition in pregnancy and, 100, 103,
        105
    obesity and, 551–552
    pathophysiology of, 387–388
    postpartum follow-up, 393–394
    potential problems of, 388, 388t
    in preeclampsia, 378
    prenatal screening and diagnosis of,
        388–390, 389t
        one-hour oral glucose tolerance
            testing, 389
        screening high-risk women, 390
        two-hour oral glucose tolerance
            testing, 389–390
    resources for health-care providers, 395
    resources for women and their
        families, 395
    risk, perspective on, 394
    risk factor classification for, 388t
    risk factors for, 551
    scope of practice issues, 394
    terminology, 387

Gestational hypertension, 376
Gestational sac, 139–140
Gestational trophoblastic disease (GTD),
        340, 343–344
    diagnosis and management, 344
    incidence of, 344
    potential problems, 344
    presentation, 344
    recurrence risk, 344
    risk factors for, 344t
    types, 343t
Gestational weeks, 125, 133, 135t–136t,
        136. See also Gestational age
        assessment
GFR (glomerular filtration rate), 39
Ghrelin, 41
Gingival edema and hyperemia, 213
Gingivitis, 40, 196
"Giving of oneself," maternal role
        attainment and, 295–296
Glomerular filtration rate (GFR), 39
Glucagon, 41
Glucocorticoids, adrenal gland release of,
        47
Glucose tolerance, 41–42
Glucosuria, 39
Glyburide, 392
Glycated hemoglobin (A1c), 567
Glycemic control, in pregestational
        diabetes, 567
Glycemic index, 397
Glycogen, 551
Glycolic acid, for melasma, 213
Goals for prenatal care, 75–77, 76t
Goat's rue, for stimulation of milk
        production, 510
Goiter, 560–561, 564
Gonadarche, 5
Gonadostat, 5
Gonadotropin-releasing hormone,
        puberty onset and, 13
Gonadotropin-releasing hormone pulse
        generator (gonadostat), 12
Gonardarche, 13
Gonorrhea, 608, 609–610
    pregnancy testing and treatment,
        609–610
    screening recommendations, 58t
Goodell's sign, 125, 129
Governmental oversight of
        pharmaceutical agents, 225, 226t
Granulosa cells, 5, 14–15
Graves' disease, 44, 560, 561t, 564
Gregg, Norman, 227
Gregg, Robin, 170
Grief, perinatal loss and, 341, 409–415
    breaking the news, 410
    care and management of women with
        stillbirth, 410–411, 411t
    case study, 414

cultural considerations, 412
etiology of stillbirth, 410, 410t
grieving and emotional care after loss,
        411–412, 412t
interconception care, 413
physical care after stillbirth, 413
postpartum follow-up, 413
resources for health-care providers, 415
resources for women and their
        families, 415
rights of parents when a baby dies, 412t
subsequent pregnancy care, 413–414
terminology, 409
Grief work, 296
Ground substance, 5, 10
Group B Streptococcus (GBS), 592–593
    assessment, 592
    incidence of infection, 592
    management, 592–593
    mortality rate in newborns, 592
    potential problems, 592
    prevalence in healthy women, 592
    in urinary tract infections, 537, 539
Group prenatal care, 314
Growth charts, 491
Growth hormone
    pituitary, 46
    placental, 46
GTD. See Gestational trophoblastic
        disease
Gums, bleeding, 196

Habitual abortion, 341
Hair
    changes during pregnancy, 213
    maternal alterations during pregnancy,
        42–43
Hamilton Anxiety Rating Scale (HAM-
        A), 627
Haploid, 19, 20
HAPO (Hyperglycemia and Adverse
        Pregnancy Outcomes), 389
Harm reduction approach to prenatal
        substance use, 240
Hart's line, 5, 8
Hashimoto thyroiditis, 560, 561t, 562–563
HAV. See Hepatitis A virus
HBV. See Hepatitis B virus
hCG. See Human chorionic
        gonadotropin
HCV (hepatitis C virus), screening
        recommendations, 58t
Headache, 202–203, 573–577, 574t–576t
    assessment, 202
    causes and symptoms, 202
    cluster, 570, 574, 576–577
    diary, 574
    migraine, 570, 574–576
    nonpharmacological management,
        574–575, 576t

Headache (*cont'd*)
    pharmacological treatment, 575–576
    postpartum, 576
    relief and preventative measures,
        202–203
    tension, 570, 574, 575*t*
    triggers, 575
Head circumference, gestational age
        estimation by, 140
Health disparity
    defined, 261
    postnatal care, 436–437
Health education, 312–323
    antenatal fetal testing, 188
    case study, 322
    childbirth education
        Bradley Method, 313
        hospital-based classes, 313
        hypnobirthing, 313
        Lamaze, 313
        prenatal visit approach to, 314
        reading material, 314
        reality television shows, 314
        sources and quality of, 312–314
    cultural considerations, 321
    developmental considerations in
        prenatal education
        adolescents, 314–315
        adults, 315
    documentation of teaching, 321
    group prenatal care, 314
    guidelines for prenatal education,
        316
    health disparities and vulnerable
        populations, 321
    issues integral to prenatal education,
        315–316
    literacy and, 316
    prenatal, 76, 88, 90–95
        alcohol use, 92
        exercise, 93–94
        illicit drugs, 92–93
        nutrition, 90–91, 91*t*
        substance abuse, 91
        throughout pregnancy, 94–95, 95*t*
        tobacco use, 91–92, 92*t*
        working and pregnancy, 94
    prioritizing prenatal education needs,
        316–317
        anticipatory guidance, 317
        discussing health and safety issues,
            317
        responding to questions, 317
    resources for health-care providers,
        322–323
    resources for women and their
        families, 323
    terminology, 312
    timing of topics, 318*t*–320*t*
    topics throughout pregnancy, 95*t*
    trimester-based approach, 317

Health history
    Environmental and Occupational
        Health History Profile, 280, 281*t*
    of obese pregnant woman, 552
    problem-focused, 552
Health literacy, 312, 316
Health promotion, prenatal, 76, 88,
        90–95
    alcohol use, 92
    exercise, 93–94
    illicit drugs, 92–93
    nutrition, 90–91, 91*t*
    substance abuse, 91
    throughout pregnancy, 94–95, 95*t*
    tobacco use, 91–92, 92*t*
    working and pregnancy, 94
Healthy People 2020 document, 316
Hearing, changes during pregnancy, 45
Heart
    disease, signs and symptoms of
        pregnancy that mimic, 37*t*
    maternal alterations during pregnancy,
        37, 37*t*
Heartburn, 40, 203–204, 398*t*
    assessment, 203
    case study, 219
    causes and symptoms, 203
    incidence and prevalence of, 203
    relief and preventative measures,
        203–204
Heart palpitations, 204
    assessment, 204
    causes and symptoms, 204
    relief and preventative measures, 204
Heart rate
    fetal (*see* Fetal heart rate)
    increased maternal during pregnancy,
        37
Heavy lifting, 286
Heavy metals, exposure to, 280, 282
Hegar's sign, 5, 10, 125, 129, 129*f*
Helicobacter pylori, 207
HELLP syndrome, 382
    laboratory manifestations of, 381*f*, 382
    symptoms of, 382
Hematocrit, during normal pregnancy,
        526*t*
Hematological disorders, 525–534
    anemia, 525–529
        diagnosis, 525–526
        folate deficiency, 527*t*, 530
        iron deficiency, 526–529, 527*t*–528*t*
        physiological changes in pregnancy,
            525–526
        unexplained maternal, 530–531
        vitamin B$_{12}$ deficiency, 527*t*, 530
    bleeding disorders, 531
    case study, 534
    coagulopathies, 531–534, 533*t*
    hematological findings during normal
        pregnancy, 526*t*

hemoglobinopathies, 527*t*, 529–530
    resource for women and their families,
        534
    resources for health-care providers,
        534
    terminology, 525
Hematologic system adaptations during
        pregnancy, 34–36, 35*t*
    clotting factors, 36, 36*t*
    folate requirements, 36
    iron requirements, 35–36
    plasma, 35
    red blood cells, 35
    white blood cells, 35
Hematoma, subchorionic, 337
Hematoma postpartum, 441, 446
Hematuria, 536, 538, 541
Heme iron. *See* Iron
Hemoglobin
    A1C, 555, 567
    findings during normal pregnancy,
        526*t*
    in hematology conditions, 527*t*
    S, 525, 529
Hemoglobinopathies, 527*t*, 529–530
    hemoglobin S, 525, 529
    laboratory findings, 527*t*
    thalassemia, 525, 527*t*, 529–530
Hemophilia A, 531
Hemophilia B, 531
Hemorrhage. *See also* Bleeding
    decidual, 367
    delayed postpartum, 441, 445–446
    postpartum, 420
    subchorionic, 337
Hemorrhoids, 204
    assessment, 204
    causes and symptoms, 204
    postnatal care, 431
    relief and preventative measures,
        204
Hemostasis, 36
Heparin, for thromboprophylaxis, 532,
        533*t*
Hepatitis A virus (HAV), 593–594
    assessment, 593
    incidence of, 593
    management, 593–594
    potential problems, 593
    prevention, 594
    risk factors, 593
Hepatitis B virus (HBV), 594–596
    assessment, 594–595
        antihepatitis Be antibody (anti-
            HBe)), 595
        antihepatitis core antibody
            (anti-HBc)), 595
        HBe antigen, 595
        hepatitis B surface antigen (HBsAg),
            594
    chronic infection, 594

management, 595
potential problems, 594
prevention, 595–596
screening recommendations, 58t
vaccination, 595
Hepatitis C virus (HBV), 596–597
assessment, 596
management, 596–597
potential problems, 596
prevalence of, 596
risk factors for, 596
Hepatitis C virus (HCV), screening
recommendations, 58t
Herbals, 224
defined, 223
for depression, 625
for stimulation of milk production,
509–510
for mood and anxiety disorders, 457
Herd immunity, 589, 599
Herpes simplex virus (HSV), 608,
610–612, 611t–612t
classification of genital, 611, 611t
congenital, 611
fetal infection, 611
neonatal, 611
pregnancy testing and treatment,
611–612, 612t
prevalence of, 610
recurrence during pregnancy, 611
screening recommendations, 58t
signs and symptoms, 611
Herpetiform, defined, 580
HG. See Hyperemesis gravidarum
Hirsutism, 193, 213
Histamine 2-receptor antagonists, 203
History
Environmental and Occupational
Health History Profile, 280,
281t
genetic risk evaluation, 161
nutritional, 112, 112t, 113f, 113t
preconception risk assessment and
screening, 53
in preeclampsia diagnosis, 379
prenatal, 82–85
family, 84
infection, 84
initial visit, 82–84
nutritional, 84
pregnancy, 82, 84
psychosocial, 84
sexual, 84
subsequent visit, 85
sexual, 285
for vaginal bleeding, 336
HIV. See Human immunodeficiency
virus
Homan's sign, 423, 447
Homelessness, poverty and, 262–263
Homicide, 266

Hormones. See also specific hormones
hypothalamic-pituitary-ovarian axis,
13
levels in menstrual cycle, 17f
stimulating gonads, 14f
teratogenicity of, 233t
Housing, poverty and, 262–263
HPV. See Human papillomavirus
HSV. See Herpes simplex virus
Human chorionic gonadotropin (hCG)
beta-human chorionic gonadotropin
(β-hCG)
discriminatory levels for, 337t
for ectopic pregnancy diagnosis,
342
in gestational trophoblastic disease,
344
for pregnancy diagnosis, 131–132
serial, 337, 342, 344
fluctuations throughout pregnancy,
561f
functions of, 25, 26t
in genetic screening, 163, 164
hyperglycosylated hCG (h-hCG), in
genetic screening, 163
placental production of, 24–25
thirst center stimulation by, 35
Human immunodeficiency virus (HIV)
breastfeeding and, 479
maternal-child transmission (MCT)
of, 77
preconception care for, 64
preconception risk assessment and
screening, 56
screening recommendations, 58t
Human papillomavirus (HPV), 612–613
pregnancy testing and treatment, 613
prevalence of, 612
vertical transmission rate, 613
Human placental lactogen, 25, 26t
Humoral immunity, 44
Hunger, in breastfed infants, 500
Hydantoins (phenytoin), teratogenicity
of, 233t
Hydatidiform mole, 19, 25, 343–344,
343t
Hydroquinone, for melasma, 213
Hydroureter, 39
Hydroxyzine, 329
FDA approved indications, 455t
side effects, 455t
Hymen, 5–6, 6f
Hyperechogenic, 589, 597
Hyperemesis gravidarum (HG), 399–401
advice for women with, 400–401
care and management, 400–401
complications of, 400
etiology of, 400, 400t
evaluation of, 400
prevalence of, 399
risk factors for, 400

Hyperglycemia and Adverse Pregnancy
Outcomes (HAPO), 389
Hyperglycosylated human chorionic
gonadotropin (h-hCG), in genetic
screening, 163
Hyperparathyroidism, physiological, 46
Hyperpigmentation, 42, 212–213, 213f
Hyperplasia, 34, 39, 419
Hypertension. See Hypertensive disorders
Hypertensive disorders, 375–385
case study, 385
chronic hypertension, 375–376, 376t
preeclampsia superimposed on,
376t, 377
classification and definitions of, 376t
decreased risk with exercise, 275
gestational hypertension, 376
maternal deaths from, 375
placental abruption and, 346
preeclampsia, 376–384
atypical presentation, 382–383, 383t
criteria for diagnosis of, 377t
diagnostic evaluation of, 379–380
HELLP syndrome, 382
incidence of, 377
interprofessional practice issues,
384
long-term sequelae of, 383–384
management of, 380–382
pathophysiology of, 377–378, 378f
potential problems due to, 378
prediction of, 383
prevention of, 383
risk factors for developing, 378–379
risk management issues in office
setting, 384
superimposed on chronic
hypertension, 376t, 377
prevalence of, 375
resources for health-care providers,
384
resources for women and their
families, 384
terminology, 375
Hyperthyroidism, 561t, 564–565
clinical presentation, 564
diagnosis, 564
Graves' disease, 561t, 564
laboratory testing, 561t, 564
management, 564–565
maternal and fetal risks, 564
preconception care for, 64
scope of practice considerations, 565
signs and symptoms, 562
subclinical, 561t, 565
thyroid storm, 561t, 565
Hypertrophy, 419
Hypnobirthing, 313
Hypomania, 621, 622t, 625–626
Hyponatremia, in hyperemesis
gravidarum, 400

Hypospadias, vegetarian diet and risk for, 117
Hypotension, in supine hypotension syndrome (SHS), 215
Hypothalamic-pituitary-ovarian axis, 13, 14f
Hypothalamus-pituitary-adrenal axis
 in mood and anxiety disorders, 449
 premature activation and preterm birth, 366
Hypothalmic-pituitary-thyroid axis, 560, 561f
Hypothyroidism, 561t, 562–564
 clinical presentation, 562
 complications of, 562
 diagnosis, 562–563
 Hashimoto thyroiditis, 560, 561t, 562–563
 laboratory testing, 561t, 562–563
 management, 562–563
 maternal and fetal risks, 562
 overt, 562–563
 preconception care in, 64, 564
 screening in pregnancy, 563–564
 signs and symptoms, 562
 subclinical, 561t, 563
Hypoxemia
 defined, 176
 prediction of, 182
Hypoxia
 defined, 176
 fetal death and, 178, 181
 prediction of, 182, 184–185, 187

IADPSG (International Association of the Diabetes in Pregnancy Study Group), 389–390
IBCLCs (International Board Certified Lactation Consultants), 479
Ibuprofen
 for afterbirth pain, 430
 after stillbirth, 413
ICP. See Intrahepatic cholestasis of pregnancy
Identification with motherhood role, 297
Idiopathic, defined, 352
Idiopathic seizure disorder, 570
Idiopathic thrombocytopenia purpura (ITP), 531
IgG antibodies, 589
IgM antibodies, 589
IH (impetigo herpetiformis), 582t, 585
Ileus, 545
Illicit drug use
 by breastfeeding mother, 493
 preconception counseling on, 60
 prenatal health promotion and education, 92–93
 prevalence of, 239

Illusion of choice, 154
Immigrants, postnatal care for, 436–437
Immune globulin
 hepatitis A virus (HAV), 593
 hepatitis B virus (HBV), 595
 varicella zoster, 603
Immune system, maternal alterations during pregnancy, 43–45
 disorders related to, 44–45
 fetus as allograft, 43–44
Immunity, herd, 589, 599
Immunization, prenatal, 88, 89f
Immunoglobulins
 classes of, 44
 defined, 589
Impetigo herpetiformis (IH), 582t, 585
Implantation
 location of, 21
 timing of, 21
Implantation bleeding, 19, 22
Implant contraception, 468–469
Incarceration, 264–265
 guidelines to consider for incarcerated pregnant women, 265
 substance abuse issues, 264
Incompetent cervix, 341
Incontinence, urinary, 39, 216
Increased warmth and perspiration, 204–205
Individual growth potential curve, 352, 359
Indomethacin, 358
Infant feeding
 bottle-feeding, 428
 breastfeeding (see Breastfeeding)
 formula-feeding, 428
 postnatal care assessment, 428
Infection history, 84
Infections/infectious diseases, 589–604
 breast abscess, 507–508
 case study, 604
 cytomegalovirus (CMV), 590–591
 food-borne, 110
 group B Streptococcus (GBS), 592–593
 hepatitis A virus (HAV), 593–594
 hepatitis B virus (HBV), 594–596
 hepatitis C virus (HBV), 596–597
 mastitis, 499, 507
 parvovirus B19, 597
 preconception counseling on, 60
 preconception risk assessment and screening, 56–57, 58t
 puerperal (postpartum) infection, 443–445
 clinical presentation, 444, 445t
 diagnosis and management, 444–445
 maternal mortality from, 443
 risk factors for, 444

 uterine infection, 443–445, 444t–445t
 resources for health-care providers, 604
 resources for women, 604
 risk with intrauterine contraception, 467–468
 rubella, 597–599
 STIs (See Sexually transmitted infections)
 terminology, 589
 toxoplasmosis, 599–602, 600f, 601t
 transplacental, 24t
 treating for preterm birth prevention, 370
 varicella zoster virus (VZV), 602–603
 wound, 445
Inferior hypogastric plexus, 8
Inflammation, preterm birth and, 366–367
Inflammatory markers increased in pregnancy, 44
Influenza, 521
 case study, 523
 treatment, 521
Informed compliance, 154, 169
Informed consent, 154–157
 components of, 169
 in genetic screening, 169–170
Inhibin, 25, 26t
Inhibin A, in genetic screening, 163–164
Innate immune system, 43–44
INR (international normalized ratio), 532t
Insomnia. See Sleep disturbances
Inspiratory capacity, 517
Institute of Medicine (IOM), 79–80, 90, 91t
 pregnancy weight gain recommendations, 107, 108t
Insufficient milk supply, 499, 508–510, 508t–509t
Insulin
 for gestational diabetes (GDM), 392
 as a growth hormone in pregnancy, 551
 metabolic alterations during pregnancy, 41–42
 for pregestational diabetes, 566
Insulin pump, 566
Insulin resistance, 41
 body mass index (BMI) and, 551
 defined, 387, 549
 in gestational diabetes, 388
 in preeclampsia, 378
Integrated screen, genetic, 163t, 164
Interconception care
 after stillbirth, 413
 defined, 51
Intercourse
 labor induction by, 405
 resumption of postpartum, 431–432

Interferon, for multiple sclerosis, 577
Internal anal sphincter, 8
Internal genitalia, anatomy of, 8–11, 9f
Internal os, 9f
Internatal care, defined, 312
International Association of the Diabetes
    in Pregnancy Study Group
    (IADPSG), 389–390
International Board Certified Lactation
    Consultants (IBCLCs), 479
International normalized ratio (INR),
    532t
Internet, as information source, 314
Interpregnancy interval, 462
    preterm birth prevention and, 370
Interval training, defined, 274
Interval-type exercise, 277–278
Intimacy, resumption of sexual
    postpartum, 431–432
Intimate partner violence, 265–266
    abdominal trauma and, 399
    assessment and planning, 266, 267t
    comorbid with substance use, 241
    cycle of, 265–266
    defined, 261
    intended pregnancy counseling,
        143
    legal action, 266
    postpartum screening for, 435, 437
    prenatal preventative care, 88, 90
    prevalence of, 265, 617
Intrahepatic cholestasis of pregnancy
    (ICP), 582t, 585–586
    assessment, 586
    collaboration, consultation, and
        referral, 586
    defining characteristics of, 582t
    differential diagnosis, 586
    fetal outcomes of, 586
    incidence of, 585
    risk factors for, 585
    treatment and management, 586
Intrauterine contraception (IUC), 462,
    467–468
    advantage of, 468
    in breastfeeding women, 492
    contraindications to use, 467–468
    copper IUD, 467–468, 475
    expulsion of device, 468
    levonorgestrel IUD, 467
Intrauterine growth restriction (IUGR),
    177, 359–361
    assessment and management, 360–361
    asymmetric, 360
    defined, 352
    risk factors for development of, 361t
    symmetric, 360
Intrauterine infection. See Uterine
    infection
Introitus, 5, 8

Introjection, in maternal role taking,
    296
Inverted nipples, 499, 503, 504t
in vitro fertilization, 305
Involution
    assessment of, 433–434
    defined, 423
Iodine, thyroid gland and, 47
Iris lesion, 580, 582
Iron
    absorption of, 106, 527
    food sources, 527–529, 528t
    hematological findings during normal
        pregnancy, 526t
    needs in pregnancy, 105–106, 106t
    requirement changes during
        pregnancy, 35–36
    in vegetarian/vegan diet, 118
Iron-deficiency anemia, 106, 526–529,
    527t–528t
    dietary counseling, 527–529, 528t
    iron supplements, 527, 527t
    laboratory findings, 527t
Iron replacement therapy, for restless leg
    syndrome, 210
Iron supplements, 106, 527, 527t
Ischiocavernosus muscle, 8f
Isotretinoin, 229, 233t
Isthmus, 5
IUC. See Intrauterine contraception
IUD. See Intrauterine device
IUGR. See Intrauterine growth
    restriction

Jacquemin's sign, 125, 129, 129f
Jaundice
    defined, 544
    intrahepatic cholestasis of pregnancy
        (ICP), 545–546

Katz-Rothman, Barbara, 171
Kava root, for mood and anxiety
    disorders, 457
Keeping Children and Families Safe Act,
    252
Kegel exercises
    for hemorrhoids, 204
    for pelvic girdle pain, 195t
    for perineal discomfort, 431
    postpartum, 429
    for urinary incontinence, 216
Kennell, Marshall, 293–294
Kessner Index, 79
Ketonuria, 325, 328
Kidney adaptations during pregnancy,
    38–39
    anatomical changes, 39
    renal function, 39
Kidney stones, 536, 541
Klaus, John, 293–294

Kleihauer-Betke test, 335, 348, 397
Known date of conception, for
    gestational age estimation, 138
K-Y Jelly, 432

Labeling women as high risk, 151
Labia
    majora, 5–6, 6f–7f
    minora, 5–6, 6f–7f
    physiological alterations during
        postnatal period, 420
Labor
    defined, 325
    dystocia, 325, 327
    in gestational diabetes (GDM), 393
    induction (see Labor induction)
    onset (see Labor onset)
    preparation for, 299–300
    preterm (see also Preterm birth)
        diagnosis, 368
        initial evaluation, 369
        management of women with,
            368–369
    psychosocial adaptation to pregnancy,
        299–300
Laboratory tests
    preconception risk assessment and
        screening, 53
    prenatal, 85–86, 86t, 87t
    for substance exposed pregnancies,
        248
    for vaginal bleeding, 337, 337t
Labor induction
    elective, 405–406
    methods
        castor oil, 405
        stripping of the membranes, 397,
            404–405
        unprotected sexual intercourse,
            405
    for post-term pregnancies, 404–406
Labor onset
    ambulation in early labor, 330
    anticipatory guidance during prenatal
        period, 327
    case study, 331
    coping strategies and comfort
        measures for early labor, 330
    data collection, 327–328
    determining active labor, 327
    determining onset of labor, 325–326
    false labor, 326–327
    plan of care, 328–329
        self-care, 329
    sleep and rest in early labor,
        329–330
    timing of admission to birth setting,
        326
Labor-stimulating activities in post-term
    pregnancy, 404–405

Lactation, 478–495. *See also*
        Breastfeeding
    anatomy and physiology of, 482–483,
        482*f*
    asthma exacerbations, management of,
        520, 520*f*
    defense agents in human milk, 482
    delayed, 489, 556
    exercise during, 491–492
    menses resumption in lactating
        women, 432, 432*t*
    milk production, 489, 490*t*
    nutritional properties of human milk,
        480–482
    nutrition for nursing mothers,
        491–492
    in obese women, 556
    terminology, 478
Lactational amenorrhea method (LAM),
        462, 463, 472, 492
Lactation consultants, 479
Lactiferous ducts, 483
Lactobacilli, 5, 614–615, 615*t*
Lactogenesis I, 482
Lactogenesis II, 464, 482, 489
Lactose, 481
Lacunae, 19, 21
Ladin's sign, 125, 129
LAM (lactational amenorrhea method),
        462–463, 472, 492
Lamaze, Fernand, 73
Lamaze method, 75, 313
Lamotrigine, maternal and fetal effects
        of, 572*t*
Language as a reflection and
        construction of social realities,
        299
Lanolin, use on nipples, 506
Lanugo, 19, 30
Laparoscopic gastric banding (LAP-
        BAND), 549, 555
LARC (long-acting reversible
        contraceptive methods), 462,
        467–469
Large for gestational age (LGA), 352,
        358, 361
    defined, 387
    in gestational diabetes (GDM), 393
    maternal obesity and, 551–552
Last menstrual period (LMP), gestational
        age estimation, 137–138
Latch, in breastfeeding, 487–488, 488*f*
Late ovulation, 397, 404
Late preterm birth, 365–366, 366*f*
Late preterm infants, breastfeeding
        problems with, 503, 504*t*
Lateral fornix, 9*f*
Laxatives, 199, 199*t*, 204
LBW. *See* Low birth weight
Lead exposure, 56, 280, 282

Lederman, Regina, 297–301
LEEP (loop electrosurgical excision
        procedure), history of prior, 368
Legal and liability issues
    fetal well-being assessment, 189–190
    in management of pregestational
        obesity, 555–556
    postnatal care, 438
Leg cramps, 205–206
    assessment, 205
    causes and symptoms, 205
    relief and preventative measures,
        205–206, 205*f*
Leg exam, postpartum, 434–435
Leg varicosities, 216–217
Leiomyoma
    defined, 335
    vaginal bleeding and, 337
Leopold's maneuvers, 85, 125, 132–133,
        134*f*, 362
Leptin, 5, 41
LES (lower esophageal sphincter), 203
Lesbian relationship
    caring for the pregnant woman in, 304
    legal issues, 305
    psychosocial adaptation and
        attachment, 304–305
Let down reflex, 482–483
Leukocyte ALP, increase in pregnancy, 44
Leukonychia, 193
Leukorrhea, 205
    assessment, 205
    causes and symptoms, 205
    defined, 193
    as presumptive sign of pregnancy, 128
    relief and preventative measures, 205
Levetiracetam, maternal and fetal effects
        of, 572*t*
Levonorgestrel
    IUD, 467
    oral, 474–475
Levothyroxine, 563, 566
LGA. *See* Large for gestational age
LH. *See* Luteinizing hormone
Libraries, as information source, 314
Life Course Perspective, 52
Lifestyle changes, for headache, 575
Light therapy, for depression, 623
Linea alba, 34
Linea nigra, 34, 212
    defined, 193
    as presumptive sign of pregnancy, 128
Lipolysis, 19, 25, 41
Lipolytic, 34
Lipoprotein, increase during pregnancy,
        41, 41*t*
Listening to Mothers II survey, 313
Listeriosis, 110, 545
Liston method of fetal movement counts,
        179

Literacy, 312, 316
Lithium
    for bipolar disorder, 626
    teratogenicity of, 233*t*
Live birth, defined, 409
Live modeling experiences, 307
Liver and biliary adaptations of
        pregnancy, 40, 40*t*
LMP (last menstrual period), gestational
        age estimation, 137–138
LMWH (low-molecular-weight heparin),
        for thromboprophylaxis, 532,
        533*t*
Lochia, 419–420
    after stillbirth, 413
    appearance of, 430*f*
    defined, 423
    flow, 430
    postpartum, 430
    in uterine infection, 444, 445*t*
Lochia alba, 420, 430
Lochia rubra, 420, 430
Lochia serosa, 420, 430
Long-acting reversible contraceptive
        methods (LARC), 462, 467–469
Loop electrosurgical excision procedure
        (LEEP), history of prior, 368
Loperamide, 545
Loratadine
    for atopic dermatitis, 581
    for pruritic urticarial papules and
        plaques of pregnancy (PUPP),
        583
Lorazepam
    FDA approved indications, 455*t*
    side effects, 455*t*
Lordosis, 34, 45
Loss of control in labor, fear of, 300
Lotus birth, 23
Low birth weight (LBW)
    caffeine linked to, 111
    defined, 352
    link to coronary heart disease,
        102–103
    nutrition in pregnancy and, 100,
        102–103
    preconception care benefits and, 52
Lower esophageal sphincter (LES), 203
Lower UTI, defined, 536
Low milk supply, 499, 508–510,
        508*t*–509*t*
Low-molecular-weight heparin
        (LMWH), for
        thromboprophylaxis, 532, 533*t*
Lumbar lordosis, 193
Luteinizing hormone (LH), 13, 14*f*
    newborn's, 12
    ovulation and, 15
    puberty onset, 13
Lymphatic breast drainage therapy, 506

Lymphatics
  uterine, 11
  vaginal, 8

Macronutrients, 99
  dietary reference intakes, 106t
  fats, 103–105
  protein, 105
  total energy, 103
Macrophages, 43–44
Macrosomia, 361–362
  assessment and management, 362
  defined, 352, 387, 397
  in gestational diabetes, 388, 393
  in post-term pregnancy, 404
  risk factors for, 361
Magnesium sulfate
  for postpartum preeclampsia/
      eclampsia, 447
  for preeclampsia management, 382
Magnesium supplements
  for headache, 574
  to reduce leg cramps, 206
Major depressive disorder (MDD), 621,
      622t
Major histocompatibility complex
      (MHC), 43
Malathion, exposure to, 283
Male condoms, 473
Male genitalia, embryonic development
      of, 7f
Male partners
  psychosocial adaptation and
      attachment, 303–304
  sexuality in pregnancy, 284–285
Male sterilization (vasectomy),
      466–467
Mania, 621, 622t, 625, 626t. See also
      Bipolar disorder
Manic depression. See Bipolar disorder
March of Dimes, 365
Marijuana
  breastfeeding and, 254t
  preconception counseling on, 60
  pregnancy implications of use, 244
  prevalence of use, 244
Marital status, trends in, 302t
Mask of pregnancy, 212, 212f
Massage, breast, 506
Massage therapy
  for depression, 623
  for headache control, 575
Massively parallel shotgun sequencing
      (MPSS), 168
Mastitis, 499, 507
  incidence of, 507
  risk factors for, 507
  signs and symptoms, 507
Material safety data sheets (MSDSs), 94,
      280, 283

Maternal attachment and adaptation,
      292–301, 426–427
  assessment of, 296
  Bowlby and Ainsworth, 293
  Brazelton, 294
  detachment as protective mechanism,
      299
  Kennell and Klaus, 293–294
  Lederman, 297–301
  Rubin, 294–297
Maternal detachment as a protective
      mechanism, 299
Maternal role attainment, 428
Maternal role development
  cognitive processes in
      dedifferentiation, 296
      fantasy, 296
      replication, 296
  indicators for, 295
  tasks for, 294–296
      acceptance of others, 295
      binding to the child, 295
      giving of oneself, 295–296
      safe passage, 295
Maternity Center Association (MCA), 74
McBurney's point, 544
McDonald's sign, 125, 130, 130f
MDD (major depressive disorder), 621,
      622t
Mean corpuscular hemoglobin (MCH),
      525–526, 526t
Mean corpuscular volume (MCV),
      525–526, 526t
Meatus, 5
MEC (medical eligibility criteria), 462,
      464–465
Meconium aspiration syndrome, 397
Meconium-stained amniotic fluid
      (MSAF), 356
Medicaid
  Medicaid for Pregnant Women
      (MPW), 263
  postpartum care visits, 463
Medical abortion, 144
Medical and psychosocial interventions
      and follow-up, in prenatal care, 76
Medical eligibility criteria (MEC), 462,
      464–465
Medication(s), 223–236. See also specific
      drugs
  breastfeeding mothers and, 493
  case study, 236
  controlled substances, 225, 226t
  environmental exposure to
      pharmaceuticals, 224
  government oversight of, 225, 226t
  off-label prescribing, 225
  pharmacokinetics and pregnancy,
      clinical implications of, 231, 234,
      235t

preconception risk assessment and
      screening, 56
prescription
  components of, 225–226
  sample, 227f
prescriptive authority, 224–225
rational use in pregnancy, 234, 235t
resources for women and their
      families, 236
risks in pregnancy, 226–227
teratology, 227–231
  critical periods in human
      development, 228–229, 230f
  drugs with minimal or no
      teratogenicity, 234t
  etiology of birth defects, 228,
      228f
  examples of teratogens, 232t–233t
  FDA categories for drugs in
      pregnancy, 229, 231, 231t
  history of, 227
  identification of a teratogen, 229
  mechanisms of teratogenic drugs,
      228–229
  Wilson's six principles of teratology,
      228, 228t, 229
terminology, 223, 224
types of pharmaceutical agents, 224
MedlinePlus Guide to Healthy Web
      Surfing, 314
Megacolon, toxic, 545
Melancholy, 621
Melanocyte-stimulating hormone
      (MSH), 42
Melasma, 212–213, 212f
  cause of, 34
  defined, 34, 193
Men, preconception care for, 65–66
  counseling, 66
  risk assessment and screening, 66
Menarche, 5
  average age for, 13, 15t
  induction of, 13
Mendelian condition, 160, 165, 167
Menses, 17
  first postpartum, 463
  postnatal resumption of, 432, 432t
Menstrual age. See Gestational weeks
Menstrual cycle physiology, 11–18
  beginnings, 11–13
  characteristics of normal cycle, 15t
  endometrial cycle, 15–17, 17f
  hormones of, 13, 14f, 15t
  hypothalamic-pituitary-ovarian axis,
      13
  onset of puberty, 13
  ovarian cycle, 13–15, 16f, 17f
Menstrual phase, of endometrial cycle,
      16
Menstrual weeks. See Gestational weeks

Mental health. *See also* Psychological disorders
    preconception care for illness, 64
    preconception risk assessment and screening, 53, 56
    prenatal care, 88
Menthol, for pruritic urticarial papules and plaques of pregnancy (PUPP), 583
Mephedrone, 244
Mercury exposure, 282
    fish consumption and, 104, 105t
    preconception counseling on, 60–61
    preconception risk assessment and screening, 56
Mesenchymal cells, 19, 28
Mesoderm, 19, 21–22, 27–28, 27f, 29f
Metabolic alterations during pregnancy, 40–42
    basal metabolic rate, 41
    carbohydrate metabolism, 41
    fat metabolism, 41, 41t
    ghrelin, 41
    insulin, 41–42
    leptin, 41
    protein metabolism, 41
Metals and metalloids, exposure to, 280, 282
Metaplasia, 5, 10
Metformin, 392
Methadone
    breastfeeding and, 254t
    drug-drug interactions and, 248
    for opioid dependence, 250–251
Methamphetamines, pregnancy implications of use, 244
Methicillin-resistant *Staphylococcus aureus* (MRSA), 248
Methimazole, 564–565
Methotrexate, 343
Methylenedioxypyrovalerone, 244
Methylergonovine
    for delayed postpartum hemorrhage, 446
    for subinvolution, 446
Methylmercury, 282
Methylone, 244
Metoclopramide, for stimulation of milk production, 509
Metritis, 441, 443. *See also* Uterine infection
Metronidazole
    for bacterial vaginosis (BV), 615
    for trichomoniasis, 614
MHC (major histocompatibility complex), 43
Micronutrients, 99
    calcium, 106t, 107
    folate, 106–107, 106t

iron, 105–106, 106t
    vitamin D, 106t, 107
Midwives, history of, 75, 303
Mifepristone, 144
Migraine headache, 570, 574–576
Milk. *See also* Breastfeeding
    defense agents in human, 482
    expressing breast milk, 493–494
    intake, assessing, 490–491
    medication transfer into breast milk, 493
    nutritional properties of human milk, 480–482
    production of, 489, 490t
Milk culture, 507
Milk duct, plugged, 506–507
Milk ejection reflex, 482–483
Milk supply, insufficient, 499, 508–510, 508t–509t
    common contributors to, 508, 508t
    interventions for, 509t
Milk thistle, for milk production stimulation, 510
Mimicry, 296
Mineralocorticoids, adrenal gland release of, 47
Minipills. *See* Progestin-only pills (POPs)
Miscarriage
    defined, 409
    fear of, 284
Misoprostol, 144, 346
    for antepartum fetal death, 410
    teratogenicity of, 233t
Mittelschmerz, 5, 15
Modeling
    live experiences, 307
    symbolic, 307
Moderate preterm birth, 365–366
Modified biophysical profile, 187, 187f, 352, 361
    defined, 352, 397
    in post-term pregnancy, 406t
MoM (multiple of the median), 161, 168
Monounsaturated fatty acids (MUFAs), 99
Monozygotic twins, 397, 401
Mons pubis, 6, 6f
Montgomery's tubercles/glands, 212, 483
Mood disorders
    postpartum, 448–457
        assessment and screening, 452
        blues, 441, 449
        management, 452–457, 453t–456t
        signs and symptoms, 450t
    prevalence of, 448
Moore method of fetal movement counts, 179
"Morning-after pill," 474
Morning sickness, 207

Mortality, maternal. *See also specific causes*
    postnatal, 442, 442f
Morula, 19–20, 21f
Mother-daughter relationships, 298
"Mothering the mother," 296
Motivational interviewing
    defined, 238
    in substance use in pregnancy, 245
Motor vehicle accidents, 399
MPSS (massively parallel shotgun sequencing), 168
MRSA (methicillin-resistant *Staphylococcus aureus*), 248
MS (multiple sclerosis), 577
MSAF (meconium-stained amniotic fluid), 356
MSDSs (material safety data sheets), 94, 280, 283
MSH (melanocyte-stimulating hormone), 42
Mucin, 5, 10
Mucolipidosis IV, genetic screening for, 167
MUFAs (monounsaturated fatty acids), 99
Multifetal pregnancy, 401–403
    anticipatory guidance, 403
    assessing fetal growth, 402
    care of women with, 402
    decreasing risk of preterm birth, 402
    diagnosis of, 402
    fetal surveillance, 402–403
    incidence of, 401
    nutritional counseling, 403, 403t
Multipara, defined, 325
Multiple of the median (MoM), 161, 168
Multiple sclerosis (MS), 577
Mupirocin, for cracked nipple infections, 506
Murphy's sign, 544, 546
Muscle glycogen, 551
Musculoskeletal system, adaptations during pregnancy, 45–46
Myasthenia gravis, 44
Myometrium, 5, 9f, 10–11
MyPlate, 114, 115t

Naegele, Franz Karl, 73, 82
Naegele's rule, 82, 137
Nail changes during pregnancy, 213
Nails, maternal alterations during pregnancy, 43
Narrow band ultraviolet B (NBUVB) phototherapy, for prurigo of pregnancy, 582
NAS. *See* Neonatal abstinence syndrome
Nasal congestion, 206
    assessment, 206
    causes and symptoms, 206
    relief and preventative measures, 206

Nasal decongestant sprays, 206
National Diabetes Data Group (NDDG), 389, 389t
National High Blood Pressure Education Program Working Group (NHBPEP), 375, 380
National Institute of Child Health and Human Development (NICHD), 180
National Institute of Health (NIH), omega-3 intake recommendations of, 104
National Patient Safety Foundation, 316
National Quitline Number, 91
National Society of Genetic Counselors (NSGC), 168
National Survey of Family Growth, 466–467
"Natural" childbirth, 299
Natural killer cells, 43–44
Nausea and vomiting of pregnancy (NVP), 207–209, 208t–209t, 209f
    assessment, 207, 208t
    case study, 218
    causes and symptoms, 207
    hyperemesis gravidarum (HG), 399–401, 400t
    incidence of, 207
    relief and preventative measures, 207–208, 208t–209t, 209f
NDDG (National Diabetes Data Group), 389, 389t
NDRI. See Norepinephrine and dopamine reuptake inhibitor
Near-poverty, defined, 261
NEC (necrotizing enterocolitis), 502
Necrotizing enterocolitis (NEC), 502
Negative feedback, 13, 14f, 15
Negative predictive value, 149, 176
Neisseria gonorrhoeae, 609–610
Neonatal abstinence syndrome (NAS), 252–253
    assessment and treatment of, 252
    breastfeeding and, 252
    defined, 238
    described, 252
    long-term implications of, 252–253
Neonatal behaviors, maternal attachment and, 294
Neonatal death, defined, 409
Neonatal intensive care units, emotional disconnect for mothers and, 293
Neonatal withdrawal
    benzodiazepines, 244
    nicotine, 242
Nephrolithiasis, 536, 541
Nerve supply
    to cervix, 10
    to uterus, 11
    to vagina, 8

Nervous system
    disorders (see Neurological disorders)
    maternal alterations during pregnancy, 45
Neural crest cells, 28
Neural tube defects (NTDs)
    defined, 34
    folate deficiency and, 106
    folate for prevention of, 36
    genetic screening test, 87t
    preconception counseling on, 59
    risk factors for, 162
    screening options for, 161–162
Neurological disorders, 570–578
    case study, 578
    headache, 573–577, 574t–576t
    multiple sclerosis (MS), 577
    resources for women and their families, 578
    seizure disorders, 570–573
    terminology, 570
Neurontin, for bipolar disorder, 626
Neurulation, 19, 28
NHBPEP (National High Blood Pressure Education Program Working Group), 375, 380
NICHD (National Institute of Child Health and Human Development), 180
Nicotine. See also Smoking
    breastfeeding and, 254t
    neonatal withdrawal, 242
    pregnancy implications of use, 242–243
    prevalence of use, 239
Nicotine replacement, 246, 492
Niemann-Pick disease, genetic screening for, 167
NIH (National Institute of Health), omega-3 intake recommendations of, 104
NIPD (noninvasive prenatal diagnosis), 168–169
Nipples
    anatomy, 483
    cracked, 505–506
    flat or inverted, 499, 503, 504t
    postnatal assessment, 428
    sore (see Sore nipples)
NIPT (noninvasive prenatal testing), 168–169
Nitric oxide, 35, 37
Nitrofurantoin, for urinary tract infection, 540t
Nocebo effects, 151
Nocturia, 536, 538
Noise exposure, 287
Noninvasive prenatal diagnosis (NIPD), 168–169

Noninvasive prenatal testing (NIPT), 168–169
Nonoxynol-9, 473
Nonrapid eye movement (NREM) sleep, 45
Nonsteroidal anti-inflammatory drugs (NSAIDs)
    for afterbirth pain, 430
    for headaches, 576
Nonstress test (NST), 180–183
    defined, 352–353, 397
    intrauterine growth restriction and, 361
    in post-term pregnancy, 406t, 407
Norepinephrine and dopamine reuptake inhibitor (NDRI)
    black box warning, 455t
    for depression, 457, 624t
    FDA approved indications, 455t
    side effects, 455t
Nosebleed, 206–207
Notochordal process, 19, 28, 29f
NREM (nonrapid eye movement) sleep, 45
NSAIDs. See Nonsteroidal anti-inflammatory drugs
NSGC (National Society of Genetic Counselors), 168
NST. See Nonstress test
NTDs. See Neural tube defects
Nuchal translucency (NT) measurement, 160, 163–164
Nugent scoring system, 614–615, 615t
Nulliparous, 5, 325
Numerical risk, 154
Nursing. See Breastfeeding
Nutrition, 99–121
    in adolescent pregnancy, 116–117
    assessment of, 112–114
        clinical signs of nutritional status, 114t
        history, 112, 112t–113t, 113f
        resource use, 112, 114
    for breastfeeding mother, 491–492
    case study, 120–121
    counseling for optimal, 114, 116
    counseling in multifetal pregnancy, 403, 403t
    deficiencies, 369
    eating disorders, 118–119
    factors influencing intake, 111–112
        culture and family, 111–112
        resource availability, 111
    food groups and subgroups, 100, 101t
    food safety, 109–111, 109t
    food units, 100
    needs in pregnancy
        calcium, 106t, 107
        carbohydrates, 105
        dietary reference intakes, 106t

Nutrition (*cont'd*)
    fats, 103–105
    fluid intake, 103
    folate, 106–107, 106*t*
    iron, 105–106, 106*t*
    macronutrients, 103–105, 106*t*
    micronutrients, 105–107, 106*t*
    omega-3 fatty acids, 104–105
    protein, 105
    total energy, 103
    vitamin D, 106*t*, 107
  nutritional properties of human milk,
    480–482
  pica, 119–120
  portion size, 100
  postpartum, 429
  poverty and, 262
  prenatal, 90–91
    health outcomes and, 100, 102–103
    prenatal flavor learning, 103
  for preterm birth prevention, 369–370
  resources for health-care providers,
    121
  resources for women and their
    families, 121
  serving size, 100, 101*t*
  terminology, 99
  for vegetarians and vegans, 117–118,
    117*t*
  weight gain, 107–108
Nutritional history, 84
Nutritional supplements, 224–225, 234
NVP. *See* Nausea and vomiting of
    pregnancy

Obesity, 549–558
  assessment, 552–553
    laboratory testing, 552
    physical examination, 552–553
    problem-focused health history, 552
  case study, 557
  comorbidities in pregnancy, 551
  cultural considerations, 550
  defined, 549
  health disparities, 550
  intrapartum issues, 556
  management of pregestational,
    552–556
    assessment, 552–553
    bariatric surgery, 555
    comfort measures, 554
    legal and liability issues, 555–556
    nondiscriminatory language, 552
    nutrition, 554
    physical activity, 554
    principles of, 553
    scope of practice considerations, 555
    weight loss, 554
  personal and family considerations,
    550

physiology, 551
postpartum issues, 556
potential problems associated with,
    551–552, 552*t*
prevalence of, 108, 305, 550
resources for health-care providers,
    556, 558
resources for women and their
    families, 556
risk factors for, 551
terminology, 549
Obesity Society, 552
Obsessive-compulsive disorder,
    postpartum, 450*t*, 451
Occupational exposures. *See also*
    Environmental exposures
  Environmental and Occupational
    Health History Profile, 280,
    281*t*
  preconception risk assessment and
    screening, 56, 57*f*
  preterm birth and, 367
Occupational Safety and Health
    Administration (OSHA), 94,
    280
Office of Child Support Enforcement,
    263
Off-labeling prescribing, 225
OLD CAARTS mnemonic, 398
Oligohydramnios, 23, 354–357
  amniotic fluid index (AFI), 354–355,
    356*f*
  causes of, 356
  defined, 19, 176, 353, 397
  diagnostic assessment and
    management, 356–357
  perinatal mortality rate (PMR), 354,
    356
  in post-term pregnancy, 404
  preterm premature rupture of
    membranes (PPROM), 354–356
Omega-3 fatty acids, 99, 104–105
  for mood and anxiety disorders, 457
  perinatal outcomes and, 104
  recommendations for intake in
    pregnancy, 104–105
  in vegetarian/vegan diet, 118
Omega-6 fatty acids, 99, 118
Oocyte, 19, 20
Oogenesis, 5, 12, 12*f*
Oogonia, 5, 11–12, 12*f*, 19, 30
Open neural tube defects, 160
Opioids
  breastfeeding and, 254*t*
  dependence, psychiatric disorders
    comorbid with, 241
  neonatal abstinence syndrome (NAS),
    252–253
    assessment and treatment of,
      252

    breastfeeding and, 252
    described, 252
    long-term implications of,
      252–253
  pregnancy implications of use, 243
  replacement therapy, 249–251
    breastfeeding and, 251
    buprenorphine, 250–251
    methadone, 250–251
Oral aversion, 499, 500
Oral glucose tolerance testing (OGTT),
    in gestational diabetes (GDM)
  Carpenter and Coustan criteria, 389,
    389*t*
  one-hour test, 389
  three-hour test, 389, 389*t*
  two-hour test, 389–390
Oral health, prenatal, 88
Oral rehydration therapy, for
    gastroenteritis, 545
Organic solvents, exposure to, 282
Organogenesis, 28–29
Organogenic, 19
Organophosphates, exposure to, 283
Os, 5
OSHA (Occupational Safety and Health
    Administration), 94, 280
OTC (over-the-counter) drug,
    223–224
Otitis media, 522
Ovarian cycle, 13–15, 16*f*–17*f*
Ovarian ligament, 9*f*, 10–11
Ovary, 9*f*
  anatomy, 11, 16
  hypothalamic-pituitary-ovarian axis,
    13, 14*f*
Over-the-counter (OTC) drug,
    223–224
Overweight
  defined, 549
  prevalence of, 108, 305
Ovo-lacto vegetarians, 99, 117
Ovulation, 12–13, 15
  after pregnancy loss, 340
  first postpartum, 463
  postnatal resumption of, 432
Oxcarbazepine, maternal and fetal effects
    of, 572*t*
Oxycodone, for restless leg syndrome,
    210–211
Oxygen therapy, for headaches, 576*t*
Oxytocin
  breastfeeding and, 430
  defined, 325
  for delayed postpartum hemorrhage,
    446
  for labor augmentation, 327
  milk ejection reflex, 482–483
  roles of, 46–47
Oxytocin challenge test (OCT), 183

P6 acupressure point for relief of nausea, 209f
Pain
    defined, 291
    fear of, 300, 301
Paling Palette, 154, 155f
Palmar erythema, 42, 128, 213
Palpation and ballottement of the fetus, as probable sign of pregnancy, 130–131
Pancreatic secretory trypsin inhibitor (PSTI), 480
Panic disorder, postpartum, 450t, 451
Panniculus, 549
Pannus, 549
Papilledema
    defined, 375
    in preeclampsia, 380
PAPP A (pregnancy-associated plasma protein-A), in genetic screening, 163
Pap smear screening, preconception, 53
Pap test, 10
Papula, defined, 580
Papule, defined, 580
Parametrium, 10
Parasympathetic nervous system, 176
Parathyroid hormone, 45
Parous, 5
Paroxetine, 624
    FDA approved indications, 453t
    side effects, 453t
Partial fetal alcohol syndrome (PFAS), 242
Partial seizure, 570
Partial thromboplastin time (PTT), 531, 532t
Partners
    adaptation and attachment, 302–305, 302t
        assessment of, 303
        lesbian partners, 304–305
        male partners, 303–304
        trends in the marital or cohabitation status of women aged 15-44, 302t
    woman's relationship with, 298–299
Partnership for Clear Health Communication, 316
Parturition envy, 304
Parvovirus B19, 597
Patient Health Questionnaire (PHQ-9), 88, 241, 452
Patient Protection and Affordable Care Act, 493
PCO₂, 34, 38, 517
PCOS. See Polycystic ovarian syndrome
PCR. See Polymerase chain reaction
PDA (Pregnancy Discrimination Act), 94
Peak expiratory flow rate, 517–518, 520f
Peak-flow meters, 517–518

Pedigree, 161
Pedometer, 274, 277
Pedunculated, 34, 42
Peer support, for mood and anxiety disorders, 457
Pelvic examination, for vaginal bleeding, 337
Pelvic floor exercises, 195, 195t. See also Kegel exercises
Pelvic girdle, defined, 193
Pelvic girdle pain, 194–196
    assessment, 195
    causes and symptoms, 194–195
    presentation of, 195
    relief and preventative measures, 195–196, 195t
Pelvic inflammatory disease, 608, 614
Pelvic rest
    after pregnancy loss, 340
    defined, 335
    for subchorionic hemorrhage, 337
Pelvic tilt exercises, 195, 195t
Pemphigoid gestationis (PG), 582t, 583–585, 584f
    assessment, 584
    collaboration, consultation, and referral, 585
    defining characteristics of, 582t
    differential diagnosis, 584
    incidence of, 583
    treatment and management, 584–585
Penicillin
    desensitization therapy, 610
    for group B Streptococcus (GBS), 592
    for Listeriosis, 545
    for syphilis, 610, 610t
Penta screen, 161, 163t, 164
Peptide, defined, 19
Peptide hormones, 24
Perception, 291
Percutaneous umbilical blood sampling (PUBS), 168
Performance accomplishment, as self-efficacy information source, 307
Perimetrium, 9f, 10
Perinatal loss and grief, 409–415
    breaking the news, 410
    care and management of women with stillbirth, 410–411, 411t
    case study, 414
    cultural considerations, 412
    etiology of stillbirth, 410, 410t
    grieving and emotional care after, 411–412, 412t
    interconception care, 413
    physical care after stillbirth, 413
    postpartum follow-up, 413
    resources for health-care providers, 415

resources for women and their families, 415
    rights of parents when a baby dies, 412t
    subsequent pregnancy care, 413–414
    terminology, 409
Perineal body, 8
Perineal discomfort, postpartum, 431
Perineal exam, postpartum, 434
Perineal wound infection, 445
Perineum
    laceration case study, 422
    physiological alterations during postnatal period, 420
Periodic health evaluation, 51
Periodontal disease, 40, 370
Peritoneum, 5
Perspiration, increased, 204–205
Pesticides, exposure to, 283
PFAS (partial fetal alcohol syndrome), 242
PFP (pruritic folliculitis of pregnancy), 582t, 583
PG. See Pemphigoid gestationis
Pharmaceuticals. See Medication(s)
Pharmacokinetics in pregnancy, 231, 234, 235t
Phenazopyridine, for urinary tract infection, 539
Phenobarbital, maternal and fetal effects of, 572t
Phenytoin, maternal and fetal effects of, 572t
Photophobia, 570, 574, 575t
PHQ-9 (Patient Health Questionnaire-9), 88, 241, 452
Phthalates, exposure to, 283
Physical abuse. See Intimate partner violence
Physical activity. See also Exercise
    in gestational diabetes (GDM) management, 391
    in obese women during pregnancy, 554
    postnatal, 428–429
Physical dependence, 239
Physical examination
    to assess nutritional status, 112
    of obese pregnant woman, 552–553
    postpartum, 433–435
        abdominal exam, 433–434
        breast exam, 433
        costovertebral angle tenderness (CVAT), 434
        leg exam, 434–435
        perineal exam, 434
        rectal exam, 434–435
        uterus exam, 434
        vaginal exam, 434
    preconception risk assessment and screening, 53
    in preeclampsia assessment, 380
    for vaginal bleeding, 336–337

Physical therapy, for headaches, 576*t*
Physiological changes of pregnancy, 34–48
  cardiovascular changes, 37–38, 37*t*
    blood pressure, 37–38
    heart changes, 37, 37*t*
    supine hypotensive syndrome, 37–38
    vascular adaptations, 37
  case study, 47
  endocrine changes, 46–47
    adrenal function changes, 47
    anatomical changes, 46
    pituitary function changes, 46–47, 46*t*
    thyroid function changes, 47
  exercise and, 274–275
  gastrointestinal adaptations, 39–40
    anatomical, 39–40
    functional changes, 40
    liver and biliary adaptations, 40, 40*t*
  hair changes, 42–43
  hematologic system adaptations, 34–36, 35*t*, 525–526
    clotting factors, 36, 36*t*
    folate requirements, 36
    iron requirements, 35–36
    plasma, 35
    red blood cells, 35
    white blood cells, 35
  immunologic changes, 43–45
    disorders related to, 44–45
    fetus as allograft, 43–44
  metabolic changes, 40–42
    basal metabolic rate, 41
    carbohydrate metabolism, 41
    fat metabolism, 41, 41*t*
    ghrelin, 41
    insulin, 41–42
    leptin, 41
    protein metabolism, 41
  musculoskeletal adaptations, 45–46
  nail changes, 43
  neurological changes, 45
  renal adaptations, 38–39
    anatomical changes, 39
    renal function, 39
  resources for health-care providers, 48
  resources for women and their families, 48
  respiratory adaptations, 38, 38*t*
    anatomical changes, 38
    pulmonary function adaptations, 38, 38*t*
  sensory changes, 45
  skin changes, 42
    connective tissue changes, 42
    pigmentation, 42
    sebaceous and sweat gland changes, 42
    vascular changes, 42

  terminology, 34
  thyroid physiology in pregnancy, 560–561, 561*f*
Physiology
  alterations during postnatal period, 419–422, 421*t*
    cardiovascular system, 421
    case study, 422
    cervix, 420
    endocrine changes, 421
    gastrointestinal tract, 421
    labia and perineum, 420
    lochia, 420
    renal system, 421
    resource for health-care providers, 422
    resource for women, 422
    uterus, 419–420
    vagina, 420
  of lactation and breastfeeding, 482–483
  obesity, 551
  of preterm birth (PTB), 366–367
  respiratory, 517
Phytoestrogens, 117
Pica, 19–120, 34, 527
Pigmentation
  changes during pregnancy, 42
    as presumptive sign of pregnancy, 128
    hyperpigmentation, 42, 212–213, 213*f*
Pinocytosis, 19, 23, 24*t*
Pitocin, for antepartum fetal death, 410
Pituitary gland, 13, 14*f*
  function changes during pregnancy, 46–47, 46*t*
  hormones, table of, 46*t*
  hypothalmic-pituitary-thyroid axis, 560, 561*f*
  size increase, 46
Placenta
  formation of, 21–22, 354, 355*f*
  functions, 23–25, 24*t*, 26*t*
    endocrine synthesis and secretion, 24–25, 26*t*
    transport, 23–24, 24*t*
  nutrition and, 102
  sociocultural uses of, 23
  structure of, 21–22
  transplacental infections, 24*t*
Placenta accreta, 20, 22
Placental abruption, 346–348
  case study, 349
  defined, 335, 346
  incidence of, 346
  potential problems, 347
  presentation, 347–348
  risk factors for, 347*t*
  types, 347, 347*f*
Placental encapsulation, 23

Placenta previa, 345–346, 346*f*, 346*t*
  defined, 335
  differential diagnosis, 346
  potential problems, 345–346
  presentation, 346
  risk factors for, 346*t*
  types, 345, 346*f*
Placentation
  defined, 34
  normal, 354
"Plant food," 244
Plasma volume changes during pregnancy, 35
Platelet-derived growth factor, 34, 36
Platelet function activity, 531
Platelets, 34, 36
Plugged ducts, 506–507
PMSS (Pregnancy Mortality Surveillance System), 442
Pneumonia, 522–523
Polycystic ovarian syndrome (PCOS)
  in gestational diabetes (GDM), 390
  metformin treatment, 392
Polyhydramnios, 22
  assessment and management, 357–358
  causes of, 357
  defined, 20, 176, 353, 357
Polymerase chain reaction (PCR)
  for CMV diagnosis, 591
  defined, 589
  for rubella virus diagnosis, 598
  for toxoplasmosis diagnosis, 600*f*, 601
  for varicella zoster diagnosis, 603–604
Polypharmacy, 223, 231, 234
Polyunsaturated fatty acids (PUFAs), 99
Polyzygotic gestation, 397, 401
Ponderal index, 353, 358
POPs (progestin-only pills), 462, 471–472
Portion size, 99, 100
Position, for breastfeeding, 484, 487, 487*f*
Position statements on prenatal substance use, 240–241
Positive feedback, 13
Positive predictive value
  antenatal fetal testing, 177, 182
  defined, 149, 160, 176
Positive signs of pregnancy, 127*t*, 132–133, 132*f*, 134*f*
  defined, 125
  fetal heart activity, 132, 132*f*
  fetal movement detection, 132–133, 134*f*
  ultrasound or X-ray detection, 132
Postbirth bonding. *See also* Attachment
  maternal pattern of behavior, 294
  prenatal preparation for, 294
Postconceptional weeks, 125
Postmortem examination, 409

Postnatal care
  activity/exercise, 428–429
  afterbirth pain, 430
  assessment of maternal physical and
      emotional adjustment, 425–428
    balance in life, 425
    family adaptation, 426–428
    infant feeding, 428
    maternal mood, 425–426
    review of birth experience, 426
  case study, 438
  components of, 423–439
  constipation, 431
  contraception, 432–433
  cultural considerations, 435–436
  depression, 435
  diaphoresis, 431
  diet and nutrition, 429
  diuresis, 431
  domestic violence screening, 435
  fourth-trimester tasks, 424
  health disparities and, 436–437
  hemorrhoids, 431
  legal issues, 438
  menses and ovulation, resumption of,
      432, 432t
  perineal discomfort, 431
  physical examination, postpartum,
      433–435
    abdominal exam, 433–434
    breast exam, 433
    costovertebral angle tenderness
        (CVAT), 434
    leg exam, 434–435
    perineal exam, 434
    rectal exam, 434–435
    uterine exam, 434
    vaginal exam, 434
  resources for health-care providers, 439
  resources for women, 439
  scope of practice considerations,
      437–438
  sexuality, 431–432
  six-week postpartum visit, 425t
  terminology, 423
  two-week postpartum visit, 424t
  vulnerable populations, 436–437
  warning signs, 435, 435t
Postnatal complications. See Postpartum
    complications
Postnatal period, physiological
    alterations during, 419–422, 421t
Postpartum
  defined, 419, 423
  maternal morbidity, 441–442
  maternal mortality, 441–442, 442f
  vaginal exam, 434
Postpartum anxiety disorders, 441. See
    also Anxiety disorders,
    postpartum

Postpartum blues, 423, 425–426, 441, 449
Postpartum complications
  case study, 458
  cultural considerations, 442–443
  delayed postpartum hemorrhage, 441,
      445–446
  hematoma, 441, 446
  mood and anxiety disorders, 441,
      448–449, 448–457
    assessment and screening, 452
    blues, 423, 425–426, 441, 449
    depression, 435, 449–450
    generalized anxiety disorder (GAD),
        451
    incidence/prevalence of, 448
    management, 452–457, 453t–456t
    obsessive-compulsive disorder, 451
    overview of, 448–449
    panic disorder, 451
    pathophysiology of, 449
    post-traumatic stress disorder
        (PTSD), 451–452
    psychosis, 451
    risk factors for, 449
    signs and symptoms, 450t
  morbidity and mortality, 442, 442f
  postpartum hematoma, 446
  preeclampsia/eclampsia, 441, 446–447
  puerperal fever (pyrexia), 443
  puerperal infection (postpartum
      infection), 443–445
    clinical presentation, 444, 445t
    diagnosis and management,
        444–445
    maternal mortality from, 443
    risk factors for, 444
    uterine infection, 443–445,
        444t–445t
  resource for health-care providers,
      458
  resource for women and their families,
      458
  subinvolution, 441, 446
  terminology, 441
  thrombophlebitis, 447
  thyroiditis, 447–448
  wound infection, 445
    abdominal, 445
    perineal, 445
Postpartum depression, defined, 441. See
    also Depression, postpartum
Postpartum Depression Screening Scale
    (PDSS), 88, 452
Postpartum headache, 576
Postpartum hematoma, 441, 446
Postpartum infection
  defined, 441
  puerperal infection, 443–445,
      444t–445t
  wound infection, 445

Postpartum preeclampsia/eclampsia,
    441, 446–447
Postpartum psychosis, 441, 448, 450t,
    451
Postpartum thyroiditis (PPT), 447–448,
    561t, 565–566
Post-term pregnancy, 403–407
  case study, 407
  complications of, 404
  defined, 397
  incidence of, 403–404
  management, 404–406
    elective labor induction, 405
    fetal surveillance, 405, 406t
    labor-stimulating activities,
        404–405
  overview, 403–404
  prevention, 404
  risk factors for, 403–404
Post-traumatic stress disorder (PTSD)
  childhood sexual abuse survivors, 268
  comorbid with substance use, 241
  postpartum, 450t, 451–452
Potassium levels in pregnancy, 39
Pouch of Douglas, 9
Poverty, 262–264
  defined, 261
  homelessness and, 262–263
  interdisciplinary care, 263
  nutrition and, 262
  thresholds by family size and number
      of adults at home, 264
PP (prurigo of pregnancy), 581–582,
    582t
PPROM (preterm premature rupture of
    membranes), 354–356
PPT (postpartum thyroiditis), 447–448,
    561t, 565–566
PRAMS (Pregnancy Risk Assessment
    Monitoring System), 436
Preconception care, 51–68
  benefits of, 52
  care for women with chronic diseases,
      61–65, 63t
    cancer survivors, 61
    chronic hypertension, 61, 64
    diabetes, 64
    epilepsy, 64
    HIV infection, 64
    mental illness, 64
    thyroid disorders, 64
  case study, 67
  challenges to providing, 51–52
  content of, 53–66
  defined, 51
  disabilities and, 65
  evidence supporting, 52, 53
  for men, 65–66
    counseling, 66
    risk assessment and screening, 66

Preconception care (*cont'd*)
  national guidelines for, 53, 54f–55f
  preconception counseling, 57–61
    conception process, 60
    diet, 57, 59
    environmental exposure to toxins,
      60–61
    exercise, 59
    infections, 60
    preparation for pregnancy and
      childbirth, 60
    substance use and abuse, 59–60
    supplementation, 59
    vaccinations, 61, 62t
    weight, 59
  with prior pregnancy history, 65
  with prior pregnancy loss, 65
  resources
    consumer brochures for office
      setting, 68
    for health-care providers, 67–68
    tools for screening, 68
    for women and families, 66–67
  risk assessment and screening, 53–57
    environmental and occupational
      exposures, 56, 57f
    genetics, 56
    history, 53
    infection, 56–57, 58t
    laboratory examination, 53
    medications, 56
    mental health issues, 53, 56
    physical examination, 53
    substance use and abuse, 53
  terminology, 51
Precursors, 20
Predictive value, 153
Prednisone
  for impetigo herpetiformis (IH), 585
  for pemphigoid gestationis (PG),
    584
Preeclampsia, 376–384
  atypical presentation, 382–383, 383t
  case study, 385
  criteria for diagnosis of, 377t
  defined, 570
  diagnostic evaluation of, 379–380
    blood pressure, 379
    edema and weight gain pattern,
      379
    history, 379
    laboratory evaluation, 380, 381f
    physical examination, 380
    proteinuria, 379, 379t
  headache and, 574
  HELLP syndrome, 382
  immunologic component of, 44
  incidence of, 377
  interprofessional practice issues, 384
  long-term sequelae of, 383–384

management of, 380–382
    education, 382
    lifestyle recommendations, 380
    maternal and fetal surveillance, 380
    medication, 380, 382
  nutrition in pregnancy and, 100
  pathophysiology of, 377–378, 378f
  postpartum, 441, 446–447
  potential problems due to, 378
  prediction of, 383
  prevention of, 383
  risk factors for developing, 378–379
  risk management issues in office
    setting, 384
  seizures and, 571
  superimposed on chronic
    hypertension, 376t, 377
Pregestational diabetes, 566–567
  adverse pregnancy outcomes and, 567
  classifications, 566
  glycemic control, 567
  perinatal risks of, 567
  preconception counseling, 567
Pregnancy-associated plasma protein-A
    (PAPP A), in genetic screening,
    163
Pregnancy dating, 82, 248
Pregnancy diagnosis, 125–145
  case study, 145
  counseling for, 140–145
    adoption counseling, 143–144
    after negative pregnancy test, 141
    after positive pregnancy test, 141
    delivery of test results, 140–141
    ethics and standards for
      reproductive options counseling,
      142
    evidence-based information about
      pregnancy options, 143
    pregnancy termination, 144–145
    steps in pregnancy options
      counseling, 143
    for unintended pregnancy, 141–143
  early, 126
  resources for health-care providers, 145
  resources for women and their
    families, 145
  signs and symptoms of pregnancy,
    127–133, 127t
    positive signs of pregnancy, 127t,
      132–133, 132f, 134f
    fetal heart activity, 132, 132f
    fetal movement detection,
      132–133, 134f
    ultrasound or X-ray detection,
      132
    presumptive signs of pregnancy,
      127–128, 127t
    amenorrhea, 128
    breast changes, 128

skin changes, 128
    subjective sensations, 128
    vaginal changes, 128
  probable signs of pregnancy, 127t,
    128–132, 129f–130f
    basal body temperatures, 131
    cervical changes, 129
    endocrine pregnancy tests,
      131–132
    enlargement of abdomen,
      128–129
    palpation and ballottement of
      fetus, 130–131
    uterine changes, 129–130,
      129f–130f
    vaginal changes, 129, 129f
  subjective symptoms, 127
  terminology, 125
Pregnancy Discrimination Act (PDA), 94
Pregnancy failures, 341
Pregnancy history, 82, 84
Pregnancy loss
  perinatal loss and grief, 409–415
    breaking the news, 410
    care and management of women
      with stillbirth, 410–411, 411t
    case study, 414
    cultural considerations, 412
    etiology of stillbirth, 410, 410t
    grieving and emotional care after
      loss, 411–412, 412t
    interconception care, 413
    physical care after stillbirth, 413
    postpartum follow-up, 413
    resources for health-care providers,
      415
    resources for women and their
      families, 415
    rights of parents when a baby dies,
      412t
    subsequent pregnancy care,
      413–414
    terminology, 409
  rate with amniocentesis, 168
  rate with chorionic villus sampling,
    168
Pregnancy Mortality Surveillance System
    (PMSS), 442
Pregnancy options counseling for
    unintended pregnancy, 141–145
  adoption, 143–144
  evidence-based information about,
    143
  pregnancy termination, 144–145
  professional ethics and standards for,
    142
  referral resources, 143
  steps in, 143
Pregnancy Risk Assessment Monitoring
    System (PRAMS), 436

Pregnancy termination counseling, 144–145
Pregnancy-Unique Quantification of Emesis (PUQE) Scale, 207, 208t
Prenatal care
  amount of, 78–79
  case study, 96
  Centering Pregnancy model, 80–81, 81t
  childbirth confidence enhancement, 306
  components of, 81–95
  diagnostic testing, 87–88
  genetic screening, 86, 87t
  goals, 75–77
  health promotion and education, 88, 90–95
    alcohol use, 92
    exercise, 93–94
    illicit drugs, 92–93
    nutrition, 90–91, 91t
    substance abuse, 91
    throughout pregnancy, 94–95, 95t
    tobacco use, 91–92, 92t
    working and pregnancy, 94
  history of, 74–75, 82, 83t, 84–85
  integrating quality into, 79–80
  laboratory studies, 85–86, 86t, 87t
  nutrition counseling, 114, 116
  physical assessment, 85
  preventative care, 88–90
    immunization, 88, 89f
    intimate partner violence, 88, 90
    mental health, 88
    oral health, 88
  resources for health-care providers, 97
  resources for women and their families, 97
  risk assessment, 81–82
  structure of, 77–80
Prenatal diagnosis, 160
Prenatal education. See Health education
Prenatal flavor learning, 102–103
Prenatal preparation
  for postbirth bonding, 294
  teaching about fetal growth and development, 294
Prenatal screening, 160
Prenatal visit schedule, 78, 78t
Preparation for pregnancy and childbirth, preconception counseling, 60
Prepuce of clitoris, 6f
Prescription
  components of, 225–226
  sample, 227f
Prescription drugs, 223, 224
Prescriptive authority, 223–225
Presumptive signs of pregnancy, 127–128, 127t
  amenorrhea, 128
  breast changes, 128

defined, 125, 127
  skin changes, 128
  subjective sensations, 128
  vaginal changes, 128
Preterm birth (PTB), 365–373
  case study, 372
  complications related to prematurity, 367, 367t
  multifetal pregnancy, decreasing risk in, 402
  nutrition in pregnancy and, 100
  physiology of, 366–367
  poor sleep quality as risk factor for, 214
  predicting, 368
    cervical length measurement, 368
    fetal fibronectin (fFN) testing, 368
  preeclampsia and, 378
  preterm labor
    diagnosis, 368
    initial evaluation, 369
    management of women with, 368–369
  prevalence of, 365
  prevention, 369–371
    cervical cerclage, 371
    fatigue reduction, 371
    interpregnancy interval, 370
    nutrition, 369–370
    progesterone therapy, 371
    sleep quality improvement, 371
    smoking cessation, 370
    treating infections, 370
  resources for women and health-care providers, 373
  risk factors for, 367–368, 367t
  sexually transmitted infections (STIs) and, 608–609
  social and racial disparities, 366
  terminology, 365
Preterm birth rate, 365
Preterm infants, breastfeeding problems in, 502–503
Preterm labor. See also Preterm birth
  diagnosis, 368
  initial evaluation, 369
  management of women with, 368–369
Preterm premature rupture of membranes (PPROM), 354–356
Preventative care, prenatal, 88–90
  immunization, 88, 89f
  intimate partner violence, 88, 90
  mental health, 88
  oral health, 88
Primary follicles, 12f, 14–15
Primary oocytes, 11–12, 12f
Primidone, maternal and fetal effects of, 572t
Primipara, defined, 325
Primitive streak, 20, 27–28, 27f, 29f

Primogeniture, 302
Primordial follicles, 12f, 14
Prior pregnancy history, preconception care for women with, 65
Prior pregnancy loss, preconception care for women with, 65
Probable signs of pregnancy, 127t, 128–132, 129f–130f
  basal body temperatures, 131
  cervical changes, 129
  defined, 125
  endocrine pregnancy tests, 131–132
  enlargement of abdomen, 128–129
  palpation and ballottement of fetus, 130–131
  uterine changes, 129–130, 129f–130f
  vaginal changes, 129, 129f
Probiotics, 545
Progesterone
  appetite stimulation by, 40
  carbonic anhydrase increase from, 38
  corpus luteum secretion of, 15, 16–17
  functions of, 25, 26t
  gastrointestinal system changes during pregnancy, 40
  gingivitis susceptibility and, 196
  postpartum levels, 421
  for preterm birth prevention, 371, 402
  stimulation of cytochrome P450 enzymes, 40
  tissue factor increase stimulated by, 36
  varicosities and, 216
  vasodilation effect of, 37–38
Progestin-only contraceptives, 462, 470–472
  depot medroxyprogesterone acetate (DMPA), 470–471
  implant contraception, 468–469
  progestin-only pills (POPs), 462, 471–472
Progestin-only pills (POPs), 462, 471–472
Progestins, in combined hormonal contraceptives (CHCs), 462, 464, 469–470
Projection, in maternal role taking, 296
Prolactin, 46, 483, 489
Proliferative phase, of endometrial cycle, 15–16
Propylthiouracil (PTU), 564–565
Prostaglandins
  for cervical ripening, 406
  defined, 325
  for delayed postpartum hemorrhage, 446
  labor and, 326
  in menstrual phase of endometrial cycle, 17
  vasodilation effect of, 37
Prostaglandin synthase inhibitor, 358

Protein
in human milk, 481
intake, 105, 106t
metabolism changes during pregnancy, 41
quality, 105
in vegetarian/vegan diet, 118
Proteinuria
defined, 375
in preeclampsia, 379, 379t
Prothrombin time (PT), 531, 532t
Protozoa
defined, 589
toxoplasmosis, 599–602, 600f, 601t
Trichomonas vaginalis, 613–614
Prurigo of pregnancy (PP), 581–582, 582t
Pruritus gravidarum. *See* Intrahepatic cholestasis of pregnancy (ICP)
Pseudoephedrine, 206
Psoriasis, 580
PSTI (pancreatic secretory trypsin inhibitor), 480
Psychiatric medications causing weight gain, 551
Psychological disorders, 621–629
bipolar disorder, 622t, 625–626, 626t
case study, 628
comorbid with substance use, 241
depression during pregnancy, 621–625, 622t, 624t
generalized anxiety disorder (GAD), 626–627
mood disorders, definition and classification of, 622t
prevalence of, 621
resources for health-care providers, 629
resources for women and their families, 629
scope of practice considerations, 627–628
terminology, 621
Psychological stress, of working during pregnancy, 287
Psychophysiology, 291
Psychosis, postpartum, 441, 448, 450t, 451
Psychosocial adaptations in pregnancy, 291–309
body image, 305–306
case study, 309
childbirth confidence, 306–308
dimensions of (Lederman's)
acceptance of pregnancy, 297
fear of loss of control in labor, 300
fear of loss of self-esteem in labor, 301
identification with a motherhood role, 297–298
preparation for labor, 299–300

relationship with own mother, 298
relationship with partner, 298–299
maternal attachment and adaptation, 292–301
assessment of, 296
Bowlby and Ainsworth, 293
Brazelton, 294
detachment as protective mechanism, 299
Kennell and Klaus, 293–294
Lederman, 297–301
Rubin, 294–297
partner adaptation and attachment, 302–305, 302t
assessment of, 303
lesbian partners, 304–305
male partners, 303–304
pregnancy as crisis, 292–293
pregnancy as developmental phase, 292–293
resources for health-care providers, 309
resources for women and their families, 308
sibling adaptation and attachment, 301–302
terminology, 291
Psychosocial assessment, of pregnant women with substance use disorders, 248
Psychosocial benefits of exercise, 275
Psychosocial effects in genetic testing, 170–171
Psychosocial history, 84
Psychosocial impacts of sexually transmitted infection diagnosis, 616–618
effects on the individual, 616–617
preventing STIs within relationships, 617–618
Psychotherapy. *See also* Cognitive-behavioral therapy (CBT)
for depression, 623
for generalized anxiety disorder, 451
interpersonal (IPT), 452, 457
for mood and anxiety disorders, 457
for panic disorder, 451
for postpartum depression, 450
for post-traumatic stress disorder, 452
Psychotropics
defined, 441
for panic disorder, 451
PT (prothrombin time), 531, 532t
PTB. *See* Preterm birth
PTSD. *See* Post-traumatic stress disorder
PTT (partial thromboplastin time), 531, 532t
PTU (propylthiouracil), 564–565
Ptyalism, 209–210
assessment, 210
causes and symptoms, 209

defined, 193, 209
in hyperemesis gravidarum, 400
relief and preventative measures, 210
Puberty
follicles present at, 11
onset of, 13
Pubic hair, 6
Pubic symphysis, 8f
Pubococcygeus muscles, 8
PUBS (percutaneous umbilical blood sampling), 168
Pudendal nerve, 8
Puerperal fever (pyrexia), 443
Puerperal infection (postpartum infection), 443–445
clinical presentation, 444, 445t
diagnosis and management, 444–445
maternal mortality from, 443
risk factors for, 444
uterine infection, 443–445, 444t–445t
Puerperium, 423, 441
PUFAs (polyunsaturated fatty acids), 99
Pulmonary embolism, 531–532
Pulmonary function adaptations during pregnancy, 38, 38t
Pulmonary function testing, 518
Pulmonary hypoplasia, 20, 23
PUQE (Pregnancy-Unique Quantification of Emesis) Scale, 207, 208t
Pruritic folliculitis of pregnancy (PFP), 582t, 583
Pruritic urticarial papules and plaques of pregnancy (PUPP), 582–583, 582f, 582t, 587
Purpura, 213
Pyelonephritis, 536, 538, 540–541
Pyrexia (puerperal fever), 443
Pyrimethamine, for toxoplasmosis, 601
Pyrosis. *See* Heartburn
Pytalism, 34, 40
Pyuria, 536, 541

Quad screen, 161, 163–164, 163t
Quality, integrating into prenatal care, 79–80
Quickening
defined, 20, 30, 125
timing of, 128
A Quick Reference Guide to Contraception, 475

RAAS (renin-angiotensin-aldosterone system), 35, 39
Racial disparities
in preterm birth rates, 366
risk of prenatal death, 189
Randomized clinical trials (RCTs), 229
Ranitidine, 203
Rapid eye movement (REM) sleep, 45

Rapport, 292
Rating of perceived exertion (RPE), 277, 277f
Reactive fetal heart rate monitoring strip, 181f
Reading level, 316
Reading list, providing, 314
Reality television shows, as information source, 314
Rebound congestion, 206
Recommended daily allowance (RDA), 99, 100
Rectal exam, postpartum, 434–435
Rectocele, 423
Rectouterine pouch, 5, 9
Rectovaginal septum, 5, 9
Recurrent pregnancy loss, 335, 341
Red blood cell indices, 525–526, 526t
Red blood cells
    antigen incompatibility, 44–45
    changes during pregnancy, 35
    in hematological conditions, 527t
Reference laboratory, 589
Rehydration therapy, for gastroenteritis, 545
Rejection, in maternal role taking, 296
Relationship-based care, 292
Relative risk, 149, 153
Relaxation treatment, for headaches, 576t
Relaxin, 45
    functions of, 25, 26t
    increased chest cartilage pliability with, 38
    sites of production, 25
REM (rapid eye movement) sleep, 45
Renal calculi, 536, 541
Renal system
    adaptations during pregnancy, 38–39
        anatomical changes, 39
        renal function, 39
    physiological alterations during postnatal period, 421
Renin-angiotensin-aldosterone system (RAAS), 35, 39
Replication, in maternal role attainment
Reproductive life plan, 141
Reproductive tract, 5–18
    anatomy of female, 6–11
        external genitalia, 6–8, 7f
        internal genitalia, 8–11, 9f
        superficial muscles of the perineum, 8, 8f
    case study, 18
    menstrual cycle physiology, 11–18
        beginnings, 11–13
        characteristics of normal cycle, 15t
        endometrial cycle, 15–17, 17f
        hormones of, 13, 14f, 15t
        hypothalamic-pituitary-ovarian axis, 13

    onset of puberty, 13
    ovarian cycle, 13–15, 16f, 17f
    oogenesis, 12, 12f
    resources for health-care providers, 18
    resources for women, 18
    terminology, 5
Requirement, 99
Reservoir, defined, 589
Residual volume, 517
Resorption, bone, 34, 45
Respiratory disorders, 517–523
    asthma, 517–521, 519t, 520f
    case study, 523
    influenza, 521, 523
    pneumonia, 522–523
    resources for health-care providers, 523
    terminology, 517
    upper respiratory infection, 521–522, 522t
Respiratory system
    adaptations during pregnancy, 38, 38t
        anatomical changes, 38
        pulmonary function adaptations, 38, 38t
    shortness of breath, 211–212
Rest
    early labor and, 329–330
    for preeclampsia management, 380
Restless leg syndrome (RLS), 210–211
    assessment, 210
    causes and symptoms, 210
    relief and preventative measures, 210–211
Retinoids, teratogenicity of, 233t
Rh antigen, 74
Rh incompatibility, 44–45
Rhinitis, 206
RhoGAM, 74, 340
Riboflavin supplements, for headache, 574
Rising, Sharon Schindler, 73
Risk, 149–157
    absolute, 149, 153
    attributable, 149, 153
    background, 223, 228
    benefits of assessment, 150
    case study, 157
    defined, 149
    disadvantages of assessment and management, 150–151
        illusion of risk control, 151
        labeling women as "high risk," 151
        normalization of technology, 151
        unnecessary interventions, 150–151
    of drugs during pregnancy, 226–227
    explaining to women, 153–154, 155f, 156t
    genetic disorders, 160–161
    of genetic screening tests, 161

    informed consent, 154–157
    limitations of assessment, 150
        lack of precision, 150
        nonmodifiable risk factors, 150
        poor predictive value, 150
    misapplication of assessment and management, 151–153
        birth fear, 153
        cost increase, 152–153
        introduction of actual risk, 152
    miscommunication, 154
        illusion of choice, 154
        informed compliance, 154
    perspective of risk and risk screening, 153
    preventions, primary and secondary, 153
    process and purpose of assessment, 149–150
    relative, 149, 153
    terminology, 149
    Resources for health-care providers and women and their families, 157
Risk assessment
    in prenatal care, 76
    prenatal care and, 81–82
Risk factors
    defined, 51, 149
    for infections in pregnancy, 58t
    nonmodifiable, 150
    for preterm birth (PTB), 367–368, 367t
Risk scoring tools, 150
Ritual
    baby shower as, 299
    fatherhood, 303
    functions of, 299
RLS. See Restless leg syndrome
Role
    conflicts, 298
    defined, 291
    fatherhood, 303–304
    identification with motherhood, 297–298
Role playing, 296
Round ligament pain, 211, 211f, 398t
    assessment, 211
    causes and symptoms, 211
    relief and preventative measures, 211
Round ligaments, 10
Roux-en-Y gastric bypass, 549, 555
RPE (rating of perceived exertion), 277, 277f
Rubella, 227, 597–599
    congenital rubella syndrome (CRS), 227, 598–599
    management, 597–599
    presentation and assessment, 598
    prevention, 599
Rubin, Reva, 294–297
Rugae, 5, 8, 9f

Saccharin, 111
Sacral nerve, 8
Sacrococcygeal teratoma, 20, 28
Sacroiliac joint pain, 194
Sadovsky method of fetal movement counts (FMCs), 179
Safety issues, discussing, 317
Salivation, excessive. *See* Ptyalism
Saturated fats, 117
Saturated fatty acids, 99
Schedule of prenatal visits, 78, 78*t*
Schedules for controlled substances, 225, 226*t*
Sciatica, 194
SCJ (squamocolumnar junction), 5
SCOFF tool to screen for eating disorders, 119
Screening, defined, 51
Seafood consumption, 104–105, 105*t*
Sebaceous gland changes during pregnancy, 42
Secobarbital, 329
Secondary oocyte, 12, 12*f*
Secondary sexual characteristics, 13
Second-degree laceration, 423
Secondhand smoke, 494
Secretory IgA, in colostrum, 480
Secretory phase, of endometrial cycle, 16
Seizure disorders, 570–573
    antiepileptic medications, 571, 572*t*, 573
    case study, 578
    preconception care for, 64
    safety precautions, 573
    types, 570–571
Selective serotonin reuptake inhibitors (SSRIs)
    for bipolar disorder, 626
    black box warning, 453*t*
    for depression, 624–625, 624*t*
    drug-drug interactions and, 248
    effect on sleep quality, 214
    FDA approved indications, 453*t*–454*t*
    for generalized anxiety disorder, 451, 627
    mechanism of action, 457
    for obsessive-compulsive disorder, 451
    for postpartum depression, 450, 452, 457
    for post-traumatic stress disorder, 452
    serotonin discontinuation syndrome, 457
    side effects, 453*t*–454*t*, 457
    withdrawal from, 625
Self-care in early labor, 329
Self-efficacy
    childbirth and, 306–308
    defined, 291
    influence of witnessing a birth on, 300

sources of information affecting beliefs, 306–307
    performance accomplishment, 307
    verbal persuasion, 307
    vicarious experience, 307
    visceral arousal, 307
    strategies to enhance, 308
Self-esteem
    defined, 291
    fear of loss in labor, 301
Self-image
    of male partners, 304
    as mother, 298
Semiallograft, 34
Sensitivity, 153
    antenatal fetal testing, 177
    defined, 149, 160, 176
Sensory changes during pregnancy, 45
Seroconversion, defined, 589
Seroprevalence, defined, 589
Serotonin discontinuation syndrome, 457
Serotonin norepinephrine reuptake inhibitors (SNRIs)
    black box warning, 454*t*
    for depression, 624, 624*t*
    FDA approved indications, 454*t*–455*t*
    for generalized anxiety disorder (GAD), 627
    mechanism of action, 457
    side effects, 454*t*–455*t*
Sertaline
    drug-drug interactions and, 248
    FDA approved indications, 454*t*
    side effects, 454*t*
Serving size, 99
    defined, 100
    guidelines and needs in pregnancy, 101*t*
Sexual history, 84, 285
Sexuality
    defined, 291
    postpartum, 431–432, 463
    in pregnancy, 284–286
        adaptations, 303–304
        contraindications to intercourse, 285
        counseling, 285–286
        pregnancy influences on sexuality, 284–285
        sexual history, 285
        types of sexual activity, 285
Sexually transmitted infections (STIs), 608–619
    case study, 619
    chlamydia, 609
    discussing diagnosis, 617
    gonorrhea, 609–610
    herpes simplex virus (HSV), 610–612, 611*t*–612*t*

human papillomavirus (HPV), 612–613
    partner treatment, 616
    preconception screening, 53
    preventing, 617–618
    psychosocial impacts of diagnosis, 616–618
        effects on the individual, 616–617
        preventing STIs within relationships, 617–618
    reportable diseases, 608, 616
    resources for health-care providers, 619
    resources for women and partners, 619
    syphilis, 610
    terminology, 608
    Trichomonas vaginalis, 613–614
SGA (small for gestational age), 353, 358–360
Sheppard-Towner Maternity and Infancy Protection Act, 73–74
Shift work, 274, 286
Shingles. *See* Varicella zoster virus (VZV)
Shortness of breath, 211–212
    assessment, 211–212
    causes and symptoms, 211
    relief and preventative measures, 212
Shoulder dystocia, in gestational diabetes, 388, 393
SHS. *See* Supine hypotension syndrome
Siblings
    adaptation and attachment, 301–302
    postnatal adjustment by, 427–428
Sickle cell disease, 525, 529
    genetic screening for, 87*t*, 165, 166*t*, 167
Sickle cell trait, 525, 529
SickleDex test, 167
Side effect, defined, 223
SIDS (sudden infant death syndrome), 242
Simethicone, 202
Simple diffusion, 20, 23, 24*t*
Sinusitis, 522
Sitz baths, for perineal discomfort, 431
Skene's glands, 6, 8
Skin
    changes, 212–214
        assessment, 213
        hair and nail changes, 213
        hyperpigmentation, 212–213, 212*f*
        presumptive signs of pregnancy, 128
        relief and preventative measures, 213–214
        striae gravidarum, 212–213, 213*f*
        vascular changes, 213
    disorders (*see* Dermatological disorders)

maternal alterations during pregnancy, 42
  connective tissue changes, 42
  pigmentation, 42
  sebaceous and sweat gland changes, 42
  vascular changes, 42
Skin tags, 42, 213
Sleep
  changing patterns during pregnancy, 45
  early labor and, 329–330
  for obese women during pregnancy, 554
  quality improvement for preterm birth prevention, 371
  recommended amount of, 287
Sleep disturbances, 214–215
  assessment, 214
  case study, 219
  causes and symptoms, 214
  relief and preventative measures, 214–215
  workplace fatigue and, 287
Sleep hygiene, 193
Sleepy baby, breastfeeding problems and, 500–501
Slow weight gain, in breastfed infant, 501–502, 501*t*–502*t*
  infant factors, 501*t*
  maternal factors, 502*t*
  supplemental feedings, 501–502
SMA. *See* Spinal muscular atrophy
Small for gestational age (SGA), 353, 358–360
Smell sensation, changes during pregnancy, 45
Smoking
  by breastfeeding mother, 492–493
  lactation, affect on, 492
  pregnancy implications, 242–243
  prevalence of, 239
  risk factor for placental abruption, 346–347
  secondhand smoke, 494
Smoking cessation, 91–92, 92*t*, 246–247
  for asthma management during pregnancy, 519
  in breastfeeding women, 253–254, 492
  bupropion, 246
  5 A's and 5 R's model of, 91, 92*t*, 246, 247*t*
  for headache control, 575
  nicotine replacement therapy, 246, 492
  for preterm birth prevention, 370
  varenicline, 246
SNAP (Supplemental Nutrition Assistance Program), 550
SNRIs. *See* Serotonin norepinephrine reuptake inhibitors

Social disparities, in preterm birth rates, 366
Social issues in pregnancy, 261–271
  case study, 269
  history of childhood sexual abuse, 266–267, 266*t*
  incarceration, 264–265
  intimate partner violence, 265–266, 266*t*
  poverty, 262–264
  resources for health-care providers, 270
  resources for women and their families, 270–271
  terminology, 261
Social systems, 291
Socioeconomic status, obesity and, 550
Sodium retention during pregnancy, 39
Soft drinks, 111
Soft markers, 151
  defined, 149
  of fetal aneuploidy, 164
Somites, 20, 28
Sore nipples, 503–506, 505*t*
  ankyloglossia, 499, 503
  causes, 503
  flat or inverted nipples, 499, 503, 504*t*
  improper positioning and latch, 503
  management of, 505–506, 505*t*
  preventing, strategies for, 505*t*
Specificity, 153
  antenatal fetal testing, 177
  defined, 149, 160, 176
Spermicides, 473–474
Spider angioma, 213
Spina bifuda occulta, 161
Spinal muscular atrophy (SMA)
  carrier screening, 167
  described, 167
  genetic screening for, 166*t*
Spiramycin, for toxoplasmosis, 601
Sponge, contraceptive, 473
Spontaneous abortion. *See* Spontaneous pregnancy loss
Spontaneous pregnancy loss, 337–341
  case study, 350
  classification of first-trimester loss, 338*t*
  defined, 335, 338
  diagnosis, 339
  differential diagnosis, 338–339, 339*t*
  family considerations, 340–341
  follow-up care, 340
  immune-related, 44
  incidence of, 338
  management, 339–340
    expectant management, 339–340
    medical, 340
    surgical, 340
  recurrent, 341

  risk factors for, 338, 339*t*
  signs and symptoms, 339*t*
  subsequent pregnancy timing, 341
Squamocolumnar junction (SCJ), 5, 10
SSRIs. *See* Selective serotonin reuptake inhibitors
St. John's wort
  for depression, 625
  for mood and anxiety disorders, 457
Standard drink, defined, 238
Standing, prolonged, 286
Staphylococcus aureus
  in abdominal wound infections, 445
  in breast abscess, 508
  in cracked nipple infections, 505
  methicillin-resistant *Staphylococcus aureus* (MRSA), 248
Starting the Conversation: diet instrument, 113*f*
Station, 325, 328
Sterilization, 462, 466–467
Steroid
  for atopic dermatitis, 581
  defined, 20
Steroid hormones, 24
Stillbirth
  breaking the news, 410
  care and management of women with, 410–411, 411*t*
  case study, 414
  components of evaluation, 411
  cultural considerations, 412
  defined, 409
  etiology of, 410, 410*t*
  in gestational diabetes, 388
  grieving and emotional care after loss, 411–412, 412*t*
  incidence of, 410
  interconception care, 413
  physical care after, 413
  postpartum follow-up, 413
  in post-term pregnancy, 404
  resources for health-care providers, 415
  resources for women and their families, 415
  rights of parents when a baby dies, 412*t*
  subsequent pregnancy care, 413–414
STIs. *See* Sexually transmitted infections
Stools of breastfed infants, 491
Strength training in pregnancy, 278
Streptococcus
  agalactiae, 592
  group B *Streptococcus* (GBS), 592–593
Stress
  defined, 291, 365
  preterm birth and, 367
  reduction in maternal by male partners, 304

Stretching, for leg cramp prevention, 205–206, 205f
Stretch marks. *See* Striae gravidarum
Striae gravidarum, 42, 193, 212–213, 213f
Stripping of the membranes, 397, 404–405
Stroke volume, increase during pregnancy, 37
Subchorionic hemorrhage, 335, 337
Subinvolution, 441, 446
Substance abuse treatment facility, referral to, 249
Substance dependence, 238–240
Substance use/abuse, 238–256
  antepartum assessment, 248–249
    anticipatory guidance, 249
    fetal assessment, 249
    pregnancy dating, 248
    prenatal laboratory testing, 248
    psychosocial assessment, 248
    screening for comorbidities, 248
    social risks, 248–249
  breastfeeding and, 253–254, 254t
  case study, 255
  commonly used substances and pregnancy implications, 241–244
    alcohol, 241–242
    amphetamines/methamphetamines, 244
    benzodiazepines, 243–244
    cocaine, 243
    designer drugs, 244
    marijuana, 244
    nicotine, 242–243
    opioids, 243
  comorbid conditions, 241
  counseling, 241, 248
  cultural considerations, 254
  defined, 238–240
  5 P's screening tool for, 93
  harm reduction approach to, 240
  historical approaches to, 240
  incarceration and, 264
  intervention and treatment
    antepartum assessment, 248–249
    care of women with substance use disorders, 247
    communication and coordination of care, 251
    initial, 246
    opioid replacement therapy, 249–251
    referral to treatment, 249
    smoking cessation, 246–247, 247t
  medical risks associated with, 241
  neonatal abstinence syndrome (NAS), 252–253
  personal and family considerations, 254

position statements on, 240–241
postpartum care, 253–254
preconception counseling on, 59–60
preconception risk assessment and screening, 53
prenatal health promotion and education, 91–93
prevalence of prenatal, 239
resources for health-care providers, 256
resources for women and their families, 256
risks of perinatal, 238–239
scope of practice considerations, 254
screening for prenatal substance abuse, 244–245, 245t
terminology, 238–240
Sudden infant death syndrome (SIDS), 242
Suicide, 450
  substance abuse and, 239
Sulfadiazine, for toxoplasmosis, 601
Sulfamethoxazole/trimethoprim, for *Listeriosis,* 545
Superficial muscles of the perineum, 8, 8f
Superficial transverse perineal muscle, 8, 8f
Superficial venous thrombosis
  defined, 441
  postpartum, 447
Supine hypotension syndrome (SHS), 37–38, 215
  assessment, 215
  causes and symptoms, 215
  relief and preventative measures, 215
Supplemental Nutrition Assistance Program (SNAP), 550
Supplements
  calcium, 383
  folic acid/folate, 59, 141, 162, 211, 224, 530
  iron, 106, 527, 527t
  magnesium, 206, 574
  for mood and anxiety disorders, 457
  nutritional, 224–225, 234
  omega-3, 104
  preconception counseling on, 59
  for preeclampsia prevention, 383
  riboflavin, 574
  thiamine, 401
Supplies for the baby, gathering of, 299
Support stockings, 447
Suspensory ligament, 9f
Swallowing by breastfeeding infant, 483
Sweat gland changes during pregnancy, 42
Sweeteners, alternative, 111
Symbolic modeling experiences, 307
Symphysis-fundus measurements, 138
Symphysis pubis diastasis, 195, 195f

Symphysis separation, 195, 195f
Symptom review, mnemonic for, 194
Syncytiotrophoblast, 20–21, 24–25
Syphilis, 608
  congenital, 610
  neonatal, 610
  pregnancy testing and treatment, 610, 610t
  screening recommendations, 58t
  signs and symptoms, 610

T-ACE Screening Tool for Alcohol Use, 92, 245t
"Talk test," 278
Tannins, 106
Targeted ultrasound, 353, 356, 360
Target lesion, 580, 583
Tay-Sachs disease, genetic screening for, 87t, 165, 166t, 167
TBG (thyroxine-binding globulin), 47
TCAs. *See* Tricyclic antidepressants
T-cytotoxic cells, 44
Technology dependency, 306
Teen pregnancy. *See* Adolescents
Telangiectasis, 34
Telephone triage tool for neonates, 486f
Telogen, 34, 43
Tension headache, 570, 574, 575t
Tentative pregnancy, 171
Teratogen, 28
  alcohol as, 242
  defined, 20, 223, 589
Teratology, 227–231
  critical periods in human development, 228–229, 230f
  drugs with minimal or no teratogenicity, 234t
  etiology of birth defects, 228, 228f
  examples of teratogens, 232t–233t
  FDA categories for drugs in pregnancy, 229, 231, 231t
  history of, 227
  identification of a teratogen, 229
  mechanisms of teratogenic drugs, 228–229
  Wilson's six principles of teratology, 228, 228t, 229
Testosterone, adrenal, 47
Tetracyclines, teratogenicity of, 233t
Thalassemia, 525, 527t, 529–530
  genetic screening for, 87t, 165, 166t, 167
Thalidomide, 75, 227, 233t
Thelarche, 5
T-helper cells, 44
Therapeutic rest, 325, 330
Therapeutic window, 223
Thiamine supplementation, for hyperemesis gravidarum, 401
Third-degree laceration, 423

Thrombocytes. *See* Platelets
Thrombocytopenia, 531
  defined, 375
  in preeclampsia, 381*t*
Thromboembolic disorders, 531–534
Thrombophilia, 525, 531–534
Thrombophlebitis
  postpartum, 447
  as sequelae to IV drug use, 241
Thromboprophylaxis, 532–534, 533*t*
Thromboxane, 34, 36
Thrombus, 36
Thyroid disorders, 560–566
  causes and expected laboratory
      findings, 561*t*
  diagnosing, 561–562
  hyperthyroidism, 561*t*, 564–565
    clinical presentation, 564
    diagnosis, 564
    Graves' disease, 561*t*, 564
    laboratory testing, 561*t*, 564
    management, 564–565
    maternal and fetal risks, 564
    scope of practice considerations, 565
    signs and symptoms, 562
    subclinical, 561*t*, 565
    thyroid storm, 561*t*, 565
  hypothyroidism, 561*t*, 562–564
    clinical presentation, 562
    complications of, 562
    diagnosis, 562–563
    Hashimoto's thyroiditis, 561*t*,
        562–563
    laboratory testing, 561*t*, 562–563
    management, 562–563
    maternal and fetal risks, 562
    overt, 562–563
    preconception care, 564
    screening in pregnancy, 563–564
    signs and symptoms, 562
    subclinical, 561*t*, 563
  postpartum thyroiditis (PPT),
      447–448, 561*t*, 565–566
  preconception care, 64
  signs and symptoms, 562
  thyroid physiology in pregnancy,
      560–561, 561*f*
Thyroidectomy, 564
Thyroid gland
  function changes during pregnancy, 47
  hypothalmic-pituitary-thyroid axis,
      560, 561*f*
  size increase, 46
  thyroid hormone fluctuations
      throughout pregnancy, 561*f*
Thyroid hormones, 47, 560–565, 561*f*,
    561*t*
Thyroiditis
  defined, 441
  postpartum, 447–448, 561*t*, 565–566

Thyroid-releasing hormone (TRH), 560,
    561*f*
Thyroid-stimulating hormone (TSH),
    46, 47, 560–565, 561*f*, 561*t*
Thyroid-stimulating immunoglobulins
    (TSIs), 564
Thyroid storm, 441, 560, 561*t*, 565
Thyrotoxicosis (thyroid storm), 441, 560,
    561*t*, 565
Thyroxine-binding globulin (TBG), 47
Tiagabine, maternal and fetal effects of,
    572*t*
Tindazole, for trichomoniasis, 614
Tissue factor, 34, 36
Tobacco use
  preconception counseling on, 59–60
  prenatal health promotion and
      education, 91–92, 92*t*
  prevalence of antepartum, 238
Tocolysis, 335, 348
Tocolytics, for preterm birth risk
      decrease, 402
Tocophobia, 153
Tolerable upper intake levels (TULs),
    99
Toluene, exposure to, 282
Tonic-clonic seizure, 570–571, 578
Topical anesthetics, for perineal
      discomfort, 431
Topiramate, maternal and fetal effects of,
    572*t*
Total energy, recommendations in
      pregnancy, 103
Total iron-binding capacity, 526*t*
Total lung capacity, 517
Total parenteral nutrition (TPN)
  defined, 397
  for hyperemesis gravidarum, 401
Toxins, exposure to, 279–284. *See also*
      Environmental exposures
Toxoplasma gondii. See Toxoplasmosis
Toxoplasmosis, 110, 599–602, 600*f*, 601*t*
  clinical presentation and assessment,
      599–601
  congenital, 599
  information for women about, 601
  life cycle of *T. gondii*, 600*f*
  management, 601
  potential problems, 599
  prevention, 602
  testing for, 601, 601*t*
TPN. *See* Total parenteral nutrition
Tramadol, for restless leg syndrome,
    210–211
Transdermal patches, for contraception,
    469
Trans-fatty acids, 99
Transferrin, 36
Transforming Maternity Care Movement,
    95–96

Transport mechanisms, 23, 24*t*
Transtheoretical stages of change, 274,
    276–277, 276*t*
Trauma, abdominal, 399
Treponema palladium, 610
Tretinoin, for melasma, 213
TRH (thyroid-releasing hormone), 560,
    561*f*
Triamcinolone, for pruritic folliculitis of
      pregnancy, 583
Trichomonas vaginalis, 608, 613–614
Trichoroacetic acid, for human
      papillomavirus, 613
Tricyclic antidepressants (TCAs)
  for anxiety disorders, 457
  black box warning, 454*t*
  for depression, 457, 624, 624*t*
  FDA approved indications, 454*t*
  side effects, 454*t*
Triglycerides, 41
Trigone, bladder, 34, 39
Trimesters, 133, 135*t*–136*t*, 136
Triptans, for headaches, 576
Trisomy 18, 162
  defined, 160
  features of, 162
  genetic screening test, 87*t*
  incidence of, 162
  screening for, 162–165, 163*t*
Trisomy 21
  defined, 160
  features of, 162
  genetic screening test, 87*t*
  incidence of, 162
  risk factors for, 162
  screening options for, 162–165, 163*t*
Trophoblast, 354
TSH. *See* Thyroid-stimulating hormone
TSIs (thyroid-stimulating
    immunoglobulins), 564
TTC SOC (transtheoretical stages of
      change), 274, 276–277, 276*t*
Tubal pregnancy, chlamydia and, 609
Tubal sterilization, 466
Tuberculosis, screening
    recommendations, 58*t*
TULs (tolerable upper intake levels), 99
Tumor necrosis factor alpha (TNFα),
    551
TWEAK screening tool, 245
Twins. *See* Multifetal pregnancy
Twin-to-twin transfusion, 397
TwoDay Method, of fertility awareness,
    474
Type 1 diabetes, 560, 566, 566*t*
Type 2 diabetes, 560, 566, 566*t*

UFH (unfractionated heparin), for
      thromboprophylaxis, 532, 533*t*
Ulipristal acetate, 474–475

Ultrasound
    amniotic fluid volume (AFV)
        assessment, 183, 184*t*
    breast, 482
    cervical length measurement for
        predicting preterm birth, 368
    for deep vein thrombosis (DVT)
        diagnosis, 532
    Doppler velocimetry for antenatal fetal
        testing, 187–188
    for estimation of gestational age, 87
    fetal age estimations, 82
    fetal heart activity detection, 132
    fetal surveillance in multifetal
        pregnancy, 402–403
    for gallstone diagnosis, 547
    for genetic screening, 87, 164–165
    gestational age estimation by,
        139–140
    for macrosomia detection, 362
    multifetal pregnancy diagnosis, 402
    obesity and, 553
    pregnancy diagnosis by, 132
    prenatal, 87–88
    serial fetal growth ultrasounds, 360
    in substance exposed pregnancies,
        249
    venous ultrasonography, 447
Ultraviolet B (UVB) therapy, for
    pruritic folliculitis of pregnancy,
    583
Umbilical cord
    formation of, 23, 355*f*
    structure of, 23
Unconjugated estriol, in genetic
    screening, 163
Underweight in pregnancy, 108
Unfractionated heparin (UFH), for
    thromboprophylaxis, 532, 533*t*
UNICEF, 480
United States Department of Agriculture
    (USDA)
    food guides, 100
    MyPlate tool, 114, 115*t*
    serving size recommendations, 100
United States Preventative Services Task
    Force (USPTF), 80
Unnecessary interventions, 150–151
Upper respiratory infection, 521–522,
    522*t*
Upper UTI, defined, 536
Ureter dilation in pregnancy, 39
Urethral meatus, 8
Uric acid levels in pregnancy, 39
Urinalysis, 538, 539*t*
Urinary frequency, 215, 536, 538
    assessment, 215
    causes and symptoms, 215
    relief and preventative measures, 215

Urinary incontinence, 216
    assessment, 216
    causes and symptoms, 216
    relief and preventative measures, 216
Urinary meatus, 6
Urinary tract disorders, 536–542
    case study, 542
    nephrolithiasis, 536, 541
    pyelonephritis, 540–541
    resources for health-care providers,
        542
    resources for women, 542
    terminology, 536
    urinary tract infection (UTI),
        536–541, 539*t*–540*t*
Urinary tract infection (UTI), 536–541,
    539*t*–540*t*
    acute cystitis, 536–538
    asymptomatic bacteriuria, 537, 542
    care of women with, 538–539, 540*t*
    common pathogens, 537
    defined, 536
    evaluation of, 538, 539*t*
        health history, 538
        laboratory testing, 538, 539*t*
        physical examination, 538
    pathophysiology, 537
    prevalence, 536
    pyelonephritis, 536, 538, 540–541
    recurrent, 540
    risk factors for, 537
    urinary frequency and, 215
Urinary urgency, 536, 538
Urine culture, 537–538, 539*t*, 541
Urogenital triangle, 8*f*
Urosepsis, 536
Ursodeoxycholic acid, for intrahepatic
    cholestasis of pregnancy (ICP),
    546, 586
Urticara, defined, 580
U.S. Preventative Services Task Force
    (USPSTF), 77, 80, 452
USDA. *See* United States Department of
    Agriculture
USDA Food Guide, 100
USPSTF (United States Preventative
    Services Task Force), 77, 80,
    452
Uterine fibroids. *See also* Leiomyoma
    types, 338*f*
    vaginal bleeding and, 337
Uterine infection, 443–445, 444*t*–445*t*
    bacteria common in, 444*t*
    clinical presentation, 444, 445*t*
    diagnosis and management, 444–445
    postpartum, 443–445, 444*t*–445*t*
    preterm births and, 44
    risk factors for, 444
Uterine (fallopian) tube, 9*f*

Uterosacral ligaments, 9–10, 9*f*
Uterotonic, 419
Uterotonic agents, for delayed
    postpartum hemorrhage, 446
Uterus
    anatomy, 9–11, 9*f*
    blood supply, 11
    changes as probable signs of
        pregnancy, 129–130, 129*f*–130*f*
    distention, pathological and preterm
        birth, 366
    fibroids, 337, 338*f*
    fundal height measurements for
        gestational age estimation,
        138–139, 139*f*
    infection (*see* Uterine infection)
    involution, 419–420, 423, 433–434
    location of the uterine fundus during
        pregnancy, 130
    perforation by IUD, 468
    physiological alterations during
        postnatal period, 419–420
    postpartum assessment of, 433–434
    postpartum examination, 434
    size and shape on bilateral
        examination, 130
    softening, 129–130
    subinvolution, 441, 446
UTI. *See* Urinary tract infection

Vaccination
    hepatitis A virus (HAV), 593–594
    hepatitis B virus (HBV), 595
    influenza, 521
    preconception, 62, 63*t*
    rubella, 598–599
    varicella zoster virus (VZV), 603
Vacuum aspiration abortion, 144
Vagina, 9*f*
    anatomy, 8–10, 9*f*
    changes in
        presumptive signs of pregnancy,
            128
        probably signs of pregnancy, 129,
            129*f*
    flora of, 615
    pH of, 9
    physiological alterations during
        postnatal period, 420
    postpartum examination, 434
Vaginal bleeding. *See* Bleeding
Vaginal candidiasis, 613, 614
Vaginal diaphragms, 473
Vaginal discharge, 5
    leukorrhea, 205
Vaginal examination, in childhood sexual
    abuse survivors, 268
Vaginal lubrication, 432
Vaginal orifice, 6*f*–8*f*

Vaginal ring, for contraception, 469
Vaginal smears, Nugent scoring system for, 614–615, 615t
Valacyclovir, for herpes simplex virus, 611–612, 612t
Valproic acid
    for bipolar disorder, 626
    maternal and fetal effects of, 572t
    teratogenicity of, 233t
Varenicline, 246, 253–254
Varicella zoster virus (VZV), 602–603
    case study, 604
    clinical presentation and assessment, 602–603
    congenital varicella syndrome (CVS), 602
    counseling on, 603
    management, 603
    neonatal varicella, 602
    potential problems, 602
Varicosities, 216–218
    leg, 216–217
    vulvar, 217–218, 217f
VAS (vibroacoustic stimulation), 182
Vasa previa, 335
Vascular changes during pregnancy, 37, 42, 213
Vascular resistance, decreased maternal during pregnancy, 37
Vascular spiders, as presumptive sign of pregnancy, 128
Vasectomy, 466–467
Vasodilation, maternal during pregnancy, 37
Vasovagal response, 5, 10
Vegetarians and vegans, nutrition for pregnant, 99, 117–118
    B vitamins, 118
    calcium, 118
    iron, 118
    nutrient sources, 117t
    omega-3 fatty acids, 118
    protein, 118
    vitamin D, 118
Veins, varicose, 216–217
Velamentous insertion, 20, 22–23
Vena cava syndrome. See Supine hypotension syndrome (SHS)
Venlafaxine, 624
    FDA approved indications, 454t
    side effects, 454t
Venous thromboembolism (VTE), 433
Venous thrombosis. See also Deep vein thrombosis (DVT)
    risk factors for, 445t
    superficial, 441, 447
Venous ultrasonography, 447
Ventilation and perfusion (V/Q) scan, for pulmonary embolism, 532

Verbal persuasion, as self-efficacy information source, 307
Vernix caseosa, 20, 30
Vertical transmission, defined, 589
Very preterm birth, 365–366
Very small for gestational age (VSGA), 358, 360
Vesicouterine pouch, 5, 9
Vesicovaginal septum, 5, 9
Vestibule, 5–6, 7f, 8
Vibroacoustic stimulation (VAS), 182
Vicarious experience, as self-efficacy information source, 307
Violence. See Intimate partner violence
Viral disease. See also specific viruses
    cytomegalovirus (CMV), 590–591
    hepatitis A virus (HAV), 593–594
    hepatitis B virus (HBV), 594–596
    hepatitis C virus (HBV), 596–597
    influenza, 521, 523
    parvovirus B19, 597
    rubella, 597–599
    sexually transmitted infections (STIs), 610–613
    upper respiratory infection, 521–522, 522t
    varicella zoster virus (VZV), 602–603
Visceral arousal, as self-efficacy information source, 307
Visual changes, 219–220
    assessment, 219
    causes and symptoms, 219
    relief and preventative measures, 220
Vitamin B$_{12}$
    deficiency and anemia, 527t, 530
    hematological findings during normal pregnancy, 526t
Vitamin D, 46
    dietary intake during pregnancy, 106t, 107
    in human milk, 481
    in vegetarian/vegan diet, 118
Vitamins, in human milk, 481
Voiding by breastfed infants, 490–491
Vomiting
    hyperemesis gravidarum (HG), 399–401, 400t
    nausea and vomiting of pregnancy (NVP), 207–209, 208t–209t, 209f
von Willebrand's disease, 531
    defined, 441
    delayed postpartum hemorrhage and, 446
VSGA (very small for gestational age), 358, 360
VTE (venous thromboembolism), 433
Vulnerable populations, postnatal care in, 436–437

Vulva, 5–6, 6f
Vulvar varicosities, 217–218, 217f
VZV. See Varicella zoster virus

Waist circumference, 549
Walking, 277
    in obese women during pregnancy, 554
    postpartum, 429
Warfarin, 532
Warmth, increased, 204–205
Warning signs, postnatal, 435, 435t
Water consumption, strategies to increase, 103
Water content of human milk, 480
Weight, preconception counseling on, 59
Weight gain, 107–108. See also Obesity
    advice for achieving healthy, 108
    body image and, 305–306
    by breastfed infants, 491
    distribution of, 107
    from fluid retention in pregnancy, 39
    in gestational diabetes (GDM) management, 391
    IOM recommended pregnancy, 90, 91t
    overweight and obesity in pregnancy, 108
    pattern in preeclampsia, 379
    psychiatric medications causing, 551
    recommendations for, 107–108, 108t
    underweight in pregnancy, 108
Weight loss
    with hyperemesis gravidarum, 399
    in obese women during pregnancy, 554
    postpartum, 429–430, 491
Wernicke's encephalopathy
    defined, 397
    in hyperemesis gravidarum, 400
Wharton's jelly, 20, 23
White blood cells, changes during pregnancy, 35
WHO. See World Health Organization
Wilson, Jim, 228–229
Witch hazel, for perineal discomfort, 431
Withdrawal
    benzodiazepines, 244, 627
    opioid, 249–252
Withdrawal, method of contraception, 474
Witnessing birth, 300
Women, Infants, and Children (WIC) nutrition program, 90, 114, 262, 550

Working during pregnancy, 94, 286–288
  data gathering and counseling,
      287–288
  discrimination, 287
  heavy lifting, 286
  long hours, 286–287
  noise exposure, 287
  psychological stress, 287
  resource on work during pregnancy
      for women, 288
  shift work, 286
Workplace, nursing mothers in, 493–494

World Health Organization (WHO)
  Baby-Friendly Hospital Initiative
      (BFHI), 480
  growth charts, 491
  medical eligibility criteria (MEC),
      464, 471
  preterm birth, report on, 365
Wound infection, postpartum, 445
  abdominal, 445
  perineal, 445

X-linked conditions, 167

X-ray, pregnancy diagnosis by, 132

Yolk sac, 22

Zolpidem, 329
Zona pellucida, 5, 14–15, 20
Zonisamide, maternal and fetal effects
      of, 572t
Zung Self-Rating Anxiety Scale
      Hamilton Anxiety Rating Scale,
      627
Zygote, 20